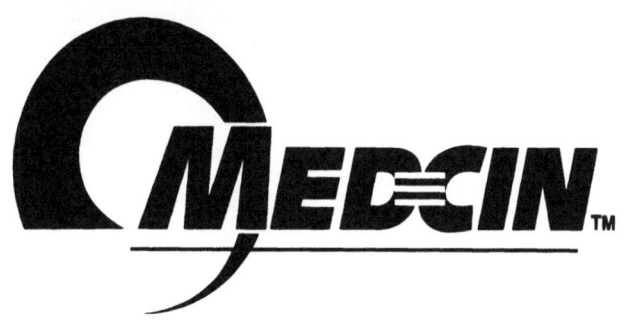

Springer
New York
Berlin
Heidelberg
Barcelona
Budapest
Hong Kong
London
Milan
Paris
Santa Clara
Singapore
Tokyo

MEDCIN
A New Nomenclature
for Clinical Medicine

Peter S. Goltra

Foreword by
Christopher G. Chute

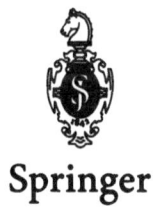

Springer

Peter S. Goltra
President
Medicomp Systems, Inc.
14500 Avion Parkway
Chantilly, VA 20151, USA

Library of Congress Cataloging-in-Publication Data
Goltra, Peter S.
    MEDCIN : a new nomenclature for clinical medicine / Peter S.
Goltra.
        p.   cm.

        ISBN-13: 978-1-4612-7487-2   e-ISBN-13: 978-1-4612-2286-6
        DOI:10.1007/978-1-4612-2286-6

    1. Medicine—Nomenclature. I. Title.
    [DNLM: 1. Clinical Medicine—nomenclature.   WB 15 G629m   1997]
    R123.G59   1997
    610′.14—dc21
DNLM/DLC   96-52993

Printed on acid-free paper.

Production managed by Karina Mikhli; manufacturing supervised by Jeff Taub.
Camera copy supplied by the author.

9 8 7 6 5 4 3 2 1

Foreword

The practice of medicine has become an information intensive profession. Pertinent and detailed information resources and references are proliferating rapidly, while the quantity of patient data gathered during an episode of care can be daunting. Identifying the best guideline and interventions which will lead to an optimal clinical outcome for an individual patient poses an increasingly difficult challenge. Matching the detailed information about a particular patient with the parameters of a guideline may be tedious. Attempting to identify or use a guideline with terms of definitions which differ from those found in a patient's record may well be impossible. Here we confront the well-known "medical vocabulary problem" which plagues nascent efforts to establish electronic medical records (EMRs) everywhere.

Efficient resource management and the adoption of cost effective strategies are of increasing importance in the new market realities of healthcare in the late 90's. Whether providers seek to describe their practice, implement continuous improvement, engage in outcomes research, or develop data driven guidelines, a way to represent patient findings and events consistently is required. The standard classifications for administrative data in healthcare, such as ICD-9-CM, have proven to be too coarse for a detailed examination of practice patterns and severity adjusted outcomes. The use of free text to represent diagnoses and procedures is unwieldy; unstructured free text cannot support information linkage and analyses without elaborate machine processing or hand abstraction and coding. So again, we engage that pesky "medical vocabulary problem"; it is clearly not going to go away.

This raises many questions. What should a medical terminology look like? How detailed should it be? What structure should it have? How can it be used? Will it map to systems for reporting or reimbursement? Does it work for a locally specific set of needs?

Despite more than three centuries of progressively improving classifications, primarily for mortality coding, it is only with the advent of EMRs that many in the healthcare field are taking a serious look at the "medical vocabulary problem." The Health Informatics Standards Board (HISB) of the American National Standards Institute (ANSI) issued a white paper during the fall of 1996 on the optimal properties and development strategies for healthcare terminologies in general.

The MEDCIN nomenclature represents a genuine contribution to the field of medical nomenclatures. It embraces many of the properties articulated in the HISB white paper (no medical terminology on the planet conforms to all the recommended properties). These include the adoption of Context Free Identifiers, Unique Identifiers, Language Independence, Explicit Uncertainty, and Mapping to Major Systems. It may well conform to other properties such as Completeness, Comprehensiveness, Non-redundancy, and reliable Synonyms (in a supplementary product). These last points have not been formally evaluated, but with the production of this volume, they can be.

The most significant aspect of the MEDCIN publication is the decision of Medicomp to make their proprietary vocabulary widely available in text and electronic form for a nominal license charge. In this characteristic, they conform most closely with the spirit of the HISB white paper, which concludes that terminologies which have significant barriers to access, including financial ones, simply cannot emerge as viable standards for EMRs. The MEDCIN nomenclature is a bold demonstration of how a commercial developer can release their terminology, retaining a focus on their primary product (an EMR system) rather than on an enabling infrastructural technology.

This openness represented by the publication of MEDCIN should result in more widespread critique and collaboration, continuously improving the nomenclature. It may contribute to the cross-terminology integration of synonyms and term variants, which the HISB document projects could lead to a coordinated set of conceptually integrated but independent terminologies in American healthcare. Conceptual convergence of privately produced and supported terminologies can only help terminology developers, users, and the healthcare-seeking public at large.

The daunting demands of this information intensive era of healthcare will require all the collaborative spirit we can bring to bear. This publication is a major step toward the virtual dialogue where we abandon the policies of Babel, and embrace an unfettered exchange by terminology developers around the concepts encountered throughout the spectrum of healthcare in the United States and the global community.

Christopher G. Chute, M.D., Dr.PH
Rochester, MN 55901; chute@mayo.edu
Head, Section of Medical Information Resource,
    Mayo Foundation
Chair, Medical Vocabulary Working Group (WG6),
    International Medical Informatics Association (IMIA)

Preface

My purpose in developing and publishing this computer-based nomenclature is to provide a common base for creating computer programs for acquisition, review and transmission of medical information independent of language.

MEDCIN assigns a permanent, unique identifying number to each finding, and includes an editable hierarchy file (not shown in this book) independent of these numbers. As medical knowledge increases and techniques improve, MEDCIN can accommodate changes in classification without ever deleting a finding. It will also facilitate the generation of narrative text, the searching of data, the use of expert system tools and interfacing with coded structures.

Each of the over 70,000 medical findings in this first edition of the MEDCIN nomenclature has a translation equivalent in French, German and Spanish. This supports international transfer of medical record data with the ability to read a patient's chart in any of the languages, irrespective of the language of acquisition.

As an adjunct to the nomenclature, MEDCIN contains three files of modifiers: status, term modifiers, and course. Used together with time parameters they will facilitate the transfer of patient data between systems[1].

For implementation of a complete system or for development of a solution for a unique need, Medicomp Systems, Inc., will supply supplemental vocabulary for each language, a narrative engine to create chart text that includes expanded phrases for the nomenclature in each language, and an expert system engine including a 420,000 planar element, multidimensional matrix of the MEDCIN nomenclature elements with 3,100 diagnoses, syndromes and conditions. The last is a resource for triage and follow-up, for intelligent prompting for support staff of additional questions based on analysis of the chart, and for building entry protocols and templates.

Through Medicomp Systems, interested readers can also obtain the MEDCIN nomenclature as a computer file. This is currently available for a

---

[1]For questions related to file structure and implementation, contact Kirby Trump at (800) 765-8080, or e-mail kirby@medicomp.com.

nominal license fee in keeping with the *pro bono* intent for this project.

I hope very much that users of MEDCIN will contribute to future updates of the nomenclature.[2]

P.S.G.

---

[2]For questions regarding the nomenclature and the information structure, Peter Goltra may be reached by phone at (703) 803-8080, by fax at (703) 803-8235, or by mail c/o Medicomp Systems, Inc., 14500 Avion Parkway, Suite 175, Chantilly, VA, 20151.

Acknowledgments

I would like to thank all the physicians who gave up evenings and weekends over the last 18 years to work with me on the development of MEDCIN. In addition to those listed as Consulting Editors, I would like to thank Deborah Birx, M.D., Catherine Eng, M.D., Michael Goldman, M.D., Darcy Hansen, M.D., Edward Illions, M.D., Philip Pierce, M.D., Bryan Raybuck, M.D., Donald Rose, M.D., and Peter Schauer, M.D.

I am most grateful to the following for the critique of the nomenclature and the expert system from which it was derived: William T. Bardsley, M.D., Stephen P. Hayden, M.D., Leo Leveridge, M.D., Michael Rolnick, M.D., and Thomas Stair, M.D.

This nomenclature would not have come into existence without the dedicated programming efforts of Richard Bayless, Adelard Brault, Jr., Arturo Gazzo, Dennis Makurat, Roy Soltoff, and Kirby Trump.

For the translations, I would like to express sincere thanks to Jean Trump for training the translators in the use of the editing systems, and the translation of MEDCIN into German; to Renee Bearse for the translation into French; to Laura Arman, Ana Darder, and Julia Morton for the translation into Spanish; and to Carlos Dias for the ongoing translation into Portuguese.

For the ideas, encouragement, and support during these years, amongst many I would especially like to thank: Charlotte P. Armstrong, J. Sinclair Armstrong, Claressa Brown, M.D., Ralph Engle, M.D., Elmer Gabrielli, M.D., Gurston Goldin, M.D., Alice Goltra, Bruce Hiland, David Lareau, Anita S. Marmaduke, Patricia Morrill, Edward S. Petersen, M.D., Harry Rositzke, Edwin A. Seipp, and Irving S. Wright, M.D.

I very much appreciate the dedication of the following during the final preparation of this manuscript: Edmund M. Herrold, M.D., Harry Lascelles, Roy Soltoff, and Jean Trump.

The methodology used to create the phrasing for the medical findings is drawn from the early writings of Ludwig Wittgenstein.

The following sources were used for tumor nomenclature and topographic site: *World Health Organization International Histological Classification of Tumors*, *World Health Organization International Classification of Diseases for Oncology*, *Armed Forces Institute of Pathology Atlas of Tumor Pathology*.

Dedication

This work is dedicated to Gail, Tad, Alexis, and Ren, without whose collective and unfailing support this 18-year effort could not have been sustained. It is also dedicated in memory of my father, William Brown Goltra, and his friend and physician, Howard S. Armstrong, M.D., whose frustrations in trying to obtain clinical study information during my father's four year battle with ALS in the 1950s were the inspiration for this work.

Consulting Editors

Robert G. Barone, M.D. Clinical Assistant Professor of Ophthalmology, Cornell University Medical College and Attending Surgeon, The New York Hospital, New York, NY

J. Gregory Cairncross, M.D. Professor, Departments of Clinical Neurological Sciences and Oncology, University of Western Ontario and London Regional Cancer Centre, London, Ontario, Canada

Richard P. Cohen, M.D. Clinical Associate Professor of Medicine, Cornell University Medical College and Associate Attending Physician, The New York Hospital, New York, NY

Bradley A. Connor, M.D. Clinical Assistant Professor of Medicine, Cornell University Medical College; Adjunct Faculty, Rockefeller University and Assistant Attending Physician, The New York Hospital, New York, NY

David R. Gastfriend, M.D. Assistant Professor in Psychiatry, Harvard Medical School and Director of Addiction Services, Massachusetts General Hospital, Boston, MA

Stephanie M. Heidelberg, M.D. Medical Director, Adult, Older Adult Programs, American Day Treatment Centers, Fairfax, VA and Psychiatrist, Adult Day Treatment Program, Northwest Mental Health Center, Reston, VA

Edmund M. Herrold, M.D., Ph.D. Associate Professor of Medicine, Director, Section of Biophysics and Biomechanics, Division of Cardiovascular Pathophysiology, Cornell University Medical College and Associate Attending Physician, The New York Hospital, New York, NY

Allan N. Houghton, M.D. Professor of Medicine and Immunology, Cornell University College and Chair, Immunology Program, Memorial Sloan-Kettering Cancer Center, New York, NY

Ralph H. Hruban, M.D. Associate Professor of Pathology, Associate Professor of Oncology, The Johns Hopkins School of Medicine and Director, Division of Cardiovascular-Respiratory Pathology, The Johns Hopkins Hospital, Baltimore, MD

Mark Lachs, M.D., MPH Assistant Professor of Medicine, Cornell University Medical College and Chief, Geriatrics Unit, Department of Medicine, The New York Hospital, New York, NY

Frederick A. McCurdy, M.D., Ph.D. Associate Professor of Pediatrics and Director of Pediatric Undergraduate Education, University of Nebraska College of Medicine, Omaha, NE

Paul F. Miskovitz, M.D. Clinical Associate Professor of Medicine, Cornell University Medical College and Associate Attending Physician, The New York Hospital, New York, NY

Preeti Pancholi, Ph.D. Staff Scientist, Department of Virology and Parasitology, Kimball Research Institute, New York Blood Center, New York, NY

Louis N. Pangaro, M.D. Associate Professor, Clinical Medicine, Vice Chairman For Educational Programs, Department of Medicine, Uniformed Services University of The Health Sciences, F. Edward Herbert School of Medicine, Bethesda, MD

Edward J. Parrish, M.D., M.S. Assistant Professor of Medicine, Cornell University Medical College; Department of Medicine, Division of Rheumatology, The New York Hospital, The Hospital for Special Surgery, New York, NY

William B. Patterson, M.D., MPH Assistant Professor of Environmental Health, Boston University School of Public Health, Boston MA and President, New England Health Center, Wilmington, MA

David Posnett, M.D. Associate Professor of Medicine, Cornell University Medical College; Division of Immunology, Department of Medicine, The New York Hospital, New York, NY

Calvin W. Roberts, M.D. Professor of Ophthalmology, Cornell University Medical College, New York, NY

Ronald C. Silvestri, M.D. Assistant Professor of Medicine, Harvard Medical School and Director, Medical Intensive Care Unit, Deaconess Hospital, Boston, MA

Michael Thorpe, M.D. Musculoskeletal Radiology Fellow, The Hospital for Special Surgery, New York, NY

Anshu Vashishtha M.D., Ph.D. Adjunct Faculty Member, Laboratory of Bacterial Pathogenesis and Immunology, The Rockefeller University and Clinical Fellow in Allergy and Immunology, The New York Hospital, New York, NY

H. Hallett Whitman III, M.D. Clinical Assistant Professor of Medicine, Cornell University Medical College; Clinical Affiliate, Hypertension Center, The New York Hospital, New York, NY and Attending Physician in Internal Medicine and Rheumatology, Summit Medical Group, Summit, NJ

E. David Wright, M.D. Clinical Assistant Professor of Medicine, Department of Dermatology, University of Virginia Health Sciences Center, Charlottesville, VA; Dermatology Associates, Inc. and Attending Physician, Winchester Medical Center, Winchester, VA

Joseph Zibrak, M.D. Assistant Professor of Medicine, Harvard Medical School and Associate Chief of Pulmonary and Critical Care Medicine, Beth Israel Deaconess Medical Center, Boston, MA

Contents

Contents

Contents

Introduction

The Challenge of Medical Nomenclature Development

The purpose of a medical computer-based nomenclature is to accommodate the acquisition, organization and analysis of clinical information. Nomenclature developers consider the need to balance the requirements of persons who acquire clinical information with those who analyze it, as well as the transfer of information between these groups.

Most clinical information (with the exception of laboratory data) is acquired by a clinician either listening to, or examining, a patient. It is the patient's own description of symptoms and history, screened through the knowledge of the clinician, that provides a starting point for the encounter.

During the patient encounter, the clinician needs to be able to concentrate on potential causes of the patient's clinical presentation. Information gathered through the patient interview, coupled with the physical examination of the patient, provides the basis for a preliminary diagnosis. From thousands of possibilities, the clinician must draw upon years of training and experience to diagnose the etiology of the patient's complaint(s).

This systematic thought process is the most important part of the clinical encounter. During the encounter, however, key clinical data must be acquired and recorded accurately and in appropriate detail for rapid analysis by basic, clinical and administrative researchers. It is at this point that a potential conflict arises between the need to record clinical information and the requirement to not interfere with the clinician's thought process.

This quandary is the central focus and challenge for developers of medical nomenclature. The nomenclature must accommodate the thought process of an individual clinician, yet be structured to capture the clinical findings needed for documentation and analysis. The only feasible solution is to have the acquisition of clinical data emulate the clinical thought processes used in interviewing, examining and treating the patient. However, the nomenclature design and structure must facilitate data analysis.

Accommodating the Clinical Thought Process

To accommodate the clinical thought process, medical nomenclature must reflect both the structure and the content of the clinician's diagnostic process. The approach used in developing MEDCIN was to organize the individual data elements (findings) into six broad categories which reflect the different types of information acquired during the clinical encounter. The categories are symptoms, history, physical examination, tests, diagnoses and treatments. These categories provide the structure for MEDCIN and have been constructed to be consistent with current clinical practice and currently available documentation standards.

It is at this level that the need for clinical detail differs between the clinician and the researcher. For the clinician, each finding must be sufficiently detailed to record clinical information with the necessary degree of specificity to support diagnoses and treatment. For the researcher, multiple levels of detail in the clinical information must be accessible. Both requirements should be accommodated during the normal course of the encounter without intruding upon the clinical thought process.

Nomenclature Design and Structure

The nature of the specific findings to be included in the nomenclature becomes the critical task of the nomenclature developer. Each finding must be organized and precisely phrased to meet the requirements of both the diagnostician and the researcher. Furthermore, the relationships between findings must be clinically logical and valid. To build such a nomenclature requires that the developer use a design which reflects the structure, hierarchy and content of the clinical thought process.

Differential Diagnosis as a Basis for Nomenclature Design

The clinical thought process is a series of repeated iterations toward a differential diagnosis and provides a useful model for defining the necessary elements of a medical nomenclature. If each item (finding) in a nomenclature is defined with a sufficient degree of sensitivity and clinical specificity to be useful for clear differential diagnoses, it will also be suitable for documentation and research.

A Structured Hierarchy of Findings

The manner in which findings are organized is a crucial consideration affecting not only the number of steps required to record a finding, but also the number of search elements needed to locate it for future analysis. To accommodate both entry and reporting, MEDCIN uses a data structure which embodies the concept of inheritance between levels in a hierarchy.

For example, "numbness" is a fairly common symptom, and can be present almost anywhere in the body. The specific location of the numbness can be crucial in making a diagnosis. MEDCIN has more than eighty findings for numbness, starting with the general finding and proceeding in a structured hierarchy through all areas of the body, increasing in detail at each level.

This structure presents two distinct advantages. First, a finding need only be recorded as a specific clinical observation. The clinician records information with only the degree of specificity needed to support diagnosis and treatment.

Second, the nomenclature hierarchy automatically passes these findings up the hierarchy by reverse inheritance to meet the needs of the researcher. Using "numbness of the first two fingers of the right hand" as an example, MEDCIN knows this includes the characteristics of "numbness of the right hand", "numbness of the extremities", and "numbness." Therefore, any future searches using MEDCIN will locate the detailed finding from the more general terms in the hierarchy above it.

Presentation of the Nomenclature

In this volume, each MEDCIN finding is presented in phrase format with its corresponding MEDCIN finding identification number. This MEDCIN finding number has no inherent meaning, structure, order or hierarchy. It is merely a computer-assigned number which never changes, and is used to record each piece of medical information as a single data element, rather than as free-text or as a composite code structure.

MEDCIN finding numbers should not be confused with other coding systems such as those issued by the American Medical Association (CPT), World Health Organization (ICD-9-CM), or others. Links to other coded structures such as CPT, ICD-O, DSM-IV, etc., are available as part of the supplemental files and tools described in Appendix B.

Applications of the Nomenclature

MEDCIN can be useful in applications requiring the capture of clinically valid coded data elements. These include outcomes studies and other research, electronic medical record systems, triage applications, risk analysis algorithms, case management, utilization review, and other patient case management and reporting functions.

MEDCIN, and its available supplemental files and tools described in the appendix, is intended to assist in the building of clinical applications. In the past, two of the major barriers to adoption of the electronic medical record have been the lack of a suitable clinical vocabulary and the difficulty of recording structured clinical data in a time-efficient and cost-effective manner. MEDCIN and its supplemental files and tools address both of these issues and provides a foundation upon which distributed patient records can be built, independent of location or language. Users of MEDCIN may also build their own supplemental files and tools.

David P. Lareau
Medicomp Systems, Inc.

Part I
SYMPTOMS

Part 1

SYMPTOMS

2900	**encounter background information**
2125	Phone Call - Chief Concern:
1718	Chief Complaint:
2062	source of patient information
2063	the patient
2064	the spouse
2065	a family member
2421	the mother
2422	the father
2423	the maternal grandmother
2424	the paternal grandmother
2425	the maternal grandfather
2426	the paternal grandfather
2427	the stepmother
2428	the stepfather
2429	a non-family caretaker
2430	a female babysitter
2431	a male babysitter
2432	a female nanny
2433	a male nanny
2434	a female guardian
2435	a male guardian
2066	a friend
2067	another physician
2068	medical records
2436	a policeman
2437	a neighbor
2438	a social worker
2439	a bystander
1878	**systemic symptoms**
1502	feeling fine
4	no symptoms
2101	completely free of symptoms between episodes
2102	generalized pain
1151	feeling poorly or tiring easily (malaise, fatigue)
1152	feel worse in the morning
1153	feel worse in the evening
5	fever
1589	over 100 F. by thermometer
6	recurrent
1590	daily
1591	every few days
1592	every week or so
7	chills
8	shake the whole body (rigor)
9	come and go (recurrent)
1879	**symptoms related to the head**
10	a headache
11	new - started recently (not a recurring headache)
12	chronic / recurring
1667	episodes worse recently
1832	chronic / unremitting
1833	getting progressively worse
2577	comes and goes (recurrent)
1863	quality
14	steady
1798	comes and goes
1796	sharp or stabbing
17	excruciating - "worst I ever had"
16	with devastating suddenness
13	throbbing or pounding
1795	dull / aching / boring
1797	burning
15	like a band around the head
18	location
19	one entire side
1758	right side
1759	left side
20	on both sides
24	in the forehead (frontal)
1768	right-sided
1769	left-sided
25	over the temple
1770	right side
1771	left side
1772	on both sides
1773	in front of the ear (over zygoma)
1776	right side
1777	left side
1781	at the center of one side (parietal)
1782	right side
1783	left side
23	at the back of the head (occipital)
1784	right side
1785	left side
27	at the top of the head (vertex)
21	generalized
28	in changing locations
1803	precipitated by
1800	by alcohol
1805	by red wine
1801	by certain foods
1802	by chocolate
1806	by cheese
1804	by Chinese foods
1821	by certain medications
1822	by oral contraceptives
1823	by indomethacin
1824	by nitroglycerin
1825	by amyl nitrite
1826	by hydralazine
1807	by sex
29	made worse by

30	by moving the eyes		63	flashing lights or wavy lines
1799	by moving the head		64	seeing a dark spot with a bright jagged outline
36	by changing body position		65	total loss of vision in one eye (anopsia)
32	by lying down		66	total loss of vision in both eyes
33	by standing or sitting up		67	loss of part of visual field (hemianopsia)
34	by bending over		68	double vision (diplopia)
35	by exertion		69	leg or arm on one side tingling or numb
31	by coughing or straining (valsalva)		70	loss of sensation or feeling in both legs
1811	by clenching the teeth		71	loss of sensation or feeling in both arms
1812	by chewing		72	weakness on one side of the body
1808	by light		73	unsteadiness when walking (ataxia)
1809	by noise		74	everything spinning around (vertigo)
1810	by odors		75	fainting (syncope)
1813	by changes in the weather		76	difficulty speaking
37	relieved by		77	accompanied by
38	by lying down		78	nausea
39	by sleep		79	vomiting
1820	by reducing stimuli		1827	diarrhea
40	by massaging the arteries in the neck or temple		1828	watery nasal discharge
41	by eating		1829	watery eyes
42	by medication		1830	red eyes
43	duration		80	skull pain
44	for a few minutes or less		22	pain behind the ear
45	for a few hours		1791	right side
46	for 1 - 3 days		1792	left side
47	for more than a week		83	facial pain
48	frequency		84	occurring on one side only
49	daily		85	occurring continuously
50	every few weeks		86	brief and excruciating
51	a few times a year		87	started by stimulation of area (trigger point)
52	many times in groups or clusters		88	facial twitching
1834	initially in groups or clusters, is now daily		89	pain over the nose
53	upon awakening		90	sinus pain
54	causing awakening from sleep		26	pain in the cheek
55	at the same time every day		1774	right side
2103	in the late afternoon		1775	left side
57	during particular seasons of the year		2901	**eye symptoms**
1819	associated with		91	worsening of vision
1814	with menarche		2904	distance
56	with menstrual cycle		2905	near
1815	with pregnancy		2906	started after prescription change
1816	with postpartum period		2907	for distance vision
1817	with menopause		2908	for near vision
1818	with jaw clicks		92	in the center of vision only
58	preceded by		93	toward the edges of vision only (peripheral)
59	by depression		94	right eye only
60	by anxiety		95	left eye only
61	by tension		96	both eyes
2104	by fatigue			
62	preceded briefly by other symptoms (aura)			

97	occurring briefly		2040	on the right
98	progressing slowly		2041	on the left
99	progressing rapidly		2042	drooping eyelid
100	started suddenly		2043	right eye
101	in one eye only		2044	left eye
102	right		2045	both eyes
103	left		2046	one eye more than the other
1603	a total loss of vision		1873	eyes are crossed
1604	in one eye only		1874	eyes are turned out
2545	right		115	pain in the eyes
2546	left		116	made worse by moving them
1602	occurring briefly		1761	right eye only
1615	in both eyes		1762	left eye only
104	loss of part of field of vision		1763	pain in both eyes
2012	suddenly		117	pain behind the eyes (retro-orbital)
2013	upper half		1764	right eye only
2014	lower half		1765	left eye only
2015	as if a curtain were being drawn		1760	pain around the eyes (periorbital)
1297	frequently bumping into things		1766	right eye only
105	blind spots (scotomata)		1767	left eye only
106	seeing double images (diplopia)		1778	pain below the eyes (infraorbital)
1668	intermittently		1779	right eye only
107	horizontal		1780	left eye only
108	vertical		2018	pain above the eyes (supraorbital)
109	diagonal		2019	right eye only
110	near		2020	left eye only
111	far		118	overflow of tears (epiphora)
2537	monocular		119	on one side only
2538	right		120	mucous discharge from the eyes
2539	left		1894	the right eye
2325	made worse by		1897	the left eye
2326	heat		2440	bilateral
2327	exercise		2514	matted eyelashes in the morning
2328	stress		121	watery discharge from the eyes
112	seeing words, letters or syllables reversed on page		1895	the right eye
			1898	the left eye
113	blurred vision		2441	bilateral
2016	as if looking through a glass of water		122	discharge of pus from the eyes
1835	flashing lights or wavy lines in the field of vision		1896	the right eye
			1899	the left eye
2017	seeing a bright light for 1-15 minutes		2442	bilateral
127	difficulty identifying colors		123	dry eyes
128	distortion of lines or objects		2021	right eye
129	seeing halos around lights		2022	left eye
130	which look yellow-green		124	itching
1862	difficulty seeing in bright light		2023	right eye
136	difficulty seeing at night		2024	left eye
140	difficulty reading		2025	scratching sensation
2047	improved by holding text further away		2026	right eye
			2027	left eye
137	difficulty closing one eye		125	gritty sensation in eyes
138	on the right		2028	right eye
139	on the left		2029	left eye
2039	difficulty opening one eye			

126	sensitivity to light (photophobia)
2030	right eye
2031	left eye
131	redness of the eyes
132	of one eye only
1901	the right eye
1902	the left eye
1900	bilaterally
2443	redness under the lower eyelid
2444	right eye
2445	left eye
2446	bilateral
2032	swollen eyes
2033	right eye
2034	left eye
2035	bilaterally
2510	right eye swollen shut
2511	left eye swollen shut
2512	both eyes swollen shut
133	puffy eyes
1903	on the right
1904	on the left
1905	bilaterally
134	eye strain (asthenopia)
2057	the eyes feel tired
135	squinting
2036	eye twitches
2037	right eye
2038	left eye
2048	difficulty with contact lenses:
2049	can only wear them for
2050	they hurt
2051	they are scratchy
2052	they are blurry
2053	they fall out
2054	they get stuck
2055	they move around in the eyes
2056	they make the eyes feel dry
2902	**otolaryngeal symptoms**
141	loss of hearing
142	getting progressively worse
143	in one ear only
144	in the right ear
145	in the left ear
1614	in both ears
1678	total
1619	temporary
1620	for a month or more
1621	difficulty understanding speech
146	high sensitivity to loud sounds (hyperacusis)
2010	hearing sounds twice (diplacusis)
2011	impairment of auditory discrimination
147	earache

1788	in the right ear
1789	in the left ear
1790	in both ears
2491	at night
1755	ears feel full
148	a discharge from the ears
152	which is chronic
2447	right ear
2448	left ear
2449	bilateral
149	clear (serous)
1906	from the right ear
1907	from the left ear
2450	bilateral
150	bloody
1908	from the right ear
1909	from the left ear
2451	bilateral
151	thick pus (purulent)
1910	from the right ear
1911	from the left ear
2452	bilateral
1754	foul smelling
2453	right ear
2454	left ear
2455	bilateral
1865	from the right ear
1866	from the left ear
1867	from both ears
2515	pulling at the ear(s)
2516	the right ear
2517	the left ear
2518	both ears
1756	popping noise in the ears
153	ringing in the ears (tinnitus)
154	occurring in
155	the right ear only
156	the left ear only
157	both ears
158	sounding like
159	clicking
160	humming
161	swooshing
162	nasal discharge
163	watery
164	containing pus (purulent)
165	blood-tinged
2456	yellow
2457	cloudy
2536	dripping down the throat
166	causing coughing
167	lasting more than 3 weeks
1868	from the right nostril

1869	from the left nostril
1870	from both nostrils
168	nose bleeds (epistaxis)
169	recurrent
170	nasal passage blockage (stuffiness)
171	gets better or worse
172	depending on the environment
173	with the change of seasons
174	with stress
175	on one side only
1730	frequently breathing through the mouth
1731	snoring
1163	loudly
177	sneezing
178	nasal itching
179	dryness of the nose
180	nasal lump or mass
181	pain in the jaw
1793	right side
1794	left side
182	jaw spasms (trismus)
184	jaw stiffness
185	jaw click
186	lump in the jaw
187	pain in the teeth
1840	teeth chip easily
188	recent tooth loss
189	loosening of teeth
190	bleeding gums
192	red gums
193	swollen gums
194	painful gums
195	sores in the gums
196	mouth sores
197	painless
198	lip abnormalities
199	swollen
200	sores
201	small dark spots
202	small bump(s)
203	soreness or pain of mouth or tongue
204	without visible sores or cuts
205	swollen tongue
206	small bump(s) on tongue
210	dryness of mouth (xerostomia)
211	excessive saliva (ptyalism)
212	frothy saliva
1720	excessive drooling
214	burning sensation in the mouth
213	metallic taste in the mouth
215	lump in the mouth
216	painless sore in the mouth
217	hoarseness

218	lasting more than 2 weeks
219	sore throat
220	lasting more than 2 weeks
221	pain radiating to the ear
225	excruciating throat pain
226	radiating to the ear
227	triggered by swallowing
222	choking
228	itching throat
230	drip or drainage down throat from above
229	lump in the throat
246	hiccups
1675	yawning
2903	**neck symptoms**
231	neck pain
232	increased by
233	swallowing
234	head movement
235	coughing
236	lying down
237	radiating
238	down the arm
239	up the back of the head
1786	on the right
1787	on the left
240	to the shoulder(s)
241	swollen glands
242	painful
1301	after consumption of alcohol
1608	more than 2 sites for more than 3 months
243	neck stiffness
224	neck enlargement under Adam's apple (goiter)
244	lump or swelling in the neck
2458	on the right
2459	on the left
2460	on the front
2461	on the back
245	growing rapidly
1884	**breast symptoms**
635	breast pain
636	in both breasts
637	occurring a few days before menstruation
638	nipple discharge
639	yellow-clear, watery (serous)
640	bloody
641	milky (abnormal lactation)
642	breast lump
643	in multiple sites
644	comes and goes
645	painful
646	growing rapidly
647	feels warm

1495	change in breast skin	2613		on the second rib
648	breasts decreasing in size	2614		between the second and third ribs
1629	breast development before age 9 (thelarche)	2615		on the third rib
649	enlargement of the breast (gynecomastia)	2616		between the third and fourth ribs
1881	**cardiovascular symptoms**	2617		on the fourth rib
279	chest pain	2618		between the fourth and fifth ribs
314	occurring	2619		on the fifth rib
315	suddenly as a new onset	2620		between the fifth and sixth ribs
313	as a recurring condition	2621		on the sixth rib
316	with increasing severity	2622		between the sixth and seventh ribs
317	more and more often	2623		on the seventh rib
307	lasting	2624		between the seventh and eighth ribs
308	1 - 15 minutes	2625		on the eighth rib
309	from 20 minutes to a day	2626		between the eighth and ninth ribs
310	continuously for several days	2627		on the ninth rib
311	continuously for several weeks or more	2628		between the ninth and tenth ribs
2578	increasingly longer	2629		along the costal margin
312	each episode	2590	posterior
2579	during the last few days	2591	lateral
2580	during the last few weeks	2584	center
2581	during the last few months	2592	anterior
280	located	2593	posterior
281	locally in the chest wall	2585	back
2582	right	282	left of the center (precordial)
2586	anterior	2630	right of the center (precordial)
2594	below the clavicle	283	centrally (substernal)
2595	on the second rib	284	in the lower chest (retrosternal)
2596	between the second and third ribs	285	on the right (hemithorax)
2597	on the third rib	286	on the left (hemithorax)
2598	between the third and fourth ribs	287	in the back between the shoulder blades
2599	on the fourth rib	288	radiating
2600	between the fourth and fifth ribs	289	to the jaw
2601	on the fifth rib	290	to the neck
2602	between the fifth and sixth ribs	291	to the right arm only (anteromedial)
2603	on the sixth rib	292	to the left arm only (anteromedial)
2604	between the sixth and seventh ribs	293	to both arms
2605	on the seventh rib	294	to the right side (hemithorax)
2606	between the seventh and eighth ribs	2631	to the left side (hemithorax)
2607	on the eighth rib	295	to the back between the shoulder blades
2608	between the eighth and ninth ribs	296	to the left shoulder
2609	on the ninth rib	297	to the right shoulder
2610	between the ninth and tenth ribs	298	to the central upper belly
2611	along the costal margin	299	changing location
2587	Posterior	300	feeling
2588	lateral	1717	of tenderness when touched
2583	left	301	dull, aching
2589	anterior		
2612	below the clavicle		

8

306	sudden, sharp, tearing	2655	throughout the body
302	sharp, shooting, knifelike	2651	right leg
303	burning	2652	left leg
304	tightness or heavy pressure	2653	right arm
305	deep, crushing	2654	left arm
1732	causing awakening from sleep	365	localized
1582	accompanied by	366	in one leg or arm
1585	stomach upset	1605	in one leg only
1584	palpitations	1606	on the right
1586	sweating	2647	upper
1583	difficulty breathing	2648	lower
325	starting	1607	on the left
326	when at rest	2649	upper
327	with exertion	2650	lower
2632	walking inside	2642	in one arm only
2633	walking on level ground	2643	right upper
2634	walking up steps and hills	2644	right lower
2635	jogging or running	2645	left upper
328	after eating (postprandial)	2646	left lower
329	with an emotional event	1588	in the hands
330	with sex	1924	right
331	when in a cold environment	1925	left
332	when lying down	1926	bilateral
333	after an injury	367	of the ankles
334	suddenly after prolonged immobility	966	foot
318	made worse by	1997	right
319	breathing or coughing	1998	left
320	body movements	1999	both
321	bending over	368	of the face
322	lying down	369	occurring
323	swallowing	370	suddenly
324	straining	371	intermittently
335	relieved	372	lower leg pain during exercise (intermittent claudication)
336	by rest		
337	by nitroglycerin	373	jaw pain during exercise
338	by antacids	388	cold hands or feet
339	by sitting up	2656	right arm
340	not relieved by rest	2657	right hand
341	rapid or irregular heartbeat (palpitation)	2658	left arm
2111	which are pounding	2659	left hand
2112	skipping beats	2660	right leg
2113	which are fast	2661	right foot
342	occurring	2662	left leg
343	15 - 30 minutes after eating	2663	left foot
344	2 - 3 hours after eating	389	sudden onset of cold hands or feet
345	lasting	2547	right arm
346	less than 1 minute	2548	right hand
347	1 to 15 minutes	2549	left arm
348	more than 15 minutes	2550	left hand
349	decreased by straining	2551	right leg
350	slow heart rate	2552	right foot
363	unexplained swelling (edema)	2553	left leg
364	generalized	2554	left foot

1880	**pulmonary symptoms**	264	yellow-green, thick (purulent)
353	difficulty breathing (dyspnea)	265	black
1858	which is new	266	foul smelling
356	started suddenly	267	large amounts (a cup or more per day)
360	rapidly getting worse	268	containing worms
357	for a long time (chronic)	1445	including hair
358	it has suddenly gotten much worse	269	clear, large amounts (bronchorrhea)
359	recurring intermittently (episodic)	270	coughing up hard particles (broncholiths)
2637	at rest (sitting up)	271	coughing up blood (hemoptysis)
354	during exertion	1298	massive (more than 1/2 cup in 4 hours)
2638	walking inside	1443	recurrent episodes
2639	walking on level ground	272	sweating heavily at night
2640	walking up steps and hills	273	wheezing
2641	jogging or running	274	only when breathing in
2636	accompanied by chest pain	275	worse at night
355	occurring only when lying down	276	worse in the morning
361	awakening at night short of breath (PND)	1308	worse during an upper respiratory infection (a cold)
362	using ___ extra pillows or sleeping upright (orthopnea)	1309	worse during cold weather
352	unusually slow breathing rate	1306	related to body position
351	rapid breathing	1307	occurring only with exercise
247	a cough	277	recurring from time to time (periodic)
248	which is	278	recurring intermittently (episodic)
1857	new	1882	**gastrointestinal symptoms**
250	chronic	390	recent loss of weight
252	worse in the morning	1722	excessive weight loss in a newborn
1512	causing awakening from sleep	391	recent gain in weight
253	repeated in spells every few minutes	1681	excessive during pregnancy
1510	occurring periodically	1490	dissatisfied with bodyweight
251	lasting > 3 mo. per yr. for > 2 consec. years	1478	feeling overweight
		1498	insufficient post-pregnancy loss
1511	occurring only with exertion	1491	feeling underweight
2522	continuous	1684	frequent weight changes of 4 or more pounds a week
249	sounding weak		
1747	sounding brassy	1411	appetite
2520	sounding like barking	1412	normal
2521	wheezy	1724	picky eater
1748	hacking	393	decreased (anorexia)
2519	loose	392	increased (polyphagia)
254	non-productive	1853	constantly hungry
2462	causing vomiting	394	extreme overeating (hyperphagia)
2463	which occurs	395	recurring with the episodes lasting 2-3 weeks
2464	during the day		
2465	during the night	1721	difficulty sucking
255	coughing up sputum	399	difficulty swallowing (dysphagia)
256	which is	1859	started recently
257	clear, mucoid or white	1860	which is chronic
258	blood-streaked	1861	is getting worse
259	pink & frothy	400	solid foods more than liquids
260	like currant jelly	401	liquids more than solid foods
261	like anchovy paste	402	particularly very hot or cold foods
262	rusty looking	403	followed by regurgitation
263	reddish brown	404	through the nose

405	accompanied by pain
406	with difficulty initiating a swallow
407	pain on swallowing
408	slow to finish meals
409	heartburn
468	belching (eructation)
1719	frequent indigestion
410	feeling full before finishing meals (early satiety)
411	nausea
412	occurring
413	15 - 30 minutes after eating
414	in the morning
1617	related to menstrual cycle
415	vomiting
416	which is
417	yellow-green (bilious)
418	clear (non-bilious)
419	containing food particles up to an hour after eating
420	containing stools
421	containing worms
422	self-induced
1587	violent and prolonged
2523	intractable
1851	projectile
1852	frequent, just after eating
1644	within a month of abdominal surgery
2466	after an injury
2467	more than twice
1701	excessive during early pregnancy
423	vomiting blood (hematemesis)
424	'coffee grounds' material
471	abdominal swelling
472	intermittent
473	occurring 20 - 30 minutes after a meal
474	occurring after milk or milk products
475	abdominal pain
500	started suddenly
1831	chronic / recurring frequently
501	chronic / constant
502	for more than 3 months
476	located
477	in the central upper belly (epigastric)
478	in the right upper belly (RUQ)
479	in the left upper belly (LUQ)
480	in the right lower belly (RLQ)
481	in the left lower belly (LLQ)
482	near the belly button (periumbilical)
483	above the pubic area (suprapubic)
484	spread evenly throughout the abdomen
2540	in multiple locations
485	radiating

486	to the upper part of the back
487	to the lower or mid region of the back
488	to the groin
489	to the left shoulder
490	to the neck & arms
491	to the right shoulder
492	changing location
493	to the right lower belly (RLQ)
494	feeling
495	steady, severe
496	crampy / colicky
497	burning
498	dull, boring or aching
499	onset
503	starting within 30 minutes after eating
504	starting 1 - 4 hours after eating
505	starting after consumption of alcohol
506	starting with exercise
507	causing awakening from sleep
508	starting in the morning upon awakening
509	seasonal, either Spring or Fall
510	starting or intensified by
511	fasting
512	coffee
513	milk
514	food
515	which is fatty
516	lying down
517	body movement or coughing
518	relieved
519	by food
520	by antacids
521	suddenly for no known reason
522	by sitting forward
523	by bowel movement
1746	by passing gas
524	by vomiting
425	regurgitation
426	through the nose
427	while sleeping
428	undigested food
1475	followed by rechewing and reswallowing
429	yellow skin or eyes (jaundice)
2492	skin only
2493	skin and eyes
2494	lower extremities
430	worsening with fasting
431	occurring after a blood transfusion
432	during the 1st week after surgery
433	occurring during pregnancy and subsiding afterwards

434	occurring intermittently
435	diarrhea
436	occurring
437	15 - 30 minutes after eating
438	after milk or milk products
439	at night (nocturnal)
440	chronic
441	watery
2468	mucous
1618	containing worms
442	bloody
443	painful
1645	within a month of abdominal surgery
444	constipation
445	chronic
446	alternating with diarrhea
469	excessive gas (flatulence)
470	unable to pass gas
447	pain when defecating
448	total stoppage of bowel movement (obstipation)
1493	change in bowel habits
449	recent increase in bowel frequency
1380	decrease in bowel frequency
450	bowel urgency with straining (tenesmus)
451	a change in the stool
452	color
453	black or tarry stools (melena)
454	red blood in bowel movement (hematochezia)
455	red blood on, rather than in the bowel movement
456	light colored bowel movement (acholic stools)
457	content
458	fat or grease (steatorrhea)
459	pus in the stool
460	mucus
461	worms
2471	white, thin worms at the rectum
2525	at night
462	size
463	has become bulky
464	has become smaller in diameter
1379	consistency
1365	looser or softer
1392	harder or firmer
465	stool has become foul smelling
2526	newborn stools
2527	meconium stools
2528	transitional stools
2469	yellow stools
2470	greenish black stools

2524	seedy stools
1728	stool retention with overflow
466	rectal pain
467	rectal sore
1883	**genitourinary symptoms**
2917	urinary
526	difficulty or pain during urination (dysuria)
527	change in urine volume
528	increased (polyuria)
529	decreased (oliguria)
530	cessation for 2 days or more (anuria)
2472	infant
2473	number of wet diapers
2474	hours since last urination
1837	urine odor
1838	foul smelling
531	change in appearance or color of urine
532	frothy
533	cloudy
534	smoky
535	dark but not cloudy
536	milky (chyluria)
537	containing pus (pyuria)
538	green
539	blood in the urine (hematuria)
540	initially
541	painful
542	occurring only at night or early morning
543	recurring over a period of years
544	occurring after exposure to cold temperature
545	starting with exercise
546	changes in urinary habits
547	incomplete emptying of bladder
548	increased in frequency
549	urinating more than once at night (nocturia)
550	feelings of urgency
551	delays in starting (hesitancy)
552	smaller urine stream, dribbling, or starting and stopping
553	urine content abnormalities
554	passage of stones or gravel
555	bubbles
556	passage of tissue
557	passage of stools
558	pain in the flank
559	radiating
560	to a testicle
561	groin symptoms (inguinal)
562	swelling

563	pain
572	genital sores
1497	penile
573	a single sore
574	with multiple sores
575	began as a small inflamed pimple
576	began as a sore
577	first looked like a small blister
578	painful
579	foul smelling
564	genital symptoms
566	testicular pain
567	occurring suddenly
1496	testicular swelling
568	scrotal swelling
1340	penile pain
569	swollen penis
2475	redness at distal end of penis
570	penile discharge
571	yellow to yellow-green, profuse
586	obstetrics and gynecology
2916	genital
581	vaginal itching or burning
582	vaginal pain during intercourse
583	vaginal lump or mass
585	vulvar itching or burning
2416	vulvar lump or mass
1455	pre-menopausal
1456	normal menstruation within the last 30 days
1500	date of last menstruation:
1630	age at first period (menarche)
587	first period (menarche) was before 9 years old
588	bleeding lasting less than 3 days
589	bleeding lasts more than 7 days
590	timing of last 2 periods
591	the most recent was late (days):
592	the previous one was late (days):
593	missed most recent period
1499	missed previous period(s) also
1687	three or more
1501	patient thinks she may be pregnant
1680	baby moving (in uterus)
594	periods have stopped for over 6 months (amenorrhea)
595	over 16 and periods haven't started
596	time between periods has increased (oligomenorrhea)
1723	periods require staying in bed
597	severe pain with periods (dysmenorrhea)

598	excessive bleeding during period (menorrhagia)
1632	frequent passing of large blood clots during periods
599	less bleeding during period (hypomenorrhea)
600	bleeding between periods (metrorrhagia)
601	irregular length of periods
1494	unexplained vaginal bleeding
1622	bleeding during pregnancy
1623	first trimester
1624	second trimester
1625	third trimester
602	using tampons regularly during period
1631	using 8 or more daily
603	fever onset during most recent period
604	birth control method
606	using rhythm method
607	condoms
608	oral contraceptives
609	an intra-uterine device (IUD)
1635	when first used
1616	can't feel string
2115	subdermal contraceptive implant
605	no use of birth control methods
610	vaginal discharge other than normal menstruation
611	white
612	worse after menstruating
613	which is yellow-green, thick
614	foul smelling
2476	mucous
2490	mucopurulent
617	bleeding occurs after sex
615	history of menopause having occurred
616	bleeding has occurred since
1642	abnormal urethral discharge
565	white
1887	**endocrine symptoms**
207	excessive thirst or water consumption (polydypsia)
1061	excessive sweating
2909	15 - 30 minutes after eating
1063	2 - 3 hours after eating
1877	colored sweat
1064	hot flashes
1065	sudden redness of the skin (flushing)
1744	mainly facial
1066	changes in body proportions or appearance
1068	size of head
1067	size of hands
1331	size of feet

1069	increasing muscle size	2675	right
1070	height is decreasing	2676	left
1503	generalized decrease in strength	2677	both
1071	feelings of weakness	1568	with cracking
1073	15 - 30 minutes after eating	1089	skin sore(s) (___cm) or a rash
1074	2 - 3 hours after eating	1090	painful
2910	relieved by food	1091	a chronic condition
1076	temperature intolerance	1092	comes and goes
1077	to heat	1601	with fever
1078	to cold	2534	appeared 1-3 days after a fever
1079	deepening of the voice	2535	and other symptoms resolved
1479	increased body odor	2544	appeared 1-3 days before a fever
1080	decreased beard growth	2542	which has gotten much worse
1081	sparse facial hair	2543	which is similar to one seen before
1839	hair breaks easily	1749	generalized
1082	excessive facial or body hair (hirsutism)	1574	localized
1083	loss of hair from head or body	2488	on the scalp
1628	growth of pubic or axillary hair before age 9	2678	towards the front
1084	eyes bulging out (exophthalmos)	2679	on top
1871	which comes and goes	2680	on the right side
1872	which is persistent	2681	on the left side
1890	sexual complaints	2682	towards the back
1139	changed sexual interest (libido)	2691	on the ears
1140	decreased	2792	right
1141	increased	2793	left
1142	premature ejaculation	1575	on the face
1336	inadequacy of penile erection	2692	forehead
1087	unable to perform sex (impotence)	2693	right
1554	lack of nocturnal erection	2694	left
1088	unable to ejaculate (but not impotent)	2695	entire forehead
1086	unable to impregnate (male infertility)	2696	between forehead and ear (temple)
1337	inadequacy of lubrication or swelling of vaginal mucosa	2697	right
		2698	left
1143	inhibited or absent female orgasm	2699	on both sides
1085	unable to conceive (infertility)	2700	cheeks
1299	hyposexuality	2701	right
1300	hypersexuality	2702	left
1888	**skin symptoms**	2703	both
1075	dry skin	2704	junction of nose and cheek (paranasal)
2477	chronic		
1563	generalized	2705	right side
1564	localized	2706	left side
1565	of the hand(s)	2707	both sides
2668	right	2708	nose
2669	left	2709	right side
2670	both	2710	left side
1566	of the face	2711	both sides
2478	of the creases of elbows, wrists, knees	2712	area around mouth (circumoral)
2671	of the shins	2713	right side
2672	right	2714	left side
2673	left	2715	both sides
2674	both	1686	around nose and mouth
1567	of the feet		

SKIN SORES OR A RASH, CONT.

2716	right side
2717	left side
2718	both sides
2719	lip
2720	upper
2721	right side
2722	left side
2723	both sides
2724	lower
2725	right side
2726	left side
2727	both sides
2728	chin
2729	right side
2730	left side
2731	both sides
2732	along the jaw line
2733	right side
2734	left side
2735	both sides
1841	on the neck
2736	right side
2742	toward the front
2743	toward the back
2737	left side
2744	toward the front
2745	toward the back
2738	both sides
2746	toward the front
2747	toward the back
1842	on the shoulders
2739	right side
2748	on the front
2749	on top
2750	on the back
2740	left side
2751	on the front
2752	on top
2753	on the back
2741	both sides
2754	on the front
2755	on top
2756	on the back
1847	within the armpits
2757	right
2758	left
2759	both
1846	on the upper extremities
1848	arms
2760	right
2761	left
2762	both
2687	elbows

2763	right
2764	on the inside
2765	on the back
2766	left
2767	on the inside
2768	on the back
2769	both
2770	on the inside
2771	on the back
1581	forearms
2772	right
2773	left
2688	wrists
2774	right
2775	on the inside
2776	on the outside
2777	left
2778	on the inside
2779	on the outside
2780	both
2781	on the inside
2782	on the outside
1576	hands
2783	right
2784	top
2785	palm
2786	left
2787	top
2788	palm
2789	both
2790	top
2791	palms
1577	fingers
2794	right thumb
2795	right index finger
2796	right middle finger
2797	right ring finger
2798	right little finger
2799	left thumb
2800	left index finger
2801	left middle finger
2802	left ring finger
2803	left little finger
2804	multiple fingers of both hands
1843	on the trunk
1844	on the chest
2805	right
2806	left
2807	entire
1573	on the belly
2808	right upper
2809	left upper
2810	right lower

SKIN SORES OR A RASH, CONT.

2811	left lower		2848	right
1845	on the back		2849	front
2812	upper		2850	back
2813	right		2851	inner aspect
2814	left		2852	outer aspect
2815	entire		2853	left
2816	middle		2854	front
2817	right		2855	back
2818	left		2856	inner aspect
2819	entire		2857	outer aspect
2820	lower		2858	both
2821	right		2859	front
2822	left		2860	back
2823	entire		2861	inner aspect
1578	in the groin		2862	outer aspect
2824	right		2684	shins
2825	left		2863	right
2826	entire area		2864	left
2479	in the diaper area		2865	both
2480	in the front		2685	calves
2481	involving buttocks		2866	right
2482	peeling		2867	left
2483	bleeding		2868	both
2484	scabs		2690	ankles
2485	raw		2869	right
2486	smooth, red		2872	inner aspect
2487	papular		2873	outer aspect
2415	vulvar		2870	left
2827	right		2874	inner aspect
2828	left		2875	outer aspect
2829	entire area		2871	both
1849	on the buttocks		2876	inner aspect
2830	right		2877	outer aspect
2831	left		1579	feet
2832	both		2878	right
2686	on the lower extremities		2879	top
1850	thighs		2880	sole
2833	right		2881	left
2834	front		2882	top
2835	back		2883	sole
2836	inner aspect		2884	both
2837	outer aspect		2885	top
2838	left		2886	soles
2839	front		1580	toes
2840	back		2887	right great toe
2841	inner aspect		2888	right second toe
2842	outer aspect		2889	right third toe
2843	both		2890	right fourth toe
2844	front		2891	right little toe
2845	back		2892	left great toe
2846	inner aspect		2893	left second toe
2847	outer aspect		2894	left third toe
2689	knees		2895	left fourth toe

SKIN SORES OR A RASH, CONT.

2896	left little toe	1594	skin stretch marks
2683	between the toes	1595	occurring after pregnancy
2897	of the right foot	1596	occurring after losing weight
2898	of the left foot	1597	occurring spontaneously
2899	of both feet	1598	in the armpit region
1750	spreading	1492	change in skin texture
1751	from face to trunk	1113	itching (pruritus)
1752	from trunk outwards	1114	generalized
2489	beginning peripherally, spreading inward	1115	localized to skin rash or sores
2529	with surrounding redness	1116	of the scalp
2531	red and splotchy	1117	of the teeth
1522	a single enlarging red patch	2503	of the ears
2500	with central clearing and scaly borders	2504	right
1302	circular in shape	2505	left
2533	lacy	2506	bilaterally
2499	bumpy	1118	in the anal region
1093	is darkening	1119	worse at night
2495	after exposure to heat	1120	of the palms and soles
2496	warm bath	1121	after warm bath or shower
2497	exposure to sun	1122	abnormal sensitivity to sunlight (photosensitivity)
1094	a loss of skin color		
1095	which doesn't heal	1123	nails break easily
2498	with blisters	1124	change in a mole
2532	which oozes	2664	lumps
1096	which bleeds	1099	in/on the skin
1570	which cracks	1100	painful
2502	with crusting	1101	lasting for months
2530	with scabs	1876	growing rapidly
2501	with yellow-white drainage	2665	under the skin
1410	unusual growth on the skin	1127	large
1097	painful skin area without rash or sore	1128	painful
1332	superficial skin pain	2666	small
1333	of the lower leg	2667	location
1334	localized skin discoloration	1889	**hematologic symptoms**
1600	blue / brown patches on legs or arms	1129	easy bleeding tendency
1335	brownish lower legs	1130	occurring
1102	change in color of skin	1131	spontaneously
1569	to red (erythema)	1132	after major surgery or trauma
1571	generalized	1133	starting
1572	localized	1134	several hours or days after an injury
1103	to white (pallor)	1135	after having stopped
1735	around the mouth	1136	recurrent
1104	episodic	1137	easy bruising tendency
1105	cyanosis	1138	occurring spontaneously
1106	of the hands or feet only	1886	**musculoskeletal symptoms**
1107	of the feet and legs	917	back pain
1108	persistent	918	in the upper back
1109	with cold temperature	2105	on the right
1110	to darker	2106	on the left
1454	to a metallic grey/blue color	920	radiating around the chest
1111	to a light lemon yellow color	919	starting suddenly
1112	greenish discoloration	921	relieved by lying down
		922	worsened by lying down

MUSCULOSKELETAL, CONT.

923	in the middle of the back		2140	MCP
2107	on the right		2143	PIP
2108	on the left		2146	DIP
925	radiating around the chest		2077	ring finger
924	starting suddenly		2141	MCP
926	relieved by lying down		2144	PIP
927	worsened by lying down		2147	DIP
928	in the lower back		2078	little finger
2109	on the right		2142	MCP
2110	on the left		2145	PIP
929	excruciating		2148	DIP
930	radiating to the legs		1921	of the fingers of both hands
931	starting suddenly		939	wrist
1534	chronic		1937	right
932	worse with coughing or sneezing		2121	radiocarpal
933	worse with bending over		2122	ulnarcarpal
934	worsened by lying down		1938	left
935	relieved by lying down		2123	radiocarpal
1757	relieved by movement		2124	ulnarcarpal
1439	precipitated by tension, depression, or anxiety		1939	bilateral
			2341	radiocarpal
936	localized joint pain		2342	ulnarcarpal
937	location		940	elbow
1916	fingers		1946	right
1919	of the right hand		2149	radiocapitellar
2069	thumb		2150	ulnartrochlear
2116	MCP joint		1947	left
2117	IP		2151	radiocapitellar
2070	index finger		2152	ulnartrochlear
2118	MCP		1948	bilateral
2119	PIP		941	shoulder
2120	DIP		1955	right
2071	middle finger		2153	glenohumeral
2126	MCP		2154	acromioclavicular
2129	PIP		2155	scapulothoracic
2132	DIP		2156	sternoclavicular
2072	ring finger		1956	left
2127	MCP		2157	glenohumeral
2130	PIP		2158	acromioclavicular
2133	DIP		2159	scapulothoracic
2073	little finger		2160	sternoclavicular
2128	MCP		1957	both
2131	PIP		942	TMJ
2134	DIP		1964	right
1920	of the left hand		1965	left
2074	thumb		1966	bilateral
2135	MCP		943	hip
2136	IP		1973	right
2075	index finger		1974	left
2137	MCP		1975	bilateral
2138	PIP		944	knee
2139	DIP		1979	right
2076	middle finger		2161	medial

MUSCULOSKELETAL, CONT.

2162	lateral	1917	fingers	
2163	posterior	1931	of the right hand	
2164	patellofemoral	2079	thumb	
1980	left	2194	MCP	
2165	medial	2196	IP	
2166	lateral	2080	index finger	
2167	posterior	2200	MCP	
2168	patellofemoral	2198	PIP	
1981	bilateral	2202	DIP	
945	ankle	2081	middle finger	
1982	right	2204	MCP	
2169	anterior	2206	PIP	
2170	posterior	2208	DIP	
2171	medial	2082	ring finger	
2172	lateral	2210	MCP	
1983	left	2212	PIP	
2173	anterior	2214	DIP	
2174	posterior	2083	little finger	
2175	medial	2216	MCP	
2176	lateral	2218	PIP	
1984	bilateral	2220	DIP	
2177	toes	1933	of the left hand	
947	great toe	2084	thumb	
1988	right	2222	MCP	
2178	MTP	2224	IP	
2179	IP	2085	index finger	
1989	left	2226	MCP	
2180	MTP	2228	PIP	
2181	IP	2230	DIP	
1990	bilateral	2086	middle finger	
2182	second toe	2232	MCP	
2186	right	2234	PIP	
2190	left	2236	DIP	
2183	middle toe	2087	ring finger	
2187	right	2238	MCP	
2191	left	2240	PIP	
2184	fourth toe	2242	DIP	
2188	right	2088	little finger	
2192	left	2244	MCP	
2185	little toe	2246	PIP	
2189	right	2248	DIP	
2193	left	1935	of the fingers of both hands	
948	occurring	960	wrist	
949	suddenly	1940	right	
950	a chronic condition	1942	left	
951	only in one joint	1944	bilateral	
952	in several joints	961	elbow	
1599	getting worse	1949	right	
953	moving from joint to joint	1951	left	
954	diffuse joint pains (arthralgias)	1953	bilateral	
957	joint swelling	962	shoulder	
958	location	1958	right	
959	hand	1960	left	

MUSCULOSKELETAL, CONT.

1962	both	2207		PIP
963	jaw	2209		DIP
1967	right	2092	ring finger	
1969	left	2211		MCP
1971	bilateral	2213		PIP
964	knee	2215		DIP
1991	right	2093	little finger	
1992	left	2217		MCP
1993	both	2219		PIP
965	ankle	2221		DIP
1994	right	1934	of the left hand	
1995	left	2094	thumb	
1996	both	2223		MCP
2250	toes	2225		IP
2252	great toe	2095	index finger	
2254	right	2227		MCP
2256	MTP	2229		PIP
2258	IP	2231		DIP
2260	left	2096	middle finger	
2262	MTP	2233		MCP
2264	IP	2235		PIP
2266	bilateral	2237		DIP
2268	second toe	2097	ring finger	
2270	right	2239		MCP
2272	left	2241		PIP
2274	middle toe	2243		DIP
2276	right	2098	little finger	
2278	left	2245		MCP
2280	fourth toe	2247		PIP
2282	right	2249		DIP
2284	left	1936	of the fingers of both hands	
2286	little toe	976	wrist	
2288	right	1941	right	
2290	left	1943	left	
967	occurring	1945	bilateral	
968	in only one joint	977	elbow	
969	in more than one joint	1950	right	
970	suddenly	1952	left	
971	a chronic condition	1954	bilateral	
972	moving from joint to joint	978	shoulder	
973	localized joint stiffness	1959	right	
974	location	1961	left	
1918	fingers	1963	both	
1932	of the right hand	979	jaw	
2089	thumb	1968	right	
2195	MCP	1970	left	
2197	IP	1972	bilateral	
2090	index finger	981	hip	
2201	MCP	1976	right	
2199	PIP	1977	left	
2203	DIP	1978	bilateral	
2091	middle finger	982	knee	
2205	MCP	2000	right	

MUSCULOSKELETAL, CONT.

2001	left		2307	medial
2002	bilateral		2308	lateral
983	ankle		2309	olecranon
2003	right		2306	left
2004	left		2310	medial
2005	bilateral		2311	lateral
2251	toes		2312	olecranon
2253	great toe		2294	in the forearm
2255	right		994	right
2257	MTP		996	left
2259	IP		2555	in the hand
2261	left		2556	right
2263	MTP		2557	left
2265	IP		2295	in the pelvic girdle
2267	bilateral		1444	on the right
2269	second toe		2298	on the left
2271	right		2292	in the hip
2273	left		2299	right
2275	middle toe		2300	left
2277	right		2296	in the thigh
2279	left		997	right
2281	fourth toe		999	left
2283	right		2313	in the knee
2285	left		2314	right
2287	little toe		2315	kneecap
2289	right		2316	in the inner side
2291	left		2317	in the outer side
985	occurring		2318	in back
986	in more than one joint		2319	left
987	suddenly		2320	kneecap
988	a chronic condition		2321	in the inner side
989	worse in the morning		2322	in the outer side
975	hand stiffness		2323	in back
1927	right		2297	in the leg (below the knee)
1928	left		998	right
1929	bilateral		1000	left
980	back stiffness		2558	in the foot
984	foot stiffness		2559	right
2006	right		2560	left
2007	left		992	diffuse
2008	bilateral		1626	within a region
990	sudden unexplained fractures		1627	in multiple sites
955	bony lump which doesn't go away		2324	neuromuscular / connective tissue symptoms
956	painless		1001	muscle aches
991	bone pain		1003	in the neck or shoulder
2301	in the clavicle		2343	in the neck
2302	right		2344	right
2303	left		2345	left
2293	in the arm		2370	bilateral
993	right		2347	in the lower neck / upper back
995	left		2348	right
2304	in the elbow		2349	left
2305	right		2346	bilateral

MUSCULOSKELETAL, CONT.

2350	in the shoulder	1020	on the front
2351	right	2375	right
2352	left	2376	left
2353	bilateral	2377	bilateral
1004	in the hip (pelvic girdle)	1021	on the back
2354	right	2378	right
2355	left	2379	left
2356	bilateral	2380	bilateral
2363	in the thigh	1022	in the inner aspect
2364	right quadriceps	2381	right
2365	left quadriceps	2382	left
2366	both quadriceps	2383	bilateral
2367	right hamstring	1023	in the outer aspect
2368	left hamstring	2384	right
2369	both hamstrings	2385	left
1005	in the leg (below the knee)	2386	bilateral
2357	front of right leg	1024	above the knee
2358	front of left leg	2387	right
2359	front of both legs	2388	left
2360	calf of right leg	2389	bilateral
2361	calf of left leg	1025	behind the knee
2362	calf of both legs	2390	right
2565	relieved by moving the leg(s)	2391	left
2566	occurring mainly at night	2392	bilateral
1002	generalized (myalgias)	2374	in the leg
374	pain in the hands	1029	right
1429	cramping	1030	left
375	occurring with hand exercise	1031	bilateral
376	relieved by rest	1026	in the shin
377	in the fingers only	1027	in the calf
378	just when cold	1028	above the heel
379	with changes in finger color	2393	right
380	in one hand only	2394	left
1912	in the right hand only	2395	bilateral
1913	in the left hand only	1032	shooting (radicular)
381	occurring often at night	1033	down the front
1007	pain in the arm(s)	2396	of the right extremity
1008	in the right arm only	2397	of the left extremity
1009	in the left arm only	2398	of both extremities
1010	shooting down the arm (radicular)	1034	down the back
1011	on the inner side of the arm	2399	of the right extremity
1012	on the outer side of the arm	2400	of the left extremity
1013	triggered by neck movement	2401	of both extremities
1014	triggered by coughing or straining	1035	down the inner side
1015	in one location only	2402	of the right extremity
1016	warmth and redness	2403	of the left extremity
1017	occurring suddenly	2404	of both extremities
1047	pain in the buttock	1036	down the outer side
2371	right	2405	of the right extremity
2372	left	2406	of the left extremity
2373	bilateral	2407	of both extremities
1018	pain in the lower extremities	2408	ending above the knee
1019	in the thigh	2409	ending below the knee

MUSCULOSKELETAL, CONT.

2410	ending below the ankle
1037	triggered by bending over
1038	triggered by coughing or sneezing
1039	triggered by lifting a heavy object
1040	only after elevation
1041	in blue swollen veins
1042	in one location only
1043	warmth and redness
1044	occurring suddenly
1045	relieved by lying down
1046	worsened by lying down
382	pain in the feet
383	occurring with exercise or relieved by rest
384	in one foot only
1914	in the right foot only
1915	in the left foot only
385	in the toes only
386	just when cold
387	pain in the hands and feet (distal)
1006	pain in both arms and legs
1048	lightning pains
1049	in the legs
1050	muscle cramps
1051	in the hands
1052	in the upper leg (thigh)
1053	in the lower leg (calf)
1054	in the feet
1055	occurring at night
1056	precipitated by exercise
1057	especially in cold weather
2567	legs feel restless
2568	mainly at night
2569	disturbs sleep
2570	relieved by movement
1058	muscle spasms
1059	in the neck
1060	in the lower back
1341	in the vagina
1342	occur with attempted penetration
912	muscles decreasing in size
913	generalized
914	in the arm
1483	in the hand
915	in the leg
916	severe pain in a wound
1745	infant flexes limbs, clenches fists and screams
1885	**neurological symptoms**
1613	lightheadedness
650	dizziness
651	while using hands or arms
652	upon bending over
653	upon standing up
2099	upon rolling over
2100	when walking up stairs
654	recurrent episodes
655	spinning dizziness (vertigo)
656	upon lying down
657	after sudden changes in position
2009	caused by noise
658	convulsions
659	recurring for a long time
660	generalized
1753	occurring with high fever
661	localized
662	progressed to involve entire side
663	fainting (syncope)
664	syncope and collapse
665	unconscious about 1 to 5 minutes
666	while using hands or arms
667	upon bending over
668	upon standing up
1524	followed by a headache
2114	preceded
1523	by sudden or severe headache
1525	by turning pale
1533	by turning blue
1532	by rapid or irregular heart beat
1593	by chest pain
1526	by sweating
1527	by flushing
1530	by sudden severe throat pain
1531	by sudden severe ear pain
1528	during urination
1529	while coughing
669	recurrent episodes
1200	decreased concentrating ability
1705	changed thought patterns
1703	rate of thinking has slowed down
1704	racing thoughts
1706	thinking two thoughts at the same time
670	staring spells
671	decreases in consciousness
672	drowsiness
2541	while driving
673	difficult to rouse (stupor)
674	coma
675	relieved by eating
676	confused or disoriented
677	delirious
678	fluctuating or waxing and waning
1676	momentary lucid intervals
2912	started recently
2913	chronic
679	steadily worsening

NEUROLOGICAL, CONT.

680	frequently become lost	719	recurrent
681	memory lapses or loss	720	causing difficulty climbing stairs (proximal)
1305	lost periods of time		
682	repeated questioning about recent events	1430	has progressed to difficulty rising from a chair
683	focal disturbances		
684	sense of smell	721	started with legs and progressed upwards
685	greatly increased or suddenly unpleasant		
		722	started with arms and progressed down to legs
686	lost (anosmia)		
687	on one side only	2329	made worse by
688	difficulty chewing	2330	heat
689	corner of the mouth drooping (facial weakness)	2331	exercise
		2332	stress
690	on the right only	723	involuntary movements
691	on the left only	724	trembling or shaking (tremor)
692	on both sides	725	occur at rest
693	taste disturbances (unusual taste of foods)	726	occur with movement
694	speech difficulties	727	on the right side only
695	slurred	728	on the left side only
696	forgetting words	729	the fingers and wrists curl up (tetany)
1482	stuttering	730	twisting
697	come and go	1476	repeated muscle twitches (tics)
1688	difficulty writing	1480	can be suppressed temporarily
698	weak or non-moving limbs (paresis / paralysis)	731	sudden, jerky
		732	come and go
699	affecting the shoulder(s)	2571	involuntary movements during sleep
700	right only	2572	which are violent
701	left only	2574	which cause awakening
702	hand(s) only	2573	with vivid dream recall
1892	right only	1477	involuntary speech or noise
1893	left only	733	abnormality of walk
703	feet only	734	wobbly or unsteady (ataxia)
704	hands and feet (distal)	735	shuffling
705	affecting both legs	1864	short steps
706	affecting all four limbs	736	waddling gait
707	developed in clockwise progression	737	limping
708	affecting one entire side only	738	dragging one foot
709	occurring temporarily (transient)	739	on the right
710	on the right	740	on the left
711	on the left	1484	frequent falling
712	affecting the right arm only	741	comes and goes
713	affecting the left arm only	742	difficulty running, but walk is normal
714	affecting the right leg only	743	difficulty keeping one's balance
715	affecting the left leg only	744	lack of coordination
716	occurring suddenly	745	on one side only
717	occurring after a starchy meal	746	on the right
718	occurring temporarily	747	on the left
1413	occurring with intense emotions (cataplexy)	1646	tingling (paresthesias)
		1609	of the tongue
1414	when falling asleep or awakening (sleep paralysis)	1610	on the right side only
		1611	on the left side only
2576	when falling asleep	1612	on both sides
2575	when awakening	748	around the mouth

NEUROLOGICAL, CONT.

749	facial	795	just of the groin
750	on one entire side	796	only on the outer side of the upper leg
751	on the right		
752	on the left	797	only on the back side of the upper leg
753	of the forehead only		
754	on the right side only	798	only of the buttock
755	on the left side only	799	only on the front of the lower leg (shin)
756	of the right cheek		
757	of the left cheek	800	only on the back of the lower leg (calf)
758	of the lip		
759	of the chin	801	just of the left leg
760	of the shoulder(s)	802	only on the front of the upper leg
761	on the right	803	only on the inner side of the upper leg
762	on the left		
763	one entire side	804	just of the groin
764	on the right	805	only on the outer side of the upper leg
765	on the left		
766	of the extremities	806	only on the back side of the upper leg
767	just of the right arm		
768	only on the inner side of the arm	807	only of the buttock
769	only on the outer side of the arm	808	only on the front of the lower leg (shin)
770	just of the left arm		
771	only on the inner side of the arm	809	only on the back of the lower leg (calf)
772	only on the outer side of the arm		
773	of both arms	810	of both legs
774	only on the inner side of the arm	811	just on both buttocks
775	only on the outer side of the arm	812	of both arms and both legs
776	just of the right hand	813	just of the right foot
777	only of the thumb	814	only on the top of the foot
778	only of the thumb and index finger	815	only on the sole of the foot
		816	just of the left foot
779	only of the thumb, index, and middle finger	817	only on the top of the foot
		818	only on the sole of the foot
780	only of the middle finger	819	of both feet
781	only of the ring (fourth), and little finger	820	hands and feet (distal)
		821	started with legs and progressed upwards
782	only of the back of the hand		
783	just of the left hand	822	occurring during exercise
784	only of the thumb	823	in the perianal region
785	only of the thumb and index finger	824	in the perineum
		2337	made worse by
786	only of the thumb, index, and middle finger	2338	heat
		2339	exercise
787	only of the middle finger	2340	stress
788	only of the ring (fourth), and little finger	825	burning sensation
		826	just in the right arm or hand
789	only of the back of the hand	827	just in the left arm or hand
790	of both hands	828	only in both arms or hands
791	from the waist down	1562	only in the fingers
792	just of the right leg	829	just in the right leg or foot
793	only on the front of the upper leg	830	just in the left leg or foot
794	only on the inner side of the upper leg	831	only in both legs or feet
		832	on one entire side

NEUROLOGICAL, CONT.

833	in the hands and feet (distal)	861	only of the ring (fourth), and little finger
834	perianal		
835	perineum	862	only on the back of the hand
1647	numbness (hypesthesia)	863	of both hands
1648	of the tongue	864	from the waist down
1649	on the right side only	865	just of the right leg
1650	on the left side only	866	only on the front of the upper leg
1651	on both sides	867	only on the inner side of the upper leg
1652	around the mouth		
1653	facial	868	just of the groin
1654	on one entire side	869	only on the outer side of the upper leg
1655	on the right		
1656	on the left	870	only on the back side of the upper leg
1657	of the forehead only		
1658	on the right side only	871	just of the buttock
1659	on the left side only	872	only on the front of the lower leg (shin)
1660	of the right cheek		
1661	of the left cheek	873	only on the back of the lower leg (calf)
1662	of the lip		
1663	of the chin	874	just of the left leg
1664	of the shoulder(s)	875	only on the front of the upper leg
1665	on the right	876	only on the inner side of the upper leg
1666	on the left		
836	one entire side	877	just of the groin
837	on the right	878	only on the outer side of the upper leg
838	on the left		
839	of the extremities	879	only on the back side of the upper leg
840	just of the right arm		
841	only on the inner side of the arm	880	just of the buttock
842	only on the outer side of the arm	881	only on the front of the lower leg (shin)
843	just of the left arm		
844	only on the inner side of the arm	882	only on the back of the lower leg (calf)
845	only on the outer side of the arm		
846	of both arms	883	of both legs
847	only on the inner side of the arm	884	just on both buttocks
848	only on the outer side of the arm	885	both arms and both legs
849	just of the right hand	886	just of the right foot
850	just of the right thumb	887	only on the top of the foot
851	only of the right thumb and index finger	888	only on the sole of the foot
		889	just of the left foot
852	only of the right thumb, index, and middle finger	890	only on the top of the foot
		891	only on the sole of the foot
853	only of the right middle finger	892	of both feet
854	only of the right ring (fourth), and little finger	893	of the hands and feet (distal)
		894	started with legs and progressed upwards
855	only on the back of the hand		
856	just of the left hand	895	occurring during exercise
857	only of the thumb	896	in the perianal region
858	only of the thumb and index finger	897	in the perineum
		2333	made worse by
859	only of the thumb, index, and middle finger	2334	heat
		2335	exercise
860	only of the middle finger	2336	stress

NEUROLOGICAL, CONT.

898	no feeling or sensation (anesthesia)	1149	homosexual experiences
899	from the neck down	1150	unwanted and persistently distressing
900	from the chest down	1154	loss of pleasure from usual activities
901	from the waist down		(anhedonia)
902	just in the legs	1155	sleep disturbances
903	increased sensitivity to touch or pain (hyperesthesia)	1156	sleeping much more than usual
		1157	recurrent episodes lasting 2-3 weeks
904	focal disturbances start with straining	1714	sleeping too much (hypersomnia)
906	difficulty starting and stopping movements	2507	infant sleeping more than 4-5 hours at a time
907	present since childhood	1158	excessive sleepiness during the day
908	unable to restrain urination		(daytime somnolence)
909	at night, while asleep	1713	suddenly falling asleep during the day
1726	during daytime	1159	insomnia
910	temporarily with sudden movement or cough	1160	difficulty falling asleep
		1856	because of pain
1836	in a previously continent child	1161	awakening in the middle of the night
2420	occurring at least twice a week	1515	have a cigarette
911	unable to restrain bowel movement	1516	have a snack
1891	**psychological symptoms**	2562	insomnia due to noise
1312	sexual behavior	2563	insomnia due to light
1145	non-vaginal intercourse	2564	insomnia due to frequent interruptions
1146	oral	1162	early morning awakening
1147	anal	1712	groggy for too long upon awakening
1144	exposure to venereal disease	1711	do not feel rested after adequate night's sleep
1338	stimulation is inadequate in duration and quality	1458	moving to parental bed in the middle of the night
1339	duration of coitus insufficient to satisfy female	1715	mismatch of sleep / wake schedule with lifestyle needs
1322	masturbation	1164	nightmares
1727	excessive / inappropriate	1165	screaming in the middle of the night
2419	anal	1485	with sense of terror but no complete dream sequences
1709	aversion to sexual intercourse	1166	sleep walking
1343	no sensation felt during intercourse	1167	periods of not breathing (sleep apnea)
1535	no sensation felt during ejaculation	1168	decreased need for sleep
1326	surreptitious observation of sexual activity or nudity	1169	increased energy
		1323	having fantasies
1313	preferred partner is same gender	1400	of unlimited success, power, adoration
1328	preference for being bound, beaten, raped, or humiliated	1324	of sexual activity with animals
		1325	of sexual activity with pre-pubertal children
1707	arousal from rubbing against non-consenting person	1327	of being bound, beaten, or raped
1330	arousal from feces, corpses, enemas, urine	1170	nervous or anxious
1708	arousal from lewdness, obscene phone calls	1171	with persistent worry
		1553	about anticipated performance
1359	arousal from watching fires	1710	about insomnia
1329	arousal only by inflicting pain on partner	1172	about homosexual encounter
1320	non-living object necessary to achieve arousal	1173	with anticipation of misfortune to self or others
1318	male breast augmentation	1457	from anticipation of separation
1148	dressing as the opposite sex	1303	with unrealistic fear of disease
1321	intense frustration when thwarted		
1317	desire to be rid of one's genitals		
1319	desire to be opposite sex when adult		

PSYCHOLOGICAL, CONT.

1174	with fear of dying, going crazy or losing self-control
1175	with difficulty breathing
1176	with chest pain or discomfort
1177	with rapid heart beat
1178	with choking or smothering sensations
1179	with dizziness, "vertigo" or unsteady feelings
1180	with feelings of unreality
1181	with tingling in hands / feet
1182	with muscle tension or jitters
1183	with stomach discomfort
1184	with frequent urination or diarrhea
1185	with hot and cold flashes
1186	with excessive sweating
2911	which comes and goes (episodic)
1187	with sudden onset, lasting minutes to hours
1189	three or more episodes occurring in a 3-week period
1188	unrelated to exertion or dangerous situation
1190	continuously for a month or more
1508	interfering with social activities
1509	interfering with work
1517	relieved by checking
1518	relieved by washing
1519	relieved by a ritual
1191	unreasonable or irrational fears
1192	of specific objects, activity or situation
1193	of being alone
1194	of being in or crossing open spaces or bridges
1513	of enclosed places, elevators, tunnels, or subways
1459	of flying
1460	of strangers
1195	of one specific social situation
1423	of being abandoned
1463	of becoming obese
1196	with a compelling desire to avoid (phobia)
1197	increasing limitation of normal activities
1734	restless
1733	fussy
2513	and inconsolable
1198	highly irritable
1295	prior to menstruation (3-10 days)
1360	hostile feelings
1361	towards authority figures
1199	feeling unique and all-powerful (grandeur)
1201	change in personality
1291	decreased effectiveness or productivity

1387	character deficiency
1388	superficial / shallow
1428	stingy / miserly
1696	evade paying debts
1389	inconsiderate of others
1397	unable to empathize with others
1424	unable to express warmth and tenderness
1431	procrastination
1426	unable to make decisions
1390	vain
1403	overly envious of others
1399	extremely self-centered, self-absorbed
1393	excessive feelings of entitlement
1425	excessive attention to detail (perfectionism)
1394	interpersonal relationship problems
1421	passive
1422	dependent
1489	unable to communicate effectively
1440	unable to express anger
1441	masochistic
1391	demanding
1521	aggressive
1691	harassing others
1402	socializing for appearances rather than for friendship
1395	exploitative
1427	domineering
1396	constant need for admiration
1398	extreme overidealization or devaluation of others
1442	turbulent and damaging
1449	marital
1448	with parent or guardian
1446	with siblings
1447	with in-laws
1450	with lover
1729	with peer group
1202	unusual behavior
1280	sharpened or unusually creative thinking
1452	hyperactive
1453	poorly organized, not goal-directed
1465	eating binges (bulimic episodes)
1467	followed by guilt and depression
1370	hypercritical or intolerant
1433	selective forgetfulness
1434	selective inefficiency
1432	oppositional
1374	social isolation
1487	ritualistic behavior
1488	mannerisms
1556	nail biting
1557	pulling out one's hair

PSYCHOLOGICAL, CONT.

1558	mouthing one's hair		1673	cocaine
1559	grinding one's teeth		1674	opioids
1281	extreme gregariousness		1685	amphetamines / sympathomimetics
1288	inappropriate laughing, joking, punning		208	salt
1682	socially inappropriate		396	unusual or non-food items (pica)
1383	a flamboyant gay male		397	earth or clay
1381	pathological lying		398	laundry starch
1382	particularly elaborate or fantastic stories		1350	impulsive behavior
1344	with temporary alterations of identity or consciousness		1451 ·	resulting in careless errors or omissions
1285	more talkative than usual		1358	resulting in serious assault or property damage
1290	less talkative than usual		1362	repeated episodes
1286	exaggeration of past achievements		1405	vandalism
1287	inflated self-esteem		1406	initiation of fights
1284	making foolish business investments		1404	running away
1371	devious, scheming		1363	sadistic behavior
1384	tantrums		1364	torturing animals
1385	being overly dramatic		1736	child's cry
1386	constantly seeking emotional stimulation		1737	angry
1555	constantly seeking reassurance		1738	frightened
1283	reckless driving		1739	sobbing
1407	irresponsible parenting		1740	whimpering
1346	behavior in pursuit of obvious goal		1741	high-pitched
1435	factitious complaints to avoid work		1743	repeated episodes
1348	factitious complaints to obtain medication		1742	weak
1436	factitious complaints to obtain financial compensation		1203	loneliness
1437	factitious complaints to avoid criminal prosecution		1633	difficulty getting going in the morning
1438	factitious complaints to avoid military duty		1634	more difficulty functioning evenings than mornings
1349	compulsive behavior		1204	depression
1464	excessive exercising		1702	chronic
1351	gambling		1536	comes and goes
1352	disrupting family or job		1205	alternating with periods of elation
1353	causing illegal or irresponsible financial activity		1537	more in the morning
1354	denial of extent of consequences		1538	more in the evening
1282	buying sprees		1560	seasonal pattern
1355	stealing unneeded objects		1539	more in the winter
1356	setting fires		1540	more in the summer
1357	just to watch		1561	few non-seasonal occurrences
1279	working unnecessarily excessive hours		1541	preceded by a high activity level
1466	concerning food		1542	accompanied
1474	surreptitious disposal		1547	by a persistent worry
1473	hoarding, concealing		1543	by eating more
1468	secretive and rapid eating of high calorie food		1544	by eating less
1670	cravings		1545	by sleeping more
1671	alcohol		1546	by sleeping less
1672	caffeine		1548	relieved
1669	nicotine		1549	by good news
			1550	by medication
			1551	by counseling
			1206	feeling pessimistic about future, or brooding about past
			1296	1-3 days prior to menstruation

PSYCHOLOGICAL, CONT.

1700	feeling more tired in morning than evening	1223	thoughts or wishes to kill someone
1207	feeling elated, euphoric	1224	thinking of a way to do it
1208	alternating with periods of depression	1225	stated intent to kill
1294	emotionally hypersensitive	1469	a fear of loss of control
1373	quick to take offense	1470	of eating
1401	overreaction to real or imagined slights or failures	1471	of emotions
		1472	of physical restraint
1226	moods change rapidly (lability of mood)	1227	illusions (altered perception of real events / objects)
1514	prior to menstruation (3-10 days)		
1293	feeling emotionally rejected	1228	hearing sounds which seem to be voices
1209	feeling emotionally detached		
1210	unresponsive to human contact	1229	seeing objects distorted in size or shape
1486	failure to develop normal attachment behavior	1230	smaller than real (micropsia)
		1231	larger than real (macropsia)
1211	loss of interest in or fear of meeting people (social with.)	1232	sense of time moving slower or faster than real
1552	loss of interest in friends and family (social withdrawal)	1689	recurring without a stimulus (flashback)
1520	feeling shy, bashful	1314	fixed beliefs contradicted by reality (delusions)
1212	feeling inadequate, low self esteem, or self-deprecating	1462	belief that one is obese when normal or thin
2914	compensated by falsely positive attitude	1693	belief that one is emitting foul odors
2561	fear of rejection	1677	belief that one is missing a limb
1366	constantly feeling jealous	1695	belief that one's body is infested with parasites
1289	feeling guilty		
1420	chronic boredom or feeling empty	1315	that sexual identity is different from one's anatomic sex
2915	unable to cope with daily activities		
1213	lacking motivation	1690	that one is loved by another
1416	identity uncertainty	1692	that one is a prominent figure
1417	about gender role	1372	shared with others
1418	about long term goals	1233	feeling that surroundings are unreal (derealization)
1419	about value systems		
1214	feeling that nothing matters (apathy)	1234	feeling that the body is unreal (depersonalization)
1215	no desire to continue living		
1216	a wish to be dead	1310	feeling that one's body is mechanical
1217	a specific means of suicide in mind (suicide plan)	1311	other people seem dead or mechanical
		1235	a new place or event seems familiar (deja vu)
1218	a stated intent to commit suicide		
1219	disturbing or unusual thoughts, feelings or sensations	1236	a familiar place is not remembered (jamais vu)
1220	having senseless or very distasteful thoughts which persist	1237	hallucinations (an imagined perception not based in reality)
1221	senseless, unpleasurable repetitive behavior (compulsion)	1238	hearing voices when no one is talking
		1239	being commanded to do something or hurt oneself
1481	complex repetitive movements		
1222	convinced the body can feel no pain	1240	seeing insects at the edge of one's vision
1683	preoccupied with religion		
2417	preoccupied with a narrowly focused interest	1241	having religious visions or experiences
		1242	seeing unusual colors
2418	preoccupied with parts of objects	1243	seeing sounds as colors
1304	preoccupied with an imagined or exaggerated physical defect	1244	seeing objects as if through colored glasses
1292	legs feel heavy		

PSYCHOLOGICAL, CONT.

1245	seeing oneself from outside the body
1246	smelling peculiar odors others can't smell
1247	peculiar tastes, unrelated to food
1248	feelings of being touched, burned or shocked
1249	feelings of bugs crawling under the skin
1250	strange body sensations or changes
1251	a sense of unexplained motion
1415	only when falling asleep or awakening
1252	feeling persecuted (paranoid ideations)
1368	requiring vigilance against treachery or threats
1367	expecting trickery
1369	concerned with hidden motives of others
1253	ordinary things have unique significance (reference)
1697	progressed rapidly over 2-4 weeks
1698	progressed slowly over months or years
1375	magical thinking
1376	clairvoyance
1377	superstitiousness
1378	telepathy
1254	disturbances of actions and reactions
1255	violent behavior

1409	child beating
2059	by parent
2060	by specified person
2061	by unspecified person
1408	spouse beating
1256	automatic behavior
1257	repetitive behavior
1258	voluntary
1643	habitual repetitive head banging
1699	rhythmic rocking or bumping
1259	frequent use of foul language
1260	unresponsiveness to questioning but awake
1261	transient
1461	refusal to speak
2509	during the first month of school
1262	chewing
1263	smacking or licking of lips
1264	blinking eyelids
1265	head turning
1266	alien urge to be in motion (akathisia)
1507	in too much discomfort to answer questions
1345	positive review of symptoms
1347	symptoms reported are inconsistent or changeable
2508	User Finding:

Part II
HISTORY

5097	**social history**
3000	coffee consumption
3851	eight or more cups a day
4065	prepared by boiling
3724	tea consumption
3852	eight or more cups a day
3741	cola consumption
3853	eight or more cans a day
3001	alcohol consumption
3732	beer consumption
3733	wine consumption
3734	hard liquor consumption
3743	a social drinker
4114	cut consumption within last 48 hours
4113	behavior changes after small amounts
3002	current drinking is denied but suspected
3003	affecting relationships with others
3004	interfering with work
3005	drinking more than friends/associates
4070	recently drinking more alcohol than usual
3744	cannot control amount
3808	considered quitting
3809	getting angry when talked to about drinking
3810	feeling guilty about drinking
4095	denial that drinking is causing problems
3006	a drink or two in the morning to get going
3007	frequent drinking before age 18
3742	stopped drinking alcohol
3008	smoking
3801	cigarettes
3834	starting upon awakening
3850	starting with the first beverage/food of the day
3835	starting only after the first meal of the day
3836	starting only in the afternoon or evening
3837	leaving a social or work setting to have a cigarette
4069	recent increase in usage
3009	over 50 pack-years
3725	cigars
3011	a pipe
3797	wishing to stop
3838	due to family pressure
3841	due to social pressure
3839	for health reasons
3840	due to urging at work

3010	unsuccessful attempt(s) to stop smoking
4335	smoking while wearing nicotine patch
3637	recently stopped smoking
3842	previous history of smoking
4142	chewing nicotine-containing substances
3012	a user of consciousness or mood-altering drugs
3015	barbiturates
3019	marijuana
3020	daily for a month or more
3013	amphetamines
3018	LSD / hallucinogens
3016	cocaine
3857	alkaloid form
4479	with heroin
3017	heroin
3021	PCP (angel dust)
4143	daily use for a month or more
3975	designer drugs
3014	MDMA ("ecstasy")
3976	fentanyl derivatives ("china white")
4013	methamphetamines
4014	powdered ("speed")
4015	powdered ("crank")
4016	powdered ("ice")
3022	with current use denied but suspected
4071	recently increased drug use
3023	to counter withdrawal or decreased effect
4141	episodic heavy use
4062	sniffing glue
4097	sniffing nitrous oxide
4480	sniffing amyl nitrite
4481	sniffing naptha
4115	using over-the-counter caffeine "stay-awake" pills
4144	difficulty understanding native language
3827	using laxatives for weight control
3025	a user of intravenous drugs
4064	sharing needles
3649	sleep
3024	a user of oral contraceptives
4072	foreign object(s) placed in the vagina
4761	recent change in cleansing materials
4762	soap
4763	bubble bath
4764	bathroom tissue
4765	female hygienic spray
3026	sexually active
3027	frequently with new partners
3028	unconcerned about painful consequences

SOCIAL HISTORY, CONT.

4905	with lack of responsibility	3781	frequent weight fluctuations (more than 10 pounds)
4906	without practicing safe sex		
3709	with persons at risk for HIV-related disease	3477	personal hygiene
		4869	change in habits
3029	with children	4870	responsible for own hygiene
3030	with animals	4868	dental hygiene
3664	preferred to human sexual contact	4871	brushing
3708	as a prostitute	4872	morning
3031	with objects	4873	night
3032	with unusual parts of the body	4874	flossing
4986	sexual activity denied	4875	child can clean teeth
4907	not currently dating	4876	seeing a dentist
4077	current diet	4877	regularly
4427	unusual	3985	recent medical examination
4078	high in fat content	3987	by a gynecologist
4773	infant	3986	by an ophthalmologist
4774	not balanced	3988	by a podiatrist
4775	low iron	4768	recent self examination
4776	pureed solid foods	4769	breast
4777	misses meals	4770	testicular
4778	inadequate fluid intake	3828	weight control
4779	low fat milk	3829	serious attempts to lose weight
4788	refuses to drink	3830	due to family pressure
4780	excessive intake of dairy products	3831	for health reasons
4781	milk	3832	due to job requirement
4924	number of ounces per day	3833	to improve social attractiveness
4782	recent changes	3843	eight or more attempts made
4783	increase	3846	on doctor-supervised diet
4784	fruits and juices	3845	on "own diet"
4785	vegetables	3780	periodic fad diets
4786	decrease	3738	exercise habits
4787	fluids	4752	frequency
4892	refuses to eat	4753	duration
4789	infant feeding	4809	recent decrease in activity
4790	breast feeding	3737	sedentary
4791	hours between feedings	3034	moderate exercising less than 3 times a week
4792	# feedings in 24 hours		
4925	the breastfeeding mother has noted sore nipples	3739	strenuous exercising less than 3 times a week
4926	the breastfeeding mother has noted itching of nipples	3740	moderate exercising 3 or more times a week
4793	bottle feeding	3554	strenuously 3 or more times/week (athletic conditioning)
4794	amount per feeding		
4795	amount in 24 hours	3993	physical activity tolerance
4796	time between feedings	3994	recently decreased
4797	# feedings in 24 hours	3772	emotional states translate to physical symptoms
4801	burping		
4802	during feedings	5023	living situations
4803	after feedings	5024	independent
4893	pulls away	5025	alone
3033	needing diet improvement	5026	with spouse
3779	refusal to maintain adequate caloric intake	5027	with parents
		5028	just one

SOCIAL HISTORY, CONT.

5043	as juvenile
5044	as an adult
5029	with relatives (other than parents)
5046	grandparent(s)
5047	with and caring for elderly parent(s) and juvenile children
5045	with adult children as elderly person
5030	in elderly assisted-living facility
5031	in handicapped assisted-living facility
5032	temporary
5033	permanent (LHA)
5039	temporary live-in rehabilitation facility
4663	activities of daily living
4664	difficulty feeding oneself
4665	difficulty dressing oneself
4666	difficulty going to the bathroom without assistance
4667	difficulty walking unassisted
4668	difficulty washing oneself
4669	difficulty getting out of bed on one's own
4670	difficulty getting out of bed to a toilet on one's own
4671	difficulty grooming oneself
4672	difficulty communicating
4673	instrumental activities of daily living
4674	unable to do one's own shopping
4675	unable to do one's own cooking
4676	unable to do one's own house cleaning
4677	unable to do one's own laundry
4678	unable to use the telephone by oneself
4679	unable to manage one's own medications
4680	unable to manage one's own money
4681	unable to drive
4682	unable to use public transportation
4683	unable to read
4684	unable to write
5137	care-giver(s) level of support sufficient and effective
5136	care-giver(s) improving their level of support
5133	care-giver(s) unable/unwilling to give adequate support
5134	care-giver(s) sabotaging support efforts
3035	recent emotional stress
5135	but coping effectively
3036	death or serious illness in the family
4160	recently widowed
3037	recently separated
4159	recently divorced
4028	having serious problems with children
3038	having serious financial problems
5132	from care-giving
3039	re-experiencing a traumatic event
3040	through dreams, actions or feelings
4634	lack of social support
4429	fears about present medical condition
4474	seriousness of illness
4475	having a communicable illness
4477	having an inheritable condition
4430	possibility of cancer
4431	possible surgery
4476	time lost from work
4432	possible loss of ability to work
4433	inability to care for family members
4434	inability to pay for medical care
4435	possible side effects of medications
4436	about dying
4437	that knowledge of condition will harm others
4478	that personal behavior caused this illness
3041	violent traumatic event
3896	mugged
3042	being a victim of rape
3646	sexually abused
3648	physically abused
3043	physically assaulted
3044	having been in military combat
3045	having been in a natural disaster
3891	having been in a plane crash
3046	having been held hostage
3047	having been in detention with torture
3784	under chronic emotional stress
3785	illness in the family
3786	financial problems
3787	broken home
3788	constant family fighting
3678	psychosocial stressor severity (Axis IV)
3679	none apparent (code 1)
3680	minimal (code 2)
3681	mild (code 3)
3682	moderate (code 4)
3683	severe (code 5)
3684	extreme (code 6)
3685	catastrophic (code 7)
3686	unspecified (code 0)
3687	best functioning level during past year (Axis V)
3688	1-Superior
3689	2-Very good
3690	3-Good
3691	4-Fair
3692	5-Poor
3693	6-Very poor

SOCIAL HISTORY, CONT.

3694	7-Grossly impaired	
3695	0-Unspecified	
3615	in a nursing home	
5034	in a hospice	
4173	in a foster home	
5035	in a juvenile group home	
5041	in an orphanage	
5042	in a reform school	
5036	in a homeless shelter	
4083	homeless	
5037	in correctional institution	
5040	temporarily in a juvenile detention center	
5038	in a halfway house (post-correctional release)	
3478	poverty conditions	
3822	difficulty understanding spoken English	
3823	difficulty reading English	
4901	difficulty understanding local (non-native) language	
4303	racial background	
4304	of father	
4305	caucasian	
4306	black	
4307	oriental	
4308	of mother	
4309	caucasian	
4310	black	
4311	oriental	
4056	happy with job	
3656	poor work performance	
4908	child does not do assigned chores	
3717	frequently changing jobs	
3718	unaccountable unemployment	
3723	multiple divorces or separations	
4489	wearing diapers	
4490	infrequently changed	
4168	daily management of child	
4810	cared for at home	
4811	cared for by a babysitter	
4172	left with a relative	
4171	home alone during day	
4169	enrolled in day care	
4903	enrolled in preschool	
4170	a "latch-key" child	
4174	child institutionalized	
3777	poor school performance	
3591	unexplained	
4196	academic failure	
4146	difficulty with arithmetic	
3659	school absenteeism	
3660	due to fear of ridicule	
3904	due to fear of criticism	

3661	due to separation anxiety	
3662	due to frequent illness	
4175	due to serious chronic illness	
3663	due to apathy or lack of motivation	
4880	# days absent	
3698	school expulsions	
3745	educational level	
3746	illiterate	
4145	preliterate	
3747	grades 1-6	
3748	grades 7-12	
3749	grades 13-16 (college)	
3750	grades 17+ (postgraduate)	
3751	trade schooling	
3752	technical schooling	
4312	highest level achieved: completed	
4292	age at completion of education	
4164	parental education limited	
4165	illiterate	
4166	through grade school only	
4167	ended with high school graduation	
4804	daily time with electronics	
4805	television	
4806	computer	
4807	video games	
4808	unsupervised	
4913	no home safety plans	
4914	in case of fire	
3710	job problems or incidents	
3713	chronically late	
3714	absent	
3735	sickness	
4150	for more than a month	
3736	because of an injury	
3715	frequently	
3716	on the first working day of the week	
3771	granted disability pay or worker's compensation	
4881	# days absent	
3791	previous occupational illness	
3707	had to leave job because of illness	
3711	previous injury	
3712	multiple	
4152	resulting in partial disability	
4153	resulting in total disability	
4242	previous employment medical examination	
4243	previous employment by this organization	
4063	concerned about work-related health problems	
3641	dysfunction resolves with hypnotic suggestion	

SOCIAL HISTORY, CONT.

3048	recent loss of job
4895	not currently employed
5048	never subtantially employed
5049	never sought employment
5050	currently on disability
5051	partial
3697	numerous lawsuits instigated
3699	criminal behavior
3700	stealing for gain
3721	fencing stolen property
3703	forgery
3719	pimping
3720	selling illegal drugs
3705	kidnapping
3701	rape
3702	homicide
3704	terrorism
4685	assault using drugs / medicinal substances
4686	assault using a handgun
4687	assault using a shotgun
4689	assault using a fire
4979	assault using motor vehicle
4688	assault by stabbing
3049	legal problems or arrests
3895	conviction for driving while intoxicated
3722	conviction for a felony
3050	wearing eye glasses
4019	wearing contact lenses
4020	soft
4021	soft extended wear
4022	hard
4055	using a hearing aid
3051	previously well
3696	preoccupied with current illness
4117	frequent illnesses
3642	frequent change of doctors
4932	previous hospitalizations
3824	recently
3640	frequent
4878	number
4934	for asthma
4935	for chest pain
4936	for ketoacidosis
4937	for drug overdose
4933	previous emergency room visits
4879	number per year
4938	for asthma
4939	for chest pain
4940	for drug overdose
3675	no response to treatment
4438	refusal of treatment
4439	for religious reasons

3673	non-compliance with treatment
4058	because of religious beliefs
4059	because of subcultural beliefs
4733	for dietary reasons
3674	non-compliance with hospital routines/regulations
3672	history of leaving the hospital against medical advice
4057	persistently denying a harmful, confirmed physical disorder
3460	slow wound healing
3461	self-mutilation
3770	wrist slashing
4331	gang member
3052	occupation
3053	medical professional
3730	medical resident
4126	lawyer
3054	miner
4991	factory worker
4992	an outdoor worker
4989	an office worker
4990	homemaker
3883	previous use of protective clothing or equipment
3884	air-supply mask
3885	air-supply respirator
4079	using safety equipment
4080	seatbelts
4081	lifejacket
4082	protective head gear
3886	workplace safety precautions
3887	overhead ventilator fan
3753	religious affiliation
3754	Protestant
3755	fundamentalist
3756	Catholic
3757	Roman
3758	Orthodox
3759	Judaism
3760	reform
3761	Orthodox
3762	Islam
3763	Sunni
3764	Shiite
4419	Mennonite
3765	Mormon
3774	Christian Scientist
3773	Jehovah's Witness
3766	Hindu
3767	Buddhism
3768	Shinto
3769	None

SOCIAL HISTORY, CONT.

3814	cannibalism	4557	in fair health
3568	eating dirt	4558	ill
3569	consumption of spicy or hot foods	4559	deceased
3570	consumption of fava beans	4279	age of child 2
3677	iodine deficient diet	4560	child 2
3647	incest	4561	in good health
3567	consanguinity	4562	in fair health
3605	previous suicide attempt	4563	ill
3905	poorly developed social responsiveness	4564	deceased
3643	assumption of new identity	4280	age of child 3
3644	after memory loss	4565	child 3
3645	after criminal conviction	4566	in good health
3606	recent high carbohydrate meal	4567	in fair health
3607	recent consumption of English walnuts	4568	ill
3608	chronic consumption of licorice	4569	deceased
3609	chronic consumption of goitrogenic foods	4281	age of child 4
3611	prolonged standing	4570	child 4
3612	prolonged kneeling	4571	in good health
5098	**family history**	4572	in fair health
4230	family health status	4573	ill
4231	father's age	4574	deceased
4232	father	4282	age of child 5
4532	in good health	4575	child 5
4533	in fair health	4576	in good health
4534	ill	4577	in fair health
4535	deceased	4578	ill
4233	mother's age	4579	deceased
4234	mother	4283	age of child 6
4536	in good health	4580	child 6
4537	in fair health	4581	in good health
4538	ill	4582	in fair health
4539	deceased	4583	ill
4540	brother's age	4584	deceased
4235	brother	4284	age of child 7
4541	in good health	4585	child 7
4542	in fair health	4586	in good health
4543	ill	4587	in fair health
4544	deceased	4588	ill
4545	sister's age	4589	deceased
4236	sister	4285	age of child 8
4546	in good health	4590	child 8
4547	in fair health	4591	in good health
4548	ill	4592	in fair health
4549	deceased	4593	ill
4550	spouse's age	4594	deceased
4241	spouse	4287	number of children
4551	in good health	4288	living
4552	in fair health	4289	deceased
4553	ill	4103	family history of cancer
4554	deceased	4100	of the colon
4555	age of child 1	3897	of the lung
4237	child 1	4101	of the breast
4556	in good health	4102	family history of leukemia

FAMILY HISTORY, CONT.

4428	family history of diabetes		3064	Tanzania
3847	family history of alcoholism		3065	Uganda
3848	the father		3066	Western
3849	the mother		3067	Northern
3893	both parents		4760	Sudan
4105	family history of mental illness (not retardation)		3068	Asia, Far East or South Pacific
			3069	Guam
4106	family history of stroke(s)		3070	Hawaii
4107	family history of epilepsy		3071	India
4109	family history of Huntington's chorea		3072	Indonesia
5093	family history of heart disease		3073	Japan
5094	ischemic heart disease		3074	Korea
3902	before age 50		3075	Malaysia
4411	congenital heart disease		3076	the Pacific Islands
3512	family history of early deaths		3077	Pakistan
4110	family history of asthma		3078	Southeastern Asia
4111	family history of arthritis		3079	Southern China
3676	family history of a goiter		3080	Taiwan
3564	family history of thyroidectomy		3081	Thailand
4104	family history of sickle cell anemia		3082	Vietnam
4017	family history of bleeding problems		3083	Australia
3551	family history of mental retardation		3084	Canada
3903	family history of kidney disease		3085	Caribbean
4108	family history of blindness		3086	Curacao
3534	family history of deafness		3087	Haiti
3514	family history of allergies		3088	Jamaica
4919	child's birth history		3089	Puerto Rico
4920	born after prolonged rupture of membranes		3090	Trinidad
			3091	Central or South America
4344	child's family history		3092	Argentina
4345	born to unwed mother		3093	Atlantic Coast
4346	born to teenage mother		3094	Bolivia
4347	product of unwanted pregnancy		3095	Brazil
4351	parent(s) having financial problems		3096	Chile
4352	parent(s) frequently unemployed		3097	Columbia
4353	parent(s) socially isolated		3098	Ecuador
4355	parent(s) abusing substance(s)		3099	French Guiana
4356	alcohol		3100	Guyana
4357	drugs		3101	Mexico
4350	parents having marital problems		3102	Panama
4348	parents separated		3103	Peru
4349	parents divorced		3104	Surinam
4354	continual stress		3105	Venezuela
5099	**travel history**		3106	Western South America
3055	travel or residence in		3107	Europe
3056	Africa		3108	Balkans
3057	Angola		3109	Eastern
3058	Central		3110	France
3059	Zaire		3111	Italy
3060	Eastern		3112	The Netherlands
3061	Kenya		3113	Switzerland
3062	Nigeria		3114	space
3063	South Africa		3115	Mediterranean Countries

TRAVEL HISTORY, CONT.

3116	the Middle East		5100	**environmental exposure**
3117	Egypt		3163	exposure
3118	Israel		3931	contact exposure to metals
3119	Lebanon		3932	aluminium
3120	Turkey		3933	arsenic
3121	Russia		3934	chromium
3122	Central		3935	magnesium
3123	Eastern Siberia		3936	mercury
3124	Omsk/Novosibirsk		3937	nickel
3125	Southern		3938	platinum
3126	Scandanavia		3939	silver
3127	The United States		3940	tin
3128	Alaska		3941	zinc
3129	California		3164	heavy metals (ingestion)
3130	the San Joaquin Valley		3165	antimony
3668	Connecticut		3166	arsenic
3131	the Eastern Seaboard		3167	barium
3132	Florida		3168	bismuth
3133	the Gulf States		3169	cadmium
3134	Indiana		3170	chromium
3135	Louisiana		3171	cobalt
3136	Midwest		3172	copper
3137	New Jersey		3173	gold
3667	rural New York state		3174	lead
3138	Ohio		3175	manganese
3139	the Ohio or Mississippi River Valleys		3176	mercury
3140	the Rocky Mountains		3177	nickel
3141	the Sierra Mountains		3178	silver
3142	Southeastern		3179	uranium
3143	Southern		3180	vanadium
3144	Southwestern		3181	metal fumes
4816	Northeastern		3182	cadmium
3145	Texas		3183	copper
3146	West		3775	lead
3147	Wisconsin		3184	magnesium oxide
3148	The United Kingdom		3185	manganese
4032	a foreign country with illness while abroad		3186	mercury
			3187	osmium tetroxide
3149	a climate which is		3188	platinum soluble salts (mist)
3150	temperate		3189	vanadium pentoxide
3151	sub-tropical		3190	zinc chloride
3152	tropical		3191	welding galvanized metal (zinc oxide)
3153	desert		3192	chemical liquids
3154	symptoms started where the local season was		3922	acids
			3923	alkalis
3155	Winter		3947	alcohols
3156	Winter-Spring		3193	antifreeze / glycols
3157	Spring		3956	chromates
3158	Spring-Summer		3195	creosote
3159	Summer		3203	diisocyanates
3160	Summer-Fall		3196	dyes
3161	Fall		4129	aniline
3162	Fall-Winter		4130	ortho-toluidine

ENVIRONMENTAL EXPOSURE, CONT.

3901	epoxy resin		4046	regularly or heavily
3919	formaldehyde		3890	gasoline
3920	gluteraldehyde		3224	halides
3967	hexachlorophene		3225	fluorides
3948	ketones		3226	chlorides
3965	oils / greases		3227	bromides
3197	pesticides		3228	iodides
4417	phenylhydrazine		3229	hydrocarbons
3198	polychlorinated biphenols		3858	benzo[a]pyrene
3921	solvents (hydrocarbons)		3231	kerosene
3194	benzene		3236	picric acid
3942	carbon disulfide		4034	chemical fumes
3946	ethylene dibromide		3237	polytetrafluoroethylene
3928	freon		3238	polyvinyl chloride
3929	glycol ethers		3240	sulfides
3930	methylene chloride		3242	trimellitic anhydride
4416	naphthalene		3239	smoke
3944	phenols		3949	gases
3943	styrene		3218	ammonia
3945	trichloroethylene		3950	anhydrous
3926	tetrachloroethylene		3219	carbon monoxide
3925	toluene		3221	chlorine
3927	1,1,1-trichloroethane		3230	hydrogen sulfide
3924	xylene		3215	liquid manure
4418	trinitrotoluene		3232	nitric oxide
4127	chemical contaminants		3233	nitrogen dioxide
4128	dioxin		4096	nitrous oxide
3199	chemical powders		3234	ozone
3200	boric acid		3235	phosgene
3201	bromates		3651	radon
3202	detergents		3241	sulphur dioxide
3204	phthalic anhydride		4035	mists
3205	rat poison		4036	acid
3206	roach powder		4037	alkali
3966	salicylanilides		4039	glycerin
3207	spanish fly		4038	oils
3208	strychnine		4041	pentachlorophenol
3879	trimellitic anhydride		3216	wood pulp
3209	vinyl chloride		3243	extreme heat
3210	chemical solids or pellets		3244	molds
3211	mothballs		3245	moldy barley malt
3212	petroleum		3246	cheese
3213	tar		3247	moldy cork dust
3957	plastics		3248	moldy hay
3958	acrylic resins		3249	moldy straw
3959	epoxy resin solids		3250	mushroom growing soil
3214	fumes		3251	moldy redwood
3217	chemical vapors		3252	moldy sugar cane
3220	carbon tetrachloride		3253	moldy wood chips or dust
3889	chloroform		4928	foreign proteins
3222	cyanide		4929	dust mites
3223	formaldehyde		4930	animal danders
4045	occasionally or lightly		4931	roach antigen

ENVIRONMENTAL EXPOSURE, CONT.

3254	dusts		3878	tragacanth
3255	aluminum powder (not stearin coated)		3288	tungsten carbide
3256	aluminum pyro flakes		3289	uranium
3257	antimony powder		3868	vanadium pentoxide
3258	asbestos		3290	vermiculite
4042	occasionally or lightly		4976	volcanic ash
4043	regularly or heavily		3872	wood
3654	anthophyllite		3874	oak
3655	amosite		3873	western red cedar
3652	crocidolite		3291	zirconium
3653	chrysotile		3880	laboratory animal dusts and danders
3259	baryte		3881	laboratory animal serums and secretions
3260	bauxite (aluminum oxide)		4766	blown into the eyes
3261	beryllium		3951	fibers
3867	cadmium		3953	ceramic
3875	castor bean		4147	erionite
3262	cement		3952	fiberglass
3866	chlorides		3954	rock wool
3870	chromium		3955	slag wool
3263	coal dust		4148	wollastonite
3264	coffee bean		4149	attapulgite
3869	coke oven emissions		3888	dusty clothing
3265	cotton or flax		3292	an air-conditioned environment
3266	diatomaceous earth		3293	possibly contaminated soil
3267	erionite		3469	recently digging for Navajo Indian relics
3268	fish meal		3470	recently spent time near a construction site
3269	flour		3474	recently clam digging
3270	fuller's earth		3471	exposure to a possibly contaminated body of water
3271	fur		3472	swimming in a pool
3863	grain		3473	swimming in a pond or stream
3272	graphite		4825	swimming in the ocean
3876	gum acacia		3790	toxic waste
3273	iron oxide		3294	contaminated inhalation therapy equipment
3274	jeweler's rouge		3295	a lot of bright sunlight
3275	kaolin		3296	weightless condition
3877	karaya gum		3297	high altitude
3276	mica		3298	environmental or occupational radiation (m.rems)
3277	mullite		4137	infrared radiation
3278	nepheline		4138	ultraviolet radiation
3871	nickel		4140	microwave radiation
4040	pentachlorophenol		4139	laser light
3864	phosphorus		4817	cleansing agents
3279	pituitary snuff		4818	new soap
3280	rare earth		4819	new detergents
3281	rope (hemp)		4820	new lotions
3282	shale		4899	bubble bath
3283	silica		4823	hot liquid
3284	sillimanite			
3915	soybean			
3865	sulfides			
3285	talc			
3286	tin			
3287	titanium			

ENVIRONMENTAL EXPOSURE, CONT.

4978	steam
4824	hot metal
3324	pets or other animals
3325	a dog
3811	dragging buttocks across floor
3326	a cat
3812	dragging buttocks across floor
3327	birds
4987	pigeons
3960	fish
3328	hamsters
3329	mice
4112	striped Korean
3330	rabbits
3331	raccoons
3332	deer
3333	wild small mammals
3334	wild game
3335	poultry
3336	dairy cows
3337	cattle
3338	horses
3339	mules
3340	donkeys
3341	pigs
3342	sheep
3343	goats
3344	foxes
3345	opossums
3346	skunks
3347	shrews
3348	rats
3349	African green monkeys
4826	leather
4827	latex
3350	plants
3351	poison ivy
3352	poison oak
3353	poison sumac
3355	nightshade
3356	roses
3354	moss
4512	meadow grass
3970	bishop's weed
3974	gas plant
3973	wild parsnip
4493	wild carrot
4494	cowslip
4497	masterwort
4498	atrillal
4499	angelica
4503	lime bergamot
4504	buttercup

4505	blind weed
4506	agrimony
4507	yarrow
4508	goose foot
4509	bavachi
4510	St. John's wort
4511	mokihana berry
3961	contact exposure to foods
4496	garden carrot
3962	celery
3963	citrus
3971	dill
3972	fennel
3968	fig
4501	limes
4502	mustard
3969	parsley
4495	garden parsnip
4500	rice
3357	contagious disease
3358	tuberculosis
3359	syphilis
3826	gonorrhea
3360	mumps
3368	measles (rubeola)
3362	viral
4828	impetigo
4830	URI
4831	mononucleosis
3366	chicken pox
3802	hepatitis
3363	herpes simplex
3364	herpes zoster
3367	German measles (rubella)
3657	HIV
4414	AZT-resistant HIV strain
4086	rabies
4087	cholera
3365	typhoid
4084	poliomyelitis
4085	smallpox
3361	leprosy
3369	whooping cough (pertussis)
4758	ebola virus
4829	bronchiolitis
5102	work related
3622	working regularly in the dark
3815	working in sealed window building with insufficient air flow
3816	working in a recently renovated building
4047	symptoms get better at home and worse at work

ENVIRONMENTAL EXPOSURE, CONT.

4050	a backache	3540	recent rat eradication
4049	a headache	3559	usually barefoot
3623	respiratory	3571	cleaning chicken coops
4048	of the skin	3572	exploring caves
4985	person with similar rash	3669	hiking through dense vegetation
4946	potentially hazardous body fluids	3573	eating out of iron pots
4821	scabies	3574	eating vegetables grown with human fertilizer
4822	lice		
4916	worms	3616	bitten by a possibly rabid animal
3299	consumed possibly contaminated / spoiled / poisonous food	3617	recent epidemic of sick horses
		3618	recent epidemic of sick birds
3300	raw / undercooked beef	3619	recently sick dog
4988	of beef contaminated by bovine spongiform encephalopathy	3620	eating or peeling water chestnuts with teeth
3301	raw / undercooked pork	3621	having used an eye poultice from an infected frog
3302	undercooked carnivores		
3303	undercooked chicken	4832	household does not have city water
3304	undercooked duck	3536	recent exposure
3305	raw liver	3537	to heat and wind
3306	raw / undercooked saltwater fish	3539	on a tropical beach
3307	raw / dried / pickled freshwater fish	3553	a member of an American Indian tribe
3308	shellfish	3860	the Pima Indians
3309	freshwater crab / crayfish	3778	a member of the Bantu tribe
3310	improperly canned foods	3414	stings, bites or scratches
3311	unpasteurized milk	3415	by a deerfly
3312	contaminated milk	3416	by bees or wasps
3313	raw / undercooked bear	3417	by lice
3314	frogmeat	3418	by mosquitoes
3315	raw honey	3419	by a tick
3316	egg-based foods	3856	ixodes damnii
3317	wild / non-store bought mushrooms	4847	pinhead size
3318	old peanuts / peanut butter	4848	1/2 inch long
3319	polar bear liver	4853	engorged
3320	water	4852	removed
3321	watercress	4898	with head intact
3322	possibly outdated drugs	4849	attached 8 hours or more
3323	antibiotics	4850	rash around bite
5014	undercooked human brains	4851	bull's eye
4088	carrier of infectious disease	3420	by a tsetse fly
4089	cholera	3421	by a sandfly
4090	typhoid	3422	by mites or midges
4091	amebiasis	3423	by a spider
4092	diphtheria	4923	by a scorpion
4093	viral hepatitis	3424	by a bat
4094	gonorrhea	3425	by fleas
5103	other exposures	3426	by a rat
4981	recently using a new skin care product	3427	by a snake
4982	recently using a new hair care product	3428	by a cat
4983	recently using a new laundry product	3429	by a dog
3533	using cosmetics	4136	by a fox or wolf
3532	oil based nose drops	3430	by a skunk
4491	using cologne	3431	by a squirrel
4492	before sun exposure	3432	by a mongoose

ENVIRONMENTAL EXPOSURE, CONT.

3433	by a weasel
3434	by a muskrat
3435	by a human
3436	tingle
3437	red and swollen
620	**pregnancy history**
621	currently pregnant
2411	for ___ weeks
622	in first trimester
623	in third trimester
1504	expected delivery date
1854	with history of abortion
2058	with history of grand multiparity
1855	unwanted
625	recently pregnant
4223	normal labor and delivery
4221	duration of labor
3599	premature rupture of membranes
4904	prolonged rupture of membranes
3598	difficult delivery
4222	precipitous delivery
4224	delivered vaginally
4225	delivered by cesarean section
4610	outcome of delivery
4611	single liveborn
4734	male child
4735	female child
4612	single stillborn
4613	twins, both liveborn
4736	males
4737	females
4738	one male and one female
4614	twins, one liveborn and one stillborn
4615	twins, both stillborn
4616	other multiple birth, all ___ liveborn
4617	other multiple birth, ___liveborn and some stillborn
4618	other multiple birth, all ___ stillborn
4739	type of birth
4622	single liveborn
4623	born in hospital
4624	born before admission to hospital
4625	born outside hospital and not hospitalized
4626	twin, mate liveborn
4627	born in hospital
4628	born before admission to hospital
4629	born outside hospital and not hospitalized
4630	twin, mate stillborn
4631	born in hospital
4632	born before admission to hospital

4633	born outside hospital and not hospitalized
4075	umbilical cord twisted or wrapped at delivery
4226	presentation
4227	normal vertex
4228	breech
4229	transverse
4408	induced birth
3596	premature birth
3597	with care under bright ambient light
4412	low birth weight
3578	baby large or post-mature at delivery
4251	congenital abnormalities present
632	milk failed to start
633	currently nursing
4909	and nipples are sore
4910	and nipples are itching
1505	stopped nursing
634	periods did not start again
1506	baby thriving
4217	duration of last pregnancy
4218	term
4219	premature delivery
4220	postterm delivery
624	history of ___ previous pregnancy(s)
3583	prolonged
626	___ routine vaginal deliveries
2412	___ premature delivery(s)
2413	___ non-hospital delivery(s)
2414	with ___ at home
627	___ Caesarean section(s)
1725	___ live births
628	___ miscarriage(s)
1636	during first trimester
1637	during second trimester
1638	subsequent change in menstrual cycle
629	___ abortion(s)
1639	during first trimester
1640	during second trimester
1641	subsequent change in menstrual cycle
630	___ stillbirth(s)
1679	___ with congenital malformation
631	with heavy blood loss at delivery
5101	**medical, surgical history**
3370	recent tests
3989	recent blood pressure check
5022	abnormal
3990	systolic above 160
3991	diastolic 90 to 100
3992	diastolic above 100
3380	recent pap smear
3381	with a (+) result

MEDICAL AND SURGICAL HISTORY, CONT.

4073	also a previous (+) result 2 or more years ago	4213	normal
3371	recent skin test for tuberculosis (PPD)	4023	recent thyroid blood tests
3372	with a (+) result	4024	thyroid level was high
3373	previously (-) within last 5 years	4025	thyroid level was low
3374	previously confirmed (+) is now negative	3517	recent immunization
		4424	for flu
3911	recent mammogram	4425	for pneumococcal pneumonia
3978	with an abnormal finding	4426	for tetanus
3375	recent chest x-ray	4918	at Health Department
3376	with an abnormal finding	4951	donating blood
4332	normal film	4952	whole
4044	recent breathing function tests	4953	stem cells
4051	recent hearing test	4642	accidental misadventure during care
4890	conducted by a physician	4643	surgical operation
4891	conducted at school	4644	infusion / transfusion
3377	recent ECG	4645	kidney dialysis
3378	with an abnormal finding	4646	injection / vaccination
4757	was normal	4647	endoscopic examination
4214	recent treadmill	4648	lumbar puncture
4215	abnormal result	4649	thoracentesis
4026	recent blood count	4650	heart catheterization
4027	low	4651	mechanical failure of instrument
4420	a recent blood sugar check	4652	during surgical operation
3979	recent home blood sugar check	4653	during infusion / transfusion
3980	a result under 80	4654	during kidney dialysis
4061	a result between 80 and 140	4655	during endoscopic examination
3981	a result between 140 and 200	3913	recently given radiographic contrast material
3982	a result over 200		
4636	before breakfast	3390	allergies
4637	before lunch	3391	hay fever
4638	before supper	3392	eczema
4639	before bedtime	3393	dermatitis
4640	2 hours after a meal	3394	to foods
4641	during symptoms	4999	to milk
3798	recent urine sugar check	5000	to cheese
3382	positive	4313	to eggs
3983	recent urine acetone check	5001	to fruit
3984	positive	5002	to peaches
3799	recent urine protein check	5003	to berries
3383	positive	5004	to citrus fruit
4423	recent test for stool blood	5005	to vegetables
4421	recent prostate examination	5006	to onions
4422	recent prostate antigen blood test	5007	to tomatoes
3384	recent lumbar puncture	5008	to corn
3385	recent VDRL was positive	5009	to beans
3386	recent white cell count	5010	to cucumbers
3387	low	5011	to peppers
4740	recent HIV positive	5012	to squash
4741	no symptoms of infection present	5013	to chocolate
3388	recent antinuclear antibody was high	3862	to shellfish
3800	recent cholesterol test	3395	to yellow food dye no. 5
3389	high	3396	to pollens
		5053	trees

MEDICAL AND SURGICAL HISTORY, CONT.

5054	grasses	4524	reaction causing
5055	weeds	4525	rash
5056	ragweed	4526	hives
3397	to dust	4527	hypotension
5057	mites	4528	bronchospasm
5058	to cockroaches	4529	anaphylaxis
4993	to animals	4530	treatment required
4994	to dogs	4531	allergy prophylaxis
4995	to cats	3403	previous severe allergic reactions
4996	to birds	4922	previous referral to an allergist
4997	to feathers	5060	previous allergy therapy
4998	to furs	5061	pollen
3398	to molds	5062	molds
5052	to latex	5063	dust mites
3399	to drugs	5064	cockroach
4927	to penicillin	4984	recent exposure
5059	to cephalosporins	3404	psychiatric treatment
4314	to nonsteroidal anti-inflammatory agents	3405	including hospitalization
		4074	feel previous medication caused problems
3861	to aspirin	4942	prior use of medications
4315	to hydantoins	4943	corticosteroids
4316	to thiazides	4944	for asthma
4317	to tetracycline	3409	taking medication currently
4318	to gold	4197	for a heart problem
4319	to horse serum	4198	for an infection (antibiotics)
3882	to animal dander	4199	for a stomach problem
4917	to bandaging tape	4200	as a blood thinner
3670	vaginal reaction to semen	4950	for a long time
3671	dermatitis reaction from vaginal secretions	4201	for high blood pressure
		4202	for anemia (low blood count)
3400	previous reaction to penicillin	4203	for headaches
4343	anaphylactic	4204	for joint pain
4833	hives	4206	to help sleep
4834	rash	4208	for diabetes
3401	previous reaction to sulfa drugs	4286	for a thyroid problem
4098	previous reaction to anesthetic agents	4205	for anxiety
4099	previous reaction to narcotic agents	4210	for depression
3402	previous reaction to blood transfusion	4212	to lose weight
3914	reaction to radiographic contrast material	5065	prophylactic aspirin
		4207	female hormones
4513	type of agent	4698	need for post-menopausal HRT
4360	iodinated contrast material	4211	steroids
4361	gadolinium contrast material	4941	for asthma
4514	Renografin-60	4209	"pep pills"
4515	Renografin-76	3410	current medication is helping
4516	Hypaque-76	4010	feel medication is causing a problem
4517	Angiovist-370	4120	over-the-counter
4518	Iohexol	4121	for colds
4519	Contrast A	4122	for allergies
4520	Contrast B	4123	for pain
4521	Hexabrix	4124	for heartburn
4522	Isovue	4125	for constipation
4523	Conray	4897	for acne

MEDICAL AND SURGICAL HISTORY, CONT.

3825	recently taking antibiotics	3892	recent severe illness or injury
4030	recently using suppositories	3412	premature cardiovascular disease
4915	recent change in medication	4132	recent episode(s) of angina
5015	dosage	4133	occurring more frequently or with more severity
5016	of antihypertensive		
5019	of antiarrhythmic medication	4134	recent insulin (hypoglycemic) reaction
5020	of anticoagulant medication	4135	occurring frequently
5017	of insulin	4371	have a staring spell
5018	of hormone replacement therapy	4370	have a seizure
5021	of antipsychotic medication	3479	recent infection
4011	stopped taking medication	4706	infection with microorganisms resistant to penicillins
3542	insulin		
4238	antidepressants	4709	infection w/ microorganisms resistant to cephalosporins / B-lactam antibiotics
4239	tranquilizers		
4240	sedatives	4716	infection with microorganisms w/ multiple drug resistance
4882	treatment for acne		
4846	time since stopped	4713	infection with microorganisms resistant to aminoglycosides
4012	ran out of medication		
4060	patient death	3480	of the ear
3413	sudden	3481	of the face
3638	violent	3482	staphylococcal
4320	accidental ingestion	3483	streptococcal
4322	of pills	3484	recent upper respiratory infection
4323	Tylenol	3490	recent mumps
4324	aspirin	3491	recent protozoal infection
4325	chewable vitamins with iron	3485	recurrent bacterial infections
4326	Imipramine	3487	neisseria
4327	of hydrocarbons	4921	group A beta hemolytic streptococcus
4328	of antifreeze	3488	streptococcus pneumoniae
4329	of a small object	3489	salmonella
4330	a coin	3486	during childhood
4321	intentional ingestion of non-food material	3492	reported prior medical history
3502	corrosive substance	3804	skin problems
3917	severe or prolonged cold exposure	3806	hearing problems
3538	recently	4302	gum disease
3459	high level of environmental noise	3726	thyroid disease
4053	at work	3493	liver disease
4054	at home	3805	stomach problems
3859	chronic vibratory tool operation	3729	bowel problems
3918	with low frequency high amplitude vibration	3807	prostate trouble
		4250	urinary disorder
3462	swallowing a small object	3494	bladder disease
3666	prolonged bedrest or sitting position	3495	gallbladder disease
3854	recent long airplane flight	3496	kidney disease
3463	recent joint dislocations	3727	arthritis
3464	recurrent joint dislocations	3792	neck trouble
3465	recent fracture	3793	back trouble
3466	open or compound	3794	shoulder trouble
3467	open surgical reduction	3795	knee trouble
4358	in an infant	3803	joint problems
4372	choke	4245	disability
3796	active illness	4154	partial
4244	currently undergoing medical treatment	4155	total

MEDICAL AND SURGICAL HISTORY, CONT.

4246	causing inability to obtain life insurance
4247	causing denial of job application
3497	pulmonary disease
4151	neurological illness
5095	stroke
3912	mental illness
4606	schizophrenia
4607	affective disorders
4608	neurosis
4609	alcoholism
3498	heart disease
4333	valvular
5096	pericardial
3995	murmur
3588	in youth
3706	coronary artery disease
4751	heart attack
4413	thromboembolic disease
4945	pulmonary embolism
4293	vein trouble
3728	venereal disease
3522	immunocompromised disease
4294	fracture
4296	of arm
4297	of spine
4295	of leg
4341	spiral
4342	multiple occurrences
3996	cancer
3997	of the skin
3998	of the lung
4597	of the larynx
3999	of the breast
4595	of the esophagus
4596	of the stomach
4000	of the colon
4001	of the prostate
4598	of the testis
4002	of the cervix
4003	of the ovary
4599	of the bladder
4600	of the kidney
4605	of the thyroid
4118	leukemia
4601	lymphoid leukemia
4602	myeloid leukemia
4603	monocytic leukemia
4119	lymphoma
4604	malignant melanoma of the skin
4004	metastasis
4005	to bone
4006	to the liver

4007	to the lung
3789	chronic illness
3639	started before age 30
4176	untreated for lack of medical insurance
3499	intermittent hypertension
4156	condition preventing travel by air
4248	medical treatment has been recommended
3406	reported prior surgical / procedural history
4031	during childhood
4299	arteriovascular
5091	carotid artery
5092	peripheral vascular
5069	diagnostic catheterization
5070	total number performed ___
5071	date of most recent:
4472	balloon angioplasty
5067	total number performed ___
5068	date of most recent:
5072	laser angioplasty
5073	total number performed ___
5074	date of most recent:
5075	stent placement
5076	total number performed ___
5077	date of most recent:
5078	atherectomy
5079	total number performed ___
5080	date of most recent:
4441	heart surgery
4754	for congenital heart disease
4298	heart valve
4755	repair
5083	aortic
5084	mitral
5085	tricuspid
5086	pulmonary
4756	replacement
5087	aortic
5088	mitral
5089	tricuspid
5090	pulmonary
5066	coronary artery bypass
5081	total operations performed ___
5082	date of most recent:
5107	details of prior grafts
5108	operation 1
5110	LIMA used
5111	RIMA used
5112	___ saphenous veins used
5109	operation 2
5113	LIMA used
5114	RIMA used

MEDICAL AND SURGICAL HISTORY, CONT.

5115	___saphenous veins used	4467	bunion removal
5116	operation 3	4742	joint replacement
5117	LIMA used	4743	shoulder
5118	RIMA used	4744	elbow
5119	___saphenous veins used	4745	wrist
5120	operation 4	4464	hip
5121	LIMA used	4746	right
5122	RIMA used	4747	left
5123	___saphenous veins used	4750	bilateral
5124	operation 5	4748	knee
5125	LIMA used	4749	ankle
5126	RIMA used	4947	larynx replacement
5127	___saphenous veins used	4948	prosthetic replacement of a breast
5128	operation 6	4949	breast implant removal
5129	LIMA used	3407	recent
5130	RIMA used	4249	surgical treatment has been recommended
5131	___saphenous veins used	4290	marital history
5106	total number of grafts ___	4291	previously married
4442	brain surgery	3501	improperly fitting dentures
4443	eye surgery	3500	having "too much blood"
4444	for cataracts	3503	recurrent upper respiratory infections
4445	facial surgery	3504	during childhood
4468	to reshape nose	3505	recurrent bronchopulmonary infections
4469	blepharoplasty	3506	drainage from a sinus tract
4470	"facelift"	3507	recent high altitude flight
3844	liposuction	3508	recent deep sea dive (ft.)
4446	jaw surgery	3894	in cold waters (below 60 F.)
4447	TMJ implant	3510	recent drowning
4473	tonsillectomy	3511	recent strangulation
4448	thyroid surgery	3513	symptoms occurring seasonally
3408	removal of an enlarged parathyroid	4902	symptoms occur at the same time most days
4449	breast surgery		
4450	for biopsy	3518	catheter in place
4451	for removal of a lump	3519	recent injection
4452	with removal of breast	3520	into buttock
4453	for reduction of size	3516	into a joint
4454	for implantation	3515	intrathecal
4732	mechanical complication due to breast prosthesis	3521	of foreign serum or serum protein
		4759	followed by bleeding from injection site
4300	kidney stone removal		
4455	gallbladder surgery	3523	swallowing air
4456	surgery for an ulcer	3524	aspiration of gastric contents
4459	surgery for diverticula	3509	a pure vegetarian
4301	intestinal polyp removal	4033	food intolerance
4457	appendectomy	3526	fatty foods
4458	surgery for tumor of intestine	3525	meat
4460	surgery for hemorrhoids	3527	eating nitrate preserved foods
4461	prostate surgery	3528	generalized pain after alcohol
4462	hysterectomy	3529	chronic cough preceded dyspnea by many years
4463	ovarian surgery		
4471	back surgery	3530	pulmonary functions were unimproved by bronchodilators
4465	knee surgery		
4466	vein stripping		

MEDICAL AND SURGICAL HISTORY, CONT.

3531	previously (< 3mo.) normal creatinine now rising daily
3541	rash appeared on the 3rd to 6th febrile day
4334	rash appeared after fever went away
3543	recent steroid withdrawal
3544	recent beta-blocker withdrawal
3821	mucous membrane exposure to possibly infected agent
3731	accidental needlestick
3546	from Hepatitis B patient's needle
3545	intimacy with person having Hepatitis B
3547	undergoing basic military training
4052	previous military service
3548	in Vietnam
4157	rejected by military service for medical reasons
4158	discharged from military service for medical reasons
3549	mentally retarded
3550	institutionalized for mental retardation
3665	repetitive exposure of genitals to unsuspecting strangers
3552	cinchonism
3813	a member of the Fore tribe (Papua New Guinea)
3555	difficult endotracheal tube intubation
3556	recent stress on vocal cords
3557	pain occurring recently with fruit juices
3558	a heavy user of analgesics
3916	using acetaminophen daily
3560	recent dental work
3561	previous uneventful tooth extraction
3562	PVC's unresponsive to therapy
3563	refractory atrial arrhythmias
3565	hypokalemic while off diuretics
3566	lump grew after thyroid hormones
3577	missed abortion
4076	recent self-induced abortion attempt
4488	mother smoked during pregnancy
3579	mother used mood altering drugs pre-partum
3855	cocaine
3776	mother regularly abused alcohol pre-partum
3820	mother was IV drug user
3580	mother had DES during pregnancy
4185	mother given phenytoin during pregnancy
4188	mother on immunosuppressives during pregnancy
4186	mother diabetic during pregnancy
4187	mother had renal insufficiency during pregnancy

3819	mother was HIV-infected during pregnancy
4181	mother was CMV-infected during pregnancy
4410	mother had genital herpes during pregnancy
3581	mother had rubella during pregnancy
4182	mother had toxoplasmosis during pregnancy
4183	mother had preeclampsia during pregnancy
4184	mother had eclampsia during pregnancy
4190	mother had abdominal trauma during pregnancy
4195	mother had radiation exposure during pregnancy
4191	mother had polyhydramnios during pregnancy
4192	mother had oligohydramnios during pregnancy
4883	mother had hypothyroidism
4193	mother was ABO incompatabile
4194	mother was Rh incompatabile
3582	mother over 35 at time of pregnancy
4179	teenage pregnancy
4180	before age 16
4619	screening for chromosomal anomolies by amniocentesis
4620	screening for malformation using ultrasonics
4621	screening for fetal growth retardation using ultrsonics
4177	poor prenatal care of mother
4178	improper nourishment
4896	mother taking medication currently
4884	maternal blood group
4885	type A positive
4886	type B positive
4887	type O positive
4888	type AB positive
3602	joint pain or swelling which responds to gammaglobulin
3603	recent cardiac arrest
3604	recent respiratory arrest
3610	dropping dishes frequently
5104	**pediatric history**
4889	infant born at home
4256	newborn remained after mother discharged
3595	neonatal jaundice
4767	age at onset
4835	treatment
4836	exposure to sun

PEDIATRIC HISTORY, CONT.

4837	phototherapy		4894	not ready
4838	duration		4812	current
4839	discontinued		4813	bladder trained
4359	nursery exposure to klebsiella		4814	bowel trained
3576	oxygen deprivation at birth		4815	toilet use refusal
4854	skin was bruised at birth		3476	an uncircumcised male
4409	delayed passage of first stool		3898	left handed
4252	difficulty feeding infant		3899	right handed
4253	by breast		3900	converted from left
4254	by bottle		4867	no hand preference
4255	solid foods		3475	fair skin
4407	failure to gain weight		4018	freckles
3587	failure to thrive		3592	unexplained growth failure
4257	difficulty weaning		3575	head or neck radiation during childhood
4258	from bottle		4029	thymus gland radiation during childhood
4259	from breast		3593	baby talk persisting beyond age 8
4260	feeding history		3658	childhood gender identity role reversal
4261	breast		3594	playing in a sandbox
4262	bottle		3586	poor growth and development without neurological deficit
4263	cow's milk formula			
4264	with iron		3585	late psychomotor development
4265	soybean milk		3584	psychomotor regression
4266	with iron		3600	precocious puberty at age
4267	goat's milk		4066	growth spurt before age 9
4799	sheep's milk		4067	no visible physical sexual development at age 14
4268	special formula (enzyme-processed)			
4911	whole cow's milk		4068	with no onset of periods
4912	after switching from formula		3601	puberty delayed to age
4269	weaned to cup at age:		3613	eating frequently to avoid tiredness
4270	solid foods introduced at age:		3614	high salt intake
4271	rice cereal		5105	**trauma**
4272	fruits		3438	physical trauma
4273	vegetables		3439	to the head
4274	meats		4008	from a fall
4275	finger-foods started at age:		4009	from being hit
4276	regular table foods started at age:		4485	forehead
4278	daily caloric intake		3440	facial
4277	particular food dislikes		4336	periorbital
4771	uses a pacifier		3441	to the eye
4772	sucks a thumb		4482	to the conjunctiva
4161	being the firstborn in family		4483	to the sclera
4162	being the secondborn in family		4484	to the cornea
4163	being the youngest in family		3442	to the jaw
3906	deficient childcare		3443	to the neck
3907	received grossly pathogenic childcare		4486	anterior
3908	disregard of basic emotional needs		4487	posterior
3909	persistent disregard of basic physical needs		3444	to the shoulder
			3445	to the arm
3910	repeated new primary caregiver precluding stable attachments		3446	to the elbow
			3447	to the wrist
4339	childcare by unrelated male		4131	from repetitive motion
3589	squatting episodes during childhood		3448	to the chest
3590	toilet training		3449	to the back

TRAUMA HISTORY, CONT.

3450	to the abdomen	3636	recent electrical shock
4189	during pregnancy	3650	hit by lightning
3451	to the pelvis	4362	patient observed / reported
3977	to the rectum	4363	to fall
3452	to the testicles	4365	striking head
3453	to the leg(s)	4364	a vertical distance of
3454	to the knee	4954	from sidewalk curb
3455	to the ankle	4656	from steps of escalator
3456	massive	4960	on a moving sidewalk
4337	unexplained	4657	from stairs
4964	from lightning	4658	from ladder
4962	from a cataclysmic event	4659	from scaffolding
4963	a hurricane	4956	into a well
4965	a typhoon	4957	into a manhole
4966	a tidal wave	4958	off a cliff
4967	a tornado	4661	from chair
4968	a flood	4955	from bed
4969	a snow storm	4959	off the toilet
4970	a dust storm	4961	from playground equipment
4971	an earthquake	4662	while playing a sport
4972	a volcanic eruption	4366	collapsed
4973	an avalanche	4375	after / during exercise
4974	a landslide	4373	clutching chest
4975	the collapse of a dam	4369	without losing consciousness
4338	nonaccidental	4368	before losing consciousness
4980	intentionally struck by a motor vehicle	4367	after losing consciousness
		4376	while holding head
4340	multiple occurrences	4374	after crying out
4866	without bleeding	4377	being beaten / mugged
4855	location of accident	4383	being stabbed
4856	at home	4384	being shot
4857	babysitter's	4378	being hit by a vehicle
4858	day care	4660	accident from diving
4859	accident witnessed by	4379	being confused
4860	parent	4380	being agitated
4861	sibling	4381	being abusive
4862	grandparent	4382	being violent
4863	babysitter	4385	patient was found
4864	day care personnel	4400	in a daze
4865	neighbor	4401	speaking / mumbling incoherently
3457	trauma at birth	4386	unresponsive
3817	accidental puncture or laceration during a procedure	4387	seizing
		4388	with vital signs absent
3818	foreign body accidentally left during a procedure	4389	bleeding
		4390	from wound(s)
4635	dehiscence of surgical wound	4394	head
3458	acoustic trauma (explosive)	4402	face
4840	injury was treated previously	4399	neck
4841	cleaned	4403	shoulder
4842	dressed	4395	chest
4843	ointment	4396	abdomen
4844	sutured	4404	pelvis
4845	number of sutures	4397	arm

TRAUMA HISTORY, CONT.

4405	hand	4415	Free text:
4398	leg	4900	User Finding:
4406	foot		
4391	from the mouth		
4392	from the nose		
4393	from the ear(s)		
4697	physical abuse		
4699	pushing, striking, slapping or pinching		
4700	force-feeding		
4701	incorrect positioning		
4702	improper use of physical restraints		
4703	improper use of medications		
4704	sexual contact or exposure without consent		
4690	physical neglect		
4691	inadequate meals		
4692	insufficient liquids		
4693	failure to provide eyeglasses		
4694	failure to provide hearing aid		
4695	failure to provide false teeth		
4696	failure to provide safety precautions		
4705	psychological neglect		
4707	left alone for long periods of time		
4708	failure to vary routine		
4710	psychological abuse		
4711	verbal berating, harassment, or intimidation		
4712	threats of punishment or deprivation		
4714	treated like an infant		
4715	isolation from family, friends or activities		
4717	material / financial neglect		
4718	failure to use available funds for healthcare		
4719	failure to use available funds for maintenance and well-being		
4720	material / financial abuse		
4721	denial of a home to live in		
4722	theft of money or possessions		
4723	coercion into signing legal documents		
4724	coercion into purchasing goods		
4725	violation of personal rights		
4726	denial of right to privacy		
4727	denial of right to make personal decisions		
4729	on healthcare		
4730	on change in marital status		
4728	forcible eviction		
4731	forcible placement in nursing home while still competent		
3535	recent wound		
3782	gunshot		
3783	knife		

Part III
Physical Findings

6000	**Physical Examination**	6038		Tachycardia
64676	Reason For Examination	6039		>160
11761	Following Surgery	6040		Slowed By Carotid Massage Or Valsalva
11762	Following Radiotherapy			
11763	Following Chemotherapy	6041		Pulse Deficit
11764	Following Treatment Of Fracture	9220		Absence Of Pulse
11765	As A Follow-up	6042		An Irregular Pulse Rhythm
6001	**Vital Signs, Weight And Height**	6043		Regularly Irregular
6002	Temperature	6044		Irregularly Irregular
6003	Oral	6045		Blood Pressure
6004	Rectal	60511		Cuff Size
62549	Axillary	60512		Regular
6005	Fever	60513		Pediatric
6006	An FUO (>101F, 38.8C for 3 weeks or more)	60514		Large
		60515		Thigh
6007	Remittent (varies, staying above normal)	6046		Systolic
		11730		At Rest
6008	Sustained (continuous)	11731		At End Of Inspiration
6009	Intermittent (within 24 hours)	11732		At End Of Expiration
11216	Ranging From Normal To 103F	11733		With Stress
6010	Relapsing (period >24 hours)	11734		Pressure While Standing
6011	Tertian (every other day)	62290		Pressure While Sitting
6012	Quartan (every third day)	62291		Pressure While Supine
6013	Pel-Epstein	11735		Orthostatic Decrease
6014	Malignant Hyperthermia (>105F)	6047		Diastolic
6015	Reversal Of Diurnal Variation (highest in AM)	11749		At Rest
		11750		At End Of Inspiration
6016	Low Grade Fever (99 - 101F)	11751		At End Of Expiration
6017	Associated With Relative Bradycardia	11752		With Stress
		9531		Pressure While Standing
6018	Hypothermia	62292		Pressure While Sitting
6019	Under 96F Or 35.6C	62293		Pressure While Supine
6020	Shaking Chill (rigor)	9264		Orthostatic Decrease
6021	Respiration Rate	6048		Left Arm Pressure
6022	Tachypnea	6049		Left / Right Discrepancy
6023	Bradypnea	6050		Leg Pressure
6024	Apnea	6051		Standing Pressure
6025	During Sleep Only	6052		Systolic Hypertension Only (diastolic <90)
6026	Respiration, Rhythm And Depth			
6027	Shallow Respiration	6053		>200
6028	Kussmaul Breathing	6054		Combined Systolic And Diastolic Hypertension
9403	Gasping (Apneustic)			
6029	Cheyne-Stokes Breathing	6055		>200/120
6030	Biot's Breathing	6056		Upper Extremities Only
6031	Sighing Respirations	62791		Labile Hypertension
6032	Painful Respirations	6057		Paroxysmal Hypertension
6033	Stridor	6058		Hypotension
6034	Pulse Rate	6059		Orthostatic Hypotension
9529	Rate While Standing	9221		Absent
9262	Orthostatic Rise	6060		Widened Pulse Pressure
6035	Bradycardia	6061		Narrowed Pulse Pressure
6036	Increased By Atropine	7325		Pulsus Paradoxus Over 10 Mm. Hg
6037	Bradycardia Relative To Activity	6062		Pulse Pressure - Mayne's Sign

62611	Venous Pressure	10010	Poorly Hydrated
6063	Weight	6369	**Head**
9257	Within Normal Limits (+- 10% ideal wt.)	10022	Circumference
		6370	Cranial Bruit
10002	Too Thin	6371	Orbital Bruit
6064	Cachectic	9404	Evidence Of Injury
11440	Loss	9405	Scalp
11441	Acute	10423	Caput Succedaneum
6065	Chronic (>7% in 1 year)	11570	Skull
11461	Under Birth Weight At Two Or More Weeks	10422	Cephalohematoma
		62348	Right
9296	Less Than 75% Of Ideal Body Weight	62349	Left
6066	Weight Gain >7% In 1 Year	62350	Bilateral
9447	Sudden (excessive) Weight Gain During The Third Trimester	9406	Forehead
		9408	Abrasion
6067	Obesity	9409	Face
6068	Symmetrical And >30% Overweight	9410	Laceration
6069	Centripetal Distribution (truncal)	9412	Penetrating Wound
6070	Centrifugal Distribution	9413	Of The Forehead
9259	Morbid (>100% over)	9414	Of The Face
60507	Skin Fold Thickness	9415	Of The Temple
60508	Abdominal	9416	Of The Back Of The Head (Occiput)
60509	Triceps	6372	Abnormality Of Appearance
60510	Axillary	6373	Of The Scalp
11729	Body Surface Area	6374	Sebaceous Cysts
9300	Body Mass Index	6375	Lipoma
62294	Body Build	6376	Cirsoid Aneurysm
62295	Mesomorphic	6377	Cavernous Hemangioma
62296	Endomorphic	6378	Pneumatocele
62297	Ectomorphic	6379	Platybasia
6071	Height	6380	Turban Tumor
6072	Span	6381	Neurofibroma
6073	Span Versus Height Ratio	6382	Cellulitis Of Scalp
6074	Upper Segment Greater Than Lower Segment	6385	Skull Mass ___ cm
		11571	Occipital ___ cm
6075	Lower Segment Greater Than Upper Segment	11572	Pulsatile ___ cm
		6386	External Swelling
6076	Excessive	6387	Skull Malformation
6077	Short Stature	6388	Craniotabes
6078	Gigantism	6389	Oxycephaly
9952	Length	6390	Brachycephalic
9307	**General Appearance**	6391	Meningocele
10023	Awake	6392	Parrot's Bosses
10011	Alert	6393	Frontal Bossing
10008	Oriented To Time, Place And Person	6394	Enlarged Malar Bones
10025	Well Developed	6395	Microcephaly
10026	Well Nourished	10424	Skull Molding
9308	Healthy Appearing	10425	Fontanelle
9310	Chronically Ill	10426	Delayed Closure
10024	In No Acute Distress	10427	Early Closure
9309	Acutely Ill	10428	Abnormally Large
10001	Uncomfortable	10429	Persistent Posterior
10009	Well Hydrated	10430	Tense

10431	Sutures	60470	Trial Frame
10432	Early Closure	60471	Phoropter
62351	Sagittal	60472	Automated Refracter
62352	Coronal	13141	Retinoscopy
62353	Lambdoid	64672	With Cycloplegia
10433	Delayed Closure	64673	Cyclopentate
6396	Skull Depression	64674	Atropine
6397	Swelling Of The Cheek	6578	On The Right (Uncorrected) 20/___
6398	Masseter Muscle Hypertrophy	64398	Missed___
6399	Lateral Deviation Of The Head	64410	Plus___
11152	To The Right	6580	Decrease Not Correctable
62354	Due To Muscle Tension	6579	Decrease Correctable By Refraction
62355	With A Mass ___ cm	11737	Diopters Of Sphere
11153	To The Left	11738	Diopters Of Cylinder
62356	Due To Muscle Tension	11739	Axis
62357	With A Mass ___ cm	9316	On The Right (Corrected) 20/___
6400	Tilted	64399	Missed___
11154	Unable To Be Supported	64411	Plus___
6401	Enlarged (Macrocephaly)	11877	Decrease Correctable By Pinhole
6402	Scar	6581	On The Left (Uncorrected) 20/___
10365	Right Side	64400	Missed___
10366	Left Side	64412	Plus___
6403	Skull Tenderness	6583	Decrease Not Correctable
6404	Scalp Tenderness	6582	Decrease Correctable By Refraction
6405	Temporal Arteries	11741	Diopters Of Sphere
6406	Dilated	11742	Diopters Of Cylinder
6407	Hard, Nodular	11743	Axis
6408	Tender	9317	On The Left (Corrected) 20/___
6409	Pulsating	64401	Missed___
6410	Inflamed	64413	Plus___
6411	Temporal Wasting	11878	Decrease Correctable By Pinhole
6412	Forehead Skin	9314	Binocular Vision (Uncorrected) 20/___
6413	Bulldog Skin (deep folds and furrows)	64402	Missed___
6414	Absence Of Forehead Wrinkling (Joffroy's sign)	64414	Plus___
		6584	< 20/200 Without Correction
11726	Facies	9319	The Right Eye Only
6415	Coarse Facial Features	9320	The Left Eye Only
6416	Moon Face	9321	Both Eyes
6417	Plethoric Face	9315	Binocular Vision (Corrected) 20/___
6418	Immobile Facies (masklike)	64403	Missed___
10902	Asymmetric Face	64432	Plus___
6420	Risus Sardonicus (distorted grin)	9318	< 20/200 With Correction
6419	Widened Philtrum	9322	The Right Eye Only
9344	Jaw Findings	9323	The Left Eye Only
6421	Prognathism (enlarged jaw)	9324	Both Eyes
6422	Micrognathia (small jaw)	6587	Non-correctable Binocular Decrease
6423	Mandibular Tumor	6588	Blindness (no light perception)
6425	**Eyes**	6589	On The Left Only
6577	Visual Acuity	6590	On The Right Only
62358	Location Of Exam	6591	Binocular
62359	Optometrist / Ophthalmologist	6592	Cortical Blindness
62360	School	6593	Deficit Denied
60469	Instrumentation	18303	Near Vision - Jaeger (at 14")

EYES, CONT.

18304	Binocular (Uncorrected)	
63298	Missed___	
63299	Plus___	
18305	Right Eye (Uncorrected)	
63300	Missed___	
63301	Plus___	
18306	Left Eye (Uncorrected)	
63302	Missed___	
63303	Plus___	
18307	Binocular (Corrected)	
63304	Missed___	
63305	Plus___	
18308	Right Eye (Corrected)	
63306	Missed___	
63307	Plus___	
18309	Left Eye (Corrected)	
63308	Missed___	
63309	Plus___	
10244	Near Vision - Snellen	
10246	Right Eye (Uncorrected) 20/__	
64404	Missed___	
64415	Plus___	
10247	Left Eye (Uncorrected) 20/__	
64405	Missed___	
64416	Plus___	
10245	Binocular (Uncorrected) 20/__	
64406	Missed___	
64417	Plus___	
10249	Right Eye (Corrected) 20/__	
64407	Missed___	
64420	Plus___	
11753	Diopters Of Sphere	
11754	Diopters Of Cylinder	
11755	Axis	
10250	Left Eye (Corrected) 20/__	
64408	Missed___	
64419	Plus___	
11756	Diopters Of Sphere	
11757	Diopters Of Cylinder	
11758	Axis	
10248	Binocular (Corrected) 20/__	
64409	Missed___	
64418	Plus___	
18227	Ortho Rater	
18228	Far Vision (Uncorrected)	
18229	Phoria	
18230	Vertical	
18231	Lateral	
18232	Acuity	
18233	Both	
18234	Right	
18235	Left	
18236	Depth	

18237	Color	
18238	Near Vision (Uncorrected)	
18239	Acuity	
18240	Both	
18241	Right	
18242	Left	
18243	Phoria	
18244	Vertical	
18245	Lateral	
18286	Far Vision (Corrected)	
18287	Phoria	
18288	Vertical	
18289	Lateral	
18290	Acuity	
18291	Both	
18292	Right	
18293	Left	
18294	Depth	
18295	Near Vision (Corrected)	
18296	Acuity	
18297	Both	
18298	Right	
18299	Left	
18300	Phoria	
18301	Vertical	
18302	Lateral	
6527	Extraocular Movements	
6556	Conjugate Movement Failure	
6557	Failure In All Directions	
6558	Failure Of Upward Gaze	
6559	Failure Of Downward Gaze	
6560	Failure Of Lateral Gaze	
6561	To The Left	
6562	To The Right	
6563	Failure Of Convergence	
6564	Conjugate Deviation	
6565	Upward	
6566	Downward	
6567	To The Left	
6568	Overcome By "doll's" Maneuver Or Calorics	
6569	Not Overcome By "doll's" Maneuver Or Calorics	
6570	To The Right	
6571	Overcome By "doll's" Maneuver Or Calorics	
6572	Not Overcome By "doll's" Maneuver Or Calorics	
6573	Oculogyric Crisis	
6574	Skew Deviation	
6575	The Left Eye Higher Than The Right	
6576	The Right Eye Higher Than The Left	
6547	Strabismus	

EYES, CONT.

62361	Right Eye		11530	Latent
62362	Left Eye		6543	Ocular Bobbing
6548	Non-paralytic		6544	Ocular Dysmetria
11879	Phoria		6545	Ocular Flutter
11880	At Distance		6546	Opsoclonus
11881	Esophoria		9439	Evaluations
11882	Exophoria		9440	Of Spontaneous Nystagmus
11883	Hyperphoria		9441	Of Positional Nystagmus
11884	At Near Gaze		9442	Of Optokinetic Nystagmus
11885	Esophoria		9443	Caloric Vestibular Test
11886	Exophoria		6498	Pupil
11887	Hyperphoria		11943	Size
11888	Tropia		11946	Subdued Light
11889	At Distance		11944	Right Eye
11890	Esophoria		11945	Left Eye
11891	Exophoria		11947	Bright Light
11892	Hyperphoria		11948	Right Eye
11893	At Near Gaze		11949	Left Eye
11894	Esophoria		11950	Accommodation
11895	Exophoria		11951	Right Eye
11896	Hyperphoria		11952	Left Eye
11897	Constant		6499	Anisocoria
11898	Intermittent		6500	Right > Left
11899	Right Eye Fixation		6501	Left > Right
11900	Left Eye Fixation		6502	Mydriasis
6549	Paralytic		6503	Unilateral
6550	Lateral Rectus (eye turned in)		6504	On The Left
6551	Medial Rectus (eye turned out)		6505	On The Right
6552	Superior Rectus (eye turned down and out)		6506	Bilaterally
			6507	Miosis
6553	Inferior Rectus (eye turned up and in)		6508	Unilateral
			6509	On The Left
6554	Inferior Oblique (eye turned down and in)		6510	On The Right
			6511	Bilaterally
6555	Superior Oblique (eye turned up and out)		6512	Non-reactive To Light
			6513	By Direct Illumination
6528	Nystagmus		6514	Unilateral
6529	Rotatory		6515	On The Left
6530	Induced Only By Sudden Position Change		6516	On The Right
			6517	Bilaterally
6531	Horizontal		6518	Non-reactive By Direct Illumination, Consensual Spared
6532	Upbeat			
6533	Downbeat		6519	On The Left
6534	Convergence (Nystagmus Retractorius)		6520	On The Right
			6526	Impaired Accommodation
6535	Opticokinetic Nystagmus Absent		6521	Adie's (large, slowly reactive to light and convergence)
6536	To The Right			
6537	To The Left		6522	Argyll-Robertson (small, react to convergence only)
6538	See-Saw			
6539	Dissociated		6523	Marcus - Gunn (pupil dilates to light)
6540	Internuclear Ophthalmoplegia		6524	On The Left
6541	Pendular		6525	On The Right
6542	Rebound		11482	Deformed

EYES, CONT.

11483	Ectopic	60145		Both Eyes
11727	On The Right	11445	Microphthalmia	
11728	On The Left	60146		Right Eye
11484	Ruptured Sphincter	60147		Left Eye
11468	Leucocoria	60148		Both Eyes
6426	External Eye	6435	Eyelids	
6427	Eyebrows	11953	Swelling	
6428	Loss Of Lateral Eyebrow	11954		Right Upper Lid
11469	Foreign Body	11955		Right Lower Lid
6429	Palpebral Fissures	11956		Left Upper Lid
6430	Exophthalmos	11957		Left Lower Lid
6431	Unilateral	11958		Both Lids
60117	Right Eye	11959	Hyperemia	
60118	Left Eye	11960		Right Upper Lid
6432	Bilaterally	11961		Right Lower Lid
11531	Pulsating	11962		Left Upper Lid
11448	With Scleral Prominence ("sunset sign")	11963		Left Lower Lid
		11964		Both Lids
6433	Enophthalmos	11965	Nodule	
60119	Right Eye	11966	Multiple	
60120	Left Eye	11967	Size	
60121	Both Eyes	11968		Right Eye
10904	Slanted Upwards	11969		Left Eye
60122	Right Eye	11970	Hard	
60123	Left Eye	11971	Soft	
60124	Both Eyes	11972	In The Medial Aspect	
10905	Slanted Downwards	11973	In The Temporal Aspect	
60125	Right Eye	11974	In The Center	
60126	Left Eye	11975	Inward-Pointing	
60127	Both Eyes	11976	Outward-Pointing	
11766	Euryblepharon	11977	Involving The Lid Margin	
60128	Right Eye	11978	Ulcerated	
60129	Left Eye	11979	Vascularized	
60130	Both Eyes	11980	Fixed	
11767	Epiblepharon	6436	Ptosis Of The Eyelid	
60131	Right Eye	6437	On The Right	
60132	Left Eye	6438	On The Left	
60133	Both Eyes	6439	Bilaterally	
11447	Short	6440	Complete	
60134	Right Eye	6441	Incomplete	
60135	Left Eye	11534	Coloboma	
60136	Both Eyes	62363	Palpebrale	
11512	Blepharophimosis	62374	Iridis	
60137	Right Eye	62375	Partial	
60138	Left Eye	62376		Right Eye
60139	Both Eyes	62377		Left Eye
11467	Hemophthalmos	62378	Complete	
60140	Right Eye	62379		Right Eye
60141	Left Eye	62380		Left Eye
60142	Both Eyes	9339	Pseudoptosis Of The Eyelid	
6434	Hypertelorism	6442	Failure Of Lid Closure	
60143	Right Eye	6443	Unilateral	
60144	Left Eye	60149		Right Eye

EYES, CONT.

60150	Left Eye	60185	Right Eye
6444	Bilateral	60186	Left Eye
11769	Lagophthalmos	6453	Nasal Upper Lid
60151	Right Eye	6454	Nasal Lower Lid
60152	Left Eye	6455	Temporal Upper Lid
60153	Both Eyes	11518	Hemorrhage
11770	Paralytic	60187	Right Eye
11771	Cicatricial	60188	Left Eye
6445	Lid Lag	6456	Heliotrope
60154	Right Eye	60189	Right Eye
60155	Left Eye	60190	Left Eye
60156	Both Eyes	6457	Palpebral Hematoma
62421	Eyes Not Open Symmetrically	60191	Right Eye
6446	Infrequent Blinking	60192	Left Eye
6447	Ectropion	6458	Palpebral Edema
60157	Right Eye	6459	Unilateral
60158	Left Eye	60193	Right Eye
6448	Entropion	60194	Left Eye
60160	Right Eye	11519	Elephantiasis
60161	Left Eye	11520	Cysts
11772	Punctal Eversion	60195	Right Eye
60162	Right Eye	60196	Left Eye
60163	Left Eye	11773	Tumors
6449	Blepharospasm	60197	Right Eye
6450	Blepharitis	60198	Left Eye
60164	Right Eye	11774	Basal Cell Appearance
60165	Left Eye	11775	Squamous Cell Appearance
60166	Both Eyes	11776	Sebaceous Cell
6451	Epicanthal Fold	11777	Melanoma
60167	Right Eye	11521	Vascular Anomalies
60168	Left Eye	60199	Right Eye
60169	Both Eyes	60200	Left Eye
11513	Xanthelasma	6460	Epiphora
60170	Right Eye	11778	Excessive Lacrimation
60171	Left Eye	11779	Deficient Drainage
60172	Both Eyes	11780	Punctal Stenosis
11514	Hyperpigmentation	11901	Veil
60173	Right Eye	11781	Canalicular Stricture
60174	Left Eye	60201	Right Eye
60175	Both Eyes	60202	Left Eye
11515	Hypopigmentation	60203	Both Eyes
60176	Right Eye	11470	Foreign Body
60177	Left Eye	60204	Right Eye
60178	Both Eyes	60205	Left Eye
11516	Hypertrichosis	11555	Laceration
60179	Right Eye	60222	Right Upper Lid
60180	Left Eye	60223	Right Lower Lid
60181	Both Eyes	60224	Left Upper Lid
11517	Hypotrichosis	60225	Left Lower Lid
60182	Right Eye	60226	Length
60183	Left Eye	60227	Superficial
60184	Both Eyes	60228	Deep
6452	Lid Hyperemia	60229	Medial

EYES, CONT.

60230	Central	11996	Left Eye
60231	Temporal	11997	Both Eyes
60232	Involving The Lid Margin	6465	Subconjunctival Hemorrhage
60233	Involving The Canaliculus	11998	Right Eye
11522	Dermatochalasis	11999	Left Eye
60206	Right Eye	60000	Both Eyes
60207	Left Eye	11471	Foreign Body
60208	Both Eyes	60001	Right Eye
9673	Infraorbital Discoloration	60002	Left Eye
60209	Right Eye	60003	Both Eyes
60210	Left Eye	6466	Ulceration
60211	Both Eyes	60004	Right Eye
9674	Periorbital Discoloration	60005	Left Eye
60212	Right Eye	60006	Both Eyes
60213	Left Eye	11557	Laceration
60214	Both Eyes	60234	Right Eye
11532	Lateral Displacement Of The Eyeball	60235	Left Eye
		60236	Both Eyes
60215	Right Eye	11656	Vesicle
60216	Left Eye	60007	Right Eye
60217	Anophthalmos	60008	Left Eye
60218	Right Eye	60009	Both Eyes
60219	With Prosthesis	11657	Scarring
60220	Left Eye	60010	Right Eye
60221	With Prosthesis	60011	Left Eye
6461	Conjunctiva	60012	Both Eyes
6470	Chemosis	6467	Pigmented Pingueculae
60025	Right Eye	60013	Right Eye
60026	Left Eye	60014	Left Eye
60027	Both Eyes	60015	Both Eyes
11981	Swelling	11782	Acquired Melanosis
11982	Right Eye	60016	Right Eye
11983	Left Eye	60017	Left Eye
11984	Both Eyes	60018	Both Eyes
6462	Hyperemia	6468	Petechiae
62364	Palpebral Conjunctiva	60019	Right Eye
11985	Right Eye	60020	Left Eye
11986	Left Eye	60021	Both Eyes
11987	Both Eyes	6469	Lacrimation Decrease
62365	Bulbar Conjunctiva	60022	Right Eye
62366	Right Eye	60023	Left Eye
62367	Left Eye	60024	Both Eyes
62368	Both Eyes	11783	Bland Edema
6463	Purulent Discharge	60028	Right Eye
11988	Right Eye	60029	Left Eye
11989	Left Eye	60030	Both Eyes
11990	Both Eyes	6471	Follicles
6464	Watery Discharge	60031	Right Eye
11991	Right Eye	60032	Left Eye
11992	Left Eye	60033	Both Eyes
11993	Both Eyes	6472	Aneurysm
11994	Mucoid Discharge	60034	Right Eye
11995	Right Eye	60035	Left Eye

EYES, CONT.

60036	Both Eyes		60072	Height
11495	Cyst		60073	Width
60037	Right Eye		60074	Central
60038	Left Eye		60075	Nasal
60039	Both Eyes		60076	Temporal
9338	Pterygium		60077	Superior
60040	Right Eye		60078	Inferior
60041	Left Eye		11924	Ulceration
60042	Both Eyes		60079	Right Eye
60043	Medial		11932	Height
60044	Lateral		60080	Width
62299	Pallor		11933	Depth
62300	Right Eye		11934	Central
62301	Left Eye		11935	Peripheral
62302	Bilateral		60081	Nasal
62499	Lacrimal Sac		60082	Temporal
62500	Edema		60083	Superior
62501	Right Eye		60084	Inferior
62502	Left Eye		60085	Left Eye
62503	Bilaterally		60086	Height
6482	Sclera		60087	Width
6483	Episcleritis (most intense at limbus, non blanching)		60088	Depth
			60089	Central
6484	Yellow (Icteric)		60090	Peripheral
6485	Blue		60091	Nasal
6486	Brown		60092	Temporal
62269	Red		60093	Superior
62270	Right Eye		60094	Inferior
62271	Left Eye		11925	Non-Infectious
62272	Bilateral		11926	Rheumatoid
6487	Scleritis		11927	Pellucid
60237	Right Eye		11928	Terrien's
60238	Left Eye		11929	Mooren's
11473	Foreign Body		11930	Sjogren's
60239	Right Eye		11931	Infectious
60240	Left Eye		11486	Abscess
11566	Abrasion		6481	With Perforation
60241	Right Eye		11559	Laceration
60242	Left Eye		60245	Right Eye
11558	Laceration		60246	Left Eye
60243	Right Eye		60247	Length
60244	Left Eye		60248	Superficial
6473	Cornea		60249	Perforating
11565	Abrasion		60250	With Uveal Prolapse
60063	Right Eye		60251	Superiorly
60064	Height		60252	Inferiorly
60065	Width		60253	Medially
60066	Central		60254	Temporally
60067	Nasal		60255	Centrally
60068	Temporal		60256	Wound Dehiscence
60069	Superior		60257	Right Eye
60070	Inferior		60258	Left Eye
60071	Left Eye		60259	Length

EYES, CONT.

60260	With Uveal Prolapse	6475	Arcus Senilis
60261	Superiorly	11936	Keratitis
60262	Inferiorly	60098	Right Eye
60263	Medially	60099	Left Eye
60264	Temporally	60100	Both Eyes
60265	Centrally	6478	Epithelial
11472	Foreign Body	11937	Dendritic
60045	Right Eye	11938	Punctate
60046	Left Eye	11939	Stromal
6474	Band Keratopathy	6479	Interstitial
60047	Right Eye	11940	Disciform
60048	Left Eye	11941	Endothelial
60049	Both Eyes	6477	Keratic Precipitates
11487	Neovascularization	9337	Edema
60053	Right Eye	60101	Right Eye
60054	Left Eye	60102	Left Eye
60055	Both Eyes	60103	Both Eyes
11463	Pannus	11904	Epithelial
60056	Right Eye	11905	Stromal
60057	Left Eye	11510	Descemet's Folds
60058	Both Eyes	11491	Pigmentation
11488	Opacity	11500	Anterior
11902	Epithelial	6476	Kayser-Fleischer Ring
11903	Stromal	60050	Right Eye
11490	Peripheral	60051	Left Eye
6480	Central	60052	Both Eyes
60059	Right Eye	11501	Stahli's Line
60060	Left Eye	11502	Stromal
60061	Both Eyes	11503	Hematocornea
11906	Dystrophy	11504	Posterior
11907	Epithelial	11505	Krukenberg Spindle
11908	Map	11492	Argentous Deposit
11909	Dot	11494	Anesthesia
11910	Fingerprint	60269	Anterior Chamber
11911	Cogan's	60270	Depth
11912	Reis-Buckler	60271	Right Eye
11913	Stromal	60273	Shallow
11914	Lattice	60274	Moderate
11915	Granular	60275	Deep
11916	Macular	60272	Left Eye
11917	Endothelial	60276	Shallow
11918	Fuchs	60277	Moderate
11919	Posterior Polymorphous	60278	Deep
60266	Right Eye	60279	Cell Grade
60267	Left Eye	60283	Right Eye
60268	Both Eyes	60284	Left Eye
11920	Degeneration	60280	Grade Of Flare
60095	Right Eye	60285	Right Eye
60096	Left Eye	60286	Left Eye
60097	Both Eyes	60281	Hyphema
11921	Keratoconus	60287	Right Eye
11922	With Hydrops	60288	Left Eye
11923	Salzmann's	19122	Angles (Gonioscopy)

EYES, CONT.

60476	Of The Right Eye	6490	Iridocyclitis
60477	Grade (0-4)	60295	Right Eye
60478	Superior Quadrant (0-4)	60296	Left Eye
60479	Inferior Quadrant (0-4)	6493	Iridodonesis
60480	Nasal Quadrant (0-4)	60297	Right Eye
60481	Temporal Quadrant (0-4)	60298	Left Eye
60482	Trabecular Meshwork	11485	Prolapse Of Iris
60483	Pigmentation (1-4)	60299	Right Eye
60484	Neovascularization	60300	Left Eye
60485	Scleral Spur	11451	Posterior Synechiae
60486	Ciliary Band	60301	Right Eye
60487	Iris Root	60302	Left Eye
60488	Schlemm's Canal	6492	Hypopyon (move this to under
60489	Blood Present		Anterior Chamber?)
60490	Mass ___ cm	60303	Right Eye
60491	Of The Left Eye	60304	Left Eye
60492	Grade (0-4)	6495	Brushfield Spots
60493	Superior Quadrant (0-4)	60305	Right Eye
60494	Inferior Quadrant (0-4)	60306	Left Eye
60495	Nasal Quadrant (0-4)	6496	Pale Blue Iris
60496	Temporal Quadrant (0-4)	60307	Right Eye
60497	Trabecular Meshwork	60308	Left Eye
60498	Pigmentation (1-4)	6497	Microfilariae
60499	Neovascularization	60309	Right Eye
60500	Scleral Spur	60310	Left Eye
60501	Ciliary Band	11481	Uveal Hemorrhage
60502	Iris Root	60311	Right Eye
60503	Schlemm's Canal	60312	Left Eye
60504	Blood Present	11222	Choroiditis
60505	Mass ___ cm	60313	Right Eye
60282	Foreign Body	60314	Left Eye
60289	Right Eye	6491	Uveitis
60290	Left Eye	60315	Right Eye
6488	Uveal Tract	60316	Left Eye
60104	Iris Color	11474	Foreign Body
60105	Blue	60317	Right Eye
60106	Right Eye	60318	Left Eye
60107	Left Eye	62422	Fundus Not Visualized
60108	Brown	62423	Right Eye
60109	Right Eye	62424	Left Eye
60110	Left Eye	62425	Bilateral
60111	Green	6619	Lens
60112	Right Eye	9340	Aphakia
60113	Left Eye	60319	Right Eye
60114	Hazel	60320	Left Eye
60115	Right Eye	60321	Both Eyes
60116	Left Eye	11784	Pseudophakia
6494	Iris Hypopigmentation	11785	Anterior Chamber
60291	Right Eye	60322	Right Eye
60292	Left Eye	60323	Left Eye
6489	Iritis	60324	Both Eyes
60293	Right Eye	11786	Posterior Chamber
60294	Left Eye	60325	Right Eye

EYES, CONT.

60326	Left Eye	60340	Left Eye
60327	Both Eyes	60341	Both Eyes
11787	Fixated Iris	11805	Membranes
60328	Right Eye	60342	Right Eye
60329	Left Eye	60343	Left Eye
62640	Both Eyes	60344	Both Eyes
62636	Secondary Cataract	11806	Strands
62637	Right Eye	60345	Right Eye
62638	Left Eye	60346	Left Eye
62639	Both Eyes	60347	Both Eyes
6620	Cataract	11807	Veils
9825	Right Eye	60348	Right Eye
9826	Left Eye	60349	Left Eye
9827	Both Eyes	60350	Both Eyes
11788	Cortical	11808	Hemorrhage
11789	Right Eye	60351	Right Eye
11790	Left Eye	60352	Left Eye
11791	Both Eyes	6622	Optic Disc
11792	Nuclear	6623	Color
11793	Right Eye	60353	Pink
11794	Left Eye	60354	Right Eye
11795	Both Eyes	60355	Left Eye
11796	Posterior Subcapsular	60356	Both Eyes
11797	Right Eye	60357	Pale
11798	Left Eye	60358	Right Eye
11799	Both Eyes	60359	Left Eye
62641	Fragments	60360	Both Eyes
62642	Right Eye	6624	White (Optic atrophy)
62643	Left Eye	9828	Right Eye
62644	Both Eyes	9829	Left Eye
11800	Grade	9830	Both Eyes
11801	Right Eye	6625	Hyperemic
11802	Left Eye	60361	Right Eye
60330	Exfoliation	60362	Left Eye
60331	Right Eye	60363	Both Eyes
60332	Left Eye	6626	Blurred Margins
6621	Dislocation	60364	Right Eye
60333	Right Eye	60365	Left Eye
60334	Left Eye	60366	Both Eyes
60335	Both Eyes	6627	Physiologic Cup
62630	Anterior Chamber	11809	Ratio
62631	Posterior Segment	11810	Right Eye
11529	Subluxation	11811	Left Eye
60336	Right Eye	6628	Increased
60337	Left Eye	6629	Obscured
60338	Both Eyes	60367	Right Eye
62632	Superior	60368	Left Eye
62633	Inferior	6630	Papilledema
62634	Temporally	9831	Of The Right Eye
62635	Nasally	9832	Of The Left Eye
11803	Vitreous	9833	Of Both Eyes
11804	Floaters	6631	Contralateral To Atrophy (Foster-Kennedy)
60339	Right Eye		

EYES, CONT.

11535	Pseudopapilledema		60390	Right Eye
11812	Right Eye		60391	Left Eye
11813	Left Eye		60392	Both Eyes
11814	Both Eyes		62426	Red Reflex Absent
11528	Drusen		62427	Right Eye
60369	Right Eye		62428	Left Eye
60370	Left Eye		62429	Bilateral
60371	Both Eyes		6640	Focal Spasm Arterioles
11533	Crater-like Holes		60393	Right Eye
60372	Right Eye		60394	Left Eye
60373	Left Eye		60395	Both Eyes
60374	Both Eyes		6641	A-V Crossing Defects
11815	Retina		6642	A-V Nicking
6632	Macula		60396	Right Eye
11816	Degeneration		60397	Left Eye
11817	Exudative		60398	Both Eyes
11818	Non-Exudative		6643	Arterial Occlusion
11819	Choroidal Neovascularization		11823	Central
11820	Right Eye		11824	Branch
11821	Left Eye		60399	Right Eye
11822	Both Eyes		60400	Left Eye
6633	Cherry Red Spot		60401	Both Eyes
60375	Right Eye		6644	Arterial Emboli
60376	Left Eye		60402	Right Eye
60377	Both Eyes		60403	Left Eye
6634	Milky-White Region		60404	Both Eyes
60378	Right Eye		11477	Hollenhorst Plaque
60379	Left Eye		6645	Venous Occlusion
60380	Both Eyes		11825	Central
11876	Drusen		11826	Branch
60381	Right Eye		60405	Right Eye
60382	Left Eye		60406	Left Eye
60383	Both Eyes		60407	Both Eyes
62612	Hole		6646	Absence Of Venous Pulsation
62613	Right Eye		60408	Right Eye
62614	Left Eye		60409	Left Eye
62615	Both Eyes		60410	Both Eyes
62616	Cyst		6647	Venous Engorgement
62617	Right Eye		60411	Right Eye
62618	Left Eye		60412	Left Eye
62619	Both Eyes		60413	Both Eyes
11478	Puckering		6648	Tortuosity
60384	Right Eye		60414	Right Eye
60385	Left Eye		60415	Left Eye
60386	Both Eyes		60416	Both Eyes
6635	Vessels		6649	Retinal Neovascularization
6636	Decreased A:V Ratio		10344	Right Only
60387	Right Eye		10345	Left Only
60388	Left Eye		10346	Bilateral
60389	Both Eyes		62620	Choroidal Neovascularization
6637	Arteriolar Light Reflex		62621	Right Only
6638	"Copper Wire"		62622	Left Only
6639	"Silver Wire"		62623	Bilateral

EYES, CONT.

6650	Microaneurysm(s)		11855	Left Eye
11827	Right Eye		11856	Both Eyes
11828	Left Eye		6664	Detachment
11829	Both Eyes		11857	Rhegmatogenous
11475	Telangiectasia		11858	Traction
11830	Right Eye		62624	Serous
11831	Left Eye		11859	Partial
11832	Both Eyes		11860	With The Macula Off
6651	Angioma		11861	Inferior
11833	Right Eye		11862	Superior
11834	Left Eye		11863	Complete
11835	Both Eyes		11864	With PVR
11476	Varices		11865	Right
11836	Right Eye		11866	Left
11837	Left Eye		11867	Both
11838	Both Eyes		6665	Chorioretinitis
6652	Hemorrhage		11868	Right Eye
6653	Flame-shaped		11869	Left Eye
6654	Subhyaloid		11870	Both Eyes
6655	Blot		11480	Chorioretinal Scar
11839	Macular		11497	Posterior Pole
11840	Posterior Pole		11498	Peripheral
11841	Periphery		11499	Disseminated
10347	Right Only		11871	Right Eye
10348	Left Only		11872	Left Eye
10349	Bilaterally		11873	Both Eyes
11942	Multiple		6666	Lipemia Retinalis
11479	Edema		60420	Right Eye
6656	Exudates		60421	Left Eye
6657	Hard 'Soapy' Exudates		60422	Both Eyes
6658	Cotton-Wool Patches		6667	Phakoma
9355	Yellow-white Patches		60423	Right Eye
6659	Granuloma		60424	Left Eye
11842	Right Eye		60425	Both Eyes
11843	Left Eye		6668	Roth's Spots
11844	Both Eyes		60426	Right Eye
6660	Pigmentation		60427	Left Eye
6661	Pigmented Retinal Spots		60428	Both Eyes
6662	Degeneration		6669	Granuloma
60417	Right Eye		62628	Choroidal
60418	Left Eye		62629	Optic Nerve
60419	Both Eyes		60429	Right Eye
6663	Angioid Streaks		60430	Left Eye
11845	Retinal Hole		60431	Both Eyes
11846	Round		6670	Intraocular Pressure
11848	With Vitreous Traction		60432	Right Eye
11849	Right Eye		60433	Left Eye
11850	Left Eye		6671	Increased
11851	Both Eyes		6672	Decreased
11852	Tear		6595	Visual Fields
11847	Horseshoe		60473	Instrumentation
11853	Giant		60474	Automated Perimeter
11854	Right Eye		60475	Goldmann Perimeter

EYES, CONT.

13138	Tangent (Bjerrum) Screen		6690	Low Set Ears
19114	Limited Examination		6691	Bat Ear(s) (lop ear)
19115	Intermediate Examination		6719	Ear Lobe Crease
19116	Extended Examination		62164	Right Ear
6596	Hemianopsia		62165	Left Ear
6597	Homonymous		62166	Bilateral
6598	On The Left		6692	Nodules And Masses ___ cm
6599	On The Right		6693	Gouty Tophus
6600	Transient		62167	Right Ear
6601	Bitemporal		62168	Left Ear
6602	Binasal		62169	Bilateral
6603	Quadrantanopsia		6694	Calcification
6604	Homonymous		62170	Right Ear
6605	In The Left Superior Quadrant		62171	Left Ear
6606	In The Left Inferior Quadrant		62172	Bilateral
6607	In The Right Superior Quadrant		6695	Painless Nodule ___ cm
6608	In The Right Inferior Quadrant		62173	Right Ear
6609	Bitemporal		62174	Left Ear
6610	Superior		62175	Bilateral
6611	Inferior		6696	Painful Nodule ___ cm
6612	Concentric Contraction Of Visual Fields		62176	Right Ear
			62177	Left Ear
6613	Central Scotomata		62178	Bilateral
60434	Right Eye		6697	Pain On Motion
60435	Left Eye		62179	Right Ear
60436	Both Eyes		62180	Left Ear
6614	Paracentral Scotoma		62181	Bilateral
60437	Right Eye		6698	Swelling Of Tragus
60438	Left Eye		62182	Right Ear
60439	Both Eyes		62183	Left Ear
6615	Enlarged Blind Spot		62184	Bilateral
60440	Right Eye		62381	Pierced Ears
60441	Left Eye		62382	Right Ear
60442	Both Eyes		62383	Infection At The Site
6616	Macular Sparing		62384	Left Ear
60443	Right Eye		62385	Infection At The Site
60444	Left Eye		62386	Bilateral
60445	Both Eyes		62387	Infection At The Sites
6673	Extraocular Muscle Motility Restricted		9341	Perichondritis
6617	Ophthalmoscopic		62391	Right Ear
9432	Extensive Initial Exam		62392	Left Ear
9433	Extensive Follow-up Exam		62393	Bilateral
9437	Ophthalmological Sensorimotor Exam		11148	Mastoid
9435	Color Vision Exam		6699	Tenderness
6594	Color Discrimination Difficulty		62257	Right Ear
9434	Pseudoisochromatic Plates		62258	Left Ear
9436	Dark Adaptation Exam		62259	Bilateral
6675	**Ears**		11149	Erythema
6688	Pinna		62260	Right Ear
6689	Malformations		62261	Left Ear
62388	Right Ear		62262	Bilateral
62389	Left Ear		11150	Swelling
62390	Bilateral		62263	Right Ear

ENT, CONT.

62264	Left Ear	62206	Right Ear
62265	Bilateral	62207	Left Ear
6700	External Auditory Meatus	62208	Bilateral
6701	A Discharge	11147	Was Retracted
6702	Ceruminous	62209	Right Ear
62185	Right Ear	62210	Left Ear
62398	Occluding The Canal	62211	Bilateral
62399	Left Ear	6712	Was Bullous
62186	Occluding The Canal	62212	Right Ear
62187	Bilateral	62213	Left Ear
62400	Occluding The Canals	62214	Bilateral
6703	Bloody	6713	Was Erythematous
62188	Right Ear	62215	Right Ear
62189	Left Ear	62216	Left Ear
62190	Bilateral	62217	Bilateral
6704	Serous	6714	Was Perforated
62191	Right Ear	62218	Right Ear
62192	Left Ear	62219	Left Ear
62193	Bilateral	62220	Bilateral
6705	Purulent	6715	Was Scarred
62194	Right Ear	62221	Right Ear
62195	Left Ear	62222	Left Ear
62196	Bilateral	62223	Bilateral
62401	Mucopurulent	11217	Was Opacified
62402	Right Ear	62224	Right Ear
62403	Left Ear	62225	Left Ear
62404	Bilateral	62226	Bilateral
62394	Cheesy Exudate	62566	Had Pressure Equalization Tube(s) In Place
62395	Right Ear		
62396	Left Ear	62567	In The Right Ear
62397	Bilateral	62568	In The Left Ear
9834	From The Right Ear	62569	In Both Ears
9835	From The Left Ear	62408	Color
9836	From Both Ears	11218	Was Blue
6706	Abnormal Wall	62227	Right Ear
6707	Reddened Epithelium	62228	Left Ear
62197	Right Ear	62229	Bilateral
62198	Left Ear	62409	Pink
62199	Bilateral	62410	Right Ear
6708	Desquamative	62411	Left Ear
62200	Right Ear	62412	Bilateral
62201	Left Ear	6716	Vesicular Eruption
62202	Bilateral	62230	Right Ear
6709	Mass ___ cm	62231	Left Ear
62203	Right Ear	62232	Bilateral
62204	Left Ear	6717	Loss Of Light Reflex
62205	Bilateral	62233	Right Ear
9417	Vascular Mass ___ cm	62234	Left Ear
62266	Right Ear	62235	Bilateral
62267	Left Ear	11146	Immobile
62268	Bilateral	62236	Right Ear
6710	Tympanic Membrane	62237	Left Ear
6711	Was Bulging	62238	Bilateral

ENT, CONT.

6718	Pus	
62239	Behind The Membrane	
62240	Right Ear	
62405	Obscurring The Canal	
62241	Left Ear	
62406	Obscurring The Canal	
62242	Bilateral	
62407	Obscurring The Canal	
62243	On The Surface	
62244	Right Ear	
62245	Left Ear	
62246	Bilateral	
62247	In The Ear Canal	
62248	Right Ear	
62249	Left Ear	
62250	Bilateral	
62417	Increased Vascularity	
62418	Right Ear	
62419	Left Ear	
62420	Bilateral	
10251	Abnormal On The Right	
10252	Abnormal On The Left	
11219	Middle Ear	
11220	White Sac-like Structure	
62251	Right Ear	
62252	Left Ear	
62253	Bilateral	
62413	Hemotympanum	
62414	Right Ear	
62415	Left Ear	
62416	Bilateral	
11221	Anomalous Carotid Artery	
62254	Right Ear	
62255	Left Ear	
62256	Bilateral	
62286	Foreign Body	
62287	Right	
62288	Left	
62289	Bilateral	
6674	Hearing	
6676	Loss	
6677	Bilaterally	
9445	Total	
6678	On The Right Only	
6679	On The Left Only	
6680	Weber's Test (tuning fork on forehead)	
6681	Tone Lateralizes To Left, Left Hearing Loss	
6682	Tone Lateralizes To Left, Right Hearing Loss	
6683	Tone Lateralizes To Right, Left Hearing Loss	

6684	Tone Lateralizes To Right, Right Hearing Loss	
6685	Rinne's Test (tuning fork on mastoid)	
6686	Air Conduction Persisting > Bone Conduction	
6687	Bone Conduction Persisting > Air Conduction	
6721	**Nose**	
6722	External Nasal Deformities	
6723	Rhinophyma	
6724	Saddle Nose	
6725	Tapir	
10903	Widened Bridge	
6726	Nasal Discharge	
6727	Epistaxis	
11212	Serosanguinous	
11214	Coryza	
6728	Rhinorrhea	
6729	Purulent	
9837	On The Right	
9838	On The Left	
9839	Bilaterally	
6730	Nasal Septum Abnormalities	
6731	Deviated	
6732	Perforated	
6733	Abscess	
6734	Nasal Membranes	
6735	Pale, Swollen, Edematous	
6736	Thick, Leathery, Blue-white	
62430	Pink	
62431	Red	
6737	Necrotic	
6738	Boggy	
62432	Crusts/sores	
62433	Excoriated	
6739	Ulcer	
10906	Prominent Superficial Veins	
6740	Granulomatous	
6741	Swollen Hypertrophied Turbinate	
6742	Black	
6743	Turbinate Atrophy	
6744	Sinus Tenderness	
62434	Maxillary	
62435	Right	
62436	Left	
62437	Bilateral	
62438	Ethmoidal	
62439	Right	
62440	Left	
62441	Bilateral	
62442	Frontal	
62443	Right	
62444	Left	

ENT, CONT.

62445	Bilateral	10912	Right Upper Lateral Incisor
6745	Intranasal Mass ___cm	10913	Right Lower Lateral Incisor
6746	Nasal Polyp ___cm	10914	Left Upper Lateral Incisor
62446	Right	10915	Left Lower Lateral Incisor
62447	Left	10916	Right Upper Cuspid
6747	Mucocele	10917	Right Lower Cuspid
6748	Pyocele	10918	Left Upper Cuspid
6749	Neoplasm	10919	Left Lower Cuspid
62583	Adenoids	10920	Right Upper First Bicuspid
62584	Hypertrophy	10921	Right Lower First Bicuspid
62585	Inflammed	10922	Left Upper First Bicuspid
62586	Obstructed Upper Airway	10923	Left Lower First Bicuspid
6751	**Oropharynx**	10924	Right Upper Second Bicuspid
6752	Odor Of Breath	10925	Right Lower Second Bicuspid
6753	Acetone Or Fruity	10926	Left Upper Second Bicuspid
6754	Fetor Hepaticus	10927	Left Lower Second Bicuspid
6755	Fetor Oris	10928	Right Upper First Molar
6756	Uremic	10929	Right Lower First Molar
6757	Alcohol	10930	Left Upper First Molar
9513	Tobacco Smoke	10931	Left Lower First Molar
6758	Lips	10932	Right Upper Second Molar
6759	Cleft Lip	10933	Right Lower Second Molar
6760	Enlarged Lips	10934	Left Upper Second Molar
11446	Thin Upper Lip	10935	Left Lower Second Molar
6761	Lip Neuroma	10936	Right Upper Third Molar
62451	Ulcer	10937	Right Lower Third Molar
6762	Upper Lip	10938	Left Upper Third Molar
6763	Lower Lip	10939	Left Lower Third Molar
6764	Nodules	10940	Multiple
62452	White Exudate	10907	At Birth
6767	Vesicle(s)	10981	False Teeth
6768	Rhagades	6785	Mandibular Erosion
6769	Cheilosis	6786	Tooth Abscess
6770	Keratosis	6787	Carious Teeth
6771	Burns	10979	Multiple
6772	Red And Swollen	11443	Enamel Chipped
6773	Gums	10941	Filling
6774	Gingival Recession	10942	Of The Right Upper Central Incisor
6775	Bleeding	10943	Of The Right Lower Central Incisor
6776	Gingival Hypertrophy	10944	Of The Left Upper Central Incisor
6777	Swollen, Spongy, Tender Gums	10945	Of The Left Lower Central Incisor
6778	Gingival Vesicle	10946	Of The Right Upper Lateral Incisor
6779	Becoming Shallow White Ulcer	10947	Of The Right Lower Lateral Incisor
	With Red Areola	10948	Of The Left Upper Lateral Incisor
6780	Gingival Line	10949	Of The Left Lower Lateral Incisor
6781	Ulceration	10950	Of The Right Upper Cuspid
6782	Teeth Findings	10951	Of The Right Lower Cuspid
6783	Widened Interdental Spaces	10952	Of The Left Upper Cuspid
6784	Absent Teeth	10953	Of The Left Lower Cuspid
10908	Right Upper Central Incisor	10954	Of The Right Upper First Bicuspid
10909	Right Lower Central Incisor	10955	Of The Right Lower First Bicuspid
10910	Left Upper Central Incisor	10956	Of The Left Upper First Bicuspid
10911	Left Lower Central Incisor	10957	Of The Left Lower First Bicuspid

ENT, CONT.

10958	Of The Right Upper Second Bicuspid	6794	Multiple Brown To Black Spots
10959	Of The Right Lower Second Bicuspid	6795	Ulcer
		6796	Burns
10960	Of The Left Upper Second Bicuspid	6797	Buccal White Spots (Koplik's)
10961	Of The Left Lower Second Bicuspid	6798	White Patch
10962	Of The Right Upper First Molar	6799	Lacelike
10963	Of The Right Lower First Molar	6800	Cheesy
10964	Of The Left Upper First Molar	6801	Ulcerated
10965	Of The Left Lower First Molar	62557	Does Not Wipe Off
10966	Of The Right Upper Second Molar	6802	Leukoplakia
10967	Of The Right Lower Second Molar	6803	Bullae
10968	Of The Left Upper Second Molar	6804	Vesicle(s)
10969	Of The Left Lower Second Molar	6805	Inflamed
10970	Of The Right Upper Third Molar	11658	Desquamation
10971	Of The Right Lower Third Molar	6806	Tongue Findings
10972	Of The Left Upper Third Molar	6807	Macroglossia
10973	Of The Left Lower Third Molar	6808	Multiple Small Nodules
10974	With Silver	6809	Dry Tongue
10975	With Gold	6810	Hairy Tongue
10976	With Ceramic	6811	Smooth Atrophic Tongue
10977	With Epoxy Resin	6812	Erythematous Edematous Tongue
10978	Multiple	6813	Strawberry Tongue
9298	Acid Erosion	6814	Red Margins And Tip, White Furred Center
6788	Loose Teeth	6815	Magenta Cobblestone Tongue
6789	Malocclusion	6816	White Patch
10980	Braces Present	62558	Does Not Wipe Off
6790	Hutchinson's Teeth	62559	Lacelike
6791	Mulberry Molar	6817	Leukoplakia
6792	Wedge-shaped	6818	Lingual Ulcer
10982	Tooth Eruption	6819	Aphthous Ulcer
10983	Of The Right Upper Central Incisor	6820	Chancre
10984	Of The Right Lower Central Incisor	6821	Condyloma Latum
10985	Of The Left Upper Central Incisor	6822	Gumma
10986	Of The Left Lower Central Incisor	6823	Tuberculous
10987	Of The Right Upper Lateral Incisor	6824	Sublingual Mass ___ cm
10988	Of The Right Lower Lateral Incisor	11007	Geographic
10989	Of The Left Upper Lateral Incisor	6825	Palate
10990	Of The Left Lower Lateral Incisor	6826	Cleft Palate
10991	Of The Right Upper Cuspid	6827	Torus Palatinus
10992	Of The Right Lower Cuspid	6828	High-arched Palate
10993	Of The Left Upper Cuspid	6829	Perforated Palate
10994	Of The Left Lower Cuspid	6830	Palatine Mass ___ cm
10995	Of The Right Upper First Molar	6831	Mixed Tumor Of Ectopic Salivary Gland
10996	Of The Right Lower First Molar	62453	White Exudate
10997	Of The Left Upper First Molar	62555	White Patch
10998	Of The Left Lower First Molar	62556	Does Not Wipe Off
10999	Of The Right Upper Second Molar	62560	Lacelike
11000	Of The Right Lower Second Molar	6832	Edematous Uvula
11001	Of The Left Upper Second Molar	11006	Cleft Uvula
11002	Of The Left Lower Second Molar	6833	Vesicle(s)
6793	Buccal Mucosa		
11003	Stensen's Duct Inflammed		

ENT, CONT.

6834	Becoming Shallow White Ulcer(s) With Red Areola	11059	Purulent
6835	Necrotic Ulcer	6865	Tenacious White Mucosal Membrane
6836	Necrotic Membrane	6866	Gray-yellow Tenacious Membrane
6837	Stops At Midline	6867	Blue Or Black Tenacious Membrane
6838	Petechiae	6868	Muscle Spasm
6839	Forchheimer's Spots	6869	Uvular Displacement
11004	Epstein's Pearls	11011	Epiglottis
11005	Bohn's Nodules	11012	Inflammation
6840	Tonsils	6870	Larynx
6841	Absent	6871	Laryngeal Dyspnea
6842	Tonsillar Hyperplasia	6872	Laryngeal Stridor
11008	Cryptic	6873	Laryngeal Edema
6843	Follicular Tonsillitis	6874	Laryngeal Membrane
6844	Erythematous	6875	Thick, Leathery, Blue-white
9343	Enlargement	6876	Gray Or Black
62455	Asymmetrically	6877	Erythematous Vocal Cords
62456	Right > Left	6878	Edematous Vocal Cords
62457	Left > Right	6879	Glottal Edema
6845	Peritonsillar Abscess	6880	Laryngeal Contact Ulcer
6846	Exudate	6881	Dull Thickened Vocal Cords
11014	Concretion	6882	Singer's Nodules
6847	White Tenacious Tonsillar Membrane	6883	Vocal Cord Polyp(s)
6848	Gray-yellow Tenacious Membrane	6884	Mass ___ cm
6849	Yellow-orange	6885	Of The Vocal Cord
6850	Firm	6886	Of The Pyriform Sinus
62454	Asymmetrical	11013	Foreign Body
11009	Anterior Tonsillar Pillar	6887	Laryngeal Leukoplakia
11010	Erythematous	6888	Unilateral Cord Paralysis, Fixed Midline
62448	Oropharynx	6889	Unilateral Cord Paralysis, Paramedian
62449	White Patches	6890	Bilateral Cord Paralysis
62450	Exudate	6891	Ulcer
6851	Pharynx	6892	Painless
6852	Retropharyngeal Abscess	6893	Salivary Gland Abnormalities
6853	Mucosal Papule	6894	Ptyalism
6854	White To Yellow With Zone Of Erythema	6895	Xerostomia
6855	Mucosal Follicles	6896	Reddened Parotid Orifice
6856	Granulomatous Mucosa	6897	Purulent Discharge Parotid Orifice
6857	Mucosal Vesicles	6898	Tender Parotid Swelling
6858	Mucosal Edema	6899	Non-tender Unilateral Parotid Swelling
6859	Mucosal Ulcer	6900	Non-tender Bilateral Parotid Swelling
6860	Grayish Center Surrounded By Red Areola	6901	Parotid Mass ___ cm
6861	Non-tender	6902	Salivary Calculus
62458	Erythematous	6903	Submaxillary Glands
6862	White Patches	6904	Wharton's Duct
6863	Red Mucosa	6905	Sublingual Glands
6864	Exudate	6906	Submandibular
62459	Clear	6908	**Neck**
62460	Yellow	6909	Suppleness
62461	Green	6910	Stiff Neck With Dorsiflexion
9863	Accumulation Of Mucous	6911	Kernig's Sign
		6912	Brudzinski's Sign
		6913	Diminished Rotation

60506	Lhermitte's Sign	6957	Tenderness
6914	Weakness	9252	Subcutaneous Crepitus
6915	Flexion	6958	Scar
6916	Extension	10367	Right Side
63327	Rotation	10368	Left Side
6917	Trachea	6959	Buffalo Hump
6918	Deviation	6960	Short, Thick
6919	Fixation	6961	Webbed
6920	Thyroid	6963	Lymph Nodes
6921	Tender	9325	Enlargement
62582	Size	6974	Generalized
6922	Diffuse Enlargement	6964	Cervical
9247	With A Dominant Nodule	10261	On The Right
6923	Rubbery	10262	On The Left
6924	Uninodular Goiter	10263	Bilaterally
10253	On The Right	10020	Anterior
10254	On The Left	10021	Posterior
6925	Hard	6965	Submental
6926	Rapidly Enlarging	6966	Submandibular
6927	Tender	10400	On The Right
6928	Multinodular Goiter	10401	On The Left
9248	With A Dominant Nodule	10402	Bilaterally
6929	Tender	6967	Supraclavicular
6930	Nontender	10258	On The Right
6931	Firm Nodule	10259	On The Left
6932	Hard Small Smooth Goiter	10260	Bilaterally
6933	Irregular	6968	Virchow's Node
6934	Fixed Nodule	6969	Preauricular
6935	Kocher's Sign	10403	On The Right
6936	Fluctuant	10404	On The Left
6937	Bruit	10405	Bilaterally
6938	Overlying Skin Darkened	6970	Postauricular
6939	Cervical Mass ___ cm	10406	On The Right
6940	Midline	10407	On The Left
6941	Suprahyoid	10408	Bilaterally
6942	Subhyoid	10416	Suboccipital
6943	Thyroid Cartilage Level	10417	On The Right
6944	Cricoid Cartilage Level	10418	On The Left
6945	Substernal Notch, Fluctuant	10419	Bilaterally
6946	Substernal Notch, Fatty	6971	Axillary
6947	Substernal Notch, Pulsatile	10264	On The Right
6948	Elevating On Tongue Protrusion	10265	On The Left
6949	Lateral	10266	Bilaterally
6950	Cystic Mass, Anterior And Deep To Upper 1/3 Of SCM	6972	Epitrochlear
		10409	On The Right
6951	Fistula	10410	On The Left
6952	Translucent	10411	Bilaterally
6953	Mobile Laterally, Restricted Vertically	6973	Inguinal
		10267	On The Right
6954	Pressure Leads To Regurgitation Of Food	10268	On The Left
		10269	Bilaterally
6955	Refilling Slowly After Compression	9730	Femoral
6956	Edematous	10413	On The Right

10414	On The Left		7003	Warmth At The Chostochondral Junction
10415	Bilaterally			
10412	Superficial		7004	Fusiform Swelling Of The Cartilage
9732	Deep		7005	Slipping Rib
62462	Popliteal		7006	Mass ___ cm
62463	Right		7007	Muscle Tenderness
62464	Left		7008	Tenderness Along The Intercostal Nerve
62465	Bilaterally		7009	Widened Retromanubrial Dullness
6975	Consistency		7065	Breast
6976	Rubbery		7066	Nipple
6977	Fluctuant		7067	Fissures
6978	Stony Hard		7068	Retraction
10421	Mobility		7069	Flattening
10420	Fixed		7070	Deviation
6979	Tender		7071	Scaling
6980	Suppurative		7072	Reddened And Excoriated
6981	Draining Sinus Tract		7073	Inflammatory Mass Beneath
6982	**Chest**		7074	Polythelia
10385	Surgical / Traumatic Scar		10434	On The Right
10386	On The Right Lateral Chest Wall		10435	On The Left
10387	On The Left Lateral Chest Wall		7075	Tender Areola Nodule
10388	Midline		7076	Abnormal Secretion
6983	Thoracic Deformity		7077	Abnormal Lactation
6984	Pectus Carinatum (pigeon breast)		7078	Serous Fluid
6985	Pectus Excavatum (funnel breast)		7079	Opalescent Fluid
6986	Barrel Chest		7080	Bloody Fluid
11156	Wide-spaced Nipples		9326	Diffuse Fibrous Tissue
6987	Harrison's Groove		9327	Bilateral
6988	Rachitic Rosary		7081	Mass ___ cm
6989	Left Sternal Bulge		7082	Fixed
11157	Accessory Nipple(s)		9270	In The Right Breast
11158	Right Side Only		9271	The Upper Outer Quarter
11159	Left Side Only		9272	The Lower Outer Quarter
11160	Bilaterally		9273	The Upper Inner Quarter
6990	Thoracic Asymmetry		9274	The Lower Inner Quarter
6991	Thoracoepigastric Cord		9265	In The Left Breast
6992	Intercostal-collateral Vessels		9266	The Upper Outer Quarter
11026	Dilated Superficial Collateral Veins		9267	The Lower Outer Quarter
11027	On The Right Side		9268	The Upper Inner Quarter
11028	On The Left Side		9269	The Lower Inner Quarter
11029	Bilaterally		7083	Multiple And Tender
6993	Soft Tissue Crepitus		7084	Solitary And Tender
6994	Hamman's Sign		7086	Multiple And Nontender
6995	Thoracic Wall Sinus		7087	Solitary And Nontender
6996	Intercostal Space Mass ___ cm		7088	With Fixation
6997	Tender Sternum		7085	Solitary And Translucent
6998	Rib Abnormalities		7090	Well Defined Margins
6999	Point Tenderness		7091	Inflammatory
7000	Compression Test For Rib Fracture		7092	During Lactation
7001	Redness At The Chostochondral Junction		7093	In A Single Breast Quadrant
			7094	In The Entire Breast
7002	Tenderness At The Costochondral Junction		7097	Cystic
			7098	Fluctuant

7095	Cordlike Structure ___cm		7127	Systolic
7096	Dimpling		7128	Apical
9422	Mastectomy Scar ___ cm		7129	2-3rd Intercostal Space - Right Parasternal Line
10369	Right			
10370	Left		7130	Carotid Artery
9423	"Clean", No Nodules		7131	Lower Sternal Border
7099	Enlargement		7132	2-3rd Left Intercostal Space - Parasternal Line
9336	Implant ___cm			
7100	Gynecomastia		7133	Suprasternal Notch
7101	Atrophy		7134	Diastolic
7102	Skin Thinned		7135	Apical
7089	Peau D'orange		7136	Left Sternal Border
7103	Dilated Superficial Veins		7137	Precordial
7104	Tenderness		7138	Supraclavicular Fossa
7105	**Cardiovascular System**		11019	Apical
7106	Apical Impulse		11020	Left Sternal Border
11707	Was Positioned		7139	Heart Borders
11168	At The 5th Left Intercostal Space In The Midclavicular Line		7140	Left Border Cardiac Dullness Shifted Right
7112	To The Left And Inferiorly		7141	Left Border Cardiac Dullness Shifted Left
11708	At The Anterior Axillary Line			
11709	At The Midaxillary Line		7142	Right Border Cardiac Dullness Shifted Right
7113	To The Right			
7114	Subxiphoid		7143	Right Border Cardiac Dullness Shifted Left
7107	Decreased			
7108	Accentuated		7144	Heart Sounds
11710	Hyperdynamic		7145	Distant
7109	Diffuse		7146	S1
7110	Dyskinetic		7147	Diminished
7111	Double Apical Thrust		7148	Accentuated
7115	Palpable S3		7149	Varying Intensity
7116	Palpable S4		7150	Split
11714	Septal Retraction		7151	S2
11721	Was Positioned		7157	Physiologic Splitting
11715	At The 5th Left Intercostal Space In The Midclavicular Line		7158	Expiratory Splitting
			7159	Fixed Splitting
11716	To The Left And Inferiorly		7160	Wide Splitting
11717	At The Anterior Axillary Line		7161	Single Sound
11718	At The Midaxillary Line		7162	Tamboric
11719	To The Right		7152	Diminished
11720	Subxiphoid		7155	Accentuated
7117	Precordial Heave		11711	The P2 Component
7118	Left Lower Parasternal Line		7153	Was Diminished
7119	Right Lower Parasternal Line		7156	Was Accentuated
7120	Pulsation At The Base Of The Heart		11712	The A2 Component
7121	2-3rd Intercostal Space - Left Sternal Border		7154	Was Diminished
			10270	Was Accentuated
7122	2-3rd Intercostal Space - Right Sternal Border		7163	Opening Snap Of Mitral Valve
			7164	Opening Snap Of Tricuspid Valve
7123	Palpable S1		7165	S3
7124	Palpable P2		7166	Left-sided
7125	Thrill		7167	Right-sided
7126	Presystolic		7168	S4

CARDIOVASCULAR, CONT.

9819	Left-sided	63387	On The Left
9820	Right-sided	63388	On The Right
7169	Gallop	63389	Along The Left Sternal Border
7170	Summation	63390	Along The Right Sternal Border
7171	Changing Timing	63391	To The Base
7172	Click	63392	To The Apex
7173	Midsystolic	63393	To The Clavicle
7174	Late Systolic	63394	On The Left
10271	Multiple	63395	On The Right
11017	Decreased With Inspiration	63396	To The Axilla
11018	Decreased With Muller Maneuver	63397	To The Interscapular Region
7175	Tumor Plop	63398	Maneuvers
7176	Ejection	63399	Heard Best In End Exhalation
7177	Louder During Expiration		While Sitting Leaning Forward
9668	Prosthetic Valve Sounds	63400	Heard Best At End Exhalation
9669	Aortic		In The Left Lateral Recumbent
9670	Mitral		Position
9671	Tricuspid	63401	Increased During Inspiration
9672	Pulmonary	63402	Increased By Handgrip
7178	Fetal	63403	Increased By Exercise
60835	Heart Rate	63404	Increased By Valsalva
11713	Single		Maneuver
9449	Multiple	63405	Increased By Squatting
7179	Pericardial Friction Rub	63406	Increased By Amyl Nitrite
7180	Murmur(s)	63407	Increased By Inotropic Agents
7185	Left Second Or Third Intercostal Space	63408	Increased By Muller Maneuver
7182	Systolic	63409	Decreased During Inspiration
9652	Early	63410	Decreased By Exercise
63329	Mid	63411	Decreased By Valsalva
9653	Late		Maneuver
63333	New	63412	Decreased By Squatting
63334	Changed	63413	Decreased By Amyl Nitrite
63335	Grade I	7183	Diastolic
63336	Grade II	63330	Early
63337	Grade III	63331	Mid
63338	Grade IV	63332	Late
63339	Grade V	63415	New
63340	Grade VI	63416	Changed
63372	Continuous	63417	Grade I
63373	Crescendo	63418	Grade II
63374	Decrescendo	63419	Grade III
63375	Crescendo-Decrescendo / Ejection	63420	Grade IV
63376	Presystolic Accentuation	63421	Continuous
63377	Holosystolic	63422	Crescendo
63378	Low-pitched	63423	Decrescendo
63379	Medium Pitched	63424	Crescendo-Decrescendo / Ejection
63380	High Pitched	63425	Presystolic Accentuation
63381	Harsh	63426	Holodiasystolic
63382	Musical	63427	Low-pitched
63383	Blowing	63428	Medium Pitched
63384	Rumbling	63429	High Pitched
63385	Transmitted	63430	Harsh
63386	Carotid Artery	63431	Musical

MURMUR, CONT.

63432	Blowing	63479	Blowing
63433	Rumbling	63743	Rumbling
63434	Transmitted	63481	Transmitted
63435	Carotid Artery	63482	Carotid Artery
63436	On The Left	63483	On The Left
63437	On The Right	63484	On The Right
63438	Along The Left Sternal Border	63485	Along The Left Sternal Border
63439	Along The Right Sternal Border	63486	Along The Right Sternal Border
63440	To The Base	63487	To The Base
63441	To The Apex	63488	To The Apex
63442	To The Clavicle	63489	To The Clavicle
63443	On The Left	63490	On The Left
63444	On The Right	63491	On The Right
63445	To The Axilla	63492	To The Axilla
63446	To The Interscapular Region	63493	To The Interscapular Region
63447	Maneuvers	63494	Maneuvers
63448	Heard Best In End Exhalation While Sitting Leaning Forward	63495	Heard Best In End Exhalation While Sitting Leaning Forward
63449	Heard Best At End Exhalation In The Left Lateral Recumbent Position	63496	Heard Best At End Exhalation In The Left Lateral Recumbent Position
63450	Increased During Inspiration	63497	Increased During Inspiration
63451	Increased By Handgrip	63498	Increased By Handgrip
63452	Increased By Exercise	63499	Increased By Exercise
63453	Increased By Valsalva Maneuver	63500	Increased By Valsalva Maneuver
63454	Increased By Squatting	63501	Increased By Squatting
63455	Increased By Amyl Nitrite	63502	Increased By Amyl Nitrite
63456	Increased By Inotropic Agents	63503	Increased By Inotropic Agents
63457	Increased By Muller Maneuver	63504	Increased By Muller Maneuver
63458	Decreased During Inspiration	63505	Decreased During Inspiration
63459	Decreased By Exercise	63506	Decreased By Exercise
63460	Decreased By Valsalva Maneuver	63507	Decreased By Valsalva Maneuver
63461	Decreased By Squatting	63508	Decreased By Squatting
63462	Decreased By Amyl Nitrite	63509	Decreased By Amyl Nitrite
7184	Continuous	7186	Right Second Or Third Intercostal Space
63463	New		
63464	Changed	9737	Systolic
63465	Grade I	9738	Early
63466	Grade II	63348	Mid
63467	Grade III	9739	Late
63468	Grade IV	63510	New
63469	Constant	63511	Changed
63470	Crescendo	63512	Grade I
63471	Decrescendo	63513	Grade II
63472	Crescendo-Decrescendo / Ejection	63514	Grade III
63473	Presystolic Accentuation	63515	Grade IV
63474	Low-pitched	63516	Grade V
63475	Medium Pitched	63517	Grade VI
63476	High Pitched	63518	Continuous
63477	Harsh	63519	Crescendo
63478	Musical	63520	Decrescendo

MURMUR, CONT.

63521	Crescendo-Decrescendo / Ejection	63565	Grade IV
63522	Presystolic Accentuation	63566	Continuous
63523	Holosystolic	63567	Crescendo
63524	Low-pitched	63568	Decrescendo
63525	Medium Pitched	63569	Crescendo-Decrescendo / Ejection
63526	High Pitched	63570	Presystolic Accentuation
63527	Harsh	63571	Holodiasystolic
63528	Musical	63572	Low-pitched
63529	Blowing	63573	Medium Pitched
63744	Rumbling	63574	High Pitched
63531	Transmitted	63575	Harsh
63532	Carotid Artery	63576	Musical
63533	On The Left	63577	Blowing
63534	On The Right	63578	Rumbling
63535	Along The Left Sternal Border	63579	Transmitted
63536	Along The Right Sternal Border	63580	Carotid Artery
63537	To The Base	63581	On The Left
63538	To The Apex	63582	On The Right
63539	To The Clavicle	63583	Along The Left Sternal Border
63540	On The Left	63584	Along The Right Sternal Border
63541	On The Right	63585	To The Base
63542	To The Axilla	63586	To The Apex
63543	To The Interscapular Region	63587	To The Clavicle
63544	Maneuvers	63588	On The Left
63545	Heard Best In End Exhalation While Sitting Leaning Forward	63589	On The Right
		63590	To The Axilla
63546	Heard Best At End Exhalation In The Left Lateral Recumbent Position	63591	To The Interscapular Region
		63592	Maneuvers
		63593	Heard Best In End Exhalation While Sitting Leaning Forward
63547	Increased During Inspiration		
63548	Increased By Handgrip	63594	Heard Best At End Exhalation In The Left Lateral Recumbent Position
63549	Increased By Exercise		
63550	Increased By Valsalva Maneuver	63595	Increased During Inspiration
		63596	Increased By Handgrip
63551	Increased By Squatting	63597	Increased By Exercise
63552	Increased By Amyl Nitrite	63598	Increased By Valsalva Maneuver
63553	Increased By Inotropic Agents		
63554	Increased By Muller Maneuver	63599	Increased By Squatting
63555	Decreased During Inspiration	63600	Increased By Amyl Nitrite
63556	Decreased By Exercise	63601	Increased By Inotropic Agents
63557	Decreased By Valsalva Maneuver	63602	Increased By Muller Maneuver
		63603	Decreased During Inspiration
63558	Decreased By Squatting	63604	Decreased By Exercise
63559	Decreased By Amyl Nitrite	63605	Decreased By Valsalva Maneuver
9740	Diastolic		
63345	Early	63606	Decreased By Squatting
63346	Mid	63607	Decreased By Amyl Nitrite
63347	Late	9741	Continuous
63560	New	63608	New
63561	Changed	63609	Changed
63562	Grade I	63610	Grade I
63563	Grade II	63611	Grade II
63564	Grade III		

MURMUR, CONT.

63612	Grade III	63654	New
63613	Grade IV	63655	Changed
63614	Constant	63656	Grade I
63615	Crescendo	63657	Grade II
63616	Decrescendo	63658	Grade III
63617	Crescendo-Decrescendo / Ejection	63659	Grade IV
63618	Presystolic Accentuation	63660	Grade V
63619	Low-pitched	63661	Grade VI
63620	Medium Pitched	63662	Continuous
63621	High Pitched	63663	Crescendo
63622	Harsh	63664	Decrescendo
63623	Musical	63665	Crescendo-Decrescendo / Ejection
63624	Blowing	63666	Presystolic Accentuation
63745	Rumbling	63667	Holosystolic
63625	Transmitted	63668	Low-pitched
63626	Carotid Artery	63669	Medium Pitched
63627	On The Left	63670	High Pitched
63628	On The Right	63671	Harsh
63629	Along The Left Sternal Border	63672	Musical
63630	Along The Right Sternal Border	63673	Blowing
63631	To The Base	63746	Rumbling
63632	To The Apex	63674	Transmitted
63633	To The Clavicle	63675	Along The Left Sternal Border
63634	On The Left	63676	To The Base
63635	On The Right	63677	To The Apex
63636	To The Axilla	63678	To The Clavicle
63637	To The Interscapular Region	63679	On The Left
63638	Maneuvers	63680	On The Right
63639	Heard Best In End Exhalation While Sitting Leaning Forward	63681	To The Axilla
		63682	To The Interscapular Region
63640	Heard Best At End Exhalation In The Left Lateral Recumbent Position	63683	Maneuvers
		63684	Heard Best In End Exhalation While Sitting Leaning Forward
63641	Increased During Inspiration	63685	Heard Best At End Exhalation In The Left Lateral Recumbent Position
63642	Increased By Handgrip		
63643	Increased By Exercise		
63644	Increased By Valsalva Maneuver	63686	Increased During Inspiration
		63687	Increased By Handgrip
63645	Increased By Squatting	63688	Increased By Exercise
63646	Increased By Amyl Nitrite	63689	Increased By Valsalva Maneuver
63647	Increased By Inotropic Agents		
63648	Increased By Muller Maneuver	63690	Increased By Squatting
63649	Decreased During Inspiration	63691	Increased By Amyl Nitrite
63650	Decreased By Exercise	63692	Increased By Inotropic Agents
63651	Decreased By Valsalva Maneuver	63693	Increased By Muller Maneuver
		63694	Decreased During Inspiration
63652	Decreased By Squatting	63695	Decreased By Exercise
63653	Decreased By Amyl Nitrite	63696	Decreased By Valsalva Maneuver
7187	Right Lower Sternal Border		
7188	Systolic	63697	Decreased By Squatting
9654	Early	63698	Decreased By Amyl Nitrite
63349	Mid	7189	Diastolic
9655	Late	63350	Early

MURMUR, CONT.

63351	Mid	63748	Changed
63352	Late	63749	Grade I
63699	New	63750	Grade II
63700	Changed	63751	Grade III
63701	Grade I	63752	Grade IV
63702	Grade II	63753	Constant
63703	Grade III	63754	Crescendo
63704	Grade IV	63755	Decrescendo
63705	Continuous	63756	Crescendo-Decrescendo / Ejection
63706	Crescendo	63757	Presystolic Accentuation
63707	Decrescendo	63758	Low-pitched
63708	Crescendo-Decrescendo / Ejection	63759	Medium Pitched
63709	Presystolic Accentuation	63760	High Pitched
63710	Holodiasystolic	63761	Harsh
63711	Low-pitched	63762	Musical
63712	Medium Pitched	63763	Blowing
63713	High Pitched	63764	Rumbling
63714	Harsh	63765	Transmitted
63715	Musical	63766	To The Left Sternal Border
63716	Blowing	63767	To The Base
63717	Rumbling	63768	To The Apex
63718	Transmitted	63769	To The Clavicle
63719	Along The Left Sternal Border	63770	On The Left
63720	To The Base	63771	On The Right
63721	To The Apex	63772	To The Axilla
63722	To The Clavicle	63773	To The Interscapular Region
63723	On The Left	63774	Maneuvers
63724	On The Right	63775	Heard Best In End Exhalation
63725	To The Axilla		While Sitting Leaning Forward
63726	To The Interscapular Region	63776	Heard Best At End Exhalation
63727	Maneuvers		In The Left Lateral Recumbent
63728	Heard Best In End Exhalation		Position
	While Sitting Leaning Forward	63777	Increased During Inspiration
63729	Heard Best At End Exhalation	63778	Increased By Handgrip
	In The Left Lateral Recumbent	63779	Increased By Exercise
	Position	63780	Increased By Valsalva
63730	Increased During Inspiration		Maneuver
63731	Increased By Handgrip	63781	Increased By Squatting
63732	Increased By Exercise	63782	Increased By Amyl Nitrite
63733	Increased By Valsalva	63783	Increased By Inotropic Agents
	Maneuver	63784	Increased By Muller Maneuver
63734	Increased By Squatting	63785	Decreased During Inspiration
63735	Increased By Amyl Nitrite	63786	Decreased By Exercise
63736	Increased By Inotropic Agents	63787	Decreased By Valsalva
63737	Increased By Muller Maneuver		Maneuver
63738	Decreased During Inspiration	63788	Decreased By Squatting
63739	Decreased By Exercise	63789	Decreased By Amyl Nitrite
63740	Decreased By Valsalva	7191	Left Lower Sternal Border
	Maneuver	7192	Systolic
63741	Decreased By Squatting	9656	Early
63742	Decreased By Amyl Nitrite	63353	Mid
7190	Continuous	9657	Late
63747	New	63790	New

MURMUR, CONT.

63791	Changed	63356	Late
63792	Grade I	63845	New
63793	Grade II	63846	Changed
63794	Grade III	63847	Grade I
63795	Grade IV	63848	Grade II
63796	Grade V	63849	Grade III
63797	Grade VI	63850	Grade IV
63798	Continuous	63851	Continuous
63799	Crescendo	63852	Crescendo
63800	Decrescendo	63853	Decrescendo
63801	Crescendo-Decrescendo / Ejection	63854	Crescendo-Decrescendo / Ejection
63802	Presystolic Accentuation	63855	Presystolic Accentuation
63803	Holosystolic	63856	Holodiasystolic
63804	Low-pitched	63857	Low-pitched
63805	Medium Pitched	63858	Medium Pitched
63806	High Pitched	63859	High Pitched
63807	Harsh	63860	Harsh
63808	Musical	63861	Musical
63809	Blowing	63862	Blowing
63810	Rumbling	63863	Rumbling
63811	Transmitted	63864	Transmitted
63812	To The Right Sternal Border	63865	To The Right Sternal Border
63813	To The Base	63866	To The Base
63814	To The Apex	63867	To The Apex
63815	To The Clavicle	63868	To The Clavicle
63816	On The Left	63869	On The Left
63817	On The Right	63870	On The Right
63818	To The Axilla	63871	To The Axilla
63819	To The Interscapular Region	63872	To The Interscapular Region
63820	Maneuvers	63873	Maneuvers
63821	Heard Best In End Exhalation While Sitting Leaning Forward	63874	Heard Best In End Exhalation While Sitting Leaning Forward
63822	Heard Best At End Exhalation In The Left Lateral Recumbent Position	63875	Heard Best At End Exhalation In The Left Lateral Recumbent Position
63823	Increased During Inspiration	63876	Increased During Inspiration
63824	Increased By Handgrip	63877	Increased By Handgrip
63825	Increased By Exercise	63878	Increased By Exercise
63826	Increased By Valsalva Maneuver	63879	Increased By Valsalva Maneuver
63827	Increased By Squatting	63880	Increased By Squatting
63828	Increased By Amyl Nitrite	63881	Increased By Amyl Nitrite
63838	Increased By Inotropic Agents	63882	Increased By Inotropic Agents
63839	Increased By Muller Maneuver	63883	Increased By Muller Maneuver
63840	Decreased During Inspiration	63884	Decreased During Inspiration
63841	Decreased By Exercise	63885	Decreased By Exercise
63842	Decreased By Valsalva Maneuver	63886	Decreased By Valsalva Maneuver
63843	Decreased By Squatting	63887	Decreased By Squatting
63844	Decreased By Amyl Nitrite	63888	Decreased By Amyl Nitrite
7193	Diastolic	7194	Continuous
63354	Early	63889	New
63355	Mid	63890	Changed

MURMUR, CONT.

63891	Grade I	63934	Grade I
63892	Grade II	63935	Grade II
63893	Grade III	63936	Grade III
63894	Grade IV	63937	Grade IV
63895	Constant	63938	Grade V
63896	Crescendo	63939	Grade VI
63897	Decrescendo	63940	Continuous
63898	Crescendo-Decrescendo / Ejection	63941	Crescendo
63899	Presystolic Accentuation	63942	Decrescendo
63900	Low-pitched	63943	Crescendo-Decrescendo / Ejection
63901	Medium Pitched	63944	Presystolic Accentuation
63902	High Pitched	63945	Holosystolic
63903	Harsh	63946	Low-pitched
63904	Musical	63947	Medium Pitched
63905	Blowing	63948	High Pitched
63906	Rumbling	63949	Harsh
63907	Transmitted	63950	Musical
63908	To The Right Sternal Border	63951	Blowing
63909	To The Base	63952	Rumbling
63910	To The Apex	63953	Transmitted
63911	To The Clavicle	63954	To The Left Sternal Border
63912	On The Left	63955	To The Right Sternal Border
63913	On The Right	63956	To The Base
63914	To The Axilla	63957	To The Clavicle
63915	To The Interscapular Region	63958	On The Left
63916	Maneuvers	63959	On The Right
63917	Heard Best In End Exhalation While Sitting Leaning Forward	63960	To The Axilla
		63961	To The Interscapular Region
63918	Heard Best At End Exhalation In The Left Lateral Recumbent Position	63962	Maneuvers
		63963	Heard Best In End Exhalation While Sitting Leaning Forward
63919	Increased During Inspiration	63964	Heard Best At End Exhalation In The Left Lateral Recumbent Position
63920	Increased By Handgrip		
63921	Increased By Exercise		
63922	Increased By Valsalva Maneuver	63965	Increased During Inspiration
		63966	Increased By Handgrip
63923	Increased By Squatting	63967	Increased By Exercise
63924	Increased By Amyl Nitrite	63968	Increased By Valsalva Maneuver
63925	Increased By Inotropic Agents		
63926	Increased By Muller Maneuver	63969	Increased By Squatting
63927	Decreased During Inspiration	63970	Increased By Amyl Nitrite
63928	Decreased By Exercise	63971	Increased By Inotropic Agents
63929	Decreased By Valsalva Maneuver	63972	Increased By Muller Maneuver
		63973	Decreased During Inspiration
63930	Decreased By Squatting	63974	Decreased By Exercise
63931	Decreased By Amyl Nitrite	63975	Decreased By Valsalva Maneuver
7195	Apical		
7196	Systolic	63976	Decreased By Squatting
9658	Early	63977	Decreased By Amyl Nitrite
63357	Mid	7198	Diastolic
7197	Late	63358	Early
63932	New	7199	Mid
63933	Changed	63359	Late

MURMUR, CONT.

63978	New	64025	Grade II
63979	Changed	64026	Grade III
63980	Grade I	64027	Grade IV
63981	Grade II	64028	Constant
63982	Grade III	64029	Crescendo
63983	Grade IV	64030	Decrescendo
63984	Continuous	64031	Crescendo-Decrescendo / Ejection
63985	Crescendo	64032	Presystolic Accentuation
63986	Decrescendo	64033	Low-pitched
63987	Crescendo-Decrescendo / Ejection	64034	Medium Pitched
63988	Presystolic Accentuation	64035	High Pitched
63989	Holodiasystolic	64036	Harsh
63990	Low-pitched	64037	Musical
63991	Medium Pitched	64038	Blowing
63992	High Pitched	64039	Rumbling
63993	Harsh	64040	Transmitted
63994	Musical	64041	To The Left Sternal Border
63995	Blowing	64042	To The Right Sternal Border
63996	Rumbling	64043	To The Base
63997	Transmitted	64044	To The Clavicle
63998	To The Left Sternal Border	64045	On The Left
63999	To The Right Sternal Border	64046	On The Right
64000	To The Base	64047	To The Axilla
64001	To The Clavicle	64048	To The Interscapular Region
64002	On The Left	64049	Maneuvers
64003	On The Right	64050	Heard Best In End Exhalation While Sitting Leaning Forward
64004	To The Axilla		
64005	To The Interscapular Region	64051	Heard Best At End Exhalation In The Left Lateral Recumbent Position
64006	Maneuvers		
64007	Heard Best In End Exhalation While Sitting Leaning Forward		
		64052	Increased During Inspiration
64008	Heard Best At End Exhalation In The Left Lateral Recumbent Position	64053	Increased By Handgrip
		64054	Increased By Exercise
		64055	Increased By Valsalva Maneuver
64009	Increased During Inspiration		
64010	Increased By Handgrip	64056	Increased By Squatting
64011	Increased By Exercise	64057	Increased By Amyl Nitrite
64012	Increased By Valsalva Maneuver	64058	Increased By Inotropic Agents
		64059	Increased By Muller Maneuver
64013	Increased By Squatting	64060	Decreased During Inspiration
64014	Increased By Amyl Nitrite	64061	Decreased By Exercise
64015	Increased By Inotropic Agents	64062	Decreased By Valsalva Maneuver
64016	Increased By Muller Maneuver		
64017	Decreased During Inspiration	64063	Decreased By Squatting
64018	Decreased By Exercise	64064	Decreased By Amyl Nitrite
64019	Decreased By Valsalva Maneuver	7201	Axilla
		7202	Systolic
64020	Decreased By Squatting	63360	Early
64021	Decreased By Amyl Nitrite	63361	Mid
7200	Continuous	63362	Late
64022	New	64065	New
64023	Changed	64066	Changed
64024	Grade I	64067	Grade I

MURMUR, CONT.

64068	Grade II	64112	Presystolic Accentuation
64069	Grade III	64113	Holodiasystolic
64070	Grade IV	64114	Low-pitched
64071	Grade V	64115	Medium Pitched
64072	Grade VI	64116	High Pitched
64073	Continuous	64117	Harsh
64074	Crescendo	64118	Musical
64075	Decrescendo	64119	Blowing
64076	Crescendo-Decrescendo / Ejection	64120	Rumbling
64077	Presystolic Accentuation	64121	Maneuvers
64078	Holosystolic	64122	Heard Best In End Exhalation While Sitting Leaning Forward
64079	Low-pitched		
64080	Medium Pitched	64123	Heard Best At End Exhalation In The Left Lateral Recumbent Position
64081	High Pitched		
64082	Harsh		
64083	Musical	64124	Increased During Inspiration
64084	Blowing	64125	Increased By Handgrip
64085	Rumbling	64126	Increased By Exercise
64086	Maneuvers	64127	Increased By Valsalva Maneuver
64087	Heard Best In End Exhalation While Sitting Leaning Forward		
		64128	Increased By Squatting
64088	Heard Best At End Exhalation In The Left Lateral Recumbent Position	64129	Increased By Amyl Nitrite
		64130	Increased By Inotropic Agents
		64131	Increased By Muller Maneuver
64089	Increased During Inspiration	64132	Decreased During Inspiration
64090	Increased By Handgrip	64133	Decreased By Exercise
64091	Increased By Exercise	64134	Decreased By Valsalva Maneuver
64092	Increased By Valsalva Maneuver		
		64135	Decreased By Squatting
64093	Increased By Squatting	64136	Decreased By Amyl Nitrite
64094	Increased By Amyl Nitrite	7204	Continuous
64095	Increased By Inotropic Agents	64137	New
64096	Increased By Muller Maneuver	64138	Changed
64097	Decreased During Inspiration	64139	Grade I
64098	Decreased By Exercise	64140	Grade II
64099	Decreased By Valsalva Maneuver	64141	Grade III
		64142	Grade IV
64100	Decreased By Squatting	64143	Constant
64101	Decreased By Amyl Nitrite	64144	Crescendo
7203	Diastolic	64145	Decrescendo
63363	Early	64146	Crescendo-Decrescendo / Ejection
63364	Mid	64147	Presystolic Accentuation
63365	Late	64149	Low-pitched
64102	New	64150	Medium Pitched
64103	Changed	64151	High Pitched
64104	Grade I	64152	Harsh
64105	Grade II	64153	Musical
64106	Grade III	64154	Blowing
64107	Grade IV	64155	Rumbling
64108	Continuous	64156	Maneuvers
64109	Crescendo	64157	Heard Best In End Exhalation While Sitting Leaning Forward
64110	Decrescendo		
64111	Crescendo-Decrescendo / Ejection		

MURMUR, CONT.

64158	Heard Best At End Exhalation In The Left Lateral Recumbent Position	64198	Increased By Exercise
		64199	Increased By Valsalva Maneuver
64159	Increased During Inspiration	64200	Increased By Squatting
64160	Increased By Handgrip	64201	Increased By Amyl Nitrite
64161	Increased By Exercise	64202	Increased By Inotropic Agents
64162	Increased By Valsalva Maneuver	64203	Increased By Muller Maneuver
		64204	Decreased During Inspiration
64163	Increased By Squatting	64205	Decreased By Exercise
64164	Increased By Amyl Nitrite	64206	Decreased By Valsalva Maneuver
64165	Increased By Inotropic Agents		
64166	Increased By Muller Maneuver	64207	Decreased By Squatting
64167	Decreased During Inspiration	64208	Decreased By Amyl Nitrite
64168	Decreased By Exercise	63343	Diastolic
64169	Decreased By Valsalva Maneuver	63369	Early
		63370	Mid
64170	Decreased By Squatting	63371	Late
64171	Decreased By Amyl Nitrite	64209	New
7205	In The Interscapular Region Of The Back	64210	Changed
		64211	Grade I
63342	Systolic	64212	Grade II
63366	Early	64213	Grade III
63367	Mid	64214	Grade IV
63368	Late	64215	Continuous
64172	New	64216	Crescendo
64173	Changed	64217	Decrescendo
64174	Grade I	64218	Crescendo-Decrescendo / Ejection
64175	Grade II	64219	Presystolic Accentuation
64176	Grade III	64220	Holodiasystolic
64177	Grade IV	64221	Low-pitched
64178	Grade V	64222	Medium Pitched
64179	Grade VI	64223	High Pitched
64180	Continuous	64224	Harsh
64181	Crescendo	64225	Musical
64182	Decrescendo	64226	Blowing
64183	Crescendo-Decrescendo / Ejection	64227	Rumbling
64184	Presystolic Accentuation	64228	Maneuvers
64185	Holosystolic	64229	Heard Best In End Exhalation While Sitting Leaning Forward
64186	Low-pitched		
64187	Medium Pitched	64230	Heard Best At End Exhalation In The Left Lateral Recumbent Position
64188	High Pitched		
64189	Harsh		
64190	Musical	64231	Increased During Inspiration
64191	Blowing	64232	Increased By Handgrip
64192	Rumbling	64233	Increased By Exercise
64193	Maneuvers	64234	Increased By Valsalva Maneuver
64194	Heard Best In End Exhalation While Sitting Leaning Forward		
		64235	Increased By Squatting
64195	Heard Best At End Exhalation In The Left Lateral Recumbent Position	64236	Increased By Amyl Nitrite
		64237	Increased By Inotropic Agents
		64238	Increased By Muller Maneuver
64196	Increased During Inspiration	64239	Decreased During Inspiration
64197	Increased By Handgrip	64240	Decreased By Exercise

MURMUR, CONT.

64241	Decreased By Valsalva Maneuver	7225	VI
64242	Decreased By Squatting	7211	Continuous
64243	Decreased By Amyl Nitrite	7206	Crescendo
63344	Continuous	7207	Decrescendo
64244	New	7208	Crescendo-Decrescendo / Ejection
64245	Changed	7209	Presystolic Accentuation
64246	Grade I	7210	Holosystolic
64247	Grade II	7212	Low-pitched
64248	Grade III	7213	Medium Pitched
64249	Grade IV	7214	High Pitched
64250	Constant	7215	Harsh
64251	Crescendo	7216	Musical
64252	Decrescendo	7217	Blowing
64253	Crescendo-Decrescendo / Ejection	7218	Rumbling
64254	Presystolic Accentuation	7226	Transmitted
64255	Low-pitched	7227	Carotid Artery
64256	Medium Pitched	7228	On The Left
64257	High Pitched	7229	On The Right
64258	Harsh	7230	To The Left Sternal Border
64259	Musical	7231	Down The Right Sternal Border
64260	Blowing	7235	To The Base
64261	Rumbling	7234	To The Apex
64262	Maneuvers	7236	To The Clavicle
64263	Heard Best In End Exhalation While Sitting Leaning Forward	7237	On The Left
64264	Heard Best At End Exhalation In The Left Lateral Recumbent Position	11722	On The Right
		7233	To The Axilla
		7232	To The Interscapular Region
64265	Increased During Inspiration	63341	Maneuvers
64266	Increased By Handgrip	7238	Heard Best In End Exhalation While Sitting Leaning Forward
64267	Increased By Exercise	7239	Heard Best At End Exhalation In The Left Lateral Recumbent Position
64268	Increased By Valsalva Maneuver	7240	Increased During Inspiration
64269	Increased By Squatting	7241	Increased By Handgrip
64270	Increased By Amyl Nitrite	7242	Increased By Exercise
64271	Increased By Inotropic Agents	7244	Increased By Valsalva Maneuver
64272	Increased By Muller Maneuver	7249	Increased By Squatting
64273	Decreased During Inspiration	7246	Increased By Amyl Nitrite
64274	Decreased By Exercise	11015	Increased By Inotropic Agents
64275	Decreased By Valsalva Maneuver	11016	Increased By Muller Maneuver
		9842	Decreased During Inspiration
64276	Decreased By Squatting	7243	Decreased By Exercise
64277	Decreased By Amyl Nitrite	7245	Decreased By Valsalva Maneuver
7248	New Or Changing	7250	Decreased By Squatting
9312	Systolic	7247	Decreased By Amyl Nitrite
9313	Diastolic	7251	Jugular Venous Pressure
7219	Grade	7253	Diminished
7220	I	9227	Elevated (estimated)
7221	II	7252	Jugular Venous Distension
7222	III	11744	Estimated Right Atrial Pressure
7223	IV	11745	At Rest
7224	V	11746	At End Of Inspiration
		11747	At End Of Expiration

CARDIOVASCULAR, CONT.

11748	With Stress		7277	Vein Findings
7254	Jugular Venous Pulsations		7278	Tender
7255	Giant A Waves		7279	Overlying Skin Erythematous And Warm
7256	Intermittent		7280	Palpable Cord
7257	A Waves Absent		9796	On The Right
7259	Prominent V Waves		9797	On The Left
7258	Deep X Descent		7281	Varicosital Changes
7260	Deep Y Descent		10272	On The Right
7261	Slow Y Descent		10273	On The Left
7262	Fibrillatory Waves		7282	Swollen And Hard
7263	Flutter Waves		7283	Brodie-Trendelenburg Test
7264	Jugular Vein		7284	Negative
7265	Swollen And Tender		7285	Positive
7266	Hepatojugular Reflux		7286	Double Positive
7267	Diffusely Distended Neck Veins		7287	Homan's Sign
9714	Abdominal Aorta		9798	On The Right
9715	Palpated Width		9799	On The Left
11723	Was Increased		7354	Superficial Collateral Veins
11130	Intensity Of Pulse (0-5)		7355	Above Diaphragm
7339	Aneurysm		11038	Dilated Superficial Collateral Veins On The Extremities
7268	Edema		11039	On The Arms
7269	Anasarca		11040	On The Right
7270	Bilateral Above Diaphragm - Nonpitting		11041	On The Left
7271	Bilateral Above Diaphragm - Pitting		11042	Bilaterally
7272	Bilateral Below Diaphragm - Nonpitting		11043	Legs
7273	Bilateral Below Diaphragm - Pitting		11044	On The Right
9659	At The Ankle		11045	On The Left
9662	Up To The Knee		11046	Bilaterally
9665	Presacral		9716	Measured Calf Circumference (10 cm below tibial tuberosity)
9331	Pretibial Non-pitting		9717	Right Leg
11031	On The Right		9718	Left Leg
11032	On The Left		9719	Right / Left Difference
11033	Bilateral		7288	Increased
9330	Pretibial Pitting		9720	Venous Filling Time
7274	Localized And Nonpitting		9721	Right Leg
7275	Unilateral Or Localized And Pitting		9722	Left Leg
9660	At The Right Ankle		6108	Localized Brownish Pigmentation
9661	At The Left Ankle		9226	In The Lower Legs
9663	At The Right Knee		9804	On The Right
9664	At The Left Knee		9805	On The Left
11030	Presacral		9806	Bilaterally
9666	On The Right		7289	Lymphatics
9667	On The Left		7290	Palpably Tender
11034	Pitting		7291	Red Streaking
11035	On The Right		11077	On The Right Forearm
11036	On The Left		11078	On The Left Forearm
11037	Bilaterally		11079	On The Right Arm
7276	Periorbital		11080	On The Left Arm
62496	Right Eye		11081	On The Right Leg Above The Knee
62497	Left Eye		11082	On The Left Leg Above The Knee
62498	Bilaterally			

CARDIOVASCULAR, CONT.

11083	On The Right Leg Below The Knee	9683	Unilaterally
11084	On The Left Leg Below The Knee	7311	Hyperactive
7292	Extending Upward From Distal	7312	Carotid
	Extremity	7313	Brachial
7293	Arterial Pulses	7314	Radial
7294	Normal	7315	Femoral
9687	Right Carotid Intensity (0-5)	7316	Popliteal
9688	Left Carotid Intensity (0-5)	7317	Posterior Tibialis
9689	Right Subclavian Intensity (0-5)	7318	Dorsalis Pedis
9690	Left Subclavian Intensity (0-5)	7319	Contour + Volume
9691	Right Brachial Intensity (0-5)	7320	Pulsus Bisferiens
9692	Left Brachial Intensity (0-5)	7321	Water Hammer
9693	Right Radial Intensity (0-5)	7322	Pulsus Tardus
9694	Left Radial Intensity (0-5)	7323	Pulsus Alternans
9695	Right Ulnar Intensity (0-5)	7324	Pulsus Bigeminus
9696	Left Ulnar Intensity (0-5)	7326	Thready Pulse
9697	Right Femoral Intensity (0-5)	7327	Quincke's Pulse
9698	Left Femoral Intensity (0-5)	7328	Auscultation
9699	Right Popliteal Intensity (0-5)	7329	Bruit
9700	Left Popliteal Intensity (0-5)	7330	Of The Carotid Artery
9701	Right Dorsalis Pedis Intensity (0-5)	7331	On The Right
9702	Left Dorsalis Pedis Intensity (0-5)	7332	On The Left
9703	Right Posterior Tibial Intensity (0-5)	7333	Bilaterally
9704	Left Posterior Tibial Intensity (0-5)	7334	Of The Subclavian Artery
7295	Absent Or Diminished	9705	On The Right
7296	Carotid	9706	On The Left
7297	Bilaterally	9707	Bilaterally
7298	Unilaterally	10448	Of The Radial Artery
11724	On The Right	10449	On The Right
11725	On The Left	10450	On The Left
9684	Subclavian	10451	Bilaterally
9685	Bilaterally	7335	Of The Femoral Artery
9686	Unilaterally	9708	On The Right
7299	Brachial	9709	On The Left
7300	Bilaterally	9710	Bilaterally
7301	Unilaterally	10452	Of The Popliteal Artery
7302	Radial	10453	On The Right
7303	Bilaterally	10454	On The Left
7304	Unilaterally	10455	Bilaterally
9675	Ulnar	7336	Pistol Shot Sound Heard Over The
9676	Bilaterally		Femoral Artery
9677	Unilaterally	7337	Duroziez's Sign
7305	Femoral	7338	Aneurysm
7306	Bilaterally	10439	Carotid Artery
7307	Unilaterally	10440	On The Right
7308	Popliteal	10441	On The Left
9678	Bilaterally	10442	Radial Artery
9679	Unilaterally	10443	On The Right
7309	Posterior Tibialis	10444	On The Left
9680	Bilaterally	7340	Femoral Artery
9681	Unilaterally	9749	On The Right
7310	Dorsalis Pedis	9750	On The Left
9682	Bilaterally	7341	Popliteal Artery

CARDIOVASCULAR, CONT.

9751	On The Right
9752	On The Left
11131	Posterial Tibial Artery
11132	On The Right
11133	On The Left
10445	Dorsalis Pedis Artery
10446	On The Right
10447	On The Left
7342	AV Fistula
7343	Other Abnormalities
7344	Pulse Discrepancy
7345	Carotid
11169	Brachial - Femoral
7346	Allen's Test
7347	Radial Artery Patent
7348	Ulnar Artery Patent
7349	Tender Artery
7350	Nodules Along Artery
7351	Adson's Test
7352	Costoclavicular Maneuver
7353	Hyperabduction Test For Subclavian Compression
7356	Branham's Bradycardiac Sign
10057	Evidence Of Embolus
10058	In The Fingers Of The Right Hand
10059	In The Thumb
10060	In The Index Finger
10061	In The Middle Finger
10062	In The Ring Finger
10063	In The Little Finger
10064	In The Fingers Of The Left Hand
10065	In The Thumb
10066	In The Index Finger
10067	In The Middle Finger
10068	In The Ring Finger
10069	In The Little Finger
10070	In The Fingers Of Both Hands
10071	In The Right Hand
10072	In The Palmar Aspect
10073	In The Dorsal Aspect
10074	In The Left Hand
10075	In The Palmar Aspect
10076	In The Dorsal Aspect
10077	In Both Hands
10098	In The Legs (below the knee)
10099	In The Right Leg
10100	In The Left Leg
10101	In Both Legs
10102	In The Right Ankle
10103	In The Left Ankle
10104	In Both Ankles
10078	In The Right Foot
10079	In The Plantar Aspect

10080	In The Dorsal Aspect
10081	In The Left Foot
10082	In The Plantar Aspect
10083	In The Dorsal Aspect
10084	In Both Feet
10085	In The Toes Of The Right Foot
10086	In The Great Toe
10087	In The Second Toe
10088	In The Middle Toe
10089	In The Fourth Toe
10090	In The Little Toe
10091	In The Toes Of The Left Foot
10092	In The Great Toe
10093	In The Second Toe
10094	In The Middle Toe
10095	In The Fourth Toe
10096	In The Little Toe
10097	In The Toes Of Both Feet
7010	**Lungs**
7012	Overinflated Chest
7013	Respiratory Movements
7014	Flaring Nasal Alae
7015	Using Accessory Muscles For Expiration
7016	Diminished Respiratory Excursion
7017	Unilaterally
10255	On The Right
10256	On The Left
10257	Bilaterally
7018	Inspiratory Retraction
7019	Localized Bulging Thorax During Expiration
7020	Localized Retracted Thorax During Inspiration
9357	Paradoxic
7021	Flail Chest
7022	Splinting
7023	Pursed Lip Breathing
7024	Vocal Fremitus
7025	Diminished
7026	Increased
7027	Percussion
7029	Low Diaphragm
7028	Elevated Diaphragm
7030	Unilaterally
7031	On The Left
7032	On The Right
7033	Bilaterally
7034	Diaphragmatic Excursion Decreased
7035	Dullness
7036	In The Apex
7037	In The Lower Lung
7038	On The Right

CARDIOVASCULAR, CONT.

7039	On The Left		62485	Midlung Fields
7040	Hyperresonance		62486	Bases
7041	Auscultation		7055	Prolonged Expiratory Time
7042	Breath Sounds / Voice Sounds		9733	Decreased Expiratory Force
7043	Bronchial Breath Sounds		7056	Adventitious Sounds
10277	On The Right		7058	Rales / Crackles
10278	On The Left		10280	On The Right
10279	Bilaterally		62487	Apex
7044	Bronchophony		62488	Midlung Field
11162	On The Right		62489	Base
11163	On The Left		10281	On The Left
11164	Bilaterally		62490	Apex
7045	Egophony		62491	Midlung Field
10283	On The Right		62492	Base
10284	On The Left		10282	Bilaterally
10285	Bilaterally		62493	Apices
7046	Whispered Pectoriloquy		62494	Midlung Fields
11165	On The Right		62495	Bases
11166	On The Left		7059	Bibasilar
11167	Bilaterally		7060	Wet
7047	Wheezing		7061	Velcro / Dry
7048	Unilaterally		7057	Post-tussive
10274	On The Right		7062	Friction Rub
62466	Apex		10436	On The Right
62467	Midlung Field		10437	On The Left
62468	Base		10438	Bilaterally
10275	On The Left		7063	Continuous Bruit
62469	Apex		7358	**Abdomen**
62470	Midlung Field		7359	Visual Inspection
62471	Base		7362	Linea Nigra
10276	Bilaterally		7363	Surgical / Traumatic Scar
62472	Apices		10371	In The RUQ
62473	Midlung Fields		10372	In The LUQ
62474	Bases		10373	In The RLQ
7049	Rhonchi		10374	In The LLQ
10286	On The Right		10375	In The Midline
62475	Apex		10376	On The Right Flank
62476	Midlung Field		10377	On The Left Flank
62477	Base		10378	Across The Lower Abdomen
10287	On The Left		9236	"Gridiron Abdomen"
62478	Apex		7364	Dilated Superficial Collateral Veins
62479	Midlung Field		7365	Caput Medusa
62480	Base		11022	RUQ
10288	Bilaterally		11021	LUQ
62481	Apices		11024	RLQ
62482	Midlung Fields		11023	LLQ
62483	Bases		11025	Periumbilical
7050	Decreased Breath Sounds		7366	Visible Epigastric Pulsation
7051	Unilaterally		7367	Visible Peristalsis
7052	In The Right Lower Lung		7368	Diastasis Recti
7053	In The Left Lower Lung		11170	Umbilical Discharge
7054	Bilateral		7369	Umbilical Nodule
62484	Apices		11573	Omphalocele

CARDIOVASCULAR, CONT.

7370	Indurated Draining Sinus Which Fails To Heal
9250	Near The Site Of A Recent Appendectomy
9251	Near The Site Of A Recent Colon Resection
7371	Cullen's Sign
7372	Grey Turner's Sign (flank erythema)
7373	Subcutaneous Crepitus
7374	Shape
7375	Scaphoid
7376	Distension
7377	Bowel Sounds
7378	Normal On Repeated Examinations
7379	Diminished Or Absent
62504	RUQ
62505	LUQ
62506	RLQ
62507	LLQ
7380	Hyperactive (Borborygmi)
7381	Percussion
7382	Tympanitic
7383	Succussion Splash
7384	Bruit
7387	Hepatic (RUQ)
7388	Splenic (LUQ)
9745	RLQ
9744	LLQ
7385	Over The Abdominal Aorta (midline)
7386	Of The Renal Artery (flank)
9711	On The Right
9712	On The Left
9713	Bilaterally
7389	Uterine Souffle
7390	Friction Rub
7391	Hepatic
7392	Splenic
9253	Muscle Guarding
7393	Muscle Rigidity
7394	Ascites
7395	Fluid Wave
7396	Shifting Dullness
9748	Tense
7397	Puddle Sign
9729	Girth
7398	Tenderness
7399	Direct
7400	Epigastric
7402	RUQ
7401	LUQ
7404	RLQ
7403	LLQ
9254	Periumbilical

7406	Suprapubic
7405	Costovertebral
7407	Rebound
7409	RUQ
7408	LUQ
7411	RLQ
7410	LLQ
9255	Periumbilical
9291	Generalized
7412	Referred Rebound
7413	Mass ___ cm
7417	Epigastric
7418	Pulsatile
11462	Non-tender, Non-pulsatile, Right Of Midline
7415	RUQ
7416	With Pointing
7414	LUQ
7420	RLQ
7419	LLQ
7422	Costovertebral
7423	On The Right
7424	On The Left
7425	Umbilical
7426	Pulsatile
7421	Suprapubic
9292	Not Present On Repeated Examination
60792	Fetal Presentation Preterm
60793	Vertex
60796	Occiput
60797	Occipitoanterior
60798	Right Occipitoanterior
60799	Left Occipitoanterior
60800	Occipitoposterior
60801	Right Occipitoposterior
60802	Left Occipitoposterior
60803	Right Occipitotransverse
60804	Left Occipitotransverse
60805	Brow
60806	Frontoanterior
60807	Right Frontoanterior
60808	Left Frontoanterior
60809	Frontoposterior
60810	Right Frontoposterior
60811	Left Frontoposterior
60812	Right Frontotransverse
60813	Left Frontotransverse
60814	Face
60815	Mentoanterior
60816	Right Mentoanterior
60817	Left Mentoanterior
60818	Mentoposterior
60819	Right Mentoposterior

CARDIOVASCULAR, CONT.

60820	Left Mentoposterior		7445	Obturator
60821	Right Frontotransverse		7446	Spigelian
60822	Left Frontotransverse		11525	Rectal Exam
60794	Breech		7630	Anus
60823	Sacroanterior		7631	Perianal Skin
60824	Right Sacroanterior		7632	Excoriated
60825	Left Sacroanterior		7633	Pilonidal Sinus
60826	Sacroposterior		7634	Ulcer
60827	Right Sacroposterior		10038	Wart
60828	Left Sacroposterior		9747	Stricture
60829	Right Sacrotransverse		7635	Fissure
60830	Left Sacrotransverse		7636	Fistula
60795	Transverse		7637	Sphincter Tone
60831	Right Scapuloanterior		7638	Tight
60832	Left Scapuloanterior		7639	Lax
60833	Right Scapuloposterior		7640	Hypertrophied Anal Papilla
60834	Left Scapuloposterior		7641	Hemorrhoids
7427	Hepatic Findings		9735	Internal
9802	Size		9736	External
7428	Enlargement		9333	Tender, Swollen And Firm
7429	Tenderness		9342	Residual Hemorrhoidal Skin Tags
7430	Pulsatile		7643	Tenderness
7431	Firm		7644	Melanosis Coli
7432	Nodular		7645	Mass ___ cm
7433	Splenic Findings		7646	Fecal Impaction
9803	Extension Below Costal Margin		7614	Rectum
7434	Enlargement		7615	Abscess
7435	Tender		7616	Prolapse
9746	Palpable Gallbladder		7617	Perirectal Abscess
7436	Hernia		7618	Stricture
7437	Incisional		7619	Fistula
7439	Umbilical		7642	Fissure
62508	Not Reducible		7620	Ulceration
7440	Paraumbilical		7621	Tenderness
7438	Ventral		7622	Subcutaneous Nodule
10297	Inguinal		7623	Mass ___ cm
10298	On The Right		10456	On The Right
10299	On The Left		10457	On The Left
10300	Bilaterally		10458	Bilaterally
7441	Indirect		9734	Palpable Shelf
11060	On The Right		7624	Perirectal Mass ___ cm
11061	On The Left		9801	Stool Visible Blood
11062	Bilaterally		7625	Stool Blood (Visible)
7442	Direct		7626	Prostate
11063	On The Right		10670	Size (Scale 0-4):
11064	On The Left		7627	Enlargement
11065	Bilaterally		7628	Tenderness
62509	Not Reducible		9651	Hard Area Or Nodule
7443	Femoral		10671	On The Right
10289	On The Right		10672	On The Left
10290	On The Left		10673	Bilaterally
10291	Bilaterally		7629	Stony Hard
7444	Scrotal		9345	Absent

7447	**Urinary System**
7448	Urethral Findings
7449	Discharge
7450	Meatal Stenosis
7451	Urethral Caruncle
7452	Prolapse
7453	Papilloma
7454	Bladder Findings
7455	Distended
7456	Exstrophy
7457	Vesicocolic Fistula
7459	**Male Genitalia**
7460	Penis
7461	Swelling
7462	Edema
7463	Priapism
7464	Lesion
7465	Ulcer
7466	Single
7467	Multiple, Uniform Size
7468	Multiple, Varying Sizes
7469	Tender
7470	With A Necrotic Base
7471	With A Beefy Red Base
7472	Indurated Edge
7473	Undermined Edge
7474	Erythematous Border
7475	Serpiginous
7476	Papules
7477	Umbilicated
7478	Verrucous
7479	Crusts
7480	Circinate Balanitis
7481	Discharge
7482	Pus
7483	Clear
11171	Phimosis
9346	Adherent Prepuce
7484	Preputial Calculus
62282	Circumcision Site
62283	Surrounding Redness
62284	Drainage
62285	Not Healed
7485	Hypospadias
7486	Epispadias
7487	Glans Growths
7488	Condyloma Latum
7489	Condyloma Acuminatum
62510	Urinary Meatus
62511	Redness And Irritation
7490	Ventral Shaft
7491	Mass ___ cm
7492	Dorsal Shaft
7493	Lateral Shaft
7494	Irregular Hard Mass ___ cm
7495	Hyperplasia
7496	Hypoplasia
7497	Scrotum
7498	Edema
11066	On The Right
11067	On The Left
11068	Bilaterally
7499	Sebaceous Cysts
7513	Hydrocele
11069	On The Right
11070	On The Left
11071	Bilaterally
7514	Varicocele
7515	On The Left Only
7500	Hematoma
7501	Laceration
7502	Firm Ulcer
7503	Gangrene
7504	Hanging Groins
7505	Testes
7506	Cryptorchism
10356	On The Right
10357	On The Left
11072	Bilaterally
7507	Atrophy
10358	On The Right
10359	On The Left
11073	Bilaterally
11172	Small For Age In An Adolescent
7508	Under 1 Cm. In An Adult
7509	Tender Testicular Swelling
7510	Nontender Testicular Swelling
7511	Translucent, Anterior To Testicle
7512	Opaque, Anterior To Testicle
9305	Mass ___ cm
10360	On The Right
10361	On The Left
11074	Bilaterally
7516	Epididymis
7517	Tender Swelling
7518	Mass ___ cm
7519	Vas Deferens / Spermatic Cord
7520	Tender Swelling
7521	Mass ___ cm
7523	**Female Genitalia**
7524	External
7525	Vulvar Atrophy
7526	Premature
7527	Vulvar Or Labial Ulcer
7528	Single
7529	Multiple, Uniform Size

7530	Multiple, Varying Sizes	7564	With A Necrotic Base
7531	Tender	7565	With Beefy Red Base
7532	With A Necrotic Base	7566	Indurated Edge
7533	With A Beefy Red Base	7567	Undermined Edge
7534	Indurated Edge	7568	Erythematous Border
7535	Undermined Edge	7569	Serpiginous
7536	Erythematous Border	7570	Papules
7537	Serpiginous	7571	Umbilicated
62512	Labia Majora	7572	Verrucous
62278	Erythema	7573	Crusts
62513	Ecchymosis	7574	Vesicle(s)
62514	Labia Minora	7575	Tenderness
62515	Erythema	7576	Neoplasm
62516	Ecchymosis	7577	Rectovaginal Fistula
62517	Fusion	7578	Colpocele
62518	Partial	7579	Cystocele
62519	Complete	7580	Rectocele
9332	Vesicle(s)	7581	Uterine Prolapse
7538	Papules	9347	Uterovaginal Prolapse
7539	Umbilicated	7582	Enlarged Introitus
7540	Verrucous	9426	Foreign Body
7541	Crusts	**7522**	**Pelvic Exam**
7542	Vulvar Tumor	7583	Cervix
7543	Condyloma Latum	7584	Discharge
7544	Condyloma Acuminatum	7585	Purulent
7545	Neoplasm	7586	With Fundus Tenderness
11173	Labial Adhesions	7587	Blood
62547	Labial Fusion	7588	Watery
9349	Scarring Of The Vulva	7589	Tissue
7546	Vulvitis	9420	Vesicular
7547	Enlarged Clitoris	7590	Softening
7548	Bartholin Gland	9424	Patent Os
7549	Inflamed	9328	Bluish Discoloration
7550	Abscess	9334	Effacement
7551	Inflammation Of Skene's Gland	9335	Dilated
7552	Vagina	7591	Erosion
7553	Mucosa	7592	Ulcer
7554	Erythematous	7593	Grouped Vesicles
7555	Dry	7594	Polyp ___ cm
7556	Atrophy	62625	Absent
9228	Imperforate Hymen	7595	Pain On Motion
11224	Hymenal Disruption	9419	Non-visualization Of IUD String
11225	Prepubertal	7596	Uterus
11226	Semen Present	7597	Position
11227	Prepubertal	9348	Retroversion
7557	Discharge	9427	Size
7558	Curds	7598	Enlargement
9245	Fecal	60790	Fundal Height
7559	Ulcer	9446	Excessive For Dates
7560	Single	9448	Insufficient Growth For Dates
7561	Multiple, Uniform Size	9329	Softening Of Corpus (Hegar's sign)
7562	Multiple, Varying Sizes	60791	Fetal Movement
7563	Tender	7599	Mass ___ cm

7600	Multiple		6081	Generalized
7601	A Smooth Contour		6082	Localized To Lesion
62626	Absent		6083	Of The Feet
7602	Tenderness		6084	Of The Hands
9425	Uterosacral Nodularity		6085	Malar
7603	Adnexa		62564	Livid
7604	Tenderness		62565	Around The Umbilicus
10354	On The Right		6087	Transitory
10355	On The Left		9258	Of The Face
62627	Absent		6086	With Swelling
7605	Frozen Pelvis		9381	With Weeping
7606	Tubal Mass ___ cm		6088	Plethora
10350	On The Right		11442	Hypopigmentation
10351	On The Left		6091	Brawny Induration
9229	Ovarian Diameter		6092	Brownish Discoloration
9230	Enlargement		11138	Pallor
7607	Ovarian Mass ___ cm		6093	Circumoral
10352	On The Right		6097	Generalized
10353	On The Left		6095	Localized
7608	Solid		6096	Of The Extremities
7609	Fluctuant		9723	Elevation Pallor
7610	Rectovaginal		9724	Right Leg (0-4)
7611	Pouch Mass ___ cm		9725	Left Leg (0-4)
6142	**Skin**		9726	Dependent Rubor
64464	Normal Except As Noted		9727	Right Leg (0-4)
10013	General Appearance		9728	Left Leg (0-4)
10014	Wrinkled		11139	Cyanosis
10015	Furrowed		6101	Generalized
11527	Weathered		6100	Localized
9380	Fissured		11452	Upper Body
11659	Horizontally Oriented, Linear		11453	Lower Body
6305	Mobility		6098	Hands And Feet
6306	Tight		6099	Circumoral
6307	Lax		6094	Gray-blue
6308	Hyperelastic		6102	Generalized Yellowish Discoloration
64465	Inelastic		6103	Without Scleral Icterus
6309	Texture		62369	Localized Yellowish Discoloration
6310	Thickened		62370	Face
6311	Over The Shins		62371	Chest
11456	Hypertrophic		62372	Abdomen
6312	Hyperkeratosis		62373	Extremities
6313	Follicular		6104	Yellow Color, Localized To A Lesion
6314	Thin		6105	Yellow Color Of Nasolabial Folds, Palms, Soles, Forehead
6315	Rough			
6316	Doughy		6106	Lemon Yellow
6317	Shiny		6107	Greenish Discoloration
6318	Smooth, Silky		9511	Brownish Discoloration
6319	Crepitant		9512	Of Fingers
6320	Friable		6114	Cherry Red
6321	Turgor		6115	Moisture
6322	Decreased		6116	Dry
6079	Color And Pigmentation		9384	Localized
6080	Erythema			

SKIN, CONT.

6118	Anhidrosis	64493		Both
6119	Localized	6153		Nose
6120	Hyperhidrosis	64494		Right
6121	Localized	64495		Left
6122	Generalized	64496		Both
6117	Sebaceous	6154		The Paranasal Folds
6123	Diaphoresis	64497		Right
6124	Mucous Membranes	64498		Left
6125	Dry	64499		Both
9214	Cold, Clammy Hands	6155		Circumorally
6126	Temperature	64500		Right
6127	Cold Extremities	64501		Left
6128	Generalized Coolness	64502		Both
6129	Localized Coolness	64503		Around Nose And Mouth
6130	Generalized Warmth	64504		Right
6131	Localized Warmth	64505		Left
6132	Feet Dependent	64506		Both
6133	Warm Skin	6156		Lip
6134	Cool With Pallor	6157		Upper
6135	Cool And Blue	64507		Right
6136	Feet Elevated	64508		Left
6137	Cool With Pallor	64509		Both
6143	Lesions	64510		Lower
6145	Location	64511		Right
6146	Generalized	64512		Left
6147	Changing	64513		Both
6148	On The Scalp	64514		Chin
64471	Frontal	64515		Right
64472	On top	64516		Left
64473	On the right side	64517		Both
64474	On the left side	64518		Along The Jaw Line
64475	Towards the back	64519		Right
6149	On The Ear	64520		Left
64476	Right	64521		Both
64477	Left	6158		A Butterfly Pattern
64478	Both	9807		Macules
6150	On The Face	9808		Papules
64479	Forehead	9811		On The Neck
64480	Right	62306		Front
64481	Left	64523		Right
64482	Entire	64524		Left
64483	On The Temple	64525		Both
64484	Right	64522		Back
64485	Left	64526		Right
64486	Both	64527		Left
6151	Upper Eyelids	64528		Both
64487	Cheeks	6159		On The Shoulders
64488	Right	64530		Front
64489	Left	64533		Right
64490	Both	64534		Left
6152	Eyebrows	64535		Both
64491	Right	64531		Top
64492	Left	64536		Right

SKIN LESIONS, CONT.

64537	Left	64589	Right Ring Finger
64538	Both	64590	Right Little Finger
64532	Back	64591	Left Thumb
64539	Right	64592	Left Index Finger
64540	Left	64594	Left Middle Finger
64541	Both	64593	Left Ring Finger
64529	Within The Armpits	64595	Left Little Finger
64543	Right	64596	Multiple Fingers Of Both
64544	Left		Hands
64545	Both	64542	On The Trunk
64546	On The Upper Extremities	64597	On The Chest
64547	Arms	64598	Right
64548	Right	64599	Left
64549	Left	64600	Entire
64550	both	64601	On The Belly
64551	Elbows	64602	Right Upper
64552	Right	64603	Left Upper
64555	Inside	64604	Right Lower
64556	Outside	64605	Left Lower
64553	Left	6160	Back
64557	Inside	64606	Upper
64558	Outside	64609	Right
64554	Both	64610	Left
64559	Inside	64611	Entire
64560	Outside	64607	Middle
64561	Forearms	64612	Right
64562	Right	64613	Left
64563	Left	64614	Entire
64564	Both	64608	Lower
64565	Wrists	64615	Right
64566	Right	64616	Left
64567	Inside	64617	Entire
64568	Outside	6161	Groin
64569	Left	64618	Right
64570	Inside	64619	Left
64571	Outside	64620	Both
64572	Both	64621	Diaper Area
64573	Inside	64622	Front
64574	Outside	64623	Buttocks
64575	Hands	64624	Peeling
64576	Right	64625	Scabs
64579	Top	64626	Raw
64580	Palm	64627	Smooth And Red
64577	Left	64628	Papular
64581	Top	64629	Vulvar
64583	Palm	64630	Right
64578	Both	64631	Left
64582	Top	64632	Both
64584	Palm	64633	Buttocks
64585	Fingers	6162	Right
64586	Right Thumb	64634	Left
64587	Right Index Finger	64635	Both
64588	Right Middle Finger	9821	Macules

SKIN LESIONS, CONT.

9822	Papules	64666	Outer Aspect
6165	Inguinal	62310	Both
6166	Christmas Tree Pattern	64667	Inner aspects
9809	Macules	64668	Outer aspects
9810	Papules	6175	Feet
6168	Anal	6173	Soles
6169	On The Lower Extremities	11049	On The Right
9382	Thighs	11050	On The Left
9823	On The Right	11051	Bilaterally
64636	Front	6174	Top
64637	Back	62312	Right
64638	Inner Aspect	62313	Left
64639	Outer Aspect	62314	Bilateral
9824	On The Left	62311	Toes
64640	Front	11052	Right Great Toe
64641	Back	11053	Right Second Toe
64642	Inner	11054	Right Third Toe
64643	Outer	11055	Right Fourth Toe
11047	Bilaterally	6178	Right Little Toe
64644	Front	6179	Left Great Toe
64645	Back	6180	Left Second Toe
64646	Inner Aspect	6181	Left Third Toe
64647	Outer Aspect	6182	Left Fourth Toe
6172	Knees	11048	Left Little Toe
64649	Right	6183	Between The Toes
64648	Front	6184	Right Foot
64650	Back	6185	Left Foot
64651	Inner Aspect	6186	Both Feet
64652	Outer Aspect	6187	Along Lymphatic Vessels
64653	Left	6188	Along Arteries
64654	Front	64669	On Sunlight Exposed Areas
64655	Back	64670	Perifollicular
64656	Inner aspect	64671	In Intertriginous Areas
64657	Outer aspect	62600	Qualities
64658	Both	6144	Tender
64659	Front	62304	Indurated
64660	Back	62601	Fluctuant
64661	Inner Aspect	62607	Crepitant
64662	Outer Aspect	62604	Pulsatile
6170	Shins	62608	Mobile
9812	Right	62609	Adherent To Adjacent Tissue
9813	Left	62602	Exudative
9814	Both	62303	Purulent-appearing
9815	Calves	62603	Warm
9816	On The Right	62605	Hot
9817	On The Left	62606	Cold
9818	Bilaterally	6254	Configuration
62307	Ankles	6255	Annular
62308	Right	9354	Erythema Chronicum Migrans
64663	Inner Aspect	6256	Polygonal
64664	Outer Aspect	6257	Serpiginous
62309	Left	62598	Bullseye
64665	Inner Aspect	6258	Iris

SKIN LESIONS, CONT.

9418	Mobilliform	11250	Knees
6259	Retiform	11251	Shins
6260	Linear	11254	Linear In Appearance
6261	Grouped	11255	Color / Age
6262	Bandlike	11256	Red-Blue / 1-2 Days
6263	Irregular	11257	Blue-Purple / 3-5 Days
6264	Spread Centripetally	11258	Green / 6-7 Days
6265	Spread Centrifugally	11259	Yellow-Brown / 8-10 Days
6266	Expanding Border	11260	Mixed
6267	Purple In Color	6275	Purpura
9358	Erythematous	6276	The Lower Half Of Body
6268	Sharply Demarcated	6277	Palpable
62315	Central Clearing	11444	"Blueberry Muffin"
62316	Central Necrosis	6207	Plaques
64463	Morphology	6208	Smooth, Shiny, Violaceous
6189	Macule(s) ___ cm	62563	With Satellite Pustules
6190	Become Crusty	6209	Nodule(s) ___ cm
6191	Brown Or Black	6210	Erythematous
9397	More Than 20	6211	Subcutaneous
6192	Variegated	6212	Tender
6193	Salmon Colored	6213	Brown Or Black
10012	Gray-blue	6214	Purple
6194	Purpuric / Petechial	6215	Variegated
6195	Become Confluent & Petechial	6219	Vesicle(s) ___ mm
6196	Erythematous	6220	Umbilicated
62593	Patch	6221	Become Shallow White
6237	White		Ulceration(s) With Red Areola
6197	Papules	6222	With Erythematous Border
6198	Brown Or Black	6223	Ruptured
6199	Variegated	6224	Tense
6200	Follicular	6225	Become Pustules
11213	Punctate	6226	Bulla ___ cm
6201	Erythematous	11652	Tense
11457	Become Pustular	11653	Flaccid
6202	Become A Vesicle	11654	Nikolsky's Sign
6203	Ulcerate	11655	Asboe-Hansen's Sign
6204	Form Black Eschar	11056	Cyst
6205	Purpuric / Petechial	11455	Which Become Nodular
6206	White Umbilicated, Expressing Cheesy Material	11464	Straw-colored
		6216	Wheal
11449	Macules And Papules	6217	Darier's Sign (appears by rubbing macule)
11450	Diffuse		
6272	Petechial Hemorrhages	6218	Dermatographia
6273	Ecchymosis	6227	Pustules
11248	Forehead	6228	At Site Of Needle Puncture
6274	Mastoid (Battle's sign)	6229	Furuncle(s)
11230	Cheeks	9352	On The Leg
11252	Upper Arm(s)	9353	On The Foot
11249	Elbows	6230	Carbuncle
11231	On The Abdomen	6765	Of The Upper Lip
11253	On The Back	6766	Of The Lower Lip
11232	On The Buttocks	9350	Of The Leg
11223	Genital	9351	Of The Foot

SKIN LESIONS, CONT.

6232	Crusts	6240	On The Legs (below the knee)
6233	Leave Scars	9767	The Right Leg
62599	Eschars	9768	The Left Leg
6234	Lichenification	9783	Both Legs
11215	Exfoliation	9769	On The Right Ankle
6235	Scales	6241	On The Medial Malleolus
11644	Thick, Silvery (micaceous)	6242	On The Lateral Malleolus
11646	Fine, Silvery, Powdery	9771	On The Left Ankle
11645	Greasy	9770	On The Medial Malleolus
11647	"Fish-like"	9772	On The Lateral Malleolus
11648	Brown, Adherent	9785	On Both Ankles
11649	Verrucous	9784	On The Medial Malleoli
11650	Large, Dark, Platelike	10051	On The Lateral Malleoli
6236	Bleeding After Scale Removed	10052	On The Right Foot
	(Auspitz's sign)	9774	On The Plantar Aspect
11660	Erosion	9775	On The Dorsal Aspect
6238	Ulcer ___ cm	10053	On The Left Foot
9753	On The Fingers Of The Right	9776	On The Plantar Aspect
	Hand	9777	On The Dorsal Aspect
10039	On The Thumb	9773	On Both Feet
10040	On The Index Finger	9778	On The Toes Of The Right Foot
10041	On The Middle Finger	9786	The Great Toe
10042	On The Ring Finger	9787	The Second Toe
10043	On The Little Finger	9788	The Middle Toe
9754	On The Fingers Of The Left Hand	9789	The Fourth Toe
10044	On The Thumb	9790	The Little Toe
10045	On The Index Finger	9779	On The Toes Of The Left Foot
10046	On The Middle Finger	9791	The Great Toe
10047	On The Ring Finger	9792	The Second Toe
10048	On The Little Finger	9793	The Middle Toe
9755	On The Fingers Of Both Hands	9794	The Fourth Toe
10050	On The Right Hand	9795	The Little Toe
9757	On The Palmar Aspect	9780	On The Toes Of Both Feet
9759	On The Dorsal Aspect	7721	Chancre (elevated, painless,
10049	On The Left Hand		indurated ulcer)
9758	On The Palmar Aspect	64467	Traumatic
9760	On The Dorsal Aspect	6269	Burn(s) ___ cm
9756	On Both Hands	6270	Covering >15% Of Body Surface
10054	On The Upper Arm		(Sec. or Tert.)
10055	On The Right	11229	Well Demarcated Border
10056	On The Left	11234	Hand(s)
10105	On The Elbow	64468	Arm(s)
10106	On The Right	64470	Shoulder(s)
10107	On The Left	11236	Buttocks
6239	On The Forearm	64469	Leg(s)
9765	On The Right	11235	Feet
9766	On The Left	11237	Poorly Demarcated Border
9761	On The Trunk	11246	Face
9763	On The Right Buttock	11241	Shoulder(s)
9764	On The Left Buttock	11244	Arm
9762	On Both Buttocks	11238	Hand(s)
9781	On The Right Thigh	11242	Chest
9782	On The Left Thigh	11243	Back

SKIN LESIONS, CONT.

11240	Buttocks
11245	Leg
11239	Feet
11247	Gradated
11228	Multiple
11692	Right Side
11693	Left Side
11694	Bilateral
11057	Abrasion
11560	Superficial
11537	Head
6384	Scalp
9411	Facial
11561	Forehead
11562	Eyebrow
11563	Eyelid
11262	Chin
11263	Shoulder
11341	On The Right
11342	On The Left
11343	Bilaterally
11264	Chest
11265	Back
11266	Upper Arm
11344	On The Right
11345	On The Left
11346	Bilaterally
11267	Elbow
11347	On The Right
11348	On The Left
11349	Bilaterally
11268	Forearm
11350	On The Right
11351	On The Left
11352	Bilaterally
11271	Hand
11353	On The Right
11354	On The Left
11355	Bilaterally
11269	Dorsum
11270	Knuckle
11272	Palm
11273	Abdomen
11274	Hip
11431	On The Right
11432	On The Left
11433	Bilaterally
11275	Buttocks
11276	Thigh
11356	On The Right
11357	On The Left
11358	Bilaterally
11277	Knee
11359	On The Right
11360	On The Left
11361	Bilaterally
11278	Lower Leg
11362	On The Right
11363	On The Left
11364	Bilaterally
11279	Ankle
11365	On The Right
11366	On The Left
11367	Bilaterally
11280	Foot
11368	On The Right
11369	On The Left
11370	Bilaterally
11281	Dorsum
11282	Sole
11337	Multiple
11058	Contusion
11538	Head
11539	Scalp
11283	Facial
11284	Chin
11285	Shoulder
11371	On The Right
11372	On The Left
11373	Bilaterally
11286	Chest
11287	Back
11288	Upper Arm
11374	On The Right
11375	On The Left
11376	Bilaterally
11289	Elbow
11377	On The Right
11378	On The Left
11379	Bilaterally
11290	Forearm
11380	On The Right
11381	On The Left
11382	Bilaterally
11293	Hand
11383	On The Right
11384	On The Left
11385	Bilaterally
11291	Dorsum
11292	Knuckles
11294	Palm
11295	Abdomen
11296	Hip
11434	On The Right
11435	On The Left
11436	Bilaterally

SKIN LESIONS, CONT.

11297	Buttocks	11405	On The Left
11298	Thigh	11406	Bilaterally
11386	On The Right	11311	Elbow
11387	On The Left	11407	On The Right
11388	Bilaterally	11408	On The Left
11299	Knee	11409	Bilaterally
11389	On The Right	11312	Forearm
11390	On The Left	11410	On The Right
11391	Bilaterally	11411	On The Left
11300	Lower Leg	11412	Bilaterally
11392	On The Right	11315	Hand
11393	On The Left	11413	On The Right
11394	Bilaterally	11414	On The Left
11301	Ankle	11415	Bilaterally
11395	On The Right	11313	Dorsum
11396	On The Left	11314	Knuckles
11397	Bilaterally	11316	Palm
11302	Foot	11317	Abdomen
11398	On The Right	11318	Hip
11399	On The Left	11437	On The Right
11400	Bilaterally	11438	On The Left
11303	Dorsum	11439	Bilaterally
11304	Sole	11319	Buttocks
11695	On The Right	11320	Thigh
11696	On The Left	11416	On The Right
11697	Bilaterally	11417	On The Left
11338	Multiple	11418	Bilaterally
6298	Laceration	11321	Knee
6299	Superficial	11419	On The Right
11536	Head	11420	On The Left
6383	Scalp	11421	Bilaterally
11574	Ear	11322	Lower Leg
62587	Right	11422	On The Right
62588	Left	11423	On The Left
62589	Bilateral	11424	Bilaterally
9407	Forehead	11323	Ankle
11554	Eyebrow	11425	On The Right
62590	Right	11426	On The Left
62591	Left	11427	Bilaterally
62592	Bilateral	11324	Foot
11556	Eye	11428	On The Right
11306	Chin	11429	On The Left
11567	Neck	11430	Bilaterally
11568	Anterior	11325	Dorsum
11569	Posterior	11326	Sole
11307	Shoulder	11698	On The Right
11401	On The Right	11699	On The Left
11402	On The Left	11700	Bilaterally
11403	Bilaterally	11339	Multiple
11308	Chest	11233	Follows The Body Contours
11309	Back	6300	With Active Blood Loss
11310	Upper Arm	62317	Shape
11404	On The Right	62318	Straight Line

SKIN LESIONS, CONT.

62319	V-shaped		11580	Eyelid
62320	Y-shaped		11581	Eye
62321	L-shaped		11582	Conjunctiva
62322	Jagged		11583	Sclera
62323	Puncture		11584	Cornea
62324	Orientation		11585	Chin
62325	Vertical		11586	Neck
62326	Horizontal		11587	Anterior
62327	Diagonal		11588	Posterior
62328	Depth		11589	Shoulder
62329	Shallow		11590	On The Right
62330	Moderate		11591	On The Left
62331	Deep		11592	Bilaterally
62332	Edges		11593	Chest
62333	Ragged		11594	Back
62334	Post-suture Approximation		11595	Upper Arm
62335	Poor		11596	On The Right
62336	Difficult		11597	On The Left
6301	Bite		11598	Bilaterally
11327	Superficial		11599	Elbow
11540	Head		11600	On The Right
11541	Scalp		11601	On The Left
11542	Forehead		11602	Bilaterally
11543	Chin		11603	Forearm
11328	Shoulder		11604	On The Right
11544	Chest		11605	On The Left
11545	Back		11606	Bilaterally
11329	Upper Arm		11607	Hand
11546	Elbow		11608	On The Right
11330	Forearm		11609	On The Left
11331	Hand		11610	Bilaterally
11332	Dorsum		11611	Dorsum
11547	Abdomen		11612	Knuckles
11548	Hip		11613	Palm
11549	Buttocks		11614	Abdomen
11333	Thigh		11615	Hip
11550	Knee		11616	On The Right
11334	Lower Leg		11617	On The Left
11335	Ankle		11618	Bilaterally
11336	Foot		11619	Buttocks
11340	Multiple		11620	Thigh
11701	On The Right		11621	On The Right
11702	On The Left		11622	On The Left
11703	Bilaterally		11623	Bilaterally
6249	Wound, NOS		11624	Knee
11551	Superficial		11625	On The Right
11552	Puncture		11626	On The Left
11553	Penetrating		11627	Bilaterally
11575	Head		11628	Lower Leg
11576	Scalp		11629	On The Right
11577	Ear		11630	On The Left
11578	Forehead		11631	Bilaterally
11579	Eyebrow		11632	Ankle

SKIN LESIONS, CONT.

11633	On The Right		6302	Needle Tracks
11634	On The Left		64466	Clinical Impressions
11635	Bilaterally		10016	Striae
11636	Foot		7360	Abdominal
11637	On The Right		7361	Purple
11638	On The Left		10017	Upper Arms
11639	Bilaterally		10019	Lower Back
11640	Dorsum		10018	Buttocks
11641	Sole		6271	Vascular
11704	On The Right		10395	Hemangioma
11705	On The Left		10396	Capillary
11706	Bilaterally		10397	Senile
11642	Multiple		10398	Verrucous
62337	Dirty		10399	Cavernous
11643	With Active Blood Loss		6278	Hematoma
62273	With Surrounding Redness		6279	Urticaria
62338	With Surrounding Induration		6280	Pulsating Tumor
6250	With A Sweet Odor		6281	Arterial Spider
62274	Purulent Drainage		6282	Telangiectasia
6251	Draining With Bubbles		6283	Livedo Reticularis
6252	Palpable Crepitus		6284	Palmar Erythema
6253	Sulfur Granules		6285	Erythromelalgia (Red burning extremities)
62339	Visible Blood Vessels			
62340	Visible Tendons		6286	Nevus Flammeus (Port Wine Nevus)
62341	Visible Foreign Body		6288	Acneiform Eruption
62342	Visible Nerve		62279	Face
62343	Visible Sutures In Place		62597	Scalp
62344	Visible Bone		62281	Trunk
62345	Fragments		62280	Back
9421	Excoriation		62594	Chest
6138	Scar		62595	Abdomen
11459	Facial		62596	Flanks
11460	Axillary		6289	Chloracne
10379	Arm		6290	Comedones (Blackheads)
10380	Right		6291	Xanthelasma
10381	Left		6292	Xanthomata
10382	Hand		6293	Tuberosum
10383	Right		6294	Tuberoeruptive
10384	Left		9249	Palmar
6140	Inguinal		6295	Calabar Swelling
10363	On The Right		6296	Wartlike
10364	On The Left		6297	Uremic Frost
6139	Bilateral		11690	Leukoderma
10392	Buttocks		6089	Vitiligo
10393	Right		6090	Albinism
10394	Left		11691	Melanoderma
10389	Leg		6109	Raynaud's Phenomenon
10390	Right		9379	Blanching With Cold Challenge
10391	Left		6110	Cafe-au-lait Spots
9260	Tattoo		6111	6 Or More Spots Of At Least 1.5 Cm.
9261	Multiple			
9843	Single		6112	Axillary Freckles
11651	With Bright Red Colors		6113	Chloasma (mask of pregnancy)

6231	Papilloma	6352	Onychorrhexis (brittle nail)
62305	Nevus Sebaceus Of Jadassohn	11669	Hapalonychia
6287	Janeway's Spots	6353	Onycholysis
62610	Sphacelus	11661	Onychauxis
6244	Abscess	11662	Onychogryphosis
11458	Sinus Tract	11663	Onychoatrophy
6248	Fistula	11664	Onychomadesis
6245	Gangrene	11667	Onychoschiza
6246	Dry	6354	Square Nails
6247	Wet	11670	Platonychia
6243	Ecthyma Gangrenosum	6355	Koilonychia (Spoon nails)
6303	Lesions In All Stages Of Development	11674	Pincer
6304	More Than 15 Lesions	11671	Pterygium
6141	Metal Splinters In The Skin	11672	Pterygium Inversum Unguis
6323	Hair	11673	Hangnail
6324	Quantity And Distribution	6356	Periungual Swelling
6325	Hirsutism, Upper Lip, Chin, Cheeks, Chest, Arms, Legs, Back	9731	Periungual Ulcers
		6357	Periungual Telangiectasia (prominent capillaries)
6326	Absence Of Axillary And Pubic Hair		
6327	Sparse Facial Hair	11665	Beau's Lines (transverse furrows)
62346	Absence Of Facial Hair	6358	Mees Lines (transverse white bands)
6328	Alopecia	11676	Discoloration
9304	Normal Male Pattern	6359	Blue-gray Nail Plates
6329	Diffuse	6360	Brown-black Nail Plates
6330	Patchy	11677	White (Leukonychia)
9428	Mixed Short And Longer Hairs	11678	Punctata
6331	Total	11679	Striata
6332	Temporal Recession Of Hairline	11680	Partialis
6333	Loss Of Hair Dorsa Toes	11681	Totalis
6334	Loss Of Hair Lower Legs	6361	Terry's Nail (white proximal nail bed)
9297	Neonatal-like (lanugo)	6363	White Bands In The Nail Bed (Muehrcke's Lines)
6335	Color		
6336	Premature Graying Of Hair	6362	Light Blue Lunulae (Nails of Wilson's disease)
6337	White Forelock		
11689	Alternating Light And Dark Banding Of The Shaft	11682	Green
		11684	Red Lunulae
6338	Texture	11686	Purple-Blue Nail Bed
6339	Thin	11685	Spotted Lunulae
6340	Coarse	11683	Staining Of The Plate
11687	Shaft	62347	Pallor Of The Nailbeds
11688	Irregularly Spaced Small White Nodes	11666	Half And Half Nails
6341	Parasites	6364	Moniliasis
6342	Lice	6365	Splinter Hemorrhages
6343	Nits	6366	Painful Red/violet Subungal Spot (Glomus tumor)
6344	Piloerection		
6345	Nails	6367	Prolonged Capillary Filling
6346	Clubbing	7649	**Musculoskeletal System**
6347	Pitting	9390	Performing Musculoskeletal Exam
6348	Absence Of Nails	9391	Range Of Motion Evaluation Of Extremity
6349	Dystrophy		
6350	Bitten Nail(s)	9392	Range Of Motion Evaluation Of Hand
11675	Onychotillomania	62650	Overall Findings
6351	Ingrowing	60771	Fingers

60773	Appearance		60962	DIP
10459	Swelling		62804	Distal Phalanx
10460	Of Fingers Of The Right Hand		62673	Diffuse
62651	MCP Joints		10470	Bilaterally
62652	IP Joints		62674	MCP
62653	PIP Joints		62805	Proximal Phalanx
62654	DIP Joints		62675	PIP
62655	Diffuse		62806	Middle Phalanx
10461	Of Fingers Of The Left Hand		62676	DIP
62656	MCP Joints		62807	Distal Phalanx
62657	IP Joints		62677	Diffuse
62658	PIP Joints		10471	Of The Middle Finger
62659	DIP Joints		10472	On The Right
62660	Diffuse		60963	MCP
10462	Of Fingers Of Both Hands		62808	Proximal Phalanx
62661	MCP Joints		60964	PIP
62662	IP Joints		62809	Middle Phalanx
62663	PIP Joints		60965	DIP
62664	DIP Joints		62810	Distal Phalanx
62665	Diffuse		62678	Diffuse
10463	Of The Thumb		10473	On The Left
10464	On The Right		60966	MCP
60953	MCP		62811	Proximal Phalanx
62793	Proximal Phalanx		60967	PIP
60954	IP		62812	Middle Phalanx
62794	Distal Phalanx		60968	DIP
62667	Diffuse		62813	Distal Phalanx
10465	On The Left		62679	Diffuse
60955	MCP		10474	Bilaterally
62795	Proximal Phalanx		62680	MCP
60956	IP		62814	Proximal Phalanx
62796	Distal Phalanx		62681	PIP
62668	Diffuse		62815	Middle Phalanx
10466	Bilaterally		62682	DIP
62669	MCP		62816	Distal Phalanx
62797	Proximal Phalanx		62683	Diffuse
62670	IP		10475	Of The Ring Finger
62798	Distal Phalanx		10476	On The Right
62671	Diffuse		60969	MCP
10467	Of The Index Finger		62817	Proximal Phalanx
10468	On The Right		60970	PIP
60957	MCP		62818	Middle Phalanx
62799	Proximal Phalanx		60971	DIP
60958	PIP		62819	Distal Phalanx
62800	Middle Phalanx		62684	Diffuse
60959	DIP		10477	On The Left
62801	Distal Phalanx		60972	MCP
62672	Diffuse		62820	Proximal Phalanx
10469	On The Left		60973	PIP
60960	MCP		62821	Middle Phalanx
62802	Proximal Phalanx		60974	DIP
60961	PIP		62822	Distal Phalanx
62803	Middle Phalanx		62685	Diffuse

FINGERS, CONT.

10478	Bilaterally	62715	On The Right
62686	MCP	62716	MCP
62823	Proximal Phalanx	62835	Proximal Phalanx
62687	PIP	62717	IP
62824	Middle Phalanx	62837	Distal Phalanx
62688	DIP	62718	Diffuse
62825	Distal Phalanx	62719	On The Left
62689	Diffuse	62720	MCP
10479	Of The Little Finger	62838	Proximal Phalanx
10480	On The Right	62721	IP
60975	MCP	62839	Distal Phalanx
62826	Proximal Phalanx	62722	Diffuse
60976	PIP	62723	Bilaterally
62827	Middle Phalanx	62724	MCP
60977	DIP	62840	Proximal Phalanx
62828	Distal Phalanx	62725	IP
62690	Diffuse	62841	Distal Phalanx
10481	On The Left	62726	Diffuse
60978	MCP	62727	Of The Index Finger
62829	Proximal Phalanx	62728	On The Right
60979	PIP	62729	MCP
62830	Middle Phalanx	62842	Proximal Phalanx
60980	DIP	62730	PIP
62831	Distal Phalanx	62843	Middle Phalanx
62691	Diffuse	62731	DIP
10482	Bilaterally	62844	Distal Phalanx
62692	MCP	62732	Diffuse
62832	Proximal Phalanx	62733	On The Left
62693	PIP	62734	MCP
62833	Middle Phalanx	62845	Proximal Phalanx
62694	DIP	62735	PIP
62834	Distal Phalanx	62846	Middle Phalanx
62695	Diffuse	62736	DIP
62666	Redness	62847	Distal Phalanx
62696	Of Fingers Of The Right Hand	62737	Diffuse
62697	MCP Joints	62738	Bilaterally
62698	IP Joints	62739	MCP
62699	PIP Joints	62848	Proximal Phalanx
62700	DIP Joints	62740	PIP
62701	Diffuse	62849	Middle Phalanx
62702	Of Fingers Of The Left Hand	62741	DIP
62703	MCP Joints	62850	Distal Phalanx
62704	IP Joints	62742	Diffuse
62705	PIP Joints	62743	Of The Middle Finger
62706	DIP Joints	62744	On The Right
62707	Diffuse	62745	MCP
62708	Of Fingers Of Both Hands	62851	Proximal Phalanx
62709	MCP Joints	62746	PIP
62710	IP Joints	62852	Middle Phalanx
62711	PIP Joints	62747	DIP
62712	DIP Joints	62853	Distal Phalanx
62713	Diffuse	62748	Diffuse
62714	Of The Thumb	62749	On The Left

FINGERS, CONT.

62750	MCP	62873	Middle Phalanx
62854	Proximal Phalanx	62784	DIP
62751	PIP	62874	Distal Phalanx
62855	Middle Phalanx	62785	Diffuse
62752	DIP	62786	Bilaterally
62856	Distal Phalanx	62787	MCP
62753	Diffuse	62875	Proximal Phalanx
62754	Bilaterally	62788	PIP
62755	MCP	62876	Middle Phalanx
62857	Proximal Phalanx	62789	DIP
62756	PIP	62877	Distal Phalanx
62858	Middle Phalanx	62790	Diffuse
62757	DIP	9215	Warmth
62859	Distal Phalanx	62792	Of Fingers Of Right Hand
62758	Diffuse	62880	MCP
62759	Of The Ring Finger	62881	IP
62760	On The Right	62882	PIP
62761	MCP	62883	DIP
62860	Proximal Phalanx	62884	Diffuse
62762	PIP	62878	Of Fingers Of Left Hand
62861	Middle Phalanx	62885	MCP
62763	DIP	62886	IP
62862	Distal Phalanx	62887	PIP
62764	Diffuse	62888	DIP
62765	On The Left	62889	Diffuse
62766	MCP	62879	Of Fingers Of Both Hands
62863	Proximal Phalanx	62890	MCP
62767	PIP	62891	IP
62864	Middle Phalanx	62892	PIP
62768	DIP	62893	DIP
62865	Distal Phalanx	62894	Diffuse
62769	Diffuse	61438	Thumb
62770	Bilaterally	61443	Right
62771	MCP	61458	MCP
62866	Proximal Phalanx	62924	Proximal Phalanx
62772	PIP	61459	IP
62867	Middle Phalanx	62925	Distal Phalanx
62773	DIP	62895	Diffuse
62868	Distal Phalanx	61444	Left
62774	Diffuse	61460	MCP
62775	Of The Little Finger	62926	Proximal Phalanx
62776	On The Right	61461	IP
62777	MCP	62927	Distal Phalanx
62869	Proximal Phalanx	62896	Diffuse
62778	PIP	61450	Bilaterally
62870	Middle Phalanx	62897	MCP
62779	DIP	62928	Proximal Phalanx
62871	Distal Phalanx	62898	IP
62780	Diffuse	62929	Distal Phalanx
62781	On The Left	62899	Diffuse
62782	MCP	61439	Index Finger
62872	Proximal Phalanx	61445	Right
62783	PIP	61462	MCP

FINGERS, CONT.

62930	Proximal Phalanx	61476	DIP
61463	PIP	62950	Distal Phalanx
62931	Middle Phalanx	62912	Diffuse
61464	DIP	61453	Left
62932	Distal Phalanx	61477	MCP
62900	Diffuse	62951	Proximal Phalanx
61446	Left	61478	PIP
61465	MCP	62952	Middle Phalanx
62933	Proximal Phalanx	61479	DIP
61466	PIP	62953	Distal Phalanx
62934	Middle Phalanx	62913	Diffuse
61467	DIP	61454	Bilaterally
62935	Distal Phalanx	62914	MCP
62901	Diffuse	62954	Proximal Phalanx
61451	Bilaterally	62915	PIP
62902	MCP	62955	Middle Phalanx
62936	Proximal Phalanx	62916	DIP
62903	PIP	62956	Distal Phalanx
62937	Middle Phalanx	62917	Diffuse
62904	DIP	61442	Little Finger
62938	Distal Phalanx	61455	Right
62905	Diffuse	61480	MCP
61440	Middle Finger	62957	Proximal Phalanx
61447	Right	61481	PIP
61468	MCP	62958	Middle Phalanx
62939	Proximal Phalanx	61482	DIP
61469	PIP	62959	Distal Phalanx
62940	Middle Phalanx	62918	Diffuse
61470	DIP	61456	Left
62941	Distal Phalanx	61483	MCP
62906	Diffuse	62960	Proximal Phalanx
61448	Left	61484	PIP
61471	MCP	62961	Middle Phalanx
62942	Proximal Phalanx	61485	DIP
61472	PIP	62962	Distal Phalanx
62943	Middle Phalanx	62919	Diffuse
61473	DIP	61457	Bilaterally
62944	Distal Phalanx	62920	MCP
62907	Diffuse	62963	Proximal Phalanx
61449	Bilaterally	62921	PIP
62908	MCP	62964	Middle Phalanx
62945	Proximal Phalanx	62922	DIP
62909	PIP	62965	Distal Phalanx
62946	Middle Phalanx	62923	Diffuse
62910	DIP	7715	Nodules
62947	Distal Phalanx	7716	Heberden's Nodes (painless nodules DIP)
62911	Diffuse		
61441	Ring Finger	7717	Bouchard's Nodes (painless nodules PIP)
61452	Right		
61474	MCP	7718	Osler's Nodes
62948	Proximal Phalanx	60981	Thumb
61475	PIP	60982	Right
62949	Middle Phalanx	60983	Left

FINGERS, CONT.

60984	Bilaterally	7709	Thumb Resembles Fingers
60985	Index Finger	62975	Right
60986	Right	62976	Left
60987	Left	62977	Bilaterally
60988	Bilaterally	7710	Short 4th & 5th Metacarpal
60989	Middle Finger	62978	Right
60990	Right	62979	Left
60991	Left	62980	Bilaterally
60992	Bilaterally	10206	Deformity
60993	Ring Finger	7708	Trigger Finger
60994	Right	60856	Thumb
60995	Left	60857	Right
60996	Bilaterally	60858	Left
60997	Little Finger	60859	Bilaterally
60998	Right	60860	Index Finger
60999	Left	60861	Right
61000	Bilaterally	60862	Left
7719	Digital Necrosis	60863	Bilaterally
62648	Dry Gangrene	60864	Middle Finger
62649	Wet Gangrene	60865	Right
61001	Thumb	60866	Left
61002	Right	60867	Bilaterally
61003	Left	60868	Ring Finger
61004	Bilaterally	60869	Right
61005	Index Finger	60870	Left
61006	Right	60871	Bilaterally
61007	Left	60872	Little Finger
61008	Bilaterally	60873	Right
61009	Middle Finger	60874	Left
61010	Right	60875	Bilaterally
61011	Left	7707	Mallet Finger (flexion deformity DIP)
61012	Bilaterally		
61013	Ring Finger	60836	Thumb
61014	Right	60837	Right
61015	Left	60838	Left
61016	Bilaterally	60839	Bilaterally
61017	Little Finger	60840	Index Finger
61018	Right	60841	Right
61019	Left	60842	Left
61020	Bilaterally	60843	Bilaterally
7702	Malformation	60844	Middle Finger
7703	Polydactyly	60845	Right
62966	Right	60846	Left
62967	Left	60847	Bilaterally
62968	Bilaterally	60848	Ring Finger
7704	Syndactyly	60849	Right
62969	Right	60850	Left
62970	Left	60851	Bilaterally
62971	Bilaterally	60852	Little Finger
62645	Bradydactyly	60853	Right
62972	Right	60854	Left
62973	Left	60855	Bilaterally
62974	Bilaterally	7711	Boutonniere Slits

FINGERS, CONT.

60876	Thumb	60927		Bilaterally
60877	Right	60928		Ring Finger
60878	Left	60929		Right
60879	Bilaterally	60930		Left
60880	Index Finger	60931		Bilaterally
60881	Right	60932		Little Finger
60882	Left	60933		Right
60883	Bilaterally	60934		Left
60884	Middle Finger	60935		Bilaterally
60885	Right	63414	Subluxation Of MCP Joints	
60886	Left	7682	Acropachy	
60887	Bilaterally	7705	Sclerodactyly	
60888	Ring Finger	10220	Of The Right Hand	
60889	Right	10221	Of The Left Hand	
60890	Left	10222	Of Both Hands	
60891	Bilaterally	10223	Of The Thumb	
60892	Little Finger	10242	On The Right	
60893	Right	10224	On The Left	
60894	Left	10225	Bilaterally	
60895	Bilaterally	10226	Of The Index Finger	
7712	Swan Neck	10227	On The Right	
60896	Thumb	10228	On The Left	
60897	Right	10229	Bilaterally	
60898	Left	10230	Of The Middle Finger	
60899	Bilaterally	10231	On The Right	
60900	Index Finger	10232	On The Left	
60901	Right	10233	Bilaterally	
60902	Left	10234	Of The Ring Finger	
60903	Bilaterally	10235	On The Right	
60904	Middle Finger	10236	On The Left	
60905	Right	10237	Bilaterally	
60906	Left	10238	Of The Little Finger	
60907	Bilaterally	10239	On The Right	
60908	Ring Finger	10240	On The Left	
60909	Right	10241	Bilaterally	
60910	Left	7679	Arachnodactyly	
60911	Bilaterally	7680	Wrist Sign	
60912	Little Finger	7681	Thumb Sign	
60913	Right	10556	Absence	
60914	Left	10557	Of Fingers Of The Right Hand	
60915	Bilaterally	10558	Of Fingers Of The Left Hand	
7713	Ulnar Deviation	10559	Of Fingers Of Both Hands	
60916	Thumb	7706	Absent Thumb	
60917	Right	10561	On The Right	
60918	Left	10562	On The Left	
60919	Bilaterally	10563	Bilaterally	
60920	Index Finger	10564	Of The Index Finger	
60921	Right	10565	On The Right	
60922	Left	10566	On The Left	
60923	Bilaterally	10567	Bilaterally	
60924	Middle Finger	10568	Of The Middle Finger	
60925	Right	10569	On The Right	
60926	Left	10570	On The Left	

FINGERS, CONT.

10571	Bilaterally		61059	Left
10572	Of The Ring Finger		61060	Bilaterally
10573	On The Right		7726	Movement
10574	On The Left		62981	Full Range Of Motion
10575	Bilaterally		62982	Except As Noted
10576	Of The Little Finger		7730	Thumb
10577	On The Right		10115	On The Right
10578	On The Left		61061	Active Motion ___degrees
10579	Bilaterally		61062	Passive Motion ___degrees
60449	Amputated Fingers		10116	On The Left
60450	Thumb		61063	Active Motion ___degrees
60451	Right		61064	Passive Motion ___degrees
60452	Left		10117	Bilaterally
60936	Bilaterally		61065	Active Motion
60937	Index Finger		61066	Passive Motion
60938	Right		7731	MCP
60939	Left		7732	Abduction
60940	Bilaterally		61067	Active Motion, Right
60941	Middle Finger			___degrees
60942	Right		61068	Active Motion, Left
60943	Left			___degrees
60944	Bilaterally		61069	Passive Motion, Right
60945	Ring Finger			___degrees
60946	Right		61070	Passive Motion, Left
60947	Left			___degrees
60948	Bilaterally		7733	Adduction
60949	Little Finger		61071	Active Motion, Right
60950	Right			___degrees
60951	Left		61072	Active Motion, Left
60952	Bilaterally			___degrees
7723	Paronychia (inflamation nail mantle and lateral nail folds)		61073	Passive Motion, Right ___degrees
7724	Felon (maximal tenderness at fingernail)		61074	Passive Motion, Left ___degrees
7722	Digital Infection		7734	Opposition (thumb to little finger)
61041	Thumb			
61042	Right		61075	Active Motion, Right
61043	Left			___degrees
61044	Bilaterally		61076	Active Motion, Left
61045	Index Finger			___degrees
61046	Right		61077	Passive Motion, Right
61047	Left			___degrees
61048	Bilaterally		61078	Passive Motion, Left
61049	Middle Finger			___degrees
61050	Right		7735	Flexion
61051	Left		61079	Active Motion, Right
61052	Bilaterally			___degrees
61053	Ring Finger		61080	Active Motion, Left
61054	Right			___degrees
61055	Left		61081	Passive Motion, Right
61056	Bilaterally			___degrees
61057	Little Finger		61082	Passive Motion, Left
61058	Right			___degrees

FINGERS, CONT.

7736	Extension	61105	Passive Motion, Right ___degrees
61083	Active Motion, Right ___degrees	61106	Passive Motion, Left ___degrees
61084	Active Motion, Left ___degrees	7744	Adduction
61085	Passive Motion, Right ___degrees	61107	Active Motion, Right ___degrees
61086	Passive Motion, Left ___degrees	61108	Active Motion, Left ___degrees
7737	Interphalangeal	61109	Passive Motion, Right ___degrees
7738	Flexion	61110	Passive Motion, Left ___degrees
61087	Active Motion, Right ___degrees	7745	Second (Index) Finger
61088	Active Motion, Left ___degrees	10118	On The Right
61089	Passive Motion, Right ___degrees	61111	Active Motion ___degrees
		61112	Passive Motion ___degrees
61090	Passive Motion, Left ___degrees	10119	On The Left
		61113	Active Motion ___degrees
7739	Extension	61114	Passive Motion ___degrees
61091	Active Motion, Right ___degrees	10120	Bilaterally
		61115	Active Motion
61092	Active Motion, Left ___degrees	61116	Passive Motion
		7746	Abduction
61093	Passive Motion, Right ___degrees	61117	Active Motion, Right ___degrees
61094	Passive Motion, Left ___degrees	61118	Active Motion, Left ___degrees
		61119	Passive Motion, Right ___degrees
7740	Carpometacarpal	61120	Passive Motion, Left ___degrees
7741	Flexion	7747	Adduction
61095	Active Motion, Right ___degrees	61121	Active Motion, Right ___degrees
61096	Active Motion, Left ___degrees	61122	Active Motion, Left ___degrees
		61123	Passive Motion, Right ___degrees
61097	Passive Motion, Right ___degrees	61124	Passive Motion, Left ___degrees
61098	Passive Motion, Left ___degrees	7748	MCP
7742	Extension	7749	Flexion
61099	Active Motion, Right ___degrees	61125	Active Motion, Right ___degrees
61100	Active Motion, Left ___degrees	61126	Active Motion, Left ___degrees
61101	Passive Motion, Right ___degrees	61127	Passive Motion, Right ___degrees
61102	Passive Motion, Left ___degrees	61128	Passive Motion, Left ___degrees
7743	Abduction	7750	Extension
61103	Active Motion, Right ___degrees	61129	Active Motion, Right ___degrees
61104	Active Motion, Left ___degrees		

FINGERS, CONT.

61130	Active Motion, Left ___degrees	
61131	Passive Motion, Right ___degrees	
61132	Passive Motion, Left ___degrees	
7751	PIP	
7752	Flexion	
61133	Active Motion, Right ___degrees	
61134	Active Motion, Left ___degrees	
61135	Passive Motion, Right ___degrees	
61136	Passive Motion, Left ___degrees	
7753	Extension	
61137	Active Motion, Right ___degrees	
61138	Active Motion, Left ___degrees	
61139	Passive Motion, Right ___degrees	
61140	Passive Motion, Left ___degrees	
7754	DIP	
7755	Flexion	
61141	Active Motion, Right ___degrees	
61142	Active Motion, Left ___degrees	
61143	Passive Motion, Right ___degrees	
61144	Passive Motion, Left ___degrees	
7756	Extension	
61145	Active Motion, Right ___degrees	
61146	Active Motion, Left ___degrees	
61147	Passive Motion, Right ___degrees	
61148	Passive Motion, Left ___degrees	
7757	Middle Finger	
10121	On The Right	
61149	Active Motion ___degrees	
61150	Passive Motion ___degrees	
10122	On The Left	
61151	Active Motion ___degrees	
61152	Passive Motion ___degrees	
10123	Bilaterally	
61153	Active Motion	

61154	Passive Motion	
7758	Abduction	
61155	Active Motion, Right ___degrees	
61156	Active Motion, Left ___degrees	
61157	Passive Motion, Right ___degrees	
61158	Passive Motion, Left ___degrees	
7759	Adduction	
61159	Active Motion, Right ___degrees	
61160	Active Motion, Left ___degrees	
61161	Passive Motion, Right ___degrees	
61162	Passive Motion, Left ___degrees	
7760	MCP	
7761	Flexion	
61163	Active Motion, Right ___degrees	
61164	Active Motion, Left ___degrees	
61165	Passive Motion, Right ___degrees	
61166	Passive Motion, Left ___degrees	
7762	Extension	
61167	Active Motion, Right ___degrees	
61168	Active Motion, Left ___degrees	
61169	Passive Motion, Right ___degrees	
61170	Passive Motion, Left ___degrees	
7763	PIP	
7764	Flexion	
61171	Active Motion, Right ___degrees	
61172	Active Motion, Left ___degrees	
61173	Passive Motion, Right ___degrees	
61174	Passive Motion, Left ___degrees	
7765	Extension	
61175	Active Motion, Right ___degrees	
61176	Active Motion, Left ___degrees	
61177	Passive Motion, Right ___degrees	

FINGERS, CONT.

61178	Passive Motion, Left ___degrees	61203	Passive Motion, Right ___degrees
7766	DIP	61204	Passive Motion, Left ___degrees
7767	Flexion		
61179	Active Motion, Right ___degrees	7774	Extension
61180	Active Motion, Left ___degrees	61205	Active Motion, Right ___degrees
61181	Passive Motion, Right ___degrees	61206	Active Motion, Left ___degrees
61182	Passive Motion, Left ___degrees	61207	Passive Motion, Right ___degrees
7768	Extension	61208	Passive Motion, Left ___degrees
61183	Active Motion, Right ___degrees	7775	PIP
61184	Active Motion, Left ___degrees	7776	Flexion
61185	Passive Motion, Right ___degrees	61209	Active Motion, Right ___degrees
61186	Passive Motion, Left ___degrees	61210	Active Motion, Left ___degrees
7769	Ring Finger	61211	Passive Motion, Right ___degrees
10124	On The Right	61212	Passive Motion, Left ___degrees
61187	Active Motion ___degrees	7777	Extension
61188	Passive Motion ___degrees	61213	Active Motion, Right ___degrees
10125	On The Left	61214	Active Motion, Left ___degrees
61189	Active Motion ___degrees		
61190	Passive Motion ___degrees	61215	Passive Motion, Right ___degrees
10126	Bilaterally	61216	Passive Motion, Left ___degrees
61191	Active Motion		
61192	Passive Motion	7778	DIP
7770	Abduction	7779	Flexion
61193	Active Motion, Right ___degrees	61217	Active Motion, Right ___degrees
61194	Active Motion, Left ___degrees	61218	Active Motion, Left ___degrees
61195	Passive Motion, Right ___degrees	61219	Passive Motion, Right ___degrees
61196	Passive Motion, Left ___degrees	61220	Passive Motion, Left ___degrees
7771	Adduction	7780	Extension
61197	Active Motion, Right ___degrees	61221	Active Motion, Right ___degrees
61198	Active Motion, Left ___degrees	61222	Active Motion, Left ___degrees
61199	Passive Motion, Right ___degrees	61223	Passive Motion, Right ___degrees
61200	Passive Motion, Left ___degrees	61224	Passive Motion, Left ___degrees
7772	MCP	7781	Little Finger
7773	Flexion	10127	On The Right
61201	Active Motion, Right ___degrees		
61202	Active Motion, Left ___degrees		

FINGERS, CONT.

61225	Active Motion ___degrees	7789	Extension
61226	Passive Motion ___degrees	61251	Active Motion, Right
10152	On The Left		___degrees
61227	Active Motion ___degrees	61252	Active Motion, Left
61228	Passive Motion ___degrees		___degrees
10128	Bilaterally	61253	Passive Motion, Right
61229	Active Motion		___degrees
61230	Passive Motion	61254	Passive Motion, Left
7782	Abduction		___degrees
61231	Active Motion, Right	7790	DIP
	___degrees	7791	Flexion
61232	Active Motion, Left ___degrees	61255	Active Motion, Right
61233	Passive Motion, Right		___degrees
	___degrees	61256	Active Motion, Left
61234	Passive Motion, Left		___degrees
	___degrees	61257	Passive Motion, Right
7783	Adduction		___degrees
61235	Active Motion, Right	61258	Passive Motion, Left
	___degrees		___degrees
61236	Active Motion, Left ___degrees	7792	Extension
61237	Passive Motion, Right	61259	Active Motion, Right
	___degrees		___degrees
61238	Passive Motion, Left	61260	Active Motion, Left
	___degrees		___degrees
7784	MCP	61261	Passive Motion, Right
7785	Flexion		___degrees
61239	Active Motion, Right	61262	Passive Motion, Left
	___degrees		___degrees
61240	Active Motion, Left	10112	Right Hand
	___degrees	61263	Active Motion ___degrees
61241	Passive Motion, Right	61264	Passive Motion ___degrees
	___degrees	10113	Left Hand
61242	Passive Motion, Left	61265	Active Motion ___degrees
	___degrees	61266	Passive Motion ___degrees
7786	Extension	10114	Both Hands
61243	Active Motion, Right	61267	Active Motion
	___degrees	61268	Passive Motion
61244	Active Motion, Left	10292	Hyperextensibility
	___degrees	10508	Tenderness On Palpation
61245	Passive Motion, Right	10509	Of The Right Hand
	___degrees	10510	Of The Left Hand
61246	Passive Motion, Left	10511	Of Both Hands
	___degrees	10512	Of The Thumb
7787	PIP	10513	On The Right
7788	Flexion	61269	MCP
61247	Active Motion, Right	61270	Ulnar
	___degrees	61271	Radial
61248	Active Motion, Left	61272	Volar
	___degrees	61273	Dorsal
61249	Passive Motion, Right	61274	Diffuse
	___degrees	62983	Proximal Phalanx
61250	Passive Motion, Left	62984	Ulnar
	___degrees	62985	Radial

FINGERS, CONT.

62986	Volar	63011	Diffuse
62987	Dorsal	61294	PIP
62988	Diffuse	61301	Ulnar
61275	IP	61302	Radial
61276	Ulnar	61303	Volar
61277	Radial	61304	Dorsal
61278	Volar	61305	Diffusely
61279	Dorsal	63012	Middle Phalanx
61280	Diffuse	63013	Ulnar
62989	Distal Phalanx	63014	Radial
62990	Ulnar	63015	Volar
62991	Radial	63016	Dorsal
62992	Volar	63017	Diffuse
62993	Nail	61295	DIP
62994	Diffuse	61306	Ulnar
10514	On The Left	61307	Radial
61281	MCP	61308	Volar
61282	Ulnar	61309	Dorsal
61283	Radial	61310	Diffusely
61284	Volar	63018	Distal Phalanx
61285	Dorsal	63019	Ulnar
61286	Diffuse	63020	Radial
62995	Proximal Phalanx	63021	Volar
62996	Ulnar	63022	Diffuse
62997	Radial	10518	On The Left
62998	Volar	61311	MCP
62999	Dorsal	61312	Ulnar
63000	Diffuse	61313	Radial
61287	IP	61314	Volar
61288	Ulnar	61315	Dorsal
61289	Radial	61316	Diffusely
61290	Volar	63023	Proximal Phalanx
61291	Dorsal	63024	Ulnar
61292	Diffuse	63025	Radial
63001	Distal Phalanx	63026	Volar
63002	Ulnar	63027	Dorsal
63003	Radial	63028	Diffuse
63004	Volar	61317	PIP
63005	Diffuse	61318	Ulnar
10515	Bilaterally	61319	Radial
10516	Of The Index Finger	61320	Volar
10517	On The Right	61321	Dorsal
61293	MCP	61322	Diffusely
61296	Ulnar	63029	Middle Phalanx
61297	Radial	63030	Ulnar
61298	Volar	63031	Radial
61299	Dorsal	63032	Volar
61300	Diffusely	63033	Dorsal
63006	Proximal Phalanx	63034	Diffuse
63007	Ulnar	61323	DIP
63008	Radial	61324	Ulnar
63009	Volar	61325	Radial
63010	Dorsal	61326	Volar

FINGERS, CONT.

61327	Dorsal	63058	Ulnar
61328	Diffusely	63059	Radial
63035	Distal Phalanx	63060	Volar
63036	Ulnar	63061	Dorsal
63037	Radial	63062	Diffuse
63038	Volar	61353	PIP
63039	Diffuse	61354	Ulnar
10519	Bilaterally	61355	Radial
10520	Of The Middle Finger	61356	Volar
10521	On The Right	61357	Dorsal
61329	MCP	61358	Diffusely
61330	Ulnar	63063	Middle Phalanx
61331	Radial	63064	Ulnar
61332	Volar	63065	Radial
61333	Dorsal	63066	Volar
61334	Diffusely	63067	Dorsal
63040	Proximal Phalanx	63068	Diffuse
63041	Ulnar	61359	DIP
63042	Radial	61360	Ulnar
63043	Volar	61361	Radial
63044	Dorsal	61362	Volar
63045	Diffuse	61363	Dorsal
61335	PIP	61364	Diffusely
61336	Ulnar	63069	Distal Phalanx
61337	Radial	63070	Ulnar
61338	Volar	63071	Radial
61339	Dorsal	63072	Volar
61340	Diffusely	63073	Diffuse
63046	Middle Phalanx	10523	Bilaterally
63047	Ulnar	10524	Of The Ring Finger
63048	Radial	10525	On The Right
63049	Volar	61365	MCP
63050	Dorsal	61366	Ulnar
63051	Diffuse	61367	Radial
61341	DIP	61368	Volar
61342	Ulnar	61369	Dorsal
61343	Radial	61370	Diffusely
61344	Volar	63074	Proximal Phalanx
61345	Dorsal	63075	Ulnar
61346	Diffusely	63076	Radial
63052	Distal Phalanx	63077	Volar
63053	Ulnar	63078	Dorsal
63054	Radial	63079	Diffuse
63055	Volar	61371	PIP
63056	Diffuse	61372	Ulnar
10522	On The Left	61373	Radial
61347	MCP	61374	Volar
61348	Ulnar	61375	Dorsal
61349	Radial	61376	Diffusely
61350	Volar	63080	Middle Phalanx
61351	Dorsal	63081	Ulnar
61352	Diffusely	63082	Radial
63057	Proximal Phalanx	63083	Volar

FINGERS, CONT.

63084	Dorsal	61403	Ulnar
63085	Diffuse	61404	Radial
61377	DIP	61405	Volar
61378	Ulnar	61406	Dorsal
61379	Radial	61407	Diffusely
61380	Volar	63108	Proximal Phalanx
61381	Dorsal	63109	Ulnar
61382	Diffusely	63110	Radial
63086	Distal Phalanx	63111	Volar
63087	Ulnar	63112	Dorsal
63088	Radial	63113	Diffuse
63089	Volar	61408	PIP
63090	Diffuse	61409	Ulnar
10526	On The Left	61410	Radial
61383	MCP	61411	Volar
61384	Ulnar	61412	Dorsal
61385	Radial	61413	Diffusely
61386	Volar	63114	Middle Phalanx
61388	Dorsal	63115	Ulnar
61389	Diffusely	63116	Radial
63091	Proximal Phalanx	63117	Volar
63092	Ulnar	63118	Dorsal
63093	Radial	63119	Diffuse
63094	Volar	61414	DIP
63095	Dorsal	61415	Ulnar
63096	Diffuse	61416	Radial
61390	PIP	61417	Volar
61391	Ulnar	61418	Dorsal
61392	Radial	61419	Diffusely
61393	Volar	63120	Distal Phalanx
61394	Dorsal	63121	Ulnar
61395	Diffusely	63122	Radial
63097	Middle Phalanx	63123	Volar
63098	Ulnar	63124	Diffuse
63099	Radial	10530	On The Left
63100	Volar	61420	MCP
63101	Dorsal	61421	Ulnar
63102	Diffuse	61422	Radial
61396	DIP	61423	Volar
61397	Ulnar	61424	Dorsal
61398	Radial	61425	Diffusely
61399	Volar	63125	Proximal Phalanx
61400	Dorsal	63126	Ulnar
61401	Diffusely	63127	Radial
63103	Distal Phalanx	63128	Volar
63104	Ulnar	63129	Dorsal
63105	Radial	63130	Diffuse
63106	Volar	61426	PIP
63107	Diffuse	61427	Ulnar
10527	Bilaterally	61428	Radial
10528	Of The Little Finger	61429	Volar
10529	On The Right	61430	Dorsal
61402	MCP	61431	Diffusely

FINGERS, CONT.

63131	Middle Phalanx	63157	MCP
63132	Ulnar	63158	PIP
63133	Radial	63159	DIP
63134	Volar	10546	On The Left
63135	Dorsal	63160	MCP
63136	Diffuse	63161	PIP
61432	DIP	63162	DIP
61433	Ulnar	10547	Bilaterally
61434	Radial	63163	MCP
61435	Volar	63164	PIP
61436	Dorsal	63165	DIP
61437	Diffusely	10548	Of The Ring Finger
63137	Distal Phalanx	10549	On The Right
63138	Ulnar	63166	MCP
63139	Radial	63167	PIP
63140	Volar	63168	DIP
63141	Diffuse	10550	On The Left
10531	Bilaterally	63169	MCP
10532	Tenderness On Motion	63170	PIP
10533	Of The Fingers Of The Right Hand	63171	DIP
64278	Active Motion	10551	Bilaterally
64279	Passive Motion	63172	MCP
10534	Of The Fingers Of The Left Hand	63173	PIP
64280	Active Motion	63174	DIP
64281	Passive Motion	10552	Of The Little Finger
10535	Of The Fingers Of Both Hands	10553	On The Right
64282	Active Motion	63175	MCP
64283	Passive Motion	63176	PIP
10536	Of The Thumb	63177	DIP
10537	On The Right	10554	On The Left
63142	MCP	63178	MCP
63143	IP	63179	PIP
10538	On The Left	63180	DIP
63144	MCP	10555	Bilaterally
63145	IP	63181	MCP
10539	Bilaterally	63182	PIP
63146	MCP	63183	DIP
63147	IP	9306	Hands
10540	Of The Index Finger	7677	Appearance
10541	On The Right	7696	Swelling Of Hands
63148	MCP	10173	On The Right
63149	PIP	10174	On The Left
63150	DIP	10175	Bilaterally
10542	On The Left	7697	Dorsal Aspect
63151	MCP	63184	Diffuse
63152	PIP	63185	Localized
63153	DIP	63186	To Anatomical Compartment
10543	Bilaterally	7698	Unilaterally
63154	MCP	10176	On The Right
63155	PIP	10177	On The Left
63156	DIP	10178	Bilaterally
10544	Of The Middle Finger	10179	Palmar Aspect
10545	On The Right	63187	Diffuse

FINGERS, CONT.

63188	Localized	63220	Malformation
63189	To Anatomical Compartment	7714	Spade Hand
10180	On The Right	61527	On The Right
10181	On The Left	61528	On The Left
10182	Bilaterally	61529	Bilaterally
7699	Swelling And Tenderness Of The Anatomical Snuffbox	7701	Simian Crease
		61524	On The Right
61520	On The Right	61525	On The Left
61521	On The Left	61526	Bilaterally
7700	Tender Palmar Edema Obliterating Normal Palmar Concavity	7683	Small Hand
		61486	On The Right
		61487	On The Left
61522	On The Right	61488	Bilaterally
61523	On The Left	10207	Deformity Of The Hands
63190	Redness Of Hands	10208	On The Right
63191	Dorsal Aspect	10209	On The Left
63192	Diffuse	10210	Bilaterally
63193	Localized	10211	Dorsal Aspect
63194	To Anatomical Compartment	10212	On The Right
63195	Right Hand	10213	On The Left
63196	Left Hand	10214	Bilaterally
63197	Bilaterally	10215	Palmar Aspect
63198	Palmar Aspect	10216	On The Right
63199	Diffuse	10217	On The Left
63200	Localized	10218	Bilaterally
63201	To Anatomical Compartment	7678	Enlargement
63202	Right Hand	7684	Muscle Atrophy
63203	Left Hand	7685	Hypothenar
63204	Bilaterally	61489	On The Right
63205	Nodules	61490	On The Left
63206	Tender	61491	Bilaterally
63207	Ulcerating	7686	Thenar
63208	Dorsal Aspect	61492	On The Right
63209	Right Hand	61493	On The Left
63210	Left Hand	61494	Bilaterally
63211	Bilaterally	7687	Interosseous
63212	Palmar Aspect	61495	On The Right
63213	Right Hand	61496	On The Left
63214	Left Hand	61497	Bilaterally
63215	Bilaterally	10580	Absence Of Hands
64284	Mass ___ cm	10581	On The Right
64285	Tender	10582	On The Left
64286	Ulcerating	10583	Bilaterally
64287	Dorsal Aspect	60446	Amputation
64288	Right Hand	60447	Right
64289	Left Hand	60448	Left
64290	Palmar Aspect	61519	Bilaterally
64291	Right Hand	7688	Localized Thickening Of Palmar Fascia
64292	Left Hand		
63216	Necrosis ___ cm	61498	On The Right
63217	Right Hand	61501	1st Ray
63218	Left Hand	61502	2nd Ray
63219	Bilaterally	61503	3rd Ray

HANDS, CONT.

61504	4th Ray	61541	On The Right
61505	5th Ray	61542	On The Left
61499	On The Left	10190	Palmar Aspect
61506	1st Ray	10191	On The Right
61507	2nd Ray	10192	On The Left
61508	3rd Ray	10205	Bilaterally
61509	4th Ray	10193	Tenderness On Movement Of Hands
61510	5th Ray	10194	On The Right
61500	Bilaterally	10195	On The Left
7692	With Dupuytren's Contracture	10196	Bilaterally
61515	On The Right	10197	Dorsal Aspect
61516	On The Left	10198	On The Right
7689	Abnormal Posture	10199	On The Left
7690	Carpal Spasm (thumb, wrist MCP flexed; IP ext. digits add.)	10200	Bilaterally
		10201	Palmar Aspect
61511	On The Right	10202	On The Right
61512	On The Left	10203	On The Left
7691	Clawhand (MCP hyperextended, IP flexed)	10204	Bilaterally
		7799	Weakness
61513	On The Right	7800	Interossei
61514	On The Left	7801	On The Right
7693	Volkmann's Ischemic Contracture (fingers flexed with slight extension possible	7802	On The Left
		7803	Bilaterally
		7804	Thumb Extension
61517	On The Right	7805	On The Right
61518	On The Left	7806	On The Left
7694	Loss Of Prominence Of Knuckle(s)	11120	Bilaterally
7695	Only One Affected	7807	Thumb Flexion
7725	Prominent Palmar Markings	7808	On The Right
61530	On The Right	7809	On The Left
61531	On The Left	11119	Bilaterally
61532	Bilaterally	61533	Thumb Opposition
10108	Limitation Of Movement Of Hands	61535	On The Right
64459	Full Range Of Motion	61536	On The Left
64460	Except As Noted	61537	Bilaterally
10109	On The Right	61534	Thumb Abduction
64293	Active Motion	61538	On The Right
64294	Passive Motion	61539	On The Left
10110	On The Left	61540	Bilaterally
64295	Active Motion	7810	Thumb Adduction
64296	Passive Motion	7811	On The Right
10111	Bilaterally	7812	On The Left
64297	Active Motion	7727	Hands Clumsy Or Awkward
64298	Passive Motion	7728	On The Right Only
7793	Tenderness On Palpation	7729	On The Left Only
10183	On The Right	7813	Wrist
10184	On The Left	7814	Appearance
10185	Bilaterally	10293	Swollen
10186	Dorsal Aspect	10294	On The Right
10187	On The Right	10295	On The Left
10188	On The Left	10296	Bilaterally
10189	Bilaterally	63221	Dorsal Aspect
7794	Palmar Prominence	63222	Right

HANDS, CONT.

63223	Left	63253	Diffuse
63224	Bilaterally	63254	Right
63225	Ventral Aspect	63255	Left
63226	Right	63256	Bilaterally
63227	Left	63257	Extensor Brevis Pollicis And
63228	Bilaterally		Abductor Pollicis
63229	Radial Aspect	63258	Right
63230	Right	63259	Left
63231	Left	63260	Bilaterally
63232	Bilaterally	63261	Longus Tendon Sheath
63233	Ulnar Aspect	63262	Right
63234	Right	63263	Left
63235	Left	63264	Bilaterally
63236	Bilaterally	63265	Nodules
7815	Diffuse	63266	Fixed
61543	On The Right	63267	Cyst-Like
61544	On The Left	63268	Dorsal Aspect
61545	Bilaterally	63269	Right
7816	Tenosynovial Compartments	63270	Left
7817	Extensor Pollicis Brevis And	63271	Bilaterally
	Abductor Pollicis	63272	Ventral Aspect
61546	On The Right	63273	Right
61547	On The Left	63274	Left
61548	Bilaterally	63275	Bilaterally
7818	Longus Tendon Sheath	63276	Radial Aspect
61549	On The Right	63277	Right
61550	On The Left	63278	Left
61551	Bilaterally	63279	Bilaterally
7819	Finkelstein's Test (forcible	63280	Ulnar Aspect
	ulnar deviation)	63281	Right
61552	On The Right	63282	Left
61553	On The Left	63283	Bilaterally
61554	Bilaterally	63284	Diffuse
7820	Redness	63285	Right
61555	On The Right	63286	Left
61556	On The Left	63287	Bilaterally
61557	Bilaterally	63288	Extensor Brevis Pollicis And
63237	Dorsal Aspect		Abductor Pollicis
63238	Right	63289	Right
63239	Left	63290	Left
63240	Bilaterally	63291	Bilaterally
63241	Ventral Aspect	63292	Longus Tendon Sheath
63242	Right	63293	Right
63243	Left	63294	Left
63244	Bilaterally	63295	Bilaterally
63245	Radial Aspect	63296	Deformity
63246	Right	63297	Subluxation
63247	Left	64299	On The Right
63248	Bilaterally	64300	On The Left
63249	Ulnar Aspect	64301	Bilaterally
63250	Right	9216	Warmth
63251	Left	61558	On The Right
63252	Bilaterally	61559	On The Left

WRIST, CONT.

61560	Bilaterally		10131	Bilaterally
7836	Tenderness On Palpation		61565	Active Motion
10483	On The Right		61566	Passive Motion
10484	On The Left		7822	Flexion
10584	Bilaterally		61567	Active Motion, Right
61583	Radial Aspect		61568	Active Motion, Left
61584	On The Right		61569	Passive Motion, Right
61585	On The Left		61570	Passive Motion, Left
61586	Bilaterally		7823	Extension
61587	Ulnar Aspect		61571	Active Motion, Right
61588	On The Right		61572	Active Motion, Left
61589	On The Left		61573	Passive Motion, Right
61590	Bilaterally		61574	Passive Motion, Left
61591	Dorsal Aspect		7824	Radial Motion
61592	On The Right		61575	Active Motion, Right
61593	On The Left		61576	Active Motion, Left
61594	Bilaterally		61577	Passive Motion, Right
61595	Volar Aspect		61578	Passive Motion, Left
61596	On The Right		7825	Ulnar Motion
61597	On The Left		61579	Active Motion, Right
61598	Bilaterally		61580	Active Motion, Left
7837	Tenderness On Motion		61581	Passive Motion, Right
10585	On The Right		61582	Passive Motion, Left
10586	On The Left		7827	Weakness
10587	Bilaterally		7828	Flexion
10588	Flexion		7829	On The Right
61599	On The Right		7830	On The Left
61600	On The Left		7831	Bilaterally
61601	Bilaterally		7832	Extension (wrist drop)
10589	Extension		7833	On The Right
61602	On The Right		7834	On The Left
61603	On The Left		7835	Bilaterally
61604	Bilaterally		9954	Abduction
10590	Radial Deviation / Abduction		9955	On The Right
61605	On The Right		9956	On The Left
61606	On The Left		9957	Bilaterally
61607	Bilaterally		9958	Adduction
10591	Ulnar Deviation / Adduction		9959	On The Right
61608	On The Right		9960	On The Left
61609	On The Left		9961	Bilaterally
61610	Bilaterally		7839	Forearm
7838	Flexion Causes Hand Pain In		7840	Appearance
	Median Nerve Distribution		10596	Swelling
9450	Phalen's Maneuver		10597	Of The Right Arm
7821	Limitation Of Movement		10598	Of The Left Arm
64302	Full Range Of Motion		10599	Of Both Arms
64303	Except As Noted		7847	Muscle Atrophy
10129	On The Right		61624	Extensor
61561	Active Motion		61625	On The Right
61562	Passive Motion		61626	On The Left
10130	On The Left		61627	Bilaterally
61563	Active Motion		61628	Flexor / Pronator
61564	Passive Motion		61629	On The Right

WRIST, CONT.

61630	On The Left	64461	Full Range Of Motion
61631	Bilaterally	64462	Except As Noted
64304	Subcutaneous Nodules	7849	Pronation
64305	Extensor Surface	61632	On The Right
64306	On The Right	61633	On The Left
64307	On The Left	61634	Bilaterally
64308	Bilaterally	7850	Supination
64309	Non-Extensor Surface	61635	On The Right
64310	On The Right	61636	On The Left
64311	On The Left	61637	Bilaterally
64312	Bilaterally	9962	Weakness
64313	Mass ___ cm	9963	Pronation
64314	Volar Aspect	9974	Of The Right Arm
64315	On The Right	9975	Of The Left Arm
64316	On The Left	9978	Of Both Arms
64317	Dorsal Aspect	9964	Supination
64318	On The Right	9976	Of The Right Arm
64319	On The Left	9977	Of The Left Arm
7841	Malformation	9979	Of Both Arms
7842	Absent Radius	7851	Tenderness On Palpation
61611	On The Right	10600	Of The Right Arm
61612	On The Left	61638	Proximal Dorsal
61613	Bilaterally	61639	Proximal Volar
7843	Shortened ___ cm	61640	Distal Dorsal
61614	On The Right	61641	Distal Volar
61615	On The Left	10601	Of The Left Arm
61616	Bilaterally	61642	Proximal Dorsal
10592	Deformity ___ cm	61643	Proximal Volar
10593	Of The Right Arm	61644	Distal Dorsal
10594	Of The Left Arm	61645	Distal Volar
10595	Of Both Arms	10602	Of Both Arms
63318	Short ___ cm	61646	Proximal Dorsal
63319	Of The Right Arm	61647	Proximal Volar
63320	Of The Left Arm	61648	Distal Dorsal
63321	Of Both Arms	61649	Distal Volar
10607	Absence	10603	Tenderness On Motion
10608	Of The Right Arm	10604	Of The Right Arm
10609	Of The Left Arm	10605	Of The Left Arm
10610	Of Both Arms	10606	Of Both Arms
60453	Amputation	7852	Elbow
60454	Right	7853	Appearance
60455	Left	7858	Swelling Of Elbow
61617	Bilaterally	10301	On The Right
7844	Volar Deviation Of Radial Head	10302	On The Left
61618	On The Right	10303	Bilaterally
61619	On The Left	7859	Fluctuant Posteriorly On Both
61620	Bilaterally		Sides Of Olecranon
7845	Bowing Of Ulna	61656	On The Right
7846	Bowing Of Radial Shaft	61657	On The Left
61621	On The Right	7860	Fluctuant Posteriorly Overlying
61622	On The Left		Olecranon
61623	Bilaterally	61658	On The Right
7848	Limitation Of Movement	61659	On The Left

FOREARM, CONT.

64320	Antecubital Fossa	61668	Passive Motion, Right
64321	On The Right	61669	Passive Motion, Left
64322	On The Left	7865	Extension
64323	Bilaterally	61670	Active Motion, Right
64324	Redness	61671	Active Motion, Left
64325	Olecranon Bursa	61672	Passive Motion, Right
64326	On The Right	61673	Passive Motion, Left
64327	On The Left	64343	Pronation
64328	Bilaterally	64344	Active Motion, Right
64329	Lateral Epicondyle	64345	Active Motion, Left
64330	On The Right	64346	Passive Motion, Right
64331	On The Left	64347	Passive Motion, Left
64332	Bilaterally	64348	Supination
64333	Medial Epicondyle	64349	Active Motion, Right
64334	On The Right	64350	Active Motion, Left
64335	On The Left	64351	Passive Motion, Right
64336	Bilaterally	64352	Passive Motion, Left
64337	Diffuse	7866	Tenderness On Palpation
64338	On The Right	10304	On The Right
64339	On The Left	10305	On The Left
64340	Bilaterally	10306	Bilaterally
7854	Olecranon Bursa Nodules	7867	Biceps Insertion
61650	On The Right	61674	On The Right
61651	On The Left	61675	On The Left
61652	Bilaterally	61676	Bilaterally
10633	Deformity	7868	Lateral Epicondyle
10634	On The Right	61677	On The Right
10635	On The Left	61678	On The Left
10636	Bilaterally	61679	Bilaterally
7855	Abnormal Carrying Angle	61680	Medial Epicondyle
7856	Cubitus Valgus	61681	On The Right
7857	Cubitus Varus	61682	On The Left
61653	On The Right	61683	Bilaterally
61654	On The Left	64353	Antecubital Fossa
61655	Bilaterally	64354	On The Right
7861	Forearm Supported By The Other Hand	64355	On The Left
		64356	Bilaterally
7862	Bony Equilateral Triangle	7869	With A Swollen Olecranon Bursa
7863	Limitation Of Movement	7870	With Supracondylar Swelling
64341	Full Range Of Motion	7871	Tenderness On Motion
64342	Except As Noted	10630	On The Right
10132	On The Right	10631	On The Left
61660	Active Motion	10632	Bilaterally
61661	Passive Motion	7872	Flexion
10133	On The Left	64358	Active Motion, Right
61662	Active Motion	64360	Against Resistance
61663	Passive Motion	64359	Active Motion, Left
10134	Bilaterally	64361	Against Resistance
61664	Active Motion	61684	Passive Motion, Right
61665	Passive Motion	61685	Passive Motion, Left
7864	Flexion	61686	Bilaterally
61666	Active Motion, Right	64357	Extension
61667	Active Motion, Left	64362	Active Motion, Right

ELBOW, CONT.

64363	Active Motion, Left		7877	Bicipital Hump
64364	Passive Motion, Right		7878	Angular Deformity
64365	Passive Motion, Left		61691	On The Right
7874	Supination		61692	On The Left
64367	Active Motion, Right		61693	Bilaterally
64368	Active Motion, Left		7879	Muscle Atrophy
61687	Passive Motion, Right		7880	Of The Biceps
61688	Passive Motion, Left		7881	On The Right
61689	Bilaterally		7882	On The Left
64366	Pronation		7883	Bilaterally
64369	Active Motion, Right		7884	Of The Triceps
64370	Active Motion, Left		7885	On The Right
64371	Passive Motion, Right		7886	On The Left
64372	Passive Motion, Left		7887	Bilaterally
7875	Arm		7889	Tenderness On Palpation
7876	Appearance		10611	On The Right
10622	Swelling		10612	On The Left
10623	Of The Right Arm		10613	Bilaterally
10624	Of The Left Arm		61694	Anterior
10625	Of Both Arms		61695	On The Right
64373	Redness		61696	On The Left
64374	Right		61697	Bilaterally
64375	Left		61698	Posterior
64376	Bilaterally		61699	On The Right
64377	Mass ___ cm		61700	On The Left
64378	Anterior		61701	Bilaterally
64379	Right		7890	Localized With Swelling
64380	Left		61702	On The Right
64381	Posterior		61703	On The Left
64382	Right		7891	With Erythema & Increased Warmth
64383	Left		61704	On The Right
64384	Medial		61705	On The Left
64385	Right		7892	Weakness
64386	Left		7893	Of The Biceps
64387	Lateral		7894	On The Right
64388	Right		7895	On The Left
64389	Left		7896	Bilaterally
10614	Deformity ___ cm		7897	Of The Triceps
10615	Of The Right Arm		7898	On The Right
10616	Of The Left Arm		7899	On The Left
10617	Of Both Arms		7900	Bilaterally
63310	Short		7901	Shoulder
63311	Of The Right Arm		7902	Appearance
63312	Of The Left Arm		10641	Swelling
63313	Of Both Arms		10642	On The Right
10618	Absence		10643	On The Left
10619	Of The Right Arm		10644	Bilaterally
10620	Of The Left Arm		64390	Redness
10621	Of Both Arms		64391	On The Right
60456	Amputation		64392	On The Left
60457	Right		64393	Bilaterally
60458	Left		64394	Mass ___ cm
61690	Bilaterally		64395	On The Right

ARM, CONT.

64396	On The Left	61728	On The Left
64397	Bilaterally	61729	Bilaterally
7914	Non-Tender	7915	Limitation Of Movement
61730	On The Right	64421	Full Range Of Motion
61731	On The Left	64422	Except As Noted
10637	Deformity	10135	On The Right
10638	On The Right ___ cm	61749	Active Motion
10639	On The Left ___ cm	61750	Passive Motion
10640	Bilaterally ___ cm	10136	On The Left
7912	Elevated Distal Clavicular End	61751	Active Motion
61706	On The Right	61752	Passive Motion
61707	On The Left	10137	Bilaterally
61708	Bilaterally	61753	Active Motion
7905	Winged Scapula	61754	Passive Motion
61709	On The Right	7916	Abduction
61710	On The Left	61755	Active Motion, Right
61711	Bilaterally	61756	Active Motion, Left
11161	Scapula High And Medially Rotated	61757	Passive Motion, Right
		61758	Passive Motion, Left
61712	On The Right	7917	Forward Flexion
61713	On The Left	61759	Active Motion, Right
61714	Bilaterally	61760	Active Motion, Left
7904	Humeral Head Displacement Anteromedially Under Coracoid	61761	Passive Motion, Right
		61762	Passive Motion, Left
61715	On The Right	7918	External Rotation
61716	On The Left	61763	At 0 Degrees Of Abduction
61717	Bilaterally	61764	Active Motion, Right
7906	Displaced Clavicular Fragment	61765	Active Motion, Left
61718	On The Right	61766	Passive Motion, Right
61719	On The Left	61767	Passive Motion, Left
7903	Minimal Elevation And Support With Contralateral Hand	61768	At 90 Degrees Of Abduction
		61770	Active Motion, Right
61720	On The Right	61769	Active Motion, Left
61721	On The Left	61771	Passive Motion, Right
7907	Muscle Atrophy	61772	Passive Motion, Left
7908	Deltoid	7919	Internal Rotation
60780	On The Right	61773	Active Motion, Right
60781	On The Left	61774	Active Motion, Left
61723	Bilaterally	61775	Passive Motion, Right
7909	Supraspinatus	61776	Passive Motion, Left
60782	On The Right	61777	Extension
60783	On The Left	61778	Active Motion, Right
61724	Bilaterally	61779	Active Motion, Left
7910	Infraspinatus	61780	Passive Motion, Right
60784	On The Right	61781	Passive Motion, Left
60785	On The Left	9965	Weakness
61725	Bilaterally	9967	Flexion
7911	Pectoralis Major	9983	Of The Right Shoulder
60786	On The Right	9984	Of The Left Shoulder
60787	On The Left	9985	Of Both Shoulders
61726	Bilaterally	63328	Extension
61722	Trapezius	64423	Of The Right Shoulder
61727	On The Right	64424	Of The Left Shoulder

SHOULDER, CONT.

64425	Of Both Shoulders	61800	On The Right
9966	Abduction	61801	On The Left
9980	Of The Right Shoulder	61802	Bilaterally
9981	Of The Left Shoulder	7928	At The Bicipital Groove
9982	Of Both Shoulders	61803	On The Right
9968	Adduction	61804	On The Left
9986	Of The Right Shoulder	61805	Bilaterally
9987	Of The Left Shoulder	7929	Of The Posterior Shoulder
9988	Of Both Shoulders	61806	On The Right
9971	Internal Rotation	61807	On The Left
9995	Of The Right Shoulder	61808	Bilaterally
9996	Of The Left Shoulder	7930	Tenderness On Motion
9997	Of Both Shoulders	10645	Of The Right Shoulder
9970	External Rotation	61809	Active Motion
9992	Of The Right Shoulder	64433	Against Resistance
64426	At 0 Degrees Of Abduction	61810	Passive Motion
64427	At 90 Degrees Of Abduction	10646	Of The Left Shoulder
9993	Of The Left Shoulder	61811	Active Motion
64428	At 0 Degrees Of Abduction	64434	Against Resistance
64429	At 90 Degrees Of Abduction	61812	Passive Motion
9994	Of Both Shoulders	10647	Of Both Shoulders
64430	At 0 Degrees Of Abduction	61813	Active Motion
64431	At 90 Degrees Of Abduction	64435	Against Resistance
7920	Tenderness On Palpation	61814	Passive Motion
10307	On The Right	7931	By Shoulder External Rotation
10308	On The Left		Against Resistance
10309	Bilaterally	64436	At 0 Degrees Of Abduction
7921	At The Acromial-clavicular Tip	64437	On The Right
61782	On The Right	64438	On The Left
61783	On The Left	64439	Bilaterally
61784	Bilaterally	64440	At 90 Degrees Of Abduction
7922	Subacromial	64441	On The Right
61785	On The Right	64442	On The Left
61786	On The Left	64443	Bilaterally
61787	Bilaterally	7932	By Shoulder Abduction Against
7923	At The Greater Tuberocity		Resistance
61788	On The Right	61815	In Internal Rotation
61789	On The Left	61817	On The Right
61790	Bilaterally	61818	On The Left
7924	With Swelling Of The Clavicle	61816	In Neutral Position
61791	On The Right	61819	On The Right
61792	On The Left	61820	On The Left
61793	Bilaterally	7933	Elbow Flexion Pain Referred To
7925	Of The Deltoid Muscle		Bicipital Origin
61794	On The Right	7934	Pain Referred To Deltoid Insertion
61795	On The Left	7936	Passive Motion 0-180 Degrees Is
61796	Bilaterally		Painless
7926	At The Pectoralis Major Insertion	7937	Muscle Weakness
	On Humerus	7938	Deltoid
61797	On The Right	7939	On The Right
61798	On The Left	7940	On The Left
61799	Bilaterally	7941	Bilaterally
7927	Of The Anterior Shoulder	7942	Supraspinatus

SHOULDER, CONT.

7943	On The Right	
7944	On The Left	
7945	Bilaterally	
7946	Infraspinatus	
7947	On The Right	
7948	On The Left	
7949	Bilaterally	
7950	Pectoralis Major	
7951	On The Right	
7952	On The Left	
7953	Bilaterally	
61732	Subscapularis	
61733	On The Right	
61734	On The Left	
61735	Bilaterally	
62525	Clavicle	
62526	Callus Formation	
62527	Right	
62528	Left	
7954	TMJ (Temporomandibular Joint)	
7955	Appearance	
7956	Oral Opening	
7957	Drooping Lower Jaw	
7958	Swelling	
7959	Movement	
7960	Click	
7961	Crepitus	
7962	Tenderness	
7963	At Angle Of Jaw	
7964	Cervical Spine	
7965	Appearance	
7966	At Trigger Point Of Cervical Muscles	
7967	Muscle Atrophy	
7968	Limitation Of Movement	
64444	Full Range Of Motion	
64445	Except As Noted	
7969	Flexion	
61821	Active Motion	
61822	Passive Motion	
7970	With Noise	
7971	Extension	
61823	Active Motion	
61824	Passive Motion	
7972	Rotation To The Left	
61825	Active Motion	
61826	Passive Motion	
7973	Rotation To The Right	
61827	Active Motion	
61828	Passive Motion	
7974	Lateral Flexion To The Left	
61829	Active Motion	
61830	Passive Motion	

7975	Lateral Flexion To The Right	
61831	Active Motion	
61832	Passive Motion	
7976	Tenderness On Palpation	
7977	To Percussion	
7978	On The Spine	
7979	On The Vertex	
7980	Of The Lower Cervical Spinous Process	
7981	Of The Trapezius Muscle	
10648	Tenderness On Motion	
11141	Right-sided	
11142	Left-sided	
7982	Weakness	
7983	Flexion	
7984	Extension	
64446	Rotation	
7985	Thoracolumbar Spine	
7986	Appearance	
62561	Normal Curvature	
7987	Scoliosis	
7988	A Single Curve	
7989	Disappearing With Extreme Spinal Flexion	
7990	A Complex Curve	
7991	Straight Back	
7992	Kyphosis	
7993	Curved	
7994	Disappearing With Extreme Spinal Flexion	
7995	Gibbus	
7996	List	
7997	Lordosis	
7998	Loss Of Normal Lumbar Lordosis	
7999	Thoracic Expansion	
8000	Rib Hump	
8001	Schoeber's Index (finger-floor distance)	
8002	Spinous Process	
8003	Stepwise Deformity L5-S1	
8004	Gap Between Two	
8005	Dorsal Spine	
8006	Dimple In The Skin Over It	
8007	Patch Of Hair Over It	
8008	Lipomatous Nevus Over It	
8009	Fluctuant Translucent Sac Over It	
8010	Fluctuant Nontranslucent Sac Over It	
8011	Mass ___ cm	
8013	Meningomyelocele	
8012	Heel-landing Test	
8014	Straight-leg Raising Test	
8015	Patrick's Test	

TMJ, CONT.

8016	Psoas Sign		61850	Passive Motion
8017	Limitation Of Movement		8186	Flexion
64447	Full Range Of Motion		61851	Active Motion, Right
64448	Except As Noted		61852	Active Motion, Left
8018	Flexion		61853	Passive Motion, Right
61833	Active Motion		61854	Passive Motion, Left
61834	Passive Motion		8187	Extension
8019	Extension		61855	Active Motion, Right
61835	Active Motion		61856	Active Motion, Left
61836	Passive Motion		61857	Passive Motion, Right
8020	Rotation To The Left		61858	Passive Motion, Left
61837	Active Motion		8188	Abduction
61838	Passive Motion		61859	Active Motion, Right
8021	Rotation To The Right		61860	Active Motion, Left
61839	Active Motion		61861	Passive Motion, Right
61840	Passive Motion		61862	Passive Motion, Left
8022	Lateral Flexion To The Left		8189	Adduction
61841	Active Motion		61863	Active Motion, Right
61842	Passive Motion		61864	Active Motion, Left
8023	Lateral Flexion To The Right		61865	Passive Motion, Right
61843	Active Motion		61866	Passive Motion, Left
61844	Passive Motion		8190	Internal Rotation
8024	Tenderness On Palpation		61867	Active Motion, Right
8025	To Percussion		61868	Active Motion, Left
8026	Sacrospinalis Spasm		61869	Passive Motion, Right
8027	At The Sciatic Notch		61870	Passive Motion, Left
8028	At The Sacroiliac Joint		8191	External Rotation
10649	Tenderness On Motion		61871	Active Motion, Right
8179	Hips		61872	Active Motion, Left
8180	Appearance		61873	Passive Motion, Right
10331	Swelling		61874	Passive Motion, Left
10332	On The Right		8192	Tenderness On Palpation
10333	On The Left		10335	On The Right
10334	Bilaterally		10336	On The Left
10653	Deformity		10337	Bilaterally
10654	On The Right		8193	Lateral
10655	On The Left		8194	Over The Groin
10656	Bilaterally		8195	Weakness
8181	Trendelenburg's Sign		10338	On The Right
8182	Iliac Horns		10339	On The Left
8183	Prominent Greater Trochanter		10340	Bilaterally
8184	Painless Bony Mass ___ cm		8196	Of The Pelvic Girdle
8185	Limitation Of Movement		8197	Of Flexion
64449	Full Range Of Motion		11121	On The Right
64450	Except As Noted		11122	On The Left
10148	On The Right		11123	Bilaterally
61845	Active Motion		8198	Of Extension
61846	Passive Motion		11124	On The Right
10149	On The Left		11125	On The Left
61847	Active Motion		11126	Bilaterally
61848	Passive Motion		8201	Tenderness On Motion
10150	Bilaterally		10650	On The Right
61849	Active Motion		10651	On The Left

Thoracolumbar Spine, cont.

10652	Bilaterally		11100	On The Right
9953	Pelvic Tilt		11101	On The Left
62529	Right Higher Than Left		11102	Bilaterally
10657	Buttocks		8200	Of Adduction
10658	Swelling		11103	On The Right
10659	On The Right		11104	On The Left
10660	On The Left		11105	Bilaterally
10661	Bilaterally		9972	Of Internal Rotation
10662	Tenderness On Palpation		9973	Of External Rotation
10663	On The Right		10689	Tenderness On Motion
10664	On The Left		10690	On The Right
10665	Bilaterally		10691	On The Left
10666	Tenderness On Motion		10692	Bilaterally
10667	On The Right		8121	Knee
10668	On The Left		8122	Appearance
10669	Bilaterally		8129	Swelling
8166	Thigh		10325	On The Right
8167	Appearance		10326	On The Left
10678	Swelling		10327	Bilaterally
10679	On The Right		8130	Fluctuant
10680	On The Left		61889	On The Right
10681	Bilaterally		61890	On The Left
10674	Deformity		61891	Bilaterally
10675	On The Right		8131	Subcutan Lower 1/2 Of Patella, Upper 1/2 Patellar Ligament
10676	On The Left		8123	Deformity
10677	Bilaterally		10697	On The Right
8168	Shortening Of The Thigh		10698	On The Left
60788	On The Right		10699	Bilaterally
60789	On The Left		8124	Genu Varum
8169	Abnormal Posture Of Thigh		61875	On The Right
63314	Short		61876	On The Left
63315	On The Right		61877	Bilaterally
63316	On The Left		8125	Genu Valgum
63317	Bilaterally		61878	On The Right
10685	Absence		61879	On The Left
10686	On The Right		61880	Bilaterally
10687	On The Left		8126	Genu Recurvatum
10688	Bilaterally		61881	On The Right
8170	Muscle		61882	On The Left
8171	Quadriceps Atrophy		61883	Bilaterally
8172	Hamstring Atrophy		8127	Of The Knee Held In Semiflexion
8173	Hypertrophy		61884	On The Right
8111	Hamstring Muscle Tightness		61885	On The Left
8174	Tenderness On Palpation		8128	Charcot's Joint
10682	On The Right		61886	On The Right
10683	On The Left		61887	On The Left
10684	Bilaterally		61888	Bilaterally
8175	Localized		8132	Cyst
8176	With Swelling		8133	Popliteal
8177	With Erythema And Increased Warmth		61892	On The Right
			61893	On The Left
8178	Weakness		8134	Of The Medial Knee
8199	Of Abduction			

THIGH, CONT.

61894	On The Right	61926	Active Motion, Left
61895	On The Left	61927	Passive Motion, Right
8135	Of The Lateral Knee	61928	Passive Motion, Left
61896	On The Right	8147	Extension
61897	On The Left	61929	Active Motion, Right
8136	Patella	61930	Active Motion, Left
8137	Crevice	61931	Passive Motion, Right
61898	On The Right	61932	Passive Motion, Left
61899	On The Left	10144	Abnormal Movement
61900	Bilaterally	8148	Hyperextension
8138	Crepitus	61933	On The Right
61901	On The Right	61934	On The Left
61902	On The Left	61935	Bilaterally
61903	Bilaterally	8149	Anterior Drawer Sign
8139	Lateral Shift	61936	On The Right
61904	On The Right	61937	On The Left
61905	On The Left	61938	Bilaterally
61906	Bilaterally	8150	Posterior Drawer Sign
8140	Increased Lateral Mobility	61939	On The Right
61907	On The Right	61940	On The Left
61908	On The Left	61941	Bilaterally
61909	Bilaterally	8151	Lateral Instability Of Knee
8141	Upward Shift	61942	On The Right
61910	On The Right	61943	On The Left
61911	On The Left	61944	Bilaterally
61912	Bilaterally	8152	Muscle Weakness
8142	Ballottement	8153	Of The Quadriceps
61913	On The Right	8154	On The Right
61914	On The Left	8155	On The Left
61915	Bilaterally	8156	Bilaterally
8143	Absent	8157	Of The Hamstring
61916	On The Right	8158	On The Right
61917	On The Left	8159	On The Left
61918	Bilaterally	8160	Bilaterally
8144	Painless Bony Mass ___ cm	8161	Tenderness On Palpation
9219	Warmth	10328	On The Right
10749	On The Right	61736	Medial
10750	On The Left	61737	Lateral
10751	Bilaterally	61738	Posterior
8145	Limitation Of Movement	61739	Patellofemoral
64451	Full Range Of Motion	10329	On The Left
64452	Except As Noted	61740	Medial
10145	On The Right	61741	Lateral
61919	Active Motion	61742	Posterior
61920	Passive Motion	61743	Patellofemoral
10146	On The Left	10330	Bilaterally
61921	Active Motion	61744	Medial
61922	Passive Motion	61745	Lateral
10147	Bilaterally	61746	Posterior
61923	Active Motion	61747	Patellofemoral
61924	Passive Motion	8162	With Swelling In The Suprapatellar
8146	Flexion		Region
61925	Active Motion, Right	61945	On The Right

KNEE, CONT.

61946	On The Left	61964		Bilaterally
61947	Bilaterally	8099		Muscle Atrophy
8163	Medial And Inferior To The Joint Line	11199		On The Right
		11200		On The Left
61948	On The Right	11201		Bilaterally
61949	On The Left	8100		Of The Tibialis Anterior
61950	Bilaterally	61965		On The Right
8164	At The Joint Line	61966		On The Left
61951	On The Right	61967		Bilaterally
61952	On The Left	8101		Of The Gastrocnemius
61953	Bilaterally	61968		On The Right
8165	Of The Patellar Tendon	61969		On The Left
61954	On The Right	61970		Bilaterally
61955	On The Left	8102		Of the quadriceps
61956	Bilaterally	8106		Distal Achilles Tendon Thickening
10693	Tenderness On Motion	61971		On The Right
10694	On The Right	61972		On The Left
10695	On The Left	61973		Bilaterally
10696	Both Knees	8108		Gap In The Distal Achilles Tendon
8097	Leg (Below Knee)	61974		On The Right
8098	Appearance	61975		On The Left
9398	Swelling	61976		Bilaterally
9399	Bilaterally	8103		Muscle Hypertrophy
9400	Unilaterally	8104		Of The Gastrocnemius
9401	On The Right	11196		On The Right
9402	On The Left	11197		On The Left
10700	Calf Swelling	11198		Bilaterally
10701	On The Right	8110		Palpable Nerves
10702	On The Left	61977		On The Right
10703	Bilaterally	61978		On The Left
10704	Deformity	61979		Bilaterally
10705	On The Right	8112		Mass ___ cm
10706	On The Left	61980		On The Right
10707	Bilaterally	61981		On The Left
8105	Short	61982		Bilaterally
61957	On The Right	8113		Tenderness On Palpation
61958	On The Left	10712		On The Right
10708	Absent	10713		On The Left
10709	On The Right	10714		Bilaterally
10710	On The Left	8114		In The Tibial Tubercle
10711	Bilaterally	61983		On The Right
10487	Amputation	61984		On The Left
10488	Right Leg Below Knee	61985		Bilaterally
10489	Right Leg Above Knee	8115		Localized In The Tibial Shaft
10490	Left Leg Below Knee	61986		On The Right
10491	Left Leg Above Knee	61987		On The Left
8107	Saber Shins	61988		Bilaterally
61959	On The Right	8116		With Erythema And Increased Warmth
61960	On The Left			
61961	Bilaterally	8117		Of The Achilles Tendon
8109	Bowed	61989		On The Right
61962	On The Right	61990		On The Left
61963	On The Left			

LEG, CONT.

61991	Bilaterally	60468	Left
8118	Of The Gastrocnemius	8079	Limitation Of Movement
61992	On The Right	64453	Full Range Of Motion
61993	On The Left	64454	Except As Noted
61994	Bilaterally	10141	On The Right
8119	Of The Anterior Tibial Muscle	62010	Active Motion
	Compartment	62011	Passive Motion
61995	On The Right	10142	On The Left
61996	On The Left	62012	Active Motion
61997	Bilaterally	62013	Passive Motion
8120	Edematous, Warm	10143	Bilaterally
10715	Calf Tenderness On Palpation	62014	Active Motion
10716	On The Right	62015	Passive Motion
10717	On The Left	8080	Dorsiflexion
10718	Bilaterally	62016	Active Motion, Right
10719	Tenderness On Motion	62017	Active Motion, Left
10720	On The Right	62018	Passive Motion, Right
10721	On The Left	62019	Passive Motion, Left
10722	Bilaterally	8081	Plantar Flexion
10723	Calf Tenderness On Motion	62020	Active Motion, Right
10724	On The Right	62021	Active Motion, Left
10725	On The Left	62022	Passive Motion, Right
10726	Bilaterally	62023	Passive Motion, Left
8072	Ankle	8082	Inversion
8073	Appearance	62024	Active Motion, Right
8074	Swelling	62025	Active Motion, Left
10316	On The Right	62026	Passive Motion, Right
10317	On The Left	62027	Passive Motion, Left
10318	Bilaterally	8083	Eversion
10727	Deformity	62028	Active Motion, Right
10728	On The Right	62029	Active Motion, Left
10729	On The Left	62030	Passive Motion, Right
10730	Bilaterally	62031	Passive Motion, Left
8075	Lateral And Posterior Displacement	8084	Tenderness On Palpation
	Of Talus	10319	On The Right
61998	On The Right	10320	On The Left
61999	On The Left	10321	Bilaterally
62000	Bilaterally	8085	Medial
8076	Increased Intermalleolar Distance	9218	Warmth
62001	On The Right	10752	On The Right
62002	On The Left	10753	On The Left
62003	Bilaterally	10754	Bilaterally
8077	Shortening Of The Malleolus To	8086	Tenderness On Motion
	Sole Distance	10322	On The Right
62004	On The Right	10323	On The Left
62005	On The Left	10324	Bilaterally
62006	Bilaterally	8087	With Dorsiflexion
8078	Charcot's Joint	8088	Weakness
62007	On The Right	8089	On Dorsiflexion
62008	On The Left	11116	On The Right
62009	Bilaterally	11117	On The Left
60466	Amputation	11118	Bilaterally
60467	Right	8090	On Plantar Flexion

LEG, CONT.

62032	On The Right		62044	On The Right
62033	On The Left		62045	On The Left
62034	Bilaterally		62046	Bilaterally
8091	On Inversion		8035	Equinovarus
62035	On The Right		62047	On The Right
62036	On The Left		62048	On The Left
62037	Bilaterally		62049	Bilaterally
8092	On Eversion		8036	Equinovalgus
62038	On The Right		62050	On The Right
62039	On The Left		62051	On The Left
62040	Bilaterally		62052	Bilaterally
8093	Foot Drop		8037	Equinus
8094	On The Right Only		62053	On The Right
8095	On The Left Only		62054	On The Left
8096	Bilaterally		62055	Bilaterally
8029	Foot		8038	Valgus
8030	Appearance		62056	On The Right
8031	Swelling		62057	On The Left
10310	On The Right		62058	Bilaterally
10311	On The Left		8039	Varus
10312	Bilaterally		62059	On The Right
10761	Plantar		62060	On The Left
10762	On The Right		62061	Bilaterally
10763	On The Left		8040	Pes
10764	Bilaterally		8041	Abductus
10765	Dorsum		62062	On The Right
10766	On The Right		62063	On The Left
10767	On The Left		62064	Bilaterally
10768	Bilaterally		8042	Adductus
10738	Deformity		62065	On The Right
10739	On The Right		62066	On The Left
10740	On The Left		62067	Bilaterally
10745	Bilaterally		8043	Cavus
10755	Plantar		62068	On The Right
10757	On The Right		62069	On The Left
10758	On The Left		62070	Bilaterally
10756	Dorsum		8044	Hippocampi
10759	On The Right		62071	On The Right
10760	On The Left		62072	On The Left
10811	Absent		62073	Bilaterally
10813	On The Right		8045	Planus (flatfoot)
10814	On The Left		62074	On The Right
10815	Bilaterally		62075	On The Left
60459	Amputated		62076	Bilaterally
60460	Right		8046	Achilles Tendon Insertion
60461	Left		8047	Swollen
61748	Bilateral		62077	On The Right
8032	Talipes		62078	On The Left
8033	Calcaneus		62079	Bilaterally
62041	On The Right		8048	Plantar
62042	On The Left		8049	Callus
62043	Bilaterally		62080	On The Right
8034	Calcaneovalgus		62081	On The Left

FOOT, CONT.

62082	Bilaterally	62113	On The Right
8050	Wart(s)	62114	On The Left
62083	On The Right	62115	Bilaterally
62084	On The Left	8069	Of Interdigital Space(s)
62085	Bilaterally	62116	On The Right
8051	Thickened Fascia	62117	On The Left
62086	On The Right	62118	Bilaterally
62087	On The Left	8070	Of The Dorsum Of The Foot
62088	Bilaterally	10731	On The Right
8053	Hallus Valgus	10732	On The Left
62089	On The Right	10733	Bilaterally
62090	On The Left	8071	Of The Instep
62091	Bilaterally	62119	On The Right
8054	Hallus Rigidus	62120	On The Left
62092	On The Right	62121	Bilaterally
62093	On The Left	10734	Plantar
62094	Bilaterally	10735	Of The Right Foot
8057	Corn(s)	10736	Of The Left Foot
62095	On The Right	10737	Both Feet
62096	On The Left	10772	Tenderness On Motion
62097	Bilaterally	10774	On The Right
8058	Dactylolysis Spontanea (Ainhum)	10775	On The Left
62098	On The Right	10776	Bilaterally
62099	On The Left	10777	Of The Dorsum Of The Foot
62100	Bilaterally	10778	On The Right
9217	Joint Warmth	10779	On The Left
8059	Limitation Of Movement	10780	Bilaterally
64455	Full Range Of Motion	10781	Plantar
64456	Except As Noted	10782	Of The Right Foot
10138	On The Right	10783	Of The Left Foot
10139	On The Left	10784	Both Feet
10140	Bilaterally	60772	Toes
8063	Tenderness On Palpation	8052	Appearance
10313	Of The Right Foot	10486	Swelling
10314	Of The Left Foot	10746	On The Right
10315	Both Feet	10747	On The Left
8064	Of The Calcaneal Tuberosity	10748	Bilaterally
62101	On The Right	10839	Great Toe
62102	On The Left	10840	On The Right
62103	Bilaterally	10841	On The Left
8065	At The Achilles Tendon Insertion	10842	Bilaterally
62104	On The Right	10843	2nd Toe
62105	On The Left	10844	On The Right
62106	Bilaterally	10845	On The Left
8066	Of The Heel	10846	Bilaterally
62107	On The Right	10847	Middle Toe
62108	On The Left	10848	On The Right
62109	Bilaterally	10849	On The Left
8067	Of The Medial Malleolus	10850	Bilaterally
62110	On The Right	10851	4th Toe
62111	On The Left	10852	On The Right
62112	Bilaterally	10853	On The Left
8068	Of The Metatarsus	10854	Bilaterally

TOES, CONT.

10855	Little Toe	60463	The Great Toe
10856	On The Right	60464	Right
10857	On The Left	60465	Left
10858	Bilaterally	8055	Hammer Toe
10741	Deformity	62122	On The Right
10742	On The Right	62123	On The Left
10743	On The Left	62124	Bilaterally
10744	Bilaterally	8056	Swelling, Erythema, Warmth Of
10859	Great Toe		Great Toe
10860	On The Right	62125	On The Right
10861	On The Left	62126	On The Left
10862	Bilaterally	62127	Bilaterally
10863	2nd Toe	10151	Limitation Of Movement
10864	On The Right	64457	Full Range Of Motion
10865	On The Left	64458	Except As Noted
10866	Bilaterally	11075	Of The Right Foot
10867	Middle Toe	11076	Of The Left Foot
10868	On The Right	10153	Great Toe
10869	On The Left	10154	On The Right
10870	Bilaterally	62128	Active Motion
10871	4th Toe	62129	Passive Motion
10872	On The Right	10155	On The Left
10873	On The Left	62130	Active Motion
10874	Bilaterally	62131	Passive Motion
10875	Little Toe	10156	Bilaterally
10876	On The Right	62132	Active Motion
10877	On The Left	62133	Passive Motion
10878	Bilaterally	10157	2nd Toe
10812	Absence	10158	On The Right
10816	On The Right	62134	Active Motion
10817	On The Left	62135	Passive Motion
10818	Bilaterally	10159	On The Left
10819	Great Toe	62136	Active Motion
10820	On The Right	62137	Passive Motion
10821	On The Left	10160	Bilaterally
10822	Bilaterally	62138	Active Motion
10823	2nd Toe	62139	Passive Motion
10824	On The Right	10161	Middle Toe
10825	On The Left	10162	On The Right
10826	Bilaterally	62140	Active Motion
10827	Middle Toe	62141	Passive Motion
10828	On The Right	10163	On The Left
10829	On The Left	62142	Active Motion
10830	Bilaterally	62143	Passive Motion
10831	4th Toe	10164	Bilaterally
10832	On The Right	62144	Active Motion
10833	On The Left	62145	Passive Motion
10834	Bilaterally	10165	4th Toe
10835	Little Toe	10166	On The Right
10836	On The Right	62146	Active Motion
10837	On The Left	62147	Passive Motion
10838	Bilaterally	10167	On The Left
60462	Amputated Toes	62148	Active Motion

TOES, CONT.

62149	Passive Motion
10168	Bilaterally
62150	Active Motion
62151	Passive Motion
10169	Little Toe
10170	On The Right
62152	Active Motion
62153	Passive Motion
10171	On The Left
62154	Active Motion
62155	Passive Motion
10172	Bilaterally
62156	Active Motion
62157	Passive Motion
8060	MTP
8061	PIP
8062	DIP
10485	Tenderness On Palpation
10769	On The Right
10770	On The Left
10771	Bilaterally
10879	Great Toe
10880	On The Right
10881	On The Left
10882	Bilaterally
10883	2nd Toe
10884	On The Right
10885	On The Left
10886	Bilaterally
10887	Middle Toe
10888	On The Right
10889	On The Left
10890	Bilaterally
10891	4th Toe
10892	On The Right
10893	On The Left
10894	Bilaterally
10895	Little Toe
10896	On The Right
10897	On The Left
10898	Bilaterally
10899	MTP
10900	PIP
10901	DIP
10773	Tenderness On Motion
10785	On The Right
10786	On The Left
10787	Bilaterally
10788	Great Toe
10789	On The Right
10790	On The Left
10791	Bilaterally
10792	2nd Toe

10793	On The Right
10794	On The Left
10795	Bilaterally
10796	Middle Toe
10797	On The Right
10798	On The Left
10799	Bilaterally
10800	4th Toe
10801	On The Right
10802	On The Left
10803	Bilaterally
10804	Little Toe
10805	On The Right
10806	On The Left
10807	Bilaterally
10808	MTP
10809	PIP
10810	DIP
11526	Other Findings
7650	Monoarticular
7651	Oligoarticular
7652	Polyarticular
7653	Asymmetric
7654	Swelling
7655	Hemarthrosis
7656	Subluxation
7657	Contracture
7658	Ankylosis
7659	Erythema
7660	Increased Warmth
7661	Tenderness
7662	In A Joint
7663	In Muscles
7664	In Bursae
7665	In Ligaments
7666	In Tendon(s)
7667	In Bone
7668	In A Bony Mass ___ cm
7669	Tendon Mass ___ cm
7670	Thickened Synovial Membrane
7671	Non-tender Bony Mass ___ cm
7672	Crepitus
7673	Click
7674	Hyperextensibility
7675	Active Motion Limited
7676	Passive Motion Limited
11140	Amputation(s)
8202	**Neurological System**
9311	Mental Status Findings
8203	Appearance
8204	Posture
8205	Stooped
8206	Rigid

NEUROLOGICAL, CONT.

8207	Erect	11203		Pulling Out Hair
8208	Opisthotonos	11204		Mouthing Hair
8209	Sitting Erect Leaning Forward	11205		Grinding Teeth
11211	Sitting Erect, Resists Being Horizontal	9243	Eccentric	
		9244		Odd Speech
11206	Extremities Flexed	9222	Multiple Patterns	
11207	Upper	8236	Chewing	
11208	Lower	8237	Smacking Or Licking Lips	
11209	Clenched Fists	8238	Blinking Eyelids	
9841	Looking Tired	8239	Head Turning	
8210	Clothing	8240	Picking	
8211	Dishevelled	8241	Waxy Flexibility	
8212	Eccentric	9301	Echokinesis (movement imitation)	
9246	Dramatic	8242	Echopraxia (repetitive movement imitation)	
8213	Revealing			
9225	Usually Worn By Opposite Sex Only	8243	Negativism	
		8244	Lethargy	
9356	Dusty	62159	Decreased Eye-to-eye Contact	
8214	Grooming	8245	Unresponsive To Questioning	
8215	Unkempt	8246		Transient
8216	Meticulous	8247	Catatonia	
8217	Excessive Cosmetics	10362	Infant Nonreactive To Parents	
8218	Older Than Stated Age	9359	Characteristics Of Cry	
8219	Younger Than Stated Age	9360	Volume	
8220	Unusual Appearing Child	9361	Weak	
8221	Effeminate	11210	Loud	
8222	Masculinized	9362	Pitch	
8223	Demonstrated Behavior	9363	Shrill	
8224	Psychomotor	9364	Harsh	
8225	Retardation	9365	Monotonous	
9293	Mild	9366	Rapidly Fluctuating	
9294	Moderate	9367	Extreme Changes	
9295	Severe	9368	Length	
9429	Profound	9369	Short Staccato	
8226	Restlessness	9370	Extended, Interfering With Inspiration	
8227	Hyperactivity			
8228	Agitation	9374	Tone	
8229	Impulsivity	9375	Flat	
8230	Violent	9376	Turbulent	
8231	Hyperalertness	9372	Threshold	
8232	Heightened Startle Reflex	9371	Delayed Response To Stimulus	
8233	Stereotypy (automatic behavior)	9373	Hypersensitive To Stimulus	
62158	Hand Wringing	9377	Cri-du-chat	
62160	Hand Flapping	8248	Attitude	
62161	Finger Twisting	8249	Distractible	
62162	Finger Flicking	8250	Inattentive	
62163	Complex Whole Body Movements	8251	Disinterested	
		9242	Indifferent	
8234	Consistent Use Of Foul Language	8252	Unable To Engage	
9256	Prevarication	8253	Guarded	
8235	Mannerisms	8254	Defensive	
9224	Typical Of Opposite Sex	8255	Evasive	
11202	Biting Nails	8256	Uncooperative	

NEUROLOGICAL, CONT.

8257	Hostile	
9237	Bitter	
8258	Uninhibited	
8259	Playful	
8260	Disinhibited	
8261	Ingratiating	
8262	Seductive	
62530	Shy	
62531	Uncommunicative	
9223	Multiple Distinct & Complex Personalities	
8263	Speech	
8264	Mute	
8265	Rate	
8266	Slowed	
8271	Rapid	
8272	Pressured	
9514	Rhythm	
9515	Erratic	
8267	Halting	
8268	Stuttering	
8269	Stammering	
8270	Tremulous	
8273	Volume	
8274	Decreased	
8275	Increased	
8276	Tone	
8277	Monotonous	
8278	Dramatic	
8279	Nasal	
9430	High-pitched	
8280	Hoarse	
8281	Articulation	
8282	Dysarthria	
8283	Paretic	
8284	Spastic	
8285	Ataxic	
8286	Lisp	
8287	Phonation	
8288	Dysphonia / Aphonia	
9303	Spastic	
9299	Involuntary	
8289	Language	
8290	Dysphasia / Aphasia	
8291	Fluent, Comprehends, Can't Repeat (Conduction)	
8292	Fluent, Doesn't Comprehend, Repeats (Transcortical Sensory)	
8293	Fluent, Doesn't Comprehend, Can't Repeat (Wernicke's)	
8294	Not Fluent, Comprehends, Repeats (Transcortical Motor)	

8295	Not Fluent, Comprehends, Can't Repeat (Broca's)
8296	Not Fluent, Doesn't Comprehend, Repeats (Isolation)
8297	Not Fluent, Doesn't Comprehend, Can't Repeat (Global)
8298	Naming Inability (Anomic)
8299	Colors
8300	Transient Impairment
8301	Difficulty Comprehending Written Word (Dyslexia)
9522	Difficulty Comprehending Spoken Word
10031	MMSE Skill Assessment
10032	Naming Pencil And Wristwatch
10033	Repeating A Sentence
10034	Following 3-stage Verbal Command
10035	Following A Written Command
10036	Writing A Sentence
10037	Copying A Design
8302	Writing
8303	Micrographia
9519	Poor Spelling
9520	Poor Grammar
9521	Poor Organization
8304	Echolalia
9302	Palilalia (repetition of own words)
8305	Using Neologisms
8306	Literal
8307	Verbal
9516	Uses Obscenities
9517	Uses Faulty Phrasing And Unrelated Word Groupings
9518	Uses Primitive Phrasing And Shortened Sentences
62532	Not Appropriate For Age
62534	Not Understood By Caregiver
62533	Frustrating The Child
8308	Affect
8309	Exuberant
8310	Excessive Laughing
8311	Elated
8312	Happy
8313	Proud
8314	Broad
8315	Full Ranging
8316	Inappropriate
8317	Silly
8318	Labile
9290	Bewildered

NEUROLOGICAL, CONT.

8319	Indifferent (la belle indifference)	8364	Level Of Consciousness
8320	Inertial	8365	Drowsy
8321	Blunted	8366	Stupor
8322	Flat	8367	Coma
9238	Restricted	62550	Glasgow Scale
9239	Unemotional	62551	Eyes Open Spontaneously (4)
9240	Humorless	62552	Eyes Open To Verbal Stimuli (3)
9241	Hard		
8323	Constricted	62553	Eyes Open To Pain Stimuli (2)
8324	Shallow	62554	Eyes Never Open (1)
8325	Anhedonic	62570	Verbal Response Oriented / Appropriate (5)
8326	Somber		
8327	Unhappy	62571	Verbal Response Disoriented / Inappropriate (4)
8328	Sad		
10006	Whimpering	62572	Verbal Response Of Inappropriate Words / Sounds (3)
8329	Tearful		
8330	Excessive Crying		
8331	Grieving	62573	Verbal Response Of Incomprehensible Sounds / Grunts (2)
8332	Pained Facies		
8333	Terrified		
8334	Frightened	62574	Verbal Response: None (1)
8335	Worried	62575	Best Motor Response: Obeys / Spontaneous (6)
8336	Irritable		
8337	Agitated	62576	Best Motor Response: Localizes Pain (5)
8338	Angered		
8339	Bizarre	62577	Best Motor Response: Flexion Withdrawal (4)
62535	Inconsolable		
62536	Quiet	62578	Best Motor Response: Flexion (Decorticate / Decerebrate Rigidity) (3)
8340	Mood		
8341	Euphoric		
8342	Expansive	62579	Best Motor Response: Decerebrate Rigidity (2)
8343	Joyous		
8344	Happy	62580	Best Motor Response: None (1)
8345	Pleased	62581	Total Score
8346	Inappropriate	8368	Intellectual Functions
8347	Lability	8369	No Cognitive Function
8348	Empty	10003	Estimated Intelligence
8349	Frustrated	10004	Low
8350	Futile	11523	Average
8351	Unhappy	10005	High
8352	Depressed	8371	Confusion
8353	Despairing	8370	Delirium
8354	In Pain	10007	Orientation
8355	Self-contemptuous	8372	Date
8356	Guilty	8374	Time
8357	Fearful	8373	Place
8358	Anxious	10000	Person
8359	Concerned	11524	Situation
8360	Irritable	8375	Memory
8361	Angry	8376	Remote
8362	Awed	8377	Recent
8363	Depressed, But Unlike Previous Grieving For A Death Or Loss	10029	Registration
		10030	Recall

NEUROLOGICAL, CONT.

8378	Confabulation	8416	Chronopsia
8379	Decreased Attention Span	8417	Depersonalization
10027	Calculation	8418	Derealization
10028	Serial Sevens	8419	Deja Vu
8380	Decrease In Concentrating Ability	8420	Jamais Vu
8381	Fund Of Knowledge	8421	Hallucinations
9523	Arithmetic Ability	8422	Auditory
9524	Difficulty Using Symbols	8423	Visual
9525	Difficulty Understanding Abstract Processes	8424	Peripheral
		8425	Religious
9526	Difficulty Performing Mental Calculations	8426	Colored
		8427	Autoscopic (vision of one's self)
9527	Difficulty Following Sequential Steps		
		8428	Olfactory
8382	Thought Processes	8429	Gustatory
8383	Thought Disorder	8430	Tactile
8384	Thought Insertion	8431	Formication
8385	Thought Withdrawal	8432	Kinesthetic
8386	Thought Broadcast	8433	Somatic
8387	Thought Control	8434	Mood Congruent
8388	Coherence (connectedness)	8435	Mood Incongruent
8389	Circumferentiality	9233	Occur Only In Presence Of Observer
8390	Tangentiality		
9232	Approximate Answering	8436	Thought Content
8391	Clang Associations	8437	Impaired Insight
8392	Thought Blocking	8438	Impaired Judgement
8393	Perserverent Thought	8439	Reduced Abstraction
8394	Loosening Of Associations	8440	Ideas Of Reference
9235	Word Salad	8441	Obsessions
8395	Incoherence	8442	Paranoid Ideations
8396	Rate Of Thought	8443	Delusions
8397	Racing Thoughts	8444	Paranoid
9528	Slowed	8445	Persecutory
8398	Poverty Of Thought	8446	Grandiose
8399	Learning Disability	8447	Somatic
8400	Reading	8448	Mood Congruent
8401	Arithmetic	8449	Mood Incongruent
8402	Language	8450	Suicidal
8403	Expressive	8451	Ideation
8404	Receptive	8452	Plan
8405	Perceptual Disturbances	8453	Intent
11759	Problems With Sight	8454	Homicidal
11760	Problems With Hearing	8455	Ideation
8406	Illusion	8456	Plan
8407	Auditory	8457	Intent
8408	Visual	8458	Examiner's Reaction To Patient
8409	Micropsia	8459	Excessive Fondness
8410	Macropsia	8460	Suspiciousness, Distrust, Or Dislike
8411	Olfactory	8461	Anxiety Or Feelings Of Intimidation
8412	Gustatory	8462	Sadness, Pity Or Compassion
8413	Tactile	8463	Lateralizing Cortical Functions
8414	Kinesthetic	11114	Right Side
8415	Somatic	11115	Left Side

NEUROLOGICAL, CONT.

8464	Right-left Disorientation	8516	On The Right Only
8465	Finger Agnosia	8517	On The Left Only
8466	Acalculia	8518	Bilaterally
8467	Visual Agnosia	8519	V2 (side of nose, infraorbital area, and upper lip)
8468	Visual Inattention (extinction)		
8469	On The Right Only	8520	On The Right Only
8470	On The Left Only	8521	On The Left Only
8471	Inability To Recognize Faces	8522	Bilaterally
8472	Drawing Apraxia	8523	V3 (chin and lower lip)
8473	Dressing Apraxia	8524	On The Right Only
8474	Constructional Apraxia	8525	On The Left Only
8475	Spatial Disorientation	8526	Bilaterally
8476	Neglect Of Body Part	8527	Corneal Reflex
8477	On The Right Only	8528	On The Right Only
8478	On The Left Only	8529	On The Left Only
8479	Tactile Inattention (extinction)	8530	Bilaterally
8480	On The Right Only	8531	Masseters
8481	On The Left Only	8535	Bilateral (Jaw droop)
8482	Stereognosis	8532	Jaw Deviation
8483	On The Right Only	8533	To The Right
8484	On The Left Only	8534	To The Left
8485	Two-point Discrimination	8536	Atrophy
8486	On The Right Only	8537	On The Right Only
8487	On The Left Only	8538	On The Left Only
8488	Graphesthesia	8539	Bilaterally
8489	On The Right Only	8540	Trismus
8490	On The Left Only	11085	On The Right
8491	Motor Apraxia	11086	On The Left
8492	Facial	11087	Bilaterally
8493	Of Gait	8541	Abducens - See Also: Eyes
8494	Cranial Nerves	8542	On The Right Only
8495	Olfactory	8543	On The Left Only
8496	Hyperosmia	8544	Bilaterally
8497	Hypoosmia / Anosmia	8545	Facial
8498	On The Right Only	8550	Peripheral (lower and upper face weak)
8499	On The Left Only		
8500	Bilaterally	8551	Right Only
8501	Optic - See Also: Eyes	8552	Left Only
8502	On The Right Only	8553	Bilaterally
8503	On The Left Only	8554	Loss Of Taste On Anterior 2/3 Of Tongue (Chorda Tympani)
8504	Bilateral		
8505	Oculomotor -See Also: Eyes	8555	On The Right Only
8506	On The Right Only	8556	On The Left Only
8507	On The Left Only	8557	Bilaterally
8508	Bilateral	8546	Central (lower face weak, upper face normal)
8509	Trochlear - See Also: Eyes		
8510	On The Right Only	8547	Right Only
8511	On The Left Only	8548	Left Only
8512	Bilateral	8549	Bilaterally
8513	Trigeminal	8558	Facial Asymmetry - See: Central/Peripheral Weakness
8514	Facial Sensation Decreased (Isolated)		
		8559	Palpebral Fissure Widened
8515	V1 (forehead and anterior scalp)	60774	Right

NEUROLOGICAL, CONT.

60775	Left
8560	Flattening Of Nasolabial Fold
60776	Right
60777	Left
8561	Mouth Droop
60778	Right
60779	Left
11088	Right-sided Weakness
11089	Left-sided Weakness
11090	Bilateral Weakness
8562	Acoustic - See Also: Ear
8563	On The Right Only
8564	On The Left Only
8565	Bilateral
8566	Glossopharyngeal
11091	Right-sided Loss
11092	Left-sided Loss
11093	Bilateral Loss
8567	Diminished Sensation On Palate & Pharynx
8568	On The Right Only
8569	On The Left Only
8570	Bilateral
8571	Loss Of Taste On Posterior 1/3 Of Tongue
8572	On The Right Only
8573	On The Left Only
8574	Bilateral
8575	Diminished Gag Reflex
8576	On The Right Only
8577	On The Left Only
8578	Bilateral
8579	Absent
8580	Vagus
8581	Diminished Palate Elevation
8582	Uvula Deviation
8583	To The Left
8584	To The Right
11094	Right-sided Loss
11095	Left-sided Loss
11096	Bilateral Loss
8585	Accessory (Cranial and Spinal)
8586	Diminished Shoulder Elevation (Trapezius)
8587	On The Right Only
8588	On The Left Only
8589	Bilateral
8590	Sternocleidomastoid Weakness
8591	On The Right Only
8592	On The Left Only
8593	Bilateral
11097	Right-sided Weakness
11098	Left-sided Weakness

11099	Bilateral Weakness
8594	Hypoglossal
8595	Tongue Protrusion
8596	Deviation
8597	To The Left
8598	To The Right
8599	Fasciculations
8600	On The Right
8601	On The Left
8602	On Both Sides
8603	Atrophy
8604	On The Left Side Only
8605	On The Right Side Only
8606	Bilateral
11127	Right-sided Loss
11128	Left-sided Loss
11129	Bilateral Loss
8607	Oculocephalic Reflexes Absent (Doll's eyes)
8608	Caloric Responses
8609	Absent
8610	Tonic Eye Deviation
8611	Nystagmus
8612	Conjugate Phasic
8613	Internuclear Ophthalmoplegia (Dissociated)
8614	Canal Paresis
8615	Sensation
8616	Pain / Temperature Decrease
8617	Of The Face
8618	On The Right Side
8619	On The Left Side
8620	On Both Sides
8621	Back Of The Head (C2 dermatome)
8622	On The Neck
8623	On The Right Side
8624	On The Left Side
8625	On Both Sides
8626	On The Shoulders
8627	On The Right Only
8628	On The Left Only
8629	On Both
8630	Of The Arm
8631	The Entire Arm
8632	On The Right
8633	On The Left
8634	Bilaterally
8635	The Outer Upper Arm (C5)
8636	The Right Only
8637	The Left Only
8638	Bilaterally
8639	The Radial Forearm, Thumb, And Index Finger (C6)

NEUROLOGICAL, CONT.

8640	The Right Only	8688	On The Knee And Medial Leg (L4)
8641	The Left Only		
8642	Bilaterally	8689	On The Right Only
8643	The Middle Finger Only (C7)	8690	On The Left Only
8644	The Right Only	8691	Bilaterally
8645	The Left Only	8692	On The Lateral Leg And Dorsum Of The Foot (L5)
8646	Bilaterally		
8647	The 4th And 5th Digits, Ulnar Hand And Distal Forearm (C8)	8693	On The Right Only
		8694	On The Left Only
8648	The Right Only	8695	Bilaterally
8649	The Left Only	8696	On The Sole Of The Foot And The Posterior Leg (S1)
8650	Bilaterally		
8651	The Ulnar Forearm And Arm (T1)	8697	On The Right Only
8652	The Right Only	8698	On The Left Only
8653	The Left Only	8699	Bilaterally
8654	Bilaterally	8700	On The Posterior Thigh (S2)
8655	The Axilla And Upper Subclavicular Chest (T2)	8701	On The Right Only
		8702	On The Left Only
8656	The Right Side Only	8703	Bilaterally
8657	The Left Side Only	8704	On The Dorsum Of The Foot Only
8658	On Both Sides		
8659	On The Hand	8705	On The Right Only
8660	On The Dorsal Aspect Of The Radial 3 1/2 Digits	8706	On The Left Only
		8707	Bilaterally
8661	On The Palmar Aspect Of The Radial 3 1/2 Digits	8708	On The Sole Of The Foot Only
		8709	On The Right Only
8662	Of The Ulnar 1 1/2 Digits	8710	On The Left Only
8663	Of The Leg / Foot	8711	Bilaterally
8664	The Entire Leg	8712	On The Buttock/perianal Region (S3,4,5)
8665	On The Right		
8666	On The Left	8713	On The Right Only
8667	Bilaterally	8714	On The Left Only
8668	On The Lateral Upper Thigh	8715	Bilaterally
8669	On The Right Only	8716	On The Distal Extremities (glove and stocking)
8670	On The Left Only		
8671	Bilaterally	9998	Peripheral Nerve Distribution
8672	On The Lower Medial Thigh And Knee	9999	Root / Radicular Distribution
		8717	Sensory Level
8673	On The Right Only	8718	At The Shoulders (C5)
8674	On The Left Only	8719	The Right Only
8675	Bilaterally	8720	The Left Only
8676	In The Inguinal Region (L1)	8721	At The Hands (C7)
8677	On The Right Side Only	8722	The Right Only
8678	On The Left Side Only	8723	The Left Only
8679	On Both Sides	8724	At The Clavicles (T2)
8680	On The Upper Thigh (L2)	8725	The Right Only
8681	On The Right Only	8726	The Left Only
8682	On The Left Only	8727	At The Nipples (T4)
8683	Bilaterally	8728	The Right Only
8684	On The Lower Thigh (L3)	8729	The Left Only
8685	On The Right Only	8730	At The Xiphisternum (T6-8)
8686	On The Left Only	8731	The Right Side Only
8687	Bilaterally		

SENSORY EXAMINATION, CONT.

8732	The Left Side Only	8779	Of The Ulnar Forearm And Arm
8733	At The Umbilicus (T10)		(T1)
8734	The Right Side Only	8780	On The Right Only
8735	The Left Side Only	8781	On The Left Only
8736	At The Symphysis Pubis (T12)	8782	Bilaterally
8737	The Right Side Only	8783	On The Axilla And Upper
8738	The Left Side Only		Subclavicular Chest (T2)
8739	Hemisensory	8784	On The Right Side Only
8740	The Entire Right Side	8785	On The Left Side Only
8741	The Right Side, Sparing The	8786	On Both Sides
	Right Face	8787	On The Hand
8742	The Entire Left Side	8788	On The Dorsal Aspect Of The
8743	The Left Side, Sparing The Left		Radial 3 1/2 Digits
	Face	8789	On The Palmar Aspect Of The
10343	Pain / Temperature Increase		Radial 3 1/2 Digits
8744	Tactile Decrease	8790	Of The Ulnar 1 1/2 Digits
8745	Of The Face	8791	Of The Leg / Foot
8746	The Entire Right Side	8792	The Entire Leg
8747	The Entire Left Side	8793	On The Right
8748	Both Entire Sides	8794	On The Left
8749	Back Of The Head (C2 dermatome)	8795	Bilaterally
8750	On The Neck	8796	On The Lateral Upper Thigh
8751	On The Right Side	8797	On The Right Only
8752	On The Left Side	8798	On The Left Only
8753	On Both Sides	8799	Bilaterally
8754	On The Shoulders	8800	On The Lower Medial Thigh And
8755	On The Right		Knee
8756	On The Left	8801	On The Right Only
8757	On Both	8802	On The Left Only
8758	Of The Arm	8803	Bilaterally
8759	The Entire Arm	8804	In The Inguinal Region (L1)
8760	On The Right	8805	On The Right Side Only
8761	On The Left	8806	On The Left Side Only
8762	Bilaterally	8807	Bilaterally
8763	The Outer Upper Arm (C5)	8808	On The Upper Thigh (L2)
8764	On The Right Only	8809	On The Right Only
8765	On The Left Only	8810	On The Left Only
8766	Bilaterally	8811	Bilaterally
8767	The Radial Forearm, Thumb, And	8812	On The Lower Thigh (L3)
	Index Finger (C6)	8813	On The Right Only
8768	On The Right Only	8814	On The Left Only
8769	On The Left Only	8815	Bilaterally
8770	Bilaterally	8816	On The Knee And Medial Leg
8771	The Middle Finger Only (C7)		(L4)
8772	On The Right Only	8817	On The Right Only
8773	On The Left Only	8818	On The Left Only
8774	Bilaterally	8819	Bilaterally
8775	The 4th And 5th Digits, Ulnar	8820	On The Lateral Leg And Dorsum
	Hand And Distal Forearm (C8)		Of The Foot (L5)
8776	On The Right Only	8821	On The Right Only
8777	On The Left Only	8822	On The Left Only
8778	Bilaterally	8823	Bilaterally

SENSORY EXAMINATION, CONT.

8824	On The Sole Of Foot And The Posterior Leg (S1)	8872	Tactile Dysesthesia / Hyperesthesia	
8825	On The Right Only	8873	Vibration Decrease	
8826	On The Left Only	8874	On The Arm / Hand	
8827	Bilaterally	8875	On The Right	
8828	On The Posterior Thigh (S2)	8876	On The Left	
8829	On The Right Only	8877	Bilaterally	
8830	On The Left Only	8878	On The Leg / Foot	
8831	Bilaterally	8879	On The Right	
8832	On The Dorsum Of Foot Only	8880	On The Left	
8833	On The Right Only	8881	Bilaterally	
8834	On The Left Only	8882	All Four Limbs	
8835	Bilaterally	8883	On The Distal Extremities (glove and stocking)	
8836	On The Sole Of Foot Only	8884	Sensory Level	
8837	On The Right Only	8885	At The Iliac Spine	
8838	On The Left Only	8886	On The Right Only	
8839	Bilaterally	8887	On The Left Only	
8840	On The Buttock/perianal Region (S3,4,5)	8888	At The Xiphisternum	
		8889	At The Clavicles	
8841	On The Right Only	8890	The Right Only	
8842	On The Left Only	8891	The Left Only	
8843	Bilaterally (saddle area)	8892	Hemisensory	
8844	On The Distal Extremities (glove and stocking)	8893	The Right Side	
		8894	The Left Side	
8845	Sensory Level	11112	Vibration Hyperesthesia	
8846	At The Shoulders (C5)	8895	Position Decrease	
8847	On The Right	8896	Of The Arm / Hand	
8848	On The Left	8897	On The Right	
8849	At The Hands (C7)	8898	On The Left	
8850	On The Right	8899	Bilaterally	
8851	On The Left	8900	Of The Leg / Foot	
8852	At The Clavicles (T2)	8901	On The Right	
8853	On The Right	8902	On The Left	
8854	On The Left	8903	Bilaterally	
8855	At The Nipples (T4)	8904	All Four Limbs	
8856	On The Right	8905	On The Distal Extremities (glove and stocking)	
8857	On The Left			
8858	At The Xiphisternum (T6-8)	8906	Hemisensory	
8859	The Right Side Only	8907	On The Right Side	
8860	The Left Side Only	8908	On The Left Side	
8861	At The Umbilicus (T10)	11113	Position Hyperesthesia	
8862	The Right Side Only	8909	Romberg's Sign (balance lost without visual clues)	
8863	The Left Side Only			
8864	At The Symphysis Pubis (T12)	8910	Hemisensory Impairment - All Modalities	
8865	The Right Side Only			
8866	The Left Side Only	8911	On The Right	
8867	Hemisensory	8912	On The Left	
8868	The Entire Right Side	9438	"Peripheral Neuropathy"	
8869	The Right Side, Sparing The Right Face	8913	Motor	
		9385	Performance Of Examination	
8870	The Entire Left Side	9386	Complete Body	
8871	The Left Side, Sparing The Left Face	9387	Body Excluding Hands	
		9388	Hand(s) Only	

SENSORY EXAMINATION, CONT.

9389	Extremity (not hand)	60581	Left
61387	Trunk	60582	Bilaterally
8914	Power	60583	Wrists
63322	Neck	60588	Flexion
63323	Flexion ___ (0-5)	60589	Right
63326	Reduced	60590	Left
63324	Extension	60591	Bilaterally
63325	Rotation	60584	Extension
60549	Upper Extremities	60585	Right
60550	Right	60586	Left
60551	Left	60587	Bilaterally
60607	Bilaterally	60677	Abduction
60552	Shoulders	60678	Right
60665	Flexion	60679	Left
60666	Right	60680	Bilaterally
60667	Left	60681	Adduction
60668	Bilaterally	60682	Right
60669	Extension	60683	Left
60674	Right	60684	Bilaterally
60675	Left	60592	Fingers
60676	Bilaterally	60597	Flexion
60553	Abduction	60598	Right
60554	Right	60599	Left
60555	Left	60600	Bilaterally
60556	Bilaterally	60593	Extension
60670	Adduction	60594	Right
60671	Right	60595	Left
60672	Left	60596	Bilaterally
60673	Bilaterally	60685	Abduction
60557	Internal Rotation	60686	Right
60558	Right	60687	Left
60559	Left	60688	Bilaterally
60560	Bilaterally	60689	Adduction
60561	External Rotation	60690	Right
60562	Right	60691	Left
60563	Left	60692	Bilaterally
60564	Bilaterally	60601	Thumbs
60565	Elbows	60693	Flexion
60566	Flexion	60694	Right
60567	Right	60695	Left
60568	Left	60696	Bilaterally
60569	Bilaterally	60697	Extension
60570	Extension	60698	Right
60571	Right	60699	Left
60572	Left	60700	Bilaterally
60573	Bilaterally	60701	Abduction
60574	Forearms	60702	Right
60575	Pronation	60703	Left
60576	Right	60704	Bilaterally
60577	Left	60705	Adduction
60578	Bilaterally	60706	Right
60579	Supination	60707	Left
60580	Right	60708	Bilaterally

SENSORY EXAMINATION, CONT.

60709	Opposition	60611	Left
60710	Right	60612	Bilaterally
60711	Left	60613	Extension
60712	Bilaterally	60614	Right
60713	Index Fingers	60615	Left
60714	Flexion	60616	Bilaterally
60715	Right	60617	Abduction
60716	Left	60618	Right
60718	Extension	60619	Left
60719	Right	60620	Bilaterally
60720	Left	60621	Adduction
60721	Abduction	60622	Right
60722	Right	60623	Left
60723	Left	60624	Bilaterally
60724	Adduction	60754	Internal Rotation
60725	Right	60755	Right
60726	Left	60756	Left
60727	Middle Fingers	60757	Bilaterally
60728	Flexion	60625	External Rotation
60729	Right	60626	Right
60730	Left	60627	Left
60731	Extension	60628	Bilaterally
60732	Right	60629	Knees
60733	Left	60634	Flexion
60734	Ring Fingers	60635	Right
60735	Flexion	60636	Left
60736	Right	60637	Bilaterally
60737	Left	60630	Extension
60738	Extension	60631	Right
60739	Right	60632	Left
60740	Left	60633	Bilaterally
60741	Little Fingers	60638	Ankles
60742	Flexion	60639	Dorsiflexion
60743	Right	60640	Right
60744	Left	60641	Left
60745	Extension	60642	Bilaterally
60746	Right	60643	Plantar Flexion
60747	Left	60644	Right
60748	Abduction	60645	Left
60749	Right	60646	Bilaterally
60750	Left	60647	Inversion
60751	Adduction	60648	Right
60752	Right	60649	Left
60753	Left	60650	Bilaterally
60602	Upper Extremities Otherwise Normal	60651	Eversion
		60652	Right
60603	Lower Extremities	60653	Left
60604	Right	60654	Bilaterally
60605	Left	60655	Toes
60606	Bilaterally	60660	Flexion
60608	Hips	60661	Right
60609	Flexion	60662	Left
60610	Right	60663	Bilaterally

SENSORY EXAMINATION, CONT.

60656	Extension	8938	Generalized
60657	Right	8939	Hemi
60658	Left	8940	Hypertrophy - See Also:
60659	Bilaterally		Musculoskeletal
60758	Abduction	8941	Hemi
60759	Right	8942	Tone
60760	Left	8943	Spasticity
60761	Bilaterally	8944	Mono
60762	Great Toes	8945	Of The Right Arm
60763	Flexion	8946	Of The Left Arm
60764	Right	8947	Of The Right Leg
60765	Left	8948	Of The Left Leg
60766	Bilaterally	8949	Of The Right Side (hemi)
60767	Extension	8950	Of The Left Side (hemi)
60768	Right	8951	Para
60769	Left	8952	Quadra
60770	Bilaterally	8953	Decorticate Rigidity
60664	Lower Extremities Otherwise Normal	8954	Only On The Right
		8955	Only On The Left
8915	Paresis / Paralysis	8956	Decerebrate Rigidity
8916	Mono	8957	Only On The Right
8917	Of The Right Upper Extermity	8958	Only On The Left
8918	Of The Left Upper Extremity	8959	Rigidity
8919	Of The Right Lower Extremity	8960	Only On The Right
8920	Of The Left Lower Extremity	8961	Only On The Left
8921	Hemi	8962	Cogwheel Rigidity
8922	On The Left	8963	Only On The Right
8923	The Leg Weaker Than The Arm And Face	8964	Only On The Left
		8965	Gegenhalten (counterholding)
8924	The Face And Arm Weaker Than The Leg	8966	Only On The Right
		8967	Only On The Left
8925	The Arm And Leg Weaker Than The Face	9378	Weak Grasp
		62539	Hypertonicity
8926	On The Right	62540	Upper Extremities
8927	The Leg Weaker Than The Face And Arm	62541	Lower Extremities
		62542	Centrally
8928	The Face And Arm Weaker Than The Leg	8968	Hypotonicity (flaccid)
		8969	Mono
8929	The Arm And Leg Weaker Than The Face	8970	Of The Right Arm
		8971	Of The Left Arm
8930	Para	8972	Of The Right Leg
11496	Diplegia	8973	Of The Left Leg
8931	Quadra	8974	On The Right Side (hemi)
8932	Distal Weaker Than Proximal	8975	On The Left Side (hemi)
8933	Proximal Weaker Than Distal	62537	Upper Extremities
8934	Proximal Only	8976	Para
8935	Increased By Repeated Movement	8977	Quadra
8936	Decreased By Repeated Movement	62538	Central
11134	On The Right	8978	Bradykinesia
11135	On The Left	8979	Involuntary Movements
11136	Bilaterally	8980	Tremor
8937	Atrophy - See Also: Musculoskeletal	8981	Fine, Rapid
10341	Localized	8982	Coarse

SENSORY EXAMINATION, CONT.

8983	Rest	
8984	Intention	
8985	Only On The Right	
8986	Only On The Left	
8987	Action	
8988	Perioral (Rabbit Syndrome)	
8989	Pill Rolling	
8990	Wing Beating	
8991	On The Right Only	
8992	On The Left Only	
8993	Dystonia	
8994	Athetosis	
8995	Chorea	
8996	On The Right Side Only	
8997	On The Left Side Only	
8998	Flailing	
11137	One-sided	
8999	On The Right Side Only	
9000	On The Left Side Only	
9001	Myoclonus	
9002	Palatal Myoclonus	
9003	Myotonia	
9004	Asterixis	
9005	Facial Grimacing	
11466	Facial Myokymia	
9006	Tics	
9007	Hiccups	
9008	Tetany	
9009	Carpal-pedal Spasm	
9010	Chvostek's Sign	
9011	Trousseau's Sign (elicited by compressing the upper arm)	
9012	Fasciculations	
9013	Generalized Seizure	
9014	Adversive Seizure	
9015	To The Right	
9016	To The Left	
9017	Focal Seizure	
11110	Right Side	
11111	Left Side	
9018	Progressive, One-sided (Jacksonian)	
9019	Staring Spell	
9020	Muscle Spasms	
9021	Coordination / Cerebellum	
9022	Right Sided Incoordination Only	
9023	Left Sided Incoordination Only	
10342	Bilateral Incoordination	
9024	Dysdiadochokinesia	
11108	On The Right	
11109	On The Left	
9025	Dysmetria	
9026	Impaired Finger-to-nose Movement	

9027	On The Right Only
9028	On The Left Only
9029	Bilaterally
9030	Impaired Heel-to-shin Movement
9031	Using The Right Heel
9032	Using The Left Heel
9033	Bilaterally
11106	On The Right
11107	On The Left
9034	Past-pointing
9035	Gait And Stance
11874	Heel Walk
11875	Toe Walk
9036	Limping
10492	On The Right
10493	On The Left
9037	Ataxic Gait
9038	Staggering / Falling To The Right
9039	Staggering / Falling To The Left
9040	Wide Based
9800	Shuffling
11143	Hemiparetic
11144	Right Side
11145	Left Side
9041	Apractic Gait
9042	Propulsive Gait (Festinating)
9043	Spastic Gait
9044	Right Sided
9045	Left Sided
9046	Bilaterally (Scissors)
9047	Steppage Gait
9048	Waddling Gait (Trendelenburg)
9049	Astasia Abasia (Hysterical)
9050	Reflexes
9051	Deep Tendon Reflexes
9052	Reflex Patterns
9053	Absent Or Diminished Overall
9054	Absent Or Diminished On One Side Only
9055	On The Right
9056	On The Left
9057	Absent Or Diminished In The Entire Arm(s)
9058	Absent Or Diminished In Arm(s) But Hyperactive In The Leg(s)
9059	Absent Or Diminished In Both Legs (Para)
9060	Absent Or Diminished In One Entire Leg
9061	On The Right
9062	On The Left
9063	Hyperactive Overall
9064	With A Normal Jaw Jerk

SENSORY EXAMINATION, CONT.

9065	Except Decreased Ankle Jerks	9110	Thigh Adductor	
9066	Hyperactive On One Side Only	10500	Right (0-4)	
9067	On The Right Side	10501	Left (0-4)	
9068	On The Left Side	9111	Absent Or Diminished (Isolated)	
9069	In The Leg More Than The Arm	9112	On The Right Only	
		9113	On The Left Only	
9070	In The Arm More Than The Leg	9114	Bilaterally	
		9115	Hyperactive (Isolated)	
9071	Hyperactive In One Entire Arm	9116	On The Right Only	
9072	On The Right	9117	On The Left Only	
9073	On The Left	9118	Bilaterally	
9074	Hyperactive In Both Legs (Para)	9119	Knee Jerk	
9075	Hyperactive In One Entire Leg	10502	Right (0-4)	
9076	On The Right	10503	Left (0-4)	
9077	On The Left	9120	Absent Or Diminished (Isolated)	
9078	Pendular Overall	9121	On The Right Only	
9079	Pendular On One Side Only	9122	On The Left Only	
9080	On The Right Side	9123	Bilaterally	
9081	On The Left Side	9124	Hyperactive (Isolated)	
9082	Delayed Relaxation (hung up)	9125	On The Right Only	
9083	Biceps	9126	On The Left Only	
10494	Right (0-4)	9127	Bilaterally	
10495	Left (0-4)	9128	Hamstring	
9084	Absent Or Diminished (Isolated)	10504	Right (0-4)	
9085	On The Right Only	10505	Left (0-4)	
9086	On The Left Only	9129	Absent Or Diminished (Isolated)	
9087	Bilaterally	9130	On The Right Only	
9088	Hyperactive (Isolated)	9131	On The Left Only	
9089	On The Right Only	9132	Bilaterally	
9090	On The Left Only	9133	Hyperactive (Isolated)	
9091	Bilaterally	9134	On The Right Only	
9092	Brachioradialis	9135	On The Left Only	
10496	Right (0-4)	9136	Bilaterally	
10497	Left (0-4)	9137	Ankle Jerk	
9093	Absent Or Diminished ('Isolated')	10506	Right (0-4)	
9094	On The Right Only	10507	Left (0-4)	
9095	On The Left Only	9138	Absent Or Diminished (Isolated)	
9096	Bilaterally	9139	On The Right Only	
9097	Hyperactive ('Isolated')	9140	On The Left Only	
9098	On The Right Only	9141	Bilaterally	
9099	On The Left Only	9142	Hyperactive (Isolated)	
9100	Bilaterally	9143	On The Right Only	
9101	Triceps	9144	On The Left Only	
10498	Right (0-4)	9145	Bilaterally	
10499	Left (0-4)	9146	Clonus Of Ankle / Knee	
9102	Absent Or Diminished (Isolated)	9147	On The Right Only	
9103	On The Right Only	9148	On The Left Only	
9104	On The Left Only	9149	Bilaterally	
9105	Bilaterally	9150	Hyperactive Jaw Jerk	
9106	Hyperactive (Isolated)	9151	Hoffman's Present (Digital reflex)	
9107	On The Right Only	9152	On The Right Only	
9108	On The Left Only	9153	On The Left Only	
9109	Bilaterally	9154	Bilateral	

SENSORY EXAMINATION, CONT.

9155	Superficial Reflexes	60525	Right
9156	Abdominal Skin Reflexes Absent	60526	Left
9157	The Upper Right	60527	Bilateral
9158	The Upper Left	60528	Tinel's Sign
9159	The Lower Right	7826	Median Nerve At Wrist (Carpal Tunnel)
9160	The Lower Left		
9161	Cremasteric Reflexes Absent	60529	Right
9162	The Right Only	60530	Left
9163	The Left Only	60531	Ulnar Nerve At Wrist
9164	Bilateral	60532	Right
9165	Absent Bulbocavernosus Reflex	60533	Left
9166	Absent Anal Reflex	60534	Ulnar Nerve At The Ulnar Groove
9167	On The Right Side	60535	Right
9168	On The Left Side	60536	Left
9169	Pathologic Reflexes	60537	Tibial Nerve At The Tarsal Tunnel
9170	Babinski Reflex	60538	Right
9171	On The Left Only	60539	Left
9172	On The Right Only	60540	Peroneal Nerve At The Fibular Head
9173	Bilateral	60541	Right
9174	Primitive Reflexes	60542	Left
9175	Snout	60543	Sural Nerve At Midcalf
9176	Suck	60544	Right
9177	Root	60545	Left
9178	To The Right	60546	Sural Nerve At The Lateral Malleolus
9179	To The Left		
9180	Palmomental	60547	Right
9181	On The Right Only	60548	Left
9182	On The Left Only	9198	Neurological Findings Inconsistent/bizarre
9183	Bilateral		
9184	Grasp	9231	Findings Do Not Support Physical Symptoms
9185	On The Right Only		
9186	On The Left Only	9234	Findings Are Psychologically Inconsistent
9187	Bilaterally		
11155	Tonic Neck	9451	**Obstetrical**
9188	Peripheral Nerves	9452	Dysfunctional Labor
9189	Palpable	9453	Protracted
9190	Postauricular	9454	Arrested
9191	Ulnar	9536	Presentation At Delivery
9192	Common Peroneal	9537	Vertex
9193	Tender	9538	Breech
9194	Radial	9539	Footling
60516	Right	9540	Frank
60517	Left	9543	Transverse Lie
60518	Bilateral	9541	Nuchal Cord
9195	Ulnar	9542	Prolapsed Cord
60519	Right	9455	Malpresentation
60520	Left	9456	Breech
60521	Bilateral	9457	Frank
9196	Sciatic	9458	Complete
60522	Right	9459	Incomplete
60523	Left	9460	Brow
60524	Bilateral	9461	Face
9197	Common Peroneal	9462	Mentum Anterior

SENSORY EXAMINATION, CONT.

9463	Mentum Posterior		9506	Dark Staining
9464	Shoulder		9507	Polyp
9465	Transverse		9508	Mass ___ cm
9466	Oblique		64677	**Neonatal**
9467	Compound		9840	Apgar Score
9468	Cord		62543	At 1 Minute
9469	Prolapse		62544	At 5 Minutes
9470	Vasa Previa		9532	Findings At Birth
9471	Short		9533	Birthweight
9472	Rupture		9534	Length
9473	Knot		9535	Head Circumference
9474	True		9544	General Inspection
9475	False		9546	Physical Abnormality
9476	Hematoma		9547	Healthy Appearing Infant
9477	Nuchal		9548	Ill Appearing Infant
9478	Entanglement		9549	Skin
9479	Abnormal Insertion		9550	Thin And Translucent With Edema (Dubowitz=0)
9480	Battledore			
9481	Velamentous		9551	Smooth, Thin, Not Translucent, No Edema (Dubowitz=1)
9482	Inflammation			
9483	Edema		9552	Pink With Few Vessels Visible (Dubowitz=2)
62275	Bleeding			
62276	Foul Smelling		9553	Pink, Pale, Some Desquamation (Dubowitz=3)
62277	Drainage			
62520	Attached		9554	Thick, Pale, Desquamation Over Entire Body (Dubowitz=4)
62521	Not Dry			
62522	Not Attached		9851	Leathery, Cracked, Wrinkled (Dubowitz=5)
62523	Not Healed			
62524	Granuloma		62298	Milia
9484	Placenta		9555	Lanugo Hair
9485	Morphology		9852	Totally Absent (Dubowitz=0)
9486	Multiple		9556	Covering Entire Body (Dubowitz=1)
9487	Accessory Lobes		9557	Covering The Entire Body Except The Face (Dubowitz=2)
9509	Circumvallate			
9510	Circummarginate		9558	Present On Shoulders Only (Dubowitz=3)
9488	Postmature			
9489	Dysmature		9559	Mostly Bald (Dubowitz=4)
9490	Size		9560	Vernix Caseosa
9491	Large		9561	Thick Layer Covering Entire Body
9492	Small		9562	On Back, Scalp And In Skin Creases
9493	Location		9563	Scant Amount In Skin Creases
9494	Previa		9564	Absent
9495	Complete		9565	Hair
9496	Partial		9566	Present On Head, Eyebrows, And Lashes
9497	Centralis			
9498	Low-lying		9567	Fine And Wolly, Bunching Out From The Head
9499	Evidence Of Abruption			
9500	Abnormal Attachment		9568	Fine And Silky, Lying Flat On The Head
9501	Placenta Accreta			
9502	Placenta Increta		9569	Receding Hairline
9503	Placenta Percreta		9570	Absent
9504	Inflammation		9571	Fingernails
9505	Necrosis		9572	Do Not Extend To Fingertip

9573	Extend To Fingertip	9601	Palpable In Inguinal Canal
9574	Extend Beyond Fingertip	9602	Palpable In Upper Scrotum
9575	Ear	9603	Palpable In Lower Scrotum
9576	Form	9604	Scrotum
9577	Flat And Shapeless	9605	Few Rugae (Dubowitz=0)
9578	Beginnings Of Incurving At The Top	9606	Rugae Anterior Only (Dubowitz=2)
9579	Incurving Of The Top Two-thirds	9607	Rugae Cover Entire Scrotum (Dubowitz=3)
9580	Well-defined Curvature To The Lobe	9608	Pendulous Scrotum (Dubowitz=4)
9581	Cartilage	9609	Female Genitalia
9582	Pinna Is Soft And Stays Folded (Dubowitz=0)	9610	Prominent Labia Minora And Clitoris (Dubowitz=0)
9583	Scant And Unfolds Slowly (Dubowitz=1)	9611	Labia Majora And Minora Equal (Dubowitz=2)
9584	Thin, But Springs Back (Dubowitz=2)	9854	Labia Majora Larger Than Minora (Dubowitz=3)
9853	Well Formed And Springs Back (Dubowitz=3)	9612	Labia Minora And Clitoris Covered (Dubowitz=4)
9585	Pinna Is Firm And Ear Stays Erect (Dubowitz=4)	9613	Neurological Development
9586	Skull Firmness	9614	Posture
9587	Bones Are Soft	9615	Completely Hypotonic (Dubowitz=0)
9588	Bones Are Firm To Within 1 Inch Of Anterior Fontanelle	9616	Beginning Of Flexion Of The Thigh (Dubowitz=1)
9589	Bones Are Spongy Along Edge Of Anterior Fontanelle	9619	Beginning Flexion Of All Four Limbs (Dubowitz=2)
9590	Bones Are Hard But Sutures Are Easily Displaced	9617	Flexion Of The Thigh To 90 Degrees (Dubowitz=3)
9591	Bones Are Hard And Sutures Cannot Be Displaced	9618	Froglike Position (Dubowitz=4)
9592	Breast Tissue And Areola	9620	Hypertonic
9593	Barely Visible (Dubowitz=0)	9621	Very Hypertonic
9594	Areola Raised, No Breast Tissue (Dubowitz=1)	9622	Heel-to-ear Maneuver
9595	Areola Raised, 1-2 Cm. Of Breast Tissue (Dubowitz=2)	9623	No Resistance (Dubowitz=0)
		9624	Slight Resistance Approaching Ear (Dubowitz=0)
9596	Areola Raised, 3-5 Cm. Of Breast Tissue (Dubowitz=3)	9625	Limited To 135 Degree Arc (Dubowitz=1)
9597	Areola Raised, 5-6 Cm. Of Breast Tissue (Dubowitz=4)	9626	Limited To 110 Degree Arc (Dubowitz=2)
9598	Areola Raised, 7-10 Cm. Of Breast Tissue (Dubowitz=4)	9627	Limited To 90 Degree Arc (Dubowitz=3)
9855	Plantar Creases	9628	Limited To Less Than 90 Degree Arc (Dubowitz=4)
9856	Absent (Dubowitz=0)	9630	Popliteal Angle
9857	Faint Red Marks (Dubowitz=1)	9631	180 Degree Angle (Dubowitz=0)
9858	Anterior Crease Only (Dubowitz=2)	9632	160 Degree Angle (Dubowitz=1)
9859	Creases On Anterior 2/3 Of Foot (Dubowitz=3)	9633	130 Degree Angle (Dubowitz=2)
		9634	110 Degree Angle (Dubowitz=3)
9860	Creases Covering Entire Foot (Dubowitz=4)	9635	90 Degree Angle (Dubowitz=4)
		9636	Less Than 90 Degree Angle (Dubowitz=5)
9599	Male Genitalia		
9600	Testes	9637	Ankle Dorsiflexion

9638	40-50 Degrees	9885	Rolls From Front Onto Back
9639	20-30 Degrees	9886	No Head Lag When Pulled To Sitting
9640	Less Than 10 Degrees		Position
9845	Square Window	9887	Brings Hands Together
9846	90 Degree Wrist Angle	9888	Reaches For Objects
	(Dubowitz=0)	9868	6 Month Milestones
9847	60 Degree Wrist Angle	9889	Babbles
	(Dubowitz=1)	9890	Rolls Over From Back To Front
9848	45 Degree Wrist Angle	9891	Sits Without Support
	(Dubowitz=2)	9904	Pulls Self To A Standing Position
9849	30 Degree Wrist Angle	9892	Passes Objects From Hand To Hand
	(Dubowitz=3)	9893	Shy With Strangers
9850	0 Degree Wrist Angle	9869	12 Month Milestones
	(Dubowitz=4)	9894	Plays Pattycake
9641	Scarf Sign	9895	Waves Bye-bye
9642	Elbow Passes Opposite Shoulder	9896	Imitates Simple Daily Tasks
	(Dubowitz=0)	9897	Rolls A Ball Back To Examiner
9643	Elbow To Opposite Shoulder	9903	Drinks From A Cup
	(Dubowitz=1)	9898	Bangs Objects Together
9844	Elbow To Opposite Mid-axillary	9899	Has A Neat Pincer Grasp
	Line (Dubowitz=2)	9900	Scribbles Spontaneously
9644	Elbow To Midline Without	9901	Says Mama Or Dada Specifically
	Resistance (Dubowitz=3)	9902	And 3 Additional Words
9645	Elbow Short Of Midline	9905	Walks Holding Onto Furniture
	(Dubowitz=4)	9906	Stands Well Alone
9646	Forearm Recoil	9907	Walks Unassisted
9647	Absent At 180 Degrees	9870	18 Month Milestones
	(Dubowitz=0)	9908	Feeds Self
9648	Weak But Easily Inhibited At	9909	Helps With Simple Tasks
	100-180 Degrees (Dubowitz=2)	9910	Removes Clothes
9649	Present And Brisk But Can Be	9911	Turns Pages Without Ripping Them
	Inhibited (Dubowitz=3)	9912	Stacks Four Or More Blocks
9650	Present And Very Strong - Less	9913	Dumps Raisins From Bottle
	Than 90 Degrees (Dubowitz=4)	9914	Combines Two Different Words
9861	Dubowitz Score	9915	Points To Body Part On Request
9862	Gestational Age	9916	Names An Animal In A Picture
64675	**Growth And Development**	9917	Vocabulary Of 7-10 Words
9864	Developmental Assessment	9918	Kicks Ball Forward
9865	2-4 Week Milestones	9919	Throws Ball Overhand
9873	Responds To Sound	9920	Walks Up Steps
9874	Fixes On Faces	9871	24 Month Milestones
9875	Extremities Move Equally	9921	Puts On Clothing
9876	Lifts Chin Off Surface	9922	Washes And Dries Hands
9866	2 Month Milestones	9923	Separates From Parent Easily
9877	Has A Social Smile	9924	Plays Interactively With Other
9878	Gaze Follows Past Midline		Children
9879	Lifts Head And Chest Off Surface	9925	Stacks 8 Or More Blocks
9880	Head Steady In Sitting Position	9926	Turns Single Pages
9881	Hands Open 50% Of The Time	9927	Colors With Crayons
9867	4 Month Milestones	9928	Imitates A Vertical Line
9882	Turns Toward Voices	9929	Uses 2-3 Word Sentences
9883	Laughs	9930	Uses Plurals
9884	Uses Arms To Push Chest Off Surface	9931	Gives First And Last Name

DEVELOPMENTAL ASSESSMENT, CONT.

9932	Balances On One Foot For 1 Second	62548	User Finding:
9933	Jumps In Place		
9934	Can Pedal Tricycle		
9935	Runs Well		
9936	Walks Up And Down Stairs		
9872	36 Month Milestones:		
9937	Buttons Clothes		
9938	Dresses With Supervision		
9939	Dresses Without Supervision		
9940	Symbolic Play		
9941	Can Copy A Circle		
9942	Drawing A Person		
9943	Comprehends Cold, Hungry, Tired		
9944	Uses Prepositions		
9945	Uses Pronouns		
9946	Recognizes 3 Of 4 Colors		
9947	Balances On One Foot For 5 Seconds		
9948	Balances On One Foot For 10 Seconds		
9949	Hops On One Foot		
9950	Alternates Feet Walking Up Stairs		
11465	Delayed Milestones		
62545	Speech		
62546	Motor		
9951	Toilet Trained		
11174	Adolescent Sexual Maturation		
11175	Testicular Development		
11176	Size		
11177	Penis Length		
11178	Male Pubic Hair		
11179	None (ages 0-9)		
11180	Barely Visible At Ages 9-12		
11181	Scant But Present At Ages 12-15		
11182	Abundant At Base Of Penis At Age 15-16		
11183	Extending Down Inner Thighs For Ages 16 On		
11184	Breast Development		
11185	None (ages 0-10)		
11186	Buds Present At Age 10-11		
11187	Small Adult Breast At Ages 11-12		
11188	Areola And Nipple Forming Secondary Mound At Ages 12-14		
11189	Fully Developed Adult Breast At Ages 14 On		
11190	Female Pubic Hair		
11191	None (ages 0-10)		
11192	Sparse Growth At Age 10-11		
11193	Growth Spreading Over Symphysis Pubis At Age 11-12		
11194	Abundant Over Labia At Ages 12-14		
11195	Extending Down Inner Thigh After Age 13		
11454	Free Text:		

Part IV
TESTS

84443	**Common Office Tests**		22100	During Catheterization
12488	**Urinalysis**		22101	During A Radionuclide Ventriculogram
22279	Routine			
22282	Without Microscopy		22102	During A Thallium Scan
81299	Automated		24894	During A Sestamibi Scan
22281	Without Microscopy		24895	During A Teboroxime Scan
81300	Results:		24896	During A Tetraphosphamide Scan
12491	pH		19203	Rhythm Strip
12492	after acid loading		19204	Interpretation and Report Only
12489	Urine Specific Gravity		19205	Performance of Tracing Only
12497	Protein		19206	Telephonic / Telemetric Transmission
12493	Glucose		19207	Interpretation And Report
12496	Bilirubin		22098	3-Lead
81302	Ketones		22103	Heart Rate
81303	Hemoglobin		25716	At Rest
19672	Urobilinogen		25717	At End of Inspiration
19670	Nitrate		25718	At End of Expiration
19669	Leukocyte Esterase		25719	With Stress
12499	WBCs		25541	Intervals
12500	Too Numerous To Count		25542	R-R interval
12501	3 Glass		25839	At Rest
12503	RBCs		25840	At End of Inspiration
18167	Crenated		25842	At End of Expiration
12504	Casts		25843	With Stress
12509	Broad		22104	Sinus Rhythm
12512	Fatty		22105	With Ectopic Beats
12510	Granular		22106	Atrial Fibrillation
12505	Hemoglobin		22107	With Ectopic Beats
12506	Hyaline		22108	Atrial Flutter
12513	Mixed		22109	With Ectopic Beats
12508	RBC		22110	First Degree Block
12514	Renal tubular cell		22111	Second Degree Block
12511	Waxy		22114	Mobitz Type I
81447	WBC		22134	Mobitz Type II
12515	Crystals		22112	Third Degree Block
19500	Bilirubin		22113	A-V Dissociation
19502	Calcium carbonate		22115	Nodal Rhythm
19503	Calcium phosphate		22116	Pacemaker In Place
19499	Cystine		22117	Demand
19498	Pyrophosphate		22118	Fully Dependent
19501	Triple phosphate		22119	A-V Sequential
19497	Uric acid		22120	Eposidic Tachycardia
81467	Occult Blood		22121	Supraventricular
12006	**Hematocrit**		22122	Ventricular
81206	Microhematocrit		22123	Wide Complex
12136	**Prothrombin Time (PT)**		22124	QRS Configuration
12133	**Partial Thromboplastin Time (PTT)**		22127	Wide Complex
81184	Plasma Fraction Substitution		22125	Left Bundle Branch Block
13256	**Electrocardiogram**		22126	Right Bundle Branch Block
19198	Interpretation And Report Only		22234	**12-Lead**
19199	Performance of Tracing Only		22235	Interval Change
24893	Concurrent Imaging Study		13258	Atrial Rate
22099	During An Echocardiogram		13259	Greater Than Ventricular Rate

ELECTROCARDIOGRAM, CONT.

13257	Ventricular Rate		13304	During chest pain only
13260	Intervals		13305	Depressed
22250	R-R interval		13306	I
13261	PR interval		13307	II
13262	Increases Until Beat Dropped		13308	III
13263	Changes Continuously		13309	aVR
13264	QRS interval		13310	aVL
13265	QTc Interval (Corrected)		13311	aVF
13266	ST interval		13312	V1
13267	Axis		13313	V2
13268	LAD (Left Axis Deviation -30 To -90)		13314	V3
			13315	V4
13269	RAD (Right Axis Deviation +120 To +180)		13316	V5
			13317	V6
13270	Indeterminate (-90 To -179.99)		13318	Scooped
13271	QRST Angle		13319	Horizontal To Downsloping
13272	P Wave		13320	During chest pain only
13273	Absent		13321	Osborne 'J' Wave
13274	Axis		13322	T Waves
13275	-90		13323	Ta Waves
13276	Diminished		13324	Inverted
13277	Increased		13325	I
13278	Inverted		13326	II
13279	I		13327	III
13280	II		13328	aVR
13281	aVF		13329	aVL
13282	V6		13330	aVF
13283	aVR		13331	V1
13284	Retrograde		13332	V2
13285	Shifting Morphology		13333	V3
13286	ST Segment		13334	V4
13287	Isoelectric Convex Upward		13335	V5
13288	Elevated		13336	V6
13289	I		29303	V3r
13290	II		29304	V4r
13291	III		29305	V5r
13292	aVR		29306	V6r
13293	aVL		13337	While ST Segment Elevated
13294	aVF		13338	While ST Segment Is Isoelectric
13295	V1		13339	Asymmetrically
13296	V2		13340	Symmetrically
13297	V3		13341	Flat
13298	V4		13342	I
13299	V5		13343	II
13300	V6		13344	III
29299	V3r		13345	aVR
29300	V4r		13346	aVL
29301	V5r		13347	aVF
29302	V6r		13348	V1
13301	Upward Concavity		13349	V2
18041	With J Point Elevation		13350	V3
13302	Upward Convexity		13351	V4
13303	Persistent (>2 weeks)		13352	V5

ELECTROCARDIOGRAM, CONT.

13353	V6		13404	Pacemaker Sensing
13354	Tall Upright		13405	Atrial Activity Failing to Inhibit
13355	I		13406	Atrial Activity Failing to Trigger
13356	II		13407	Ventricular Activity Failing to Inhibit
13357	III			
13358	aVR		13408	Ventricular Activity Failing to Trigger
13359	aVL			
13360	aVF		13409	Intermittent Failure
13361	V1		13410	Constant Failure
13362	V2		13411	Left Atrial Hypertrophy (LAH)
13363	V3		13412	Broad Notched P Wave in I
13364	V4		13413	Broad Notched P Wave in II
13365	V5		13414	Diphasic P Wave in V1
13366	V6		13415	Right Atrial Hypertrophy (RAH)
13367	Symmetrical		13416	Tall Peaked P Waves in II
13368	Nonspecific ST-T Wave Changes		13417	Tall Peaked P Wave in III
13369	QRS		13418	Tall Peaked P Wave in aVF
13370	Low Voltage		13419	Peaked P Wave in V1
18043	High Voltage		13420	Diphasic P Wave in V1
13371	Wide Slurred		13421	Inverted P Wave in V1
13372	Q Waves		13422	Left Ventricular Hypertrophy (LVH)
13373	I		13423	R in V5-6 Greater Than 27mm.
13374	II		13424	S in V1 + R in V5-6 Greater Than 35mm.
13375	III			
13376	aVR		13425	QRS Greater Than 0.1 Sec. in V5-6
13377	aVL		13426	VAT Greater Than 0.5 Sec. in V5-6
13378	aVF		13427	R in aVL Greater Than 13mm.
13379	V1		13428	R in I and S in III Greater Than 26mm.
13380	V2			
13381	V3		13429	Right Ventricular Hypertrophy (RVH)
13382	V4		13430	R Greater Than S in V1
13383	V5		13431	Rs or qR in V1
13384	V6		13432	VAT Greater than 0.3 Sec in V1
13385	Tall R Wave V1		13433	Persistent S in V5-6
13386	Poor R Wave Progression		18045	Combined Ventricular Hypertrophy
18042	Early Transition		13434	Left Bundle Branch Block (LBBB)
13387	Absent		29350	Heart Rate Dependent
13388	Intermittently Absent		13435	RsR' rsR' or Broad Slurred R Wave in V4-6
13389	Sine Wave			
13390	U Wave		13436	VAT Greater Than 0.9 Sec. in V4-6
13391	Positive		13437	rSR' or Broad Notched R in I, II
13392	Negative		13438	Left Anterior Hemiblock
13393	Electrical Alternans		13439	qR in I, aVL
13394	Pacemaker Rhythm		13440	rS in II, III, aVF
13395	Excessively Fast		13441	Left Posterior Hemiblock
13396	Excessively Slow		13442	RS in I
13397	Pacemaker Capture		13443	qR in II, III, aVF
13398	Right Ventricular		13444	Incomplete LBBB
13399	Threshold Level		13445	RsR', rsR' Or Broad Slurred R Wave in V4-6
13400	Left Ventricular			
13401	Atrial		13446	VAT Less Than 0.9 Sec.
13402	Failure to Capture		13447	rsR' Or Broad Notched R in I, II
13403	Intermittent		13448	Right Bundle Branch Block (RBBB)

ELECTROCARDIOGRAM, CONT.

29351	Heart Rate Dependent	81011	Conduction Rate 4:1
13452	RSR', rsR' in V1-2	13522	Complete Heart Block
13449	Broad S Waves V5-6	13521	Constant AV Block
13450	VAT 0.06 Seconds or more in V1-2	13523	Paroxysmal Supraventricular tachycardia
13451	Broad S in I		
13453	Incomplete RBBB	13524	A-V Junctional Rhythms
13454	rSr' in V1	13525	Escape Beats
13455	VAT Less Than 0.06 Sec. in V1	13526	Premature Beats
13456	Intraventricular Conduction Delay (IVCD)	13527	Bigeminal
		13528	Trigeminal
13457	Alternating RBBB And LBBB	13529	Frequent
13458	Bifasicular Bundle Branch Block	13530	Consecutive
13459	Trifascicular Block	13531	Aberrant Conduction
13486	Sinus Rhythms	13532	Tachycardia
28559	Normal	24877	Bradycardia
13487	Tachycardia	13533	Ventricular Arrhythmias
13488	Bradycardia	13534	Escape Beats
13489	Arrhythmia	13535	Premature Depolarization
13490	Arrest	13536	Multifocal
13491	Sinus Node Wenckebach	13537	Superimposed on T Wave
13492	Sinoatrial Exit Block	13538	>5 per Minute
24874	Mobitz	13539	>30 per Hour
13495	Wandering Pacemaker	13540	Consecutive
13496	Atrial Arrhythmias	13541	Couplet
13497	Escape Beats	13542	Non-sustained ventricular tachycardia (3-6 beats)
13498	Atrial Premature Depolarization		
13499	Bigeminal	13543	Sustained ventricular tachycardia (7 or more beats)
13500	Trigeminal		
13501	Frequent	13544	Fusion Beats
13502	Consecutive	13545	Bigeminal
13503	With Aberrant Intraventricular Conduction (IVCD)	13546	Trigeminal
		13547	Tachycardia
13504	With block	13548	Accelerated Idioventricular Rhythm
24875	Atrial Tachycardia	13549	Fibrillation
13505	Automatic Atrial Tachycardia	18471	Asystole
22236	Paroxysmal Atrial Tachycardia	18000	Ventriculo-atrial conduction
13506	With Block	13550	Pararrhythmias
13507	Chaotic Atrial Rhythm	13551	Parasystole
13508	Bradycardia-Tachycardia Syndrome	13552	A-V Dissociation
13509	Flutter	13553	Preexcitation
13511	QRS Complexes in 2:1 to 8:1 ratio	13554	QRS Wide and Slurred
13512	Fibrillation	13555	Delta R Wave
13513	With Slow Ventricular Response	13556	Tall R in V1
13514	With Rapid Ventricular Response	13557	Tall R in V6
13510	with F Waves	13558	Negative QRS in V1
13515	1:1 A-V Conduction	13559	P-J Interval Normal
13516	Atrioventricular Block	13560	P-J Interval Shortened
13517	First Degree	22001	Fetal Findings
13518	Second Degree	22002	Arrythmias
13519	Mobitz Type I	22003	Sinus Rhythms
13520	Mobitz Type II	22004	Atrial Rhythms
81009	Conduction Rate 2:1	22005	Fibrillation
81010	Conduction Rate 3:1	22006	Flutter

ELECTROCARDIOGRAM, CONT.

22007	Premature Depolarization
22008	Ventricular Arrhythmias
22009	Premature Depolarization
22010	Atrioventricular Block
22011	First Degree
22012	Second Degree
22013	Mobitz Type I
22014	Mobitz Type II
22015	Complete Heart Block
13658	**Chest X-Ray**
84847	Views
22570	Single View, Frontal
22571	Stereo, Frontal
22572	Frontal And Lateral Views
22573	With Apical Lordotic Procedure
22574	With Oblique Projections
22575	With Fluoroscopy
22576	Complete, Four Or More Views
22577	With Fluoroscopy
22578	Lateral Decubitis View
22579	Bucky Study
84882	Hila
13716	Hilar Lymphadenopathy
13718	Unilateral
13717	Bilateral
18275	Symmetrical
18276	Asymmetrical
13719	Hilar Calcification
13720	Hilar "Eggshell" Calcification
84881	Lungs
13659	Infiltrate
13660	Unilateral
13661	Bilateral
13664	Apical predominance
13667	Basilar predominance
13663	Perihilar predominance
13665	Peripheral predominance
13672	Interstitial
13673	Nodular
13674	Reticular
13675	Reticular-Nodular
13686	Honeycomb Pattern
13681	Scarring
13682	Apical
13683	Basilar
17928	Peripheral
13678	Alveolar
13679	Lobar / localized
13680	Diffuse / patchy
18032	Air Bronchogram
13676	Miliary
13677	Pulmonary Calcification
18369	Diffuse Microcalcification

13685	Bowed Fissure
13684	Increased bronchovascular markings
13687	Solitary Pulmonary Nodule (cm.)
17929	Calcified
18111	"Popcorn" Pattern
13688	Multiple Pulmonary Nodules
18117	Calcified
18116	"Buckshot" Pattern
18109	Linear Strands Extending from Nodule(s) Towards Pleura
13691	Mass Lesion ___ cm
13692	Apical
13693	Hilar
13694	Peripheral
13695	Pleural Based
13696	Basal
13697	Mediastinal
18118	Anterior
18119	Middle
18120	Posterior
18121	Superior
18166	Containing calcified elements
13698	Cavitary Lesion
13699	Thin Walled
13700	Thick Walled
13701	Multiple
13702	Partially Filled with Air Meniscus
13689	Cyst(s)
13690	Bulla(e)
17926	Upper lobe
17927	Lower lobe
13703	Pneumatocele
13704	Hyperinflation
13705	Increased retrosternal air space
13712	Atelectasis
18219	Lobar
18220	Platelike
18218	Upper Lobe
18221	Bilateral
13713	Pneumothorax
18270	Air Containing Structure
13731	Pulmonary Edema
13732	Cardiogenic
13733	Noncardiogenic
84905	Pulmonary Vasculature
13780	Pulmonary Veins
13781	Superior Veins Dilated
13782	Inferior Veins Constricted
13783	Kerley A Lines (Central densities rad. outward)
13784	Present
13785	Absent

CHEST X-RAY, CONT.

13786	Kerley B Lines (Linear densities + pleura)	13765		Tumor
13787	Present	13766		Pericardial
13788	Absent	13767		Diaphragmatic
13789	Kerley C Lines	13768		Atria
13790	Present	13769		A-V Groove
13791	Absent	13770		Myocardial
13792	Congested	13771		Apical
13793	Pulmonary Arteries	13772		Valvular
13794	Central	13773		Mitral
13795	Dilated	13774		Aortic
13796	Diminished	13775		Annular
13797	Absent	13776		Smooth
13798	Peripheral	13777		Dense
13799	Dilated	13778		J-Shaped
13800	Diminished	13779		U-Shaped
13801	Absent	84907		Diaphragm
13722	Esophagus	13730		Flattened Diaphragm
13723	Widened	13725		Elevated Diaphragm
13724	Air fluid level present	13726		Unilateral
84906	Heart	13727		On The Right
13734	Heart Size, Shape	13728		On The Left
13735	Cardiomegaly	13729		Bilaterally
13736	LVE	85016		Pleura And Thoracic Wall
13737	LAE	18408		Subcutaneous air
13738	RVE	13706		Pleural Effusion
13739	RAE	13707		On The Right Only
13740	Cardiac Mass ___ cm	13708		On The Left Only
13741	Small	13709		Bilaterally
13742	Abnormal Shape	13710		Pleural Thickening
13743	Lengthened and narrowed	19076		On The Right Only
13744	Boot	19077		On The Left Only
13745	Waterbottle	19078		Bilaterally
82025	Dextrocardia	18217		Plaques
13746	Aorta	13711		Pleural Calcification
13747	Root	85018		Mass ___ cm
13748	Dilated	85346		Pleura ___ cm
13749	Decreased	85347		right ___ cm)
13750	Calcification Present	85353		Superior ___ cm
13754	Ascending	85357		Anterior ___ cm
13755	Dilated	85358		Lateral ___ cm
13756	Calcification Present	85362		Posterior ___ cm
13757	Prominent Knob	85366		Inferior ___ cm
13751	Descending	85367		Anterior ___ cm
13752	Dilated	85368		Lateral ___ cm
13753	Calcification Present	85369		Posterior ___ cm
13758	Right-sided	85373		Left ___ cm
13759	Cardiac Calcification	85374		Superior ___ cm
13760	Coronary Artery	85375		Anterior ___ cm
13761	Small Flecks	85376		Lateral ___ cm
13762	Tubular Flecks	85377		Posterior ___ cm
13763	Left Atrial	85379		Inferior ___ cm
13764	Curvilineal Density	85380		Anterior ___ cm
		85381		Lateral ___ cm

CHEST X-RAY, CONT.

85382	Posterior ___ cm		81207	Eosinophils
85617	Thoracic all ___ cm		81230	Manual Blood Smear (Without Diff)
85618	Right ___ cm		81211	Buffy Coat Smear
85619	Superior ___ cm		28602	Hemogram
85620	Anterior ___ cm		81143	With Platelet Count
85621	Lateral ___ cm		81145	With Manual Diff
85623	Posterior ___ cm		81212	Hemogram Indices
85624	Inferior ___ cm		81213	Red Cell Distribution Width
85625	Anterior ___ cm		81214	Mean Corpuscular Volume
85627	Lateral ___ cm		81215	Mean Corpuscular Hemoglobin Concentration
85629	Posterior ___ cm			
85630	Left ___ cm		81216	Mean Corpuscular Hemoglobin
85631	Superior ___ cm		81217	Stained Red Cell Examination
85632	Anterior ___ cm		81237	Fetal Red Cells
85633	Lateral ___ cm		81219	Mean Platelet Volume
85634	Posterior ___ cm		81220	Red Blood Cell Histogram
85635	Inferior ___ cm		81221	White Blood Cell Histogram
85639	Anterior ___ cm		81222	Platelet Histogram
85640	Lateral ___ cm		81224	One To Three Indices (Billing)
85644	Posterior ___ cm		81225	Four Or More Indices (Billing)
85017	Mediastinum		81236	Hemoglobin Studies
13714	Pneumomediastinum		12004	Hemoglobin
18029	Mediastinal Widening		12315	Electrophoretic Analysis
18222	Anterior		12316	Hgb A
18223	Middle		12317	Hgb A2
18224	Posterior		12318	Hgb C
13715	Mediastinal Lymphadenopathy		12319	Hgb D
18261	Unilateral		12320	Hgb F
18262	Bilateral		12321	Hgb H
18266	Symmetric		12322	Hgb M
18265	Asymmetric		12323	Hgb S
13721	Paratracheal		12324	Ratio HgbS/HbgA
18263	Containing Calcified Elements		81199	Copper Sulfate Method
18264	Mediastinal "Eggshell" Calcification		22547	Hemoglobin F, By Alkali Denaturation
84452	No Radiographic Evidence Of Osteoarticular Abnormalities Is Seen		81238	Fetal Hemoglobin (RBC) Stain
			81239	Rosette Screen
12001	**Hematology**		81203	Unstable Hemoglobin Screen
12002	Blood Cell Counts		81204	Thermolabile Hemoglobin
81209	CBC		12108	Methemoglobin
81146	With Differential		81200	Methemoglobin Screen
29342	With Manual Differential		81201	Plasma Methemoglobin
28605	With Partial Differential		12452	Sulfhemoglobin
81144	Manual CBC With Diff & Indices		81202	Qualitative Sulfhemoglobin
12003	RBC Count		27089	Iron Deficiency Anemia, Screening Exam
12114	Reticulocyte Count			
84451	Manual		12110	Iron Turnover Rate
81210	Automated		12365	Iron Binding Capacity (TIBC)
12012	WBC Count		12366	Saturation
81147	Manual Differential		12367	Iron / TIBC Ratio
12013	Neutrophils		12326	Ferritin
12016	Basophils		12331	Folate, Serum
12018	Lymphocytes		12332	Folate, RBC
12021	Monocytes		12113	Acidified Serum Lysis Test

HEMATOLOGY, CONT.

81426	Methemalbumin	12134	Bleeding Time (Ivy Method)
81240	Erythrocyte Tests	12135	Bleeding Time (Duke)
81151	Erythrocyte Sedimentation Rate	12132	Clotting Time
81152	Non-Automated	81160	Lee-White
12123	Wintrobe Method	81161	Activated
18052	Westergren Method	81162	Other Methods
22541	ZETA Method	12138	Clot Urea Solubility
81153	Automated	12139	Clot Retraction Time
81231	Heinz Body Stain	81163	Clot Lysis Time
81232	Heinz Body Induction	12149	Specific Clotting Factor Assays
12093	RBC Osmotic Fragility	81164	Factor II
22480	Incubated	12150	Factor V
81243	Autohemolysis	22518	Factor VII
81241	RBC Mechanical Fragility	12151	Factor VIII
12449	Sickle Cell Test	18512	Below 50%
12112	RBC Protoporphyrin	81165	Ristocetin-Willebrand Factor
81261	Screening	81166	Von Willebrand's Factor
81244	Acid Hemolysin Test	12152	Factor IX
12436	RBC Enzymes	22519	Factor X
12437	Glucose 6-Phosphate Dehydrogenase (G6PD)	22520	Factor XI
		22521	Factor XII
12438	Screening	22522	Factor XIII
12439	Glucose Phosphate Isomerase	81167	Screen Solubility
81260	Glutathione Reductase	81168	Fletcher Factor
81404	Glutathione	81169	Fitzgerald Factor
12440	Hexokinase	81186	Fibrinogen Antigen
12441	Phosphoglycerate Kinase	81188	Fibrin Split Products (By Agglutination)
81431	6-, Phosphogluconate Dehydrogenase	81187	Paracoagulation Test
12442	Pyruvate Kinase	12329	Screen
12443	Triose Phosphate Isomerase	81190	Fibrin Split Products (D-Dimer)
81150	Coagulation Studies	81189	Screen
81155	Plasma Fraction Substitution	81899	Factor Inhibitor Test
12137	Thrombin Time	12153	Factor Antigen Assays
81185	Titer	12154	Factor VIII
81257	Reptilase Time	81170	Von Willebrand
81154	Activated Partial Thromboplastin Time (APTT)	12155	Factor IX
		12156	Factor XI
81258	Russell Viper Venom Time	12157	Factor XII
81259	Diluted	12158	Factor XIII
12147	Platelet Adhesion	81193	Coagulopathy Screen
81242	Platelet Neutralization	81171	Anticoagulant Assays
12146	Platelet Retention	81172	Antithrombin III
12140	Platelet Aggregation	81173	Antithrombin III Antigen
12145	To Ristocetin	81174	Protein C Antigen
12141	To ADP	81175	Protein C
12143	To Collagen	81176	Total Protein S
12144	To Epinephrine	81177	Free Protein S
81156	Platelet Counts	81178	Thrombomodulin Test
81157	Manual Count	81196	Plasminogen Activator
81159	Automated Count	81179	Thromboplastin Inhibition (Tissue)
81158	Estimation From Smear	81198	Plasminogen Antigen Assay
81149	Bleeding Time	81180	Heparin Assay

HEMATOLOGY, CONT.

81181	Heparin Neutralization	81131	Pooling Of Platelets
22500	Tourniquet Test	81132	Preparation Of RBC's For Testing
81191	Euglobulin Lysis	81133	Chemical Incubation
81182	Heparin-Protamine Tolerance Test	81134	Enzymatic Incubation
12327	Plasma Fibrinogen	81135	Density Gradient Separation
81194	Plasmin Level	81136	Preparation Of Serum For RBC
81195	Alpha-2 Antiplasmin		Testing
81197	Plasminogen	81137	Chemical Incubation
81478	Cryofibrinogen	81138	Dilution
81192	Unlisted Coagulation Study	81139	Inhibitory Incubation
81103	Transfusion Tests And Procedures	81140	Differential Absorbtion
81104	RBC Antibody Screen	81141	Splitting Of Blood Products
81109	RBC Antibody Elution	81142	Unlisted Transfusion Procedure
81110	RBC Antibody Identification	81247	Hematopoietic Nuclear Studies
12290	Coombs Test	18064	Platelet Survival Test
12291	Direct	81253	Localized Platelet Survival Test
12292	Indirect - Qualitative	12103	RBC Clearance
81102	Indirect - Titer	12104	RBC Survival Time Test
81100	Blood Typing	81248	Sequestered RBC Survival Time
81106	ABO		Test
12464	Type A	81249	RBC Seqestration Test
12465	Type B	12107	Red Cell Mass
12466	Type AB	81250	Radioiron RBC Utilization
12467	Type O	22489	RBC Volume
81105	Duffy	28544	Multiple Samples
22617	Rh	12111	Plasma Volume
81108	Complete Rh Phenotyping	28542	Multiple Samples
81107	Other RBC Antigens	81251	Plasma Radioiron Turnover Rate
81113	Antigen Screen For Compatible	22516	Total Blood Volume
	Blood - Using Donor Serum	81254	Radioiron Oral Absorption
81118	Crossmatch	81255	Chelatable Iron Test
81119	Immediate Spin Method	81252	Unlisted Hematopoietic Nuclear Study
81121	Incubation Method	81256	Chromogenic Substrate Assay
81122	Antiglobulin Method	12122	Leukocyte Alkaline Phosphatase Stain
81114	Antigen Screen For Compatible	12161	Blood Viscosity
	Blood - Using Recipient Serum	12096	Blood Spectrophotometry
81115	Paternity Testing	12308	Lysozyme
81120	ABO, Rh, and MN	81229	Peripheral Blood Smear
81116	Additional Antigens	81233	Iron Stain
81111	Collection Of Predeposited Autologous	12039	Platelet Morphology
	Blood Components	12040	Atypical Forms
81112	Intra- Or Postoperative Collection Of	12041	Large Platelets
	Autologous Blood Components	12042	RBC Morphology
81117	Bone Marrow Cell Elimination	12043	Anisocytosis
81123	Thawing Of Fresh Frozen Plasma	12044	Acanthocytosis
81124	Freezing of Blood	12045	Basophilic Stippling
81125	Thawing Of Blood	12046	Burr Cells
81126	Freezing And Thawing Of Blood	12047	Cigar-shaped RBCs
81127	Hemolysins And Agglutinins	12048	Erythroblasts
	Screening	12049	Elliptocytes
81128	Auto	12051	Hypochromic / Microcytic RBCs
81129	Incubated	12052	Howell-Jolly Bodies
81130	Irradiation Of A Blood Product	12053	Macrocytes

HEMATOLOGY, CONT.

12054	Macroovalocytes
12055	Microovalocytes
12056	Nucleated RBCs
12057	Normochromic / Normocytic
12058	Poikilocytes
12059	Polychromatophilia
12060	Rouleaux Formation
12061	RBC Fragments
12062	Sickled RBCs
12063	Spherocytosis
12064	Spiculocytes
12065	Stomatocytes
12066	Target Cells
12067	Teardrop
12068	WBC Morphology
12069	Auer Rods
12070	Hypersegmented WBCs
12071	Myeloid Precursors
12072	Myeloblasts
12073	Metamyelocytes
12074	Myelocytes
12075	Promyelocytes
12076	Toxic Granulations
12077	Lymphoblasts
12078	Mast Cells
12079	Smudge Cells
12080	Giant Granules
18321	Hairy Cells
81245	Unlisted Hematology Study

Blood Gas Analyses

81318	**Blood Gas Analyses**
12404	Arterial Blood Gases
12194	ABG Panel
81319	With SaO2
12195	pH
12209	HCO3
81325	SaO2
12166	CO2 Content
12196	PaCO2
12198	After Hyperventilation
18434	After Exercise
12405	O2 Content
12274	CO2 Content
12199	PaO2
18435	After Exercise
12082	CO
12276	CO, Qualitative
81500	Hemoglobin-Oxygen Affinity
12903	A-aDO2 Gradient
81324	a/A Ratio
22469	Lactic Acid
12371	Post-exercise With Tourniquet
12266	Total serum base
81323	Venous Blood Gases

81326	Panel
81327	With SvO2
81328	pH
81329	HCO3
81330	SvO2
81332	CO2 Content
81331	PvCO2
12211	O2 Content
81333	PvO2
81334	CO
81335	CO, Qualitative
12170	Anion Gap
22470	Lactic Acid
12212	Arteriovenous Oxygen Content Difference
12200	Oxygen Saturation
12201	Inferior Vena Cava
12202	Superior Vena Cava
12203	Right Atrium
12204	Right Ventricle
12205	Pulmonary Artery
12206	Left Atrium
12207	Left Ventricle
12208	Brachial Artery
81320	Radial Artery
81321	Femoral Artery

12213	**Blood Chemistry**
22607	Test Panels
22608	General Health
22609	Obstetric
22610	Liver Function
22611	Hepatitis
22612	Lipids
22613	Arthritis
22614	TORCH
81885	Screening Tests
13096	Drug Screen
22272	Single Class Procedure
22273	Multiple Class Procedure
22274	Chromatography Confirmation
81093	Using Tissue Preparation
18278	Amphetamines
18279	Barbiturates
18280	Benzodiazepines
18281	Cocaine
19112	LSD
18282	Marijuana
18511	Methamphetamines
18284	PCP
18285	Phenothiazines
22275	Propoxyphenes
13097	Sulfonylurea
22276	Tricyclic Antidepressants

BLOOD CHEMISTRY, CONT.

22592	Automated Multichannel Tests
22593	1 Or 2 Tests
22594	3 Tests
22595	4 Tests
22596	5 Tests
22597	6 Tests
22606	7 Tests
22598	8 Tests
22599	9 Tests
22600	10 Tests
22601	11 Tests
22602	12 Tests
22603	13 - 16 Tests
22604	17 Or 18 Tests
22605	19 Or More Tests
12162	SMA-6
12171	SMA-12
81263	Electrolytes
12163	Sodium
12164	Potassium
12416	Potassium, Total Body
12188	Calcium, Total
12271	Calcium, Ionized
12396	Magnesium
12165	Chloride
12189	Phosphate
12402	Osmolality Of Serum
13022	Water Load Test
81265	Vitamin Levels
12455	Vitamin A
12277	Carotene
22497	Vitamin B1
81296	Vitamin B2
12456	Vitamin B6
12457	Vitamin B12
12458	Binding Capacity
12261	Vitamin C
12262	In Leukocytes
81266	Vitamin D
81267	Vitamin D3
12460	1,25-Dihydroxy Vitamin D
12459	25-Hydroxy Vitamin D2
12343	25-Hydroxycholecalciferol
12453	Vitamin E
81268	Vitamin K
12412	Pantothenate
81269	Trace Minerals
81270	Serum Aluminum
13075	Serum Arsenic
81294	Serum Bismuth
81276	Serum Boran
81277	Serum Cadmium
81280	Serum Chromium

81281	Serum Cyanide
81282	Serum Cobalt
12293	Serum Copper
81283	Serum Fluoride
81099	Serum Gold
12360	Serum Iron
12373	Serum Lead
12395	Serum Manganese
81285	Serum Mercury
81286	Serum Nickel
22496	Serum Selenium
81287	Serum Silver
81288	Serum Thallium
12462	Serum Zinc
12711	Endocrine Laboratory Tests
81308	Blood Sugar Studies
12168	Blood Glucose
81309	Reagent Strip
19083	Fingerstick
12337	Fasting - Whole Blood
12334	2 hour postprandial
12341	After Epinephrine
12336	Glucagon Level
81310	Glucagon Level With Tolerance Test
81316	Glucagon Tolerance Panel For Insulinoma
19355	Glucose Level With 1-Hour Glucola Test
81317	Tolbutamide Glucose Tolerance Test
12790	Oral Glucose Tolerance Test - 2 Hours
81311	Fasting Value
19339	30 Min. Interim Value
19340	60 Min. Interim Value
19341	90 Min. Interim Value
19342	2-Hour Interim Value
18447	Additional Specimens After Three
19344	Oral Glucose Tolerance Test - 3 Hour Prenatal
19345	Fasting Value
19336	1-Hour Value
19346	2-Hour Value
19335	3-Hour Value
12736	Glycosylated Hemoglobin
12749	Insulin / Glucose Ratio
12755	C-Peptide Level
12750	Proinsulin Level
12746	Fasting Insulin Level
12748	72-Hour Fasting Insulin Level
81314	Free Insulin Level
81315	Insulin Induced C-peptide Suppression Panel

BLOOD CHEMISTRY, CONT.

12751	Provocative Tests for Insulin Secretion	12722	% of Baseline After 4 hr. of Ambulation
12752	Using Glucagon	12718	Aldosterone Suppression Panel
81313	Using Glucose	12713	Androstenedione
12753	Using Leucine	12714	Postmenopausal Females
12754	Using Tolbutamide	81354	Androsterone
22551	30 Min. Interim Value	81355	Androstanediol Glucuronide
22552	1 Hour Interim Value	12724	Angiotensin II (supine)
22553	2 Hour Interim Value	81453	Anterior Pituitary Evaluation Panel
22554	3 Hour Interim Value	12725	Anti-Diuretic Hormone (ADH)
81338	**Thyroid Function Tests**	81451	Chorionic Gonadotropin Stimulation Panel
22615	Thyroid Function Panel (Without TSH)	81452	Estradiol Response
22616	Thyroid Function Panel With TSH	81898	Testosterone Response
81339	TRH Stimulation Panel - 1 Hr	12294	Corticosteroids (Porter-Silber)
81340	TRH Stimulation Panel - 2 Hour	81356	Corticosterone
12806	T4 Levels	12728	Cortisol (RIA)
12808	Total T4	12729	AM
81344	Total T4 By RIA	12730	PM
12809	Free T4	12731	AM following dexamethasone
12810	Free Thyroxine Index	19068	CRH Stimulation Panel
81343	Neonatal T4 screen	22306	Dehydroepiandrosterone (DHEA)
81342	Triiodothyronine (T3)	12733	Dehydroepiandrosterone Sulfate (DHEA-S)
12812	Total T3		
81345	Total T3 By RIA	12734	11-Deoxycortisol
22506	Free T3	81358	11-Deoxycorticosterone
12813	Reverse T3	81357	Dexamethasone Suppression Panel
12804	T3 Uptake	81361	Dihydrotestosterone
12805	T3 Uptake Ratio	81365	Erythropoietin
12816	T3 Suppression Test	22543	By Hemagglutination
12814	TSH	22544	Bioassay
18044	Super Sensitive TSH	12788	Estradiol
12815	20 Min. After TRH Stimulation	81366	Estrogens, Fractionated
82027	Neonatal TSH	22337	Estrogen, Total
12239	TSI	22338	Preovulatory Females
12817	Thyroglobulin	22339	Ovulatory Females
18051	Thyroxine Binding Globulin	22340	Postovulatory Females
12272	Calcitonin Level	81381	Estrogen Receptor Assay
12273	Stimulation Panel - Calcium	22311	Estriol, Free
81341	Stimulation Panel - Pentagastrin	22313	At 25 Weeks
12800	Protein-Bound Iodine	22314	At 28 Weeks
81353	**Hormone Levels**	22315	At 30 Weeks
12715	ACTH	22316	At 32 Weeks
81458	ACTH Stimulation Panels	22317	At 34 Weeks
12732	For Adrenal Insufficiency	22318	At 36 Weeks
81459	For 21 Hydroxylase Deficiency	22319	At 37 Weeks
81460	For 3 Beta-Hydroxydehydogenase Deficiency	22320	At 38 Weeks
		22321	At 39 Weeks
12745	Metyrapone Test	22322	At 40 Weeks
12717	Aldosterone	22323	Estriol, Total
12719	With 2L NS IV Over 4 Hours	22324	24-28 Weeks
12720	100 mEq Na Diet	22325	28-32 Weeks
12721	After ACTH	22326	32-36 Weeks

BLOOD CHEMISTRY, CONT.

22327	36-40 Weeks	12798	> 200 ng./ml
81367	Etiocholanolone	81380	Prostaglandin
12759	FSH	12792	PTH
12773	Prepubertal Male	22474	Intact
81370	Prepubertal Female	81375	C-terminal
12770	Postpubertal Male	22475	N-terminal
12761	Postpubertal Female	22476	Ca/PTH Ratio
12764	During Ovulation	22490	Renin Activity
12767	Postmenopausal Female	22491	Normal Sodium Diet
12775	After LH-RH Provocation	12756	Supine
12333	Gastrin	12757	Standing
22284	After Secretin Stimulation	22492	Low Sodium Diet
81454	Glucagon Tolerance - For	22493	Supine
	Pheochromocytoma	22494	Standing
81461	Gonadotropin Releasing Hormone	81455	Renin Stimulation Panels
	Stimulation Panel	81456	Renal Vein
18996	Human Chorionic Gonadotropin	81457	Peripheral Vein
12777	Human Growth Hormone	12783	Sex Hormone Binding Globulin
12778	Glucose Suppression	81860	Somatomedin-C
12780	After Exercise	81384	Somatostatin
12781	L-Dopa Stimulation	12758	Testosterone, Total
12782	Arginine Stimulation	22308	Testosterone, Free
81264	Calcium Infusion Test	22501	Transcortin
81373	Human Placental Lactogen	22502	Luteal Phase
81462	Insulin Tolerance Panel	22503	2nd Trimester Pregnancy
81463	For HGH Deficiency	22504	3rd Trimester Pregnancy
12738	For ACTH Deficiency	81465	TRH Stimulation Panel For
81378	17-Hydroxypregnenolone		Hyperprolactinemia
81371	17-Hydroxyprogesterone	81383	Other Endocrine Receptor Assay
81372	20-Hydroxyprogesterone	81347	Metabolic Tests
12723	18-Hydroxycorticosterone	81406	Acetaldehyde
81838	Ketogenic Steroids, Fractionation	22510	Acetone
81368	LH	12214	Acetone, Qualitative
12774	Prepubertal Male	19071	Acetoacetate
81369	Prepubertal Females	81858	Acetylcholine, Receptor Assay
12771	Postpubertal Male	12923	Aminolevulinic Acid (ALA)
12762	Postpubertal Females	12218	Ammonia, Blood
12765	During Ovulation	22512	Ammonia, Plasma
12768	Postmenopausal Female	12267	Bile Acids - Total
81374	LRH	22515	2-Hour Postprandial
81464	Metyrapone Panel	81412	Cholylglycine
81385	Ovulation Tests By Color	12181	Bilirubin, Total Serum
	Comparison	12182	Bilirubin, Direct (Conjugated)
81377	Pregnenolone	12183	Monoconjugated
81376	Pregnanetriol	12184	Diconjugated
12784	Progesterone	81351	Bilirubin, Total AND Direct
22485	Luteal Phase	12185	Bilirubin, Indirect (Unconjugated)
12785	Preovulatory Females	81350	Bilirubin, Newborn
12786	Postovulatory Females	81469	Bradykinin
12787	Prepubertal Males	12726	BMR
81379	Postmenopausal Females	12167	BUN
81382	Progesterone Receptor Assay	81946	Pre-Procedure
12797	Prolactin	81348	BUN, Using Reagent Strip

BLOOD CHEMISTRY, CONT.

12739	Catecholamines, Total	81438	Albumin-Globulin Capacity
81466	Catecholamines, Fractionated	18573	Beta 2-Microglobulin
12740	Norepinephrine	81434	Alpha-1-antitrypsin
12741	Supine	81882	Phenotype Z/Z
12742	Standing	81883	Phenotype Z/A
12743	After Oral Clonidine	12309	WBC Enzyme Assay
22302	Plasma Epinephrine	12310	Arylsulfatase A
22303	Supine	18124	Hexosaminidase A Assay
22304	Standing	18380	Hexosaminidase B Assay
22305	Dopamine	12098	Lymphoblast Terminal
81482	Citrate		Deoxyriboxidyl Transferase
12187	Creatinine	81884	RBC Enzyme Assays
81945	Pre-Procedural	81352	Cholinesterase, RBC
12727	Cyclic AMP, Nephrogenous	12312	Erythrocyte Transketolase
81420	Cyclic GMP		Activity
19069	Fructosamine	12313	with Thiamine Pyrophosphate
22341	Galactose	12305	Blood Enzyme Assays
12344	Hemoglobin	81407	Acetylcholinesterase
19072	Hydroxybutyrate, Beta	12414	Acid Phosphatase - Total
22467	Hypoxanthine	81390	Prostatic
81836	Intrinsic Factor	12215	Aldolase
12372	Lactose Tolerance Test	12180	Alkaline Phosphatase
81417	Metanephrine	81391	Heat Stable
81880	Nitrogen Studies	81392	Isoenzymes
12216	Alpha-amino Nitrogen	12193	ALT (SGPT)
22513	Ammonia Nitrogen, Serum	22514	Amylase (Beckman)
12398	Nonprotein Nitrogen	12220	Amylase (Somogyi)
12413	Phenylalanine	12306	Angiotensin-Converting Enzyme
81856	Pyruvate	12307	Arylsulfatase A
12444	Pyruvic Acid	12172	AST (SGOT)
18110	Serotonin	12173	AST Persistently Higher Than
81862	Sialic Acid		ALT
12454	Teichoic Acid	81504	Beta Glucosidase
81866	Thiocyanate	81349	Cholinesterase, Plasma
22507	Tyrosine	81474	Cathepsin-D
12186	Uric Acid	12302	Creatine
12835	Xylose Absorption Test	12296	Creatine Kinase (Total CK)
12836	5-Hour Urine (25-gram Dose)	81393	Creatine Phosphokinase (CPK)
22509	5-Hour Urine (0.5-gram/kg Dose)	81394	CPK Isoenzymes
12837	2-Hour Blood	12297	CPK-BB
81386	Protein Studies	12298	CPK-MB
12191	Protein - Total	12299	CPK-MM
81433	By Refractometry	12300	CPK Isoenzymes After Exercise
12417	Protein Electrophoresis	81395	CPK MB Fraction Only
12418	Albumin	81396	CPK Isoforms
12419	Globulin	81402	Gamma Glutamyl Transferase
12420	Alpha 1	81401	Gamma Glutamyl Transpeptidase
12422	Alpha 2	22343	Galactose-1-Phosphate Uridyl
12423	Beta		Transferase
12424	Gamma	81397	Galactosemia Screen
12425	Monoclonal Spike	81398	Galactokinase
12192	Albumin	12311	Galactocerebroside Beta-
81437	Albumin/Globulin Ratio		Galactosidase

BLOOD CHEMISTRY, CONT.

81399	Glutamate Dehydrogenase	22429	Isoleucine
18378	Hexosaminidase, Total	22430	Leucine
18122	Hexosaminidase A	22431	Tyrosine
18123	Less than 15%	22432	Phenylalanine
18379	Hexosaminidase B	22433	Homocystine
81405	Isocitric dehydrogenase	22434	Tryptophan
12174	LDH	22435	Ornithine
81413	Electrophoresis Of LDH	22436	Lysine
	Isoenzymes	22437	1-Methylhistidine
12175	LDH - Fraction I	22438	3-Methylhistidine
12176	LDH - Fraction II	22439	Histidine
12177	LDH - Fraction III	22440	Arginine
12178	LDH - Fraction IV	22481	Prealbumin
12179	LDH - Fraction V	81873	Vasoactive Intestinal Peptide
81414	Leucine Aminopeptidase	12376	Serum Lipoproteins
12375	Lipase	12190	Total Cholesterol
81415	Malate Dehydrogenase	18184	HDL Cholesterol
12397	NADH Methemoglobin Reductase	18185	LDL Cholesterol
12400	5'-Nucleotidase	18186	VLDL Cholesterol
81432	Phosphohexose Isomerase	18187	Total Cholesterol/HDL Ratio
18248	Guthrie Microbiologic	18188	LDL/HDL Ratio
18250	Maple Syrup Urine Disease	12393	Triglycerides
18251	Homocystinuria	12394	12 Hour Fasting
18252	Tyrosinemia	81425	Fatty Acids, Free
18253	Galactosemia	12325	Fatty Acids
18249	Phenylalanine	18205	Unesterified Cholesterol
22495	Retinol Binding Protein	18660	Hexacosanoic Acid
22505	Transferrin	12387	Type X
12278	Ceruloplasmin	22479	Phospholipids
12097	Haptoglobin	12377	Electrophoresis
81419	Haptoglobin Phenotypes	81422	VLDL
12403	Myoglobin	81421	LDL
81429	Osteocalcin	81423	HDL
22346	Plasma Amino Acids	81424	Chylomicrons
81444	Qualitative Analysis	12381	Ultracentrifugation
22369	Chromatographic Fractionation	12382	VLDL
22412	Phosphoserine	12383	LDL
22413	Taurine	12384	IDL
22414	Aspartic Acid	12385	HDL
22415	Hydroxyproline	12386	Chylomicrons
22416	Threonine	18168	Apolipoproteins
22417	Serine	18169	A-I
22418	Asparagine	18176	A-II
22419	Glutamic Acid	18170	A-IV
22420	Glutamine	18183	Total B
22421	Proline	18171	B-100
22422	Glycine	18172	B-48
22423	Alanine	18182	Apo B/Apo A-I Ratio
22424	Citrulline	18173	C-I
22425	2-Aminobutyric Acid	18174	C-II
22426	Valine	18175	C-III
22427	Cystine	18177	D
22428	Methionine	18178	E

BLOOD CHEMISTRY, CONT.

18179	F	81416	Meprobamate
18180	G	81845	Morphine
18181	H	81098	Nortriptyline
22591	Drug Assays	20905	Phenobarbital
81911	Therapeutic Drug Assays	20912	Primidone
18545	Acetaminophen	20906	Procainamide
20918	Amikacin	81096	Procainamide With NAPA
81900	Peak		Metabolite
81901	Trough	20903	Quinidine
20913	Amitriptyline	81857	Quinine
81409	Amphetamine	12446	Salicylate
81410	Dextroamphetamine Sulfate	20922	Sulfamethoxazole
81411	Methamphetamine Sulfate	20907	Theophylline
20908	Amphotericin	81095	Tobramycin
12263	Barbiturates	81907	Peak
12264	Long Acting	81908	Trough
81914	Intermediate Acting	20923	Trimethoprim
12265	Short Acting	20911	Valproic Acid
12268	Bromide	20919	Vancomycin
20910	Carbamazepine	81912	Unlisted Therapeutic Drug Assay
20924	Chloramphenicol	81909	Toxic Drug Assays
81430	Chlorpromazine	81910	Acetaminophen
20916	Clonazepam	81913	Amphetamine
20917	Cyclosporin	81915	Barbiturates
20915	Desipramine	81916	Long Acting
81481	Dibucaine Number	81917	Intermediate Acting
12301	Digoxin	81918	Short Acting
12295	Digitoxin	81484	Cocaine
12304	Dilantin	81359	Hydrocodone
81097	Dilantin, Free	81922	LSD
81362	Dimethadione	81428	Nicotine
20909	Disopyramide	81847	Phencyclidine (PCP)
81094	Doxepin	81921	Strychnine
81364	Ethchlorvynol	81874	Volatiles
20925	Ethosuximide	12314	Ethanol
20921	Flucytosine	81493	Ethylene Glycol
81498	Flurazepam	81920	Isopropyl Alcohol
20904	Gentamicin	81919	Methanol
81902	Peak	81876	Unlisted Chemistry Study
81903	Trough	87003	**Laboratory-Based Chemistry**
81403	Glutethimide	19303	**Immunology Studies**
81284	Gold	12352	Serum Immunoglobulins
81360	Hydromorphone	12353	IgG
20914	Imipramine	18589	Subclasses (IRMA)
81904	Kanamycin	18590	G1
81905	Peak	18591	G2
81906	Trough	18592	G3
20920	Ketoconazole	18593	G4
22277	Lidocaine	12354	IgA
12369	Lithium	12355	IgD
81418	Methadone	12356	IgE
81427	Methsuximide	12357	IgM
81844	Meperidine	12358	Sia Test

IMMUNOLOGY STUDIES, CONT.

12475	Histocompatibility Antigen	12286	C5
12476	HL-A - B1	82151	Antigen ___ug/ml
12477	HL-A - B7	82150	Functional Activity ___%
12478	HL-A - B8	12287	C6
12479	HL-A - B13	82152	Antigen ___ug/ml
18206	HL-A - B14	82153	Functional Activity ___%
12480	HL-A - B27	12288	C7
12481	HL-A - B35	82154	Antigen ___ug/ml
12482	HL-A - BW15	82155	Functional Activity ___%
12483	HL-A - BW17	12289	C8
18207	HL-A - A3	82156	Antigen ___ug/ml
12484	HL-A - A10	82157	Functional Activity ___%
20093	HL-A - DR4	17993	C9
20094	HL-A - DR5	82158	Antigen ___ug/ml
20095	HL-A - DRW6	82159	Functional Activity ___%
20096	HL-A - DRW8	17994	Factor B
12485	HL-A - DW2	17995	Factor D
12486	HL-A - DW3	17996	Factor I
12487	HL-A - DW4	17997	Factor H
12426	Immunoelectrophoresis	17998	Factor P (Properdin)
82172	Crossed	12303	Serum Cryoglobulin
12427	Heavy Chain	12227	Heterophil
12428	Gamma	82169	Titre 1:___
12429	Alpha	82170	Titre After Beef Cells, Guinea Pig
12430	Delta		Kidney Absorption 1:___
12431	Epsilon	12789	Histamine Test
12432	Mu	18574	Serum Neopterin
12433	Light Chain	12243	Serum Precipitating Antibody
12434	Kappa	81520	Autoantibodies
12435	Lambda	82033	Antiplatelet
82175	Immunofixation Electrophoresis	82034	Platelet Associated Immunoglobulin
82174	Immune Complex Assay		Assay
12279	Serum Complement	12223	Adrenal
22254	Total Hemolytic	12224	Antimyocardial
22255	Serum	12230	Anti-RNP
22256	Plasma	12231	Antinuclear (ANA)
12280	CH50	12232	Nucleolar Pattern
12281	C1	82035	Titre 1:___
82142	Antigen ___ug/ml	12234	Anti-Salivary Duct (ASDA)
82143	Functional Activity ___%	19300	Anticardiolipin
17990	C1q	19301	Antihistone
17991	C1r	82032	Antileukocyte
17992	C1s (Esterase)	18441	Antineutrophilic Cytoplasmic
12282	inhibitor	18442	Bright Coarsely Granular Pattern
12283	C2	18443	Bright Nongranular Pattern
82144	Antigen ___ug/ml	18444	Weak Diffuse Pattern
82145	Functional Activity ___%	81521	Antineutrophilic Perinuclear
12284	C3	19299	Anti-La (SSB)
82146	Antigen ___ug/ml	19298	Anti-Ro (SSA)
82147	Functional Activity ___%	12241	Single-Stranded DNA
12285	C4	12242	Double-Stranded DNA %
82148	Antigen ___ug/ml	12240	Glomerular Basement Membrane
82149	Functional Activity ___%	82162	Growth Hormone Antibody

IMMUNOLOGY STUDIES, CONT.

82176	Insulin	13109	candida albicans
12222	Intrinsic Factor	13110	dinitrochlorobenzene
82177	Islet Cells	13111	mumps
12374	LE Prep	13112	tetanus
12392	Latex Fixation	13113	tuberculin
12450	Rheumatoid Factor	22292	Intradermal
12451	IgG ___ mg/ml	22293	Tine Test
12229	Mitochondrial	13114	trichophytin
12411	Parietal Cell Antibody	13115	Kveim
12226	Parietal Cell	13116	Direct Immunofluorescence of Perilesional Skin
12233	Sm Antigen		
12235	Smooth Muscle	27083	Screening examination for pulmonary tuberculosis
12236	Thyroid		
12237	Microsomal	13117	Tuberculin PPD
18065	Titre (1:X)	81523	Tine
12238	Thyroglobulin	25053	Induration ___ mm
18066	Titre (1:X)	81524	Positive Interpretation
12221	Serum Antibody (NOC)	81522	Device
12225	Frei Skin Test	13118	Skin test
12228	Isohemagglutinins titer 1:	13119	cat scratch disease
18582	Lymphocyte Enumeration	13120	aspergillus
12027	T Cells (CD3 +)	13121	coccidioides immitis
12028	Thymocytes (T6 +)	13122	histoplasma capsulatum
12029	Helper T Cells (T4 +)	13123	clonorchis sinensis
12030	Suppressor T Cells (T8 +)	13124	leishmania tropica
12031	Helper / Suppressor Cell (T4/T8) Ratio	13125	schistosoma
		13126	schistosoma haemotobium
12032	Activated (IL-2, HLA-DR +)	13127	wuchereria bancrofti
12033	Natural Killer Cells (LGL)	13128	wuchereria malayai
12034	Null Cells (CD3, CD19, CD20 -)	13129	DICK Test
12035	B Cells (CD19, CD20 +)	27081	Screening for chemical poisoning and other contamination
12036	immature (CD10, CALLA +)		
12037	Monocyte Cell Markers (Leu-M1, Leu-M2 +)	81476	For Chlorinated Hydrocarbons
		18448	Allergy Sensitivity Testing
82138	Leukocyte Studies	18449	Percutaneous tests with allergenic extracts
19464	Lymphocyte Studies		
82180	Antigen-Induced Blastogenesis	18450	Percutaneous tests with drugs, biologicals or venoms
82181	Mitogen-Induced Blastogenesis		
18548	Beryllium-Stimulated Lymphocyte Transformation	18451	Intradermal tests with drug, biologicals, venoms (immediate)
19465	Polymerase Chain Reaction	18452	Intradermal tests with allergenic extracts (immediate)
19466	Mutation in B-cardiac myosin heavy-chain gene	18453	Intradermal tests with allergenic extracts (delayed)
82139	Neutrophil Studies	81897	Radio-Allergen-Sorbent Test (RAST)
82140	Chemotaxis Assay	82031	Multiallergen Screen
82178	Phagocytosis	13130	Patch Testing
82182	Nitroblue Tetrazolium Dye Test	13131	Beryllium
82183	Migration Inhibitory Factor Test	13132	Chromates
82179	Histamine Release Test	13133	Cobalt
82160	Fc Receptor	13134	Neomycin
13107	Skin Test	13135	Nickel
18572	Hypoergic (1 of panel reactive)	13136	Parabens
13108	Anergy		

IMMUNOLOGY STUDIES, CONT.

22296	Up To 10 Tests		81547	Maple Mix	
22297	11 To 20 Tests		81650	Induration ___mm	
22298	21 To 30 Tests		81651	Erythema ___mm	
22299	Over 30 Tests		82045	Specific IgE ___ng/ml	
18454	Photo Patch Tests		81548	Oak Mix (Red & White)	
22300	Up To 10 Tests		81652	Induration ___mm	
22301	Over 10 Tests		81653	Erythema ___mm	
18455	Allergy Photo Testing		82046	Specific IgE ___ng/ml	
81538	Antigens		81549	Sycamore	
81525	Diluent Control		81654	Induration ___mm	
82028	Induration ___mm		81655	Erythema ___mm	
82029	Erythema ___mm		82047	Specific IgE ___ng/ml	
81537	Histamine		81550	Black Walnut	
81804	Induration ___mm		81656	Induration ___mm	
81805	Erythema ___mm		81657	Erythema ___mm	
81890	Drugs		82048	Specific IgE ___ng/ml	
81891	Penicillin G		81551	Sweet Gum	
81892	Induration ___mm		81658	Induration ___mm	
81893	Erythema ___mm		81659	Erythema ___mm	
82030	Specific IgE ___ng/ml		82049	Specific IgE ___ng/ml	
81894	Pre-Penicillin		81552	Mulberry (Red)	
81895	Induration ___mm		81660	Induration ___mm	
81896	Erythema ___mm		81661	Erythema ___mm	
82037	Specific IgE ___ng/ml		82050	Specific IgE ___ng/ml	
81526	Tree Mix		81553	Cedar (Red)	
81631	Induration ___mm		81662	Induration ___mm	
81632	Erythema ___mm		81663	Erythema ___mm	
82038	Specific IgE ___ng/ml		82051	Specific IgE ___ng/ml	
81633	Individual Trees		81554	Juniper	
81540	Alder		81664	Induration ___mm	
81638	Induration ___mm		81665	Erythema ___mm	
81639	Erythema ___mm		82052	Specific IgE ___ng/ml	
82039	Specific IgE ___ng/ml		81555	Pecan	
81542	American Beech		81666	Induration ___mm	
81640	Induration ___mm		81667	Erythema ___mm	
81641	Erythema ___mm		82053	Specific IgE ___ng/ml	
82040	Specific IgE ___ng/ml		81556	Aspen	
81543	Red Birch		81668	Induration ___mm	
81642	Induration ___mm		81669	Erythema ___mm	
81643	Erythema ___mm		82054	Specific IgE ___ng/ml	
82041	Specific IgE ___ng/ml		81557	Black Willow	
81544	Cottonwood		81670	Induration ___mm	
81644	Induration ___mm		81671	Erythema ___mm	
81645	Erythema ___mm		82055	Specific IgE ___ng/ml	
82042	Specific IgE ___ng/ml		81558	Boxelder	
81545	American Elm		81672	Induration ___mm	
81646	Induration ___mm		81673	Erythema ___mm	
81647	Erythema ___mm		82056	Specific IgE ___ng/ml	
82043	Specific IgE ___ng/ml		81559	Cypress	
81546	Shagbark Hickory		81674	Induration ___mm	
81648	Induration ___mm		81675	Erythema ___mm	
81649	Erythema ___mm		82057	Specific IgE ___ng/ml	
82044	Specific IgE ___ng/ml		81560	Olive	

IMMUNOLOGY STUDIES, CONT.

81676	Induration ___mm		81702	Induration ___mm
81677	Erythema ___mm		81703	Erythema ___mm
82058	Specific IgE ___ng/ml		82071	Specific IgE ___ng/ml
81561	Poplar		81581	Meadow Fescue
81678	Induration ___mm		81704	Induration ___mm
81679	Erythema ___mm		81705	Erythema ___mm
82059	Specific IgE ___ng/ml		82072	Specific IgE ___ng/ml
81562	Black Locust		81582	Orchard Grass
81680	Induration ___mm		81706	Induration ___mm
81681	Erythema ___mm		81707	Erythema ___mm
82060	Specific IgE ___ng/ml		82073	Specific IgE ___ng/ml
81563	Douglass Fir		81583	Velvet Grass
81682	Induration ___mm		81708	Induration ___mm
81683	Erythema ___mm		81709	Erythema ___mm
82061	Specific IgE ___ng/ml		82074	Specific IgE ___ng/ml
81564	Red Spruce		81584	Bent Grass
81684	Induration ___mm		81710	Induration ___mm
81685	Erythema ___mm		81711	Erythema ___mm
82062	Specific IgE ___ng/ml		82075	Specific IgE ___ng/ml
81565	Pine		81585	Bermuda Grass
81686	Induration ___mm		81712	Induration ___mm
81687	Erythema ___mm		81713	Erythema ___mm
82063	Specific IgE ___ng/ml		82076	Specific IgE ___ng/ml
81566	Hazelnut		81586	Johnson Grass
81688	Induration ___mm		81714	Induration ___mm
81689	Erythema ___mm		81715	Erythema ___mm
82064	Specific IgE ___ng/ml		82077	Specific IgE ___ng/ml
81567	Privet		81587	Salt Grass
81690	Induration ___mm		81716	Induration ___mm
81691	Erythema ___mm		81717	Erythema ___mm
82065	Specific IgE ___ng/ml		82078	Specific IgE ___ng/ml
81527	Grass Mix		81588	Bahia Grass
81692	Induration ___mm		81718	Induration ___mm
81693	Erythema ___mm		81719	Erythema ___mm
82066	Specific IgE ___ng/ml		82079	Specific IgE ___ng/ml
81634	Individual Grasses		81528	Ragweed
81576	Timothy		81720	Induration ___mm
81694	Induration ___mm		81721	Erythema ___mm
81695	Erythema ___mm		82080	Specific IgE ___ng/ml
82067	Specific IgE ___ng/ml		81529	Weed Mix
81577	Sweet Vernal		81722	Induration ___mm
81696	Induration ___mm		81723	Erythema ___mm
81697	Erythema ___mm		82081	Specific IgE ___ng/ml
82068	Specific IgE ___ng/ml		81635	Individual Weeds
81578	Rye		81589	Pigweed
81698	Induration ___mm		81724	Induration ___mm
81699	Erythema ___mm		81725	Erythema ___mm
82069	Specific IgE ___ng/ml		82082	Specific IgE ___ng/ml
81579	Red Top		81590	Lamb's Quarter
81700	Induration ___mm		81726	Induration ___mm
81701	Erythema ___mm		81727	Erythema ___mm
82070	Specific IgE ___ng/ml		82083	Specific IgE ___ng/ml
81580	Kentucky Blue Grass		81591	Russian Thistle

IMMUNOLOGY STUDIES, CONT.

81728	Induration ___mm		81754	Induration ___mm
81729	Erythema ___mm		81755	Erythema ___mm
82084	Specific IgE ___ng/ml		82097	Specific IgE ___ng/ml
81592	Fire Bush		81604	Epicoccum
81730	Induration ___mm		81756	Induration ___mm
81731	Erythema ___mm		81757	Erythema ___mm
82085	Specific IgE ___ng/ml		82098	Specific IgE ___ng/ml
81593	Wing Scale		81605	Fusarium
81732	Induration ___mm		81758	Induration ___mm
81733	Erythema ___mm		81759	Erythema ___mm
82086	Specific IgE ___ng/ml		82099	Specific IgE ___ng/ml
81594	Cocklebur		81606	Penicillium (mixed)
81734	Induration ___mm		81760	Induration ___mm
81735	Erythema ___mm		81761	Erythema ___mm
82087	Specific IgE ___ng/ml		82100	Specific IgE ___ng/ml
81595	Marshelder		81607	Aspergillus (mix)
81736	Induration ___mm		81762	Induration ___mm
81737	Erythema ___mm		81763	Erythema ___mm
82088	Specific IgE ___ng/ml		82101	Specific IgE ___ng/ml
81596	Sage		81531	Animals
81738	Induration ___mm		81532	Cat
81739	Erythema ___mm		81764	Induration ___mm
82089	Specific IgE ___ng/ml		81765	Erythema ___mm
81597	Mugwort		82102	Specific IgE ___ng/ml
81740	Induration ___mm		81539	Dog
81741	Erythema ___mm		81766	Induration ___mm
82090	Specific IgE ___ng/ml		81767	Erythema ___mm
81598	Dock		82103	Specific IgE ___ng/ml
81742	Induration ___mm		81608	Goat
81743	Erythema ___mm		81768	Induration ___mm
82091	Specific IgE ___ng/ml		81769	Erythema ___mm
81599	Sheep Sorrel		82104	Specific IgE ___ng/ml
81744	Induration ___mm		81609	Pig
81745	Erythema ___mm		81770	Induration ___mm
82092	Specific IgE ___ng/ml		81771	Erythema ___mm
81600	English Plantain		82105	Specific IgE ___ng/ml
81746	Induration ___mm		81610	Monkey
81747	Erythema ___mm		81772	Induration ___mm
82093	Specific IgE ___ng/ml		81773	Erythema ___mm
81530	Fungal Mix		82106	Specific IgE ___ng/ml
81748	Induration ___mm		81611	Rabbit
81749	Erythema ___mm		81774	Induration ___mm
82094	Specific IgE ___ng/ml		81775	Erythema ___mm
81636	Individual Fungi		82107	Specific IgE ___ng/ml
81601	Alternaria		81612	Guinea pig
81750	Induration ___mm		81776	Induration ___mm
81751	Erythema ___mm		81777	Erythema ___mm
82095	Specific IgE ___ng/ml		82108	Specific IgE ___ng/ml
81602	Cladosporium		81613	Rat
81752	Induration ___mm		81778	Induration ___mm
81753	Erythema ___mm		81779	Erythema ___mm
82096	Specific IgE ___ng/ml		82109	Specific IgE ___ng/ml
81603	Aspergillus Fumigatus		81614	Mouse

IMMUNOLOGY STUDIES, CONT.

81780	Induration ___mm		81808	Induration ___mm
81781	Erythema ___mm		81809	Erythema ___mm
82110	Specific IgE ___ng/ml		82123	Specific IgE ___ng/ml
81615	Gerbil		81625	Caddis Fly
81782	Induration ___mm		81810	Induration ___mm
81783	Erythema ___mm		81811	Erythema ___mm
82111	Specific IgE ___ng/ml		82124	Specific IgE ___ng/ml
81616	Hamster		81626	Deer Fly
81784	Induration ___mm		81812	Induration ___mm
81785	Erythema ___mm		81813	Erythema ___mm
82112	Specific IgE ___ng/ml		82125	Specific IgE ___ng/ml
81617	Sheep (Crude Wool)		81627	Horse Fly
81786	Induration ___mm		81814	Induration ___mm
81787	Erythema ___mm		81815	Erythema ___mm
82113	Specific IgE ___ng/ml		82126	Specific IgE ___ng/ml
81618	Silk		81628	May Fly
81788	Induration ___mm		81816	Induration ___mm
81789	Erythema ___mm		81817	Erythema ___mm
82114	Specific IgE ___ng/ml		82127	Specific IgE ___ng/ml
81619	Cow		81629	Ant Mix (Black & Red)
81790	Induration ___mm		81818	Induration ___mm
81791	Erythema ___mm		81819	Erythema ___mm
82115	Specific IgE ___ng/ml		82128	Specific IgE ___ng/ml
81620	Horse		81630	Mosquito Mix
81792	Induration ___mm		81820	Induration ___mm
81793	Erythema ___mm		81821	Erythema ___mm
82116	Specific IgE ___ng/ml		82129	Specific IgE ___ng/ml
81621	Parakeet		81568	Other
81794	Induration ___mm		81887	Latex
81795	Erythema ___mm		81888	Induration ___mm
82117	Specific IgE ___ng/ml		81889	Erythema ___mm
81533	Cockroach		82130	Specific IgE ___ng/ml
81796	Induration ___mm		81569	Kapok
81797	Erythema ___mm		81822	Induration ___mm
82118	Specific IgE ___ng/ml		81823	Erythema ___mm
81534	Dust Mite		82131	Specific IgE ___ng/ml
81798	Induration ___mm		81570	Pyrethrum
81799	Erythema ___mm		81824	Induration ___mm
82119	Specific IgE ___ng/ml		81825	Erythema ___mm
81535	Mixed Feathers		82132	Specific IgE ___ng/ml
81800	Induration ___mm		81571	Cotton Seed
81801	Erythema ___mm		81826	Induration ___mm
82120	Specific IgE ___ng/ml		81827	Erythema ___mm
81536	Pigeon		82133	Specific IgE ___ng/ml
81802	Induration ___mm		81572	Acacia Gum
81803	Erythema ___mm		81828	Induration ___mm
82121	Specific IgE ___ng/ml		81829	Erythema ___mm
81622	Insects		82134	Specific IgE ___ng/ml
81623	Aphid		81573	Carragheen Gum
81806	Induration ___mm		81830	Induration ___mm
81807	Erythema ___mm		81831	Erythema ___mm
82122	Specific IgE ___ng/ml		82135	Specific IgE ___ng/ml
81624	Black Fly		81574	Karaya Gum

IMMUNOLOGY STUDIES, CONT.

81832	Induration ___mm	81479	Homocystine, Qualitative
81833	Erythema ___mm	22403	Hydroxylysine
82136	Specific IgE ___ng/ml	22375	Hydroxyproline
81575	Tragacanth Gum	22392	Isoleucine
81834	Induration ___mm	22393	Leucine
81835	Erythema ___mm	22405	Lysine
82137	Specific IgE ___ng/ml	22389	Methionine
22295	Skin End Point Titration	22406	1-Methylhistidine
18457	Direct Nasal Mucous Membrane	22407	3-Methylhistidine
18458	Inhalation Bronchial Challenge With Drugs	22404	Ornithine
		22395	Phenylalanine
18459	Inhalation Bronchial Challenge With Antigens	22373	Phosphoethanolamine
		22371	Phosphoserine
18456	Ophthalmic Mucous Membrane	22382	Proline
18460	Ingestion Challenge	22381	Sarcosine
18461	Rinkel Test	22377	Serine
81473	Tumor Markers	22372	Taurine
19353	Prostate-specific Antigen (PSA)	22376	Threonine
12254	Carcinoembryonic Antigen (CEA)	22394	Tyrosine
12217	Alpha-fetoprotein	22402	Tryptophan
29284	CA-125	22387	Valine
81519	CA-19-9	12984	Aminolevulinic Acid (ALA)
84444	**Urine Tests**	12942	Ammonia Nitrogen
12936	Acidity, Titratable	19668	Appearance, Gross
22562	Albumin, Total	12999	Arylsulfatase A
81442	Alkaloids	12948	Ascorbate
12937	Alpha Amino Nitrogen	19671	Ascorbic acid
22347	Amino Acids	12946	Amylase Excretion (Somogyi Units)
22370	Chromatographic Fractionation And Quantitation	12947	Amylase / Creatinine Clearance Ratio (%)
		22278	Bacteria Screen (Non-Culture)
81443	Qualitative Analysis	12943	Bence-Jones Protein
22384	Alanine	12944	Kappa Light Chain
22396	B-Alanine	12945	Lambda Light Chain
22386	2-Aminobutyric Acid	18576	Beta 2-Microglobulin
22397	3-Aminoisobutyric Acid	18277	Blood, Hemolyzed
22398	4-Aminoisobutyric Acid	12494	Blood, Occult (0-4+)
22409	Anserine	81301	Calcium
22411	Arginine	12956	Catecholamines, Free
22400	Argininosuccinic Acid	18401	Epinephrine
22378	Asparagine	18402	Norepinephrine
22374	Aspartic Acid	12957	Metanephrine, Total
22410	Carnosine	12958	Vanillyl Mandelic Acid
22385	Citrulline	22549	Pediatric
22391	Cystathionine	18403	Methoxy-4-Hydroxyphenylglycol (MHPG)
22388	Cystine		
81480	Cystine, Qualitative	18404	Homovanillic Acid
22401	Ethanolamine	22548	Pediatric
22379	Glutamic Acid	12963	Chloride
22380	Glutamine	12953	Per Gram of Creatinine
22383	Glycine	12954	Calcium/Creatinine Ratio
22408	Histidine	12964	Cocaine (Quantitative)
22390	Homocitrulline	12962	Coproporphyrins, Types I & III
22399	Homocystine	12971	Creatine

12982	Creatinine	
12983	Urine : Plasma Ratio	
81441	Cyclic AMP	
18446	Digitoxin	
18400	Dopamine Excretion	
81448	Drug Screens	
81926	Acetaminophen	
12940	Amphetamines	
12949	Barbiturates	
12950	Benzodiazepines	
81483	Cocaine	
81924	Heroin	
12974	LSD	
12975	Marijuana	
81923	Methadone	
81927	Methoqualone	
81925	Morphine	
12977	Phencyclidine (PCP)	
81928	Phenothiazine	
81932	Phenytoin	
81933	Propoxyphenes	
81930	Tricyclic Antidepressants	
81875	Volatiles	
12998	Enzyme Assay	
81491	Erythropoietin	
12961	Ferric Chloride Test	
22546	Fibrin Split Products	
13001	Glucose, True (Oxidase Method)	
22285	Heavy Metal Screen	
22290	Antimony Levels	
81271	Arsenic Levels	
81273	Barium Levels	
81272	Beryllium Levels	
81274	Bismuth Levels	
81275	Mercury Levels	
13002	Hemoglobin	
13005	Hemosiderin	
81515	Hemosiderin, Screen	
12929	Histamine (24 hr.)	
81363	Hormone Levels	
12938	Aldosterone	
12939	After 100 mEq Na Diet	
12970	Cortisol, Free	
18661	after ACTH Stimulation	
81485	Epiandrosterone	
12985	Estrogens (Brown Method)	
81486	Estrogens, Total	
22336	Males & Prepubertal Females	
22335	Postmenopausal Females	
22332	During Ovulation	
22333	At Luteal Peak	
22334	Gravid Female	
81490	Estrogens, Fractionated	

81487	Estrone	
12995	Males & Prepubertal Females	
12991	Postmenopausal Females	
12987	Postpubertal/Premenopausal Females	
22545	During ovulation	
81488	Estradiol	
12992	Postmenopausal Females	
12996	Males & Prepubertal Females	
12988	Postpubertal/Premenopausal	
22309	During Ovulation	
22310	During Follicular Stage	
81489	Estriol	
12997	Males & Prepubertal Females	
12993	Postmenopausal Females	
12989	Prepubertal/Postmenopausal Females	
22328	30 Weeks Gestation	
22329	35 Weeks Gestation	
22330	40 Weeks Gestation	
12959	HCG, Quantitative	
12776	HCG, Pregnancy Test	
81506	FSH	
81507	Post-Menopausal	
81508	At Midcycle Peak	
81509	LH	
81510	LH (Male)	
81511	LH (Postmenopausal Female)	
81512	LH (During Follicular Stage)	
81513	LH (Midcycle Peak Value)	
22482	Pregnanediol	
22483	Luteal Peak	
22484	Pregnancy Peak	
13031	Pregnanetriol	
13039	Testosterone	
13040	Tetrahydro 11-Deoxycortisol	
13041	Male	
13042	Female	
12965	17-Hydroxycorticosteroids	
18662	after 8-hr. ACTH Stimulation	
13004	5-Hydroxyindolacetic Acid	
81516	Hydroxyproline, Free	
13008	Hydroxyproline, Total	
12966	Iodine	
12930	Immunoelectrophoresis	
12931	IgG	
12932	IgA	
12933	IgM	
12934	Excessive Light Chains	
12928	Iron (24hr.), After Desferrioxamine	
13006	Kallikrein	
12495	Ketones	
13007	Ketones, Total (1 SD)	

12967	17-Ketosteroids, Total		22453	Pyroglutamic
81837	17-Ketosteroids, Fractionation		22448	Succinic
12968	17-Ketosteroids		22464	Suberic
12969	>40		22473	Orotic Acid
12518	Kidney Stone Analysis		13017	Osmolality
12519	Oxalate		13018	>1000
12520	Phosphate		13019	Urine : Serum Ratio
12521	Urate		13020	After Dehydration Test
12522	Cystine		13021	Followed by Vasopressin (ADH) With Osmolality Increase >15%
81470	Quantitative Analysis			
81471	Infrared Spectroscopy		13048	Output
81472	X-ray Diffraction		81846	Oxalate
13009	Lactic Dehydrogenase		12926	pCO2
81839	Lactose, Quantitative		12927	Urine : Plasma Ratio
81840	Lactose, Qualitative		18663	Pentachlorophenol
12924	Lipids		22478	Phenylalanine
81878	Lysozyme		81848	Phenylketones, Qualitative
22559	Magnesium		81850	Phosphate
12516	Maltese cross		13028	Phosphate Clearance
13015	Methylmalonate		13029	Ratio to Creatinine Clearance
13013	N'-Methylnicotinamide		13030	After PTH Injection
28613	Microalbumin		12935	Phytamic Acid
28614	Microalbumin Dipstick		13016	Porphobilinogen, Qualitative
81842	Mucopolysaccharides, Screen		81851	Porphobilinogen, Quantitative
22472	Mucopolysaccharides, Quantitative		81852	Porphyrins, Black Light Screen
13010	Myoglobin		81853	Porphyrins, Quantitation
18575	Neopterin		13023	Potassium
22344	Niacin		22561	24-hour
13003	Nitrite		13014	Protein, Total
12976	Opiates		12978	Protein Electrophoresis
22345	Organic Acids		12981	Albumin
22457	cis-Aconitic		22563	Alpha 1 Globulin
22451	Adipic		12979	Alpha 2 Globulin
22458	Azeleic		12980	B Globulin
22460	Citric		22564	Gamma Globulin
22447	Ethylmalonic		19667	Reducing Substance
22449	Fumaric		13034	Renal Failure Index
22450	Glutaric		12517	Renal Tubular Cells
22442	Glycolic		13024	Riboflavin
22443	3-Hydroxybutyric		12125	Schilling Test
22446	4-Hydroxybutyric		12126	Increase With Intrinsic Factor
22455	2-Hydroxyglutaric		12127	Increase After Antibiotics
22463	5-Hydroxyindoleacetic		12128	Increase After Antihelminthics
22444	3-Hydroxyisobutyric		12129	Increase After Pancreatic Extract
22445	3-Hydroxyisovaleric		81859	Serotonin
22465	3-Hydry-3-Methylglutaric		13025	Sodium (24 hour)
22456	p-Hydroxyphenylacetic		13026	Sodium
22461	4-Hydroxyphenyl Lactic		13027	Fractional Excretion Na (FENA - UNa/UCr x PCr/PNa)
22459	Isocitric			
22441	Lactic		13036	Sucrose, 24 Hour Test
22454	Mevalonic		81865	Sulfate
22462	2-Oxoglutaric		13035	Sulfatides
22452	Pyruvic		81278	Trace Minerals - Urine

81289	Boran	18344		Strongyloides
81279	Cadmium	12882		Saline Purge
18445	Chromium	22477	pH	
12960	Copper	81854	Porphyrins, Qualitative	
81290	Fluoride	81855	Porphyrins, Quantitative	
13011	Lead	12883	Protein Content	
13012	Increased After Calcium (EDTA)	81868	Trypsin, Quantitative	
81291	Nickel	81869	Trypsin, Qualitative	
81292	Selenium	12884	Urobilinogen	
81293	Thallium	12885	Water	
22508	Zinc	12869	Wet Weight	
13037	Tryptophan Load Test	12890	I-131 Labeled Albumin Recovery	
13043	Urea Nitrogen	12634	**CSF Analysis**	
13044	Urine : Plasma Ratio	22214	Lumbar Puncture	
81870	Urea Nitrogen Clearance	12635	Opening Pressure	
13046	Uric Acid	12636	Clarity & Color	
13047	Urobilinogen, 24 Hour	81863	Clear, Colorless	
81871	Urobilinogen, 2 Hour	12637	Xanthrochromia	
81872	Urobilinogen, Random	12638	Sanguinous	
81295	Vitamin Levels	12639	Cloudy	
13045	Vitamin B1	81468	Occult Blood	
81297	Vitamin B2	81864	Specific Gravity	
81298	Vitamin B6	12640	Viscous	
22283	Volume Measurement For Timed Collection	12641	Cells	
13038	Xanthurenic Acid	12642	RBC	
81877	Unlisted Urine Test	12643	WBC	
81449	**Fecal Analysis**	12644	% Lymphocytes + Monocytes	
81450	Bilirubin	12645	% Monocytes	
18256	Blood, Occult	12646	% Lymphocytes	
18257	1 Of 3 Cards Positive	12647	% Neutrophils	
18258	2 Of 3 Cards Positive	12648	% Eosinophils	
18259	3 Of 3 Cards Positive	12649	% Basophils	
12868	Bulk	12650	Malignant Cells	
12880	Calcium	12651	Astrocytes	
12871	Coproporphyrin	12652	Lymphoblasts	
81496	Culture For Enteric Pathogens	12653	Adenocarcinoma Cells	
12889	Clostridium Difficile Toxin Assay	22486	Protein	
12870	Dry Weight	12654	Lumbar	
12872	Fat Content	12655	% Gamma-Globulin	
81495	Fat Differential	18577	IgG	
81497	Qualitative Fat Analysis	18578	IgG Index	
12873	3-Day Collection	18580	IgG Daily Synthesis	
12874	% Of Dry Weight	22511	Albumin	
12875	Coefficient of Fecal Fat Absorption	18579	Albumin CSF/Serum Ratio	
12876	Fatty Acids	18581	Beta 2-Microglobulin	
12877	Free	12656	Oligoclonal Bands	
12878	Fatty Acid Soap Level	22487	Cisternal	
81514	Fetal Hemoglobin	22488	Ventricular	
12886	Leukocytes	12657	Glucose	
12888	Monocytes	12658	Chloride	
12887	Neutrophils, Segmented	22517	Calcium	
12881	Ova & Parasites	81505	Glutamine	
		12659	Myelin Basic Protein	

CSF ANALYSIS, CONT.

12660	VDRL
12661	Cryptococcal Antigen
12662	Intracranial Pressure Monitor
22468	Hypoxanthine
22348	Amino Acids
22349	Taurine
22350	Aspartic Acid
22351	Threonine
22352	Serine + Asparagine
22353	Glutamine
22354	Proline
22355	Glutamic Acid
22356	Glycine
22357	Alanine
22358	Valine
22359	Half Cystine
22360	Methionine
22361	Isoleucine
22366	Lysine
22367	Histidine
22368	Arginine
22362	Leucine
22363	Tyrosine
22364	Phenylalanine
22365	Ornithine
12614	**Synovial Fluid Analysis**
12615	RBC
12616	Leukocytes
12617	>100,000
12618	Segmented Neutrophils (%)
12619	Polymorphonuclear %
12620	Monocytes
12621	Complement
12622	Glucose
12623	Protein
12624	Appearance
12625	Cloudy
12626	Purulent
12627	Sanguinous
81843	Mucin Coagulation
12628	Calcium Pyrophosphate Crystals
12629	Uric Acid Crystals
12630	Bursal Fluid
12631	Leukocytes
12632	Polymorphonuclear
12633	Purulent
13063	**Semen Analysis**
13064	Sperm Count
13065	Azoospermia
13066	Motility
13067	Abnormal Forms
81499	Semen Fructose
19286	**Fetal Testing**

19290	Non-stress Test
19287	Stress Test
19288	Oxytocin
19289	Nipple Stimulation
19291	Scalp Blood Sampling
13068	Chromosome Studies
13069	Barr Body
13071	Trisomy of #21 (Denver)
22555	Amniotic Fluid Analysis
22466	Alpha-fetoprotein
81477	Creatinine
22556	Lecithin Phosphorus
22557	Lecithin-Sphingomyelin Ratio
22558	Foam Stability Test
81849	Phosphatidylglycerol
81445	Spectrophotometric Scan
12529	**Peritoneal Fluid**
12530	Gross Appearance
12531	Bile-Stained
12532	Chylous
12533	Gelatinous
12534	Hemorrhagic
12535	Mucinous
12536	Purulent
12537	Straw-Colored
12538	Turbid
12539	Specific Gravity
12540	Glucose
12541	Protein
12542	Amylase
12543	RBC
12544	WBC
12545	Neutrophils predominate
12546	Mononuclear predominate
12547	Eosinophils
12548	Lymphocytes
12549	LDH
12550	Sudan Staining
12551	Ether Extraction
12552	Cytology
12575	**Bone Marrow**
81227	Aspiration
81234	Smear
81235	Iron Stain
12576	Dry Tap
12577	Hypercellular
12578	Hypocellular With Fat
12579	Neoplastic Cells
12580	Foam Cells
12581	Gaucher's Cells
12582	Histiocytes
12583	Fibrosis
12584	Megaloblastic

12585	Myeloid		12831	Gastrointestinal Lab Tests
12586	Neutrophilic Series		12832	Esophageal
12587	Myeloblast		12838	Vitamin A
12588	Promyelocyte		12839	Gastric Juice
12589	Myelocyte		12840	Volume
12590	Metamyelocyte		12841	Nocturnal
12591	Band		12842	Fasting Basal
12592	Segmented		12843	24 hour
12593	Eosinophilic Series		12844	Reaction
12594	Basophilic Series		12845	As pH
12595	Myeloid / Erythroid Ratio		81503	Gastric Acid, Free AND Total
12596	Erythroid		12847	Acid Output
12597	Erythroblasts		12846	Titratable Acidity
12598	Pronormoblasts		81501	Gastric Acid, Free
12599	Basophilic Normoblasts		81502	Gastric Acid, Total
12600	Polychromatophilic Normoblasts		12849	Basal
12601	Orthochromatic Normoblasts		12850	Maximal (Pentagastrin)
12602	Megakaryocytes /50 LPF		12848	Achlorhydria
12603	Lymphoreticular		12852	Basal/Maximal Ratio
12604	Lymphocytes		12853	Pancreatic Functions
12605	Plasma Cells		12854	Amylase
12606	Reticulum Cells		12855	Juice Analysis
12607	Siderotic Granules		12856	Lipase
12608	Erythrophagocytosis		12857	Azure A Dye
12609	Lymphoblasts		12858	Secretin Stimulation Test
12610	Mast Cells		12859	PAS Positive Macrophage
12611	Iron		12860	Bile Acid Breath Test
12612	Sideroblast		12861	51 Chromium Labeled Albumin
12613	Ringed		81389	Other Laboratory Tests
18550	Serum Inhibin		12473	Karyotype
18551	Follicular		12474	Philadelphia Chromosome
18552	Mid-Follicular		19082	Fetus
18553	Ovulatory Surge		18514	Restriction Fragment Length
18554	Postmenopausal			Polymorphisms (RFLIP)
12791	Phentolamine		18526	Alpha 1 Antitrypsin Deficiency
12793	Urinary Cyclic AMP		18533	Antithrombin III Deficiency
12794	after PTH Injection		18518	Cystic Fibrosis
12795	Pancreatic Islet Cell Antibody		18527	Familial Hypercholesterolemia
12796	Catecholamine 24 hr. Urine Test		18522	Fragile X Syndrome
12818	Venous Sampling		18515	Hemophilia A
12819	For ACTH		18516	Hemophilia B
12820	Right vs. Left Gradient Present		18517	Huntington's Disease
12821	Pituitary vs. Peripheral Gradient		18528	Lesch-Nyhan Syndrome
	Present		18531	Myotonic Dystrophy
12822	For PTH		18529	Ornithine Transcarbamylase
12823	Right vs. Left Gradient Present			Deficiency
12824	Local vs. Peripheral Gradient Present		18530	Carbamyl Phosphate Synthetase
12825	For Aldosterone			Deficiency
12826	Right vs. Left Gradient Present		18525	Phenylketonuria
12827	Local vs. Peripheral Gradient Present		18519	Adult Polycystic Kidney Disease
12828	For Cortisol		18520	Retinoblastoma
12829	Right vs. Left Gradient Present		18521	X-Linked Retinitis Pigmentosa
12830	Local vs. Peripheral Gradient Present		18524	Alpha Thalassemia

194

18523	Beta Thalassemia		18355	RV
18532	Molecular Detection of Mutation		12896	RV/TLC
18543	Alpha 1-Antitrypsin Deficiency		18360	MVV
18542	Antithrombin III Deficiency		12901	reduced commensurate with FEV1 decrease (MVV>30xFEV1)
18541	Familial Hypercholesterolemia			
18540	Hemophilia A		18361	reduced more than the FEV1 decrease (MVV<30xFEV1)
18539	Hemophilia B			
18538	Lesch-Nyhan Syndrome		12902	Carbon Monoxide Diffusion % (DLCO)
18537	Ornithine Transcarbamylase Deficiency		12904	CO2 Sensitivity
			18433	Response to hypoxia
18544	Sickle Cell Anemia		12905	Minute Ventilation
18535	Alpha Thalassemia		12906	Increased
18534	Beta Thalassemia		12907	Decreased
81886	Screening		18432	Flow Volume Loop
27084	for venereal disease		12908	Static Compliance (dV/dP)(l/cm H2O)
27085	for malignant rectal neoplasm		18436	Airway Resistance (cm H2O/l/sec)
27086	for thyroid disorders		18437	CO2 Expired Gas Determination
27087	for diabetes mellitus		18438	O2 Uptake - Expired Gas Determination
27088	for malnutrition		18439	Including CO2 Output
27090	for sickle-cell disease or trait		25489	Oxygen Consumption
27092	for alcoholism		25507	Oxygen Consumption Index
27082	Multiphasic Screening		25490	Oxygen Assumed
81388	Forensic Exam For Acid Phosphatase		19513	Transcutaneous Oximetry
81440	Breathalyzer For Blood Alcohol Content		19514	With Ankle / Brachial Index
81475	Sweat Test For Chloride		19515	With Multiple Determinations
12270	BSP Retention		19516	With Continuous Overnight Monitoring
81881	Tissue Prep For Drug Analysis			
24891	**Laboratory Studies**		12909	Renal Function
12891	**Pulmonary Function Tests**		12910	Creatinine Clearance
29376	Peak Flow		12911	Para-aminohippuric Acid Clearance
29377	% Of Baseline		12912	Concentration & Dilution
29378	Spirometry		12913	Specific Gravity
29379	Pre-bronchodilator		12914	12 Hour Fluid Restriction
29380	Post-bronchodilator		12915	12 Hour Fluid Intake
29375	Methacholine		12916	Phenosulfonphthalein Excretion
12893	VC		12917	2 Hours After IM Injection
12900	% change after bronchodilator		12918	15 Minutes After IV Injection
12894	FVC		12919	2 Hours After IV Injection
12897	FEV1		12920	Phosphorous Tubular Reabsorption
18356	% change after bronchodilator		12921	Renal Venous Renin Asymmetry
18430	% change persisting after bronchodilator on prolonged test		19094	Gastrointestinal Studies
			19098	Esophageal Intubation For Cytology
18431	% change persisting after antigen provocation		19095	Esophageal Motility Study
			19096	With Mecholyl
18358	Methacholine dose required to provoke 20% decrease		19097	With Acid Perfusion
			12833	Bernstein Test
18359	Histamine dose required to provoke 20% decrease		13147	Esophageal Intraluminal pH
			19093	With Prolonged Recording
12898	FEV1% (FEV1/FVC)		12863	Gastric Washing
12899	FEF (25 - 75%)		12864	blood
18357	% change after bronchodilator		12865	pills
12892	TLC		12866	capsules
12895	FRC		19099	Gastric Intubation For Cytology

19100	Analysis Following Stimulant Of Gastric Secretion	19387	Through Established Nephrostomy
		19388	With Biopsy
19101	Gastric Secretory Studies	19389	Through Nephrotomy
19102	Basal Collection - One Hour	19390	With Biopsy
19103	Basal Collection - Two Hours	19433	Ureteral Endoscopy
19104	Two Hour Collection With Stimulation	19434	Through Established Ureterostomy
19105	Three Hour Collection With Stimulation	19435	With Biopsy
		19436	Through Ureterotomy
19106	Gastric Saline Load Test	19437	With Biopsy
19107	Duodenal Intubation	19277	Culdoscopy
19109	For Bleeding	19278	With Biopsy
12862	Washing And Aspiration	19279	With Adhesiolysis
19108	Fractional Collection After Stimulation	19280	With Tubal Sterilization
		16426	Laparoscopy
81867	Trypsin	19334	Fallopian Tube Dilation
19375	Proctosigmoidoscopy (Rigid)	19409	Peritoneal
19376	For Cytology	19410	With Biopsy
19377	For Microbiologic Testing	19411	With Transhepatic Cholangiography
19379	For Biopsy	19412	With Biopsy
16420	**Fiberoptic Examinations**	19284	Hysteroscopy
16421	Esophagoscopy	16427	Bronchoscopy
16445	Gastroscopy	19482	Flexible
19363	Enteroscopy	19483	Rigid
19364	For Biopsy	19484	Through Established Tracheostomy
19365	Ileoscopy	19485	With Biopsy
19366	For Biopsy	19486	With Transbronchial Lung Biopsy
19367	Kock Pouch Endoscopy	19487	With Transbronchial Needle Aspiration Biopsy
19368	For Biopsy		
16442	Complete Colonoscopy	19488	With Contrast Injection For Bronchography
16443	Forceps Biopsy		
16444	CMV Inclusions	18113	Endobronchial Lesions
19378	Intraoperative Colonoscopy	18114	Purpuric
19369	Colonoscopy Via Colostomy	16428	Bronchoalveolar Lavage
19370	For Biopsy	16429	Total Cells
16422	Sigmoidoscopy	16430	Macrophages
19380	For Cytology	16431	Lymphocytes
19381	For Microbiologic Testing	16432	T Cells
16423	Proctoscopy	16433	Activated T Cells
16447	Cystoscopy	16434	B Cells
16448	With Biopsy	16435	Neutrophils
19458	With Ureteral Catheterization	16436	Eosinophils
19459	With Brush Biopsy	16437	Basophils
19460	With Ejaculatory Duct Catheterization	16438	Total Protein (mg)
19461	With Ureteroscopy For Biopsy	16439	IgG (mg/mg albumin)
19462	With Pyeloscopy For Biopsy	16440	IgM
16424	Anoscopy	16441	Collagenase
19392	For Cytology	19470	Nasal Endoscopy
19393	For Microbiologic Testing	19471	Maxillary Sinus
19394	For Biopsy	19472	Sphenoid Sinus
19399	Percutaneous Biliary Endoscopy	19473	Multiple
19400	For Biopsy	16449	Laryngoscopy
16425	Endoscopy	19475	Indirect Laryngoscopy
19386	Renal Endoscopy	19476	With Biopsy

19477	Direct Laryngoscopy		22199	Function
19478	Of Newborn		22200	Systolic
19479	With Operating Microscope		22201	Diastolic
44578	With Biopsy		22202	Ejection Fraction
89044	Flexible		22203	Left Atrium
19480	With Biopsy		22204	Size
19481	With Stroboscopy		22205	Right Atrium
16450	Mediastinoscopy		22206	Size
19468	Thoracoscopy		22237	Right Heart Pressure
28300	Of The Lungs And Pleural Space		22208	Ascending Aorta
19469	With Biopsy		22243	For Source Of Emboli
28301	Of The Pericardial Sac		22244	For Clots Or Thrombi
28303	With Biopsy		22245	For Masses
28302	Of The Mediastinal Space		13059	Curettage
28304	With Biopsy		22621	Corneal
18330	Arthroscopy (Diagnostic Only)		18246	Skin Fold Thickness Increased
82001	Temporomandibular Joint		13060	Cold Hemolysis (Donath-Landsteiner Test)
82002	Right			
82003	Left		13061	Intrabursa Injection Test
82019	With Biopsy		13062	Renal Stone Analysis
82004	Shoulder		13072	Dark Field Examination
82005	Right		13073	Donovan Bodies
82006	Left		13074	Woods Light
82020	With Biopsy		13076	Toxin Assay
82007	Elbow		13077	Culdocentesis
82008	Right		13078	Pregnancy Test
82009	Left		13080	Carotid Sinus Massage
82021	With Biopsy		13081	Increases 2nd Degree Block
82010	Wrist		13082	Stops Tachycardia
82011	Right		13083	Paroxysmal Atrial
82012	Left		13084	A-V Nodal Re-entry
82022	With Biopsy		13085	Slows Sinus Tachycardia
82013	Knee		13086	Initiates Bradycardia
82014	Right		13087	Initiates Hypotension
82015	Left		13088	Initiates Hypertension
82023	With Biopsy		13091	Breath Test
82016	Ankle		13092	Hydrogen For Lactose Absorption
82017	Right		13093	Sputum Eosinophils
82018	Left		13094	Sputum Fat
82024	With Biopsy		13095	Sputum Asbestos Fibers
16446	Colposcopy		18050	Sleep Penile Tumescence Test
19281	With Biopsy		13103	Tensilon Test
22190	Cardiac Evaluation		18481	With EMG recording
22242	Preoperative		13104	Arthrogram
22191	Left Ventricle		13105	Knee
22192	Size		13106	Shoulder
22193	Function		22619	Determination Of Refractive State
22194	Systolic		19117	Tonometry
22195	Diastolic		19121	After Provocation
22196	Ejection Fraction		27077	Screening for Glaucoma
22207	Ventricular Wall Thickness		19118	Tonography
22197	Right Ventricle		28615	Coefficient Of Outflow
22198	Size		19120	Glaucoma Index

19119	Water Provocation Test	22222	Threshold Shift
28616	Intraocular Pressure Change	22223	Lower Frequencies
19129	Slit Lamp Examination With Photography	22224	Higher Frequencies
		19150	Air And Bone
19130	Gonioscopy With Photography	19151	Speech Threshold
13139	Visual Fields Test	19152	With Discrimination
13140	Schirmer's Test	19153	Comprehensive
28617	With Anesthesia	19154	Group Testing
28618	Wetting Of The Right Eye	19155	Bekesy Screening
28619	After (Time)	19156	Bekesy Diagnostic
28620	Wetting Of The Left Eye	19157	Loudness Balance Test
28621	After (Time)	19158	Tone Decay Test
19125	Fluorescein Angioscopy	19159	Short Increment Sensitivity Index
19127	Anterior Segment Photography With Specular Microscopy	19160	Stenger Test (Pure Tone)
		26217	Recruitment
19128	Anterior Segment Photography With Fluorescein Angiography	19161	Audiologic Impedance Testing
		19162	Tympanometry
19131	External Ocular Photography	19163	Acoustic Reflex Testing
19126	Extensive Color Vision Testing	18053	Obtain & evaluate previous medical records
19132	Electroretinography		
19133	Electro-oculography	19164	Acoustic Reflex Decay Test
19134	Oculoelectromyography	19165	Filtered Speech Test
19138	Nasal Function Studies (Rhinomanometry)	19166	Staggered Spondaic Word Test
		19167	Lombard Test
19140	Laryngeal Function Studies	19169	Sensorineural Acuity Level Test
19139	Facial Nerve Function Studies	19170	Synthetic Sentence Identification Test
19141	Vestibular Evaluation With Recording	19171	Stenger Test (Speech)
19142	Spontaneous Nystagmus Test	19175	Conditioning Play Audiometry
19143	Positional Nystagmus Test	19176	Select Picture Audiometry
19144	Optokinetic Nystagmus Test	19177	Electrocochleography
13098	Caloric	19178	Brainstem Auditory Evoked Response Recording
19145	Oscillating Tracking Test		
19146	Torsion Swing Test	19179	Central Auditory Function Testing
19147	Utilizing Vertical Electrodes	13153	**Psychometric**
19149	Audiometry	22628	Developmental
13099	Screening Audiogram	18255	Cattell Infant Intelligence Scale (CIIS)
19148	Threshold Pure Tone Audiogram	22625	Bayley Scales Of Infant Development
18189	Right Ear	22629	Illinois Test Of Psycholinguistic Ability (ITPA)
18190	dB at 1K		
18191	dB at 2K	22633	Vineland Social Maturity Scale
18192	dB at 3K	13154	Intelligence quotient (IQ)
18193	dB at 4K	13155	Wechsler Adult Intelligence Scale, Revised (WAIS-R)
18194	dB at 6K		
18195	dB at 500 Hz	13156	Wechsler Pre-school Pre-primary Scale (WPPSI)
18196	dB at 1K on retest		
18197	Left Ear	13157	Wechsler Intelligence Scale for Children, Revised (WISC-R)
18198	dB at 1K		
18199	dB at 2K	13158	Stanford-Binet
18200	dB at 3K	13159	Otis - Lennon
18201	dB at 4K	13160	Beta
18202	dB at 6K	13161	Slosson
18203	dB at 500 Hz	13162	Achievement
18204	dB at 1K on retest	13163	Wide Range (WRAT)

198

13164	Personality		22268	24-Hour Monitoring With 16+ Channel Telemetry
13165	Minnesota Multiphasic Personality Inventory (MMPI)		18477	Prolonged Monitoring With Drug Stimulation
13166	California Psychiatric Inventory (CPI)		18478	Hemispheric Evaluation (Wada Test)
13167	Millon Clinical Multi-Axial Inventory		22269	Cortical Mapping By Brain Surface Electrode Stimulation
22626	Perception		22270	Initial Hour
22627	Frostig Developmental Test Of Visual Perception		22271	Additional Hour
13171	Projective		18474	Placement Of Sphenoid Electrodes
13174	Rorschach Test		18476	Intraoperative (nonintracranial surgery)
13172	Thematic Apperception Test (TAT)		13187	Disorganization
13173	Children's Apperception Test (CAT)		13188	Excessive Fast (Beta) Activity
22631	Senior Apperception Test (SAT)		13189	Theta Slowing (4-7 hz)
13168	Draw-A-Person Test		13190	Unilaterally
13170	House-Tree-Person Test		13191	On The Right
13169	Human Figure Drawing Test		13192	On The Left
13175	Incomplete Sentence Test		13193	Bilaterally
22630	Michigan Picture Stories		13194	Delta Slowing (1-3 hz)
22632	Tasks Of Emotional Development (TED)		13195	Unilaterally
27091	Screening examination for depression		13196	On The Right
13176	Depression Scale		13197	On The Left
13177	Beck		13198	Bilaterally
17989	Hamilton Depression Rating Scale (HDRS)		13199	Triphasic Waves
13178	Organic		13200	Paroxysmal Activity
13179	Bender-Gestalt		13201	3 Per Second Spike and Wave
13180	Benton Visual Retention Test		13202	Polyspike and Wave
13181	Memory For Designs		13203	Hypsarrythmia
13182	Hooper		13204	PLEDS (Paroxysmal Lateralizing Epileptiform Discharges)
13183	Luria-Nebraska		13205	On The Right Only
13184	Halstead Reitan		13206	On The Left Only
21499	Outflow Muscular		13207	Bilaterally
13185	Neuro-Electrical Functions		13208	Sharp Waves
13186	**EEG**		13209	Frontal, right
18463	Administration		13210	Frontal, left
22263	Exam Recording Awake And Drowsy		13211	Temporal, right
22264	Portable To Different Facility		13212	Temporal, left
18464	Exam Recording Awake And Asleep		13213	Parietal, right
18465	Portable To Different Facility		13214	Parietal, left
18466	During Sleep Only		13215	Occipital, right
18468	Evaluation For Brain Death		13216	Occipital, left
18469	Intracerebral Only		13217	Bilateral Waves
18470	All Night Sleep Only		13218	Spikes
18472	24-Hour 8-Channel Monitoring With Interpretation		13219	Frontal, right
18473	24-Hour Monitoring With Videotaping		13220	Frontal, left
22267	24-Hour Monitoring With 16-Channel Computerized Portable EEG		13221	Temporal, right
			13222	Temporal, left
			13223	Parietal, right
			13224	Parietal, left
			13225	Occipital, right
			13226	Occipital, left

13227	Bilateral Spikes		18499	Sensory Pathway
13228	Electrical Status		13251	Velocity Sciatic Nerve
13229	Burst Suppression		18493	Motor Pathway
13230	Alpha Coma		18500	Sensory Pathway
13231	Isoelectric		13252	Velocity Ulnar Nerve
13232	Evoked Responses (Potentials)		18494	Motor Pathway
13233	Visual		18501	Sensory Pathway
13234	Auditory		13253	Velocity Brachial Plexus
13235	Tactile ("Sensory")		18495	Motor Pathway
22226	Electronic Analysis Of Implanted Neurostimulator		18502	Sensory Pathway
			19457	Bulbocavernosus Reflex
22227	With Reprogramming Of Pulse Generator		13254	Decreased Velocity Overall
			18503	H Reflex Testing
13236	**EMG**		18504	F Response Testing
18482	Extremities and Paraspinal Areas		18505	Repetitive Stimulation Tests
22259	One Extremity		22265	Sleep Testing
22260	Two Extremities		22266	Multiple Sleep Latency Testing
22261	Three Extremities		13102	Sleep Study
22262	Four Extremities		18115	Reversal of REM/NREM order
18483	Cranial Nerve Distribution		18479	Polysomnography
22257	Unilateral		29374	With Four Or More Additional Sleep Parameters
22258	Bilateral			
18484	Specific Truncal Group		18480	Electrooculogram (EOG)
18485	Single Fiber		13638	Vectorcardiogram
18486	After Ischemic Limb Exercise, With Lactic Acid Determination		19221	Tracing Only
			19222	Analysis And Report
13237	Fibrillation Potentials		19208	**Continuous EKG Monitoring**
13238	Fasiculation		19209	Visual Superimposition Scanning
13239	Action Potentials - Decreased Amplitude & Duration		19210	Recording Only
			19211	Analysis & Report
13240	Action Potentials - Large Amplitude and Duration		19212	Physician Interpretation
			19213	With Microprocessor Analysis
13241	Decreased Motor Units		19214	Recording Only
13242	Recruitment		19215	Analysis & Report
13243	Repetitive Stimulation Decrement		19216	Physician Interpretation
13244	Myotonia		19217	With Realtime Data Analysis
19455	Anal Sphincter		19218	With Report
19456	Urethral Sphincter		19219	Physician Interpretation
13245	**Nerve Conduction Studies**		19220	Patient Demand Event Recording
13246	Velocity Tibiae		28305	Hookup, Recording, And Disconnection Only
18487	Motor Pathway			
18488	Sensory Pathway		28306	Monitoring, Receive Transmission, And Analysis
13247	Velocity Anterior Tibiae			
18489	Motor Pathway		28307	Physician Review And Interpretation Only
18496	Sensory Pathway			
13248	Velocity Median Nerve		19673	Signal-averaged (SAECG)
18490	Motor Pathway		13561	Holter monitor
18497	Sensory Pathway		13562	12 Hour
13249	Velocity Peroneal Nerve		13563	24 Hour
18491	Motor Pathway		13564	72 Hour
18498	Sensory Pathway		17974	QRS
13250	Velocity Radial Nerve		17975	Absent
18492	Motor Pathway		17976	Intermittently Absent

17977	Pacemaker Rhythm		13599	Complete Heart Block
17978	Excessively Fast		13596	Constant AV Block
17979	Excessively Slow		13600	Paroxysmal Supraventricular tachycardia
17980	Failure to Capture		13601	A-V Junctional Rhythms
17981	Intermittent		13602	Escape Beats
17982	Pacemaker Sensing		13603	Premature Beats
17983	Atrial Activity Failing to Inhibit		13604	Bigeminal
17984	Atrial Activity Failing to Trigger		13605	Trigeminal
17985	Ventricular Activity Failing to Inhibit		13606	Frequent
17986	Ventricular Activity Failing to Trigger		13607	Consecutive
17987	Intermittent Failure		13608	Aberrant Conduction
17988	Constant Failure		13609	Tachycardia
13565	Sinus Rhythms		13610	Ventricular Arrhythmias
13566	Tachycardia		13611	Escape Beats
13567	Bradycardia		13612	Premature Depolarization
13568	Arrhythmia		13613	Multifocal
13569	Arrest		13614	Superimposed on T Wave
13570	Sinus Node Wenckebach		13615	>5 per Minute
13571	Sinoatrial Exit Block		13616	>30 per Hour
13493	Type I		13617	Consecutive
13494	Type II		13618	Couplet
13572	Wandering Pacemaker		13619	Non-sustained ventricular tachycardia (3-6 beats)
13573	Atrial Rhythms			
13574	Escape Beats		13620	Sustained ventricular tachycardia (7 or more beats)
13575	Atrial Premature Depolarization			
13576	Bigeminal		13621	Fusion Beats
13577	Trigeminal		13622	Bigeminal
13578	Frequent		13623	Trigeminal
13579	Consecutive		13624	Tachycardia
13580	With Aberrant Intraventricular Conduction (IVCD)		13625	Accelerated Idioventricular Rhythm
			13626	Fibrillation
13581	With Block		17999	Ventriculo-atrial conduction
24876	Atrial Tachycardia		13627	Pararrhythmias
13582	Automatic Atrial Tachycardia		13628	Parasystole
13583	Paroxysmal Atrial Tachycardia With Block		13629	A-V Dissociation
			13630	Preexcitation
13584	Chaotic Atrial Rhythm		13631	QRS Wide and Slurred
13585	Bradycardia-Tachycardia Syndrome		13632	Delta R Wave
13586	Flutter		13633	P-J Interval Normal
13588	QRS Complexes in 2:1 to 8:1 ratio		13634	P-J Interval Shortened
13589	Fibrillation		82026	Electrophysiology
13590	With Slow Ventricular Response		19257	Comprehensive Electrophysiologic Evaluation
13591	With Rapid Ventricular Response			
13587	with F Waves		22703	With Induction Of Arrhythmia
13592	1:1 A-V Conduction		19258	With Left Atrial Recording
13593	Atrioventricular Block		19259	With Left Ventricular Recording
13594	First Degree		13635	His Bundle Electrocardiography
13595	Second Degree		13636	A-H Interval (msec.)
13597	Mobitz Type I		13637	H-V Interval (msec.)
13598	Mobitz Type II		18048	Early His Bundle Depolarization
81012	Conduction Rate 2:1		19242	Intra-atrial Electrophysiologic Recording
81013	Conduction Rate 3:1		19243	Right Ventricular Electrophysiologic Recording
81014	Conduction Rate 4:1			

19244	Left Ventricular Electrophysiologic Recording	12557	Pus
		12558	Sanguinous
19245	Intracardiac Mapping Of Tachycardia	12559	Straw-Colored
19246	Intracardiac Pacing	12560	Protein (as % of serum value)
19247	Intra-atrial	12561	RBC
19248	Intraventricular	12562	WBC
19249	For Induction of Arrhythmia	12563	neutrophils predominate
19250	Intra-operative With Mapping	12564	lymphocytes predominate
19251	Follow-up For Therapy Effectiveness	12565	mononuclear cells predominate
19254	Programmed Stimulation After IV Medication	12566	Elevated LDH
		12567	pH
19252	Esophageal Recording Of Atrial Electrogram	12568	Specific Gravity
		12569	Glucose
19253	With Intracardiac Pacing	12570	Amylase
19255	Evaluation Of Cardioverter-defibrillator	18112	Hyaluronic Acid
28308	With Testing Of Pulse Generator	12571	Cytology
29393	Subsequent Therapeutic Evaluation	12572	Cholesterol
29394	Electronic Analysis	12573	Triglycerides
29395	With Reprogramming	12574	Chylomicrons
19263	Electronic Analysis Of Pacemaker	18327	Venipuncture
19264	Dual-chamber	18407	Chorionic Villus Sampling
19265	With Reprogramming	27078	Screening for Ischemic Heart Disease
19266	Telephonic Analysis	27079	Screening for Hypertension
19267	Single-chamber	19347	Vascular Procedures
19268	With Reprogramming	18328	Arterial puncture
19269	Telephonic Analysis	19349	Arterial Cannulation For Monitoring (Percutaneous)
18325	Arthrocentesis		
18326	Amniocentesis	19350	Arterial Cannulation For Monitoring (Cutdown)
19285	Cordocentesis		
18324	Paracentesis	19352	Umbilical Artery Catheterization
18323	Pericardiocentesis	13143	Manometry
22062	Echo-Guided	13144	Biliary
22061	Unsuccessful Attempt	13145	Sphincter of Oddi
22068	Fluid Volume	13146	Esophageal
12523	Gross Appearance	13148	Bladder
22059	Serosanguinous	13149	Cystometrogram
22060	Bloody	19448	Simple
12524	Cytology	19449	Complex
12525	RBC / HPF	13049	Flow Rate Studies
12526	Protein	19450	Simple
12527	LDH	19451	Complex
12528	pO2	19385	Through Pyelostomy Tube
19495	Pneumocentesis	19438	Through Ureterostomy Or Ureteral Catheter
22079	culture for klebsiella pneumoniae		
13090	Thoracentesis	19454	Urethral
22067	Echo-Guided	19452	Intra-abdominal Voiding Pressure
22069	CT-Guided	13150	CSF
22071	Unsuccessful Attempt	13151	Gastric
12553	Pleural Fluid	13152	Rectal
22070	Volume	19413	Pneumoperitoneum (Diagnostic)
12554	Gross Appearance	19414	Initial
12555	Chocolate Color	19415	Subsequent
12556	Milky	16452	Esophageal

16453	Bougeniage
16454	Eder-Peustow
16455	Hurst
16456	Maloney
16457	Savary
16458	Pneumatic
72114	Dental Procedures (Diagnostic)
19002	Home Environment Testing
19003	Air Sampling
19062	Particulate Matter (Annual Mean)
19063	Carbon Monoxide (Max. 8-Hr.)
19064	Hydrocarbons
19065	Nitrogen Oxides
19066	Photochemical Oxidants
19073	Radon
19067	Sulfur Dioxide
19004	Drinking Water Sampling
19020	Inorganic Chemicals
19010	Arsenic
19011	Barium
19012	Cadmium
19013	Chromium (As hexavalent ion)
19014	Fluoride
19015	Lead
19016	Mercury
19017	Nitrates as Nitrogen
19018	Selenium
19019	Silver
19032	Insecticides
19033	Endrin
19034	Lindane
19035	Methoxychlor
19036	Toxaphene
19037	Weed Killers
19038	2-4-D
19039	2-4-5TP
19005	Noise Measurement
19006	**Work Environment Testing**
19007	Air Sampling
19048	Particulate Matter (Annual Mean)
19049	Benzene (TWA)
19050	Carbon Monoxide (TWA)
19051	Gasoline (TWA)
19052	Hydrocarbons
19053	Hydrogen Fluoride (Ceiling Limit)
19054	Hydrogen Sulfide (TWA)
19055	Light Napthas (TWA)
19056	Heavy Napthas (TWA)
19057	Nitrogen Oxides
19058	Oil Vapor (TWA)
19059	Petroleum Coke (TWA)
19060	Photochemical Oxidants
19061	Sulfur Dioxide
19009	Noise Measurement
19293	Discharge Testing
19294	Air For
19297	Particulate Matter (Annual Mean)
19304	Benzene (TWA)
19305	Carbon Monoxide (TWA)
19306	Gasoline (TWA)
19307	Hydrocarbons
19308	Hydrogen Sulfide (TWA)
19309	Nitrogen Oxides
19310	Petroleum Coke (TWA)
19311	Sulfur Dioxide
19008	Water Sampling
19021	Inorganic Chemicals
19022	Arsenic
19023	Barium
19024	Cadmium
19025	Chromium (As hexavalent ion)
19026	Fluoride
19027	Lead
19028	Mercury
19029	Nitrates as Nitrogen
19030	Selenium
19031	Silver
19040	Insecticides
19041	Endrin
19042	Lindane
19043	Methoxychlor
19044	Toxaphene
19045	Weed Killers
19046	2-4-D
19047	2-4-5TP
19295	Soil Sampling
19315	Arsenic
19316	Cadmium
19317	Chromium (As hexavalent ion)
19318	Lead
19319	Mercury
19320	Selenium
19321	Silver
19322	Insecticides
19323	Endrin
19324	Lindane
19325	Methoxychlor
19326	Toxaphene
19327	Weed Killers
19328	2-4-D
19329	2-4-5TP
19312	Benzene
19313	Gasoline
19314	Hydrocarbons
19296	Noise Measurement
84442	**Surgical Studies**

84437	Cranial Procedures		19374	With Nephrotomy
22149	Cranial Tap		24890	**Imaging Studies**
22150	Subdural		13142	Fluorescein Angiography
22151	Inital		19123	With Fundus Photography
22152	Subsequent		19124	With Ophthalmodynamometry
22153	Ventricular		29476	Hyperfluorescence
22154	With Injection Of Diagnostic Substance		29480	Right Eye
			29481	Left Eye
22155	Cisternal (C1-C2)		29482	Bilateral
22156	With Injection Of Diagnostic Substance		29492	Leak
			29495	And Pooling
22157	Lateral Cervical (C1-C2)		29497	In The Subretinal Space
22158	With Injection Of Diagnostic Substance		29511	From A Neurosensory Detachment
22159	Of Shunt Tubing		29512	From An RPE Detachment
22160	Of Reservoir		29498	Within The Retina
22161	Burr Hole		29496	And Staining
22162	Subdural		29499	In The Subretinal Space
22164	For Implanting Pressure Recording Device		29500	Within The Retina
			29515	Noncystoid
22177	With Implantation For Seizure Monitoring		29516	Perivascular
			29493	Increased Transmission
22163	Ventricular		29494	Abnormal Vessels
22165	For Implanting Pressure Recording Device		29501	In The Subretinal Space
			29513	Due To Neovascularization
22166	Intracerebral		29514	Within A Scar
22167	For Implanting Pressure Recording Device		29502	Within The Retina
			29504	Due To Neovascularization
22168	Supratentorial, Exploratory		29505	Due To Telangiectasias
22169	Infratentorial		29506	With Microaneurysm(s)
22170	On The Right		29507	With Macroaneurysm(s)
22171	On The Left		29508	With Dilation And Tortuosity
22172	Bilaterally		29509	With Shunt(s)
22173	Craniotomy		29510	With Collateral Vessel(s)
22174	Supratentorial		29503	Associated With A Mass
22175	Infratentorial		29477	Hypofluorescence
22176	Transcranial Exploration Of Orbit		29483	Right Eye
22178	Bone Flap Elevation, Implant Strip Elect For Seizure Monitor		29484	Left Eye
			29485	Bilateral
22180	Stereotactic Implant Depth Electrodes For Seizure Monitoring		29517	Due To Blockage
			29522	By Hemorrhage
22179	Removal Of Electrode Array		29530	Within The Retina
18475	Intraoperative Electrocorticogram		29531	In The Subretinal Space
28597	Aspiration Of Intraocular Fluids		29532	In The Vitreous
28598	Aqueous Humor		29533	Preretinal
49241	Removal Of Vitreous - Anterior Chamber		29520	By Exudates
49242	Including Air Injection		29528	Hard
49329	Release Of Vitreous Fluid By Pars Plana Approach - Posterior Segment		29529	Soft
			29521	By Edema
19474	Laryngotomy		29519	By Melanin
17893	Exploratory Laparotomy		29526	By Drusen
19404	Surgical Retroperitoneal Exploration		29523	By Foreign Body
19373	Renal Exploration		29524	By Myelin

29525	By Lipofuscin		29254	Epinephrine
29527	By Xanthophyll		29255	Norepinephrine
29518	Due To A Filling Defect		21918	Infusion Duration
29534	In The Retina		21919	Up To 5 Minutes
29536	Artery		21920	5-10 Minutes
29537	Vein(s)		21921	10-15 Minutes
29538	Capillaries		21922	15-20 Minutes
29535	In The Choroid		28735	Studies / Measurements Performed
29478	Pseudofluorescence		21882	ECG
29486	Right Eye		25212	At Rest
29487	Left Eye		25213	At Peak Exercise
29488	Bilateral		25214	Post Exercise
29539	Due To Mismatched Filters		28736	ST / Heart Rate Slope Done
29479	Autofluorescence		28737	Wall Motion Was Studied
29489	Right Eye		28738	The Ejection Fraction Was Calculated
29490	Left Eye		28739	Perfusion Was Studied
29491	Bilateral		28740	Infarct Size Was Quantitated
29540	From Myelinated Nerve Fibers		28741	Regurgitation Fraction Was Calculated
29541	From Optic Disc Drusen		28742	Oxygen Consumption Was Determined
29543	From Retinal Drusen		21923	Interval Measurements
29542	From Scars		24897	Measurements At Rest
21874	**Cardiac Stress Test**		29066	Sitting
80918	Services Performed		27350	Feet Down
13460	With Physician Supervision, Interpretation And Report		27351	Feet Up
			29067	Supine
19200	Interpretation And Report Only		29068	Standing
19201	Performance of Tracing Only		29069	Hyperventilating
29389	Physician Supervision Only		21924	Heart Rate
21888	Type Of Stress		21925	Systolic BP
21875	Treadmill		21926	Diastolic BP
21991	Bruce Protocol		24991	ECG Findings
21992	Modified Bruce Protocol		24992	P Wave Axis
25638	Mayo Protocol		24993	PR Interval
28338	Modified Mayo Protocol		24994	QRS Interval
25054	Cornell Protocol		29360	Repolarization Normal
25055	Naughton Protocol		24995	ST Segment (mm.)
25659	O2 Uptake Protocol		29358	elevation < 1mm
28339	Balke Protocol		29359	elevation > or = 1mm
21876	Ergometer		24996	ST Segment Slope
25632	Arm		24997	T Wave Axis
25635	Upright Bicycle		29361	T Wave Inversion(s)
25636	Supine Bicycle		29362	during ST elevation
21877	Pharmacologic Challenge		29363	T Wave Pseudo Normalization
21879	Dipyridamole		24998	U Wave
25685	Adenosine		24999	Rhythm
28494	Calculated Total Dose		28558	Atrial Abnormality
28495	Total Dose Given		28556	Right
28496	Aminophylline Given		28557	Left
28497	Total Dose		28624	Other Findings
28498	Time Following Challenge		28625	Borg Scale
21878	Dobutamine		28626	Ectopic Count Last Minute
21880	Dopamine		28627	QRS Duration
25686	Arbutamine		28628	X Axis

CARDIAC STRESS TEST, CONT.

28629	Y Axis	28680	V5
28630	Z Axis	28681	V6
28631	Q-Wave Duration	28685	X
28632	T-Wave Amplitude	28686	Y
28633	X-Axis	28687	Z
28634	Y-Axis	28827	Sinus Rhythm
28635	Z-Axis	28828	Arrhythmia
28636	R-Wave Amplitude	28829	Ventriculophasic Arrhythmia
28637	X-Axis	28830	Bradycardia
28638	Y-Axis	28831	Tachycardia
28639	Z-Axis	28832	Arrest
28640	R-Max Cosine Vector	28833	Sinoatrial Exit Block
28641	X-Axis	28834	Ectopic Atrial Rhythm
28642	Y-Axis	28835	Wandering Atrial Pacemaker
28643	Z-Axis	28836	Atrial Premature Depolarization
28644	R-Max Amplitude	28837	Abnormal Conduction
28645	ST Slope	28838	Nonconduction
28646	X-Axis	28839	Aberrant Conduction
28647	Y-Axis	28840	Atrial Tachycardia
28648	Z-Axis	28841	Sustained
28649	3-D ST Segment Vector Magnitude @ 60 msec.	28842	1:1 Conduction
		28843	Short Paroxysms
29070	3-D ST Segment Vector Angle In The XY Plane	28844	Multifocal
		28845	With AV Block
29071	3-D ST Segment Vector Angle In The XZ Plane	28846	Supraventricular Tachycardia
		28847	Paroxysmal Supraventricular Tachycardia
28653	ST Segment Changes		
28654	I	28848	Atrial Flutter
28655	II	28849	Atrial Fibrillation
28656	III	28850	Retrograde Atrial Activation
28657	aVR	28851	A-V Junctional Rhythms
28658	aVL	28852	Premature Beats
28659	aVF	28853	Escape Beats
28660	V1	28854	Accelerated
28661	V2	28855	Ventricular Premature Depolarization
28662	V3		
28663	V4	28856	Uniform, Fixed Coupling
28664	V5	28857	Uniform, Non-Fixed Coupling
28665	V6		
28666	X	28858	Multiform
28667	Y	28859	In Pairs
28668	Z	28860	Ventricular Parasystole
28669	ST / Heart Rate Slope	28861	Ventricular Tachycardia
28670	I	28862	Accelerated Idioventricular Rhythm
28671	II		
28672	III	28863	Ventricular Escape Beats
28673	aVR	28864	Ventricular Fibrillation
28674	aVL	28865	AV Block
28675	aVF	28866	1st Degree
28676	V1	28867	2nd Degree Mobitz Type I
28677	V2	28868	2nd Degree Mobitz Type II
28678	V3	28869	3rd Degree
28679	V4	28870	2:1

CARDIAC STRESS TEST, CONT.

28871	Variable		21891	Speed
28872	P-R Interval		21892	Grade
28873	Wolff-Parkinson-White Pattern		21910	Load
28874	Fusion Beats		25153	Infusion Rate
28875	Re-Entrant Ventricular Beats		26414	Dosage
28876	AV Dissociation		21930	Heart Rate
28877	QRS Axis Deviation		21931	Systolic BP
28878	Left		21932	Diastolic BP
28879	Right		25238	ST Segment
28880	Electrical Alternans		29080	X-axis Component
28881	Left Ventricular Hypertrophy		29109	Y-axis Component
28882	By Voltage		29138	Z-axis Component
28883	By Strain		29167	3-D Vector Magnitude
28884	Right Ventricular Hypertrophy		29196	3-D Vector Angle In XY Plane
28885	Combined Ventricular Hypertrophy		29225	3-D Vector Angle In XZ Plane
			25121	Oxygen Consumption
28886	Ventricular Conduction Delay		28705	Peak Stress Level
28887	Right		24900	3rd Interval Measurements
28888	Left Anterior Hemiblock		25183	Elapsed Time
28889	Left Posterior Hemiblock		21893	Speed
28890	Left Branch Bundle Block		21894	Grade
28891	ST-T Waves of Acute MI		21911	Load
28892	Complete		25154	Infusion Rate
28893	Incomplete		26415	Dosage
29352	Onset Rate		21933	Heart Rate
28897	Right Branch Bundle Block		24963	Systolic BP
28894	Intraventricular Conduction Delay		24964	Diastolic BP
			25239	ST Segment
28895	Nonspecific		29081	X-axis Component
28896	With Aberrancy		29110	Y-axis Component
29353	Onset Rate		29139	Z-axis Component
25000	Oxygen Consumption		29168	3-D Vector Magnitude
24898	1st Interval Measurements		29197	3-D Vector Angle In XY Plane
25152	Elapsed Time		29226	3-D Vector Angle In XZ Plane
21889	Speed		25122	Oxygen Consumption
21890	Grade		28706	Peak Stress Level
21909	Load		24901	4th Interval Measurements
25151	Infusion Rate		25184	Elapsed Time
26413	Dosage		21895	Speed
21927	Heart Rate		21896	Grade
24961	Systolic BP		21912	Load
24962	Diastolic BP		25155	Infusion Rate
25237	ST Segment		26416	Dosage
29074	X-axis Component		21936	Heart Rate
29075	Y-axis Component		21937	Systolic BP
29076	Z-axis Component		21938	Diastolic BP
29077	3-D Vector Magnitude		25240	ST Segment
29078	3-D Vector Angle In XY Plane		29082	X-axis Component
29079	3-D Vector Angle In XZ Plane		29111	Y-axis Component
25120	Oxygen Consumption		29140	Z-axis Component
28704	Peak Stress Level		29169	3-D Vector Magnitude
24899	2nd Interval Measurements		29198	3-D Vector Angle In XY Plane
25182	Elapsed Time		29227	3-D Vector Angle In XZ Plane

CARDIAC STRESS TEST, CONT.

25123	Oxygen Consumption		29143	Z-axis Component
28707	Peak Stress Level		29172	3-D Vector Magnitude
24902	5th Interval Measurements		29201	3-D Vector Angle In XY Plane
25185	Elapsed Time		29230	3-D Vector Angle In XZ Plane
21897	Speed		25126	Oxygen Consumption
21898	Grade		28710	Peak Stress Level
21913	Load		24905	8th Interval Measurements
25156	Infusion Rate		25188	Elapsed Time
26417	Dosage		21903	Speed
21939	Heart Rate		21904	Grade
24965	Systolic BP		21916	Load
24966	Diastolic BP		25159	Infusion Rate
25241	ST Segment		26420	Dosage
29083	X-axis Component		21944	Heart Rate
29112	Y-axis Component		21945	Systolic BP
29141	Z-axis Component		21946	Diastolic BP
29170	3-D Vector Magnitude		25244	ST Segment
29199	3-D Vector Angle In XY Plane		29086	X-axis Component
29228	3-D Vector Angle In XZ Plane		29115	Y-axis Component
25124	Oxygen Consumption		29144	Z-axis Component
28708	Peak Stress Level		29173	3-D Vector Magnitude
24903	6th Interval Measurements		29202	3-D Vector Angle In XY Plane
25186	Elapsed Time		29231	3-D Vector Angle In XZ Plane
21899	Speed		25127	Oxygen Consumption
21900	Grade		28711	Peak Stress Level
21914	Load		24906	9th Interval Measurements
25157	Infusion Rate		25189	Elapsed Time
26418	Dosage		21905	Speed
21940	Heart Rate		21906	Grade
21941	Systolic BP		21917	Load
21942	Diastolic BP		25160	Infusion Rate
25242	ST Segment		26421	Dosage
29084	X-axis Component		21947	Heart Rate
29113	Y-axis Component		24969	Systolic BP
29142	Z-axis Component		24970	Diastolic BP
29171	3-D Vector Magnitude		25245	ST Segment
29200	3-D Vector Angle In XY Plane		29087	X-axis Component
29229	3-D Vector Angle In XZ Plane		29116	Y-axis Component
25125	Oxygen Consumption		29145	Z-axis Component
28709	Peak Stress Level		29174	3-D Vector Magnitude
24904	7th Interval Measurements		29203	3-D Vector Angle In XY Plane
25187	Elapsed Time		29232	3-D Vector Angle In XZ Plane
21901	Speed		25128	Oxygen Consumption
21902	Grade		28712	Peak Stress Level
21915	Load		24907	10th Interval Measurements
25158	Infusion Rate		25190	Elapsed Time
26419	Dosage		21907	Speed
21943	Heart Rate		21908	Grade
24967	Systolic BP		25056	Load
24968	Diastolic BP		25161	Infusion Rate
25243	ST Segment		26422	Dosage
29085	X-axis Component		21948	Heart Rate
29114	Y-axis Component		21949	Systolic BP

CARDIAC STRESS TEST, CONT.

21950	Diastolic BP		25164	Infusion Rate
25246	ST Segment		26425	Dosage
29088	X-axis Component		21955	Heart Rate
29117	Y-axis Component		24973	Systolic BP
29146	Z-axis Component		24974	Diastolic BP
29175	3-D Vector Magnitude		25249	ST Segment (mm.)
29204	3-D Vector Angle In XY Plane		29091	X-axis Component
29233	3-D Vector Angle In XZ Plane		29120	Y-axis Component
25129	Oxygen Consumption		29149	Z-axis Component
28713	Peak Stress Level		29178	3-D Vector Magnitude
24908	11th Interval Measurements		29207	3-D Vector Angle In XY Plane
25191	Elapsed Time		29236	3-D Vector Angle In XZ Plane
25078	Speed		25132	Oxygen Consumption
25099	Grade		28716	Peak Stress Level
25057	Load		24911	14th Interval Measurements
25162	Infusion Rate		25194	Elapsed Time
26423	Dosage		25081	Speed
21951	Heart Rate		25102	Grade
24971	Systolic BP		25060	Load
24972	Diastolic BP		25211	Infusion Rate
25247	ST Segment		26426	Dosage
29089	X-axis Component		21956	Heart Rate
29118	Y-axis Component		21957	Systolic BP
29147	Z-axis Component		21958	Diastolic BP
29176	3-D Vector Magnitude		25250	ST Segment (mm.)
29205	3-D Vector Angle In XY Plane		29092	X-axis Component
29234	3-D Vector Angle In XZ Plane		29121	Y-axis Component
25130	Oxygen Consumption		29150	Z-axis Component
28714	Peak Stress Level		29179	3-D Vector Magnitude
24909	12th Interval Measurements		29208	3-D Vector Angle In XY Plane
25192	Elapsed Time		29237	3-D Vector Angle In XZ Plane
25079	Speed		25133	Oxygen Consumption
25100	Grade		28717	Peak Stress Level
25058	Load		24912	15th Interval Measurements
25163	Infusion Rate		25195	Elapsed Time
26424	Dosage		25082	Speed
21952	Heart Rate		25103	Grade
21953	Systolic BP		25061	Load
21954	Diastolic BP		25165	Infusion Rate
25248	ST Segment (mm.)		26427	Dosage
29090	X-axis Component		21959	Heart Rate
29119	Y-axis Component		24975	Systolic BP
29148	Z-axis Component		24976	Diastolic BP
29177	3-D Vector Magnitude		25251	ST Segment (mm.)
29206	3-D Vector Angle In XY Plane		29093	X-axis Component
29235	3-D Vector Angle In XZ Plane		29122	Y-axis Component
25131	Oxygen Consumption		29151	Z-axis Component
28715	Peak Stress Level		29180	3-D Vector Magnitude
24910	13th Interval Measurements		29209	3-D Vector Angle In XY Plane
25193	Elapsed Time		29238	3-D Vector Angle In XZ Plane
25080	Speed		25134	Oxygen Consumption
25101	Grade		28718	Peak Stress Level
25059	Load		24913	16th Interval Measurements

CARDIAC STRESS TEST, CONT.

25196	Elapsed Time		29241	3-D Vector Angle In XZ Plane
25083	Speed		25137	Oxygen Consumption
25104	Grade		28721	Peak Stress Level
25062	Load		24916	19th Interval Measurements
25166	Infusion Rate		25199	Elapsed Time
26428	Dosage		25086	Speed
21960	Heart Rate		25107	Grade
21961	Systolic BP		25065	Load
21962	Diastolic BP		25169	Infusion Rate
25252	ST Segment (mm.)		26431	Dosage
29094	X-axis Component		21967	Heart Rate
29123	Y-axis Component		24979	Systolic BP
29152	Z-axis Component		24980	Diastolic BP
29181	3-D Vector Magnitude		25255	ST Segment (mm.)
29210	3-D Vector Angle In XY Plane		29097	X-axis Component
29239	3-D Vector Angle In XZ Plane		29126	Y-axis Component
25135	Oxygen Consumption		29155	Z-axis Component
28719	Peak Stress Level		29184	3-D Vector Magnitude
24914	17th Interval Measurements		29213	3-D Vector Angle In XY Plane
25197	Elapsed Time		29242	3-D Vector Angle In XZ Plane
25084	Speed		25138	Oxygen Consumption
25105	Grade		28722	Peak Stress Level
25063	Load		24917	20th Interval Measurements
25167	Infusion Rate		25200	Elapsed Time
26429	Dosage		25087	Speed
21963	Heart Rate		25108	Grade
24977	Systolic BP		25066	Load
24978	Diastolic BP		25170	Infusion Rate
25253	ST Segment (mm.)		26432	Dosage
29095	X-axis Component		21968	Heart Rate
29124	Y-axis Component		21969	Systolic BP
29153	Z-axis Component		21970	Diastolic BP
29182	3-D Vector Magnitude		25256	ST Segment (mm.)
29211	3-D Vector Angle In XY Plane		29098	X-axis Component
29240	3-D Vector Angle In XZ Plane		29127	Y-axis Component
25136	Oxygen Consumption		29156	Z-axis Component
28720	Peak Stress Level		29185	3-D Vector Magnitude
24915	18th Interval Measurements		29214	3-D Vector Angle In XY Plane
25198	Elapsed Time		29243	3-D Vector Angle In XZ Plane
25085	Speed		25139	Oxygen Consumption
25106	Grade		28723	Peak Stress Level
25064	Load		24918	21st Interval Measurements
25168	Infusion Rate		25201	Elapsed Time
26430	Dosage		25088	Speed
21964	Heart Rate		25109	Grade
21965	Systolic BP		25067	Load
21966	Diastolic BP		25171	Infusion Rate
25254	ST Segment (mm.)		26433	Dosage
29096	X-axis Component		21971	Heart Rate
29125	Y-axis Component		24981	Systolic BP
29154	Z-axis Component		24982	Diastolic BP
29183	3-D Vector Magnitude		25257	ST Segment (mm.)
29212	3-D Vector Angle In XY Plane		29099	X-axis Component

CARDIAC STRESS TEST, CONT.

29128	Y-axis Component	21977	Systolic BP
29157	Z-axis Component	21978	Diastolic BP
29186	3-D Vector Magnitude	25260	ST Segment (mm.)
29215	3-D Vector Angle In XY Plane	29102	X-axis Component
29244	3-D Vector Angle In XZ Plane	29131	Y-axis Component
25140	Oxygen Consumption	29160	Z-axis Component
28724	Peak Stress Level	29189	3-D Vector Magnitude
24919	22nd Interval Measurements	29218	3-D Vector Angle In XY Plane
25202	Elapsed Time	29247	3-D Vector Angle In XZ Plane
25089	Speed	25143	Oxygen Consumption
25110	Grade	28727	Peak Stress Level
25068	Load	24922	25th Interval Measurements
25172	Infusion Rate	25205	Elapsed Time
26434	Dosage	25092	Speed
21972	Heart Rate	25113	Grade
21973	Systolic BP	25071	Load
21974	Diastolic BP	25175	Infusion Rate
25258	ST Segment (mm.)	26437	Dosage
29100	X-axis Component	21979	Heart Rate
29129	Y-axis Component	24985	Systolic BP
29158	Z-axis Component	24986	Diastolic BP
29187	3-D Vector Magnitude	25261	ST Segment (mm.)
29216	3-D Vector Angle In XY Plane	29103	X-axis Component
29245	3-D Vector Angle In XZ Plane	29132	Y-axis Component
25141	Oxygen Consumption	29161	Z-axis Component
28725	Peak Stress Level	29190	3-D Vector Magnitude
24920	23rd Interval Measurements	29219	3-D Vector Angle In XY Plane
25203	Elapsed Time	29248	3-D Vector Angle In XZ Plane
25090	Speed	25144	Oxygen Consumption
25111	Grade	28728	Peak Stress Level
25069	Load	24923	26th Interval Measurements
25173	Infusion Rate	25206	Elapsed Time
26435	Dosage	25093	Speed
21975	Heart Rate	25114	Grade
24983	Systolic BP	25072	Load
24984	Diastolic BP	25176	Infusion Rate
25259	ST Segment (mm.)	26438	Dosage
29101	X-axis Component	21980	Heart Rate
29130	Y-axis Component	21981	Systolic BP
29159	Z-axis Component	21982	Diastolic BP
29188	3-D Vector Magnitude	25262	ST Segment (mm.)
29217	3-D Vector Angle In XY Plane	29104	X-axis Component
29246	3-D Vector Angle In XZ Plane	29133	Y-axis Component
25142	Oxygen Consumption	29162	Z-axis Component
28726	Peak Stress Level	29191	3-D Vector Magnitude
24921	24th Interval Measurements	29220	3-D Vector Angle In XY Plane
25204	Elapsed Time	29249	3-D Vector Angle In XZ Plane
25091	Speed	25145	Oxygen Consumption
25112	Grade	28729	Peak Stress Level
25070	Load	24924	27th Interval Measurements
25174	Infusion Rate	25207	Elapsed Time
26436	Dosage	25094	Speed
21976	Heart Rate	25115	Grade

CARDIAC STRESS TEST, CONT.

25073	Load	24927	30th Interval Measurements
25177	Infusion Rate	25210	Elapsed Time
26439	Dosage	25097	Speed
21983	Heart Rate	25118	Grade
24987	Systolic BP	25076	Load
24988	Diastolic BP	25180	Infusion Rate
25263	ST Segment (mm.)	26442	Dosage
29105	X-axis Component	21988	Heart Rate
29134	Y-axis Component	21989	Systolic BP
29163	Z-axis Component	21990	Diastolic BP
29192	3-D Vector Magnitude	25266	ST Segment (mm.)
29221	3-D Vector Angle In XY Plane	29108	X-axis Component
29250	3-D Vector Angle In XZ Plane	29137	Y-axis Component
25146	Oxygen Consumption	29166	Z-axis Component
28730	Peak Stress Level	29195	3-D Vector Magnitude
24925	28th Interval Measurements	29224	3-D Vector Angle In XY Plane
25208	Elapsed Time	29253	3-D Vector Angle In XZ Plane
25095	Speed	25149	Oxygen Consumption
25116	Grade	28733	Peak Stress Level
25074	Load	25679	Number of Levels Completed
25178	Infusion Rate	28909	Interim Stress ECG
26440	Dosage	28911	Sinus Rhythm
21984	Heart Rate	28912	Sinus Arrhythmia
21985	Systolic BP	28913	Sinus Bradycardia
21986	Diastolic BP	28914	Sinus Tachycardia
25264	ST Segment (mm.)	28915	Sinus Pause
29106	X-axis Component	28916	Sinoatrial Exit Block
29135	Y-axis Component	28917	Ectopic Atrial Rhythm
29164	Z-axis Component	28918	Wandering Atrial Pacemaker
29193	3-D Vector Magnitude	28919	Premature Atrial Contractions
29222	3-D Vector Angle In XY Plane	28922	Normally Conducted
29251	3-D Vector Angle In XZ Plane	28920	Nonconducted
25147	Oxygen Consumption	28921	Aberrantly Conducted
28731	Peak Stress Level	28923	Atrial Tachycardia
24926	29th Interval Measurements	28924	Sustained With 1:1 Conduction
25209	Elapsed Time	28925	With Short Paroxysms
25096	Speed	28926	Multifocal
25117	Grade	28927	With A-V Block
25075	Load	28928	Supraventricular Tachycardia
25179	Infusion Rate	28929	Paroxysmal
26441	Dosage	28930	Atrial Flutter
21987	Heart Rate	28931	Atrial Fibrillation
24989	Systolic BP	28932	Retrograde Atrial Activation
24990	Diastolic BP	28933	A-V Junction Conduction
25265	ST Segment (mm.)		Abnormalities
29107	X-axis Component	28934	Premature Beats
29136	Y-axis Component	28935	Escape Beats
29165	Z-axis Component	28936	Accelerated Rhythm
29194	3-D Vector Magnitude	28937	Junctional Rhythm
29223	3-D Vector Angle In XY Plane	28938	Premature Ventricular Contractions
29252	3-D Vector Angle In XZ Plane	28939	With Uniform Fixed Coupling
25148	Oxygen Consumption	28940	With Non-Fixed Coupling
28732	Peak Stress Level	28941	Multiform

CARDIAC STRESS TEST, CONT.

28942	In Pairs	28986	Early Repolarization, Normal Variant Pattern
28943	Ventricular Parasystole		
28944	Ventricular Tachycardia	28987	Juvenile T-waves, Normal Variant Pattern
28945	Accelerated Idioventricular Rhythm		
28946	Ventricular Escape Complexes	28988	ST-T Wave Changes
28947	Ventricular Fibrillation	28910	Non-specific
28948	A-V Block	28989	Consistent With Myocardial Ischemia
28949	1st Degree		
28950	2nd Degree	28990	Consistent With Myocardial Injury
28951	Mobitz I		
28952	Mobitz II	28991	Consistent With Acute Pericarditis
28953	2:1 Block	28992	Consistent With Intraventricular Conduction Delay
28954	3rd Degree		
28955	Variable	28993	ST Segment Depression
28956	Short P-R Interval	28994	Less Than 1 millimeter
28957	WPW Pattern	28995	Equal To Or Greater Than 1 millimeter
28958	Fusion Complexes		
28959	Reciprocal Complexes	28996	Increased R Wave Voltage
28960	Ventricular Capture Beats	28997	Absent Septal Q Waves
28961	A-V Dissociation	28998	Inverted U Waves
28962	Ventriculophasic Sinus Arrhythmia	28999	Prominent U Waves
28963	Low Voltage Leads	29000	Post Extrasystolic T Wave Abnormality
28964	Limb Leads		
28965	Limb And Precordial Leads	29001	Isolated J Point Depression
28966	Left Axis Deviation	29002	Peaked T Waves
28967	Right Axis Deviation	29003	Prolonged Q-T Interval
28968	Electrical Alternans	29004	Pacing Patterns
28969	Left Ventricular Hypertrophy	29005	Atrial Or Coronary Pacing Pattern
28970	By Voltage Criteria	29006	Ventricular Demand Pacing Pattern
28971	By Voltage Criteria And Strain Pattern		
		29007	A-V Sequential Pacing Pattern
28972	Right Ventricular Hypertrophy	29008	100% Ventricular Pacing Pattern
28973	Combined Ventricular Hypertrophy	29009	Dual Chamber, Atrial Pacing Pattern
28974	Right Bundle Branch Block		
28975	With An Incomplete Block Pattern	29010	Pacemaker Malfunction
28976	With A Complete Block Pattern	29011	Failure To Capture
29354	Onset Rate	29012	Failure To Sense
29355	Offset Rate	29013	Not Firing
28977	Left Bundle Branch Block	29014	Pacing Too Slowly
28978	With Left Anterior Fasicular Block Pattern	21993	Peak Exercise Response
		21994	Heart Rate
28979	With Left Posterior Fasicular Block Pattern	22058	Peak
		13461	Heart Rate >85% Of Target
28980	With ST-T Wave Consistent With An Acute Myocardial Infarction	13462	METS Attained
		28195	Double Product
28981	With A Complete Block Pattern	25695	Functional Aerobic Capacity
28982	With An Incomplete Block Pattern	28592	Bruce
29356	Onset Rate	28593	Mayo
29357	Offset Rate	21995	Blood Pressure
28983	Intraventricular Conduction Delay	28623	Systolic
28984	With A Nonspecific Pattern	28622	Diastolic
28985	SV With Aberrant Pattern	21996	Hypertensive

CARDIAC STRESS TEST, CONT.

13482	Falling Systolic Pressure of 10mm. or greater	13472	V3
		13473	V4
28594	ST Segment - Heart Rate Curve	13474	V5
28196	Integral ST Segment	13475	V6
13483	Exercise Duration (standard Bruce protocol)	13476	Duration 0.08 sec. or more
		13477	Horizontal For 0.08 seconds or more
21997	ECG		
28551	Artifact Present	13478	Horizontal To Downsloping For 0.08 sec. or more
28552	Muscle Tremor		
28553	Respiratory Motion	13479	Sloping Upwards Towards Baseline For 0.08 sec. or more
28554	Loose Lead		
28555	Electrical Noise	28734	Other Findings
28560	ST Segment Changes	13480	ST Depression of 2mm. or more
28561	I	28490	ST Elevation of 1mm. or more
28562	II	13481	J - Point Depression 1mm. or more
28563	III	13484	Reversal T Waves
28564	aVR	28491	Normalization Of T Waves
28566	aVL	28492	Time To Onset Of Positive ST Segments
28567	aVF		
28568	V1	28493	Heart Rate At Onset Of Positive ST Segments
28569	V2		
28570	V3	28350	Time To Reversion Of Positive ST Segments
28571	V4		
28572	V5	24928	Sinus Rhythm
28573	V6	28743	Arrhythmia
28650	X	28778	Ventriculophasic
28651	Y	28744	Bradycardia
28652	Z	13463	Tachycardia
28574	ST / Heart Rate Slope	28745	Arrest
28575	I	28746	Sinoatrial Exit Block
28576	II	13485	Dysrhythmia
28577	III	24929	Atrial Premature Depolarization
28578	aVR	24930	Present At Rest
28580	aVL	24931	Appeared During Exercise
28581	aVF	24932	Disappeared During Exercise
28582	V1	28749	Abnormal Conduction
28583	V2	28750	Nonconduction
28584	V3	28751	Aberrant Conduction
28585	V4	28349	A-V Junctional Rhythms
28586	V5	28760	Premature Beats
28587	V6	28761	Escape Beats
28682	X	28762	Accelerated
28683	Y	24933	Ventricular Premature Depolarization
28684	Z		
13464	ST Depression of 1mm. or more	24934	Present At Rest
13465	I	24935	Appeared During Exercise
13466	II	24936	Disappeared During Exercise
13467	III	28763	Uniform, Fixed Coupling
28565	aVR	28764	Uniform, Non-Fixed Coupling
13468	aVL	28765	Multiform
13469	aVF	28766	In Pairs
13470	V1	24937	Atrial Tachycardia
13471	V2	28752	Sustained

CARDIAC STRESS TEST, CONT.

28753	1:1 Conduction		28807	Ectopic Count Last Minute
28754	Short Paroxysms		28808	QRS Duration
28755	Multifocal		28809	X Axis
28756	With AV Block		28810	Y Axis
24938	Supraventricular Tachycardia		28811	Z Axis
24939	Atrial Fibrillation		28812	Q-Wave Duration
24940	Ventricular Tachycardia		28813	T-Wave Amplitude
24941	Conduction Abnormalities		28814	X-Axis
28771	AV Block		28815	Y-Axis
24944	1st Degree		28816	Z-Axis
24945	2nd Degree		28817	R-Wave Amplitude
24946	Mobitz Type I		28818	X-Axis
24947	Mobitz Type II		28819	Y-Axis
24948	3rd Degree		28820	Z-Axis
28772	2:1		28821	R-Max Cosine Vector
28773	Variable		28822	X-Axis
28747	Ectopic Atrial Rhythm		28823	Y-Axis
28748	Wandering Atrial Pacemaker		28824	Z-Axis
28757	Paroxysmal Supraventricular		28825	R-Max Amplitude
	Tachycardia		28826	3-D ST Segment Vector Magnitude
28758	Atrial Flutter			@ 60 msec.
28759	Retrograde Atrial Activation		29072	3-D ST Segment Vector Angle In
28767	Ventricular Parasystole			The XY Plane
28768	Accelerated Idioventricular Rhythm		29073	3-D ST Segment Vector Angle In
28769	Ventricular Escape Beats			The XZ Plane
28770	Ventricular Fibrillation		28688	Maximum ST Segment Change
28774	P-R Interval		28689	I
28775	Fusion Beats		28690	II
28776	Re-Entrant Ventricular Beats		28691	III
28777	AV Dissociation		28692	aVR
28779	Axis Deviation		28693	aVL
28780	Left		28694	aVF
28781	Right		28695	V1
28782	Electrical Alternans		28696	V2
28803	Left Ventricular Hypertrophy		28697	V3
28783	By Voltage		28698	V4
28784	By Strain		28699	V5
28785	Right Ventricular Hypertrophy		28700	V6
28786	Combined Ventricular Hypertrophy		28701	X
28787	Ventricular Conduction Delay		28702	Y
28788	Right		28703	Z
28791	Left		24942	Stress-induced Symptoms
28792	Left Anterior Hemiblock		24949	Fatigue
28793	Left Posterior Hemiblock		24950	Chest Pain
28794	Intraventricular Conduction Delay		28589	Resolved
28795	Nonspecific		28518	Headache
28796	With Aberrancy		28335	Palpitations
28804	Left Branch Bundle Block		28591	Resolved
28797	ST-T Waves of Acute MI		24951	Dyspnea
28798	Complete		28590	Resolved
28799	Incomplete		24952	Leg Distress
28805	Right Branch Bundle Block		24953	Claudication
28806	Borg Scale		28588	Anxiety

CARDIAC STRESS TEST, CONT.

28520	Light Headedness	21999	Negative Response For Ischemia
24954	Syncope	22000	Non-Diagnostic
28336	Change In Mental Status	28036	Because of
24955	Hysteria	28348	Inadequate Exercise
28519	Nausea / Vomiting	28037	Left Bundle Branch Block
24943	Stress-induced Signs	28038	Digoxin Effect
24956	Hypertension	28039	Left Ventricular Hypertrophy
24957	Hypotension	28040	Pre-existing ST Segment
24960	Requiring Medication		Abnormalities
24958	S3	28041	Paced QRS
24959	S4	28042	Wolff-Parkinson-White Syndrome
28337	New Murmur	28550	Incorrect Electrode Placement
29364	Wheezing	80917	Severe Artifact
29371	Rales	14540	**Echocardiogram**
29372	Absent Pedal Pulse	19506	M-mode
29365	Stress-induced Conditions	14539	With Contrast
29366	Atypical Angina	22228	Strip
29367	Non-cardiac Chest Pain	22229	Video
29369	Orthopedic Limitation	14634	2-D Mode
29368	Hysteria	14635	With Contrast
29370	CNS Changes	19519	Complete
25701	Post Exercise Recovery	19237	Follow-up Or Limited Exam
25702	Time Of Image Acquisition	19238	Transesophageal
25703	Heart Rate	22141	Biplane
25742	Termination of Stress Test	22142	Multiplane
25757	Due to Protocol Being Fulfilled	22137	Placement Of Probe Only
27331	Target Heart Rate	19518	Interpretation And Report Only
27332	METS attained	19239	During Stress Test
28595	100% Functional Aerobic Capacity	19517	With Pharmacologic Stress
	Achieved	14636	Doppler Mode
25743	Due to Patient Fatigue	19240	Color Flow Velocity Mapping
25744	Due to Chest Pain	19241	Follow-up Or Limited Study
25753	Due to Dyspnea	22046	With Amyl Nitrite
25754	Due to Leg Distress	22230	Strip
27333	Fatigue	22231	Video
27334	Pain	27095	Intra-Coronary
25755	Due to ECG Changes	21738	Intraoperative
25756	Due to Dysrhythmia	22232	Epicardial
27335	Due to Brachycardia	22143	Bedside
25766	Due to Ventricular Arrhythmia	22136	Precardioversion
25767	Due to Supraventricular Arrhythmia	22047	Post-Pericardiocentesis Follow-Up
25758	MD / RN Discontinued the test	22135	Unsatisfactory Exam
25760	The Target Heart Rate was Achieved	22138	Outside Echo Interpretation
25762	Due to Region Wall Motion	22233	Digitize To Disk
	Abnormalities	14558	Aortic Valve
25764	The Peak Dose was Administered	25325	Diameter
25768	Due to Intolerable Symptoms	25326	Valve Opening
28596	Due to Anxiety	25327	At Rest
27336	Due to Hysteria	25328	At End of Inspiration
25769	Due to Hypotension	25329	At End of Expiration
25770	Due to Hypertension	25330	With Stress
80916	ECG Conclusions	25331	Eccentricity
21998	Positive Response For Ischemia	25332	At Rest

ECHOCARDIOGRAM, CONT.

25333	At End of Inspiration
25334	At End of Expiration
25335	With Stress
25336	PEP (msec)
25339	At Rest
25340	At End of Inspiration
25341	At End of Expiration
25342	With Stress
25337	LVET (msec)
25343	At Rest
25344	At End of Inspiration
25345	At End of Expiration
25346	With Stress
25338	STI
25347	At Rest
25348	At End of Inspiration
25349	At End of Expiration
25350	With Stress
19547	Anatomy
19685	Contour
14559	Cusps
20140	Unicuspid
20141	Bicuspid
20142	Deformed Tricuspid
20143	Quadracuspid
20144	Indeterminate Number
14560	Thickening
20343	Left Cusp
20344	Right Cusp
20345	Non-Coronary Cusp
19761	Multiple Echoes
20274	Left Cusp
20275	Right Cusp
20276	Non-Coronary
14565	Vegetation Present
20277	Left Cusp
20278	Right Cusp
20279	Non-Coronary
14566	Calcification Present
20280	Left Cusp
20281	Right Cusp
20282	Non-Coronary
19754	Bowing
20283	Left Cusp
20284	Right Cusp
20285	Non-Coronary
19755	Rupture
20286	Left Cusp
20287	Right Cusp
20288	Non-Coronary
19756	Perforation
20289	Left Cusp
20290	Right Cusp

20291	Non-Coronary
20223	Fenestration
20292	Left Cusp
20293	Right Cusp
20294	Non-Coronary
14568	Absent
14569	Opening (cm.)
14567	Prolapsed
14570	Amplitude
14571	Subvalvular Membrane
21211	Discrete
21212	Anomalous Subaortic Muscle Bundle
14572	Supravalvular Membrane
20192	Doming
20207	Overriding
20233	Hypoplasia
21213	Atresia
21215	Subvalvular
21189	Mass ___ cm
21190	Papilloma ___ cm
81934	Echogenicity ___ cm
14633	Aortic - Mitral Continuity Abnormal
20234	Annulus
25500	Dimension (mm)
25622	Area
20232	Calcification Present
20235	Hypoplasia
21231	Annuloplasty Ring
19548	Function
14561	Premature Closure
14562	Trapezoid Configuration
19750	Tapered
14563	Eccentric Closure
19751	Incomplete Coaptation
14564	Flutter
19752	Systolic
19753	Diastolic
20259	Stenosis
20260	Valvular
20261	Calcific Etiology
20262	Rheumatic Etiology
20263	Critical
20264	Congenital Etiology
20295	Hypertrophic
20296	Subvalvular
20297	Discrete
20298	Tunnel
20299	Dynamic
20300	Supravalvular
20301	Discrete
20302	Tunnel
20303	Dynamic
21739	Residual (Postoperative)

ECHOCARDIOGRAM, CONT.

20251	Regurgitation		25855	At Rest
20313	Concentric		25856	At End of Inspiration
20314	Eccentric		25857	At End of Expiration
21740	Residual (Postoperative)		25858	With Stress
19757	Flow Velocity		25509	Peak Aortic Time Velocity
19758	Systolic			Integral
21233	Peak Flow		25664	At Rest
25631	At Rest		25665	At End of Inspiration
25633	At End of Inspiration		25666	At End of Expiration
25634	At End of Expiration		25667	With Stress
25637	With Stress		25510	TVI1/TVI2 Ratio
26567	Acceleration Time		25672	At Rest
26568	At Rest		25673	At End of Inspiration
26569	At End of Inspiration		25674	At End of Expiration
26570	At End of Expiration		25675	With Stress
26571	With Stress		19759	Diastolic
26572	Peak Acceleration Rate		25516	Regurgitant Half Time
26573	At Rest		25819	At Rest
26574	At End of Inspiration		25820	At End of Inspiration
26575	At End of Expiration		25821	At End of Expiration
26576	With Stress		25822	With Stress
26577	Deceleration Time		21239	Early Peak Flow
26578	At Rest		25798	At Rest
26579	At End of Inspiration		25800	At End of Inspiration
26580	At End of Expiration		25801	At End of Expiration
26581	With Stress		25802	With Stress
25494	V1/V2 Ratio		25508	Late Peak Flow
25639	At Rest		25807	At Rest
25640	At End of Inspiration		25808	At End of Inspiration
25641	At End of Expiration		25809	At End of Expiration
25642	With Stress		25810	With Stress
21235	Calculated Peak Flow Gradient		21240	Calculated Peak Flow Gradient
25643	At Rest		21241	Mean Flow
25644	At End of Inspiration		21242	Calculated Mean Flow Gradient
25645	At End of Expiration		21814	Residual Gradient (Postoperative)
25646	With Stress		25511	Regurgitant TVI
21236	Mean Flow		25831	At Rest
21238	Calculated Mean Flow Gradient		25832	At End of Inspiration
25647	At Rest		25834	At End of Expiration
25648	At End of Inspiration		25836	With Stress
25649	At End of Expiration		25514	Deceleration Time
25650	With Stress		25811	At Rest
21813	Residual Gradient (Postoperative)		25812	At End of Inspiration
22082	Residual Peak Gradient		25813	At End of Expiration
	(Postoperative)		25814	With Stress
22083	Residual Mean Gradient		25515	Deceleration Slope
	(Postoperative)		25823	At Rest
25512	Ejection Time		25824	At End of Inspiration
25847	At Rest		25826	At End of Expiration
25848	At End of Inspiration		25828	With Stress
25849	At End of Expiration		21361	Doppler Derived Valve Area
25850	With Stress		25517	Aortic Valve Area By Velocity
25513	Ejection Time (Corrected)		25655	At Rest

ECHOCARDIOGRAM, CONT.

25656	At End of Inspiration	14643		Low Frequency
25657	At End of Expiration	14541	Mitral Valve	
25658	With Stress	19549	Anatomy	
25518	Aortic Valve Area By TVI	19760	Contour	
25681	At Rest	20157	Bowing	
25682	At End of Inspiration	14544	Thick Leaflet(s)	
25683	At End of Expiration	20346	Anterior	
25684	With Stress	20347	Posterior	
25550	Regurgitant Fraction	20164	Flailing	
26101	At Rest	20165	Anterior Leaflet	
26102	At End of Inspiration	20166	Posterior Leaflet	
26103	At End of Expiration	22129	Bileaflet	
26104	With Stress	20167	Ruptured Chordae	
25551	Regurgitant Volume	20348	Anterior Leaflet	
26105	At Rest	20349	Posterior Leaflet	
26106	At End of Inspiration	20168	Perforation	
26107	At End of Expiration	20350	Anterior Leaflet	
26109	With Stress	20351	Posterior Leaflet	
25552	Effective Regurgitant Orifice	14549	Systolic Prolapse	
26113	At Rest	14550	Anterior Leaflet	
26115	At End of Inspiration	14551	Posterior Leaflet	
26117	At End of Expiration	22128	Bileaflet	
26119	With Stress	14554	Prominent B-Point	
25519	Doppler Derived Valve Area Indices	14555	Vegetation Present	
25520	Aortic Valve Area By Velocity	20352	Anterior Leaflet	
	Index	20353	Posterior Leaflet	
25689	At Rest	14556	Calcification Present	
25691	At End of Inspiration	20354	Anterior Leaflet	
25693	At End of Expiration	20355	Posterior Leaflet	
25694	With Stress	14557	Diastolic Density Present	
25521	Aortic Valve Area By TVI Index	20185	Cleft	
25708	At Rest	20193	Doming	
25709	At End of Inspiration	20199	Parachute	
25710	At End of Expiration	20203	Double Orifice	
25711	With Stress	20212	Straddling	
25522	Doppler Derived Flow Rates	20224	Fenestration	
25523	Left Ventricular Stroke Volume	20356	Anterior Leaflet	
25863	At Rest	20357	Posterior Leaflet	
25865	At End of Inspiration	20241	Hypoplasia	
25867	At End of Expiration	21214	Atresia	
25870	With Stress	21191	Mass	
25525	Systolic Aortic Pressure	21192	Papilloma	
25526	Systemic Vascular Resistance	81947	Echogenicity	
25883	At Rest	14631	Annulus	
25884	At End of Inspiration	25543	Diameter (cm)	
25885	At End of Expiration	26064	At Rest	
25886	With Stress	26065	At End of Inspiration	
14637	Turbulence	26066	At End of Expiration	
14638	Systolic	26067	With Stress	
14639	High Frequency	25351	Dimension (mm)	
14640	Low Frequency	26599	At Rest	
14641	Diastolic	26600	At End of Inspiration	
14642	High Frequency	26601	At End of Expiration	

ECHOCARDIOGRAM, CONT.

26602	With Stress
25623	Area
14632	Calcification Present
20521	Dilation
20236	Hypoplasia
21369	Abscess
21370	Supravalvular Ring
20231	Chordae
19767	Calcification Present
19550	Function
20265	Stenosis
20266	Valvular
20267	Calcific Etiology
20268	Rheumatic Etiology
20304	Congenital Etiology
20305	Subvalvular
20306	Discrete
20307	Tunnel
20308	Dynamic
20309	Supravalvular
20310	Discrete
20311	Tunnel
20312	Dynamic
21741	Residual (Postoperative)
20252	Regurgitation
20315	Concentric
20316	Eccentric
21742	Residual (Postoperative)
14545	Parallel Leaflet Motion
14542	Excursion
19762	Decreased
14546	Premature Closure
19763	Interrupted Closure
19764	Blunted
14547	Absent A-kick
20182	Incomplete Coaptation
14548	Fluttering Anterior Leaflet
14552	Systolic Anterior Motion
14553	E-point to Septal Distance >1.0cm.
26595	At Rest
26596	At End of Inspiration
26597	At End of Expiration
26598	With Stress
25352	D-E Excursion
25353	At Rest
25354	At End of Inspiration
25355	At End of Expiration
25356	With Stress
25357	E-E Opening
25361	At Rest
25362	At End of Inspiration
25363	At End of Expiration
25364	With Stress

25495	E-F Slope
25496	At Rest
25497	At End of Inspiration
25498	At End of Expiration
25499	With Stress
25358	A-C Slope
25365	At Rest
25366	At End of Inspiration
25367	At End of Expiration
25368	With Stress
25359	A-C Duration
25369	At Rest
25370	At End of Inspiration
25371	At End of Expiration
25372	With Stress
25360	Mitral Leaf Velocity (D-E)
25373	At Rest
25374	At End of Inspiration
25375	At End of Expiration
25376	With Stress
19768	Flow Velocity
19769	Systolic
21243	Peak Flow
25891	At Rest
25894	At End of Inspiration
25896	At End of Expiration
25898	With Stress
25530	Regurgitant Time
25932	At Rest
25934	At End of Inspiration
25937	At End of Expiration
25938	With Stress
25531	Regurgitant Time Velocity Integral
25951	At Rest
25952	At End of Inspiration
25953	At End of Expiration
25954	With Stress
25532	Peak Acceleration Rate
25915	At Rest
25916	At End of Inspiration
25919	At End of Expiration
25921	With Stress
25533	Acceleration Time
25908	At Rest
25910	At End of Inspiration
25911	At End of Expiration
25914	With Stress
25534	Deceleration Time
25923	At Rest
25926	At End of Inspiration
25928	At End of Expiration
25930	With Stress

ECHOCARDIOGRAM, CONT.

21244	Calculated Peak Flow Gradient	26012		At End of Inspiration
25899	At Rest	26013		At End of Expiration
25900	At End of Inspiration	26015		With Stress
25901	At End of Expiration	25538		Pressure Half Time
25902	With Stress	26023		At Rest
21245	Mean Flow	26024		At End of Inspiration
21246	Calculated Mean Flow Gradient	26025		At End of Expiration
21815	Residual Gradient (Postoperative)	26026		With Stress
19770	Diastolic	25539		1/3 Diastolic Filling Period
21247	Peak Flow E	26044		At Rest
25956	At Rest	26045		At End of Inspiration
25959	At End of Inspiration	26046		At End of Expiration
25961	At End of Expiration	26049		With Stress
25962	With Stress	25540		1/2 Diastolic Filling Period
25527	Peak Flow A	26056		At Rest
25971	At Rest	26057		At End of Inspiration
25972	At End of Inspiration	26058		At End of Expiration
25973	At End of Expiration	26059		With Stress
25974	With Stress	21816		Residual Gradient (Postoperative)
25528	E/A Ratio	22084		Residual Peak Gradient (Postoperative)
25975	At Rest			
25976	At End of Inspiration	22085		Residual Mean Gradient (Postoperative)
25977	At End of Expiration			
25978	With Stress	25544		Regurgitant TVI
25529	Regurgitant Velocity	26129		At Rest
25939	At Rest	26131		At End of Inspiration
25941	At End of Inspiration	26132		At End of Expiration
25944	At End of Expiration	26134		With Stress
25946	With Stress	25545		LV Inflow Stroke Volume
25535	Acceleration Time	26072		At Rest
25991	At Rest	26073		At End of Inspiration
25993	At End of Inspiration	26074		At End of Expiration
25995	At End of Expiration	26075		With Stress
25998	With Stress	25546		LV Inflow Cardiac Output
25536	Deceleration Time	26089		At Rest
26003	At Rest	26092		At End of Inspiration
26004	At End of Inspiration	26095		At End of Expiration
26005	At End of Expiration	26096		With Stress
26006	With Stress	21362	Doppler Derived Valve Area	
21248	Calculated Peak Flow Gradient	26031	At Rest	
21249	Mean Flow	26033	At End of Inspiration	
26586	Inflow Time Velocity Integral	26034	At End of Expiration	
26587	At Rest	26036	With Stress	
26588	At End of Inspiration	25547	Regurgitant Fraction (%)	
26589	At End of Expiration	26080	At Rest	
26590	With Stress	26081	At End of Inspiration	
21250	Calculated Mean Flow Gradient	26082	At End of Expiration	
25983	At Rest	26083	With Stress	
25984	At End of Inspiration	25548	Regurgitant Volume	
25985	At End of Expiration	26122	At Rest	
25987	With Stress	26123	At End of Inspiration	
25537	Isovolumetric Relaxation Period	26126	At End of Expiration	
26011	At Rest	26128	With Stress	

ECHOCARDIOGRAM, CONT.

25549	Effective Regurgitant Orifice		20243	Hypoplasia
26137	At Rest		19552	Function
26138	At End of Inspiration		20269	Stenosis
26139	At End of Expiration		28216	Valvular
26140	With Stress		20373	Infundibular
14644	Turbulence		20374	Subvalvular
14645	Systolic		20375	Discrete
14646	High Frequency		20376	Tunnel
14647	Low Frequency		20377	Dynamic
14648	Diastolic		20378	Supravalvular
14649	High Frequency		20379	Discrete
14650	Low Frequency		20380	Tunnel
14589	Pulmonary Valve		20381	Dynamic
19551	Anatomy		21743	Residual (Postoperative)
19774	Contour		20253	Regurgitation
20158	Bowing		20317	Concentric
20184	Thick Cusps		20318	Eccentric
20358	Left Cusp		21744	Residual (Postoperative)
20359	Right Cusp		20183	Incomplete Coaptation
20360	Anterior Cusp		20147	Leaflet Flutter
20170	Rupture		20148	Systolic
20361	Left Cusp		19771	Flow Velocity
20362	Right Cusp		19772	Systolic
20363	Anterior Cusp		21251	Peak Flow
19775	Prolapse		25554	Early
20364	Left Cusp		25660	At Rest
20365	Right Cusp		25661	At End of Inspiration
20366	Anterior Cusp		25662	At End of Expiration
21148	Vegetation Present		25663	With Stress
21573	Abscess		25555	Late
20189	Calcification Present		25668	At Rest
20367	Left Cusp		25669	At End of Inspiration
20368	Right Cusp		25670	At End of Expiration
20369	Anterior Cusp		25671	With Stress
20194	Doming		25556	Time To Peak Velocity
20208	Overriding		26191	At Rest
20225	Fenestration		26195	At End of Inspiration
20370	Left Cusp		26197	At End of Expiration
20371	Right Cusp		26198	With Stress
20372	Anterior Cusp		25553	V1/V2 Ratio
20242	Hypoplasia		26163	At Rest
21216	Atresia		26164	At End of Inspiration
21217	Subvalvular		26165	At End of Expiration
21193	Mass ___ cm		26166	With Stress
21194	Papilloma ___ cm		21252	Calculated Peak Flow Gradient
81948	Echogenicity		26167	At Rest
20237	Annulus		26168	At End of Inspiration
25377	Dimension (mm)		26169	At End of Expiration
26603	At Rest		26170	With Stress
26604	At End of Inspiration		21253	Mean Flow
26605	At End of Expiration		21254	Calculated Mean Flow Gradient
26606	With Stress		26175	At Rest
25624	Area		26176	At End of Inspiration

ECHOCARDIOGRAM, CONT.

26177	At End of Expiration	26187	With Stress
26178	With Stress	25563	RV Stroke Volume
21817	Residual Gradient (Postoperative)	25712	At Rest
22086	Residual Peak Gradient	25713	At End of Inspiration
	(Postoperative)	25714	At End of Expiration
22087	Residual Mean Gradient	25715	With Stress
	(Postoperative)	25564	RV Cardiac Output
26199	Ejection Time	25720	At Rest
26200	At Rest	25721	At End of Inspiration
26201	At End of Inspiration	25722	At End of Expiration
26202	At End of Expiration	25723	With Stress
26203	With Stress	25565	RV Cardiac Index
26204	Ejection Time (Corrected)	25724	At Rest
26205	At Rest	25725	At End of Inspiration
26206	At End of Inspiration	25726	At End of Expiration
26207	At End of Expiration	25727	With Stress
26208	With Stress	25566	RV/LV Cardiac Output Ratio
25557	RV Outflow Tract Time Velocity	25735	At Rest
	Integral	25736	At End of Inspiration
26171	At Rest	25737	At End of Expiration
26172	At End of Inspiration	25738	With Stress
26173	At End of Expiration	14658	Turbulence
26174	With Stress	14659	Systolic
25559	Peak Acceleration Rate	14660	High Frequency
26192	At Rest	14661	Low Frequency
26193	At End of Inspiration	14662	Diastolic
26194	At End of Expiration	14663	High Frequency
26196	With Stress	14664	Low Frequency
25560	Deceleration Time	14590	A Dip
26186	At Rest	14591	Absent
26188	At End of Inspiration	14592	Increased
26189	At End of Expiration	14578	Tricuspid Valve
26190	With Stress	19553	Anatomy
19773	Diastolic	19776	Contour
21255	Peak Flow	14579	Enlarged
21256	Calculated Peak Flow Gradient	20159	Bowing
21257	Mean Flow	20169	Flailing
21258	Calculated Mean Flow Gradient	20403	Anterior Leaflet
21818	Residual Gradient (Postoperative)	20404	Posterior Leaflet
25562	Regurgitant Half Time	20405	Septal Leaflet
25687	At Rest	14580	Systolic Prolapse
25688	At End of Inspiration	14581	Anterior Leaflet
25690	At End of Expiration	14582	Posterior Leaflet
25692	With Stress	20390	Septal Leaflet
25561	Deceleration Time	14586	Vegetation Present
25676	At Rest	20393	Anterior Leaflet
25677	At End of Inspiration	20394	Posterior Leaflet
25678	At End of Expiration	20395	Septal Leaflet
25680	With Stress	19779	Calcification Present
21363	Doppler Derived Valve Area	19780	Anterior Leaflet
26183	At Rest	20391	Posterior Leaflet
26184	At End of Inspiration	20392	Septal Leaflet
26185	At End of Expiration	20186	Cleft

ECHOCARDIOGRAM, CONT.

20195	Doming		19777	Incomplete Coaptation
20200	Parachute		14584	Delayed Closure
20204	Double Orifice		19778	Interrupted Closure
20213	Straddling		14585	Increased Excursion
20396	Perforation		19782	Flow Velocity
20397	Anterior Leaflet		19783	Systolic
20398	Posterior Leaflet		21259	Peak Flow
20399	Septal Leaflet		25745	At Rest
20226	Fenestration		25746	At End of Inspiration
20400	Anterior Leaflet		25747	At End of Expiration
20401	Posterior Leaflet		25748	With Stress
20402	Septal Leaflet		25570	Regurgitant Time
20244	Hypoplasia		25779	At Rest
21218	Atresia		25780	At End of Inspiration
21219	with pulmonary atresia (Type I-a)		25781	At End of Expiration
21220	with pulmonary stenosis (Type I-b)		25782	With Stress
21221	without pulmonary stenosis (Type I-c)		25571	Regurgitant Time Velocity Integral
21222	with transposed great arteries and pulmonary atresia (Type II-a)		25795	At Rest
			25796	At End of Inspiration
21223	with transposed great arteries and pulmonary stenosis (Type II-b)		25797	At End of Expiration
			25799	With Stress
21224	with transposed great arteries but no pulmonary stenosis (Type II-c)		25572	Peak Acceleration Rate
			25771	At Rest
21195	Mass ___ cm		25772	At End of Inspiration
21196	Papilloma ___ cm		25773	At End of Expiration
81949	Echogenicity		25774	With Stress
14587	Absent		25573	Acceleration Time
14588	Thick Leaflets		25759	At Rest
20238	Annulus		25761	At End of Inspiration
25378	Dimension (mm)		25763	At End of Expiration
25625	Area		25765	With Stress
19781	Calcification Present		25574	Deceleration Time
20522	Dilation		25775	At Rest
20245	Hypoplasia		25776	At End of Inspiration
21572	Abscess		25777	At End of Expiration
21232	Annuloplasty Ring		25778	With Stress
19554	Function		21260	Calculated Peak Flow Gradient
20270	Stenosis		25749	At Rest
20382	Subvalvular		25750	At End of Inspiration
20383	Discrete		25751	At End of Expiration
20384	Tunnel		25752	With Stress
20385	Dynamic		21261	Mean Flow
20386	Supravalvular		21262	Calculated Mean Flow Gradient
20387	Discrete		21819	Residual Gradient (Postoperative)
20388	Tunnel		19784	Diastolic
20389	Dynamic		21263	Peak Flow E
21745	Residual (Postoperative)		25803	At Rest
20254	Regurgitation		25804	At End of Inspiration
20319	Concentric		25805	At End of Expiration
20320	Eccentric		25806	With Stress
21746	Residual (Postoperative)		25567	Peak Flow A
14583	EF Slope Decreased		25815	At Rest

ECHOCARDIOGRAM, CONT.

25816	At End of Inspiration	22089	Residual Mean Gradient
25817	At End of Expiration		(Postoperative)
25818	With Stress	25577	RA Pressure
25568	E/A Ratio	25787	At Rest
25825	At Rest	25788	At End of Inspiration
25827	At End of Inspiration	25789	At End of Expiration
25829	At End of Expiration	25790	With Stress
25830	With Stress	25578	RV Pressure
25569	Regurgitant Velocity	25791	At Rest
25783	At Rest	25792	At End of Inspiration
25784	At End of Inspiration	25793	At End of Expiration
25785	At End of Expiration	25794	With Stress
25786	With Stress	21364	Doppler Derived Valve Area
25575	Acceleration Time	25871	At Rest
25841	At Rest	25872	At End of Inspiration
25844	At End of Inspiration	25873	At End of Expiration
25845	At End of Expiration	25874	With Stress
25846	With Stress	14651	Turbulence
25576	Deceleration Time	14652	Systolic
25851	At Rest	14653	High Frequency
25852	At End of Inspiration	14654	Low Frequency
25853	At End of Expiration	14655	Diastolic
25854	With Stress	14656	High Frequency
21264	Calculated Peak Flow Gradient	14657	Low Frequency
21265	Mean Flow	19527	Left A-V Valve
21266	Calculated Mean Flow Gradient	19555	Anatomy
25833	At Rest	20149	Contour
25835	At End of Inspiration	20160	Bowing
25837	At End of Expiration	20171	Flailing
25838	With Stress	20172	Ruptured Chordae
25579	Isovolumetric Relaxation Period	20173	Perforation
25859	At Rest	19931	Prolapse
25860	At End of Inspiration	21153	Vegetation Present
25861	At End of Expiration	19932	Calcification Present
25862	With Stress	19933	Thick Leaflets
25580	Pressure Half Time	20150	Accessory Tissue
25864	At Rest	20187	Cleft
25866	At End of Inspiration	20196	Doming
25868	At End of Expiration	20201	Parachute
25869	With Stress	20205	Double Orifice
25581	1/3 Filling Fraction Period	20209	Overriding
25875	At Rest	20214	Straddling
25876	At End of Inspiration	20215	Type A
25877	At End of Expiration	20216	Type B
25878	With Stress	20217	Type C
25582	1/2 Filling Fraction Period	20227	Fenestration
25879	At Rest	20246	Hypoplasia
25880	At End of Inspiration	21225	Atresia
25881	At End of Expiration	20239	Annulus
25882	With Stress	20247	Hypoplasia
21820	Residual Gradient (Postoperative)	19556	Function
22088	Residual Peak Gradient	20271	Stenosis
	(Postoperative)	20255	Regurgitation

ECHOCARDIOGRAM, CONT.

20321	Concentric		21276	Calculated Peak Flow Gradient
20322	Eccentric		21277	Mean Flow
19934	Flow Velocity		21278	Calculated Mean Flow Gradient
19935	Systolic		19949	Diastolic
21267	Peak Flow		21279	Peak Flow
21268	Calculated Peak Flow Gradient		21280	Calculated Peak Flow Gradient
21269	Mean Flow		21281	Mean Flow
21270	Calculated Mean Flow Gradient		21282	Calculated Mean Flow Gradient
19936	Diastolic		19950	Turbulence
21271	Peak Flow		19951	Systolic
21272	Calculated Peak Flow Gradient		19952	High Frequency
21273	Mean Flow		19953	Low Frequency
21274	Calculated Mean Flow Gradient		19954	Diastolic
19937	Turbulence		19955	High Frequency
19938	Systolic		19956	Low Frequency
19939	High Frequency		19680	Common A-V Valve
19940	Low Frequency		19785	Anatomy
19941	Diastolic		20152	Contour
19942	High Frequency		20162	Bowing
19943	Low Frequency		20177	Flailing
19528	Right A-V Valve		19786	Prolapse
19557	Anatomy		21155	Vegetation Present
20151	Contour		19787	Calcification Present
20161	Bowing		19788	Thick Leaflets
20174	Flailing		20229	Fenestration
20175	Ruptured Chordae		19789	Function
20176	Perforation		20257	Regurgitation
19944	Prolapse		20325	Concentric
21154	Vegetation Present		20326	Eccentric
19945	Calcification Present		19790	Flow Velocity
19946	Thick Leaflets		19791	Systolic
20191	Cleft		21283	Peak Flow
20197	Doming		21284	Calculated Peak Flow Gradient
20202	Parachute		21285	Mean Flow
20206	Double Orifice		21286	Calculated Mean Flow Gradient
20210	Overriding		19792	Diastolic
20218	Straddling		21287	Peak Flow
20219	Type A		21288	Calculated Peak Flow Gradient
20220	Type B		21289	Mean Flow
20221	Type C		21290	Calculated Mean Flow Gradient
20228	Fenestration		19793	Turbulence
20248	Hypoplasia		19794	Systolic
21226	Atresia		19795	High Frequency
20240	Annulus		19796	Low Frequency
20249	Hypoplasia		19797	Diastolic
19558	Function		19798	High Frequency
20272	Stenosis		19799	Low Frequency
20256	Regurgitation		19800	Truncal Valve
20323	Concentric		20153	Contour
20324	Eccentric		20163	Bowing
19947	Flow Velocity		20188	Thick Leaflets
19948	Systolic		20178	Perforation
21275	Peak Flow		20156	Prolapse

ECHOCARDIOGRAM, CONT.

21156	Vegetation Present	26446	With Stress
20190	Calcification Present	26796	Acceleration Time
20198	Doming	26797	At Rest
20211	Overriding	26798	At End of Inspiration
20230	Fenestration	26799	At End of Expiration
20250	Hypoplasia	26800	With Stress
20273	Stenosis	26801	Peak Acceleration Rate
20258	Regurgitation	26802	At Rest
20327	Concentric	26803	At End of Inspiration
20328	Eccentric	26804	At End of Expiration
21356	Flow Velocity	26805	With Stress
21357	Systolic	26806	Deceleration Time
21291	Peak Flow	26807	At Rest
21292	Calculated Peak Flow Gradient	26808	At End of Inspiration
21293	Mean Flow	26809	At End of Expiration
21294	Calculated Mean Flow Gradient	26810	With Stress
21358	Diastolic	26447	V1/V2 Ratio
21295	Peak Flow	26448	At Rest
21296	Calculated Peak Flow Gradient	26449	At End of Inspiration
21297	Mean Flow	26450	At End of Expiration
21298	Calculated Mean Flow Gradient	26451	With Stress
20474	Criss-Cross A-V Valve	21301	Calculated Peak Flow Gradient
20475	Hypoplasia	26452	At Rest
14593	Prosthetic Valve	26453	At End of Inspiration
19559	Prosthetic Aortic Valve	26454	At End of Expiration
19561	Tissue	26455	With Stress
19562	Homograft	21302	Mean Flow
19563	Porcine	21303	Calculated Mean Flow Gradient
19564	Mechanical	26456	At Rest
19565	Anatomy	26457	At End of Inspiration
19567	Thrombosed	26458	At End of Expiration
19568	Dehisced sewing ring	26459	With Stress
19569	Thickened	22048	Residual Gradient (Postoperative)
19570	Calcified	22090	Residual Peak Gradient (Postoperative)
21149	Vegetation		
19566	Function	22091	Residual Mean Gradient (Postoperative)
19571	Loosening / Rocking		
19572	Motion pattern	26460	Ejection Time
19653	Stenosis	26461	At Rest
21747	Residual (Postoperative)	26462	At End of Inspiration
19654	Regurgitation	26463	At End of Expiration
20329	Concentric	26464	With Stress
20330	Eccentric	26465	Ejection Time (Corrected)
20406	Paravalvular (Localized)	26466	At Rest
20407	Perivalvular (Circumferential)	26467	At End of Inspiration
21748	Residual (Postoperative)	26468	At End of Expiration
19573	Uncertain	26469	With Stress
19801	Flow Velocity	26470	Peak Aortic Time Velocity Integral
19802	Systolic		
21300	Peak Flow	26471	At Rest
26443	At Rest	26472	At End of Inspiration
26444	At End of Inspiration	26473	At End of Expiration
26445	At End of Expiration	26474	With Stress

ECHOCARDIOGRAM, CONT.

26475	TVI1/TVI2 Ratio		26521	At End of Inspiration	
26476	At Rest		26522	At End of Expiration	
26477	At End of Inspiration		26523	With Stress	
26478	At End of Expiration		26524	Regurgitant Volume	
26479	With Stress		26525	At Rest	
21299	Diastolic		26526	At End of Inspiration	
26480	Regurgitant Half Time		26527	At End of Expiration	
26481	At Rest		26528	With Stress	
26482	At End of Inspiration		26529	Effective Regurgitant Orifice	
26483	At End of Expiration		26530	At Rest	
26484	With Stress		26531	At End of Inspiration	
21304	Early Peak Flow		26532	At End of Expiration	
26485	At Rest		26533	With Stress	
26486	At End of Inspiration		26534	Doppler Derived Valve Area Indices	
26487	At End of Expiration		26535	Aortic Valve Area By Velocity Index	
26488	With Stress				
26489	Late Peak Flow		26536	At Rest	
26490	At Rest		26537	At End of Inspiration	
26491	At End of Inspiration		26538	At End of Expiration	
26492	At End of Expiration		26539	With Stress	
26493	With Stress		26540	Aortic Valve Area By TVI Index	
21305	Calculated Peak Flow Gradient		26541	At Rest	
21306	Mean Flow		26542	At End of Inspiration	
21307	Calculated Mean Flow Gradient		26543	At End of Expiration	
22049	Residual Gradient (Postoperative)		26544	With Stress	
26494	Regurgitant TVI		26545	Doppler Derived Flow Rates	
26495	At Rest		26546	Left Ventricular Stroke Volume	
26496	At End of Inspiration		26547	At Rest	
26497	At End of Expiration		26548	At End of Inspiration	
26498	With Stress		26549	At End of Expiration	
26499	Deceleration Time		26550	With Stress	
26500	At Rest		26551	Left Ventricular Cardiac Output	
26501	At End of Inspiration		26552	At Rest	
26502	At End of Expiration		26553	At End of Inspiration	
26503	With Stress		26554	At End of Expiration	
26504	Deceleration Slope		26555	With Stress	
26505	At Rest		26556	Systolic Aortic Pressure	
26506	At End of Inspiration		26557	Systemic Vascular Resistance	
26507	At End of Expiration		26558	At Rest	
26508	With Stress		26559	At End of Inspiration	
21365	Doppler Derived Valve Area		26560	At End of Expiration	
26509	Aortic Valve Area By Velocity		26561	With Stress	
26510	At Rest		19803	Turbulence	
26511	At End of Inspiration		19804	Systolic	
26512	At End of Expiration		19805	High Frequency	
26513	With Stress		19806	Low Frequency	
26514	Aortic Valve Area By TVI		19807	Diastolic	
26515	At Rest		19808	High Frequency	
26516	At End of Inspiration		19809	Low Frequency	
26517	At End of Expiration		19560	Prosthetic Mitral Valve	
26518	With Stress		19574	Tissue	
26519	Regurgitant Fraction		19575	Homograft	
26520	At Rest		19576	Porcine	

ECHOCARDIOGRAM, CONT.

19577	Mechanical		26650	At End of Expiration
19578	Anatomy		26651	With Stress
19580	Thrombosed		26652	A-C Duration
19581	Dehisced sewing ring		26653	At Rest
19582	Thickened		26654	At End of Inspiration
19583	Calcified		26655	At End of Expiration
14594	Vegetation		26656	With Stress
14595	Loosening / Rocking		26657	Mitral Leaf Velocity (D-E)
26816	Annulus		26658	At Rest
26817	Diameter		26659	At End of Inspiration
26818	At Rest		26660	At End of Expiration
26819	At End of Inspiration		26661	With Stress
26820	At End of Expiration		19810	Flow Velocity
26821	With Stress		19811	Systolic
26822	Dimension		21308	Peak Flow
26823	At Rest		26662	At Rest
26824	At End of Inspiration		26663	At End of Inspiration
26825	At End of Expiration		26664	At End of Expiration
26826	With Stress		26665	With Stress
19579	Function		26666	Regurgitant Time
19585	Motion pattern		26667	At Rest
19655	Stenosis		26668	At End of Inspiration
21749	Residual (Postoperative)		26669	At End of Expiration
19656	Regurgitation		26670	With Stress
20331	Concentric		26671	Regurgitant Time Velocity
20332	Eccentric			Integral
20408	Paravalvular (Localized)		26672	At Rest
20409	Perivalvular (Circumferential)		26673	At End of Inspiration
21750	Residual (Postoperative)		26674	At End of Expiration
19586	Uncertain		26675	With Stress
26627	E-point to Septal Distance >1.0cm.		26676	Peak Acceleration Rate
26628	At Rest		26677	At Rest
26629	At End of Inspiration		26678	At End of Inspiration
26630	At End of Expiration		26679	At End of Expiration
26631	With Stress		26680	With Stress
26632	D-E Excursion		26681	Acceleration Time
26633	At Rest		26682	At Rest
26634	At End of Inspiration		26683	At End of Inspiration
26635	At End of Expiration		26684	At End of Expiration
26636	With Stress		26685	With Stress
26637	E-E Opening		26686	Deceleration Time
26638	At Rest		26687	At Rest
26639	At End of Inspiration		26688	At End of Inspiration
26640	At End of Expiration		26689	At End of Expiration
26641	With Stress		26690	With Stress
26642	E-F Slope		21309	Calculated Peak Flow Gradient
26643	At Rest		26691	At Rest
26644	At End of Inspiration		26692	At End of Inspiration
26645	At End of Expiration		26693	At End of Expiration
26646	With Stress		26694	With Stress
26647	A-C Slope		21310	Mean Flow
26648	At Rest		21311	Calculated Mean Flow Gradient
26649	At End of Inspiration		22050	Residual Gradient (Postoperative)

ECHOCARDIOGRAM, CONT.

19812	Diastolic	26738	1/3 Diastolic Filling Period
21312	Peak Flow E	26739	At Rest
26695	At Rest	26740	At End of Inspiration
26696	At End of Inspiration	26741	At End of Expiration
26697	At End of Expiration	26742	With Stress
26698	With Stress	26743	1/2 Diastolic Filling Period
26699	Peak Flow A	26744	At Rest
26700	At Rest	26745	At End of Inspiration
26701	At End of Inspiration	26746	At End of Expiration
26702	At End of Expiration	26747	With Stress
26703	With Stress	22051	Residual Gradient (Postoperative)
26704	E/A Ratio	22092	Residual Peak Gradient
26705	At Rest		(Postoperative)
26706	At End of Inspiration	22093	Residual Mean Gradient
26707	At End of Expiration		(Postoperative)
26708	With Stress	26748	Regurgitant TVI
26709	Regurgitant Velocity	26749	At Rest
26710	At Rest	26750	At End of Inspiration
26711	At End of Inspiration	26751	At End of Expiration
26712	At End of Expiration	26752	With Stress
26713	With Stress	26753	LV Inflow Stroke Volume
26714	Acceleration Time	26754	At Rest
26715	At Rest	26755	At End of Inspiration
26716	At End of Inspiration	26756	At End of Expiration
26717	At End of Expiration	26757	With Stress
26718	With Stress	26758	LV Inflow Cardiac Output
26719	Deceleration Time	26759	At Rest
26720	At Rest	26760	At End of Inspiration
26721	At End of Inspiration	26761	At End of Expiration
26722	At End of Expiration	26762	With Stress
26723	With Stress	21366	Doppler Derived Valve Area
21313	Calculated Peak Flow Gradient	26763	At Rest
21314	Mean Flow	26764	At End of Inspiration
26811	Inflow Time Velocity Integral	26765	At End of Expiration
26812	At Rest	26766	With Stress
26813	At End of Inspiration	26767	Regurgitant Fraction (%)
26814	At End of Expiration	26768	At Rest
26815	With Stress	26769	At End of Inspiration
21315	Calculated Mean Flow Gradient	26770	At End of Expiration
26724	At Rest	26771	With Stress
26725	At End of Inspiration	26772	Regurgitant Volume
26726	At End of Expiration	26773	At Rest
26727	With Stress	26774	At End of Inspiration
26728	Isovolumetric Relaxation Period	26775	At End of Expiration
26729	At Rest	26776	With Stress
26730	At End of Inspiration	26777	Effective Regurgitant Orifice
26731	At End of Expiration	26778	At Rest
26732	With Stress	26779	At End of Inspiration
26733	Pressure Half Time	26780	At End of Expiration
26734	At Rest	26781	With Stress
26735	At End of Inspiration	19813	Turbulence
26736	At End of Expiration	19814	Systolic
26737	With Stress	19815	High Frequency

ECHOCARDIOGRAM, CONT.

19816	Low Frequency	26271	At End of Expiration
19817	Diastolic	26272	With Stress
19818	High Frequency	21318	Mean Flow
19819	Low Frequency	21319	Calculated Mean Flow Gradient
19587	Prosthetic Pulmonary Valve	26278	At Rest
19588	Tissue	26279	At End of Inspiration
19589	Homograft	26281	At End of Expiration
19590	Porcine	26283	With Stress
19591	Mechanical	22054	Residual Gradient (Postoperative)
19592	Anatomy	26289	Residual Peak Gradient (Postoperative)
19594	Thrombosed		
19595	Dehisced sewing ring	26290	Residual Mean Gradient (Postoperative)
19596	Thickened		
19597	Calcified	26291	Ejection Time
21150	Vegetation	26292	At Rest
19593	Function	26293	At End of Inspiration
19598	Loosening / Rocking	26294	At End of Expiration
19599	Motion pattern	26296	With Stress
19657	Stenosis	26298	Ejection Time (Corrected)
21751	Residual (Postoperative)	26300	At Rest
19658	Regurgitation	26302	At End of Inspiration
20333	Concentric	26304	At End of Expiration
20334	Eccentric	26305	With Stress
20410	Paravalvular (Localized)	26308	RV Outflow Tract Time Velocity Integral
20411	Perivalvular (Circumferential)		
21752	Residual (Postoperative)	26311	At Rest
19600	Uncertain	26314	At End of Inspiration
19820	Flow Velocity	26316	At End of Expiration
19821	Systolic	26318	With Stress
21316	Peak Flow	26319	Peak Acceleration Rate
26220	Early	26322	At Rest
26222	At Rest	26324	At End of Inspiration
26227	At End of Inspiration	26326	At End of Expiration
26232	At End of Expiration	26327	With Stress
26234	With Stress	26328	Deceleration Time
26235	Late	26329	At Rest
26239	At Rest	26330	At End of Inspiration
26241	At End of Inspiration	26331	At End of Expiration
26243	At End of Expiration	26332	With Stress
26244	With Stress	19822	Diastolic
26245	Time To Peak Velocity	21320	Peak Flow
26251	At Rest	21321	Calculated Peak Flow Gradient
26253	At End of Inspiration	21322	Mean Flow
26255	At End of Expiration	21323	Calculated Mean Flow Gradient
26258	With Stress	22055	Residual Gradient (Postoperative)
26260	V1/V2 Ratio	26339	Regurgitant Half Time
26263	At Rest	26343	At Rest
26265	At End of Inspiration	26345	At End of Inspiration
26267	At End of Expiration	26346	At End of Expiration
26268	With Stress	26348	With Stress
21317	Calculated Peak Flow Gradient	26350	Deceleration Time
26269	At Rest	26353	At Rest
26270	At End of Inspiration	26355	At End of Inspiration

ECHOCARDIOGRAM, CONT.

26356	At End of Expiration		20412	Paravalvular (Localized)
26357	With Stress		20413	Perivalvular (Circumferential)
26359	Doppler Derived Valve Area		21754	Residual (Postoperative)
26363	At Rest		19610	Uncertain
26365	At End of Inspiration		19831	Flow Velocity
26366	At End of Expiration		19832	Systolic
26367	With Stress		21324	Peak Flow
26370	RV Stroke Volume		21325	Calculated Peak Flow Gradient
26373	At Rest		21326	Mean Flow
26374	At End of Inspiration		21327	Calculated Mean Flow Gradient
26375	At End of Expiration		22052	Residual Gradient (Postoperative)
26376	With Stress		22094	Residual Peak Gradient (Postoperative)
26377	RV Cardiac Output			
26379	At Rest		22095	Residual Mean Gradient (Postoperative)
26380	At End of Inspiration			
26382	At End of Expiration		19833	Diastolic
26384	With Stress		21328	Peak Flow
26387	RV Cardiac Index		21329	Calculated Peak Flow Gradient
26389	At Rest		21330	Mean Flow
26392	At End of Inspiration		21331	Calculated Mean Flow Gradient
26394	At End of Expiration		22053	Residual Gradient (Postoperative)
26396	With Stress		21367	Doppler Derived Valve Area
26397	RV/LV Cardiac Output Ratio		19834	Turbulence
26398	At Rest		19835	Systolic
26399	At End of Inspiration		19836	High Frequency
26400	At End of Expiration		19837	Low Frequency
26401	With Stress		19838	Diastolic
19823	Turbulence		19839	High Frequency
19824	Systolic		19840	Low Frequency
19825	High Frequency		19611	Prosthetic Tricuspid Valve
19826	Low Frequency		19612	Tissue
19827	Diastolic		19613	Homograft
19828	High Frequency		19614	Porcine
19829	Low Frequency		19615	Mechanical
26406	A Dip		19616	Anatomy
26407	Absent		19618	Thrombosed
26408	Increased		19619	Dehisced sewing ring
19601	Pulmonary Conduit		19620	Thickened
19602	Anatomy		19621	Calcified
19604	Thrombosed		21152	Vegetation
19605	Dehisced sewing ring		19617	Function
19606	Thickened		19622	Loosening / Rocking
19607	Calcified		19623	Motion pattern
21151	Vegetation		19661	Stenosis
21371	Pseudoaneurysm		21755	Residual (Postoperative)
19603	Function		19662	Regurgitation
19608	Loosening / Rocking		20337	Concentric
19609	Motion pattern		20338	Eccentric
19659	Stenosis		20414	Paravalvular (Localized)
21753	Residual (Postoperative)		20415	Perivalvular (Circumferential)
19660	Regurgitation		21756	Residual (Postoperative)
20335	Concentric		19624	Uncertain
20336	Eccentric		19841	Flow Velocity

ECHOCARDIOGRAM, CONT.

19842	Systolic		26288	At End of Inspiration
21332	Peak Flow		26295	At End of Expiration
26221	At Rest		26297	With Stress
26223	At End of Inspiration		26299	Regurgitant Velocity
26224	At End of Expiration		26301	At Rest
26225	With Stress		26303	At End of Inspiration
26226	Regurgitant Time		26306	At End of Expiration
26228	At Rest		26307	With Stress
26229	At End of Inspiration		26309	Acceleration Time
26230	At End of Expiration		26310	At Rest
26231	With Stress		26312	At End of Inspiration
26233	Regurgitant Time Velocity		26313	At End of Expiration
	Integral		26315	With Stress
26236	At Rest		26317	Deceleration Time
26237	At End of Inspiration		26320	At Rest
26238	At End of Expiration		26321	At End of Inspiration
26240	With Stress		26323	At End of Expiration
26242	Peak Acceleration Rate		26325	With Stress
26246	At Rest		21337	Calculated Peak Flow Gradient
26247	At End of Inspiration		21338	Mean Flow
26248	At End of Expiration		21339	Calculated Mean Flow Gradient
26249	With Stress		26333	At Rest
26250	Acceleration Time		26334	At End of Inspiration
26252	At Rest		26335	At End of Expiration
26254	At End of Inspiration		26336	With Stress
26256	At End of Expiration		26337	Isovolumetric Relaxation Period
26257	With Stress		26338	At Rest
26259	Deceleration Time		26340	At End of Inspiration
26261	At Rest		26341	At End of Expiration
26262	At End of Inspiration		26342	With Stress
26264	At End of Expiration		26344	Pressure Half Time
26266	With Stress		26347	At Rest
21333	Calculated Peak Flow Gradient		26349	At End of Inspiration
26409	At Rest		26351	At End of Expiration
26410	At End Of Inspiration		26352	With Stress
26411	At End of Expiration		26354	1/3 Filling Fraction Period
26412	With Stress		26358	At Rest
21334	Mean Flow		26360	At End of Inspiration
21335	Calculated Mean Flow Gradient		26361	At End of Expiration
22056	Residual Gradient (Postoperative)		26362	With Stress
19843	Diastolic		26364	1/2 Filling Fraction Period
21336	Peak Flow E		26368	At Rest
26273	At Rest		26369	At End of Inspiration
26274	At End of Inspiration		26371	At End of Expiration
26275	At End of Expiration		26372	With Stress
26276	With Stress		22057	Residual Gradient (Postoperative)
26277	Peak Flow A		22096	Residual Peak Gradient (Postoperative)
26280	At Rest			
26282	At End of Inspiration		22097	Residual Mean Gradient (Postoperative)
26284	At End of Expiration			
26285	With Stress		26378	RA Pressure
26286	E/A Ratio		26381	At Rest
26287	At Rest		26383	At End of Inspiration

ECHOCARDIOGRAM, CONT.

26385	At End of Expiration		19643	Mechanical
26386	With Stress		19644	Anatomy
26388	RV Pressure		19646	Thrombosed
26390	At Rest		19647	Dehisced sewing ring
26391	At End of Inspiration		19648	Thickened
26393	At End of Expiration		19649	Calcified
26395	With Stress		19645	Function
21368	Doppler Derived Valve Area		19650	Loosening / Rocking
26402	At Rest		19651	Motion pattern
26403	At End of Inspiration		19665	Stenosis
26404	At End of Expiration		19666	Regurgitation
26405	With Stress		20341	Concentric
19844	Turbulence		20342	Eccentric
19845	Systolic		20418	Paravalvular (Localized)
19846	High Frequency		20419	Perivalvular (Circumferential)
19847	Low Frequency		19652	Uncertain
19848	Diastolic		19870	Flow Velocity
19849	High Frequency		19861	Systolic
19850	Low Frequency		19862	Diastolic
19625	Prosthetic Left A-V Valve		19863	Turbulence
19626	Tissue		19864	Systolic
19627	Homograft		19865	High Frequency
19628	Porcine		19866	Low Frequency
19629	Mechanical		19867	Diastolic
19630	Anatomy		19868	High Frequency
19632	Thrombosed		19869	Low Frequency
19633	Dehisced sewing ring		20420	Prosthetic Common A-V Valve
19634	Thickened		20421	Tissue
19635	Calcified		20422	Homograft
19631	Function		20423	Porcine
19636	Loosening / Rocking		20424	Mechanical
19637	Motion pattern		20425	Anatomy
19663	Stenosis		20426	Thrombosed
19664	Regurgitation		20427	Dehisced sewing ring
20339	Concentric		20428	Thickened
20340	Eccentric		20429	Calcified
20416	Paravalvular (Localized)		20430	Function
20417	Perivalvular (Circumferential)		20431	Loosening / Rocking
19638	Uncertain		20432	Motion pattern
19851	Flow Velocity		20433	Stenosis
19852	Systolic		20470	Regurgitation
19853	Diastolic		20434	Concentric
19854	Turbulence		20435	Eccentric
19855	Systolic		20436	Paravalvular (Localized)
19856	High Frequency		20437	Perivalvular (Circumferential)
19857	Low Frequency		20438	Uncertain
19858	Diastolic		20439	Flow Velocity
19859	High Frequency		20440	Systolic
19860	Low Frequency		20441	Diastolic
19639	Prosthetic Right A-V Valve		20442	Turbulence
19640	Tissue		20443	Systolic
19641	Homograft		20444	Diastolic
19642	Porcine		20445	Prosthetic Truncal A-V Valve

ECHOCARDIOGRAM, CONT.

20446	Tissue		20222	Straddling
20447	Homograft		21574	Mass ___ cm
20448	Porcine		21575	Rhabdomyoma ___ cm
20449	Mechanical		81935	Echogenicity
20450	Anatomy		21635	Hypoplasia
20451	Thrombosed		14573	Root
20452	Dehisced sewing ring		14574	Diameter
20453	Thickened		28330	Diastolic
20454	Calcified		28331	Systolic
20455	Function		14575	Dilated Sinuses
20456	Loosening / Rocking		20858	Aneurysm
20457	Motion pattern		14576	Thickened (>1mm.)
20458	Stenosis		14577	Overriding the Septum
20471	Regurgitation		20145	Multiple Echoes
20459	Concentric		20146	Vegetation
20460	Eccentric		21188	Abscess
20461	Paravalvular (Localized)		19686	Aortic Sinus of Valsalva
20462	Perivalvular (Circumferential)		25379	Diameter (mm)
20463	Uncertain		20492	Dilation
20464	Flow Velocity		20859	Aneurysm
20465	Systolic		27002	Conduit Present
20466	Diastolic		25380	Sino-tubular Junction
20467	Turbulence		25381	Diameter (mm)
20468	Systolic		19687	Ascending Aorta
20469	Diastolic		21866	Internal Diameter
19525	Periprosthetic		25382	Proximal
19679	Great Arteries		25383	Distal
19692	Relationships		20596	Wall Thickness
21372	Malpositioned		20599	Increased
21378	Aorta Anterior To Pulmonary Artery		21382	Atherosclerosis
21373	Aorta Anterior And Right Of Pulmonary		21383	Mobile
			21384	Immobile
21374	Aorta Anterior And Left Of Pulmonary		21385	Pedunculated
			21386	Laminated
21379	Aorta Posterior To Pulmonary Artery		21141	Mass ___ cm
			21387	Rhabdomyoma ___ cm
21375	Arteries Side By Side		81951	Echogenicity
21376	Aorta On Right		21174	Thrombus Formation ___ cm
21377	Aorta On Left		20107	Hypoplasia
21227	Transposition		20108	Interrupted
21228	Corrected		20106	Collateral Aortic Arteries
19526	Aorta		20504	Dilation
20857	Generalized Wall Thickening		20523	Post-Stenotic
21205	Atherosclerosis		20860	Aneurysm
21206	Mobile		27003	Conduit Present
21207	Immobile		21721	Spontaneous Echo Contrast
21208	Pedunculated		19872	Turbulence
21209	Laminated		19903	Systolic
21210	Debris		19904	Diastolic
19871	Intimal Flap / Dissection		19688	Aortic Arch
20116	Type I (Ascending / Descending)		21867	Internal Diameter
20117	Type II (Ascending)		20597	Wall Thickness
20118	Type III (Descending)		20600	Increased

ECHOCARDIOGRAM, CONT.

20102	Right-Sided		28091	Hypoplasia
20101	Left-Sided		28092	Interrupted
21394	Atherosclerosis		28093	Collateral Aortic Arteries
21395	Mobile		28094	Dilation
21396	Immobile		28095	Post-Stenotic
21397	Pedunculated		28096	Aneurysm
21398	Laminated		28097	Turbulence
20103	Double Arch		28098	Systolic
20104	Both Patent		28099	Diastolic
20105	One Atretic		20852	Right Carotid Artery
21142	Mass ___ cm		28100	Wall Thickness
21399	Rhabdomyoma ___ cm		28101	Increased
81952	Echogenicity		28102	Atherosclerosis
21175	Thrombus Formation ___ cm		28103	Mobile
20505	Dilation		28104	Immobile
20524	Post-Stenotic		28105	Pedunculated
20861	Aneurysm		28106	Laminated
27004	Conduit Present		28107	Mass ___ cm
21722	Spontaneous Echo Contrast		28108	Rhabdomyoma ___ cm
19873	Turbulence		81954	Echogenicity
19905	Systolic		28109	Thrombus Formation
20850	Aortic Arch Vessels		28110	Hypoplasia
20862	Wall Thickness		28111	Interrupted
20863	Increased		28112	Collateral Aortic Arteries
21388	Atherosclerosis		28113	Dilation
21389	Mobile		28114	Post-Stenotic
21390	Immobile		28115	Aneurysm
21391	Pedunculated		28116	Turbulence
21392	Laminated		28117	Systolic
21143	Mass ___ cm		28118	Diastolic
21393	Rhabdomyoma ___ cm		20853	Right Vertebral Artery
21176	Thrombus Formation ___ cm		28119	Wall Thickness
20864	Hypoplasia		28120	Increased
20865	Interrupted		28121	Atherosclerosis
20866	Collateral Aortic Arteries		28122	Mobile
20867	Dilation		28123	Immobile
20868	Post-Stenotic		28124	Pedunculated
20869	Aneurysm		28125	Laminated
20870	Turbulence		28126	Mass ___ cm
20871	Systolic		28127	Rhabdomyoma ___ cm
20872	Diastolic		81955	Echogenicity
20851	Brachiocephalic Artery		28128	Thrombus Formation
28082	Wall Thickness		28129	Hypoplasia
28083	Increased		28130	Interrupted
28084	Atherosclerosis		28131	Collateral Aortic Arteries
28085	Mobile		28132	Dilation
28086	Immobile		28133	Post-Stenotic
28087	Pedunculated		28134	Aneurysm
28088	Laminated		28135	Turbulence
28089	Mass ___ cm		28136	Systolic
28090	Rhabdomyoma ___ cm		28137	Diastolic
81953	Echogenicity		20856	Left Subclavian Artery
21542	Thrombus Formation		28138	Wall Thickness

ECHOCARDIOGRAM, CONT.

28139	Increased	28187	Interrupted
28140	Atherosclerosis	28188	Collateral Aortic Arteries
28141	Mobile	28189	Dilation
28142	Immobile	28190	Post-Stenotic
28143	Pedunculated	28191	Aneurysm
28144	Laminated	28192	Turbulence
28145	Mass ___ cm	28193	Systolic
28146	Rhabdomyoma ___ cm	28194	Diastolic
81956	Echogenicity	19689	Descending Thoracic Aorta
28147	Thrombus Formation	21868	Internal Diameter
28148	Hypoplasia	25384	Upper
28149	Interrupted	25385	Middle
28150	Collateral Aortic Arteries	25386	Lower
28151	Dilation	20598	Wall Thickness
28152	Post-Stenotic	20601	Increased
28153	Aneurysm	21400	Atherosclerosis
28154	Turbulence	21401	Mobile
28155	Systolic	21402	Immobile
28156	Diastolic	21403	Pedunculated
20854	Left Carotid Artery	21404	Laminated
28157	Wall Thickness	21144	Mass ___ cm
28158	Increased	21405	Rhabdomyoma ___ cm
28159	Atherosclerosis	81959	Echogenicity
28160	Mobile	21177	Thrombus Formation ___ cm
28161	Immobile	20109	Ductus Arteriosus
28162	Pedunculated	20110	Coarctation
28163	Laminated	21850	Systolic Flow Velocity
28164	Mass ___ cm	26121	At Rest
28165	Rhabdomyoma ___ cm	26124	At End of Inspiration
81957	Echogenicity	26125	At End of Expiration
28166	Thrombus Formation	26127	With Stress
28167	Hypoplasia	21851	Systolic Peak Flow Velocity
28168	Interrupted	26114	At Rest
28169	Collateral Aortic Arteries	26116	At End of Inspiration
28170	Dilation	26118	At End of Expiration
28171	Post-Stenotic	26120	With Stress
28172	Aneurysm	21852	Systolic Calculated Peak Flow Gradient
28173	Turbulence		
28174	Systolic	26130	At Rest
28175	Diastolic	26133	At End of Inspiration
20855	Left Vertebral Artery	26135	At End of Expiration
28176	Wall Thickness	26136	With Stress
28177	Increased	21853	Systolic Mean Flow Velocity
28178	Atherosclerosis	21854	Systolic Calculated Mean Flow Gradient
28179	Mobile		
28180	Immobile	26141	At Rest
28181	Pedunculated	26142	At End of Inspiration
28182	Laminated	26143	At End of Expiration
28183	Mass ___ cm	26144	With Stress
28184	Rhabdomyoma ___ cm	25619	Systolic TVI
81958	Echogenicity	26147	At Rest
28185	Thrombus Formation	26148	At End of Inspiration
28186	Hypoplasia	26150	At End of Expiration

ECHOCARDIOGRAM, CONT.

26152	With Stress	19907	Flow Velocity
25620	Diastolic TVI	19908	Systolic
26153	At Rest	19909	Diastolic
26154	At End of Inspiration	21724	Spontaneous Echo Contrast
26157	At End of Expiration	19910	Turbulence
26158	With Stress	19911	Systolic
25621	Diastolic/Systolic TVI Ratio	19912	Diastolic
26159	At Rest	19691	Main
26160	At End of Inspiration	19741	Anatomy
26161	At End of Expiration	21870	Internal Diameter
26162	With Stress	26623	At Rest
20506	Dilation	26624	At End of Inspiration
20525	Post-Stenotic	26625	At End of Expiration
20873	Aneurysm	26626	With Stress
27005	Conduit Present	25387	Pulmonary / Aortic Artery Index
21723	Spontaneous Echo Contrast	26615	At Rest
19874	Turbulence	26616	At End of Inspiration
19906	Systolic	26617	At End of Expiration
19690	Abdominal Aorta	26618	With Stress
21869	Internal Diameter	25388	% of Predicted
21406	Atherosclerosis	26619	At Rest
21407	Mobile	26620	At End of Inspiration
21408	Immobile	26621	At End of Expiration
21409	Pedunculated	26622	With Stress
21410	Laminated	20509	Dilation
21145	Mass ___cm	20877	Aneurysm
21411	Rhabdomyoma ___ cm	27008	Conduit Present
81960	Echogenicity	20112	Hypoplasia
21178	Thrombus Formation ___cm	21180	Thrombus Formation ___cm
20507	Dilation	19744	Function
20874	Aneurysm	20485	Stenosis
27006	Conduit Present	19913	Flow Velocity
19529	Pulmonary Artery	19914	Systolic
19729	Anatomy	21846	Systolic Peak Flow
20111	Hypoplasia	21847	Systolic Calculated Peak Flow
20508	Dilation		Gradient
20875	Post-Stenotic	21848	Systolic Mean Flow
20876	Aneurysm	21849	Systolic Calculated Mean Flow
27007	Conduit Present		Gradient
21380	Atresia	19915	Diastolic
21381	Confluent	21725	Spontaneous Echo Contrast
20115	Non-Confluent	19916	Turbulence
21576	Mass ___cm	19917	Systolic
21577	Rhabdomyoma ___ cm	19918	Diastolic
81961	Echogenicity	20060	Systolic Pressure
21179	Thrombus Formation ___ cm	19693	Left Branch
21412	Catheter	19742	Anatomy
21413	Monitoring	21871	Internal Diameter
21414	Infusion	26607	At Rest
21160	Vegetation	26608	At End of Inspiration
21415	Thrombus	26609	At End of Expiration
21736	Foreign Object	26610	With Stress
19747	Function	20510	Dilation

ECHOCARDIOGRAM, CONT.

20878	Aneurysm	19749	Function	
27009	Conduit Present	19877	Flow Velocity	
20113	Hypoplasia	19878	Systolic	
21181	Thrombus Formation ___ cm	21834	Systolic Peak Flow	
19745	Function	21835	Systolic Calculated Peak Flow	
20486	Stenosis		Gradient	
19919	Flow Velocity	21836	Systolic Mean Flow	
19920	Systolic	21837	Systolic Calculated Mean Flow	
21842	Systolic Peak Flow		Gradient	
21843	Systolic Calculated Peak Flow	19879	Diastolic	
	Gradient	19880	Turbulence	
21844	Systolic Mean Flow	19881	Systolic	
21845	Systolic Calculated Mean Flow	19882	Diastolic	
	Gradient	20484	Stenosis	
19921	Diastolic	21862	Doppler Derived Pressure	
21726	Spontaneous Echo Contrast	21863	Systolic	
19922	Turbulence	26209	At Rest	
19694	Right Branch	26210	At End of Inspiration	
19743	Anatomy	26211	At End of Expiration	
21872	Internal Diameter	26212	With Stress	
26611	At Rest	21864	Diastolic	
26612	At End of Inspiration	26213	At Rest	
26613	At End of Expiration	26214	At End of Inspiration	
26614	With Stress	26215	At End of Expiration	
20511	Dilation	26216	With Stress	
20879	Aneurysm	21865	Mean	
27010	Conduit Present	26179	At Rest	
20114	Hypoplasia	26180	At End of Inspiration	
21182	Thrombus Formation ___ cm	26181	At End of Expiration	
19746	Function	26182	With Stress	
20487	Stenosis	19696	Left Ventricular Outflow Tract	
19923	Flow Velocity	25501	Internal Diameter	
19924	Systolic	25651	At Rest	
21838	Systolic Peak Flow	25652	At End of Inspiration	
21839	Systolic Calculated Peak Flow	25653	At End of Expiration	
	Gradient	25654	With Stress	
21840	Systolic Mean Flow	20513	Dilation	
21841	Systolic Calculated Mean Flow	20880	Narrowing	
	Gradient	21229	Double Outlet	
19925	Diastolic	21633	Hypoplasia	
21727	Spontaneous Echo Contrast	20478	Stenosis	
19926	Turbulence	20882	Dynamic Obstruction	
19695	Branch	19883	Flow Velocity	
19875	Anatomy	19884	Systolic	
20512	Dilation	21340	Peak Flow	
19876	Function	25626	At Rest	
20489	Stenosis	25627	At End of Inspiration	
19927	Flow Velocity	25628	At End of Expiration	
19928	Systolic	25629	With Stress	
19929	Diastolic	21341	Calculated Peak Flow Gradient	
19930	Turbulence	21342	Mean Flow	
19740	Band	21343	Calculated Mean Flow Gradient	
19748	Anatomy	26562	Time Velocity Integral	

ECHOCARDIOGRAM, CONT.

26563	At Rest	25698	At End of Expiration
26564	At End of Inspiration	25699	With Stress
26565	At End of Expiration	19895	Diastolic
26566	With Stress	21352	Peak Flow
19885	Diastolic	21353	Calculated Peak Flow Gradient
21344	Peak Flow	21354	Mean Flow
21345	Calculated Peak Flow Gradient	21355	Calculated Mean Flow Gradient
21346	Mean Flow	19896	Turbulence
21347	Calculated Mean Flow Gradient	19897	Systolic
21824	After Amyl Nitrite	19898	High Frequency
21825	Calculated Peak Flow Gradient	19899	Low Frequency
21826	Recovery Peak Flow Gradient	19900	Diastolic
21827	Calculated Mean Flow Gradient	19901	High Frequency
21828	Recovery Mean Flow Gradient	19902	Low Frequency
21829	With Valsalva	20059	Systolic Pressure
21830	Calculated Peak Flow Gradient	14596	Left Ventricle
21831	Recovery Peak Flow Gradient	19700	Anatomy
21832	Calculated Mean Flow Gradient	19698	Dimension
21833	Recovery Mean Flow Gradient	14597	Systolic
19886	Turbulence	25389	At Rest
19887	Systolic	25390	At End of Inspiration
19888	High Frequency	25391	At End of Expiration
19889	Low Frequency	25392	With Stress
19890	Diastolic	14598	Diastolic
19891	High Frequency	25393	At Rest
19892	Low Frequency	25394	At End of Inspiration
19697	Right Ventricular Outflow Tract	25395	At End of Expiration
25502	Internal Diameter	25396	With Stress
25704	At Rest	20493	Was Enlarged
25705	At End of Inspiration	20494	Was Decreased
25706	At End of Expiration	19711	Global Wall Thickness
25707	With Stress	20636	Increased
20514	Dilation	20833	Decreased
20881	Narrowing	25397	Wall Mass
21230	Double Outlet	81962	Echogenicity
21634	Hypoplasia	25398	Mass Index
20515	Stenosis	25399	Chamber Volume
20476	Obstruction	25400	Diastolic
20477	Deviated Septum	25401	Systolic
20883	Dynamic Obstruction	20637	Localized Wall Thickness Increase
19893	Flow Velocity	20638	Anterior
19894	Systolic	20895	Antero-Lateral
21348	Peak Flow	20639	Lateral
26145	At Rest	20896	Infero-Lateral
26146	At End of Inspiration	20640	Inferior
26149	At End of Expiration	20897	Antero-Septal
26151	With Stress	20898	Infero-Septal
21349	Calculated Peak Flow Gradient	20645	Apical
21350	Mean Flow	20894	Localized Wall Thickness Decrease
21351	Calculated Mean Flow Gradient	28197	Anterior
25558	Time Velocity Integral	28198	Antero-lateral
25696	At Rest	28199	Lateral
25697	At End of Inspiration	28200	Infero-lateral

ECHOCARDIOGRAM, CONT.

28201	Inferior	21091		Well Demarcated
28202	Antero-septal	21092		Poorly Demarcated
28203	Infero-septal	21093	Infero-Lateral-Basal	
28204	Apical	21094		Well Demarcated
14599	Posterior Wall	21095		Poorly Demarcated
14600	Thickness	21096	Infero-Septal	
19958	Diastolic	21097		Well Demarcated
25402	At Rest	21098		Poorly Demarcated
25403	At End of Inspiration	29262	Posterior	
25404	At End of Expiration	29263		Well Demarcated
25405	With Stress	29264		Poorly Demarcated
19959	Systolic	21099	Postero-Basal	
25406	At Rest	21100		Well Demarcated
25407	At End of Inspiration	21101		Poorly Demarcated
25408	At End of Expiration	21102	Postero-Lateral	
25409	With Stress	21103		Well Demarcated
20567	Increased	21104		Poorly Demarcated
20604	Thin	29265	Lateral	
14617	Aneurysm	29266		Well Demarcated
29256	Anterior	29267		Poorly Demarcated
29257	Well Demarcated	29268	Septal	
29258	Poorly Demarcated	29269		Well Demarcated
21063	Antero-Apical	29270		Poorly Demarcated
21064	Well Demarcated	21105	Ruptured	
21065	Poorly Demarcated	21106	Pseudoaneurysm	
21066	Antero-Lateral	21107	Apical Bulge	
21067	Well Demarcated	14618	Mass ___cm	
21068	Poorly Demarcated	21556	Infiltrative ___cm	
21069	Antero-Lateral-Apical	21557	Myxoma ___cm	
21070	Well Demarcated	21197	Rhabdomyoma ___cm	
21071	Poorly Demarcated	21201	Extracardiac, Adjacent To LV Wall	
21072	Antero-Septal		___cm	
21073	Well Demarcated	81950	Echogenicity	
21074	Poorly Demarcated	18058	Thrombus Formation ___cm	
21075	Antero-Septal-Apical	21163	Laminated ___cm	
21076	Well Demarcated	21164	Pedunculated ___cm	
21077	Poorly Demarcated	21165	At The Apex	
21078	Apical	21558	Contusion	
21079	Well Demarcated	21628	Hypoplasia	
21080	Poorly Demarcated	19701	Function	
21081	Apical-Septal	20526	Systolic Performance	
21082	Well Demarcated	20527	Hyperdynamic	
21083	Poorly Demarcated	20528	Hypodynamic	
29259	Inferior	20529	Indeterminate	
29260	Well Demarcated	28212	Diastolic Performance	
29261	Poorly Demarcated	20633	Contraction Lags IVS Contraction	
21084	Infero-Apical	20479	Obstruction	
21085	Well Demarcated	20480	Mid-Chamber	
21086	Poorly Demarcated	20481	Dynamic	
21087	Infero-Basal	20482	Apex	
21088	Well Demarcated	20483	Dynamic	
21089	Poorly Demarcated	20930	Systolic Global Wall Thickening	
21090	Infero-Lateral	20931	Reduced	

ECHOCARDIOGRAM, CONT.

20932	Increased	14603	Rapid Early Diastolic Relaxation
20933	Systolic Global Wall Thinning	14604	Diastolic Motion Decreased
20891	Local Wall Systolic Thickening	20630	Conduction Abnormality
20892	Reduced	20631	Abnormal Pacing
20942	Anterior	20632	Postoperative State
20943	Antero-Lateral	20647	Anterior Wall Motion
20944	Lateral	20664	Hypokinetic
20945	Infero-Lateral	20665	At The Base
20946	Inferior	20666	Base To Mid-Wall
20947	Antero-Septal	20667	Base To Apex
20948	Infero-Septal	20668	Mid-Wall
20949	Apex	20669	Mid-Wall To Apex
20893	Increased	20670	At The Apex
20950	Anterior	20671	Akinetic
20951	Antero-Lateral	20673	At The Base
20952	Lateral	20674	Base To Mid-Wall
20953	Infero-Lateral	20675	Base To Apical
20954	Inferior	20676	Mid-Wall
20955	Antero-Septal	20677	Mid-Wall To Apex
20956	Infero-Septal	20678	At The Apex
20957	Apex	20679	Dyskinetic
20889	Posterior Wall Systolic Thickening	20680	At The Base
25410	At Rest	20681	Base To Mid-Wall
25411	At End of Inspiration	20682	Base To Apex
25412	At End of Expiration	20683	Mid-Wall
25413	With Stress	20684	Mid-Wall To Apex
20607	Reduced	20685	At The Apex
20890	Increased	20648	Antero-Lateral Wall Motion
20655	Systolic Regional Wall Thinning	20686	Hypokinetic
20656	Anterior	20687	At The Base
20657	Antero-Lateral	20688	Base To Mid-Wall
20658	Lateral	20689	Base To Apex
20659	Infero-Lateral	20690	Mid-Wall
20660	Inferior	20691	Mid-Wall To Apex
20661	Antero-Septal	20692	At The Apex
20662	Infero-Septal	20693	Akinetic
20663	Apex	20694	At The Base
20610	Posterior Wall Systolic Thinning	20695	Base To Mid-Wall
20884	Global Wall Motion	20696	Base To Apex
20885	Hyperkinetic	20697	Mid-Wall
20886	Hypokinetic	20698	Mid-Wall To Apex
20887	Akinetic	20699	At The Apex
20888	Dyskinetic	20700	Dyskinetic
20899	Conduction Abnormality	20701	At The Base
20900	Abnormal due to Pacing	20702	Base To Mid-Wall
20901	Postoperative State	20703	Base To Apex
19719	Posterior Wall Motion	20704	Mid-Wall
20621	Hyperkinetic	20705	Mid-Wall To Apex
20622	Hypokinetic	20706	At The Apex
20623	Akinetic	20649	Lateral Wall Motion
20624	Dyskinetic	20707	Hypokinetic
14601	Systolic Motion Increased	20708	Basal
14602	Systolic Motion Decreased	20709	Base To Mid-Wall

ECHOCARDIOGRAM, CONT.

20710	Base To Apex		20761	Dyskinetic
20711	Mid-Wall		20762	Base To Mid-Wall
20712	Mid-Wall To Apex		20763	Base To Apex
20713	Apical		20764	Mid-Wall
20714	Akinetic		20765	Mid-Wall To Apex
20715	At The Base		20766	At The Apex
20716	Base To Mid-Wall		20672	Septal Wall Motion
20717	Base To Apex		20767	Hypokinetic
20718	Mid-Wall		20768	At The Base
20719	Mid-Wall To Apex		20769	Base To Mid-Wall
20720	At The Apex		20770	Base To Apex
20721	Dyskinetic		20772	Mid-Wall To Apex
20722	At The Base		20773	At The Apex
20723	Base To Mid-Wall		20774	Akinetic
20724	Base To Apex		20775	At The Base
20725	Mid-Wall		20776	Base To Mid-Wall
20726	Mid-Wall To Apex		20777	Base To Apex
20727	At The Apex		20779	Mid-Wall To Apex
20650	Infero-Lateral Wall Motion		20780	At The Apex
20728	Hypokinetic		20781	Dyskinetic
20729	At The Base		20782	At The Base
20730	Base To Mid-Wall		20783	Base To Mid-Wall
20731	Base To Apex		20784	Base To Apex
20732	Mid-Wall		20786	Mid-Wall To Apex
20733	Mid-Wall To Apex		20787	At The Apex
20734	At The Apex		20652	Antero-Septal Wall Motion
20735	Akinetic		20788	Hypokinetic
20736	At The Base		20789	At The Base
20737	Base To Mid-Wall		20790	Base To Mid-Wall
20738	Base To Apex		20791	Base To Apex
20739	Mid-Wall		20792	Mid-Wall
20740	Mid-Wall To Apex		20793	Mid-Wall To Apex
20741	At The Apex		20794	At The Apex
20742	Dyskinetic		20795	Akinetic
20743	At The Base		20796	At The Base
20744	Base To Mid-Wall		20797	Base To Mid-Wall
20745	Base To Apex		20798	Base To Apex
20746	Mid-Wall		20799	Mid-Wall
20747	Mid-Wall To Apex		20800	Mid-Wall To Apex
20748	At The Apex		20801	At The Apex
20651	Inferior Wall Motion		20802	Dyskinetic
20749	Hypokinetic		20803	At The Base
20750	Base To Mid-Wall		20804	Base To Mid-Wall
20751	Base To Apex		20805	Base To Apex
20752	Mid-Wall		20806	Mid-Wall
20753	Mid-Wall To Apex		20807	Mid-Wall To Apex
20754	At The Apex		20808	At The Apex
20755	Akinetic		20653	Infero-Septal Wall Motion
20756	Base To Mid-Wall		20809	Hypokinetic
20757	Base To Apex		20810	At The Base
20758	Mid-Wall		20811	Base To Mid-Wall
20759	Mid-Wall To Apex		20812	Base To Apex
20760	At The Apex		20813	Mid-Wall

ECHOCARDIOGRAM, CONT.

20814	Mid-Wall To Apex		26585	With Stress
20815	At The Apex		19963	Filling Rate
20816	Akinetic		19960	Flow Velocity
20817	At The Base		19961	Systolic
20818	Base To Mid-Wall		19962	Diastolic
20819	Base To Apex		21359	Doppler Derived Systolic Pressure
20820	Mid-Wall		21562	Spontaneous Echo Contrast
20821	Mid-Wall To Apex		14665	Ventricular Turbulence
20822	At The Apex		14666	Systolic
20823	Dyskinetic		14667	High Frequency
20824	At The Base		14668	Low Frequency
20825	Base To Mid-Wall		14669	Diastolic
20826	Base To Apex		14670	High Frequency
20827	Mid-Wall		14671	Low Frequency
20828	Mid-Wall To Apex		19732	Morphologic Left Ventricle
20829	At The Apex		19733	Anatomy
20654	Apical Wall Motion		19734	Dimension
20830	Hypokinetic		20498	Enlarged
20831	Akinetic		20499	Decreased
20832	Dyskinetic		21563	Aneurysm
19957	Circumferential Fiber Shortening		21138	Mass ___ cm
25414	At Rest		81963	Echogenicity
25415	At End of Inspiration		21167	Thrombus Formation ___ cm
25416	At End of Expiration		21631	Hypoplasia
25417	With Stress		19735	Function
14605	Increased		20530	Systolic Performance
14606	Decreased		20531	Hyperdynamic
14615	Fractional Shortening (%)		20532	Hypodynamic
20593	Pressure		20533	Indeterminate
80912	Ejection Fraction		28213	Diastolic Performance
20546	Calculated		20569	Pressure
14616	Estimated		20551	Ejection Fraction
25418	At Rest		80919	Estimated
25419	At End of Inspiration		20552	Calculated
25420	At End of Expiration		20553	Non-Estimable
25421	With Stress		20570	Filling Rate
20547	Non-Estimable		20571	Flow Velocity
21559	Stroke Volume		20572	Systolic
26591	At Rest		20573	Diastolic
26592	At End of Inspiration		21713	Spontaneous Echo Contrast
26593	At End of Expiration		20574	Ventricular Turbulence
26594	With Stress		20575	Systolic
21560	Cardiac Output		20576	High Frequency
80913	SV x HR		20577	Low Frequency
80914	Aortic Valve		20578	Diastolic
25728	At Rest		20579	High Frequency
25729	At End of Inspiration		20580	Low Frequency
25730	At End of Expiration		14607	Ventricular Septum
25731	With Stress		19702	Anatomy
21561	Cardiac Index		14608	Thickness
26582	At Rest		25422	Diastolic
26583	At End of Inspiration		25423	At Rest
26584	At End of Expiration		25424	At End of Inspiration

ECHOCARDIOGRAM, CONT.

25425	At End of Expiration	20628	Abnormal Pacing
25426	With Stress	20629	Postoperative State
25427	Systolic	20609	Systolic Thinning
25428	At Rest	20834	Abnormality Due To Conduction
25429	At End of Inspiration	20835	Abnormality Due To Pacing
25430	At End of Expiration	20836	Postoperative Abnormality
25431	With Stress	19716	Motion
25432	Pre A-Wave	20625	Hyperkinetic
25433	At Rest	20626	Hypokinetic
25434	At End of Inspiration	20619	Akinetic
25435	At End of Expiration	20620	Dyskinetic
25436	With Stress	14610	Paradoxic
20565	Increased	14612	Accentuated
20566	Basal	14611	Flattened
20642	Upper	21855	VSD Flow Velocity
20643	Middle	21856	Systolic
20644	Apex	21857	Peak Flow
20641	Assymetric	21858	Calculated Peak Flow Gradient
20602	Thin	21859	Mean Flow
25437	Excursion	21860	Calculated Mean Flow Gradient
25438	At Rest	21861	Diastolic
25439	At End of Inspiration	14619	Right Ventricle
25440	At End of Expiration	19703	Anatomy
25441	With Stress	14621	Dimension
20634	Patch Present	25442	At Rest
20635	Dehisced	25443	At End of Inspiration
21496	Defect	25444	At End of Expiration
14613	Absent	25445	With Stress
14614	Partial Absence	14620	Enlarged
21497	Inflow Muscular	20495	Decreased
21498	Trabecular Muscular	20837	Global Wall Thickness
21500	Paramembranous Muscular	25446	Diastolic
21501	Supracristal	25447	At Rest
21502	Paramembranous Restrictive	25448	At End of Inspiration
21503	Outflow Restrictive	25449	At End of Expiration
21504	Malalignment Inflow	25450	With Stress
21505	Malalignment Outflow	20838	Increased
21506	Multiple	20839	Decreased
21507	Residual / Recurrent	25451	Systolic
14609	Ratio to Posterior Wall >1.3	25452	At Rest
20929	Aneurysm	25453	At End of Inspiration
21494	Membranous	25454	At End of Expiration
21495	Muscular	25455	With Stress
21508	Function	25456	Pre A-Wave Thickness
20926	Systolic Thickening	25457	At Rest
25503	At Rest	25458	At End of Inspiration
25504	At End Of Inspiration	25459	At End of Expiration
25505	At End Of Expiration	25460	With Stress
25506	With Stress	25461	Excursion
20605	Reduced	25462	At Rest
20927	Increased	25463	At End of Inspiration
20928	Assymetrical	25464	At End of Expiration
20627	Conduction Abnormality	25465	With Stress

ECHOCARDIOGRAM, CONT.

20615	Anterior Wall		20966	Mid-Chamber
19714	Thickness		20967	Anterior
20564	Increased		20968	Apex
20603	Thin		20934	Anterior Wall Systolic Thickening
20616	Conduction Abnormality		20606	Reduced
20617	Abnormal Pacing		20935	Increased
20618	Postoperative State		20969	Local Wall Systolic Thinning
21509	Prominent Moderator Band		20970	Inferior
21510	Anomalous Subpulmonary Muscle Bundle		20971	Mid-Chamber
			20608	Anterior Wall
21511	Trabeculation Prominent		20973	Apex
21061	Aneurysm		19715	Global Wall Motion
21062	Apical Bulge		20611	Hyperkinetic
20974	Vegetation		20612	Hypokinetic
21419	Pacemaker Wire		20613	Akinetic
20975	Vegetation		20614	Dyskinetic
21420	Thrombus		20939	Conduction Abnormality
21416	Catheter		20940	Abnormal Pacing
21417	Monitoring		20941	Postoperative State
21418	Infusion		20840	Regional Wall Motion
20976	Vegetation		21042	Hypokinetic
21421	Thrombus		21043	Akinetic
21732	Foreign Object		21044	Dyskinetic
21135	Mass ___ cm		21045	Inferior Wall Motion
21564	Infiltrative ___ cm		21046	Hypokinetic
21565	Myxoma ___ cm		21047	Akinetic
21198	Rhabdomyoma ___ cm		21048	Dyskinetic
21202	Extracardiac, Adjacent To RV Wall ___ cm		21049	Mid-Chamber Wall Motion
			21050	Hypokinetic
81964	Echogenicity		21051	Akinetic
21166	Thrombus Formation ___ cm		21052	Dyskinetic
21629	Hypoplasia		21053	Anterior Wall Motion
19705	Function		21054	Hypokinetic
20534	Systolic Performance		21055	Akinetic
20535	Hyperdynamic		21056	Dyskinetic
20536	Hypodynamic		21057	Apical Wall Motion
20537	Indeterminate		21058	Hypokinetic
20646	Systolic Global Wall Thickening		21059	Akinetic
25963	At Rest		21060	Dyskinetic
25964	At End of Inspiration		20581	Pressure
25965	At End of Expiration		20548	Ejection Fraction
25967	With Stress		80920	Estimated
20936	Reduced		20549	Calculated
20937	Increased		20550	Non-Estimable
20938	Systolic Global Wall Thinning		20582	Filling Rate
20958	Local Wall Systolic Thickening		20583	Flow Velocity
20959	Reduced		20584	Systolic
20960	Inferior		20585	Diastolic
20961	Mid-Chamber		21360	Doppler Derived Systolic Pressure
20962	Anterior		21714	Spontaneous Echo Contrast
20963	Apex		20586	Ventricular Turbulence
20964	Increased		20587	Systolic
20965	Inferior		20588	High Frequency

ECHOCARDIOGRAM, CONT.

20589	Low Frequency		80922	Estimated
20590	Diastolic		20558	Calculated
20591	High Frequency		20559	Non-Estimable
20592	Low Frequency		21716	Spontaneous Echo Contrast
19736	Morphologic Right Ventricle		20560	Systemic Ventricle
19737	Anatomy		20561	Ejection Fraction
19738	Dimension		80923	Estimated
20500	Enlarged		20562	Calculated
20501	Decreased		20563	Non-Estimable
21512	Aneurysm		14622	Left Atrium
21139	Mass ___ cm		19712	Anatomy
81965	Echogenicity		14623	Dimension
21168	Thrombus Formation ___ cm		28332	Systolic Diameter
21632	Hypoplasia ___ cm		28333	Diastolic Diameter
19739	Function		25466	Normalized to Aortic Diameter
20538	Systolic Performance		25467	At Rest
20539	Hyperdynamic		25468	At End of Inspiration
20540	Hypodynamic		25469	At End of Expiration
20541	Indeterminate		25470	With Stress
28214	Diastolic Performance		25471	Four Chamber Area
19965	Pressure		25472	At Rest
20554	Ejection Fraction		25473	At End of Inspiration
80921	Estimated		25474	At End of Expiration
20555	Calculated		25475	With Stress
20556	Non-Estimable		25476	Two Chamber Area
19964	Filling Rate		25477	At Rest
19966	Flow Velocity		25478	At End of Inspiration
19967	Systolic		25479	At End of Expiration
19968	Diastolic		25480	With Stress
21715	Spontaneous Echo Contrast		25481	Left Atrial Length
19969	Ventricular Turbulence		25482	Left Atrial Volume
19970	Systolic		20472	Showed Enlargement
19971	High Frequency		20473	Was Decreased
19972	Low Frequency		14624	Abnormal Intra-Atrial Echoes Present
19973	Diastolic		14625	Ratio to Aorta
19974	High Frequency		21626	Double Outlet
19975	Low Frequency		21513	Membrane
19681	Common Ventricle		21514	Cor Triatriatum
19706	Anatomy		21515	Obstructing Pulmonary Venous Entry
19707	Dimension			
20502	Enlarged		21136	Mass ___ cm
20503	Decreased		21566	Myxoma ___ cm
21140	Mass ___ cm		21199	Rhabdomyoma ___ cm
81966	Echogenicity		21203	Extracardiac, Adjacent To LA Wall ___ cm
21169	Thrombus Formation ___ cm			
21630	Hypoplasia		81967	Echogenicity
19708	Function		21172	Thrombus ___ cm
20542	Systolic Performance		21516	Prosthetic Material
20543	Hyperdynamic		19720	Atrial Appendage
20544	Hypodynamic		19730	Dilated
20545	Indeterminate		20977	Aneurysm
28215	Diastolic Performance		21171	Thrombus Formation ___ cm
20557	Ejection Fraction		21719	Spontaneous Echo Contrast

ECHOCARDIOGRAM, CONT.

19713	Function	19983	Flattened
20978	Systolic Performance	19536	Right Atrium
19979	Hyperdynamic	19721	Anatomy
20980	Hypodynamic	19723	Diameter
19978	Indeterminate	20496	Enlarged
20981	Systolic Wall Thickening	20497	Decreased
20982	Reduced	20594	Wall Thickness
20983	Increased	20595	Increased
20984	Systolic Wall Thinning	21157	Vegetation
20979	Global Wall Motion	21422	Pacemaker Wire
19976	Hypokinetic	21158	Vegetation
19977	Akinetic	21423	Thrombus
21717	Spontaneous Echo Contrast	21424	Catheter
19535	Atrial Septum	21425	Monitoring
19717	Anatomy	21426	Infusion
19718	Thickness	21159	Vegetation
20568	Increased	21427	Thrombus
20996	Aneurysm	21733	Foreign Object
20986	Redundant Flap	21627	Double Outlet
21517	Congenital Defect	21585	Membrane
25583	Diameter	21586	Cor Triatriatum Dexter
25887	At Rest	21137	Mass ___ cm
25888	At End of Inspiration	21567	Myxoma ___ cm
25889	At End of Expiration	21200	Rhabdomyoma ___ cm
25890	With Stress	21204	Extracardiac, Adjacent To RA Wall ___ cm
21518	Secundum		
21519	Primum	81968	Echogenicity
21520	Sinus Venosus	21173	Thrombus ___ cm
21521	Coronary Sinus	19722	Atrial Appendage
21522	Patent Foramen Ovale	19731	Dilated
21523	Fenestrated	21002	Aneurysm
21524	Restrictive	21170	Thrombus Formation ___ cm
21525	Residual	21720	Spontaneous Echo Contrast
21526	Recurrent	19724	Function
21527	Common Atrium	21003	Systolic Performance
20985	Lipomatous	19987	Hyperdynamic
20987	Function	21004	Hypodynamic
20988	Systolic Performance	19986	Indeterinate
20989	Hyperdynamic	21005	Systolic Wall Thickening
20990	Hypodynamic	21006	Reduced
20991	Indeterminate	21007	Increased
20992	Systolic Wall Thickening	21008	Systolic Wall Thinning
20993	Reduced	21009	Wall Motion
20994	Increased	19984	Hypokinetic
20995	Systolic Wall Thinning	19985	Akinetic
20997	Motion	21718	Spontaneous Echo Contrast
20998	Hyperkinetic	20124	Juxtaposed Atrial Appendages
20999	Hypokinetic	21528	Atrioventricular Canal
21000	Akinetic	21529	Double Inlet Atrioventricular Valve
21001	Dyskinetic	21530	Chamber Relationships
19980	Motion	21531	Atrioventricular
19981	Paradoxic	21532	Concordance
19982	Accentuated	21533	Discordance

ECHOCARDIOGRAM, CONT.

21534	Ambiguous	21639	Bidirectional Flow	
21535	Ventriculoatrial	21640	Ventricular Shunt	
21536	Concordance	21641	Left To Right Flow	
21537	Discordance	21642	Right To Left Flow	
21538	Congenital Chamber Abnormality	21643	Bidirectional Flow	
21587	Double Inlet Ventricle	21644	Shunt Across A-V Canal	
21588	Left	21645	Left To Right Flow	
21589	Right	21646	Right To Left Flow	
21590	Accessory Chamber	21647	Bidirectional Flow	
21591	Indeterminate	21648	LV To RA Shunt	
21592	Rudimentary RV Chamber	21649	Left To Right Flow	
21593	Anterior	21650	Right To Left Flow	
21594	To The Left	21651	Bidirectional Flow	
21595	To The Right	21821	Coronary Artery Fistula	
21596	Posterior	21822	Pulmonary Arteriovenous Fistula	
21597	To The Left	21823	Systemic Arteriovenous Fistula	
21598	To The Right	21540	Postoperative Congenital Findings	
21599	RV Chamber Outlet	21652	Balloon Septostomy	
21600	Anterior	21653	Patent	
21601	To The Left	21654	Obstructed	
21602	To The Right	21655	Restrictive	
21603	Posterior	21656	Blalock-Hanlon Septostomy	
21604	To The Left	21657	Patent	
21605	To The Right	21658	Obstructed	
21606	Rudimentary LV Chamber	21659	Restrictive	
21607	Anterior	21687	Transeptal Septostomy	
21608	To The Left	21688	Patent	
21609	To The Right	21689	Obstructed	
21610	Posterior	21690	Restrictive	
21611	To The Left	21660	Blalock-Taussig Shunt	
21612	To The Right	21661	Patent	
21613	LV Chamber Outlet	21662	Obstructed	
21614	Anterior	21663	Restrictive	
21615	To The Left	21757	Flow Velocity	
21616	To The Right	21758	Systolic Flow Velocity	
21617	Posterior	21759	Peak Flow	
21618	To The Left	21760	Calculated Peak Flow Gradient	
21619	To The Right	21761	Mean Flow	
21620	Two Chamber Ventricle	21762	Calculated Mean Flow Gradient	
21621	Two Chamber Atrium	21763	Diastolic Flow Velocity	
21622	Two Chamber Ventricle / Atrium	21764	Peak Flow	
21623	Inverted Ventricular Chambers	21765	Calculated Peak Flow Gradient	
21624	Criss-cross Ventricles	21766	Mean Flow	
21625	Upstairs / Downstairs Ventricles	21767	Calculated Mean Flow Gradient	
21539	Congenital Flow Abnormality	21691	Waterston Shunt	
21636	Atrial Shunt	21692	Patent	
25584	Shunt Velocity	21693	Obstructed	
25892	At Rest	21694	Restrictive	
25893	At End of Inspiration	21768	Flow Velocity	
25895	At End of Expiration	21769	Systolic Flow Velocity	
25897	With Stress	21770	Peak Flow	
21637	Left To Right Flow	21771	Calculated Peak Flow Gradient	
21638	Right To Left Flow	21772	Mean Flow	

ECHOCARDIOGRAM, CONT.

21773	Calculated Mean Flow Gradient
21774	Diastolic Flow Velocity
21775	Peak Flow
21776	Calculated Peak Flow Gradient
21777	Mean Flow
21778	Calculated Mean Flow Gradient
21709	Pott's Shunt
21710	Patent
21779	Flow Velocity
21780	Systolic Flow Velocity
21781	Peak Flow
21782	Calculated Peak Flow Gradient
21783	Mean Flow
21784	Calculated Mean Flow Gradient
21785	Diastolic Flow Velocity
21786	Peak Flow
21787	Calculated Peak Flow Gradient
21788	Mean Flow
21789	Calculated Mean Flow Gradient
21711	Goretex Interpositional Shunt
21712	Patent
21790	Flow Velocity
21791	Systolic Flow Velocity
21792	Peak Flow
21793	Calculated Peak Flow Gradient
21794	Mean Flow
21796	Calculated Mean Flow Gradient
21797	Diastolic Flow Velocity
21798	Peak Flow
21799	Calculated Peak Flow Gradient
21800	Mean Flow
21801	Calculated Mean Flow Gradient
21664	Fontan
21665	Patent
21666	Obstructed
21667	Restrictive
21668	Glenn Anastamosis
21669	Patent
21670	Obstructed
21671	Restrictive
21672	Mustard Baffle
21673	Patent
21674	Venous Obstruction
21675	Systemic Obstruction
21676	Restrictive
21677	Senning Baffle
21678	Patent
21679	Pulmonary Venous Obstruction
21680	Systemic Obstruction
21681	Restrictive
21682	Rastelli Conduit
21683	Patent
21684	Obstructed

21685	With Obstructed VSD
21686	Restrictive
21695	Surgically Created Defect
21696	Patent
21697	Obstructed
21802	Flow Velocity
21803	Systolic Flow Velocity
21804	Peak Flow
21805	Calculated Peak Flow Gradient
21806	Mean Flow
21807	Calculated Mean Flow Gradient
21808	Diastolic Flow Velocity
21809	Peak Flow
21810	Calculated Peak Flow Gradient
21811	Mean Flow
21812	Calculated Mean Flow Gradient
21698	Jatene Arterial Switch
21699	Auber Arterial Switch
21700	Ventricular Septation
21701	Septal Myectomy
21702	Patch Closure Of Defect
21703	Atrial
21704	Intact
21705	Dehisced
21706	Ventricular
21707	Intact
21708	Dehisced
22130	Residual Shunt
22131	Atrial (ASD)
22132	Ventricular (VSD)
22133	Extracardiac
21584	Aortopulmonary Window
19531	Papillary Muscles
80924	Normal
19988	Mitral Valve
80926	Normal
19989	Hypertrophy
19990	Transected
19991	Partial
19992	Complete
29307	Anterolateral
29308	Posteromedial
21541	Anomalous Left Ventricular Chord
21010	Function
21011	Systolic Thickening
21012	Antero-Lateral
21013	Postero-Medial
19993	Dysfunction
19994	Tricuspid Valve
80925	Normal
19995	Hypertrophy
19996	Transected
19997	Partial

ECHOCARDIOGRAM, CONT.

19998	Complete	14630	"Swinging" Heart
29309	Anterolateral	21547	Mass ___ cm
29310	Posteromedial	21548	Right Ventricular Region ___ cm
21014	Function	21549	Left Ventricular Region ___ cm
21015	Systolic Thickening	21550	Region Of Both Ventricles ___ cm
21016	Antero-Lateral	81969	Echogenicity
21017	Postero-Medial	21551	Cyst
19999	Dysfunction	20019	Epicardial Fat Layer
20000	Left A-V Valve	20070	Anterior
80930	Normal	20071	Posterior
20001	Hypertrophy	20072	Circumferential
20002	Transected	19534	Atrial Connections
20003	Partial	20097	Anomalous Pulmonary-Venous Return
20004	Complete	20098	Partial
20005	Multiple Muscles	20099	Total
20006	Dysfunction	20100	Anomalous Right Systemic-Venous
20007	Right A-V Valve		Return
80931	Normal	20045	Atrial Baffle
20008	Hypertrophy	20046	Turbulence
20009	Transected	20488	Obstruction
20010	Partial	20020	Jugular Vein
20011	Complete	20088	Valve In Vein
20012	Multiple Muscles	21552	Mass ___ cm
20013	Dysfunction	81970	Echogenicity
20014	Single A-V Valve Muscle	21553	Thrombus ___ cm
20015	Multiple A-V Valve Muscles	20021	Subclavian Vein
20016	Hypoplastic A-V Chordae	20087	Valve In Vein
21543	Muscle In A-V Valve Connected To	21554	Mass ___ cm
	Conus	81971	Echogenicity
19532	Extracardiac & Thoracic Anatomy	21555	Thrombus ___ cm
14626	Pericardium	19537	Superior Vena Cava
14627	Thick	20089	Absent
19766	Calcification Present	20090	Persistent Left SVC
21544	Absent	20091	Bilateral SVC
21545	Congenital	20092	Anomalous Connection
21546	Surgical	20119	Anomalous Drainage
20018	Effusion	21428	Pacemaker Wire
20128	Anterior	21161	Vegetation
20139	Lateral	21429	Thrombus
20129	Posterior	21430	Catheter
20130	Circumferential	21431	Monitoring
20131	Apical	21432	Infusion
20134	Localized	21162	Vegetation
20135	Around Left Ventricle	21433	Thrombus
20136	Around Right Ventricle	21734	Foreign Object
20137	Around Left Atrium	21146	Mass ___ cm
20138	Around Right Atrium	21569	Infiltrative ___ cm
20132	Loculated	21578	Rhabdomyoma ___ cm
20133	Strands	81972	Echogenicity
20017	Echo Free Space	21183	Thrombus Formation ___ cm
14628	Anterior	20516	Dilation
14629	Posterior	20490	Stenosis
20069	Circumferential	20047	Flow Velocity

ECHOCARDIOGRAM, CONT.

20048	Systolic		20051	Systolic
26040	At Rest		20052	Diastolic
26041	At End of Inspiration		20022	Brachiocephalic Veins
26042	At End of Expiration		80927	Normal
26043	With Stress		20085	Absent
25611	Systolic TVI		20086	Anomalous Course
26047	At Rest		21436	Pacemaker Wire
26048	At End of Inspiration		21186	Vegetation
26050	At End of Expiration		21437	Thrombus
26051	With Stress		21438	Catheter
25612	Peak Systolic Reversal Velocity		21439	Monitoring
26052	At Rest		21440	Infusion
26053	At End of Inspiration		21187	Vegetation
26054	At End of Expiration		21441	Thrombus
26055	With Stress		21580	Mass ___ cm
25613	Systolic Reversal TVI		21581	Rhabdomyoma ___ cm
26060	At Rest		81973	Echogenicity
26061	At End of Inspiration		21184	Thrombus Formation ___ cm
26062	At End of Expiration		21442	Left Vein
26063	With Stress		21443	Absent
20049	Diastolic		21444	Anomalous Course
26068	At Rest		21445	Pacemaker Wire
26069	At End of Inspiration		21446	Vegetation
26070	At End of Expiration		21447	Thrombus
26071	With Stress		21448	Catheter
25614	Peak Diastolic Velocity (D2)		21449	Monitoring
26097	At Rest		21450	Infusion
26098	At End of Inspiration		21451	Vegetation
26099	At End of Expiration		21452	Thrombus
26100	With Stress		81976	Mass ___ cm
25615	Peak Diastolic Velocity (D2) from TVI		81983	Echogenicity ___ cm
			21453	Thrombus Formation ___ cm
26108	At Rest		21730	Spontaneous Echo Contrast
26110	At End of Inspiration		21454	Right Vein
26111	At End of Expiration		21455	Absent
26112	With Stress		21456	Anomalous Course
25616	Diastolic TVI		21457	Pacemaker Wire
26076	At Rest		21458	Vegetation
26077	At End of Inspiration		21459	Thrombus
26078	At End of Expiration		21460	Catheter
26079	With Stress		21461	Monitoring
25617	Peak Atrial Reversal Velocity		21462	Infusion
26084	At Rest		21463	Vegetation
26085	At End of Inspiration		21464	Thrombus
26086	At End of Expiration		81977	Mass ___ cm
26087	With Stress		81984	Echogenicity ___ cm
25618	Atrial Reversal TVI		21465	Thrombus Formation ___ cm
26090	At Rest		21731	Spontaneous Echo Contrast
26091	At End of Inspiration		19538	Inferior Vena Cava
26093	At End of Expiration		21873	Internal Diameter
26094	With Stress		20073	Absent
21728	Spontaneous Echo Contrast		20074	Anomalous Connection
20050	Turbulence		20120	Anomalous Drainage

ECHOCARDIOGRAM, CONT.

20075	Azygous Vein Continues To IVC		20035	Dimension
21735	Foreign Object		81981	Mass ___cm
21147	Mass ___cm		81986	Echogenicity ___cm
21568	Infiltrative ___cm		25593	Peak Systolic Velocity
21579	Rhabdomyoma ___cm		25903	At Rest
81974	Echogenicity		25904	At End of Inspiration
21185	Thrombus Formation ___cm		25905	At End of Expiration
20517	Dilation		25906	With Stress
20491	Stenosis		25594	Systolic TVI
20053	Flow Velocity		25907	At Rest
20054	Systolic		25909	At End of Inspiration
20055	Diastolic		25912	At End of Expiration
21729	Spontaneous Echo Contrast		25913	With Stress
20056	Turbulence		25595	Peak Diastolic Velocity
20057	Systolic		25917	At Rest
20058	Diastolic		25918	At End of Inspiration
19539	Coronary Sinus		25920	At End of Expiration
20121	Absent		25922	With Stress
20122	Anomalous		25596	Diastolic TVI
20518	Dilation		25924	At Rest
19540	Pulmonary Veins		25925	At End of Inspiration
20023	Dimensions		25927	At End of Expiration
20519	Dilation		25929	With Stress
20123	Malpositioned		25597	Peak Atrial Reversal Velocity
20024	Turbulence		25931	At Rest
21570	Mass ___cm		25933	At End of Inspiration
21571	Infiltrative ___cm		25935	At End of Expiration
21583	Rhabdomyoma ___cm		25936	With Stress
81975	Echogenicity		25598	Atrial Reversal TVI
20025	Proximal Left Superior		25940	At Rest
20026	Dimension		25942	At End of Inspiration
81978	Mass ___cm		25943	At End of Expiration
81982	Echogenicity ___cm		25945	With Stress
20027	Turbulence		25599	Peak Diastolic Velocity (D2)
20028	Distal Left Superior		25947	At Rest
20029	Dimension		25948	At End of Inspiration
81979	Mass ___cm		25949	At End of Expiration
81985	Echogenicity ___cm		25950	With Stress
25585	Peak Systolic Velocity		25600	Peak Diastolic Velocity (D2) TVI
25586	Systolic TVI		25955	At Rest
25587	Peak Diastolic Velocity		25957	At End of Inspiration
25588	Diastolic TVI		25958	At End of Expiration
25589	Peak Atrial Reversal Velocity		25960	With Stress
25590	Atrial Reversal TVI		20036	Turbulence
25591	Peak Diastolic Velocity (D2)		19541	Coronary Arteries
25592	Peak Diastolic Velocity (D2) TVI		20126	Malpositioned
20030	Turbulence		20125	Anomalous Origin Of Artery
20031	Proximal Right Superior		20127	Ambiguous Connection Of Artery
20032	Dimension		21466	Compression Due To Pulmonary Conduit
81980	Mass ___cm			
81987	Echogenicity ___cm		21467	Collateral Circulation Established
20033	Turbulence		21018	Aneurysm
20034	Distal Right Superior		21022	Left Main

ECHOCARDIOGRAM, CONT.

21023	Stenosis	81988		Echogenicity
21024	Dilation	19682	Pleura	
21025	Aneurysm	20040	Effusion Present	
21026	Ectasia	20041		On The Right Side
21027	Left Anterior Descending	20042		On The Left Side
21028	Stenosis	20043		Bilateral
21029	Dilation	19533	Abdominal Anatomy	
21030	Aneurysm	19543	Hepatic Veins	
21031	Ectasia	20037		Dimensions
21032	Circumflex	20520		Dilation
21033	Stenosis	20038		Thrombosis
21034	Dilation	20079		Anomalous Connection
21035	Aneurysm	20080		Direct Connection To Right Atrium
21036	Ectasia	21491		Mass ___ cm
21037	Right Coronary	81989		Echogenicity
21038	Stenosis	21492		Cyst
21039	Dilation	25601	Peak Systolic Velocity	
21040	Aneurysm	25966		At Rest
21041	Ectasia	25968		At End of Inspiration
21468	Doppler Hemodynamic Interpretations	25969		At End of Expiration
21469	Extracardiac Shunt	25970		With Stress
21470	Abnormal Diastolic Relaxation	25602	Systolic TVI	
21471	Restrictive Hemodynamics	25979		At Rest
21472	Constrictive Hemodynamics	25980		At End of Inspiration
21473	Pseudonormalized Hemodynamics	25981		At End of Expiration
21474	Hemodynamics Of Tamponade	25982		With Stress
21475	Systolic Flow Reversal	25603	Peak Systolic Reversal Velocity	
21476	Arterial	25986		At Rest
21477	Venous	25988		At End of Inspiration
21478	Intracardiac	25989		At End of Expiration
21479	Diastolic Flow Reversal	25990		With Stress
21480	Arterial	25604	Systolic Reversal TVI	
21481	Venous	25992		At Rest
21482	Intracardiac	25994		At End of Inspiration
21483	Increased Derived Systolic Pressure	25996		At End of Expiration
21484	Right Ventricle	25997		With Stress
21485	Pulmonary Artery	25605	Peak Diastolic Velocity	
19542	Visceral & Heart Position	25999		At Rest
20061	Situs Solitus	26000		At End of Inspiration
20062	Situs Inversus	26001		At End of Expiration
20063	Situs Ambiguous	26002		With Stress
20064	Levocardia	25606	Diastolic TVI	
20065	Dextrocardia	26007		At Rest
20066	Isolated Dextrocardia / Levocardia	26008		At End of Inspiration
20067	Mesocardia	26009		At End of Expiration
20068	Heterotaxia	26010		With Stress
22248	Thorax	25607	Peak Atrial Reversal Velocity	
22249	Hematoma	26014		At Rest
21486	Mediastinum	26016		At End of Inspiration
21487	Mass ___ cm	26017		At End of Expiration
21488	Anterior ___ cm	26018		With Stress
21489	Posterior ___ cm	25608	Atrial Reversal TVI	
21490	Superior ___ cm	26019		At Rest

ECHOCARDIOGRAM, CONT.

26020	At End of Inspiration	22040	Mitral Regurgitation
26021	At End of Expiration	22041	Increased
26022	With Stress	22042	Decreased
25609	Peak Diastolic Velocity (D2)	22043	Tricuspid Regurgitation
26027	At Rest	22044	Increased
26028	At End of Inspiration	22045	Decreased
26029	At End of Expiration	22246	Pre-Ablation
26030	With Stress	22247	Follow-Up After Ablation
25610	Peak Diastolic Velocity (D2) TVI	21493	Fetal
26032	At Rest	22016	Anatomy
26035	At End of Inspiration	22017	Cardiac Dimensions
26037	At End of Expiration	22139	Arrhythmias
26038	With Stress	22018	Doppler Flow Velocities
20039	Turbulence	21108	Equipment Type
19544	Liver	21109	Acuson
80928	Normal	21110	ADR
20076	Enlarged	21111	Aloka
22238	Infaract	21112	Model 860
22239	Mass ___cm	21113	Model 870
81990	Echogenicity	21114	Model 880
20077	Cystic	21115	ATL
20078	A-V Fistula	21116	Model 300
19545	Spleen	21117	Model 600
80929	Normal	21118	Hewlett-Packard
20083	Enlargement	21119	Color
22240	Infarct	21120	Sonos
22241	Mass ___cm	21121	Interspec
81991	Echogenicity	21122	Irex Meridian
20081	Absent	21123	Siemens
20082	Multiple	21124	Toshiba
19546	Ascites	21125	Model 65
20044	Strands	21126	Model 140
19683	Diaphragm	21127	Model 160
20084	Hernia	21128	Ultramark
19684	Noncardiac Echo Free Space	21129	Model 4
29388	Conclusions	21130	Model 6
21737	Stress Echo	21131	Model 7
22027	Relative Wall Motion Abnormality	21132	Model 8
22028	At Rest	21133	Model 9
22029	During Stress	21134	Vingmed
22030	New Abnormality	80915	**Cardiac Isotope Imaging**
22031	Change In Previous Abnormality	21881	Image Acquisition
22032	Worsened	27337	Protocol
22033	Improved	29456	Rest only
22034	During Recovery	27338	Rest-Rest
22035	Worsened	29457	Stress Only
22036	Improved	27339	Stress-Rest
22037	New Abnormality	27340	3 Hours
22038	Measurements	27341	4 Hours
22251	Ejection Fraction	27342	24 Hours
22252	Start	27343	Stress-Rest-Rest
22253	Peak Value	27344	Rest 1 at 3 Hours
22039	Response	27345	Rest 1 at 4 Hours

CARDIAC ISOTOPE IMAGING, CONT.

27347	Radionuclide Utilizing Isotope	28221	Anterobasal wall
16170	Thallium	27324	Anteroseptal wall
27349	Technetium-Labelled Red Blood	28224	Septal wall
	Cells	27325	Lateral wall
21886	Technetium-Labelled MIBI	27326	Anterolateral wall
21887	Technetium-Labelled Teboroxime	27327	Anteroapical wall
24892	Technetium-Labelled Tetrofosmin	28227	Apical wall
29450	18-fluoro-deoxyglucose	27328	Inferior wall
29451	C-11-Labelled Palmitate	28230	Inferoapical wall
29452	Krypton	27329	Posterior wall
29453	O-15-Labelled H2O	27330	Global
29454	N-13-Labelled NH3	16150	Hypokinetic wall motion
29455	C-11-Labelled Leucine	28367	Regional
27348	Technetium Pyrophosphate	16151	Anterior wall
29776	Planar	28217	Anterobasal wall
29775	With A First Pass Ejection	16152	Anteroseptal wall
	Fraction	28220	Septal wall
29777	SPECT	16153	Lateral wall
16138	Ventriculography	16154	Anterolateral wall
27352	Equilibrium	16155	Anteroapical wall
29458	Single Study	28218	Apical wall
29459	Multiple Studies	16156	Inferior wall
29443	With Gamma Camera	28219	Inferoapical wall
29444	With Nuclear Probe	16157	Posterior wall
29445	With Nuclear Stethoscope	16158	Global
29446	With Nuclear Vest	16142	Akinetic wall motion
29447	Cardiac Shunt Detection	16143	Anterior wall
27353	First Pass	28222	Anterobasal wall
29460	Single Study	16144	Anteroseptal wall
29461	Multiple Studies	28225	Septal wall
27354	Views	16145	Lateral wall
27355	Planar	16146	Anterolateral wall
27356	LAO	16147	Anteroapical wall
27357	RAO	28228	Apical wall
27358	Anterior	16148	Inferior wall
27359	SPECT	28231	Inferoapical wall
25215	Rest Image - Feet Down	16149	Posterior wall
27360	Left Ventricle	28043	Global
16139	Ejection Fraction	16159	Dyskinetic Wall Motion
27363	Global	28044	Anterior wall
27364	Septal	28223	Anterobasal wall
27365	Inferoapical	16160	Anteroseptal wall
27366	Lateral	28226	Septal wall
27361	End Diastolic Volume	28045	Lateral wall
27362	End Systolic Volume	28046	Anterolateral wall
28353	Function Compared With	16161	Anteroapical wall
	Previous Study	28229	Apical wall
28354	Unchanged	16162	Inferior wall
28355	Improved	28232	Inferoapical wall
28356	Worse	28047	Posterior wall
27367	Wall Motion	28048	Global
27322	Hyperkinetic wall motion	16164	Hypertrophy
27323	Anterior wall	16165	Concentric

CARDIAC ISOTOPE IMAGING, CONT.

16166	Asymmetric	28434	Anteroseptal wall
29298	Eccentric	28435	Septal wall
16167	Dilation	28436	Lateral wall
28351	Mural Thrombus	28437	Anterolateral wall
28352	Aneurysm	28438	Anteroapical wall
29272	Anterior	28439	Apical wall
29273	Inferior	28440	Inferior wall
29274	Lateral	28441	Inferoapical wall
29275	Posterior	28442	Posterior wall
29276	Apical	28443	Global
27368	Right Ventricle	28444	Akinetic wall motion
16141	Ejection Fraction	28445	Anterior wall
29311	Wall Motion	28446	Anterobasal wall
16163	Global Hypokinetic wall motion	28447	Anteroseptal wall
		28448	Septal wall
16168	Hypertrophy	28449	Lateral wall
28049	Concentric	28450	Anterolateral wall
28050	Asymmetric	28451	Anteroapical wall
16169	Dilation	28452	Apical wall
28483	Regurgitant Fraction	28453	Inferior wall
28403	Rest Image - Feet Up	28454	Inferoapical wall
28404	Left Ventricle	28455	Posterior wall
28407	Ejection Fraction	28456	Global
28408	Global	28457	Dyskinetic wall motion
28409	Septal	28458	Anterior wall
28410	Inferoapical	28459	Anterobasal wall
28411	Lateral	28460	Anteroseptal wall
28405	End Diastolic Volume	28461	Septal wall
28406	End Systolic Volume	28462	Lateral wall
28899	Function	28463	Anterolateral wall
28412	Function Compared With Previous Study	28464	Anteroapical wall
		28465	Apical wall
28413	Unchanged	28466	Inferior wall
28414	Improved	28467	Inferoapical wall
28415	Worse	28468	Posterior wall
28416	Wall Motion	28469	Global
28417	Hyperkinetic wall motion	28470	Hypertrophy
28418	Anterior wall	28471	Concentric
28419	Anterobasal wall	28472	Asymmetric
28420	Anteroseptal wall	29318	Eccentric
28421	Septal wall	28473	Dilation
28422	Lateral wall	28474	Mural Thrombus
28423	Anterolateral wall	28475	Aneurysm
28424	Anteroapical wall	29277	Anterior
28425	Apical wall	29278	Inferior
28426	Inferior wall	29279	Lateral
28427	Inferoapical wall	29280	Posterior
28428	Posterior wall	29281	Apical
28429	Global	28476	Right Ventricle
28430	Hypokinetic wall motion	28477	Ejection Fraction
28431	Regional	28900	Function
28432	Anterior wall	29312	Wall Motion
28433	Anterobasal wall		

CARDIAC ISOTOPE IMAGING, CONT.

28478	Global Hypokinetic wall motion		27403	Inferior wall
			28243	Inferoapical wall
28479	Hypertrophy		27404	Posterior wall
28480	Concentric		28051	Global
28481	Asymmetric		27405	Dyskinetic wall motion
28482	Dilation		28052	Anterior wall
28484	Regurgitant Fraction		28235	Anterobasal wall
25217	Stress Image 1		27406	Anteroseptal wall
27369	Time		28238	Septal wall
27370	Left Ventricle		28053	Lateral wall
27373	Ejection Fraction		28054	Anterolateral wall
27374	Global		27407	Anteroapical wall
27375	Septal		28241	Apical wall
27376	Inferoapical		27408	Inferior wall
27377	Lateral		28244	Inferoapical wall
27371	End Diastolic Volume		28055	Posterior wall
27372	End Systolic Volume		28056	Global
27378	Wall Motion		27409	Right Ventricle
27379	Hyperkinetic wall motion		27410	Ejection Fraction
27380	Anterior wall		29313	Wall Motion
28233	Anterobasal wall		27411	Global Hypokinetic
27381	Anteroseptal wall		28485	Regurgitant Fraction
28236	Septal wall		25218	Stress Image 2
27382	Lateral wall		27412	Time
27383	Anterolateral wall		27413	Left Ventricle
27384	Anteroapical wall		27416	Ejection Fraction
28239	Apical wall		27417	Global
27385	Inferior wall		27418	Septal
28242	Inferoapical wall		27419	Inferoapical
27386	Posterior wall		27420	Lateral
27387	Global		27414	End Diastolic Volume
27388	Hypokinetic wall motion		27415	End Systolic Volume
27389	Anterior wall		27421	Wall Motion
28309	Anterobasal wall		27422	Hyperkinetic wall motion
27390	Anteroseptal wall		27423	Anterior wall
28314	Septal wall		28245	Anterobasal wall
27391	Lateral wall		27424	Anteroseptal wall
27392	Anterolateral wall		28248	Septal wall
27393	Anteroapical wall		27425	Lateral wall
28319	Apical wall		27426	Anterolateral wall
27394	Inferior wall		27427	Anteroapical wall
28324	Inferoapical wall		28251	Apical wall
27395	Posterior wall		27428	Inferior wall
27396	Global		28254	Inferoapical wall
27397	Akinetic wall motion		27429	Posterior wall
27398	Anterior wall		27430	Global
28234	Anterobasal wall		27431	Hypokinetic wall motion
27399	Anteroseptal wall		27432	Anterior wall
28237	Septal wall		28310	Anterobasal wall
27400	Lateral wall		27433	Anteroseptal wall
27401	Anterolateral wall		28315	Septal wall
27402	Anteroapical wall		27434	Lateral wall
28240	Apical wall		27435	Anterolateral wall

CARDIAC ISOTOPE IMAGING, CONT.

27436	Anteroapical wall		27468	Lateral wall
28320	Apical wall		27469	Anterolateral wall
27437	Inferior wall		27470	Anteroapical wall
28325	Inferoapical wall		28263	Apical wall
27438	Posterior wall		27471	Inferior wall
27439	Global		28266	Inferoapical wall
27440	Akinetic wall motion		27472	Posterior wall
27441	Anterior wall		27473	Global
28246	Anterobasal wall		27474	Hypokinetic wall motion
27442	Anteroseptal wall		27475	Anterior wall
28249	Septal wall		28311	Anterobasal wall
27443	Lateral wall		27476	Anteroseptal wall
27444	Anterolateral wall		28316	Septal wall
27445	Anteroapical wall		27477	Lateral wall
28252	Apical wall		27478	Anterolateral wall
27446	Inferior wall		27479	Anteroapical wall
28255	Inferoapical wall		28321	Apical wall
27447	Posterior wall		27480	Inferior wall
28057	Global		28326	Inferoapical wall
27448	Dyskinetic wall motion		27481	Posterior wall
28058	Anterior wall		27482	Global
28247	Anterobasal wall		27483	Akinetic wall motion
27449	Anteroseptal wall		27484	Anterior wall
28250	Septal wall		28258	Anterobasal wall
28059	Lateral wall		27485	Anteroseptal wall
28060	Anterolateral wall		28261	Septal wall
27450	Anteroapical wall		27486	Lateral wall
28253	Apical wall		27487	Anterolateral wall
27451	Inferior wall		27488	Anteroapical wall
28256	Inferoapical wall		28264	Apical wall
28061	Posterior wall		27489	Inferior wall
28062	Global		28267	Inferoapical wall
27452	Right Ventricle		27490	Posterior wall
27453	Ejection Fraction		28063	Global
29314	Wall Motion		27491	Dyskinetic wall motion
27454	Global Hypokinetic		28064	Anterior wall
28486	Regurgitant Fraction		28259	Anterobasal wall
25219	Stress Image 3		27492	Anteroseptal wall
27455	Time		28262	Septal wall
27456	Left Ventricle		28065	Lateral wall
27459	Ejection Fraction		28066	Anterolateral wall
27460	Global		27493	Anteroapical wall
27461	Septal		28265	Apical wall
27462	Inferoapical		27494	Inferior wall
27463	Lateral		28268	Inferoapical wall
27457	End Diastolic Volume		28067	Posterior wall
27458	End Systolic Volume		28068	Global
27464	Wall Motion		27495	Right Ventricle
27465	Hyperkinetic wall motion		27496	Ejection Fraction
27466	Anterior wall		29315	Wall Motion
28257	Anterobasal wall		27497	Global Hypokinetic Wall Motion
27467	Anteroseptal wall			
28260	Septal wall		28487	Regurgitant Fraction

CARDIAC ISOTOPE IMAGING, CONT.

25220	Peak Stress Image	28279		Inferoapical wall
27498	Time	27533		Posterior wall
27499	Left Ventricle	28069		Global
27502	Ejection Fraction	27534		Dyskinetic wall motion
27503	Global	28070		Anterior wall
27504	Septal	28271		Anterobasal wall
27505	Inferoapical	27535		Anteroseptal wall
27506	Lateral	28274		Septal wall
27500	End Diastolic Volume	28071		Lateral wall
27501	End Systolic Volume	28072		Anterolateral wall
28901	Function	27536		Anteroapical wall
28902	Function Compared With	28277		Apical wall
	Previous Study	27537		Inferior wall
28903	Unchanged	28280		Inferoapical wall
28904	Improved	28073		Posterior wall
28905	Worse	28074		Global
27507	Wall Motion	27538	Right Ventricle	
27508	Hyperkinetic wall motion	27539	Ejection Fraction	
27509	Anterior wall	28906	Function	
28269	Anterobasal wall	29316	Wall Motion	
27510	Anteroseptal wall	27540	Global Hypokinetic	
28272	Septal wall	28488	Regurgitant Fraction	
27511	Lateral wall	25221	Post-Peak Stress Image	
27512	Anterolateral wall	27541	Time	
27513	Anteroapical wall	27542	Left Ventricle	
28275	Apical wall	27545	Ejection Fraction	
27514	Inferior wall	27546	Global	
28278	Inferoapical wall	27547	Septal	
27515	Posterior wall	27548	Inferoapical	
27516	Global	27549	Lateral	
27517	Hypokinetic wall motion	27543	End Diastolic Volume	
27518	Anterior wall	27544	End Systolic Volume	
28312	Anterobasal wall	27550	Wall Motion	
27519	Anteroseptal wall	27551	Hyperkinetic wall motion	
28317	Septal wall	27552	Anterior wall	
27520	Lateral wall	28281	Anterobasal wall	
27521	Anterolateral wall	27553	Anteroseptal wall	
27522	Anteroapical wall	28284	Septal wall	
28322	Apical wall	27554	Lateral wall	
27523	Inferior wall	27555	Anterolateral wall	
28327	Inferoapical wall	27556	Anteroapical wall	
27524	Posterior wall	28287	Apical wall	
27525	Global	27557	Inferior wall	
27526	Akinetic wall motion	28290	Inferoapical wall	
27527	Anterior wall	27558	Posterior wall	
28270	Anterobasal wall	27559	Global	
27528	Anteroseptal wall	27560	Hypokinetic wall motion	
28273	Septal wall	27561	Anterior wall	
27529	Lateral wall	28313	Anterobasal wall	
27530	Anterolateral wall	27562	Anteroseptal wall	
27531	Anteroapical wall	28318	Septal wall	
28276	Apical wall	27563	Lateral wall	
27532	Inferior wall	27564	Anterolateral wall	

CARDIAC ISOTOPE IMAGING, CONT.

27565	Anteroapical wall
28323	Apical wall
27566	Inferior wall
28328	Inferoapical wall
27567	Posterior wall
27568	Global
27569	Akinetic wall motion
27570	Anterior wall
28282	Anterobasal wall
27571	Anteroseptal wall
28285	Septal wall
27572	Lateral wall
27573	Anterolateral wall
27574	Anteroapical wall
28288	Apical wall
27575	Inferior wall
28291	Inferoapical wall
27576	Posterior wall
28075	Global
27577	Dyskinetic wall motion
28076	Anterior wall
28283	Anterobasal wall
27578	Anteroseptal wall
28286	Septal wall
28077	Lateral wall
28078	Anterolateral wall
27579	Anteroapical wall
28289	Apical wall
27580	Inferior wall
28292	Inferoapical wall
28079	Posterior wall
28080	Global
27581	Right Ventricle
27582	Ejection Fraction
29317	Wall Motion
27583	Global Hypokinetic
28489	Regurgitant Fraction
25732	Systolic Volume Change
28357	Rest To Peak Stress
25733	Increase
25734	Decrease
28358	Compared With Previous Study
28365	Unchanged
28359	Increase
28360	Decrease
25739	Ejection Fraction Change
28361	Rest To Peak Stress
16140	Increase
25741	Decrease
28364	Compared With Previous Study
28366	Unchanged
28362	Increase
28363	Decrease

27346	Perfusion
29462	Single Study
29463	Planar
29464	With Wall Motion Analysis
29465	With Ejection Fraction
29466	SPECT
29467	With Wall Motion Analysis
29468	With Ejection Fraction
29469	Multiple Studies
29470	Planar
29471	With Wall Motion Analysis
29472	With Ejection Fraction
29473	SPECT
29474	With Wall Motion Analysis
29475	With Ejection Fraction
27584	Image 1
27585	Time
27586	Planar Views Showed Decreased Uptake
27587	LAO
27588	Septum
27589	Inferoapical
27590	Posterolateral
27591	Left Lateral
27592	Anteroseptal
27593	Apical
27594	Inferior
27595	Basal
27596	Anterior
27597	Septum
27598	Apical
27599	Anterolateral
27600	Anterobasal
27601	RAO
27602	Anterolateral
27603	Apical
27604	Inferior
27605	Basal
27606	SPECT
27607	Short Axis
27608	Apex
27609	Anterior
27610	Septum
27611	Inferior
27612	Lateral
27613	Mid-Wall
27614	Anterior
27615	Anteroseptal
27616	Septum
27617	Inferoseptal
27618	Inferior
27619	Lateral
27620	Base

CARDIAC ISOTOPE IMAGING, CONT.

27621	Anterior	27674	Inferoapical
27622	Anteroseptal	27675	Inferior
27623	Septum	27676	Inferobasal
27624	Inferoseptal	27677	Composite Circumferential
27625	Inferior	27678	Apex
27626	Lateral	27679	Anterior
27627	Horizontal Long Axis	27680	Septum
27628	Inferior	27681	Inferior
27629	Apical Septum	27682	Lateral
27630	Septum	27683	Mid-Wall
27631	Basal Septum	27684	Anterior
27632	Apex	27685	Anteroseptal
27633	Anterolateral	27686	Septum
27634	Lateral	27687	Inferoseptal
27635	Basal Lateral	27688	Inferior
27636	Mid-Wall	27689	Lateral
27637	Apical Septum	27690	Base
27638	Septum	27691	Anterior
27639	Basal Septum	27692	Anteroseptal
27640	Apex	27693	Septum
27641	Anterolateral	27694	Inferoseptal
27642	Lateral	27695	Inferior
27643	Basal Lateral	27696	Lateral
27644	Anterior	28340	Relative Decrease In Isotope Activity Compared To A Reference Image
27645	Apical Septum		
27646	Septum		
27647	Basal Septum	27697	Image 2
27648	Apex	27698	Time
27649	Anterolateral	27699	Planar Views Showed Decreased Uptake
27650	Lateral		
27651	Basal Lateral	27700	LAO
27652	Vertical Long Axis	27701	Septum
27653	Septum	27702	Inferoapical
27654	Anterobasal	27703	Posterolateral
27655	Anterior	27704	Left Lateral
27656	Anteroapical	27705	Anteroseptal
27657	Apex	27706	Apical
27658	Inferoapical	27707	Inferior
27659	Inferior	27708	Basal
27660	Inferobasal	27709	Anterior
27661	Mid-Wall	27710	Septum
27662	Anterobasal	27711	Apical
27663	Anterior	27712	Anterolateral
27664	Anteroapical	27713	Anterobasal
27665	Apex	27714	RAO
27666	Inferoapical	27715	Anterolateral
27667	Inferior	27716	Apical
27668	Inferobasal	27717	Inferior
27669	Lateral	27718	Basal
27670	Anterobasal	27719	SPECT
27671	Anterior	27720	Short Axis
27672	Anteroapical	27721	Apex
27673	Apex	27722	Anterior

27723	Septum	27776	Anterior
27724	Inferior	27777	Anteroapical
27725	Lateral	27778	Apex
27726	Mid-Wall	27779	Inferoapical
27727	Anterior	27780	Inferior
27728	Anteroseptal	27781	Inferobasal
27729	Septum	27782	Lateral
27730	Inferoseptal	27783	Anterobasal
27731	Inferior	27784	Anterior
27732	Lateral	27785	Anteroapical
27733	Base	27786	Apex
27734	Anterior	27787	Inferoapical
27735	Anteroseptal	27788	Inferior
27736	Septum	27789	Inferobasal
27737	Inferoseptal	27790	Composite Circumferential
27738	Inferior	27791	Apex
27739	Lateral	27792	Anterior
27740	Horizontal Long Axis	27793	Septum
27741	Inferior	27794	Inferior
27742	Apical Septum	27795	Lateral
27743	Septum	27796	Mid-Wall
27744	Basal Septum	27797	Anterior
27745	Apex	27798	Anteroseptal
27746	Anterolateral	27799	Septum
27747	Lateral	27800	Inferoseptal
27748	Basal Lateral	27801	Inferior
27749	Mid-Wall	27802	Lateral
27750	Apical Septum	27803	Base
27751	Septum	27804	Anterior
27752	Basal Septum	27805	Anteroseptal
27753	Apex	27806	Septum
27754	Anterolateral	27807	Inferoseptal
27755	Lateral	27808	Inferior
27756	Basal Lateral	27809	Lateral
27757	Anterior	28341	Relative Decrease In Isotope Activity Compared To A Reference Image
27758	Apical Septum		
27759	Septum		
27760	Basal Septum	27810	Image 3
27761	Apex	27811	Time
27762	Anterolateral	27812	Planar Views Showed Decreased Uptake
27763	Lateral		
27764	Basal Lateral	27813	LAO
27765	Vertical Long Axis	27814	Septum
27766	Septum	27815	Inferoapical
27767	Anterobasal	27816	Posterolateral
27768	Anterior	27817	Left Lateral
27769	Anteroapical	27818	Anteroseptal
27770	Apex	27819	Apical
27771	Inferoapical	27820	Inferior
27772	Inferior	27821	Basal
27773	Inferobasal	27822	Anterior
27774	Mid-Wall	27823	Septum
27775	Anterobasal	27824	Apical

27825	Anterolateral	27878	Vertical Long Axis
27826	Anterobasal	27879	Septum
27827	RAO	27880	Anterobasal
27828	Anterolateral	27881	Anterior
27829	Apical	27882	Anteroapical
27830	Inferior	27883	Apex
27831	Basal	27884	Inferoapical
27832	SPECT	27885	Inferior
27833	Short Axis	27886	Inferobasal
27834	Apex	27887	Mid-Wall
27835	Anterior	27888	Anterobasal
27836	Septum	27889	Anterior
27837	Inferior	27890	Anteroapical
27838	Lateral	27891	Apex
27839	Mid-Wall	27892	Inferoapical
27840	Anterior	27893	Inferior
27841	Anteroseptal	27894	Inferobasal
27842	Septum	27895	Lateral
27843	Inferoseptal	27896	Anterobasal
27844	Inferior	27897	Anterior
27845	Lateral	27898	Anteroapical
27846	Base	27899	Apex
27847	Anterior	27900	Inferoapical
27848	Anteroseptal	27901	Inferior
27849	Septum	27902	Inferobasal
27850	Inferoseptal	27903	Composite Circumferential
27851	Inferior	27904	Apex
27852	Lateral	27905	Anterior
27853	Horizontal Long Axis	27906	Septum
27854	Inferior	27907	Inferior
27855	Apical Septum	27908	Lateral
27856	Septum	27909	Mid-Wall
27857	Basal Septum	27910	Anterior
27858	Apex	27911	Anteroseptal
27859	Anterolateral	27912	Septum
27860	Lateral	27913	Inferoseptal
27861	Basal Lateral	27914	Inferior
27862	Mid-Wall	27915	Lateral
27863	Apical Septum	27916	Base
27864	Septum	27917	Anterior
27865	Basal Septum	27918	Anteroseptal
27866	Apex	27919	Septum
27867	Anterolateral	27920	Inferoseptal
27868	Lateral	27921	Inferior
27869	Basal Lateral	27922	Lateral
27870	Anterior	28342	Relative Decrease In Isotope Activity Compared To A Reference Image
27871	Apical Septum		
27872	Septum		
27873	Basal Septum	27923	Image 4
27874	Apex	27924	Time
27875	Anterolateral	27925	Planar Views Showed Decreased Uptake
27876	Lateral		
27877	Basal Lateral	27926	LAO

264

CARDIAC ISOTOPE IMAGING, CONT.

27927	Septum	27980	Anterolateral
27928	Inferoapical	27981	Lateral
27929	Posterolateral	27982	Basal Lateral
27930	Left Lateral	27983	Anterior
27931	Anteroseptal	27984	Apical Septum
27932	Apical	27985	Septum
27933	Inferior	27986	Basal Septum
27934	Basal	27987	Apex
27935	Anterior	27988	Anterolateral
27936	Septum	27989	Lateral
27937	Apical	27990	Basal Lateral
27938	Anterolateral	27991	Vertical Long Axis
27939	Anterobasal	27992	Septum
27940	RAO	27993	Anterobasal
27941	Anterolateral	27994	Anterior
27942	Apical	27995	Anteroapical
27943	Inferior	27996	Apex
27944	Basal	27997	Inferoapical
27945	SPECT	27998	Inferior
27946	Short Axis	27999	Inferobasal
27947	Apex	28000	Mid-Wall
27948	Anterior	28001	Anterobasal
27949	Septum	28002	Anterior
27950	Inferior	28003	Anteroapical
27951	Lateral	28004	Apex
27952	Mid-Wall	28005	Inferoapical
27953	Anterior	28006	Inferior
27954	Anteroseptal	28007	Inferobasal
27955	Septum	28008	Lateral
27956	Inferoseptal	28009	Anterobasal
27957	Inferior	28010	Anterior
27958	Lateral	28011	Anteroapical
27959	Base	28012	Apex
27960	Anterior	28013	Inferoapical
27961	Anteroseptal	28014	Inferior
27962	Septum	28015	Inferobasal
27963	Inferoseptal	28016	Composite Circumferential
27964	Inferior	28017	Apex
27965	Lateral	28018	Anterior
27966	Horizontal Long Axis	28019	Septum
27967	Inferior	28020	Inferior
27968	Apical Septum	28021	Lateral
27969	Septum	28022	Mid-Wall
27970	Basal Septum	28023	Anterior
27971	Apex	28024	Anteroseptal
27972	Anterolateral	28025	Septum
27973	Lateral	28026	Inferoseptal
27974	Basal Lateral	28027	Inferior
27975	Mid-Wall	28028	Lateral
27976	Apical Septum	28029	Base
27977	Septum	28030	Anterior
27978	Basal Septum	28031	Anteroseptal
27979	Apex	28032	Septum

CARDIAC ISOTOPE IMAGING, CONT.

28033	Inferoseptal
28034	Inferior
28035	Lateral
28343	Relative Decrease In Isotope Activity Compared To A Reference Image
28907	Increased Regional Wall Uptake
28908	In The Lateral Wall
28512	Coronary Perfusion Summary:
28513	Normal Study
28514	Ischemia Of One Coronary Distribution
28515	Ischemia Of Two Or More Coronary Distributions
28516	Infarct In One Coronary Distribution
29016	The Left Anterior Coronary Distribution
29017	The Right Coronary Distribution
29018	The Circumflex Coronary Distribution
28517	Infarct In Two Or More Coronary Distributions
29019	The Left Anterior And Right Coronary Distribution
29020	The Left Anterior And Circumflex Coronary Distribution
29021	The Right And Circumflex Coronary Distribution
29022	The Left Anterior, Circumflex And Right Coronary Distribution
28800	Infarct And Ischemia Of The Same Coronary Distribution
28801	Infarct And Ischemia Of Different Coronary Distributions
28802	Nonspecific Abnormality Of Uncertain Significance
28499	Technical Quality Of The Images
28500	Satisfactory
28501	Unsatisfactory
28502	Due To Bad Injection
28503	Due To Poor Counting Statistics
28504	Due To Acquisition Difficulties
28505	Conclusions
28506	Normal Study
28507	Abnormal Study
28508	Cardiac Enlargement
28509	Increased Pulmonary Uptake
28510	Increased Right Ventricular Uptake
28511	Reversible Right Ventricular Uptake
28898	Increased Uptake In Other Organs
29373	Chronotropic Incompetence
13100	Phonocardiogram
19223	Interpretation And Report Only

19224	Tracing Only
19225	With Artery, Vein, Or Apical Tracing
19226	Analysis & Report Only
19227	Tracing Only
19228	Intracardiac
19270	24-Hour Ambulatory Blood Pressure Monitoring
19271	Recording Only
19272	Scanning Analysis
19273	Physician Interpretation
14532	**Ultrasound**
80951	Ophthalmic
80952	A-Scan
80953	For Calculation Of IOL Power
80954	For Axial Measurements
80958	A-P Length
80959	Anterior Chamber Depth
80955	B-Scan
80956	With Immersion
80957	For Localization Of Foreign Body
80960	With A-Scan
80961	Ciliary Body
80970	Mass ___mm
80971	Right
80973	At __ O'Clock
80972	Left
80974	At __ O'Clock
81051	Detachment
81052	Right
81053	At __ O'Clock
81054	Left
81055	At __ O'Clock
80962	Iris
80975	Mass
80976	Right
80978	At __ O'Clock
80977	Left
80979	At __ O'Clock
80963	Lens
80980	Mass ___mm
80981	Right
80983	At __ O'Clock
80982	Left
80984	At __ O'Clock
81056	Dislocation
81057	Right
81058	Posterior
81059	Anterior
81060	Inferior
81061	Nasal
81062	Temporal
81063	Extraocular

ULTRASOUND, CONT.

81064	Left	
81065	Posterior	
81066	Anterior	
81067	Inferior	
81068	Nasal	
81069	Temporal	
81070	Extraocular	
81071	Rupture	
81072	Right	
81073	Left	
80964	Vitreous	
81024	Opacity	
81025	Right	
81026	Left	
80965	Retina	
80985	Mass ___ mm	
80986	Right	
80988	At __ O'Clock	
80987	Left	
80989	At __ O'Clock	
81015	Detachment	
81016	Superiorly In The Right Eye	
81018	Inferiorly In The Right Eye	
81020	Temporal Aspect Of The Right Eye	
81022	Nasal Aspect Of The Right Eye	
81017	Superiorly In The Left Eye	
81019	Inferiorly In The Left Eye	
81021	Temporal Aspect Of The Left Eye	
81023	Nasal Aspect Of The Left Eye	
80966	Optic Nerve	
80995	Mass ___ mm	
80996	Right	
80997	Left	
80967	Choroid	
80990	Mass ___ mm	
80991	Right	
80993	At __ O'Clock	
80992	Left	
80994	At __ O'Clock	
81027	Detachment	
81028	Superiorly In The Right Eye	
81030	Inferiorly In The Right Eye	
81032	Temporal Aspect Of The Right Eye	
81034	Nasal Aspect Of The Right Eye	
81029	Superiorly In The Left Eye	
81031	Inferiorly In The Left Eye	
81033	Temporal Aspect Of The Left Eye	
81035	Nasal Aspect Of The Left Eye	
81036	Hemorrhage	

81037	Superiorly In The Right Eye	
81039	Inferiorly In The Right Eye	
81041	Temporal Aspect Of The Right Eye	
81043	Nasal Aspect Of The Right Eye	
81038	Superiorly In The Left Eye	
81040	Inferiorly In The Left Eye	
81042	Temporal Aspect Of The Left Eye	
81044	Nasal Aspect Of The Left Eye	
81074	Thickening	
81075	Superiorly In The Right Eye	
81077	Inferiorly In The Right Eye	
81079	Temporal Aspect Of The Right Eye	
81081	Nasal Aspect Of The Right Eye	
81076	Superiorly In The Left Eye	
81078	Inferiorly In The Left Eye	
81080	Temporal Aspect Of The Left Eye	
81082	Nasal Aspect Of The Left Eye	
81083	Sclera	
81084	Thickening	
81085	Superiorly In The Right Eye	
81087	Inferiorly In The Right Eye	
81089	Temporal Aspect Of The Right Eye	
81091	Nasal Aspect Of The Right Eye	
81086	Superiorly In The Left Eye	
81088	Inferiorly In The Left Eye	
81090	Temporal Aspect Of The Left Eye	
81092	Nasal Aspect Of The Left Eye	
80968	Orbit	
80998	Mass	
80999	Superior, Right	
81001	Inferior, Right	
81003	Temporal, Right	
81005	Nasal, Right	
81007	Posterior, Right	
81000	Superior, Left	
81002	Inferior, Left	
81004	Temporal, Left	
81006	Nasal, Left	
81008	Posterior, Left	
80969	Extraocular Muscles	
14533	Abdominal	
22565	Gastric	
22566	Dilation	
22567	Thickened Pyloric Muscle	
22568	Intestinal	
18069	Adrenal Gland	
18070	Diffuse Enlargement	

ULTRASOUND, CONT.

18071	Right Only		14534	Liver
18072	Left Only		14535	Enlarged
18073	Bilateral		14536	Fluid-filled cavity
18074	Focal Mass Lesion ___ cm		14537	Multiple cysts
24759	Solitary ___ cm		80932	Common Bile Duct
18075	On The Right ___ cm		14538	Echoencephalography
18076	On The Left ___ cm		14672	Renal
18077	Bilaterally ___ cm		14673	Absent Kidney
24760	Multiple ___ cm		14674	On The Right Only
18078	On The Right ___ cm		14675	On The Left Only
18079	On The Left ___ cm		14676	Bilaterally
18080	Bilaterally ___ cm		14677	Large Kidney
81992	echogenicity		14678	On The Right Only
18081	Cyst		14679	On The Left Only
24761	Solitary		14680	Bilaterally
18082	On The Right		14681	Small Kidney
18083	On The Left		14682	On The Right Only
18084	Bilaterally		14683	On The Left Only
24762	Multiple		14684	Bilaterally
18085	On The Right		14685	Extrinsic Compression of Kidney
18086	On The Left		14686	From Above
18087	Bilaterally		14687	From Below
18088	Calcification		14688	Right Kidney Only
18089	On The Right Only		14689	Left Kidney Only
18090	On The Left Only		14690	Both Kidneys
18091	Bilaterally		14691	Fusion of Kidneys
18092	Pancreas		14692	Ectopic Kidney
18093	Mass ___ cm		14693	Kidney Mass Lesion ___ cm
18094	Body		14694	Solitary
18095	Tail		14695	On The Right Only
18096	Uncinate		14696	On The Left Only
81993	Echogenicity		14697	Bilaterally
18097	Diffuse Enlargement		14698	Multiple
18098	Cyst		14699	On The Right Only
18099	Head		14700	On The Left Only
18100	Body		14701	Bilaterally
18101	Tail		14702	Calcified
18102	Uncinate		81994	Echogenicity
18103	Calcification		14703	Kidney Cyst
18104	Focal		14704	Solitary
18105	Diffuse		14705	On The Right Only
18106	Pancreatic Duct		14706	On The Left Only
18107	Dilated		14707	Bilaterally
18108	Calculi		14708	Multiple
18965	Gallbladder		14709	On The Right Only
18966	Calculi		14710	On The Left Only
18967	Solitary		14711	Bilaterally
18968	Multiple		14712	Calcification of Wall
18969	Sludge		14713	Papillary Necrosis
18970	Polyp		14714	On The Right Only
18971	Wall Thickened		14715	On The Left Only
18972	Soft Tissue Mass ___ cm		14716	Bilaterally
18973	Septated		14717	Nephrocalcinosis

ULTRASOUND, CONT.

14718	On The Right Only	14753	Solitary
14719	On The Left Only	14754	Multiple
14720	Bilaterally	14755	Biparietal Diameter
14721	Obstructive Pattern	14756	Placenta Previa
14722	On The Right Only	18310	Polyhydramnios
14723	On The Left Only	19337	Macrosomia
14724	Bilaterally	18311	Intrauterine Growth Retardation
14725	Solitary Kidney Calculus	18313	Anencephaly
14726	On The Right Only	18314	Hydrocephaly
14727	On The Left Only	18315	Spina Bifida
14728	Bilaterally	18316	Meningocele
14729	Multiple Kidney Calculi	18317	Omphalocele
14730	On The Right Only	19338	Absence of Sacrum
14731	On The Left Only	18318	"snowstorm" pattern
14732	Bilaterally	14757	Ovaries
14733	Pelvic	14758	Enlargement
22682	Follow-Up Study	14759	On The Right Only
22684	For Pregnancy	14760	On The Left Only
22683	Complete Evaluation	14761	Bilaterally
22685	For Multiple Gestation	14762	Atrophied
22686	Limited Evaluation	14763	On The Right Only
22687	Follow-Up	14764	On The Left Only
22140	Gestational Duration	14765	Bilaterally
22019	Multiple Fetuses	14766	Absence
22020	Polyhydramnios	14767	On The Right Only
22021	Oligohydramnios	14768	On The Left Only
22022	Omphalocele	14769	Bilaterally
22023	Spina Bifida	14770	Mass ___ cm
22024	Hydrocephalus	14771	On The Right Only
22025	Polycystic Kidneys	14772	On The Left Only
22026	Umbilical Cord Abnormality	14773	Bilaterally
14734	Bladder	14774	Calcified
14735	Wall Thickened	81996	Echogenicity
14736	Focal	14775	Cystic Lesion
14737	Diffuse	14776	On The Right Only
14738	Calculi	14777	On The Left Only
14739	Solitary	14778	Bilaterally
14740	Multiple	14779	Calcified
14741	Post-Surgical Changes	14780	Fallopian Tubes
14742	Uterus	14781	Absence
14743	Enlarged	14782	On The Right Only
14744	Atrophied	14783	On The Left Only
14745	And Calcified	14784	Bilaterally
14746	Absence	14785	Mass ___ cm
14747	Mass Lesion ___ cm	14786	On The Right Only
14748	Solitary	14787	On The Left Only
14749	Multiple	14788	Bilaterally
14750	Calcified	81997	Echogenicity
81995	Echogenicity	19332	Fetus
14751	Bicornate	14789	Intraabdominal Pregnancy
19331	Gestational Sac	18506	Trans-Vaginal
14752	Fetus	18597	Bladder
18312	Abnormal Morphology	18598	Wall Thickened

ULTRASOUND, CONT.

18599	Focal
18600	Diffuse
18601	Calculi
18602	Solitary
18603	Multiple
18604	Post-Surgical Changes
18605	Uterus
18606	Enlarged
18607	Atrophied
18608	And Calcified
18609	Absence
18610	Mass Lesion ___ cm
18611	Solitary
18612	Multiple
18613	Calcified
81998	Echogenicity
18614	Bicornate
19330	Gestational Sac
18615	Fetus
18617	Abnormal Morphology
18616	Solitary
18618	Multiple
18619	Placenta Previa
18620	Polyhydramnios
18621	Anencephaly
18622	Hydrocephaly
18623	Spina Bifida
18624	Meningocele
18625	Omphalocele
18626	"snowstorm" pattern
18627	Ovaries
18628	Enlargement
18629	On The Right Only
18630	On The Left Only
18631	Bilaterally
18632	Atrophied
18633	On The Right Only
18634	On The Left Only
18635	Bilaterally
18636	Absence
18637	On The Right Only
18638	On The Left Only
18639	Bilaterally
18640	Mass ___ cm
18641	On The Right Only
18642	On The Left Only
18643	Bilaterally
18644	Calcified
81999	Echogenicity
18645	Cystic Lesion
18646	On The Right Only
18647	On The Left Only
18648	Bilaterally

18649	Calcified
18650	Fallopian Tubes
18651	Absence
18652	On The Right Only
18653	On The Left Only
18654	Bilaterally
18655	Mass ___ cm
18656	On The Right Only
18657	On The Left Only
18658	Bilaterally
82000	Echogenicity
19333	Fetus
18659	Intraabdominal Pregnancy
14790	Trans-Rectal Sonogram of Prostate
14791	Enlargement
14792	Atrophy
14793	Nodules
14794	Solitary
14795	Multiple
14796	Calcification
14797	Focal
14798	Diffuse
14799	Seminal Vesicles
14800	Enlarged
14801	On The Right Only
14802	On The Left Only
14803	Bilaterally
14804	Doppler
18416	Arterial
18420	Cerebral
29399	Duplex Scan Of Extracranial Arteries
29400	Bilateral
29401	Unilateral
29402	Transcranial Doppler Study Of Intracranial Arteries
29403	Limited Study
18417	Upper Extremity
19507	With Exercise
19508	With Digital Temperature Measurement
29408	Duplex Scan
29409	Of Bypass Graft
29410	Unilateral
29411	Limited
19510	Thoracic Outlet
18418	Lower Extremity
19511	With Exercise And ECG
29404	Duplex Scan
29405	Of Bypass Graft
29406	Unilateral
29407	Limited
19512	With Transcutaneous Oximetry

ULTRASOUND, CONT.

19674	Rest And Post Exercise
18419	Venous of Extremity
18555	Lower
18556	Proximal
18557	Distal
18365	Pulsed Velocimeter
18372	B-Mode
18421	Arterial
18423	Cerebral
18424	Upper Extremity
18425	Lower Extremity
18422	Venous
18373	Common Femoral Vein
18374	Echogenic band
18375	Popliteal Vein
18376	Echogenic band
18558	Doppler Duplex Color-Flow
18559	Venous of Extremity
29412	Unilateral
29413	Limited
18560	Lower
18561	Proximal
18562	Distal
29420	Abdominal / Pelvic Vasculature
29421	Aorta
29422	Bypass Graft(s)
29427	Unilateral
29428	Limited
29423	IVC
29424	Bypass Graft(s)
29429	Unilateral
29430	Limited
29425	Iliac Vasculature
29426	Bypass Graft(s)
29431	Unilateral
29432	Limited
29414	Abdominal Organs
29417	Limited
29415	Pelvic Organs
29418	Limited
29416	Retroperitoneal Organs
29419	Limited
29433	Penile Vessels
29434	Limited
29435	Hemodialysis Access
14806	Thyroid
14807	Solid Mass ___ cm
14808	Pure Cyst
14809	Mixed/Solid Cystic Mass ___ cm
14810	Parathyroid
14811	Uniform Hypodense Mass ___ cm
14812	Irregular Solid Mass ___ cm
14813	Cyst

14805	Thoracic
18426	Quantative Venous Flow Studies
13639	**X-Ray**
13640	**Skull**
13641	Mastoid
13642	Internal Auditory Canals
18011	Frontal
18012	Bossing
18013	Internal hyperostosis
22638	Occipital Bone
22639	Meningocele
13643	Sinus
29349	Complete, Three Or More Views
13644	Mucosal thickening
13645	Air fluid levels
13646	Bone destruction
13647	Clouding
13648	Orbits
82201	Hypoplasia
82202	Right
82203	Left
82204	Erosion
82205	Orbit Canal
82209	Right
82210	Left
82206	Roof
82211	Right
82212	Left
82207	Lateral Wall
82213	Right
82214	Left
82208	Floor
82215	Right
82216	Left
28344	Eyes
28345	For Foreign Body
28346	Present
28347	Optic Foramina
13649	Coned View of Sella
13650	Enlarged
13651	Double Floor
13652	Erosion
13653	Base
102877	Fracture
82194	Orbital
82195	Right
82196	Lateral Wall
82197	Floor
82198	Left
82199	Lateral Wall
82200	Floor
102878	Sinus Bones
102879	Right

X-RAY, CONT.

102880	Left	84697	AP (anteroposteriorly) ___ cm
102881	Bilateral	84698	Pattern
82187	Frontal	84699	Geographic
82188	Linear	84700	Moth-eaten
82189	Right	84701	Permeative
82190	Left	84702	Zone Of Transition
82191	Depressed	84703	Narrow
82192	Right	84704	Wide
82193	Left	84705	Margin
102882	Parietal	84706	Sclerotic
102883	Right	84707	Non-Sclerotic
102884	Left	84708	Cortex
102885	Bilateral	84709	Intact
102886	Occipital	84710	Destruction
102887	Right	84711	Endosteal Scalloping
102888	Left	84712	Expansion
102889	Bilateral	84713	Thickening
102890	Sella	84714	Thinning
102891	Right	84715	Soft Tissue Mass
102892	Left	84716	Suspected
102893	Bilateral	84717	Seen
102894	Mastoid	84718	Periosteal Reaction
102895	Right	84719	Thick
102896	Left	84720	Thin
102897	Bilateral	84721	Uniform
13654	Lytic lesion(s)	84722	Irregular
84686	Location	84723	Dense
84687	Superior	84724	Amorphous
84688	Inferior	84725	Wavy
84689	Medial	84726	Lamellated
84690	Lateral	84727	Sunburst
84691	Anterior	84728	Spiculated
84692	Posterior	84729	Codman Triangle
84693	Central	84730	Matrix
84849	Frontal	84731	Osteoid
84856	Right	84732	Chondral
84857	Left	84733	Septation
84858	Both	84734	Trabecular
84850	Parietal	84735	Prominence
84853	Right	84736	Thickening
84854	Left	84737	Sequestrum
84855	Both	84738	Ground Glass Appearence
84851	Occipital	84739	Sclerotic Lesion
84859	Right	84740	Location
84860	Left	84741	Superior
84861	Both	84742	Inferior
84852	Temporal	84743	Medial
84862	Right	84744	Lateral
84863	Left	84745	Anterior
84864	Both	84746	Posterior
84694	Dimensions	84747	Central
84695	Height ___ cm	84865	Frontal
84696	Transversely ___ cm	84866	Right

X-RAY, CONT.

84867	Left	84781	Sunburst
84868	Both	84782	Spiculated
84869	Parietal	84783	Codman Triangle
84870	Right	84784	Matrix
84871	Left	84785	Osteoid
84872	Both	84786	Chondral
84873	Occipital	84787	Septation
84874	Right	84788	Trabecular
84883	Left	84789	Prominence
84884	Both	84790	Thickening
84885	Temporal	84791	Sequestrum
84886	Right	84792	Ground Glass Appearence
84887	Left	84793	Mixed Lytic / Sclerotic Lesion
84888	Both	84794	Location
84748	Dimensions	84795	Superior
84749	Height ___ cm	84796	Inferior
84875	Left	84797	Medial
84750	Transversely ___ cm	84798	Lateral
84876	Both	84799	Anterior
84751	AP (anteroposteriorly) ___ cm	84800	Posterior
84877	Temporal	84801	Central
84878	Right	84889	Frontal
84879	Left	84890	Right
84880	Both	84891	Left
84752	Pattern	84892	Both
84753	Geographic	84893	Parietal
84754	Moth-eaten	84894	Right
84755	Permeative	84895	Left
84756	Zone Of Transition	84896	Both
84757	Narrow	84897	Occipital
84758	Wide	84898	Right
84759	Margin	84899	Left
84760	Sclerotic	84900	Both
84761	Non-Sclerotic	84901	Temporal
84762	Cortex	84902	Right
84763	Intact	84903	Left
84764	Destruction	84904	Both
84765	Endosteal Scalloping	84802	Dimensions
84766	Expansion	84803	Height ___ cm
84767	Thickening	84804	Transversely ___ cm
84768	Thinning	84805	AP (anteroposteriorly) ___ cm
84769	Soft Tissue Mass	84806	Pattern
84770	Suspected	84807	Geographic
84771	Seen	84808	Moth-eaten
84772	Periosteal Reaction	84809	Permeative
84773	Thick	84810	Zone Of Transition
84774	Thin	84811	Narrow
84775	Uniform	84812	Wide
84776	Irregular	84813	Margin
84777	Dense	84814	Sclerotic
84778	Amorphous	84815	Non-Sclerotic
84779	Wavy	84816	Cortex
84780	Lamellated	84817	Intact

X-RAY, CONT.

84818	Destruction	29547	Fracture
84819	Endosteal Scalloping	29548	Open
84820	Expansion	29549	Closed
84821	Thickening	29550	Acute
84822	Thinning	29551	Old
84823	Soft Tissue Mass	29552	Stress
84824	Suspected	29553	Complete
84825	Seen	29554	Incomplete
84596	Thick	29555	Pathologic
84597	Thin	29556	Pediatric
84598	Uniform	29557	Torus
84599	Irregular	29558	Greenstick
84600	Dense	29559	Salter Type I
84601	Amorphous	29560	Salter Type II
84602	Wavy	29561	Salter Type III
84603	Lamellated	29562	Salter Type IV
84604	Sunburst	29563	Intra-articular
84605	Spiculated	29564	Extra-articular
84606	Codman Triangle	29565	Comminuted
84607	Matrix	29566	Minimally
84839	Osteoid	29567	Moderately
84840	Chondral	29568	Severely
84841	Septation	29569	Simple
84842	Trabecular	29570	Displaced
84843	Prominence	29573	Non-displaced
84844	Thickening	29581	Pattern
84845	Sequestrum	29574	Angulated
84846	Ground Glass Appearence	29575	Spiral
18014	Osteopenia	29576	Oblique
18015	Suggestive Of Osteoporosis	29577	Transverse
	Circumscripta	29578	Butterfly Component
18019	"Salt-and-pepper"	29579	Complex
18016	Calvarial thickening	29580	Avulsion
18017	Suggestive Of Osteosclerosis	29582	Location
18018	Leontiasis ossea	29583	Proximal
18020	Calcification	29584	Middle
18022	Basal Ganglia	29585	Medial
18021	Suprasellar	29586	Lateral
80948	Developmental Bone Age	29587	Anterior
80949	Retarded	29588	Posterior
80950	Advanced	29589	Section
13809	**TMJ Joint**	29590	Metaphyseal
29319	Arthrography	29591	Diaphyseal
28386	Right	29592	Epiphyseal
28387	Left	80384	Right Thumb
28388	Bilateral	80385	Proximal Phalanx
28371	**Fingers**	80386	Distal Phalanx
102840	Views	80387	Right Index Finger
102839	Two Or More	80388	Proximal Phalanx
84445	Of The Right Hand	80389	Middle Phalanx
84446	Of The Left Hand	80390	Distal Phalanx
102841	No Radiographic Evidence Of Any	80391	Right Middle Finger
	Osteoarticular Abnormality	80392	Proximal Phalanx

80393	Middle Phalanx		80723	PIP
80394	Distal Phalanx		80724	DIP
80395	Right Ring Finger		80725	Left Thumb
80396	Proximal Phalanx		80726	MCP
80397	Middle Phalanx		80727	IP
80398	Distal Phalanx		80728	Left Index Finger Joint
80399	Right Little Finger		80729	MCP
80400	Proximal Phalanx		80730	PIP
80401	Middle Phalanx		80731	DIP
80402	Distal Phalanx		80732	Left Middle Finger Joint
80403	Left Thumb		80733	MCP
80404	Proximal Phalanx		80734	PIP
80422	Middle Phalanx		80735	DIP
80405	Distal Phalanx		80736	Left Ring Finger Joint
80406	Left Index Finger		80737	MCP
80407	Proximal Phalanx		80738	PIP
80408	Middle Phalanx		80739	DIP
80409	Distal Phalanx		80740	Left Little Finger Joint
80410	Left Middle Finger		80741	MCP
80411	Proximal Phalanx		80742	PIP
80412	Middle Phalanx		80743	DIP
80413	Distal Phalanx		83215	Lytic Lesion
80414	Left Ring Finger		83216	Septated
80415	Proximal Phalanx		83217	Non-Septated
80416	Middle Phalanx		83218	Dimensions
80417	Distal Phalanx		83219	Height ___cm
80418	Left Little Finger		83220	Transverse ___ cm
80419	Proximal Phalanx		83221	AP ___ cm
80420	Middle Phalanx		83222	Location
80421	Distal Phalanx		83223	Cortical
80700	Dislocation		83224	Medullary
80701	Partial		83225	Central
80702	Complete		83226	Eccentric
80703	Acute		83227	Epiphyseal
80704	Old		83228	Proximal
80705	Recurrent		83229	Distal
80706	Right Thumb		83230	Metaphyseal
80707	MCP		83231	Proximal
80708	IP		83232	Distal
80709	Right Index Finger Joint		83233	Diaphyseal
80710	MCP		83327	Proximal Phalanx
80711	PIP		83328	R Thumb
80712	DIP		83329	R Middle Finger
80713	Right Middle Finger Joint		83330	R Index Finger
80714	MCP		83331	R Ring Finger
80715	PIP		83332	R Little Finger
80716	DIP		83333	L Thumb
80717	Right Ring Finger Joint		83334	L Index Finger
80718	MCP		83335	L Middle Finger
80719	PIP		83336	L Ring Finger
80720	DIP		83337	L Little Finger
80721	Right Little Finger Joint		83338	Middle Phalanx
80722	MCP		83339	R Index Finger

X-RAY, CONT.

83340	R Middle Finger	85823	Matrix
83341	R Ring Finger	85824	Osteoid
83342	R Little Finger	85825	Chondral
83343	L Index Finger	85826	Soft Tissue Mass
83344	L Middle Finger	85827	Suspected
83345	L Ring Finger	85828	Seen
83346	L Little Finger	85829	Superior
83347	Distal Phalanx	85830	Inferior
83348	R Thumb	85831	Medial
83349	R Index Finger	85832	Lateral
83350	R Middle Finger	85833	Anterior
83351	R Ring Finger	85834	Trabecular
83352	R Little Finger	85835	Prominence
83353	L Thumb	85836	Thickening
83354	L Index Finger	85837	Sequestrum
83355	L Middle Finger	85838	Ground Glass Appearence
83356	L Ring Finger	83234	Sclerotic Lesion
83357	L Little Finger	83237	Dimensions
85788	Pattern	83238	Height ___ cm
85789	Geographic	83239	Transverse ___ cm
85790	Moth-eaten	83240	AP ___ cm
85791	Permeative	83241	Location
85792	Zone Of Transition	83242	Cortical
85793	Narrow	83243	Medullary
85794	Wide	83244	Central
85795	Margin	83245	Eccentric
85796	Sclerotic	83246	Epiphyseal
85797	Non-Sclerotic	83247	Proximal
85798	Cortex	83248	Distal
85799	Intact	83249	Metaphyseal
85800	Destruction	83250	Proximal
85801	Endosteal Scalloping	83251	Distal
85802	Expansion	83252	Diaphyseal
85803	Thickening	83254	Proximal Phalanx
85804	Thinning	83255	Right Thumb
85805	Superior	83256	Right Middle Finger
85806	Inferior	83257	Right Index Finger
85807	Medial	83258	Right Ring Finger
85808	Lateral	83259	Right Little Finger
85809	Anterior	83260	Left Thumb
85810	Posterior	83261	Left Index Finger
85811	Periosteal Reaction	83262	Left Middle Finger
85812	Thick	83263	Left Ring Finger
85813	Thin	83264	Left Little Finger
85814	Uniform	83265	Middle Phalanx
85815	Irregular	83266	Right Index Finger
85816	Dense	83267	Right Middle Finger
85817	Amorphous	83268	Right Ring Finger
85818	Wavy	83269	Right Little Finger
85819	Lamellated	83270	Left Index Finger
85820	Sunburst	83271	Left Middle Finger
85821	Spiculated	83273	Left Ring Finger
85822	Codman Triangle	83274	Left Little Finger

X-RAY, CONT.

83275	Distal Phalanx	85779		Inferior
83276	Right Thumb	85780		Medial
83277	Right Index Finger	85781		Lateral
83278	Right Middle Finger	85782		Anterior
83279	Right Ring Finger	85783	Trabecular
83280	Right Little Finger	85784		Prominence
83281	Left Thumb	85785		Thickening
83282	Left Index Finger	85786	Sequestrum
83283	Left Middle Finger	85787	Ground Glass Appearence
83284	Left Ring Finger	83032	Mixed Lytic / Sclerotic Lesion
83285	Left Little Finger	83033		Septated
85737	Pattern	83034		Non-Septated
85738	Geographic	83035		Dimensions
85739	Moth-eaten	83036		Height ___ cm
85740	Permeative	83037		Transverse ___ cm
85741	Zone Of Transition	83038		AP ___ cm
85742	Narrow	83039		Location
85743	Wide	83040		Cortical
85744	Margin	83041		Medullary
85745	Sclerotic	83042		Central
85746	Non-Sclerotic	83043		Eccentric
85747	Cortex	83044		Epiphyseal
85748	Intact	83077		Proximal
85749	Destruction	83078		Distal
85750	Endosteal Scalloping	83079		Metaphyseal
85751	Expansion	83080		Proximal
85752	Thickening	83081		Distal
85753	Thinning	83045		Diaphyseal
85754	Superior	84447		Proximal
85755	Inferior	84448		Distal
85756	Medial	83046	Proximal Phalanx
85757	Lateral	83047		Right Thumb
85758	Anterior	83048		Right Middle Finger
85759	Posterior	83049		Right Index Finger
85760	Periosteal Reaction	83050		Right Ring Finger
85761	Thick	83051		Right Little Finger
85762	Thin	83052		Left Thumb
85763	Uniform	83053		Left Index Finger
85764	Irregular	83054		Left Middle Finger
85765	Dense	83055		Left Ring Finger
85766	Amorphous	83056		Left Little Finger
85767	Wavy	83057	Middle Phalanx
85768	Lamellated	83058		Right Index Finger
85769	Sunburst	83059		Right Middle Finger
85770	Spiculated	83060		Right Ring Finger
85771	Codman Triangle	83061		Right Little Finger
85772	Matrix	83062		Left Index Finger
85773	Osteoid	83063		Left Middle Finger
85774	Chondral	83064		Left Ring Finger
85775	Soft Tissue Mass	83065		Left Little Finger
85776	Suspected	83066	Distal Phalanx
85777	Seen	83067		Right Thumb
85778	Superior	83068		Right Index Finger

X-Ray, cont.

83069	Right Middle Finger	85884	Anterior
83070	Right Ring Finger	85885	Trabecular
83071	Right Little Finger	85886	Prominence
83072	Left Thumb	85887	Thickening
83073	Left Index Finger	85888	Sequestrum
83074	Left Middle Finger	85889	Ground Glass Appearence
83075	Left Ring Finger	101900	Osteopenia
83076	Left Little Finger	101925	Generalized
85839	Pattern	101926	Juxta-Articular
85840	Geographic	101931	Right
85841	Moth-eaten	102493	1st IP Joint
85842	Permeative	102494	2nd DIP Joint
85843	Zone Of Transition	102495	3rd DIP Joint
85844	Narrow	102496	4th DIP Joint
85845	Wide	102497	5th DIP Joint
85846	Margin	102498	2nd PIP Joint
85847	Sclerotic	102499	3rd PIP Joint
85848	Non-Sclerotic	102500	4th PIP Joint
85849	Cortex	102501	5th PIP Joint
85850	Intact	102502	1st MCP Joint
85851	Destruction	102503	2nd MCP Joint
85852	Endosteal Scalloping	102504	3rd MCP Joint
85853	Expansion	102505	4th MCP Joint
85854	Thickening	102506	5th MCP Joint
85855	Thinning	102158	Left
85856	Superior	102507	1st IP Joint
85857	Inferior	102508	2nd DIP Joint
85858	Medial	102509	3rd DIP Joint
85859	Lateral	102510	4th DIP Joint
85860	Anterior	102511	5th DIP Joint
85861	Posterior	102512	2nd PIP Joint
85862	Periosteal Reaction	102513	3rd PIP Joint
85863	Thick	102514	4th PIP Joint
85864	Thin	102515	5th PIP Joint
85865	Uniform	102516	1st MCP Joint
85866	Irregular	102517	2nd MCP Joint
85867	Dense	102518	3rd MCP Joint
85868	Amorphous	102519	4th MCP Joint
85869	Wavy	102520	5th MCP Joint
85870	Lamellated	101901	Soft Tissue Swelling
85871	Sunburst	102159	Diffuse
85872	Spiculated	102163	Periarticular
85873	Codman Triangle	102313	Right
85874	Matrix	102521	1st IP Joint
85875	Osteoid	102522	2nd DIP Joint
85876	Chondral	102523	3rd DIP Joint
85877	Soft Tissue Mass	102524	4th DIP Joint
85878	Suspected	102525	5th DIP Joint
85879	Seen	102526	2nd PIP Joint
85880	Superior	102527	3rd PIP Joint
85881	Inferior	102528	4th PIP Joint
85882	Medial	102529	5th PIP Joint
85883	Lateral	102530	1st MCP Joint

X-RAY, CONT.

102531	2nd MCP Joint
102532	3rd MCP Joint
102533	4th MCP Joint
102534	5th MCP Joint
102340	Left
102535	1st IP Joint
102536	2nd DIP Joint
102537	3rd DIP Joint
102538	4th DIP Joint
102539	5th DIP Joint
102540	2nd PIP Joint
102541	3rd PIP Joint
102542	4th PIP Joint
102543	5th PIP Joint
102544	1st MCP Joint
102545	2nd MCP Joint
102546	3rd MCP Joint
102547	4th MCP Joint
102548	5th MCP Joint
102168	Fusiform
102341	Right
102549	1st Digit
102550	2nd Digit
102551	3rd Digit
102552	4th Digit
102553	5th Digit
102342	Left
102554	1st Digit
102555	2nd Digit
102556	3rd Digit
102557	4th Digit
102558	5th Digit
101902	Joint Space Abnormality
102369	Right
102559	1st IP Joint
102560	2nd DIP Joint
102561	3rd DIP Joint
102562	4th DIP Joint
102563	5th DIP Joint
102564	2nd PIP Joint
102565	3rd PIP Joint
102566	4th PIP Joint
102567	5th PIP Joint
102568	1st MCP Joint
102569	2nd MCP Joint
102570	3rd MCP Joint
102571	4th MCP Joint
102572	5th MCP Joint
102370	Left
102573	1st IP Joint
102574	2nd DIP Joint
102575	3rd DIP Joint
102576	4th DIP Joint

102577	5th DIP Joint
102578	2nd PIP Joint
102579	3rd PIP Joint
102580	4th PIP Joint
102581	5th PIP Joint
102582	1st MCP Joint
102583	2nd MCP Joint
102584	3rd MCP Joint
102585	4th MCP Joint
102586	5th MCP Joint
102172	Narrowing
102173	Sclerosis
102174	Osteophytes
102191	Subchondral Cysts
101903	Erosions
102371	Right
102587	1st IP Joint
102588	Base Of Distal Phalanx
102589	Distal End Of Proximal Phalanx
102590	2nd DIP Joint
102591	Base Of Distal Phalanx
102592	Distal End Of Middle Phalanx
102593	3rd DIP Joint
102594	Base Of Distal Phalanx
102595	Distal End Of Middle Phalanx
102596	4th DIP Joint
102597	Base Of Distal Phalanx
102598	Distal End Of Middle Phalanx
102599	5th DIP Joint
102600	Base Of Distal Phalanx
102601	Distal End Of Middle Phalanx
102602	2nd PIP Joint
102603	Base Of Middle Phalanx
102604	Distal End Of Proximal Phalanx
102605	3rd PIP Joint
102606	Base Of Middle Phalanx
102607	Distal End Of Proximal Phalanx
102608	4th PIP Joint
102609	Base Of Middle Phalanx
102610	Distal End Of Proximal Phalanx
102611	5th PIP Joint
102612	Base Of Middle Phalanx
102613	Distal End Of Proximal Phalanx
102614	1st MCP Joint
102615	Base Of Proximal Phalanx
102616	Metacarpal Head
102617	2nd MCP Joint
102618	Base Of Proximal Phalanx
102619	Metacarpal Head
102620	3rd MCP Joint
102621	Base Of Proximal Phalanx
102622	Metacarpal Head
102623	4th MCP Joint

X-RAY, CONT.

102624	Base Of Proximal Phalanx	101904	Periosteal Reaction
102625	Metacarpal Head	102223	Amorphous
102665	5th MCP Joint	102250	Solid
102666	Base Of Proximal Phalanx	102373	Right
102667	Metacarpal Head	102671	1st Distal Phalanx
102372	Left	102672	2nd Distal Phalanx
102626	1st IP Joint	102673	3rd Distal Phalanx
102627	Base Of Distal Phalanx	102674	4th Distal Phalanx
102628	Distal End Of Proximal Phalanx	102675	5th Distal Phalanx
102629	2nd DIP Joint	102676	2nd Middle Phalanx
102630	Base Of Distal Phalanx	102677	3rd Middle Phalanx
102631	Distal End Of Middle Phalanx	102678	4th Middle Phalanx
102632	3rd DIP Joint	102679	5th Middle Phalanx
102633	Base Of Distal Phalanx	102680	1st Proximal Phalanx
102634	Distal End Of Middle Phalanx	102681	2nd Proximal Phalanx
102635	4th DIP Joint	102682	3rd Proximal Phalanx
102636	Base Of Distal Phalanx	102683	4th Proximal Phalanx
102637	Distal End Of Middle Phalanx	102684	5th Proximal Phalanx
102638	5th DIP Joint	102374	Left
102639	Base Of Distal Phalanx	102685	1st Distal Phalanx
102640	Distal End Of Middle Phalanx	102686	2nd Distal Phalanx
102641	2nd PIP Joint	102687	3rd Distal Phalanx
102642	Base Of Middle Phalanx	102688	4th Distal Phalanx
102643	Distal End Of Proximal Phalanx	102689	5th Distal Phalanx
102644	3rd PIP Joint	102690	2nd Middle Phalanx
102645	Base Of Middle Phalanx	102691	3rd Middle Phalanx
102646	Distal End Of Proximal Phalanx	102692	4th Middle Phalanx
102647	4th PIP Joint	102693	5th Middle Phalanx
102648	Base Of Middle Phalanx	102694	1st Proximal Phalanx
102649	Distal End Of Proximal Phalanx	102695	2nd Proximal Phalanx
102650	5th PIP Joint	102696	3rd Proximal Phalanx
102651	Base Of Middle Phalanx	102697	4th Proximal Phalanx
102652	Distal End Of Proximal Phalanx	102698	5th Proximal Phalanx
102653	1st MCP Joint	102251	Radial Side
102654	Base Of Proximal Phalanx	102252	Ulnar Side
102655	Metacarpal Head	102257	Proximal
102656	2nd MCP Joint	102272	Distal
102657	Base Of Proximal Phalanx	101905	Bony Ankylosis
102658	Metacarpal Head	102375	Right
102659	3rd MCP Joint	102699	1st IP Joint
102660	Base Of Proximal Phalanx	102700	2nd DIP Joint
102661	Metacarpal Head	102701	3rd DIP Joint
102662	4th MCP Joint	102702	4th DIP Joint
102663	Base Of Proximal Phalanx	102703	5th DIP Joint
102664	Metacarpal Head	102704	2nd PIP Joint
102668	5th MCP Joint	102705	3rd PIP Joint
102669	Base Of Proximal Phalanx	102706	4th PIP Joint
102670	Metacarpal Head	102707	5th PIP Joint
102192	Overhanging Edge	102708	1st MCP Joint
102214	Marginal	102709	2nd MCP Joint
102220	Central	102710	3rd MCP Joint
102221	Radial Side	102711	4th MCP Joint
102222	Ulnar Side	102712	5th MCP Joint

X-RAY, CONT.

102376	Left		102759	2nd PIP Joint
102713	1st IP Joint		102760	3rd PIP Joint
102714	2nd DIP Joint		102761	4th PIP Joint
102715	3rd DIP Joint		102762	5th PIP Joint
102716	4th DIP Joint		101916	Soft Tissue Calcification
102717	5th DIP Joint		102485	Right
102718	2nd PIP Joint		102783	1st IP Joint
102719	3rd PIP Joint		102784	2nd DIP Joint
102720	4th PIP Joint		102785	3rd DIP Joint
102721	5th PIP Joint		102786	4th DIP Joint
102722	1st MCP Joint		102787	5th DIP Joint
102723	2nd MCP Joint		102788	2nd PIP Joint
102724	3rd MCP Joint		102789	3rd PIP Joint
102725	4th MCP Joint		102790	4th PIP Joint
102726	5th MCP Joint		102791	5th PIP Joint
101908	Pencil-In-Cup Deformity		102792	2nd MCP Joint
102377	Right		102793	3rd MCP Joint
102727	1st IP Joint		102794	4th MCP Joint
102728	2nd DIP Joint		102795	5th MCP Joint
102729	3rd DIP Joint		102796	1st Distal Phalanx
102730	4th DIP Joint		102797	2nd Distal Phalanx
102731	5th DIP Joint		102798	3rd Distal Phalanx
102732	2nd PIP Joint		102799	4th Distal Phalanx
102733	3rd PIP Joint		102800	5th Distal Phalanx
102734	4th PIP Joint		102801	2nd Middle Phalanx
102735	5th PIP Joint		102802	3rd Middle Phalanx
102378	Left		102803	4th Middle Phalanx
102736	1st IP Joint		102804	5th Middle Phalanx
102737	2nd DIP Joint		102805	1st Proximal Phalanx
102738	3rd DIP Joint		102806	2nd Proximal Phalanx
102739	4th DIP Joint		102807	3rd Proximal Phalanx
102740	5th DIP Joint		102808	4th Proximal Phalanx
102741	2nd PIP Joint		102809	5th Proximal Phalanx
102742	3rd PIP Joint		102486	Left
102743	4th PIP Joint		102810	1st IP Joint
102744	5th PIP Joint		102811	2nd DIP Joint
101913	Seagull Wing Deformity		102812	3rd DIP Joint
102379	Right		102813	4th DIP Joint
102745	1st IP Joint		102814	5th DIP Joint
102746	2nd DIP Joint		102815	2nd PIP Joint
102747	3rd DIP Joint		102816	3rd PIP Joint
102748	4th DIP Joint		102817	4th PIP Joint
102749	5th DIP Joint		102818	5th PIP Joint
102750	2nd PIP Joint		102819	2nd MCP Joint
102751	3rd PIP Joint		102820	3rd MCP Joint
102752	4th PIP Joint		102821	4th MCP Joint
102753	5th PIP Joint		102822	5th MCP Joint
102484	Left		102823	1st Distal Phalanx
102754	1st IP Joint		102824	2nd Distal Phalanx
102755	2nd DIP Joint		102825	3rd Distal Phalanx
102756	3rd DIP Joint		102826	4th Distal Phalanx
102757	4th DIP Joint		102827	5th Distal Phalanx
102758	5th DIP Joint		102828	2nd Middle Phalanx

X-RAY, CONT.

102829	3rd Middle Phalanx	29596	Acute
102830	4th Middle Phalanx	29597	Old
102831	5th Middle Phalanx	29598	Stress
102832	1st Proximal Phalanx	29599	Complete
102833	2nd Proximal Phalanx	29600	Incomplete
102834	3rd Proximal Phalanx	29601	Pathologic
102835	4th Proximal Phalanx	29602	Pediatric
102836	5th Proximal Phalanx	29603	Torus
102281	Radial Side	29604	Greenstick
102282	Ulnar Side	29605	Salter Type I
101919	Chondrocalcinosis	29606	Salter Type II
102487	Right	29607	Salter Type III
102488	Left	29608	Salter Type IV
17939	Acroosteolysis	29609	Intra-articular
102489	Right	29610	Extra-articular
102773	1st Distal Phalanx	29611	Comminuted
102774	2nd Distal Phalanx	29612	Minimally
102775	3rd Distal Phalanx	29613	Moderately
102776	4th Distal Phalanx	29614	Severely
102777	5th Distal Phalanx	29615	Simple
102490	Left	29616	Displaced
102778	1st Distal Phalanx	29619	Non-displaced
102779	2nd Distal Phalanx	29627	Pattern
102780	3rd Distal Phalanx	29620	Angulated
102781	4th Distal Phalanx	29621	Spiral
102782	5th Distal Phalanx	29622	Oblique
101920	Distribution	29623	Transverse
102311	Bilaterally Symmetrical	29624	Butterfly Component
102312	Bilaterally Asymmetrical	29625	Complex
102491	Right	29626	Avulsion
102763	1st Digit	29628	Location
102764	2nd Digit	29629	Proximal
102765	3rd Digit	29630	Middle
102766	4th Digit	29631	Medial
102767	5th Digit	29632	Lateral
102492	Left	29633	Anterior
102768	1st Digit	29634	Posterior
102769	2nd Digit	29635	Section
102770	3rd Digit	29636	Metaphyseal
102771	4th Digit	29637	Diaphyseal
102772	5th Digit	29638	Epiphyseal
84450	**Hands**	80423	First Metacarpal Of The Right Hand
102837	Views	80424	Second Metacarpal Of The Right Hand
84449	2 Views		
28373	3 Or More Views	80425	Third Metacarpal Of The Right Hand
27044	Right Hand		
27045	Left Hand	80426	Fourth Metacarpal Of The Right Hand
27046	Both Hands		
102838	No Radiographic Evidence Of Any	80427	First Metacarpal Of The Left Hand
	Osteoarticular Abnormality	80428	Second Metacarpal Of The Left Hand
29593	Fracture		
29594	Open	80429	Third Metacarpal Of The Left Hand
29595	Closed	80430	Fourth Metacarpal Of The Left Hand

X-RAY, CONT.

Code	Description	Code	Description
80744	Dislocation	101325	Right
80745	Partial	101328	1st CM Joint
80746	Complete	101330	2nd CM Joint
80747	Acute	101331	3rd CM Joint
80748	Old	101332	4th CM Joint
80749	Recurrent	101333	5th CM Joint
80798	Right First Carpometacarpal	101335	Left
80799	Right Second Carpometacarpal	101339	1st CM Joint
80800	Right Third Carpometacarpal	101340	2nd CM Joint
80801	Right Fourth Carpometacarpal	101341	3rd CM Joint
80802	Right Fifth Carpometacarpal	101343	4th CM Joint
80803	Right First Metacarpophalangeal	101344	5th CM Joint
80804	Right Second Metacarpophalangeal	17932	Soft Tissue Swelling
80805	Right Third Metacarpophalangeal	101318	Right
80806	Right Fourth Metacarpophalangeal	101319	Left
80807	Right Fifth Metacarpophalangeal	101303	Diffuse
80808	Left First Carpometacarpal	101307	Periarticular
80809	Left Second Carpometacarpal	101309	Fusiform
80810	Left Third Carpometacarpal	17933	Erosions
80811	Left Fourth Carpometacarpal	101375	Right Hand
80812	Left Fifth Carpometacarpal	101376	1st CM Joint
80813	Left First Metacarpophalangeal	101377	2nd CM Joint
80814	Left Second Metacarpophalangeal	101378	3rd CM Joint
80815	Left Third Metacarpophalangeal	101379	4th CM Joint
80816	Left Fourth Metacarpophalangeal	101380	5th CM Joint
80817	Left Fifth Metacarpophalangeal	101388	Intercarpal Joints
82981	Sclerotic Lesion	101394	Scaphoid
17930	Joint Space	101395	Lunate
101312	Narrowing	101396	Triquetral
101315	Sclerosis	101397	Pisiform
17934	Osteophytes	101398	Trapezium
18412	Subchondral Cysts	101402	Capitate
101352	Right Hand	101403	Hamate
101353	1st CM Joint	101407	Radiocarpal Joint
101354	2nd CM Joint	101408	Distal Radioulnar Joint
101355	3rd CM Joint	101411	Ulnar Styloid Process
101356	4th CM Joint	101381	Left Hand
101357	5th CM Joint	101383	1st CM Joint
101358	Intercarpal Joints	101384	2nd CM Joint
101359	Radiocarpal Joint	101385	3rd CM Joint
101360	Distal Radioulnar Joint	101386	4th CM Joint
101361	Left Hand	101387	5th CM Joint
101362	1st CM Joint	101413	Intercarpal Joints
101363	2nd CM Joint	101414	Scaphoid
101364	3rd CM Joint	101415	Lunate
101365	4th CM Joint	101416	Triquetral
101366	5th CM Joint	101419	Pisiform
101367	Intercarpal Joints	101421	Trapezium
101368	Radiocarpal Joint	101422	Capitate
101369	Distal Radioulnar Joint	101423	Hamate
17931	Osteopenia	101424	Radiocarpal Joint
101282	Generalized	101425	Distal Radioulnar Joint
18413	Juxtaarticular	101426	Ulnar Styloid Process

X-RAY, CONT.

101370	Overhanging Edge	101558	3rd Metacarpal
101371	Marginal	101559	4th Metacarpal
101372	Central	101560	5th Metacarpal
101373	Radial Side	101561	Distal Radius
101374	Ulnar Side	101562	Distal Ulna
18411	Subchondral	101578	Left Hand
17935	Chondrocalcinosis	101579	1st CM Joint
101728	Right Hand	101580	2nd CM Joint
101729	Left Hand	101581	3rd CM Joint
101730	Triangular Fibrocartilage	101582	4th CM Joint
17937	"Pencil-in-Cup" Deformity	101583	5th CM Joint
17938	Bony Ankylosis	101584	Intercarpal Joints
101513	Right Hand	101585	Radiocarpal Joint
101514	1st CM Joint	101586	Distal Radioulnar Joint
101515	2nd CM Joint	101587	1st Metacarpal
101516	3rd CM Joint	101588	2nd Metacarpal
101520	4th CM Joint	101589	3rd Metacarpal
101521	5th CM Joint	101593	4th Metacarpal
101522	Intercarpal Joints	101605	5th Metacarpal
101523	Radiocarpal Joint	101612	Distal Radius
101524	Distal Radioulnar Joint	101622	Distal Ulna
101525	Left Hand	102283	Radial Side
101526	1st CM Joint	102284	Ulnar Side
101527	2nd CM Joint	101727	Chondrocalcinosis
101528	3rd CM Joint	101754	Acro-osteolysis
101529	4th CM Joint	101774	Right Hand
101530	5th CM Joint	101859	Left Hand
101531	Intercarpal Joints	101860	Distribution
101532	Radiocarpal Joint	101861	Bilaterally Symmetrical
101533	Distal Radioulnar Joint	101862	Bilaterally Asymmetrical
101427	Periosteal Reaction	80933	Developmental Bone Age
101506	Right Hand	80934	Retarded
101508	Left Hand	80935	Advanced
101431	Amorphous	83287	Lytic Lesion
101432	Solid	83288	Septated
101509	Radial Side	83289	Non-Septated
101510	Ulnar Side	83290	Dimensions
101511	Proximal	83291	Height ___cm
101512	Distal	83292	Transverse ___ cm
17936	Periosteal Bone Resorption	83293	AP ___cm
17940	Periosteal New Bone Formation	83294	Location
101536	Soft Tissue Calcification	83295	Cortical
101544	Right Hand	83296	Medullary
101545	1st CM Joint	83297	Central
101549	2nd CM Joint	83298	Eccentric
101550	3rd CM Joint	83299	Epiphyseal
101551	4th CM Joint	83300	Proximal
101552	5th CM Joint	83301	Distal
101553	Intercarpal Joints	83302	Metaphyseal
101554	Radiocarpal Joint	83303	Proximal
101555	Distal Radioulnar Joint	83304	Distal
101556	1st Metacarpal	83305	Diaphyseal
101557	2nd Metacarpal	83984	Right

X-RAY, CONT.

83985	First Metacarpal	85932		Inferior
83986	Second Metacarpal	85933		Medial
83987	Third Metacarpal	85934		Lateral
83988	Fourth Metacarpal	85935		Anterior
83989	Fifth Metacarpal	85936	Trabecular
83990	Left	85937		Prominence
83991	First Metacarpal	85938		Thickening
83992	Second Metacarpal	85939	Sequestrum
83993	Third Metacarpal	85940	Ground Glass Appearence
83994	Fourth Metacarpal	83306	Sclerotic Lesion
83995	Fifth Metacarpal	83307	Septated
85890	Pattern	83308	Non-Septated
85891	Geographic	83309	Dimensions
85892	Moth-eaten	83310	Height ___ cm
85893	Permeative	83311	Transverse ___ cm
85894	Zone Of Transition	83312	AP ___ cm
85895	Narrow	83313	Location
85896	Wide	83314	Cortical
85897	Margin	83315	Medullary
85898	Sclerotic	83316	Central
85899	Non-Sclerotic	83317	Eccentric
85900	Cortex	83318	Epiphyseal
85901	Intact	83319	Proximal
85902	Destruction	83320	Distal
85903	Endosteal Scalloping	83321	Metaphyseal
85904	Expansion	83322	Proximal
85905	Thickening	83323	Distal
85906	Thinning	83324	Diaphyseal
85907	Superior	83983	Right
85908	Inferior	83972	First Metacarpal
85909	Medial	83973	Second Metacarpal
85910	Lateral	83974	Third Metacarpal
85911	Anterior	83975	Fourth Metacarpal
85912	Posterior	83976	Fifth Metacarpal
85913	Periosteal Reaction	83977	Left
85914	Thick	83978	First Metacarpal
85915	Thin	83979	Second Metacarpal
85916	Uniform	83980	Third Metacarpal
85917	Irregular	83981	Fourth Metacarpal
85918	Dense	83982	Fifth Metacarpal
85919	Amorphous	85941	Pattern
85920	Wavy	85942	Geographic
85921	Lamellated	85943	Moth-eaten
85922	Sunburst	85944	Permeative
85923	Spiculated	85945	Zone Of Transition
85924	Codman Triangle	85946	Narrow
85925	Matrix	85947	Wide
85926	Osteoid	85948	Margin
85927	Chondral	85949	Sclerotic
85928	Soft Tissue Mass	85950	Non-Sclerotic
85929	Suspected	85951	Cortex
85930	Seen	85952	Intact
85931	Superior	85953	Destruction

X-RAY, CONT.

85954	Endosteal Scalloping		83097	Metaphyseal
85955	Expansion		83098	Proximal
85956	Thickening		83099	Distal
85957	Thinning		83100	Diaphyseal
85958	Superior		83960	Right
85959	Inferior		83961	First Metacarpal
85960	Medial		83962	Second Metacarpal
85961	Lateral		83963	Third Metacarpal
85962	Anterior		83964	Fourth Metacarpal
85963	Posterior		83965	Fifth Metacarpal
85964	Periosteal Reaction		83966	Left
85965	Thick		83967	First Metacarpal
85966	Thin		83968	Second Metacarpal
85967	Uniform		83969	Third Metacarpal
85968	Irregular		83970	Fourth Metacarpal
85969	Dense		83971	Fifth Metacarpal
85970	Amorphous		85992	Pattern
85971	Wavy		85993	Geographic
85972	Lamellated		85994	Moth-eaten
85973	Sunburst		85995	Permeative
85974	Spiculated		85996	Zone Of Transition
85975	Codman Triangle		85997	Narrow
85976	Matrix		85998	Wide
85977	Osteoid		85999	Margin
85978	Chondral		86000	Sclerotic
85979	Soft Tissue Mass		86001	Non-Sclerotic
85980	Suspected		86002	Cortex
85981	Seen		86003	Intact
85982	Superior		86004	Destruction
85983	Inferior		86005	Endosteal Scalloping
85984	Medial		86006	Expansion
85985	Lateral		86007	Thickening
85986	Anterior		86008	Thinning
85987	Trabecular		86009	Superior
85988	Prominence		86010	Inferior
85989	Thickening		86011	Medial
85990	Sequestrum		86012	Lateral
85991	Ground Glass Appearence		86013	Anterior
83082	Mixed Lytic/Sclerotic Lesion		86014	Posterior
83083	Septated		86015	Periosteal Reaction
83084	Non-Septated		86016	Thick
83085	Dimensions		86017	Thin
83086	Height ___ cm		86018	Uniform
83087	Transverse ___ cm		86019	Irregular
83088	AP ___ cm		86020	Dense
83089	Location		86021	Amorphous
83090	Cortical		86022	Wavy
83091	Medullary		86023	Lamellated
83092	Central		86024	Sunburst
83093	Eccentric		86025	Spiculated
83094	Epiphyseal		86026	Codman Triangle
83095	Proximal		86027	Matrix
83096	Distal		86028	Osteoid

X-RAY, CONT.

86029	Chondral	29668	Butterfly Component
86030	Soft Tissue Mass	29669	Complex
86031	Suspected	29670	Avulsion
86032	Seen	29672	Location
86033	Superior	29673	Proximal
86034	Inferior	29674	Middle
86035	Medial	29675	Medial
86036	Lateral	29676	Lateral
86037	Anterior	29677	Anterior
86038	Trabecular	29678	Posterior
86039	Prominence	29679	Section
86040	Thickening	29680	Metaphyseal
86041	Sequestrum	29681	Diaphyseal
86042	Ground Glass Appearence	29682	Epiphyseal
13804	**Wrist**	80431	Right Carpal
102842	Views	80432	Scaphoid
28368	Anteroposterior And Lateral Views	80433	Capitate
28369	Complete - Three Or More Views	80434	Hamate
28370	Arthrography	80435	Lunate
29322	Supervision And Interpretation	80436	Piciform
27047	Right Wrist	80437	Triquetrum
27048	Left Wrist	80438	Trapezoid
27049	Both Wrists	80439	Trapezium
102843	No Radiographic Evidence Of Any Osteoarticular Abnormality	80440	Right Distal Radius
		80441	Right Distal Ulna
29639	Fracture	80442	Left Carpal
29640	Open	80443	Scaphoid
29641	Closed	80444	Capitate
29642	Acute	80445	Hamate
29643	Old	80446	Lunate
29644	Stress	80447	Piciform
29645	Complete	80448	Triquetrum
29646	Incomplete	80449	Trapezoid
29647	Pathologic	80450	Trapezium
29648	Pediatric	80451	Left Distal Radius
29649	Salter Type I	80452	Left Distal Ulna
29650	Salter Type II	80750	Dislocation
29651	Salter Type III	80751	Partial
29652	Salter Type IV	80752	Complete
29653	Intra-articular	80753	Acute
29654	Extra-articular	80754	Old
29655	Comminuted	80755	Recurrent
29656	Minimally	80818	Right Perilunate Dissociation
29657	Moderately	80819	Right Radiocarpal Joint
29658	Severely	80820	Right Distal Radioulnar Joint
29659	Simple	80822	Left Perilunate Dissociation
29660	Displaced	80823	Left Radiocarpal Joint
29663	Non-displaced	80821	Left Distal Radioulnar Joint
29671	Pattern	17942	Joint Space Narrowing
29664	Angulated	17943	Juxtaarticular Osteopenia
29665	Spiral	17944	Soft Tissue Swelling
29666	Oblique	17945	Subchondral Bone Erosion
29667	Transverse	17946	Subchondral Bone Cysts

X-RAY, CONT.

17947	Osteophytes	84032	Periosteal Reaction
17948	Chondrocalcinosis	84033	Thick
17949	Periosteal Bone Resorption	84034	Thin
17950	Periosteal New Bone Formation	84035	Uniform
17952	Ankylosis	84036	Irregular
80939	Developmental Bone Age	84037	Dense
80940	Retarded	84038	Amorphous
80941	Advanced	84039	Wavy
83996	Lytic Lesion	84040	Lamellated
83997	Location	84041	Sunburst
83998	Superior	84042	Spiculated
83999	Inferior	84043	Codman Triangle
84000	Medial	84044	Matrix
84001	Lateral	84045	Osteoid
84002	Anterior	84046	Chondral
84003	Posterior	84047	Septation
84004	Central	84029	Trabecular
84050	Right	84030	Prominence
84052	First Carpal	84031	Thickening
84053	Second Carpal	84048	Sequestrum
84054	Third Carpal	84049	Ground Glass Appearence
84055	Fourth Carpal	84062	Sclerotic Lesion
84056	Fifth Carpal	84063	Location
84051	Left	84064	Superior
84057	First Carpal	84065	Inferior
84058	Second Carpal	84066	Medial
84059	Third Carpal	84067	Lateral
84060	Fourth Carpal	84068	Anterior
84061	Fifth Carpal	84069	Posterior
84005	Dimensions	84070	Central
84006	Height ___cm	84116	Right
84007	Transversely ___cm	84117	First Carpal
84008	AP (anteroposteriorly) ___cm	84118	Second Carpal
84009	Pattern	84119	Third Carpal
84010	Geographic	84120	Fourth Carpal
84011	Moth-eaten	84121	Fifth Carpal
84012	Permeative	84122	Left
84013	Zone Of Transition	84123	First Carpal
84014	Narrow	84124	Second Carpal
84015	Wide	84125	Third Carpal
84016	Margin	84126	Fourth Carpal
84017	Sclerotic	84127	Fifth Carpal
84018	Non-Sclerotic	84071	Dimensions
84019	Cortex	84072	Height ___cm
84020	Intact	84073	Transversely ___cm
84021	Destruction	84074	AP (anteroposteriorly) ___cm
84022	Endosteal Scalloping	84075	Pattern
84023	Expansion	84076	Geographic
84024	Thickening	84077	Moth-eaten
84025	Thinning	84078	Permeative
84026	Soft Tissue Mass	84079	Zone Of Transition
84027	Suspected	84080	Narrow
84028	Seen	84081	Wide

X-RAY, CONT.

84082	Margin	84192		Fourth Carpal
84083	Sclerotic	84193		Fifth Carpal
84084	Non-Sclerotic	84137	Dimensions	
84085	Cortex	84138		Height ___cm
84086	Intact	84139		Transversely ___cm
84087	Destruction	84140		AP (anteroposteriorly) ___cm
84088	Endosteal Scalloping	84141	Pattern	
84089	Expansion	84142		Geographic
84090	Thickening	84143		Moth-eaten
84091	Thinning	84144		Permeative
84092	Soft Tissue Mass	84145	Zone Of Transition	
84093	Suspected	84146		Narrow
84094	Seen	84147		Wide
84095	Periosteal Reaction	84148	Margin	
84096	Thick	84149		Sclerotic
84097	Thin	84150		Non-Sclerotic
84098	Uniform	84151	Cortex	
84099	Irregular	84152		Intact
84100	Dense	84153		Destruction
84101	Amorphous	84154		Endosteal Scalloping
84102	Wavy	84155		Expansion
84103	Lamellated	84156		Thickening
84104	Sunburst	84157		Thinning
84105	Spiculated	84158	Soft Tissue Mass	
84106	Codman Triangle	84159		Suspected
84107	Matrix	84160		Seen
84108	Osteoid	84161	Periosteal Reaction	
84109	Chondral	84162		Thick
84110	Septation	84163		Thin
84111	Trabecular	84164		Uniform
84112	Prominence	84165		Irregular
84113	Thickening	84166		Dense
84114	Sequestrum	84167		Amorphous
84115	Ground Glass Appearence	84168		Wavy
84128	Mixed Lytic / Sclerotic Lesion	84169		Lamellated
84129	Location	84170		Sunburst
84130	Superior	84171		Spiculated
84131	Inferior	84172		Codman Triangle
84132	Medial	84173	Matrix	
84133	Lateral	84174		Osteoid
84134	Anterior	84175		Chondral
84135	Posterior	84176	Septation	
84136	Central	84177	Trabecular	
84182	Right	84178		Prominence
84183	First Carpal	84179		Thickening
84184	Second Carpal	84180	Sequestrum	
84185	Third Carpal	84181	Ground Glass Appearence	
84186	Fourth Carpal	13805	**Forearm**	
84187	Fifth Carpal	102900	Views	
84188	Left	28536		Anteroposterior And Lateral Views
84189	First Carpal	27050		Right Forearm
84190	Second Carpal	27051		Left Forearm
84191	Third Carpal	27052		Both Forearms

X-RAY, CONT.

102844	No Radiographic Evidence Of Any Osteoarticular Abnormality	83361	Non-Septated
21021	Fracture Dislocation Of The Epiphysis	83362	Dimensions
29774	Fracture	83363	Height ___cm
29683	Open	83364	Transverse ___cm
29684	Closed	83365	AP ___cm
29685	Acute	83366	Location
29686	Old	83367	Cortical
29687	Stress	83368	Medullary
29688	Complete	83369	Central
29689	Incomplete	83370	Eccentric
29690	Pathologic	83371	Epiphyseal
29691	Pediatric	83372	Proximal
29692	Torus	83373	Distal
29693	Greenstick	83374	Metaphyseal
29694	Salter Type I	83375	Proximal
29695	Salter Type II	83376	Distal
29696	Salter Type III	83377	Diaphyseal
29697	Salter Type IV	83604	Left Radius
29698	Intra-articular	83606	Right Radius
29699	Extra-articular	83608	Left Ulna
29700	Comminuted	83609	Right Ulna
29701	Minimally	86043	Pattern
29702	Moderately	86044	Geographic
29703	Severely	86045	Moth-eaten
29704	Simple	86046	Permeative
29705	Displaced	86047	Zone Of Transition
29708	Non-displaced	86048	Narrow
29716	Pattern	86049	Wide
29709	Angulated	86050	Margin
29710	Spiral	86051	Sclerotic
29711	Oblique	86052	Non-Sclerotic
29712	Transverse	86053	Cortex
29713	Butterfly Component	86054	Intact
29714	Complex	86055	Destruction
29715	Avulsion	86056	Endosteal Scalloping
29717	Location	86057	Expansion
29718	Proximal	86058	Thickening
29719	Middle	86059	Thinning
29720	Medial	86060	Superior
29721	Lateral	86061	Inferior
29722	Anterior	86062	Medial
29723	Posterior	86063	Lateral
29724	Section	86064	Anterior
29725	Metaphyseal	86065	Posterior
29726	Diaphyseal	86066	Periosteal Reaction
29727	Epiphyseal	86067	Thick
80457	Right Radius	86068	Thin
80458	Right Ulna	86069	Uniform
80459	Left Radius	86070	Irregular
80460	Left Ulna	86071	Dense
83359	Lytic Lesion	86072	Amorphous
83360	Septated	86073	Wavy
		86074	Lamellated

X-RAY, CONT.

86075	Sunburst
86076	Spiculated
86077	Codman Triangle
86078	Matrix
86079	Osteoid
86080	Chondral
86081	Soft Tissue Mass
86082	Suspected
86083	Seen
86084	Superior
86085	Inferior
86086	Medial
86087	Lateral
86088	Anterior
86089	Trabecular
86090	Prominence
86091	Thickening
86092	Sequestrum
86093	Ground Glass Appearence
83378	Sclerotic Lesion
83381	Dimensions
83382	Height ___cm
83383	Transverse ___cm
83384	AP ___cm
83385	Location
83386	Cortical
83387	Medullary
83388	Central
83389	Eccentric
83390	Epiphyseal
83391	Proximal
83392	Distal
83393	Metaphyseal
83394	Proximal
83395	Distal
83396	Diaphyseal
83626	Left Radius
83627	Proximal
83628	Middle
83629	Distal
83630	Right Radius
83631	Proximal
83632	Middle
83633	Distal
83634	Left Ulna
83635	Proximal
83636	Middle
83638	Distal
83639	Right Ulna
83640	Proximal
83641	Middle
83642	Distal
86094	Pattern

86095	Geographic
86096	Moth-eaten
86097	Permeative
86098	Zone Of Transition
86099	Narrow
86100	Wide
86101	Margin
86102	Sclerotic
86103	Non-Sclerotic
86104	Cortex
86105	Intact
86106	Destruction
86107	Endosteal Scalloping
86108	Expansion
86109	Thickening
86110	Thinning
86111	Superior
86112	Inferior
86113	Medial
86114	Lateral
86115	Anterior
86116	Posterior
86117	Periosteal Reaction
86118	Thick
86119	Thin
86120	Uniform
86121	Irregular
86122	Dense
86123	Amorphous
86124	Wavy
86125	Lamellated
86126	Sunburst
86127	Spiculated
86128	Codman Triangle
86129	Matrix
86130	Osteoid
86131	Chondral
86132	Soft Tissue Mass
86133	Suspected
86134	Seen
86135	Superior
86136	Inferior
86137	Medial
86138	Lateral
86139	Anterior
86140	Trabecular
86141	Prominence
86142	Thickening
86143	Sequestrum
86144	Ground Glass Appearence
83101	Mixed Lytic/Sclerotic Lesion
83102	Septated
83103	Non-Septated

X-Ray, CONT.

83104	Dimensions		86167	Anterior
83105	Height ___ cm		86168	Posterior
83106	Transverse ___ cm		86169	Periosteal Reaction
83107	AP ___ cm		86170	Thick
83108	Location		86171	Thin
83109	Cortical		86172	Uniform
83110	Medullary		86173	Irregular
83111	Central		86174	Dense
83112	Eccentric		86175	Amorphous
83113	Epiphyseal		86176	Wavy
83114	Proximal		86177	Lamellated
83115	Distal		86178	Sunburst
83116	Metaphyseal		86179	Spiculated
83117	Proximal		86180	Codman Triangle
83118	Distal		86181	Matrix
83119	Diaphyseal		86182	Osteoid
83644	Left Radius		86183	Chondral
83645	Proximal		86184	Soft Tissue Mass
83646	Middle		86185	Suspected
83647	Distal		86186	Seen
83648	Right Radius		86187	Superior
83649	Proximal		86188	Inferior
83650	Middle		86189	Medial
83651	Distal		86190	Lateral
83652	Left Ulna		86191	Anterior
83653	Proximal		86192	Trabecular
83654	Middle		86193	Prominence
83655	Distal		86194	Thickening
83656	Right Ulna		86195	Sequestrum
83657	Proximal		86196	Ground Glass Appearence
83658	Middle		**13806**	**Elbow**
83659	Distal		102845	Views
86146	Pattern		28534	Anteroposterior And Lateral Views
86147	Geographic		28535	Complete, Three Or More Views
86148	Moth-eaten		29321	Arthrography
86149	Permeative		27053	Right Elbow
86150	Zone Of Transition		27054	Left Elbow
86151	Narrow		27055	Both Elbows
86152	Wide		102846	No Radiographic Evidence Of Any
86153	Margin			Osteoarticular Abnormality
86154	Sclerotic		29728	Fracture
86155	Non-Sclerotic		29729	Open
86156	Cortex		29730	Closed
86157	Intact		29731	Acute
86158	Destruction		29732	Old
86159	Endosteal Scalloping		29733	Stress
86160	Expansion		29734	Complete
86161	Thickening		29735	Incomplete
86162	Thinning		29736	Pathologic
86163	Superior		29737	Pediatric
86164	Inferior		29738	Torus
86165	Medial		29739	Greenstick
86166	Lateral		29740	Salter Type I

X-RAY, CONT.

29741	Salter Type II
29742	Salter Type III
29743	Salter Type IV
29744	Intra-articular
29745	Extra-articular
29746	Comminuted
29747	Minimally
29748	Moderately
29749	Severely
29750	Simple
29751	Displaced
29754	Non-displaced
29762	Pattern
29755	Angulated
29756	Spiral
29757	Oblique
29758	Transverse
29759	Butterfly Component
29760	Complex
29761	Avulsion
29763	Location
29764	Proximal
29765	Middle
29766	Medial
29767	Lateral
29768	Anterior
29769	Posterior
29770	Section
29771	Metaphyseal
29772	Diaphyseal
29773	Epiphyseal
80461	Right Proximal Radius
80462	Radial Head
80463	Radial Neck
80464	Right Proximal Ulna
80465	Olecranon
80466	Right Distal Humerus
80467	Coronoid
80468	Condylar
80469	Left Proximal Radius
80470	Radial Head
80471	Radial Neck
80472	Left Proximal Ulna
80473	Olecranon
80474	Left Distal Humerus
80475	Coronoid
80476	Condylar
80756	Dislocation
80757	Partial
80758	Complete
80759	Acute
80760	Old
80761	Recurrent

80824	Right Radial Head
80825	Right Elbow Joint
80826	Left Radial Head
80827	Left Elbow Joint
101168	Osteopenia
101169	Right
101170	Left
101171	Juxta-Articular
101172	Generalized
101173	Joint Effusion
101177	Right
101178	Left
101174	Displaced Fat Pad
101175	Anterior
101176	Posterior
101179	Narrowing Of Joint Space
101180	Right
101181	Left
101182	Proliferative Changes
101183	Sclerosis
101184	Right
101185	Left
101186	Radial Head
101187	Capitellum
101188	Trochlea
101189	Olecranon
101190	Osteophytes
101194	Single
101195	Multiple
101191	Right
101192	Left
101193	Radial Head
101196	Capitellum
101197	Trochlea
101198	Coronoid Process
101199	Bony Overgrowth
101200	Right
101201	Left
101202	Radial Head
101203	Epiphysis
101204	Capitellum
101205	Epiphysis
101206	Trochlea
101207	Epiphysis
101208	Coronoid Process
101209	Epiphysis
101210	Subchondral Cysts
101211	Single
101212	Multiple
101213	Right
101214	Left
101215	Radial Head
101216	Capitellum

X-RAY, CONT.

101217	Trochlea	29813		Moderately
101218	Coronoid Process	29814		Severely
101219	Erosions	29815	Simple	
101220	Right	29816	Displaced	
101221	Left	29819	Non-displaced	
101222	Radial Head	29827	Pattern	
101223	Capitellum	29820		Angulated
101224	Trochlea	29821		Spiral
101225	Coronoid Process	29822		Oblique
101226	Soft Tissue Calcification	29823		Transverse
101227	Right	29824		Butterfly Component
101228	Left	29825		Complex
101229	Lateral	29826		Avulsion
101230	Medial	29828	Location	
101231	Anterior	29829		Proximal
101232	Posterior	29830		Middle
101233	Radiodense Loose Bodies	29831		Medial
101234	Single	29832		Lateral
101235	Multiple	29833		Anterior
101236	Right	29834		Posterior
101237	Left	29835	Section	
101238	Lateral	29836		Metaphyseal
101239	Medial	29837		Diaphyseal
101240	Anterior	29838		Epiphyseal
101241	Posterior	80477	Right Humerus	
13807	**Arm**	80478	Left Humerus	
102901	Views	80936	Developmental Bone Age	
29344	Two Or More Views	80937	Retarded	
27056	Right Arm	80938	Advanced	
27057	Left Arm	83398	Lytic Lesion	
27058	Both Arms	83399	Septated	
102847	No Radiographic Evidence Of Any Osteoarticular Abnormality	83400	Non-Septated	
		83401	Dimensions	
29793	Fracture	83402	Height ___ cm	
29794	Open	83403	Transverse ___ cm	
29795	Closed	83404	AP ___ cm	
29796	Acute	83405	Location	
29797	Old	83406	Cortical	
29798	Stress	83407	Medullary	
29799	Complete	83408	Central	
29800	Incomplete	83409	Eccentric	
29801	Pathologic	83410	Epiphyseal	
29802	Pediatric	83411		Proximal
29803	Torus	83412		Distal
29804	Greenstick	83413	Metaphyseal	
29805	Salter Type I	83414		Proximal
29806	Salter Type II	83415		Distal
29807	Salter Type III	83416	Diaphyseal	
29808	Salter Type IV	83662	Left Humerus	
29809	Intra-articular	83663	Proximal	
29810	Extra-articular	83664	Middle	
29811	Comminuted	83665	Distal	
29812	Minimally	83666	Right Humerus	

X-RAY, CONT.

83667	Proximal		86247	Ground Glass Appearence
83668	Middle		83417	Sclerotic Lesion
83669	Distal		83420	Dimensions
86197	Pattern		83421	Height ___ cm
86198	Geographic		83422	Transverse ___ cm
86199	Moth-eaten		83423	AP ___ cm
86200	Permeative		83424	Location
86201	Zone Of Transition		83425	Cortical
86202	Narrow		83426	Medullary
86203	Wide		83427	Central
86204	Margin		83428	Eccentric
86205	Sclerotic		83429	Epiphyseal
86206	Non-Sclerotic		83430	Proximal
86207	Cortex		83431	Distal
86208	Intact		83432	Metaphyseal
86209	Destruction		83433	Proximal
86210	Endosteal Scalloping		83434	Distal
86211	Expansion		83435	Diaphyseal
86212	Thickening		83672	Left Humerus
86213	Thinning		83673	Proximal
86214	Superior		83674	Middle
86215	Inferior		83675	Distal
86216	Medial		83676	Right Humerus
86217	Lateral		83677	Proximal
86218	Anterior		83678	Middle
86219	Posterior		83679	Distal
86220	Periosteal Reaction		86248	Pattern
86221	Thick		86249	Geographic
86222	Thin		86250	Moth-eaten
86223	Uniform		86251	Permeative
86224	Irregular		86252	Zone Of Transition
86225	Dense		86253	Narrow
86226	Amorphous		86254	Wide
86227	Wavy		86255	Margin
86228	Lamellated		86256	Sclerotic
86229	Sunburst		86257	Non-Sclerotic
86230	Spiculated		86258	Cortex
86231	Codman Triangle		86259	Intact
86232	Matrix		86260	Destruction
86233	Osteoid		86261	Endosteal Scalloping
86234	Chondral		86262	Expansion
86235	Soft Tissue Mass		86263	Thickening
86236	Suspected		86264	Thinning
86237	Seen		86265	Superior
86238	Superior		86266	Inferior
86239	Inferior		86267	Medial
86240	Medial		86268	Lateral
86241	Lateral		86269	Anterior
86242	Anterior		86270	Posterior
86243	Trabecular		86271	Periosteal Reaction
86244	Prominence		86272	Thick
86245	Thickening		86273	Thin
86246	Sequestrum		86274	Uniform

X-RAY, CONT.

86275	Irregular		86301	Moth-eaten
86276	Dense		86302	Permeative
86277	Amorphous		86303	Zone Of Transition
86278	Wavy		86304	Narrow
86279	Lamellated		86305	Wide
86280	Sunburst		86306	Margin
86281	Spiculated		86307	Sclerotic
86282	Codman Triangle		86308	Non-Sclerotic
86283	Matrix		86309	Cortex
86284	Osteoid		86310	Intact
86285	Chondral		86311	Destruction
86286	Soft Tissue Mass		86312	Endosteal Scalloping
86287	Suspected		86313	Expansion
86288	Seen		86314	Thickening
86289	Superior		86315	Thinning
86290	Inferior		86316	Superior
86291	Medial		86317	Inferior
86292	Lateral		86318	Medial
86293	Anterior		86319	Lateral
86294	Trabecular		86320	Anterior
86295	Prominence		86321	Posterior
86296	Thickening		86322	Periosteal Reaction
86297	Sequestrum		86323	Thick
86298	Ground Glass Appearence		86324	Thin
83120	Mixed Lytic / Sclerotic Lesion		86325	Uniform
83121	Septated		86326	Irregular
83122	Non-Septated		86327	Dense
83123	Dimensions		86328	Amorphous
83124	Height ___ cm		86329	Wavy
83125	Transverse ___ cm		86330	Lamellated
83126	AP ___ cm		86331	Sunburst
83127	Location		86332	Spiculated
83128	Cortical		86333	Codman Triangle
83129	Medullary		86334	Matrix
83130	Central		86335	Osteoid
83131	Eccentric		86336	Chondral
83132	Epiphyseal		86337	Soft Tissue Mass
83133	Proximal		86338	Suspected
83134	Distal		86339	Seen
83135	Metaphyseal		86340	Superior
83136	Proximal		86341	Inferior
83137	Distal		86342	Medial
83138	Diaphyseal		86343	Lateral
83681	Left Humerus		86344	Anterior
83682	Proximal		86345	Trabecular
83683	Middle		86346	Prominence
83684	Distal		86347	Thickening
83685	Right Humerus		86348	Sequestrum
83686	Proximal		86349	Ground Glass Appearence
83687	Middle		13808	**Shoulder**
83688	Distal		102848	Views
86299	Pattern		28532	One View
86300	Geographic		28533	Complete, Two Or More Views

X-RAY, CONT.

29320	Arthrography	80481	Glenoid
27059	Right Shoulder	80482	Blade
27060	Left Shoulder	80483	Coracoid
27061	Both Shoulders	80484	Acromium
102849	No Radiographic Evidence Of Any	80485	Right Clavicle
	Osteoarticular Abnormality	80486	Left Proximal Humerus
29839	Fracture	80487	Left Scapula
29840	Open	80488	Glenoid
29841	Closed	80489	Blade
29842	Acute	80490	Coracoid
29843	Old	80491	Acromium
29844	Stress	80492	Left Clavicle
29845	Complete	80762	Dislocation
29846	Incomplete	80763	Partial
29847	Pathologic	80764	Complete
29848	Pediatric	80765	Acute
29849	Torus	80766	Old
29850	Greenstick	80767	Recurrent
29851	Salter Type I	80828	Anterior Displacement
29852	Salter Type II	80829	Anteroinferior Displacement
29853	Salter Type III	80830	Posterior Displacement
29854	Salter Type IV	80831	Posteroinferior Displacement
29855	Intra-articular	80832	Inferior Displacement
29856	Extra-articular	80833	Multidirectional Displacement
29857	Comminuted	80834	Right Glenohumeral Joint
29858	Minimally	80835	Right Acromioclavicular Joint
29859	Moderately	80836	Right Sternoclavicular Joint
29860	Severely	80837	Left Glenohumeral Joint
29861	Simple	80838	Left Acromioclavicular Joint
29862	Displaced	80839	Left Sternoclavicular Joint
29865	Non-displaced	101053	Osteopenia
29873	Pattern	101090	Right
29866	Angulated	101091	Left
29867	Spiral	101062	Juxta-Articular
29868	Oblique	101063	Generalized
29869	Transverse	101064	Narrowing of Joint Space
29928	Stellate	101092	Right
29870	Butterfly Component	101093	Left
29871	Complex	101065	Glenohumeral Joint
29872	Avulsion	101066	Acromio-Clavicular Joint
29874	Location	101067	Superior Migration
29875	Proximal	101094	Right
29876	Middle	101095	Left
29877	Medial	101068	Proliferative Changes
29878	Lateral	101069	Sclerosis
29879	Anterior	101096	Right
29880	Posterior	101097	Left
29881	Section	101070	Humeral Head
29882	Metaphyseal	101071	Glenoid
29883	Diaphyseal	101072	Osteophytes
29884	Epiphyseal	101098	Right
80479	Right Proximal Humerus	101099	Left
80480	Right Scapula	101073	Humeral Head

X-RAY, CONT.

101075	Lateral Aspect	101154	Left	
101076	Medial Aspect	101155	Superior	
101074	Acromio-Clavicular Joint	101156	Lateral	
101077	Inferior Aspect	101157	Medial	
101078	Subchondral Cysts	101158	Anterior	
101100	Right	101159	Posterior	
101101	Left	101160	Neuropathic Joint Appearance	
101079	Single	101162	Destruction	
101081	Multiple	101163	Right	
101082	Humeral Head	101164	Left	
101104	Erosion	101165	Debris	
101105	Right	101166	Right	
101106	Left	101167	Left	
101107	Humeral Head	85019	**Clavicle**	
101108	Lateral Aspect	102850	No Radiographic Evidence Of Any	
101109	Medial Aspect		Osteoarticular Abnormality	
101110	Glenoid	85020	Lytic Lesion	
101111	Distal Clavicle	85021	Location	
101112	Undersurface	85022	Superior	
101113	Soft Tissue Calcification	85023	Inferior	
101114	Right	85024	Medial	
101115	Left	85025	Lateral	
101116	Superior	85026	Anterior	
101117	Lateral	85027	Posterior	
101118	Radiodense Loose Bodies	85028	Central	
101133	Single	85359	Right	
101134	Multiple	85360	Left	
101119	Right	85361	Both	
101120	Left	85191	Dimensions	
101121	Superior	85192	Height ___ cm	
101122	Lateral	85031	Transversely ___ cm	
101123	Medial	85032	AP (anteroposteriorly) ___ cm	
101124	Anterior	85033	Pattern	
101125	Posterior	85034	Geographic	
101135	Osteonecrosis	85035	Moth-eaten	
101136	Sclerosis	85036	Permeative	
101137	Right	85037	Zone Of Transition	
101138	Left	85038	Narrow	
101139	Superior	85039	Wide	
101140	Lateral	85040	Margin	
101141	Medial	85041	Sclerotic	
101142	Anterior	85042	Non-Sclerotic	
101143	Posterior	85043	Cortex	
101144	Subchondral Lucency	85044	Intact	
101145	Right	85045	Destruction	
101146	Left	85046	Endosteal Scalloping	
101147	Superior	85047	Expansion	
101148	Lateral	85048	Thickening	
101149	Medial	85049	Thinning	
101150	Anterior	85050	Soft Tissue Mass	
101151	Posterior	85051	Suspected	
101152	Flattening	85052	Seen	
101153	Right	85053	Periosteal Reaction	

X-RAY, CONT.

85054	Thick
85055	Thin
85056	Uniform
85057	Irregular
85058	Dense
85059	Amorphous
85060	Wavy
85061	Lamellated
85062	Sunburst
85063	Spiculated
85064	Codman Triangle
85065	Matrix
85066	Osteoid
85067	Chondral
85068	Septation
85069	Trabecular
85070	Prominence
85071	Thickening
85072	Sequestrum
85073	Ground Glass Appearence
85074	Sclerotic Lesion
85075	Location
85076	Superior
85077	Inferior
85078	Medial
85079	Lateral
85080	Anterior
85081	Posterior
85082	Central
85363	Right
85364	Left
85365	Both
85083	Dimensions
85084	Height ___cm
85085	Transversely ___cm
85086	AP (anteroposteriorly) ___cm
85087	Pattern
85088	Geographic
85089	Moth-eaten
85090	Permeative
85091	Zone Of Transition
85092	Narrow
85093	Wide
85094	Margin
85095	Sclerotic
85096	Non-Sclerotic
85097	Cortex
85098	Intact
85099	Destruction
85100	Endosteal Scalloping
85101	Expansion
85102	Thickening
85103	Thinning

85104	Soft Tissue Mass
85105	Suspected
85106	Seen
85107	Periosteal Reaction
85108	Thick
85109	Thin
85110	Uniform
85111	Irregular
85112	Dense
85113	Amorphous
85114	Wavy
85115	Lamellated
85116	Sunburst
85117	Spiculated
85118	Codman Triangle
85119	Matrix
85120	Osteoid
85121	Chondral
85122	Septation
85123	Trabecular
85124	Prominence
85125	Thickening
85126	Sequestrum
85127	Ground Glass Appearence
85128	Mixed Lytic / Sclerotic Lesion
85129	Location
85130	Superior
85131	Inferior
85132	Medial
85133	Lateral
85134	Anterior
85135	Posterior
85136	Central
85370	Right
85371	Left
85372	Both
85137	Dimensions
85138	Height ___cm
85139	Transversely ___cm
85140	AP (anteroposteriorly) ___cm
85141	Pattern
85142	Geographic
85143	Moth-eaten
85144	Permeative
85145	Zone Of Transition
85146	Narrow
85147	Wide
85148	Margin
85149	Sclerotic
85150	Non-Sclerotic
85151	Cortex
85152	Intact
85153	Destruction

X-RAY, CONT.

85154	Endosteal Scalloping		85201	Wide
85155	Expansion		85202	Margin
85156	Thickening		85203	Sclerotic
85157	Thinning		85204	Non-Sclerotic
85158	Soft Tissue Mass		85205	Cortex
85159	Suspected		85206	Intact
85160	Seen		85207	Destruction
85161	Periosteal Reaction		85208	Endosteal Scalloping
85162	Thick		85209	Expansion
85163	Thin		85210	Thickening
85164	Uniform		85211	Thinning
85165	Irregular		85212	Soft Tissue Mass
85166	Dense		85213	Suspected
85167	Amorphous		85214	Seen
85168	Wavy		85215	Periosteal Reaction
85169	Lamellated		85216	Thick
85170	Sunburst		85217	Thin
85171	Spiculated		85218	Uniform
85172	Codman Triangle		85219	Irregular
85173	Matrix		85220	Dense
85174	Osteoid		85221	Amorphous
85175	Chondral		85222	Wavy
85176	Septation		85223	Lamellated
85177	Trabecular		85224	Sunburst
85178	Prominence		85225	Spiculated
85179	Thickening		85226	Codman Triangle
85180	Sequestrum		85227	Matrix
85181	Ground Glass Appearence		85228	Osteoid
85344	**Scapula**		85229	Chondral
102851	No Radiographic Evidence Of Any		85230	Septation
	Osteoarticular Abnormality		85231	Trabecular
85182	Lytic Lesion		85232	Prominence
85183	Location		85233	Thickening
85184	Superior		85234	Sequestrum
85185	Inferior		85235	Ground Glass Appearence
85186	Medial		85236	Sclerotic Lesion
85187	Lateral		85237	Location
85188	Anterior		85238	Superior
85189	Posterior		85239	Inferior
85190	Central		85240	Medial
85345	Right		85241	Lateral
85348	Left		85242	Anterior
85349	Both		85243	Posterior
85029	Dimensions		85244	Central
85030	Height ___cm		85350	Right
85193	Transversely ___cm		85351	Left
85194	AP (anteroposteriorly) ___cm		85352	Both
85195	Pattern		85245	Dimensions
85196	Geographic		85246	Height ___cm
85197	Moth-eaten		85247	Transversely ___cm
85198	Permeative		85248	AP (anteroposteriorly) ___cm
85199	Zone Of Transition		85249	Pattern
85200	Narrow		85250	Geographic

X-RAY, CONT.

85251	Moth-eaten		85301	Transversely ___ cm
85252	Permeative		85302	AP (anteroposteriorly) ___ cm
85253	Zone Of Transition		85303	Pattern
85254	Narrow		85304	Geographic
85255	Wide		85305	Moth-eaten
85256	Margin		85306	Permeative
85257	Sclerotic		85307	Zone Of Transition
85258	Non-Sclerotic		85308	Narrow
85259	Cortex		85309	Wide
85260	Intact		85310	Margin
85261	Destruction		85311	Sclerotic
85262	Endosteal Scalloping		85312	Non-Sclerotic
85263	Expansion		85313	Cortex
85264	Thickening		85314	Intact
85265	Thinning		85315	Destruction
85266	Soft Tissue Mass		85316	Endosteal Scalloping
85267	Suspected		85317	Expansion
85268	Seen		85318	Thickening
85269	Periosteal Reaction		85319	Thinning
85270	Thick		85320	Soft Tissue Mass
85271	Thin		85321	Suspected
85272	Uniform		85322	Seen
85273	Irregular		85323	Periosteal Reaction
85274	Dense		85324	Thick
85275	Amorphous		85325	Thin
85276	Wavy		85326	Uniform
85277	Lamellated		85327	Irregular
85278	Sunburst		85328	Dense
85279	Spiculated		85329	Amorphous
85280	Codman Triangle		85330	Wavy
85281	Matrix		85331	Lamellated
85282	Osteoid		85332	Sunburst
85283	Chondral		85333	Spiculated
85284	Septation		85334	Codman Triangle
85285	Trabecular		85335	Matrix
85286	Prominence		85336	Osteoid
85287	Thickening		85337	Chondral
85288	Sequestrum		85338	Septation
85289	Ground Glass Appearence		85339	Trabecular
85290	Mixed Lytic / Sclerotic Lesion		85340	Prominence
85291	Location		85341	Thickening
85292	Superior		85342	Sequestrum
85293	Inferior		85343	Ground Glass Appearence
85294	Medial		28395	Survey Study Of Entire Spine
85295	Lateral		28396	Single View Of Spine
85296	Anterior		13851	**Ribs**
85297	Posterior		102902	Views
85298	Central		22580	Unilateral
85354	Right		22581	Two Views
85355	Left		22582	Three Or More Views Including
85356	Both			Posteroanterior Chest
85299	Dimensions		22583	Bilateral
85300	Height ___ cm		22584	Three Views

X-Ray, cont.

22585	Four Or More Views Including		80538	Right Manubrium
	Posteroanterior Chest		80539	Left Sternum
22586	Sternum		80540	Left Manubrium
22587	Two Or More Views		18028	Bone Erosion
22588	Three Or More Views Including		84303	Lytic Lesion
	Sternoclavicular Joint(s)		84304	Location
102852	No Radiographic Evidence Of Any		84305	Superior
	Osteoarticular Abnormality		84306	Inferior
18225	Fracture		84307	Medial
80493	Open		84308	Lateral
80494	Closed		84309	Anterior
18226	Multiple Ribs		84310	Posterior
80495	Acute		84311	Central
80496	Old		84656	Right
80497	Stress		84657	Rib 1st
80498	Complete		84658	Rib 2nd
80499	Incomplete		84659	Rib 3rd
80500	Pathologic		84660	Rib 4th
80501	Pediatric		84661	Rib 5th
80502	Greenstick		84662	Rib 6th
80503	Salter Type I		84663	Rib 7th
80504	Salter Type II		84664	Rib 8th
80505	Salter Type III		84665	Rib 9th
80506	Salter Type IV		84666	Rib 10th
80507	Intra-articular		84667	Rib 11th
80508	Extra-articular		84668	Rib 12th
80509	Comminuted		84669	Left
80510	Minimally		84670	Rib 1st
80511	Moderately		84671	Rib 2nd
80512	Severely		84672	Rib 3rd
80513	Simple		84673	Rib 4th
80514	Displaced		84674	Rib 5th
80517	Non-displaced		84675	Rib 6th
80525	Pattern		84676	Rib 7th
80518	Angulated		84677	Rib 8th
80519	Spiral		84678	Rib 9th
80520	Oblique		84679	Rib 10th
80521	Transverse		84680	Rib 11th
80522	Butterfly Component		84681	Rib 12th
80523	Complex		84682	Both
80524	Avulsion		84312	Dimensions
80526	Location		84313	Height ___cm
80527	Proximal		84314	Transversely ___cm
80528	Middle		84315	AP (anteroposteriorly) ___ cm
80529	Medial		84316	Pattern
80530	Lateral		84317	Geographic
80531	Anterior		84318	Moth-eaten
80532	Posterior		84319	Permeative
80533	Section		84320	Zone Of Transition
80534	Metaphyseal		84321	Narrow
80535	Diaphyseal		84322	Wide
80536	Epiphyseal		84323	Margin
80537	Right Sternum		84324	Sclerotic

X-RAY, CONT.

84325	Non-Sclerotic		84641	Rib 12th
84326	Cortex		84642	Left
84327	Intact		84643	Rib 1st
84328	Destruction		84644	Rib 2nd
84329	Endosteal Scalloping		84645	Rib 3rd
84330	Expansion		84646	Rib 4th
84331	Thickening		84647	Rib 5th
84332	Thinning		84648	Rib 6th
84333	Soft Tissue Mass		84649	Rib 7th
84334	Suspected		84650	Rib 8th
84335	Seen		84651	Rib 9th
84336	Periosteal Reaction		84652	Rib 10th
84337	Thick		84653	Rib 11th
84338	Thin		84654	Rib 12th
84339	Uniform		84655	Both
84340	Irregular		84258	Dimensions
84341	Dense		84259	Height ___cm
84342	Amorphous		84260	Transversely ___cm
84343	Wavy		84261	AP (anteroposteriorly) ___cm
84344	Lamellated		84262	Pattern
84345	Sunburst		84263	Geographic
84346	Spiculated		84264	Moth-eaten
84347	Codman Triangle		84265	Permeative
84348	Matrix		84266	Zone Of Transition
84349	Osteoid		84267	Narrow
84350	Chondral		84268	Wide
84351	Septation		84269	Margin
84352	Trabecular		84270	Sclerotic
84353	Prominence		84271	Non-Sclerotic
84354	Thickening		84272	Cortex
84355	Sequestrum		84273	Intact
84356	Ground Glass Appearence		84274	Destruction
84249	Sclerotic Lesion		84275	Endosteal Scalloping
84250	Location		84276	Expansion
84251	Superior		84277	Thickening
84252	Inferior		84278	Thinning
84253	Medial		84279	Soft Tissue Mass
84254	Lateral		84280	Suspected
84255	Anterior		84281	Seen
84256	Posterior		84282	Periosteal Reaction
84257	Central		84283	Thick
84629	Right		84284	Thin
84630	Rib 1st		84285	Uniform
84631	Rib 2nd		84286	Irregular
84632	Rib 3rd		84287	Dense
84633	Rib 4th		84288	Amorphous
84634	Rib 5th		84289	Wavy
84635	Rib 6th		84290	Lamellated
84636	Rib 7th		84291	Sunburst
84637	Rib 8th		84292	Spiculated
84638	Rib 9th		84293	Codman Triangle
84639	Rib 10th		84294	Matrix
84640	Rib 11th		84295	Osteoid

X-RAY, CONT.

84296	Chondral	84213	Wide
84297	Septation	84214	Margin
84298	Trabecular	84215	Sclerotic
84299	Prominence	84216	Non-Sclerotic
84300	Thickening	84217	Cortex
84301	Sequestrum	84218	Intact
84302	Ground Glass Appearence	84219	Destruction
84194	Mixed Lytic / Sclerotic Lesion	84220	Endosteal Scalloping
84195	Location	84221	Expansion
84196	Superior	84222	Thickening
84197	Inferior	84223	Thinning
84198	Medial	84224	Soft Tissue Mass
84199	Lateral	84225	Suspected
84200	Anterior	84226	Seen
84201	Posterior	84227	Periosteal Reaction
84202	Central	84228	Thick
84248	Right	84229	Thin
84357	Rib 1st	84230	Uniform
84360	Rib 2nd	84231	Irregular
84361	Rib 3rd	84232	Dense
84362	Rib 4th	84233	Amorphous
84363	Rib 5th	84234	Wavy
84364	Rib 6th	84235	Lamellated
84365	Rib 7th	84236	Sunburst
84366	Rib 8th	84237	Spiculated
84367	Rib 9th	84238	Codman Triangle
84368	Rib 10th	84239	Matrix
84369	Rib 11th	84240	Osteoid
84370	Rib 12th	84241	Chondral
84358	Left	84242	Septation
84617	Rib 1st	84243	Trabecular
84618	Rib 2nd	84244	Prominence
84619	Rib 3rd	84245	Thickening
84620	Rib 4th	84246	Sequestrum
84621	Rib 5th	84247	Ground Glass Appearence
84622	Rib 6th	13810	**Cervical Spine**
84623	Rib 7th	102853	Views
84624	Rib 8th	28389	Anteroposterior And Lateral Views
84625	Rib 9th	28392	Including Oblique And Flexion Studies
84626	Rib 10th		
84627	Rib 11th	28394	And Extension Studies
84628	Rib 12th	28390	Four Or More Views
84359	Both	28391	Complete
84203	Dimensions	28393	Including Oblique And Extension Studies
84204	Height ___cm		
84205	Transversely ___cm	102854	No Radiographic Evidence Of Any Osteoarticular Abnormality
84206	AP (anteroposteriorly) ___cm		
84207	Pattern	13811	Fracture
84208	Geographic	29885	Open
84209	Moth-eaten	29886	Closed
84210	Permeative	29887	Acute
84211	Zone Of Transition	29888	Old
84212	Narrow	29889	Stress

X-RAY, CONT.

29890	Complete	89269	At C3 - C4
29891	Incomplete	89265	At C4 - C5
29892	Pathologic	13819	At C5 - C6
13812	Compression	13820	At C6 - C7
29544	Burst	89266	At C7 - T1
13813	Pars Interarticularis	89284	Endplate Abnormality
13815	Odontoid	89288	Sclerosis
29893	Pediatric	89291	Inferior Endplate Of C1
29894	Torus	89292	Superior Endplate Of C2
29895	Greenstick	89293	Inferior Endplate Of C2
29896	Salter Type I	89294	Superior Endplate Of C3
29897	Salter Type II	89295	Inferior Endplate Of C3
29898	Salter Type III	89296	Superior Endplate Of C4
29899	Salter Type IV	89297	Inferior Endplate Of C4
29900	Comminuted	89298	Superior Endplate Of C5
29901	Minimally	89299	Inferior Endplate Of C5
29902	Moderately	89300	Superior Endplate Of C6
29903	Severely	89301	Inferior Endplate Of C6
29904	Simple	89302	Superior Endplate Of C7
29905	Displaced	89303	Inferior Endplate Of C7
29908	Non-displaced	89304	Superior Endplate Of T1
29916	Pattern	89289	Irregularity
29909	Angulated	89305	Inferior Endplate Of C1
29910	Spiral	89306	Superior Endplate Of C2
29911	Oblique	89307	Inferior Endplate Of C2
13814	transverse process	89308	Superior Endplate Of C3
29913	Butterfly Component	89309	Inferior Endplate Of C3
29914	Complex	89310	Superior Endplate Of C4
29915	Avulsion	89311	Inferior Endplate Of C4
29917	Location	89312	Superior Endplate Of C5
29918	Proximal	89313	Inferior Endplate Of C5
29919	Middle	89314	Superior Endplate Of C6
29920	Medial	89315	Inferior Endplate Of C6
29921	Lateral	89316	Superior Endplate Of C7
29922	Anterior	89317	Inferior Endplate Of C7
29923	Posterior	89318	Superior Endplate Of T1
29924	Section	89290	Destruction
29925	Metaphyseal	89319	Inferior Endplate Of C1
29926	Diaphyseal	89320	Superior Endplate Of C2
29927	Epiphyseal	89321	Inferior Endplate Of C2
80541	C1	89322	Superior Endplate Of C3
80542	C2	89323	Inferior Endplate Of C3
80543	C3	89324	Superior Endplate Of C4
80544	C4	89325	Inferior Endplate Of C4
80545	C5	89326	Superior Endplate Of C5
80546	C6	89327	Inferior Endplate Of C5
80547	C7	89328	Superior Endplate Of C6
13816	Subluxation	89329	Inferior Endplate Of C6
13817	Atlanto-Axial	89330	Superior Endplate Of C7
89261	Osteopenia	89331	Inferior Endplate Of C7
13818	Disc Space Narrowing	89332	Superior Endplate Of T1
89267	At C1 - C2	89423	Apophyseal Joints
89268	At C2 - C3	89424	Narrowing

X-RAY, CONT.

89426	At C1 - C2		89471	Superior Endplate Of T1
89427	At C2 - C3		89510	Posterior Vertebral Bodies
89428	At C3 - C4		89511	At C1 - C2
89429	At C4 - C5		89512	At C2 - C3
89430	At C5 - C6		89513	At C3 - C4
89431	At C6 - C7		89514	At C4 - C5
89432	At C7 - T1		89515	At C5 - C6
89425	Sclerosis		89516	At C6 - C7
89433	At C1 - C2		89517	At C7 - T1
89434	At C2 - C3		89534	Flowing Ossification
89435	At C3 - C4		89536	At C1 - C2
89436	At C4 - C5		89537	At C2 - C3
89437	At C5 - C6		89538	At C3 - C4
89438	At C6 - C7		89539	At C4 - C5
89439	At C7 - T1		89540	At C5 - C6
13821	Osteophytes		89541	At C6 - C7
89442	Anterior		89542	At C7 - T1
89444	Inferior Endplate Of C1		89535	Bony Ankylosis
89445	Superior Endplate Of C2		89550	Vertebral Bodies
89446	Inferior Endplate Of C2		89543	C1 and C2
89447	Superior Endplate Of C3		89544	C2 and C3
89448	Inferior Endplate Of C3		89545	C3 and C4
89449	Superior Endplate Of C4		89546	C4 and C5
89450	Inferior Endplate Of C4		89547	C5 and C6
89451	Superior Endplate Of C5		89548	C6 and C7
89452	Inferior Endplate Of C5		89549	C7 and T1
89453	Superior Endplate Of C6		89555	Posterior Elements
89454	Inferior Endplate Of C6		89566	At C1 - C2
89455	Superior Endplate Of C7		89567	At C2 - C3
89456	Inferior Endplate Of C7		89568	At C3 - C4
89457	Superior Endplate Of T1		89569	At C4 - C5
89509	Anterior Vertebral Bodies		89570	At C5 - C6
89502	At C1 - C2		89571	At C6 - C7
89503	At C2 - C3		89572	At C7 - T1
89504	At C3 - C4		89578	Apophyseal Joints
89505	At C4 - C5		89579	At C1 - C2
89506	At C5 - C6		89581	At C2 - C3
89507	At C6 - C7		89582	At C3 - C4
89508	At C7 - T1		89583	At C4 - C5
89443	Posterior		89584	At C5 - C6
89458	Inferior Endplate Of C1		89585	At C6 - C7
89459	Superior Endplate Of C2		89586	At C7 - T1
89460	Inferior Endplate Of C2		89589	Odontoid Erosion
89461	Superior Endplate Of C3		89590	Mild
89462	Inferior Endplate Of C3		89591	Moderate
89463	Superior Endplate Of C4		89592	Severe
89464	Inferior Endplate Of C4		89593	Atlanto-Dental Widening
89465	Superior Endplate Of C5		89595	Flexion
89466	Inferior Endplate Of C5		89602	Distance ___mm
89467	Superior Endplate Of C6		89598	Flexion and Extension
89468	Inferior Endplate Of C6		89603	Distance ___mm
89469	Superior Endplate Of C7		89600	Improves With Extension ___mm
89470	Inferior Endplate Of C7		89604	Neural Foraminal Narrowing

X-RAY, CONT.

89609	Right	87021	C5 Vertebral Body
89610	At C1 - C2	87022	C6 Vertebral Body
89611	At C2 - C3	87023	C7 Vertebral Body
89612	At C3 - C4	86991	Anterior
89613	At C4 - C5	87037	C1 Vertebral Body
89614	At C5 - C6	87031	C2 Vertebral Body
89615	At C6 - C7	87032	C3 Vertebral Body
89616	At C7 - T1	87033	C4 Vertebral Body
89608	Left	87034	C5 Vertebral Body
89617	At C1 - C2	87035	C6 Vertebral Body
89618	At C2 - C3	87036	C7 Vertebral Body
89619	At C3 - C4	86992	Posterior
89620	At C4 - C5	87024	C1 Vertebral Body
89621	At C5 - C6	87025	C2 Vertebral Body
89622	At C6 - C7	87026	C3 Vertebral Body
89623	At C7 - T1	87027	C4 Vertebral Body
89654	Both	87028	C5 Vertebral Body
89655	At C1 - C2	87029	C6 Vertebral Body
89656	At C2 - C3	87030	C7 Vertebral Body
89657	At C3 - C4	86993	Right
89658	At C4 - C5	87010	C1 Vertebral Body
89659	At C5 - C6	87011	C2 Vertebral Body
89660	At C6 - C7	87012	C3 Vertebral Body
89661	At C7 - T1	87013	C4 Vertebral Body
13822	Bone Erosion	87014	C5 Vertebral Body
13823	Subchondral Bone Plate	87015	C6 Vertebral Body
13824	Vertebral Body	87016	C7 Vertebral Body
13825	Pedicle	86994	Left
13826	Transverse Process	87038	C1 Vertebral Body
13827	Lamina	87039	C2 Vertebral Body
13828	Spinous Process	87040	C3 Vertebral Body
13829	Bone Density Decreased	87041	C4 Vertebral Body
13830	Bone Density Increased	87042	C5 Vertebral Body
18005	Diffuse	87043	C6 Vertebral Body
18006	Localized	87044	C7 Vertebral Body
18038	Spina Bifida	87045	Right Pedicle
13831	Calcifications	87073	C1 Pedicle On The Right
13832	Disc Space	87074	C2 Pedicle On The Right
86987	Lytic Lesion	87075	C3 Pedicle On The Right
86988	Location	87076	C4 Pedicle On The Right
86989	Superior	87077	C5 Pedicle On The Right
87001	C1 Vertebral Body	87078	C6 Pedicle On The Right
87004	C2 Vertebral Body	87079	C7 Pedicle On The Right
87005	C3 Vertebral Body	87048	Left Pedicle
87006	C4 Vertebral Body	87080	C1 Pedicle On The Left
87007	C5 Vertebral Body	87081	C2 Pedicle On The Left
87008	C6 Vertebral Body	87082	C3 Pedicle On The Left
87009	C7 Vertebral Body	87083	C4 Pedicle On The Left
86990	Inferior	87084	C5 Pedicle On The Left
87017	C1 Vertebral Body	87085	C6 Pedicle On The Left
87018	C2 Vertebral Body	87086	C7 Pedicle On The Left
87019	C3 Vertebral Body	87049	Both Pedicles
87020	C4 Vertebral Body	87087	C1 Pedicle On Both Sides

X-RAY, CONT.

87088	C2 Pedicle On Both Sides	86976	Destruction
87089	C3 Pedicle On Both Sides	87102	Superior
87090	C4 Pedicle On Both Sides	87103	Inferior
87091	C5 Pedicle On Both Sides	87104	Anterior
87092	C6 Pedicle On Both Sides	87105	Posterior
87093	C7 Pedicle On Both Sides	87106	Right
87046	Right Lamina	87107	Left
87052	C1 Lamina On The Right	86977	Expansion
87053	C2 Lamina On The Right	87108	Superior
87054	C3 Lamina On The Right	87109	Inferior
87055	C4 Lamina On The Right	87110	Anterior
87056	C5 Lamina On The Right	87111	Posterior
87057	C6 Lamina On The Right	87112	Right
87058	C7 Lamina On The Right	87113	Left
87050	Left Lamina	86978	Thickening
87059	C1 Lamina On The Left	87114	Superior
87060	C2 Lamina On The Left	87115	Inferior
87061	C3 Lamina On The Left	87116	Anterior
87062	C4 Lamina On The Left	87117	Posterior
87063	C5 Lamina On The Left	87118	Right
87064	C6 Lamina On The Left	87119	Left
87065	C7 Lamina On The Left	86979	Thinning
87051	Both Lamina	87120	Superior
87066	C1 Lamina On Both Sides	87121	Inferior
87067	C2 Lamina On Both Sides	87122	Anterior
87068	C3 Lamina On Both Sides	87123	Posterior
87069	C4 Lamina On Both Sides	87124	Right
87070	C5 Lamina On Both Sides	87125	Left
87071	C6 Lamina On Both Sides	86980	Soft Tissue Mass
87072	C7 Lamina On Both Sides	86981	Suspected
87047	Spinous Process	87126	Superior
87094	C1 Spinous Process	87127	Inferior
87095	C2 Spinous Process	87128	Anterior
87096	C3 Spinous Process	87129	Posterior
87097	C4 Spinous Process	87130	Right
87098	C5 Spinous Process	87131	Left
87099	C6 Spinous Process	86982	Seen
87100	C7 Spinous Process	87132	Superior
87101	Bone Expansion	87133	Inferior
86968	Zone Of Transition	87134	Anterior
86969	Narrow	87135	Posterior
86970	Wide	87136	Right
86971	Margin	87137	Left
86972	Sclerotic	87138	Displaced Bone Fragment
86973	Non-Sclerotic	87139	___cm
86974	Cortex	87141	Superior
86975	Intact	87142	Inferior
86995	Superior	87143	Anterior
86996	Inferior	87144	Posterior
86997	Anterior	87145	Right
86998	Posterior	87146	Left
86999	Right	87140	Central Canal
87267	Left	86983	Trabecular

X-RAY, CONT.

86984	Prominence	87551	Right Pedicle
86985	Thickening	87552	C1 Pedicle On The Right
86986	Sequestrum	87553	C2 Pedicle On The Right
87501	Sclerotic Lesion	87554	C3 Pedicle On The Right
87502	Location	87555	C4 Pedicle On The Right
87503	Superior	87556	C5 Pedicle On The Right
87504	C1 Vertebral Body	87557	C6 Pedicle On The Right
87505	C2 Vertebral Body	87558	C7 Pedicle On The Right
87506	C3 Vertebral Body	87559	Left Pedicle
87507	C4 Vertebral Body	87560	C1 Pedicle On The Left
87508	C5 Vertebral Body	87561	C2 Pedicle On The Left
87509	C6 Vertebral Body	87562	C3 Pedicle On The Left
87510	C7 Vertebral Body	87563	C4 Pedicle On The Left
87511	Inferior	87564	C5 Pedicle On The Left
87512	C1 Vertebral Body	87565	C6 Pedicle On The Left
87513	C2 Vertebral Body	87566	C7 Pedicle On The Left
87514	C3 Vertebral Body	87567	Both Pedicles
87515	C4 Vertebral Body	87568	C1 Pedicle On Both Sides
87516	C5 Vertebral Body	87569	C2 Pedicle On Both Sides
87517	C6 Vertebral Body	87570	C3 Pedicle On Both Sides
87518	C7 Vertebral Body	87571	C4 Pedicle On Both Sides
87519	Anterior	87572	C5 Pedicle On Both Sides
87520	C1 Vertebral Body	87573	C6 Pedicle On Both Sides
87521	C2 Vertebral Body	87574	C7 Pedicle On Both Sides
87522	C3 Vertebral Body	87575	Right Lamina
87523	C4 Vertebral Body	87576	C1 Lamina On The Right
87524	C5 Vertebral Body	87577	C2 Lamina On The Right
87525	C6 Vertebral Body	87578	C3 Lamina On The Right
87526	C7 Vertebral Body	87579	C4 Lamina On The Right
87527	Posterior	87580	C5 Lamina On The Right
87528	C1 Vertebral Body	87581	C6 Lamina On The Right
87529	C2 Vertebral Body	87582	C7 Lamina On The Right
87530	C3 Vertebral Body	87583	Left Lamina
87531	C4 Vertebral Body	87584	C1 Lamina On The Left
87532	C5 Vertebral Body	87585	C2 Lamina On The Left
87533	C6 Vertebral Body	87586	C3 Lamina On The Left
87534	C7 Vertebral Body	87587	C4 Lamina On The Left
87535	Right	87588	C5 Lamina On The Left
87536	C1 Vertebral Body	87589	C6 Lamina On The Left
87537	C2 Vertebral Body	87590	C7 Lamina On The Left
87538	C3 Vertebral Body	87591	Both Lamina
87539	C4 Vertebral Body	87592	C1 Lamina On Both Sides
87540	C5 Vertebral Body	87593	C2 Lamina On Both Sides
87541	C6 Vertebral Body	87594	C3 Lamina On Both Sides
87542	C7 Vertebral Body	87595	C4 Lamina On Both Sides
87543	Left	87596	C5 Lamina On Both Sides
87544	C1 Vertebral Body	87597	C6 Lamina On Both Sides
87545	C2 Vertebral Body	87598	C7 Lamina On Both Sides
87546	C3 Vertebral Body	87599	Spinous Process
87547	C4 Vertebral Body	87600	C1 Spinous Process
87548	C5 Vertebral Body	87601	C2 Spinous Process
87549	C6 Vertebral Body	87602	C3 Spinous Process
87550	C7 Vertebral Body	87603	C4 Spinous Process

X-RAY, CONT.

87604	C5 Spinous Process	87657	Left
87605	C6 Spinous Process	87658	Seen
87606	C7 Spinous Process	87659	Superior
87607	Bone Expansion	87660	Inferior
87608	Zone Of Transition	87661	Anterior
87609	Narrow	87662	Posterior
87610	Wide	87663	Right
87611	Margin	87664	Left
87612	Sclerotic	87665	Displaced Bone Fragment
87613	Non-Sclerotic	87666	___cm
87614	Cortex	87667	Superior
87615	Intact	87668	Inferior
87616	Superior	87669	Anterior
87617	Inferior	87670	Posterior
87618	Anterior	87671	Right
87619	Posterior	87672	Left
87620	Right	87673	Central Canal
87621	Left	87674	Trabecular
87622	Destruction	87675	Prominence
87623	Superior	87676	Thickening
87624	Inferior	87677	Sequestrum
87625	Anterior	87678	Mixed Lytic / Sclerotic Lesion
87626	Posterior	87679	Location
87627	Right	87680	Superior
87628	Left	87681	C1 Vertebral Body
87629	Expansion	87682	C2 Vertebral Body
87630	Superior	87683	C3 Vertebral Body
87631	Inferior	87684	C4 Vertebral Body
87632	Anterior	87685	C5 Vertebral Body
87633	Posterior	87686	C6 Vertebral Body
87634	Right	87687	C7 Vertebral Body
87635	Left	87688	Inferior
87636	Thickening	87689	C1 Vertebral Body
87637	Superior	87690	C2 Vertebral Body
87638	Inferior	87691	C3 Vertebral Body
87639	Anterior	87692	C4 Vertebral Body
87640	Posterior	87693	C5 Vertebral Body
87641	Right	87694	C6 Vertebral Body
87642	Left	87695	C7 Vertebral Body
87643	Thinning	87696	Anterior
87644	Superior	87697	C1 Vertebral Body
87645	Inferior	87698	C2 Vertebral Body
87646	Anterior	87699	C3 Vertebral Body
87647	Posterior	87700	C4 Vertebral Body
87648	Right	87701	C5 Vertebral Body
87649	Left	87702	C6 Vertebral Body
87650	Soft Tissue Mass	87703	C7 Vertebral Body
87651	Suspected	87704	Posterior
87652	Superior	87705	C1 Vertebral Body
87653	Inferior	87706	C2 Vertebral Body
87654	Anterior	87707	C3 Vertebral Body
87655	Posterior	87708	C4 Vertebral Body
87656	Right	87709	C5 Vertebral Body

X-RAY, CONT.

87710	C6 Vertebral Body	87763	C3 Lamina On The Left
87711	C7 Vertebral Body	87764	C4 Lamina On The Left
87712	Right	87765	C5 Lamina On The Left
87713	C1 Vertebral Body	87766	C6 Lamina On The Left
87714	C2 Vertebral Body	87767	C7 Lamina On The Left
87715	C3 Vertebral Body	87768	Both Lamina
87716	C4 Vertebral Body	87769	C1 Lamina On Both Sides
87717	C5 Vertebral Body	87770	C2 Lamina On Both Sides
87718	C6 Vertebral Body	87771	C3 Lamina On Both Sides
87719	C7 Vertebral Body	87772	C4 Lamina On Both Sides
87720	Left	87773	C5 Lamina On Both Sides
87721	C1 Vertebral Body	87774	C6 Lamina On Both Sides
87722	C2 Vertebral Body	87775	C7 Lamina On Both Sides
87723	C3 Vertebral Body	87776	Spinous Process
87724	C4 Vertebral Body	87777	C1 Spinous Process
87725	C5 Vertebral Body	87778	C2 Spinous Process
87726	C6 Vertebral Body	87779	C3 Spinous Process
87727	C7 Vertebral Body	87780	C4 Spinous Process
87728	Right Pedicle	87781	C5 Spinous Process
87729	C1 Pedicle On The Right	87782	C6 Spinous Process
87730	C2 Pedicle On The Right	87783	C7 Spinous Process
87731	C3 Pedicle On The Right	87784	Bone Expansion
87732	C4 Pedicle On The Right	87785	Zone Of Transition
87733	C5 Pedicle On The Right	87786	Narrow
87734	C6 Pedicle On The Right	87787	Wide
87735	C7 Pedicle On The Right	87788	Margin
87736	Left Pedicle	87789	Sclerotic
87737	C1 Pedicle On The Left	87790	Non-Sclerotic
87738	C2 Pedicle On The Left	87791	Cortex
87739	C3 Pedicle On The Left	87792	Intact
87740	C4 Pedicle On The Left	87793	Superior
87741	C5 Pedicle On The Left	87794	Inferior
87742	C6 Pedicle On The Left	87795	Anterior
87743	C7 Pedicle On The Left	87796	Posterior
87744	Both Pedicles	87797	Right
87745	C1 Pedicle On Both Sides	87798	Left
87746	C2 Pedicle On Both Sides	87799	Destruction
87747	C3 Pedicle On Both Sides	87800	Superior
87748	C4 Pedicle On Both Sides	87801	Inferior
87749	C5 Pedicle On Both Sides	87802	Anterior
87750	C6 Pedicle On Both Sides	87803	Posterior
87751	C7 Pedicle On Both Sides	87804	Right
87752	Right Lamina	87805	Left
87753	C1 Lamina On The Right	87806	Expansion
87754	C2 Lamina On The Right	87807	Superior
87755	C3 Lamina On The Right	87808	Inferior
87756	C4 Lamina On The Right	87809	Anterior
87757	C5 Lamina On The Right	87810	Posterior
87758	C6 Lamina On The Right	87811	Right
87759	C7 Lamina On The Right	87812	Left
87760	Left Lamina	87813	Thickening
87761	C1 Lamina On The Left	87814	Superior
87762	C2 Lamina On The Left	87815	Inferior

X-RAY, CONT.

87816	Anterior	29932	Old
87817	Posterior	29933	Stress
87818	Right	29934	Complete
87819	Left	29935	Incomplete
87820	Thinning	29936	Pathologic
87821	Superior	13835	Compression
87822	Inferior	29545	Burst
87823	Anterior	13836	Transverse Process
87824	Posterior	29937	Pediatric
87825	Right	29938	Torus
87826	Left	29939	Greenstick
87827	Soft Tissue Mass	29940	Salter Type I
87828	Suspected	29941	Salter Type II
87829	Superior	29942	Salter Type III
87830	Inferior	29943	Salter Type IV
87831	Anterior	29944	Comminuted
87832	Posterior	29945	Minimally
87833	Right	29946	Moderately
87834	Left	29947	Severely
87835	Seen	29948	Simple
87836	Superior	29949	Displaced
87837	Inferior	29952	Non-displaced
87838	Anterior	29960	Pattern
87839	Posterior	29953	Angulated
87840	Right	29954	Spiral
87841	Left	29955	Oblique
87842	Displaced Bone Fragment	29956	Transverse
87843	___cm	29957	Butterfly Component
87844	Superior	29958	Complex
87845	Inferior	29959	Avulsion
87846	Anterior	29961	Location
87847	Posterior	29962	Proximal
87848	Right	29963	Middle
87849	Left	29964	Medial
87850	Central Canal	29965	Lateral
87851	Trabecular	29966	Anterior
87852	Prominence	29967	Posterior
87853	Thickening	29968	Section
87854	Sequestrum	29969	Metaphyseal
13833	**Thoracic Spine**	29970	Diaphyseal
102855	Views	29971	Epiphyseal
28400	Anteroposterior And Lateral	80548	T1
28401	Including Swimmer's View Of	80549	T2
	The Cervicothoracic Junction	80550	T3
28402	Complete, Including Obliques - 4 Or	80551	T4
	More Views	80552	T5
102856	No Radiographic Evidence Of Any	80553	T6
	Osteoarticular Abnormality	80554	T7
18395	Kyphosis	80555	T8
13834	Fracture	80556	T9
29929	Open	80557	T10
29930	Closed	80558	T11
29931	Acute	80559	T12

X-RAY, CONT.

13837	Subluxation	89733	Superior Endplate Of T7
89678	Osteopenia	89734	Inferior Endplate Of T7
89679	Disc Space Narrowing	100017	Superior Endplate Of T8
89681	At T1 - T2	100018	Inferior Endplate Of T8
89682	At T2 - T3	100019	Superior Endplate Of T9
89683	At T3 - T4	100020	Inferior Endplate Of T9
89684	At T4 - T5	100021	Superior Endplate Of T10
89685	At T5 - T6	100022	Inferior Endplate Of T10
89686	At T6 - T7	100023	Superior Endplate Of T11
89687	At T7 - T8	100024	Inferior Endplate Of T11
89982	At T8 - T9	100025	Superior Endplate Of T12
89983	At T9 - T10	100026	Inferior Endplate Of T12
89984	At T10 - T11	89735	Superior Endplate Of L1
89985	At T11 - T12	89736	Destruction
89986	At T12 - L1	89737	Inferior Endplate Of T1
89704	Endplate Abnormality	89738	Superior Endplate Of T2
89706	Sclerosis	89739	Inferior Endplate Of T2
89707	Inferior Endplate Of T1	89740	Superior Endplate Of T3
89708	Superior Endplate Of T2	89741	Inferior Endplate Of T3
89709	Inferior Endplate Of T2	89742	Superior Endplate Of T4
89710	Superior Endplate Of T3	89743	Inferior Endplate Of T4
89711	Inferior Endplate Of T3	89744	Superior Endplate Of T5
89712	Superior Endplate Of T4	89745	Inferior Endplate Of T5
89713	Inferior Endplate Of T4	89746	Superior Endplate Of T6
89714	Superior Endplate Of T5	89747	Inferior Endplate Of T6
89715	Inferior Endplate Of T5	89748	Superior Endplate Of T7
89716	Superior Endplate Of T6	89749	Inferior Endplate Of T7
89717	Inferior Endplate Of T6	100027	Superior Endplate Of T8
89718	Superior Endplate Of T7	100028	Inferior Endplate Of T8
89719	Inferior Endplate Of T7	100029	Superior Endplate Of T9
100007	Superior Endplate Of T8	100030	Inferior Endplate Of T9
100008	Inferior Endplate Of T8	100031	Superior Endplate Of T10
100009	Superior Endplate Of T9	100032	Inferior Endplate Of T10
100010	Inferior Endplate Of T9	100033	Superior Endplate Of T11
100011	Superior Endplate Of T10	100034	Inferior Endplate Of T11
100012	Inferior Endplate Of T10	100035	Superior Endplate Of T12
100013	Superior Endplate Of T11	100036	Inferior Endplate Of T12
100014	Inferior Endplate Of T11	89750	Superior Endplate Of L1
100015	Superior Endplate Of T12	89844	Osteophytes
100016	Inferior Endplate Of T12	89846	Anterior
89720	Superior Endplate Of L1	89847	Inferior Endplate Of T1
89721	Irregularity	89848	Superior Endplate Of T2
89722	Inferior Endplate Of T1	89849	Inferior Endplate Of T2
89723	Superior Endplate Of T2	89850	Superior Endplate Of T3
89724	Inferior Endplate Of T2	89851	Inferior Endplate Of T3
89725	Superior Endplate Of T3	89852	Superior Endplate Of T4
89726	Inferior Endplate Of T3	89853	Inferior Endplate Of T4
89727	Superior Endplate Of T4	89854	Superior Endplate Of T5
89728	Inferior Endplate Of T4	89855	Inferior Endplate Of T5
89729	Superior Endplate Of T5	89856	Superior Endplate Of T6
89730	Inferior Endplate Of T5	89857	Inferior Endplate Of T6
89731	Superior Endplate Of T6	89858	Superior Endplate Of T7
89732	Inferior Endplate Of T6	89859	Inferior Endplate Of T7

X-RAY, CONT.

100111	Superior Endplate Of T8	89888	At T4 - T5
100112	Inferior Endplate Of T8	89889	At T5 - T6
100113	Superior Endplate Of T9	89890	At T6 - T7
100114	Inferior Endplate Of T9	89891	At T7 - T8
100115	Superior Endplate Of T10	100156	At T8 - T9
100116	Inferior Endplate Of T10	100157	At T9 - T10
100117	Superior Endplate Of T11	100158	At T10 - T11
100118	Inferior Endplate Of T11	100159	At T11 - T12
100119	Superior Endplate Of T12	100160	At T12 - L1
100120	Inferior Endplate Of T12	89939	Flowing Ossification
89860	Superior Endplate Of L1	89940	At T1 - T2
89861	Anterior Vertebral Bodies	89941	At T2 - T3
89862	At T1 - T2	89942	At T3 - T4
89863	At T2 - T3	89943	At T4 - T5
89864	At T3 - T4	89944	At T5 - T6
89865	At T4 - T5	89945	At T6 - T7
89866	At T5 - T6	89946	At T7 - T8
89867	At T6 - T7	100171	At T8 - T9
89868	At T7 - T8	100172	At T9 - T10
100151	At T8 - T9	100173	At T10 - T11
100152	At T9 - T10	100174	At T11 - T12
100153	At T10 - T11	100175	At T12 - L1
100154	At T11 - T12	89947	Bony Ankylosis
100155	At T12 - L1	89948	Vertebral Bodies
89869	Posterior	89949	T1 and T2
89870	Inferior Endplate Of T1	89950	T2 and T3
89871	Superior Endplate Of T2	89951	T3 and T4
89872	Inferior Endplate Of T2	89952	T4 and T5
89873	Superior Endplate Of T3	89953	T5 and T6
89874	Inferior Endplate Of T3	89954	T6 and T7
89875	Superior Endplate Of T4	89955	T7 and T8
89876	Inferior Endplate Of T4	100190	T8 and T9
89877	Superior Endplate Of T5	100186	T9 and T10
89878	Inferior Endplate Of T5	100187	T10 and T11
89879	Superior Endplate Of T6	100188	T11 and T12
89880	Inferior Endplate Of T6	100189	T12 and L1
89881	Superior Endplate Of T7	89956	Posterior Elements
89882	Inferior Endplate Of T7	89957	At T1 - T2
100121	Superior Endplate Of T8	89958	At T2 - T3
100122	Inferior Endplate Of T8	89959	At T3 - T4
100123	Superior Endplate Of T9	89960	At T4 - T5
100124	Inferior Endplate Of T9	89961	At T5 - T6
100125	Superior Endplate Of T10	89962	At T6 - T7
100126	Inferior Endplate Of T10	89963	At T7 - T8
100127	Superior Endplate Of T11	100176	At T8 - T9
100128	Inferior Endplate Of T11	100177	At T9 - T10
100129	Superior Endplate Of T12	100178	At T10 - T11
100130	Inferior Endplate Of T12	100179	At T11 - T12
89883	Superior Endplate Of L1	100180	At T12 - L1
89884	Posterior Vertebral Bodies	89965	Apophyseal Joints
89885	At T1 - T2	89966	At T1 - T2
89886	At T2 - T3	89967	At T2 - T3
89887	At T3 - T4	89968	At T3 - T4

X-RAY, CONT.

89969	At T4 - T5	88242	T1 Vertebral Body
89970	At T5 - T6	88243	T2 Vertebral Body
89971	At T6 - T7	88244	T3 Vertebral Body
89972	At T7 - T8	88245	T4 Vertebral Body
100181	At T8 - T9	88246	T5 Vertebral Body
100182	At T9 - T10	88247	T6 Vertebral Body
100183	At T10 - T11	88248	T7 Vertebral Body
100184	At T11 - T12	89068	T8 Vertebral Body
100185	At T12 - L1	89069	T9 Vertebral Body
18003	Syndesmophytes	89070	T10 Vertebral Body
13840	Bone Erosion	89071	T11 Vertebral Body
13841	Subchondral Bone Plate	89072	T12 Vertebral Body
13842	Vertebral Body	87173	Posterior
13843	Pedicle	88249	T1 Vertebral Body
13844	Transverse Process	88250	T2 Vertebral Body
13845	Lamina	88251	T3 Vertebral Body
13846	Spinous Process	88252	T4 Vertebral Body
13847	Bone Density Decreased	88253	T5 Vertebral Body
13848	Bone Density Increased	88254	T6 Vertebral Body
18007	Diffuse	88255	T7 Vertebral Body
18008	Localized	89073	T8 Vertebral Body
18039	Spina Bifida	89075	T9 Vertebral Body
13849	Calcifications	89076	T10 Vertebral Body
13850	Disc Space	89077	T11 Vertebral Body
87147	Lytic Lesion	89078	T12 Vertebral Body
87148	Location	87181	Right
87149	Superior	88256	T1 Vertebral Body
87150	T1 Vertebral Body	88257	T2 Vertebral Body
87151	T2 Vertebral Body	88258	T3 Vertebral Body
87152	T3 Vertebral Body	88259	T4 Vertebral Body
87153	T4 Vertebral Body	88260	T5 Vertebral Body
87154	T5 Vertebral Body	88261	T6 Vertebral Body
87155	T6 Vertebral Body	88262	T7 Vertebral Body
89052	T7 Vertebral Body	89080	T8 Vertebral Body
89046	T8 Vertebral Body	89081	T9 Vertebral Body
89047	T9 Vertebral Body	89082	T10 Vertebral Body
89048	T10 Vertebral Body	89083	T11 Vertebral Body
89049	T11 Vertebral Body	89084	T12 Vertebral Body
89050	T12 Vertebral Body	87189	Left
87157	Inferior	88263	T1 Vertebral Body
88235	T1 Vertebral Body	88264	T2 Vertebral Body
88236	T2 Vertebral Body	88265	T3 Vertebral Body
88237	T3 Vertebral Body	88266	T4 Vertebral Body
88238	T4 Vertebral Body	88267	T5 Vertebral Body
88239	T5 Vertebral Body	88268	T6 Vertebral Body
88240	T6 Vertebral Body	88269	T7 Vertebral Body
88241	T7 Vertebral Body	89085	T8 Vertebral Body
89062	T8 Vertebral Body	89086	T9 Vertebral Body
89063	T9 Vertebral Body	89087	T10 Vertebral Body
89064	T10 Vertebral Body	89088	T11 Vertebral Body
89065	T11 Vertebral Body	89089	T12 Vertebral Body
89066	T12 Vertebral Body	87197	Right Pedicle
87165	Anterior	87198	T1 Pedicle On The Right

X-RAY, CONT.

87199	T2 Pedicle On The Right	87232	T3 Lamina On The Left
87200	T3 Pedicle On The Right	87233	T4 Lamina On The Left
87201	T4 Pedicle On The Right	87234	T5 Lamina On The Left
87202	T5 Pedicle On The Right	87235	T6 Lamina On The Left
87203	T6 Pedicle On The Right	87236	T7 Lamina On The Left
87204	T7 Pedicle On The Right	89196	T8 Lamina On The Left
89096	T8 Pedicle On The Right	89197	T9 Lamina On The Left
89097	T9 Pedicle On The Right	89198	T10 Lamina On The Left
89098	T10 Pedicle On The Right	89199	T11 Lamina On The Left
89099	T11 Pedicle On The Right	89200	T12 Lamina On The Left
89100	T12 Pedicle On The Right	87237	Both Lamina
87205	Left Pedicle	87238	T1 Lamina On Both Sides
87206	T1 Pedicle On The Left	87239	T2 Lamina On Both Sides
87207	T2 Pedicle On The Left	87240	T3 Lamina On Both Sides
87208	T3 Pedicle On The Left	87241	T4 Lamina On Both Sides
87209	T4 Pedicle On The Left	87242	T5 Lamina On Both Sides
87210	T5 Pedicle On The Left	87243	T6 Lamina On Both Sides
87211	T6 Pedicle On The Left	87244	T7 Lamina On Both Sides
87212	T7 Pedicle On The Left	89201	T8 Lamina On Both Sides
89101	T8 Pedicle On The Left	89202	T9 Lamina On Both Sides
89102	T9 Pedicle On The Left	89203	T10 Lamina On Both Sides
89103	T10 Pedicle On The Left	89204	T11 Lamina On Both Sides
89104	T11 Pedicle On The Left	89205	T12 Lamina On Both Sides
89105	T12 Pedicle On The Left	87245	Spinous Process
87213	Both Pedicles	87246	T1 Spinous Process
87214	T1 Pedicle On Both Sides	87247	T2 Spinous Process
87215	T2 Pedicle On Both Sides	87248	T3 Spinous Process
87216	T3 Pedicle On Both Sides	87249	T4 Spinous Process
87217	T4 Pedicle On Both Sides	87250	T5 Spinous Process
87218	T5 Pedicle On Both Sides	87251	T6 Spinous Process
87219	T6 Pedicle On Both Sides	87252	T7 Spinous Process
89106	T7 Pedicle On Both Sides	89206	T8 Spinous Process
89107	T8 Pedicle On Both Sides	89207	T9 Spinous Process
87220	T9 Pedicle On Both Sides	89208	T10 Spinous Process
89108	T10 Pedicle On Both Sides	89209	T11 Spinous Process
89109	T11 Pedicle On Both Sides	89210	T12 Spinous Process
89110	T12 Pedicle On Both Sides	87253	Bone Expansion
87221	Right Lamina	87254	Zone Of Transition
87222	T1 Lamina On The Right	87255	Narrow
87223	T2 Lamina On The Right	87256	Wide
87224	T3 Lamina On The Right	87257	Margin
87225	T4 Lamina On The Right	87258	Sclerotic
87226	T5 Lamina On The Right	87259	Non-Sclerotic
87227	T6 Lamina On The Right	87260	Cortex
87228	T7 Lamina On The Right	87261	Intact
89191	T8 Lamina On The Right	87262	Superior
89192	T9 Lamina On The Right	87263	Inferior
89193	T10 Lamina On The Right	87264	Anterior
89194	T11 Lamina On The Right	87265	Posterior
89195	T12 Lamina On The Right	87266	Right
87229	Left Lamina	87000	Left
87230	T1 Lamina On The Left	87268	Destruction
87231	T2 Lamina On The Left	87269	Superior

X-RAY, CONT.

87270	Inferior	87323	Sequestrum
87271	Anterior	88270	Sclerotic lesion
87272	Posterior	88271	Location
87273	Right	88272	Superior
87274	Left	88273	T1 Vertebral Body
87275	Expansion	88274	T2 Vertebral Body
87276	Superior	88275	T3 Vertebral Body
87277	Inferior	88276	T4 Vertebral Body
87278	Anterior	88277	T5 Vertebral Body
87279	Posterior	88278	T6 Vertebral Body
87280	Right	88279	T7 Vertebral Body
87281	Left	89111	T8 Vertebral Body
87282	Thickening	89112	T9 Vertebral Body
87283	Superior	89113	T10 Vertebral Body
87284	Inferior	89114	T11 Vertebral Body
87285	Anterior	89115	T12 Vertebral Body
87286	Posterior	88280	Inferior
87287	Right	88281	T1 Vertebral Body
87288	Left	88282	T2 Vertebral Body
87289	Thinning	88283	T3 Vertebral Body
87290	Superior	88284	T4 Vertebral Body
87291	Inferior	88285	T5 Vertebral Body
87292	Anterior	88286	T6 Vertebral Body
87293	Posterior	88287	T7 Vertebral Body
87294	Right	89116	T8 Vertebral Body
87295	Left	89117	T9 Vertebral Body
87296	Soft Tissue Mass	89118	T10 Vertebral Body
87297	Suspected	89119	T11 Vertebral Body
87298	Superior	89120	T12 Vertebral Body
87299	Inferior	88288	Anterior
87300	Anterior	88289	T1 Vertebral Body
87301	Posterior	88290	T2 Vertebral Body
87302	Right	88291	T3 Vertebral Body
87303	Left	88292	T4 Vertebral Body
87304	Seen	88293	T5 Vertebral Body
87305	Superior	88294	T6 Vertebral Body
87306	Inferior	88295	T7 Vertebral Body
87307	Anterior	89121	T8 Vertebral Body
87308	Posterior	89122	T9 Vertebral Body
87309	Right	89123	T10 Vertebral Body
87310	Left	89124	T11 Vertebral Body
87311	Displaced Bone Fragment	89125	T12 Vertebral Body
87312	___cm	88296	Posterior
87313	Superior	88297	T1 Vertebral Body
87314	Inferior	88298	T2 Vertebral Body
87315	Anterior	88299	T3 Vertebral Body
87316	Posterior	88300	T4 Vertebral Body
87317	Right	88301	T5 Vertebral Body
87318	Left	88302	T6 Vertebral Body
87319	Central Canal	88303	T7 Vertebral Body
87320	Trabecular	89126	T8 Vertebral Body
87321	Prominence	89127	T9 Vertebral Body
87322	Thickening	89128	T10 Vertebral Body

X-RAY, CONT.

89129	T11 Vertebral Body	89150	T12 Pedicle On The Left
89130	T12 Vertebral Body	88336	Both Pedicles
88304	Right	88337	T1 Pedicle On Both Sides
88305	T1 Vertebral Body	88338	T2 Pedicle On Both Sides
88306	T2 Vertebral Body	88339	T3 Pedicle On Both Sides
88307	T3 Vertebral Body	88340	T4 Pedicle On Both Sides
88308	T4 Vertebral Body	88341	T5 Pedicle On Both Sides
88309	T5 Vertebral Body	88342	T6 Pedicle On Both Sides
88310	T6 Vertebral Body	88343	T7 Pedicle On Both Sides
88311	T7 Vertebral Body	89236	T8 Pedicle On Both Sides
89131	T8 Vertebral Body	89237	T9 Pedicle On Both Sides
89132	T9 Vertebral Body	89238	T10 Pedicle On Both Sides
89133	T10 Vertebral Body	89239	T11 Pedicle On Both Sides
89134	T11 Vertebral Body	89240	T12 Pedicle On Both Sides
89135	T12 Vertebral Body	88344	Right Lamina
88312	Left	88345	T1 Lamina On The Right
88313	T1 Vertebral Body	88346	T2 Lamina On The Right
88314	T2 Vertebral Body	88347	T3 Lamina On The Right
88315	T3 Vertebral Body	88348	T4 Lamina On The Right
88316	T4 Vertebral Body	88349	T5 Lamina On The Right
88317	T5 Vertebral Body	88350	T6 Lamina On The Right
88318	T6 Vertebral Body	88351	T7 Lamina On The Right
88319	T7 Vertebral Body	89241	T8 Lamina On The Right
89136	T8 Vertebral Body	89242	T9 Lamina On The Right
89137	T9 Vertebral Body	89243	T10 Lamina On The Right
89138	T10 Vertebral Body	89244	T11 Lamina On The Right
89139	T11 Vertebral Body	89245	T12 Lamina On The Right
89140	T12 Vertebral Body	88352	Left Lamina
88320	Right Pedicle	88353	T1 Lamina On The Left
88321	T1 Pedicle On The Right	88354	T2 Lamina On The Left
88322	T2 Pedicle On The Right	88355	T3 Lamina On The Left
88323	T3 Pedicle On The Right	88356	T4 Lamina On The Left
88324	T4 Pedicle On The Right	88357	T5 Lamina On The Left
88325	T5 Pedicle On The Right	88358	T6 Lamina On The Left
88326	T6 Pedicle On The Right	88359	T7 Lamina On The Left
88327	T7 Pedicle On The Right	89246	T8 Lamina On The Left
89141	T8 Pedicle On The Right	89247	T9 Lamina On The Left
89142	T9 Pedicle On The Right	89248	T10 Lamina On The Left
89143	T10 Pedicle On The Right	89249	T11 Lamina On The Left
89144	T11 Pedicle On The Right	89250	T12 Lamina On The Left
89145	T12 Pedicle On The Right	88360	Both Lamina
88328	Left Pedicle	88361	T1 Lamina On Both Sides
88329	T1 Pedicle On The Left	88362	T2 Lamina On Both Sides
88330	T2 Pedicle On The Left	88363	T3 Lamina On Both Sides
88331	T3 Pedicle On The Left	88364	T4 Lamina On Both Sides
88332	T4 Pedicle On The Left	88365	T5 Lamina On Both Sides
88333	T5 Pedicle On The Left	88366	T6 Lamina On Both Sides
88334	T6 Pedicle On The Left	88367	T7 Lamina On Both Sides
88335	T7 Pedicle On The Left	89251	T8 Lamina On Both Sides
89146	T8 Pedicle On The Left	89252	T9 Lamina On Both Sides
89147	T9 Pedicle On The Left	89253	T10 Lamina On Both Sides
89148	T10 Pedicle On The Left	89254	T11 Lamina On Both Sides
89149	T11 Pedicle On The Left	89255	T12 Lamina On Both Sides

X-RAY, CONT.

88368	Spinous Process
88369	T1 Spinous Process
88370	T2 Spinous Process
88371	T3 Spinous Process
88372	T4 Spinous Process
88373	T5 Spinous Process
88374	T6 Spinous Process
88375	T7 Spinous Process
89256	T8 Spinous Process
89257	T9 Spinous Process
89258	T10 Spinous Process
89259	T11 Spinous Process
89260	T12 Spinous Process
88376	Bone Expansion
88377	Zone Of Transition
88378	Narrow
88379	Wide
88380	Margin
88381	Sclerotic
88382	Non-Sclerotic
88383	Cortex
88384	Intact
88385	Superior
88386	Inferior
88387	Anterior
88388	Posterior
88389	Right
88390	Left
88391	Destruction
88392	Superior
88393	Inferior
88394	Anterior
88395	Posterior
88396	Right
88397	Left
88398	Expansion
88399	Superior
88400	Inferior
88401	Anterior
88402	Posterior
88403	Right
88404	Left
88405	Thickening
88406	Superior
88407	Inferior
88408	Anterior
88409	Posterior
88410	Right
88411	Left
88412	Thinning
88413	Superior
88414	Inferior
88415	Anterior

88416	Posterior
88417	Right
88418	Left
88419	Soft Tissue Mass
88420	Suspected
88421	Superior
88422	Inferior
88423	Anterior
88424	Posterior
88425	Right
88426	Left
88427	Seen
88428	Superior
88429	Inferior
88430	Anterior
88431	Posterior
88432	Right
88433	Left
88434	Displaced Bone Fragment
88435	___ cm
88436	Superior
88437	Inferior
88438	Anterior
88439	Posterior
88440	Right
88441	Left
88442	Central Canal
88443	Trabecular
88444	Prominence
88445	Thickening
88446	Sequestrum
88483	Mixed Lytic / Sclerotic Lesion
88484	Location
88485	Superior
88486	T1 Vertebral Body
88487	T2 Vertebral Body
88488	T3 Vertebral Body
88489	T4 Vertebral Body
88490	T5 Vertebral Body
88491	T6 Vertebral Body
88492	T7 Vertebral Body
89151	T8 Vertebral Body
89152	T9 Vertebral Body
89153	T10 Vertebral Body
89154	T11 Vertebral Body
89155	T12 Vertebral Body
88493	Inferior
88494	T1 Vertebral Body
88495	T2 Vertebral Body
88496	T3 Vertebral Body
88497	T4 Vertebral Body
88498	T5 Vertebral Body
88499	T6 Vertebral Body

X-Ray, cont.

88500	T7 Vertebral Body	89176	T8 Vertebral Body
89156	T8 Vertebral Body	89177	T9 Vertebral Body
89157	T9 Vertebral Body	89178	T10 Vertebral Body
89158	T10 Vertebral Body	89179	T11 Vertebral Body
89159	T11 Vertebral Body	89180	T12 Vertebral Body
89160	T12 Vertebral Body	88533	Right Pedicle
88501	Anterior	88534	T1 Pedicle On The Right
88502	T1 Vertebral Body	88535	T2 Pedicle On The Right
88503	T2 Vertebral Body	88536	T3 Pedicle On The Right
88504	T3 Vertebral Body	88537	T4 Pedicle On The Right
88505	T4 Vertebral Body	88538	T5 Pedicle On The Right
88506	T5 Vertebral Body	88539	T6 Pedicle On The Right
88507	T6 Vertebral Body	88540	T7 Pedicle On The Right
88508	T7 Vertebral Body	89181	T8 Pedicle On The Right
89161	T8 Vertebral Body	89182	T9 Pedicle On The Right
89162	T9 Vertebral Body	89183	T10 Pedicle On The Right
89163	T10 Vertebral Body	89184	T11 Pedicle On The Right
89164	T11 Vertebral Body	89185	T12 Pedicle On The Right
89165	T12 Vertebral Body	88541	Left Pedicle
88509	Posterior	88542	T1 Pedicle On The Left
88510	T1 Vertebral Body	88543	T2 Pedicle On The Left
88511	T2 Vertebral Body	88544	T3 Pedicle On The Left
88512	T3 Vertebral Body	88545	T4 Pedicle On The Left
88513	T4 Vertebral Body	88546	T5 Pedicle On The Left
88514	T5 Vertebral Body	88547	T6 Pedicle On The Left
88515	T6 Vertebral Body	88548	T7 Pedicle On The Left
88516	T7 Vertebral Body	89186	T8 Pedicle On The Left
89166	T8 Vertebral Body	89187	T9 Pedicle On The Left
89167	T9 Vertebral Body	89188	T10 Pedicle On The Left
89168	T10 Vertebral Body	89189	T11 Pedicle On The Left
89169	T11 Vertebral Body	89190	T12 Pedicle On The Left
89170	T12 Vertebral Body	88549	Both Pedicles
88517	Right	88550	T1 Pedicle On Both Sides
88518	T1 Vertebral Body	88551	T2 Pedicle On Both Sides
88519	T2 Vertebral Body	88552	T3 Pedicle On Both Sides
88520	T3 Vertebral Body	88553	T4 Pedicle On Both Sides
88521	T4 Vertebral Body	88554	T5 Pedicle On Both Sides
88522	T5 Vertebral Body	88555	T6 Pedicle On Both Sides
88523	T6 Vertebral Body	88556	T7 Pedicle On Both Sides
88524	T7 Vertebral Body	89211	T8 Pedicle On Both Sides
89171	T8 Vertebral Body	89212	T9 Pedicle On Both Sides
89172	T9 Vertebral Body	89213	T10 Pedicle On Both Sides
89173	T10 Vertebral Body	89214	T11 Pedicle On Both Sides
89174	T11 Vertebral Body	89215	T12 Pedicle On Both Sides
89175	T12 Vertebral Body	88557	Right Lamina
88525	Left	88558	T1 Lamina On The Right
88526	T1 Vertebral Body	88559	T2 Lamina On The Right
88527	T2 Vertebral Body	88560	T3 Lamina On The Right
88528	T3 Vertebral Body	88561	T4 Lamina On The Right
88529	T4 Vertebral Body	88562	T5 Lamina On The Right
88530	T5 Vertebral Body	88563	T6 Lamina On The Right
88531	T6 Vertebral Body	88564	T7 Lamina On The Right
88532	T7 Vertebral Body	89216	T8 Lamina On The Right

X-Ray, cont.

89217	T9 Lamina On The Right	88599	Inferior
89218	T10 Lamina On The Right	88600	Anterior
89219	T11 Lamina On The Right	88601	Posterior
89220	T12 Lamina On The Right	88602	Right
88565	Left Lamina	88603	Left
88566	T1 Lamina On The Left	88604	Destruction
88567	T2 Lamina On The Left	88605	Superior
88568	T3 Lamina On The Left	88606	Inferior
88569	T4 Lamina On The Left	88607	Anterior
88570	T5 Lamina On The Left	88608	Posterior
88571	T6 Lamina On The Left	88609	Right
88572	T7 Lamina On The Left	88610	Left
89221	T8 Lamina On The Left	88611	Expansion
89222	T9 Lamina On The Left	88612	Superior
89223	T10 Lamina On The Left	88613	Inferior
89224	T11 Lamina On The Left	88614	Anterior
89225	T12 Lamina On The Left	88615	Posterior
88573	Both Lamina	88616	Right
88574	T1 Lamina On Both Sides	88617	Left
88575	T2 Lamina On Both Sides	88618	Thickening
88576	T3 Lamina On Both Sides	88619	Superior
88577	T4 Lamina On Both Sides	88620	Inferior
88578	T5 Lamina On Both Sides	88621	Anterior
88579	T6 Lamina On Both Sides	88622	Posterior
88580	T7 Lamina On Both Sides	88623	Right
89226	T8 Lamina On Both Sides	88624	Left
89227	T9 Lamina On Both Sides	88625	Thinning
89228	T10 Lamina On Both Sides	88626	Superior
89229	T11 Lamina On Both Sides	88627	Inferior
89230	T12 Lamina On Both Sides	88628	Anterior
88581	Spinous Process	88629	Posterior
88582	T1 Spinous Process	88630	Right
88583	T2 Spinous Process	88631	Left
88584	T3 Spinous Process	88632	Soft Tissue Mass
88585	T4 Spinous Process	88633	Suspected
88586	T5 Spinous Process	88634	Superior
88587	T6 Spinous Process	88635	Inferior
88588	T7 Spinous Process	88636	Anterior
89231	T8 Spinous Process	88637	Posterior
89232	T9 Spinous Process	88638	Right
89233	T10 Spinous Process	88639	Left
89234	T11 Spinous Process	88640	Seen
89235	T12 Spinous Process	88641	Superior
88589	Bone Expansion	88642	Inferior
88590	Zone Of Transition	88643	Anterior
88591	Narrow	88644	Posterior
88592	Wide	88645	Right
88593	Margin	88646	Left
88594	Sclerotic	88647	Displaced Bone Fragment
88595	Non-Sclerotic	88648	___ cm
88596	Cortex	88649	Superior
88597	Intact	88650	Inferior
88598	Superior	88651	Anterior

X-RAY, CONT.

88652	Posterior	29992	Displaced
88653	Right	29995	Non-displaced
88654	Left	80003	Pattern
88655	Central Canal	29996	Angulated
88656	Trabecular	29997	Spiral
88657	Prominence	29998	Oblique
88658	Thickening	29999	Transverse
88659	Sequestrum	80000	Butterfly Component
28397	**Thoracolumbar Spine**	80001	Complex
28398	Anteroposterior And Lateral	80002	Avulsion
102857	No Radiographic Evidence Of Any Osteoarticular Abnormality	80004	Location
		80005	Proximal
13854	For Scoliosis	80006	Middle
13852	**Lumbosacral Spine**	80007	Medial
102859	Views	80008	Lateral
28399	Anteroposterior And Lateral	80009	Anterior
28523	Complete, With Oblique Views	80010	Posterior
28524	Complete, Including Bending Views	80011	Section
28525	Bending Views Only, Four Or More Views	80012	Metaphyseal
		80013	Diaphyseal
102858	No Radiographic Evidence Of Any Osteoarticular Abnormality	80014	Epiphyseal
		80560	L1
13853	Loss of Lordosis	80561	L2
13855	Spondylolisthesis	80562	L3
13856	Grade 1	80563	L4
13857	Grade 2	80564	L5
13858	Grade 3	80567	S1
13859	Grade 4	13864	Disc Space Narrowing
13860	Fracture	13865	at L3 - L4
29972	Open	13866	at L4 - L5
29973	Closed	13867	at L5 - S1
29974	Acute	100191	Osteopenia
29975	Old	100192	Disc Space Narrowing
29976	Stress	100199	At T12 - L1
29977	Complete	100194	At L1 - L2
29978	Incomplete	100195	At L2 - L3
29979	Pathologic	100196	At L3 - L4
13861	Compression	100197	At L4 - L5
29546	Burst	100198	At L5 - S1
13862	Pars Interarticularis	100214	Endplate Abnormality
13863	Transverse Process	100216	Sclerosis
29980	Pediatric	100382	Inferior Endplate Of T12
29981	Torus	100383	Superior Endplate Of L1
29982	Greenstick	100384	Inferior Endplate Of L1
29983	Salter Type I	100385	Superior Endplate Of L2
29984	Salter Type II	100386	Inferior Endplate Of L2
29985	Salter Type III	100387	Superior Endplate Of L3
29986	Salter Type IV	100388	Inferior Endplate Of L3
29987	Comminuted	100389	Superior Endplate Of L4
29988	Minimally	100390	Inferior Endplate Of L4
29989	Moderately	100391	Superior Endplate Of L5
29990	Severely	100392	Inferior Endplate Of L5
29991	Simple	100393	Superior Endplate Of S1

X-RAY, CONT.

100229	Irregularity	100503	Superior Endplate Of L3
100430	Inferior Endplate Of T12	100504	Inferior Endplate Of L3
100431	Superior Endplate Of L1	100505	Superior Endplate Of L4
100432	Inferior Endplate Of L1	100506	Inferior Endplate Of L4
100433	Superior Endplate Of L2	100507	Superior Endplate Of L5
100434	Inferior Endplate Of L2	100508	Inferior Endplate Of L5
100435	Superior Endplate Of L3	100509	Superior Endplate Of S1
100436	Inferior Endplate Of L3	100497	Posterior
100437	Superior Endplate Of L4	100510	Inferior Endplate Of T12
100438	Inferior Endplate Of L4	100511	Superior Endplate Of L1
100439	Superior Endplate Of L5	100512	Inferior Endplate Of L1
100440	Inferior Endplate Of L5	100513	Superior Endplate Of L2
100441	Superior Endplate Of S1	100514	Inferior Endplate Of L2
100242	Destruction	100515	Superior Endplate Of L3
100406	Inferior Endplate Of T12	100516	Inferior Endplate Of L3
100407	Superior Endplate Of L1	100517	Superior Endplate Of L4
100408	Inferior Endplate Of L1	100518	Inferior Endplate Of L4
100409	Superior Endplate Of L2	100519	Superior Endplate Of L5
100410	Inferior Endplate Of L2	100520	Inferior Endplate Of L5
100411	Superior Endplate Of L3	100521	Superior Endplate Of S1
100412	Inferior Endplate Of L3	100359	Posterior Vertebral Bodies
100413	Superior Endplate Of L4	100522	Inferior Endplate Of T12
100414	Inferior Endplate Of L4	100523	Superior Endplate Of L1
100415	Superior Endplate Of L5	100524	Inferior Endplate Of L1
100416	Inferior Endplate Of L5	100525	Superior Endplate Of L2
100417	Superior Endplate Of S1	100526	Inferior Endplate Of L2
100490	Vacuum Disc	100527	Superior Endplate Of L3
100491	At T12 - L1	100528	Inferior Endplate Of L3
100492	At L1 - L2	100529	Superior Endplate Of L4
100493	At L2 - L3	100530	Inferior Endplate Of L4
100494	At L3 - L4	100531	Superior Endplate Of L5
100495	At L4 - L5	100532	Inferior Endplate Of L5
100496	At L5 - S1	100533	Superior Endplate Of S1
100336	Osteophytes	18004	Syndesmophytes
100338	Anterior	100583	Right Marginal
100349	Inferior Endplate Of T12	100592	Inferior Endplate Of T12
100350	Superior Endplate Of L1	100593	Superior Endplate Of L1
100339	Inferior Endplate Of L1	100594	Inferior Endplate Of L1
100340	Superior Endplate Of L2	100595	Superior Endplate Of L2
100341	Inferior Endplate Of L2	100596	Inferior Endplate Of L2
100342	Superior Endplate Of L3	100597	Superior Endplate Of L3
100343	Inferior Endplate Of L3	100598	Inferior Endplate Of L3
100344	Superior Endplate Of L4	100599	Superior Endplate Of L4
100345	Inferior Endplate Of L4	100600	Inferior Endplate Of L4
100346	Superior Endplate Of L5	100601	Superior Endplate Of L5
100347	Inferior Endplate Of L5	100602	Inferior Endplate Of L5
100348	Superior Endplate Of S1	100603	Superior Endplate Of S1
100351	Anterior Vertebral Bodies	100584	Left Marginal
100498	Inferior Endplate Of T12	100604	Inferior Endplate Of T12
100499	Superior Endplate Of L1	100605	Superior Endplate Of L1
100500	Inferior Endplate Of L1	100606	Inferior Endplate Of L1
100501	Superior Endplate Of L2	100607	Superior Endplate Of L2
100502	Inferior Endplate Of L2	100608	Inferior Endplate Of L2

X-RAY, CONT.

100609	Superior Endplate Of L3	100714	Inferior Endplate Of L3
100610	Inferior Endplate Of L3	100715	Superior Endplate Of L4
100611	Superior Endplate Of L4	100716	Inferior Endplate Of L4
100612	Inferior Endplate Of L4	100717	Superior Endplate Of L5
100613	Superior Endplate Of L5	100718	Inferior Endplate Of L5
100614	Inferior Endplate Of L5	100719	Superior Endplate Of S1
100615	Superior Endplate Of S1	100690	Right Non-Bridging
100586	Left Non-Marginal	100720	Inferior Endplate Of T12
100616	Inferior Endplate Of T12	100721	Superior Endplate Of L1
100617	Superior Endplate Of L1	100722	Inferior Endplate Of L1
100618	Inferior Endplate Of L1	100723	Superior Endplate Of L2
100619	Superior Endplate Of L2	100724	Inferior Endplate Of L2
100620	Inferior Endplate Of L2	100725	Superior Endplate Of L3
100621	Superior Endplate Of L3	100726	Inferior Endplate Of L3
100622	Inferior Endplate Of L3	100727	Superior Endplate Of L4
100623	Superior Endplate Of L4	100728	Inferior Endplate Of L4
100624	Inferior Endplate Of L4	100729	Superior Endplate Of L5
100625	Superior Endplate Of L5	100730	Inferior Endplate Of L5
100626	Inferior Endplate Of L5	100731	Superior Endplate Of S1
100627	Superior Endplate Of S1	100691	Left Non-Bridging
100585	Right Non-Marginal	100732	Inferior Endplate Of T12
100628	Inferior Endplate Of T12	100733	Superior Endplate Of L1
100629	Superior Endplate Of L1	100734	Inferior Endplate Of L1
100630	Inferior Endplate Of L1	100735	Superior Endplate Of L2
100631	Superior Endplate Of L2	100736	Inferior Endplate Of L2
100632	Inferior Endplate Of L2	100737	Superior Endplate Of L3
100633	Superior Endplate Of L3	100738	Inferior Endplate Of L3
100634	Inferior Endplate Of L3	100739	Superior Endplate Of L4
100635	Superior Endplate Of L4	100740	Inferior Endplate Of L4
100636	Inferior Endplate Of L4	100741	Superior Endplate Of L5
100637	Superior Endplate Of L5	100742	Inferior Endplate Of L5
100638	Inferior Endplate Of L5	100743	Superior Endplate Of S1
100639	Superior Endplate Of S1	100365	Flowing Ossification
100688	Right Bridging	100792	At T12 - L1
100696	Inferior Endplate Of T12	100793	At L1 - L2
100697	Superior Endplate Of L1	100794	At L2 - L3
100698	Inferior Endplate Of L1	100795	At L3 - L4
100699	Superior Endplate Of L2	100796	At L4 - L5
100700	Inferior Endplate Of L2	100797	At L5 - S1
100701	Superior Endplate Of L3	100798	Bamboo Appeerence
100702	Inferior Endplate Of L3	100366	Bony Ankylosis
100703	Superior Endplate Of L4		Vertebral Bodies
100704	Inferior Endplate Of L4	100804	T12 and L1
100705	Superior Endplate Of L5	100799	L1 and L2
100706	Inferior Endplate Of L5	100800	L2 and L3
100707	Superior Endplate Of S1	100802	L4 and L5
100689	Left Bridging	100801	L3 and L4
100708	Inferior Endplate Of T12	100803	L5 and S1
100709	Superior Endplate Of L1	100368	Posterior Elements
100710	Inferior Endplate Of L1	100810	At T12 - L1
100711	Superior Endplate Of L2	100805	At L1 - L2
100712	Inferior Endplate Of L2	100806	At L2 - L3
100713	Superior Endplate Of L3	100807	At L3 - L4

X-RAY, CONT.

100808	At L4 - L5		100914	At L4 - L5
100809	At L5 - S1		100915	At L5 - S1
100369	Both		100916	Both
100811	At T12 - L1		100917	At T12 - L1
100812	At L1 - L2		100918	At L1 - L2
100813	At L2 - L3		100919	At L2 - L3
100814	At L3 - L4		100920	At L3 - L4
100815	At L4 - L5		100921	At L4 - L5
100816	At L5 - S1		100922	At L5 - S1
13878	Calcifications		100842	Hypertrophy
13879	Disc Space		100965	Right
100817	At T12 - L1		100966	At T12 - L1
100818	At L1 - L2		100967	At L1 - L2
100819	At L2 - L3		100968	At L2 - L3
100820	At L3 - L4		100969	At L3 - L4
100821	At L4 - L5		100970	At L4 - L5
100822	At L5 - S1		100971	At L5 - S1
100823	Facet Joints		100972	Left
100824	Narrowing		100973	At T12 - L1
100845	Right		100974	At T12 - L1
100825	At T12 - L1		100975	At L2 - L3
100826	At L1 - L2		100976	At L3 - L4
100827	At L2 - L3		100977	At L4 - L5
100828	At L3 - L4		100978	At L5 - S1
100829	At L4 - L5		100979	Both
100830	At L5 - S1		100980	At T12 - L1
100846	Left		100981	At L1 - L2
100848	At T12 - L1		100982	At L2 - L3
100849	At T12 - L1		100983	At L3 - L4
100850	At L2 - L3		100984	At L4 - L5
100851	At L3 - L4		100985	At L5 - S1
100852	At L4 - L5		13868	Osteophytes
100853	At L5 - S1		13869	Bone Erosion
100847	Both		13870	Subchondral Bone Plate
100854	At T12 - L1		13871	Vertebral Body
100855	At L1 - L2		13872	Pedicle
100856	At L2 - L3		13873	Transverse Process
100857	At L3 - L4		13874	Lamina
100858	At L4 - L5		13875	Spinous Process
100859	At L5 - S1		13876	Bone Density Decreased
100839	Sclerosis		13877	Bone Density Increased
100902	Right		18009	Diffuse
100903	At T12 - L1		18010	Localized
100904	At L1 - L2		18040	Spina Bifida
100905	At L2 - L3		87324	Lytic Lesion
100906	At L3 - L4		87325	Location
100907	At L4 - L5		87326	Superior
100908	At L5 - S1		87327	L1 Vertebral Body
100909	Left		87328	L2 Vertebral Body
100910	At T12 - L1		87329	L3 Vertebral Body
100911	At T12 - L1		87330	L4 Vertebral Body
100912	At L2 - L3		87331	L5 Vertebral Body
100913	At L3 - L4		87334	Inferior

X-RAY, CONT.

87335	L1 Vertebral Body	87406	Left Lamina
87336	L2 Vertebral Body	87407	L1 Lamina On The Left
87337	L3 Vertebral Body	87408	L2 Lamina On The Left
87338	L4 Vertebral Body	87409	L3 Lamina On The Left
87339	L5 Vertebral Body	87410	L4 Lamina On The Left
87342	Anterior	87411	L5 Lamina On The Left
87343	L1 Vertebral Body	87414	Both Lamina
87344	L2 Vertebral Body	87415	L1 Lamina On Both Sides
87345	L3 Vertebral Body	87416	L2 Lamina On Both Sides
87346	L4 Vertebral Body	87417	L3 Lamina On Both Sides
87347	L5 Vertebral Body	87418	L4 Lamina On Both Sides
87350	Posterior	87419	L5 Lamina On Both Sides
87351	L1 Vertebral Body	87422	Spinous Process
87352	L2 Vertebral Body	87423	L1 Spinous Process
87353	L3 Vertebral Body	87424	L2 Spinous Process
87354	L4 Vertebral Body	87425	L3 Spinous Process
87355	L5 Vertebral Body	87426	L4 Spinous Process
87358	Right	87427	L5 Spinous Process
87359	L1 Vertebral Body	87430	Bone Expansion
87360	L2 Vertebral Body	87431	Zone Of Transition
87361	L3 Vertebral Body	87432	Narrow
87362	L4 Vertebral Body	87433	Wide
87363	L5 Vertebral Body	87434	Margin
87366	Left	87435	Sclerotic
87367	L1 Vertebral Body	87436	Non-Sclerotic
87368	L2 Vertebral Body	87437	Cortex
87369	L3 Vertebral Body	87438	Intact
87370	L4 Vertebral Body	87439	Superior
87371	L5 Vertebral Body	87440	Inferior
87374	Right Pedicle	87441	Anterior
87375	L1 Pedicle On The Right	87442	Posterior
87376	L2 Pedicle On The Right	87443	Right
87377	L3 Pedicle On The Right	87444	Left
87378	L4 Pedicle On The Right	87445	Destruction
87379	L5 Pedicle On The Right	87446	Superior
87382	Left Pedicle	87447	Inferior
87383	L1 Pedicle On The Left	87448	Anterior
87384	L2 Pedicle On The Left	87449	Posterior
87385	L3 Pedicle On The Left	87450	Right
87386	L4 Pedicle On The Left	87451	Left
87387	L5 Pedicle On The Left	87452	Expansion
87390	Both Pedicles	87453	Superior
87391	L1 Pedicle On Both Sides	87454	Inferior
87392	L2 Pedicle On Both Sides	87455	Anterior
87393	L3 Pedicle On Both Sides	87456	Posterior
87394	L4 Pedicle On Both Sides	87457	Right
87395	L5 Pedicle On Both Sides	87458	Left
87398	Right Lamina	87459	Thickening
87399	L1 Lamina On The Right	87460	Superior
87400	L2 Lamina On The Right	87461	Inferior
87401	L3 Lamina On The Right	87462	Anterior
87402	L4 Lamina On The Right	87463	Posterior
87403	L5 Lamina On The Right	87464	Right

X-RAY, CONT.

87465	Left		88684	L3 Vertebral Body
87466	Thinning		88685	L4 Vertebral Body
87467	Superior		88686	L5 Vertebral Body
87468	Inferior		88689	Posterior
87469	Anterior		88690	L1 Vertebral Body
87470	Posterior		88692	L2 Vertebral Body
87471	Right		88693	L3 Vertebral Body
87472	Left		88694	L4 Vertebral Body
87473	Soft Tissue Mass		88695	L5 Vertebral Body
87474	Suspected		88698	Right
87475	Superior		88699	L1 Vertebral Body
87476	Inferior		88700	L2 Vertebral Body
87477	Anterior		88701	L3 Vertebral Body
87478	Posterior		88702	L4 Vertebral Body
87479	Right		88703	L5 Vertebral Body
87480	Left		88706	Left
87481	Seen		88707	L1 Vertebral Body
87482	Superior		88708	L2 Vertebral Body
87483	Inferior		88709	L3 Vertebral Body
87484	Anterior		88710	L4 Vertebral Body
87485	Posterior		88711	L5 Vertebral Body
87486	Right		88714	Right Pedicle
87487	Left		88715	L1 Pedicle On The Right
87488	Displaced Bone Fragment		88716	L2 Pedicle On The Right
87489	___cm		88717	L3 Pedicle On The Right
87490	Superior		88718	L4 Pedicle On The Right
87491	Inferior		88719	L5 Pedicle On The Right
87492	Anterior		88722	Left Pedicle
87493	Posterior		88723	L1 Pedicle On The Left
87494	Right		88724	L2 Pedicle On The Left
87495	Left		88725	L3 Pedicle On The Left
87496	Central Canal		88726	L4 Pedicle On The Left
87497	Trabecular		88727	L5 Pedicle On The Left
87498	Prominence		88730	Both Pedicles
87499	Thickening		88731	L1 Pedicle On Both Sides
87500	Sequestrum		88732	L2 Pedicle On Both Sides
88663	Sclerotic Lesion		88733	L3 Pedicle On Both Sides
88664	Location		88734	L4 Pedicle On Both Sides
88665	Superior		88735	L5 Pedicle On Both Sides
88666	L1 Vertebral Body		88738	Right Lamina
88667	L2 Vertebral Body		88739	L1 Lamina On The Right
88668	L3 Vertebral Body		88740	L2 Lamina On The Right
88669	L4 Vertebral Body		88741	L3 Lamina On The Right
88670	L5 Vertebral Body		88742	L4 Lamina On The Right
88673	Inferior		88743	L5 Lamina On The Right
88674	L1 Vertebral Body		88746	Left Lamina
88675	L2 Vertebral Body		88747	L1 Lamina On The Left
88676	L3 Vertebral Body		88748	L2 Lamina On The Left
88677	L4 Vertebral Body		88749	L3 Lamina On The Left
88678	L5 Vertebral Body		88750	L4 Lamina On The Left
88681	Anterior		88751	L5 Lamina On The Left
88682	L1 Vertebral Body		88754	Both Lamina
88683	L2 Vertebral Body		88755	L1 Lamina On Both Sides

X-RAY, CONT.

88756	L2 Lamina On Both Sides	88814	Soft Tissue Mass
88757	L3 Lamina On Both Sides	88816	Suspected
88758	L4 Lamina On Both Sides	88817	Superior
88759	L5 Lamina On Both Sides	88818	Inferior
88762	Spinous Process	88825	Anterior
88763	L1 Spinous Process	88826	Posterior
88764	L2 Spinous Process	88827	Right
88765	L3 Spinous Process	88828	Left
88767	L4 Spinous Process	88829	Seen
88768	L5 Spinous Process	88830	Superior
88771	Bone Expansion	88831	Inferior
88772	Zone Of Transition	88832	Anterior
88773	Narrow	88833	Posterior
88774	Wide	88834	Right
88775	Margin	88835	Left
88776	Sclerotic	88836	Displaced Bone Fragment
88777	Non-Sclerotic	88837	___cm
88778	Cortex	88838	Superior
88779	Intact	88839	Inferior
88780	Superior	88840	Anterior
88781	Inferior	88841	Posterior
88782	Anterior	88842	Right
88783	Posterior	88843	Left
88784	Right	88844	Central Canal
88785	Left	88845	Trabecular
88786	Destruction	88846	Prominence
88787	Superior	88847	Thickening
88788	Inferior	88848	Sequestrum
88789	Anterior	88853	Mixed Lytic / Sclerotic Lesion
88790	Posterior	88854	Location
88791	Right	88855	Superior
88792	Left	88856	L1 Vertebral Body
88793	Expansion	88857	L2 Vertebral Body
88794	Superior	88858	L3 Vertebral Body
88795	Inferior	88859	L4 Vertebral Body
88796	Anterior	88860	L5 Vertebral Body
88797	Posterior	88863	Inferior
88798	Right	88864	L1 Vertebral Body
88799	Left	88865	L2 Vertebral Body
88800	Thickening	88866	L3 Vertebral Body
88801	Superior	88867	L4 Vertebral Body
88802	Inferior	88868	L5 Vertebral Body
88803	Anterior	88871	Anterior
88804	Posterior	88872	L1 Vertebral Body
88805	Right	88873	L2 Vertebral Body
88806	Left	88874	L3 Vertebral Body
88807	Thinning	88875	L4 Vertebral Body
88808	Superior	88876	L5 Vertebral Body
88809	Inferior	88879	Posterior
88810	Anterior	88880	L1 Vertebral Body
88811	Posterior	88881	L2 Vertebral Body
88812	Right	88882	L3 Vertebral Body
88813	Left	88883	L4 Vertebral Body

X-RAY, CONT.

88884	L5 Vertebral Body	88955	L4 Spinous Process
88887	Right	88956	L5 Spinous Process
88888	L1 Vertebral Body	88959	Bone Expansion
88889	L2 Vertebral Body	88960	Zone Of Transition
88890	L3 Vertebral Body	88961	Narrow
88891	L4 Vertebral Body	88962	Wide
88892	L5 Vertebral Body	88963	Margin
88895	Left	88964	Sclerotic
88896	L1 Vertebral Body	88965	Non-Sclerotic
88897	L2 Vertebral Body	88966	Cortex
88898	L3 Vertebral Body	88967	Intact
88899	L4 Vertebral Body	88968	Superior
88900	L5 Vertebral Body	88969	Inferior
88903	Right Pedicle	88970	Anterior
88904	L1 Pedicle On The Right	88971	Posterior
88905	L2 Pedicle On The Right	88972	Right
88906	L3 Pedicle On The Right	88973	Left
88907	L4 Pedicle On The Right	88974	Destruction
88908	L5 Pedicle On The Right	88975	Superior
88911	Left Pedicle	88976	Inferior
88912	L1 Pedicle On The Left	88977	Anterior
88913	L2 Pedicle On The Left	88978	Posterior
88914	L3 Pedicle On The Left	88979	Right
88915	L4 Pedicle On The Left	88980	Left
88916	L5 Pedicle On The Left	88981	Expansion
88919	Both Pedicles	88982	Superior
88920	L1 Pedicle On Both Sides	88983	Inferior
88921	L2 Pedicle On Both Sides	88984	Anterior
88922	L3 Pedicle On Both Sides	88985	Posterior
88923	L4 Pedicle On Both Sides	88986	Right
88924	L5 Pedicle On Both Sides	88987	Left
88927	Right Lamina	88988	Thickening
88928	L1 Lamina On The Right	88989	Superior
88929	L2 Lamina On The Right	88990	Inferior
88930	L3 Lamina On The Right	88991	Anterior
88931	L4 Lamina On The Right	88992	Posterior
88932	L5 Lamina On The Right	88993	Right
88935	Left Lamina	88994	Left
88936	L1 Lamina On The Left	88995	Thinning
88937	L2 Lamina On The Left	88996	Superior
88938	L3 Lamina On The Left	88997	Inferior
88939	L4 Lamina On The Left	88998	Anterior
88940	L5 Lamina On The Left	88999	Posterior
88943	Both Lamina	89000	Right
88944	L1 Lamina On Both Sides	89001	Left
88945	L2 Lamina On Both Sides	89002	Soft Tissue Mass
88946	L3 Lamina On Both Sides	89003	Suspected
88947	L4 Lamina On Both Sides	89004	Superior
88948	L5 Lamina On Both Sides	89005	Inferior
88951	Spinous Process	89006	Anterior
88952	L1 Spinous Process	89007	Posterior
88953	L2 Spinous Process	89008	Right
88954	L3 Spinous Process	89009	Left

X-RAY, cont.

89010	Seen	80577	Pathologic
89011	Superior	80578	Pediatric
89012	Inferior	80579	Torus
89013	Anterior	80580	Greenstick
89014	Posterior	80581	Salter Type I
89015	Right	80582	Salter Type II
89016	Left	80583	Salter Type III
89017	Displaced Bone Fragment	80584	Salter Type IV
89018	___cm	80585	Intra-articular
89019	Superior	80586	Extra-articular
89020	Inferior	80587	Comminuted
89021	Anterior	80588	Minimally
89022	Posterior	80589	Moderately
89023	Right	80590	Severely
89024	Left	80591	Simple
89025	Central Canal	80592	Displaced
89026	Trabecular	80595	Non-displaced
89027	Prominence	80603	Pattern
89028	Thickening	80596	Angulated
89029	Sequestrum	80597	Spiral
13880	**Sacroiliac**	80598	Oblique
102860	No Radiographic Evidence Of Any	80599	Transverse
	Osteoarticular Abnormality	80600	Butterfly Component
18001	Joint Space	80601	Complex
101253	Widened	80602	Avulsion
101255	Narrowed	80604	Location
101256	Irregular	80605	Proximal
18002	Sclerosis	80606	Middle
101260	Sacral Side	80607	Medial
101261	Iliac Side	80608	Lateral
101262	Indistinct Cortex	80609	Anterior
101263	Sacral Side	80610	Posterior
101265	Iliac Side	80611	Section
101266	Erosions	80612	Metaphyseal
101267	Sacral Side	80613	Diaphyseal
101268	Iliac Side	80614	Epiphyseal
101270	Osteophytes	13881	**Pelvic**
101271	Inferior	102862	Views
101272	Bony Ankylosis	29347	Anteroposterior
101273	Distribution	29348	Complete, Two Or More Views
101275	Bilaterally Symmetrical	102863	No Radiographic Evidence Of Any
101277	Bilaterally Asymmetrical		Osteoarticular Abnormality
80565	**Coccyx**	80015	Fracture
102861	No Radiographic Evidence Of Any	80016	Open
	Osteoarticular Abnormality	80017	Closed
80569	Fracture	80018	Acute
80570	Open	80019	Old
80571	Closed	80020	Stress
80572	Acute	80021	Complete
80573	Old	80022	Incomplete
80574	Stress	80023	Pathologic
80575	Complete	18024	Blastic lesion
80576	Incomplete	18025	Bony remodeling

X-RAY, CONT.

80024	Pediatric	85411	Right
80025	Torus	85412	Left
80026	Greenstick	85413	Both
80027	Salter Type I	85414	Superior Pubic Ramus
80028	Salter Type II	85415	Right
80029	Salter Type III	85416	Left
80030	Salter Type IV	85417	Both
80031	Intra-articular	85418	Inferior Pubic Ramus
80032	Extra-articular	85419	Right
80033	Comminuted	85420	Left
80034	Minimally	85421	Both
80035	Moderately	85422	Pubic Symphysis
80036	Severely	85423	Right
80037	Simple	85424	Left
80038	Displaced	85425	Both
80041	Non-displaced	85426	Acetabulum
80049	Pattern	85427	Right
80042	Angulated	85428	Left
80043	Spiral	85429	Both
80044	Oblique	84463	Dimensions
80045	Transverse	84464	Height ___ cm
80046	Butterfly Component	84465	Transversely ___ cm
80047	Complex	84466	AP (anteroposteriorly) ___ cm
80048	Avulsion	84467	Pattern
80050	Location	84468	Geographic
80051	Proximal	84469	Moth-eaten
80052	Middle	84470	Permeative
80053	Medial	84471	Zone Of Transition
80054	Lateral	84472	Narrow
80055	Anterior	84473	Wide
80056	Posterior	84474	Margin
80057	Section	84475	Sclerotic
80058	Metaphyseal	84476	Non-Sclerotic
80059	Diaphyseal	84477	Cortex
80060	Epiphyseal	84478	Intact
80615	Ilium	84479	Destruction
80616	Ischium	84480	Endosteal Scalloping
80617	Pubis	84481	Expansion
18026	Brim thickening	84482	Thickening
84454	Lytic Lesion	84483	Thinning
84455	Location	84484	Soft Tissue Mass
84456	Superior	84485	Suspected
84457	Inferior	84486	Seen
84458	Medial	84487	Periosteal Reaction
84459	Lateral	84488	Thick
84460	Anterior	84489	Thin
84461	Posterior	84490	Uniform
84462	Central	84491	Irregular
85406	Ilium	84492	Dense
85407	Right	84493	Amorphous
85408	Left	84494	Wavy
85409	Both	84495	Lamellated
85410	Ischium	84496	Sunburst

X-RAY, CONT.

84497	Spiculated	84526	Narrow
84498	Codman Triangle	84527	Wide
84499	Matrix	84528	Margin
84500	Osteoid	84529	Sclerotic
84501	Chondral	84530	Non-Sclerotic
84502	Septation	84531	Cortex
84503	Trabecular	84532	Intact
84504	Prominence	84533	Destruction
84505	Thickening	84534	Endosteal Scalloping
84506	Sequestrum	84535	Expansion
84507	Ground Glass Appearence	84536	Thickening
84508	Sclerotic Lesion	84537	Thinning
84509	Location	84538	Soft Tissue Mass
84510	Superior	84539	Suspected
84511	Inferior	84540	Seen
84512	Medial	84541	Periosteal Reaction
84513	Lateral	84542	Thick
84514	Anterior	84543	Thin
84515	Posterior	84544	Uniform
84516	Central	84545	Irregular
85378	Ilium	84546	Dense
85388	Right	84547	Amorphous
85389	Left	84548	Wavy
85390	Both	84549	Lamellated
85383	Ischium	84550	Sunburst
85391	Right	84551	Spiculated
85392	Left	84552	Codman Triangle
85393	Both	84553	Matrix
85384	Superior Pubic Ramus	84554	Osteoid
85394	Right	84555	Chondral
85395	Left	84556	Septation
85396	Both	84557	Trabecular
85385	Inferior Pubic Ramus	84558	Prominence
85397	Right	84559	Thickening
85398	Left	84560	Sequestrum
85399	Both	84561	Ground Glass Appearence
85386	Pubic Symphysis	84562	Mixed Lytic / Sclerotic Lesion
85400	Right	84563	Location
85401	Left	84564	Superior
85402	Both	84565	Inferior
85387	Acetabulum	84566	Medial
85403	Right	84567	Lateral
85404	Left	84568	Anterior
85405	Both	84569	Posterior
84517	Dimensions	84570	Central
84518	Height ___ cm	85430	Ilium
84519	Transversely ___ cm	85431	Right
84520	AP (anteroposteriorly) ___ cm	85432	Left
84521	Pattern	85433	Both
84522	Geographic	85434	Ischium
84523	Moth-eaten	85435	Right
84524	Permeative	85436	Left
84525	Zone Of Transition	85437	Both

X-RAY, CONT.

85438	Superior Pubic Ramus		84608	Osteoid
85439	Right		84609	Chondral
85440	Left		84610	Septation
85441	Both		84611	Trabecular
85442	Inferior Pubic Ramus		84612	Prominence
85443	Right		84613	Thickening
85444	Left		84614	Sequestrum
85445	Both		84615	Ground Glass Appearence
85446	Pubic Symphysis		85454	**Sacrum**
85447	Right		102864	No Radiographic Evidence Of Any Osteoarticular Abnormality
85448	Left			
85449	Both		85455	Lytic Lesion
85450	Acetabulum		85456	Location
85451	Right		85457	Superior
85452	Left		85458	Inferior
85453	Both		85459	Medial
84571	Dimensions		85460	Lateral
84572	Height ___cm		85461	Anterior
84573	Transversely ___cm		85462	Posterior
84574	AP (anteroposteriorly) ___cm		85463	Central
84575	Pattern		85622	Right
84576	Geographic		85626	Left
84577	Moth-eaten		85628	Both
84578	Permeative		85464	Dimensions
84579	Zone Of Transition		85465	Height ___cm
84580	Narrow		85466	Transversely ___cm
84581	Wide		85467	AP (anteroposteriorly) ___cm
84582	Margin		85468	Pattern
84583	Sclerotic		85469	Geographic
84584	Non-Sclerotic		85470	Moth-eaten
84585	Cortex		85471	Permeative
84586	Intact		85472	Zone Of Transition
84587	Destruction		85473	Narrow
84588	Endosteal Scalloping		85474	Wide
84589	Expansion		85475	Margin
84590	Thickening		85476	Sclerotic
84591	Thinning		85477	Non-Sclerotic
84592	Soft Tissue Mass		85478	Cortex
84593	Suspected		85479	Intact
84594	Seen		85480	Destruction
84595	Periosteal Reaction		85481	Endosteal Scalloping
84827	Thick		85482	Expansion
84828	Thin		85483	Thickening
84829	Uniform		85484	Thinning
84830	Irregular		85485	Soft Tissue Mass
84831	Dense		85486	Suspected
84832	Amorphous		85487	Seen
84833	Wavy		85488	Periosteal Reaction
84834	Lamellated		85489	Thick
84835	Sunburst		85490	Thin
84836	Spiculated		85491	Uniform
84837	Codman Triangle		85492	Irregular
84838	Matrix		85493	Dense

X-RAY, CONT.

85494	Amorphous	85544	Thin
85495	Wavy	85545	Uniform
85496	Lamellated	85546	Irregular
85497	Sunburst	85547	Dense
85498	Spiculated	85548	Amorphous
85499	Codman Triangle	85549	Wavy
85500	Matrix	85550	Lamellated
85501	Osteoid	85551	Sunburst
85502	Chondral	85552	Spiculated
85503	Septation	85553	Codman Triangle
85504	Trabecular	85554	Matrix
85505	Prominence	85555	Osteoid
85506	Thickening	85556	Chondral
85507	Sequestrum	85557	Septation
85508	Ground Glass Appearence	85558	Trabecular
85509	Sclerotic Lesion	85559	Prominence
85510	Location	85560	Thickening
85511	Superior	85561	Sequestrum
85512	Inferior	85562	Ground Glass Appearence
85513	Medial	85563	Mixed Lytic / Sclerotic Lesion
85514	Lateral	85564	Location
85515	Anterior	85565	Superior
85516	Posterior	85566	Inferior
85517	Central	85567	Medial
85636	Right	85568	Lateral
85637	Left	85569	Anterior
85638	Both	85570	Posterior
85518	Dimensions	85571	Central
85519	Height ___ cm	85641	Right
85520	Transversely ___ cm	85642	Left
85521	AP (anteroposteriorly) ___ cm	85643	Both
85522	Pattern	85572	Dimensions
85523	Geographic	85573	Height ___ cm
85524	Moth-eaten	85574	Transversely ___ cm
85525	Permeative	85575	AP (anteroposteriorly) ___ cm
85526	Zone Of Transition	85576	Pattern
85527	Narrow	85577	Geographic
85528	Wide	85578	Moth-eaten
85529	Margin	85579	Permeative
85530	Sclerotic	85580	Zone Of Transition
85531	Non-Sclerotic	85581	Narrow
85532	Cortex	85582	Wide
85533	Intact	85583	Margin
85534	Destruction	85584	Sclerotic
85535	Endosteal Scalloping	85585	Non-Sclerotic
85536	Expansion	85586	Cortex
85537	Thickening	85587	Intact
85538	Thinning	85588	Destruction
85539	Soft Tissue Mass	85589	Endosteal Scalloping
85540	Suspected	85590	Expansion
85541	Seen	85591	Thickening
85542	Periosteal Reaction	85592	Thinning
85543	Thick	85593	Soft Tissue Mass

X-RAY, CONT.

85594	Suspected	80077	Salter Type IV
85595	Seen	80078	Intra-articular
85596	Periosteal Reaction	80079	Extra-articular
85597	Thick	80080	Comminuted
85598	Thin	80081	Minimally
85599	Uniform	80082	Moderately
85600	Irregular	80083	Severely
85601	Dense	80084	Simple
85602	Amorphous	80085	Displaced
85603	Wavy	80088	Non-displaced
85604	Lamellated	80096	Pattern
85605	Sunburst	80089	Angulated
85606	Spiculated	80090	Spiral
85607	Codman Triangle	80091	Oblique
85608	Matrix	80092	Transverse
85609	Osteoid	80061	Stellate
85610	Chondral	80093	Butterfly Component
85611	Septation	80094	Complex
85612	Trabecular	80095	Avulsion
85613	Prominence	80097	Location
85614	Thickening	80098	Proximal
85615	Sequestrum	80099	Middle
85616	Ground Glass Appearence	80100	Medial
13882	**Hip**	80101	Lateral
102865	Views	80102	Anterior
28537	One View	80103	Posterior
28538	Complete, Two Or More Views	80104	Section
27080	Screening for Congenital Dislocation of Hip	80105	Metaphyseal
		80106	Diaphyseal
27062	Right Hip	80107	Epiphyseal
27063	Left Hip	80618	Right Acetabulum
88447	Both Hips	80619	Right Proximal Femur
27064	Complete, With Anteroposterior View Of Pelvis	80620	Head
		80621	Neck
29323	Arthrography	80623	Left Acetabulum
29324	With Anesthesia	80624	Left Proximal Femur
102866	No Radiographic Evidence Of Any Osteoarticular Abnormality	80625	Head
		80626	Neck
80062	Fracture	80768	Dislocation
80063	Open	80769	Partial
80064	Closed	80770	Complete
80065	Acute	80771	Acute
80066	Old	80772	Old
80067	Stress	80773	Recurrent
80068	Complete	80840	Anterior Displacement Of The Right Hip
80069	Incomplete		
80070	Pathologic	80841	Posterior Displacement Of The Right Hip
80071	Pediatric		
80072	Torus	80842	Intrapelvic Displacement Of The Right Hip
80073	Greenstick		
80074	Salter Type I	80843	Anterior Displacement Of The Left Hip
80075	Salter Type II		
80076	Salter Type III		

X-RAY, CONT.

80844	Posterior Displacement Of The Left Hip	100106	Anterior
		100107	Posterior
80845	Intrapelvic Displacement Of The Left Hip	100108	Medial
		100109	Lateral
89095	Osteopenia	100110	Femoral Neck
89551	Right	101030	Scalloped Appearance
89552	Left	101031	Anterior Aspect
89553	Juxta-articular	101032	Posterior Aspect
89554	Generalized	101033	Medial Aspect
89563	Joint Effusion	101034	Lateral Aspect
89564	Narrowing Of Joint Space	101035	Chondrocalcinosis
89565	Right	101036	Superolateral
89573	Left	101037	Inferomedial
89574	Superolateral	101038	Radiodense Loose Bodies
89575	Medial	101039	Medial
89576	Axial	101040	Lateral
89577	Protrusio Acetabuli	101041	Superior
89580	Right	101042	Inferior
89587	Left	101043	Acetabulum
89588	Proliferative Changes	101044	Femoral Head
89594	Sclerosis	101045	Osteonecrosis
89596	Right	101046	Sclerosis
89597	Left	101047	Subchondral Lucency
89599	Acetabulum	101048	Flattening
89601	Femoral Head	101049	Secondary Osteoarthritic Changes
89813	Osteophytes	101050	Distribution
89964	Medial	101051	Bilaterally Symmetrical
89973	Lateral	101052	Bilaterally Asymmetrical
89974	Acetabulum	13883	**Femur**
89975	Femoral Head	102903	Views
89976	Bony Ankylosis	29343	Anteroposterior And Lateral Views Of Femur
89977	Right		
89978	Left	27065	Right Femur
89979	Subchondral Cyst(s)	27066	Left Femur
89987	Single	27067	Both Femurs
89994	Multiple	102867	No Radiographic Evidence Of Any Osteoarticular Abnormality
89980	Right		
89981	Left	80108	Fracture
100001	Anterior	80109	Open
100002	Posterior	80110	Closed
100003	Medial	80111	Acute
100004	Lateral	80112	Old
100005	Acetabulum	80113	Stress
100006	Femoral Head	80114	Complete
100067	Erosion	80115	Incomplete
100071	Right	80116	Pathologic
100079	Left	80117	Pediatric
100100	Acetabulum	80118	Torus
100101	Anterior	80119	Greenstick
100102	Posterior	80120	Salter Type I
100103	Medial	80121	Salter Type II
100104	Lateral	80122	Salter Type III
100105	Femoral Head	80123	Salter Type IV

X-RAY, CONT.

80124	Intra-articular	83690	Proximal
80125	Extra-articular	83691	Middle
80126	Comminuted	83692	Distal
80127	Minimally	83693	Right Femur
80128	Moderately	83694	Proximal
80129	Severely	83695	Middle
80130	Simple	83696	Distal
80131	Displaced	86350	Pattern
80134	Non-displaced	86351	Geographic
80142	Pattern	86352	Moth-eaten
80135	Angulated	86353	Permeative
80136	Spiral	86354	Zone Of Transition
80137	Oblique	86355	Narrow
80138	Transverse	86356	Wide
80139	Butterfly Component	86357	Margin
80140	Complex	86358	Sclerotic
80141	Avulsion	86359	Non-Sclerotic
80143	Location	86360	Cortex
80144	Proximal	86361	Intact
80145	Middle	86362	Destruction
80146	Medial	86363	Endosteal Scalloping
80147	Lateral	86364	Expansion
80148	Anterior	86365	Thickening
80149	Posterior	86366	Thinning
80150	Section	86367	Superior
80151	Metaphyseal	86368	Inferior
80152	Diaphyseal	86369	Medial
80153	Epiphyseal	86370	Lateral
80622	Right Femur	86371	Anterior
80627	Left Femur	86372	Posterior
80942	Developmental Bone Age	86373	Periosteal Reaction
80943	Retarded	86374	Thick
80944	Advanced	86375	Thin
83439	Lytic Lesion	86376	Uniform
83440	Septated	86377	Irregular
83441	Non-Septated	86378	Dense
83442	Dimensions	86379	Amorphous
83443	Height ___ cm	86380	Wavy
83444	Transverse ___ cm	86381	Lamellated
83445	AP ___ cm	86382	Sunburst
83446	Location	86383	Spiculated
83447	Cortical	86384	Codman Triangle
83448	Medullary	86385	Matrix
83449	Central	86386	Osteoid
83450	Eccentric	86387	Chondral
83451	Epiphyseal	86388	Soft Tissue Mass
83452	Proximal	86389	Suspected
83453	Distal	86390	Seen
83454	Metaphyseal	86391	Superior
83455	Proximal	86392	Inferior
83456	Distal	86393	Medial
83457	Diaphyseal	86394	Lateral
83689	Left Femur	86395	Anterior

X-RAY, CONT.

86396	Trabecular
86397	Prominence
86398	Thickening
86399	Sequestrum
86400	Ground Glass Appearence
83458	Sclerotic Lesion
83461	Dimensions
83462	Height ___cm
83463	Transverse ___ cm
83464	AP ___ cm
83465	Location
83466	Cortical
83467	Medullary
83468	Central
83469	Eccentric
83470	Epiphyseal
83471	Proximal
83472	Distal
83473	Metaphyseal
83474	Proximal
83475	Distal
83476	Diaphyseal
83698	Left Femur
83699	Proximal
83700	Middle
83701	Distal
83702	Right Femur
83703	Proximal
83704	Middle
83705	Distal
86401	Pattern
86402	Geographic
86403	Moth-eaten
86404	Permeative
86405	Zone Of Transition
86406	Narrow
86407	Wide
86408	Margin
86409	Sclerotic
86410	Non-Sclerotic
86411	Cortex
86412	Intact
86413	Destruction
86414	Endosteal Scalloping
86415	Expansion
86416	Thickening
86417	Thinning
86418	Superior
86419	Inferior
86420	Medial
86421	Lateral
86422	Anterior
86423	Posterior

86424	Periosteal Reaction
86425	Thick
86426	Thin
86427	Uniform
86428	Irregular
86429	Dense
86430	Amorphous
86431	Wavy
86432	Lamellated
86433	Sunburst
86434	Spiculated
86435	Codman Triangle
86436	Matrix
86437	Osteoid
86438	Chondral
86439	Soft Tissue Mass
86440	Suspected
86441	Seen
86442	Superior
86443	Inferior
86444	Medial
86445	Lateral
86446	Anterior
86447	Trabecular
86448	Prominence
86449	Thickening
86450	Sequestrum
86451	Ground Glass Appearence
83139	Mixed Lytic / Sclerotic Lesion
83140	Septated
83141	Non-Septated
83142	Dimensions
83143	Height ___cm
83144	Transverse ___ cm
83145	AP ___ cm
83146	Location
83147	Cortical
83148	Medullary
83149	Central
83150	Eccentric
83151	Epiphyseal
83152	Proximal
83153	Distal
83154	Metaphyseal
83155	Proximal
83156	Distal
83157	Diaphyseal
83706	Left Femur
83707	Proximal
83708	Middle
83709	Distal
83710	Right Femur
83711	Proximal

X-Ray, cont.

83712	Middle	13884	**Knee**
83713	Distal	102868	Views
86452	Pattern	28539	Anteroposterior And Lateral Views
86453	Geographic	28540	With Oblique(s), Three Or More
86454	Moth-eaten		Views
86455	Permeative	27068	Right Knee
86456	Zone Of Transition	27069	Left Knee
86457	Narrow	27070	Both Knees
86458	Wide	29325	Arthrography
86459	Margin	102869	No Radiographic Evidence Of Any
86460	Sclerotic		Osteoarticular Abnormality
86461	Non-Sclerotic	80154	Fracture
86462	Cortex	80155	Open
86463	Intact	80156	Closed
86464	Destruction	80157	Acute
86465	Endosteal Scalloping	80158	Old
86466	Expansion	80159	Stress
86467	Thickening	80160	Complete
86468	Thinning	80161	Incomplete
86469	Superior	80162	Pathologic
86470	Inferior	80163	Pediatric
86471	Medial	80164	Torus
86472	Lateral	80165	Greenstick
86473	Anterior	80166	Salter Type I
86474	Posterior	80167	Salter Type II
86475	Periosteal Reaction	80168	Salter Type III
86476	Thick	80169	Salter Type IV
86477	Thin	80170	Intra-articular
86478	Uniform	80171	Extra-articular
86479	Irregular	80172	Comminuted
86480	Dense	80173	Minimally
86481	Amorphous	80174	Moderately
86482	Wavy	80175	Severely
86483	Lamellated	80176	Simple
86484	Sunburst	80177	Displaced
86485	Spiculated	80180	Non-displaced
86486	Codman Triangle	80188	Pattern
86487	Matrix	80181	Angulated
86488	Osteoid	80182	Spiral
86489	Chondral	80183	Oblique
86490	Soft Tissue Mass	80184	Transverse
86491	Suspected	80185	Butterfly Component
86492	Seen	80186	Complex
86493	Superior	80187	Avulsion
86494	Inferior	80189	Location
86495	Medial	80190	Proximal
86496	Lateral	80191	Middle
86497	Anterior	80192	Medial
86498	Trabecular	80193	Lateral
86499	Prominence	80194	Anterior
86500	Thickening	80195	Posterior
86501	Sequestrum	80196	Section
86502	Ground Glass Appearence	80197	Metaphyseal

X-RAY, CONT.

80198	Diaphyseal	88457	Medial Femoral Condyle
80199	Epiphyseal	88458	Medial Tibial Plateau
80628	Right Distal Femur	88460	Lateral Femoral Condyle
80629	Right Patella	88459	Lateral Tibial Plateau
80630	Right Proximal Tibia	89034	Proliferative Changes
80631	Left Distal Femur	88475	Sclerosis
80632	Left Patella	88476	Right
80633	Left Proximal Tibia	88477	Left
80774	Dislocation	88478	Medial Femoral Condyle
80775	Partial	88479	Medial Tibial Plateau
80776	Complete	88480	Lateral Femoral Condyle
80777	Acute	88481	Lateral Tibial Plateau
80778	Old	88482	Patella
80779	Recurrent	88660	Superior
80846	Anterior Displacement	88661	Inferior
80847	Posterior Displacement	17959	Osteophytes
80848	Medial Displacement	88461	Right
80849	Lateral Displacement	88462	Left
80850	Right Tibiofemoral Joint	88463	Medial Femoral Condyle
80851	Right Patella	88464	Medial Tibial Plateau
80852	Right Proximal Tibiofibular Joint	88466	Lateral Femoral Condyle
80853	Left Tibiofemoral Joint	88465	Lateral Tibial Plateau
80854	Left Patella	88467	Patella
80855	Left Proximal Tibiofibular Joint	88468	Superior
17954	Joint Space Narrowing	88469	Inferior
88038	Right	89035	Pointing Of Tibial Spines
88085	Left	89036	Right
87950	Medial	89037	Left
88120	Lateral	17960	Chondrocalcinosis
88155	Patellofemoral	88470	Right
89030	Joint Effusion	88471	Left
89031	Right	88472	Medial Joint Space
89032	Left	88473	Lateral Joint Space
17955	Osteopenia	88474	Patellofemoral Joint Space
88230	Right	88662	Loose Bodies
88231	Left	88691	Number
88225	Juxtaarticular	88766	Size
88232	Generalized	88815	Medial Femoral Condyle
17956	Soft Tissue Swelling	88819	Medial Tibial Plateau
17957	Subchondral Bone Erosion	88820	Lateral Femoral Condyle
88233	Right	88821	Lateral Tibial Plateau
88234	Left	88822	Patella
101029	Lateral Aspect	88823	Superior
88448	Medial Femoral Condyle	88824	Inferior
88449	Medial Tibial Plateau	89033	Suprapatellar Bursa
88450	Lateral Femoral Condyle	88849	Lateral
88451	Lateral Tibial Plateau	88850	Medial
88452	Patella	88851	Anterior
88453	Superior	88852	Posterior
88454	Inferior	17961	Periosteal Bone Resorption
17958	Subchondral Bone Cysts	17962	Periosteal New Bone Formation
88455	Right	17963	Ankylosis
88456	Left	89038	Osteonecrotic Appearance

X-RAY, CONT.

89039	Subchondral Lucency		80229	Oblique
89040	Crescent-Shaped		80230	Transverse
89041	Flattening		80231	Butterfly Component
89042	Squaring		80232	Complex
89043	Bony Overgrowth		80233	Avulsion
89053	Medial Femoral Condyle		80235	Location
89054	Epiphysis		80236	Proximal
89055	Medial Tibial Plateau		80237	Middle
89056	Epiphysis		80238	Medial
89057	Lateral Femoral Condyle		80239	Lateral
89058	Epiphysis		80240	Anterior
89060	Lateral Tibial Plateau		80241	Posterior
89061	Epiphysis		80242	Section
89067	Distribution		80243	Metaphyseal
89074	Bilaterally Symmetrical		80244	Diaphyseal
89079	Bilaterally Asymmetrical		80245	Epiphyseal
13885	**Leg**		80453	Right Tibia
102870	Views		80454	Right Fibula
29345	Anteroposterior And Lateral Views		80455	Left Tibia
29346	Infant, Two Views		80456	Left Fibula
28374	Right		21020	Fracture Dislocation Of The Epiphysis
28375	Left		22189	Longitudinal Areas of Increased Density In Metaphysis
28376	Both Legs			
102871	No Radiographic Evidence Of Any Osteoarticular Abnormality		22188	"Celery Stalk" Appearance Of Distal Femur
80200	Fracture		80945	Developmental Bone Age
80201	Open		80946	Retarded
80202	Closed		80947	Advanced
80203	Acute		83480	Lytic Lesion
80204	Old		83481	Septated
80205	Stress		83482	Non-Septated
80206	Complete		83483	Dimensions
80207	Incomplete		83484	Height ___cm
80208	Pathologic		83485	Transverse ___ cm
80209	Pediatric		83486	AP ___ cm
80210	Torus		83487	Location
80211	Greenstick		83488	Cortical
80212	Salter Type I		83489	Medullary
80213	Salter Type II		83490	Central
80214	Salter Type III		83491	Eccentric
80215	Salter Type IV		83492	Epiphyseal
80216	Intra-articular		83493	Proximal
80217	Extra-articular		83494	Distal
80218	Comminuted		83495	Metaphyseal
80219	Minimally		83496	Proximal
80220	Moderately		83497	Distal
80221	Severely		83498	Diaphyseal
80222	Simple		83733	Left Tibia
80223	Displaced		83734	Proximal
80226	Non-displaced		83735	Middle
80234	Pattern		83736	Distal
80227	Angulated		83737	Right Tibia
80228	Spiral		83738	Proximal

X-RAY, CONT.

83739	Middle	86648	Medial
83740	Distal	86649	Lateral
83741	Left Fibia	86650	Anterior
83742	Proximal	86651	Trabecular
83743	Middle	86652	Prominence
83744	Distal	86653	Thickening
83745	Right Fibia	86654	Sequestrum
83746	Proximal	86655	Ground Glass Appearence
83747	Middle	83499	Sclerotic Lesion
83748	Distal	83502	Dimensions
86605	Pattern	83503	Height ___cm
86606	Geographic	83504	Transverse ___ cm
86607	Moth-eaten	83505	AP ___ cm
86608	Permeative	83506	Location
86609	Zone Of Transition	83507	Cortical
86610	Narrow	83508	Medullary
86611	Wide	83509	Central
86612	Margin	83510	Eccentric
86613	Sclerotic	83511	Epiphyseal
86614	Non-Sclerotic	83512	Proximal
86615	Cortex	83513	Distal
86616	Intact	83514	Metaphyseal
86617	Destruction	83515	Proximal
86618	Endosteal Scalloping	83516	Distal
86619	Expansion	83517	Diaphyseal
86620	Thickening	83715	Left Tibia
86621	Thinning	83716	Proximal
86622	Superior	83717	Middle
86623	Inferior	83718	Distal
86624	Medial	83719	Right Tibia
86625	Lateral	83720	Proximal
86626	Anterior	83721	Middle
86627	Posterior	83722	Distal
86628	Periosteal Reaction	83723	Left Fibia
86629	Thick	83724	Proximal
86630	Thin	83725	Middle
86631	Uniform	83726	Distal
86632	Irregular	83727	Right Fibia
86633	Dense	83728	Proximal
86634	Amorphous	83729	Middle
86635	Wavy	83730	Distal
86636	Lamellated	86554	Pattern
86637	Sunburst	86555	Geographic
86638	Spiculated	86556	Moth-eaten
86639	Codman Triangle	86557	Permeative
86640	Matrix	86558	Zone Of Transition
86641	Osteoid	86559	Narrow
86642	Chondral	86560	Wide
86643	Soft Tissue Mass	86561	Margin
86644	Suspected	86562	Sclerotic
86645	Seen	86563	Non-Sclerotic
86646	Superior	86564	Cortex
86647	Inferior	86565	Intact

X-RAY, CONT.

86566	Destruction	83172	Distal
86567	Endosteal Scalloping	83173	Metaphyseal
86568	Expansion	83174	Proximal
86569	Thickening	83175	Distal
86570	Thinning	83176	Diaphyseal
86571	Superior	83750	Left Tibia
86572	Inferior	83751	Proximal
86573	Medial	83752	Middle
86574	Lateral	83753	Distal
86575	Anterior	83754	Right Tibia
86576	Posterior	83755	Proximal
86577	Periosteal Reaction	83756	Middle
86578	Thick	83757	Distal
86579	Thin	83758	Left Fibia
86580	Uniform	83759	Proximal
86581	Irregular	83760	Middle
86582	Dense	83761	Distal
86583	Amorphous	83762	Right Fibia
86584	Wavy	83763	Proximal
86585	Lamellated	83764	Middle
86586	Sunburst	83765	Distal
86587	Spiculated	86503	Pattern
86588	Codman Triangle	86504	Geographic
86589	Matrix	86505	Moth-eaten
86590	Osteoid	86506	Permeative
86591	Chondral	86507	Zone Of Transition
86592	Soft Tissue Mass	86508	Narrow
86593	Suspected	86509	Wide
86594	Seen	86510	Margin
86595	Superior	86511	Sclerotic
86596	Inferior	86512	Non-Sclerotic
86597	Medial	86513	Cortex
86598	Lateral	86514	Intact
86599	Anterior	86515	Destruction
86600	Trabecular	86516	Endosteal Scalloping
86601	Prominence	86517	Expansion
86602	Thickening	86518	Thickening
86603	Sequestrum	86519	Thinning
86604	Ground Glass Appearence	86520	Superior
83158	Mixed Lytic / Sclerotic Lesion	86521	Inferior
83159	Septated	86522	Medial
83160	Non-Septated	86523	Lateral
83161	Dimensions	86524	Anterior
83162	Height ___ cm	86525	Posterior
83163	Transverse ___ cm	86526	Periosteal Reaction
83164	AP ___ cm	86527	Thick
83165	Location	86528	Thin
83166	Cortical	86529	Uniform
83167	Medullary	86530	Irregular
83168	Central	86531	Dense
83169	Eccentric	86532	Amorphous
83170	Epiphyseal	86533	Wavy
83171	Proximal	86534	Lamellated

X-RAY, CONT.

86535	Sunburst	80269	Displaced
86536	Spiculated	80272	Non-displaced
86537	Codman Triangle	80280	Pattern
86538	Matrix	80273	Angulated
86539	Osteoid	80274	Spiral
86540	Chondral	80275	Oblique
86541	Soft Tissue Mass	80276	Transverse
86542	Suspected	80277	Butterfly Component
86543	Seen	80278	Complex
86544	Superior	80279	Avulsion
86545	Inferior	80281	Location
86546	Medial	80282	Proximal
86547	Lateral	80283	Middle
86548	Anterior	80284	Medial
86549	Trabecular	80285	Lateral
86550	Prominence	80286	Anterior
86551	Thickening	80287	Posterior
86552	Sequestrum	80288	Section
86553	Ground Glass Appearence	80289	Metaphyseal
13886	**Ankle**	80290	Diaphyseal
102872	Views	80291	Epiphyseal
28383	Anteroposterior And Lateral Views	80634	Right Distal Tibia
28384	Complete - Three Or More Views	80635	Right Lateral Malleolus
27071	Right Ankle	80636	Right Talus
27072	Left Ankle	80637	Left Distal Tibia
27073	Both Ankles	80638	Left Lateral Malleolus
28385	Arthrography	80639	Left Talus
29326	Supervision And Interpretation	80780	Dislocation
102873	No Radiographic Evidence Of Any Osteoarticular Abnormality	80781	Partial
		80782	Complete
80246	Fracture	80783	Acute
80247	Open	80784	Old
80248	Closed	80785	Recurrent
80249	Acute	80856	Right Tibiotalar Joint
80250	Old	80857	Right Subtalar Joint
80251	Stress	80858	Left Tibiotalar Joint
80252	Complete	80859	Left Subtalar Joint
80253	Incomplete	84383	Lytic Lesion
80254	Pathologic	84384	Location
80255	Pediatric	84385	Superior
80256	Torus	84386	Inferior
80257	Greenstick	84387	Medial
80258	Salter Type I	84388	Lateral
80259	Salter Type II	84389	Anterior
80260	Salter Type III	84390	Posterior
80261	Salter Type IV	84391	Central
80262	Intra-articular	85645	Right
80263	Extra-articular	85646	First tarsal
80264	Comminuted	85647	Second tarsal
80265	Minimally	85648	Third tarsal
80266	Moderately	85649	Fourth tarsal
80267	Severely	85650	Fifth tarsal
80268	Simple	85651	Left

X-RAY, CONT.

85652	First tarsal	84911	Inferior
85653	Second tarsal	84912	Medial
85654	Third tarsal	84913	Lateral
85655	Fourth tarsal	84914	Anterior
85656	Fifth tarsal	84915	Posterior
84392	Dimensions	84916	Central
84393	Height ___cm	85657	Right
84394	Transversely ___cm	85658	First tarsal
84395	AP (anteroposteriorly) ___cm	85659	Second tarsal
84396	Pattern	85660	Third tarsal
84397	Geographic	85661	Fourth tarsal
84398	Moth-eaten	85662	Fifth tarsal
84399	Permeative	85663	Left
84400	Zone Of Transition	85664	First tarsal
84401	Narrow	85665	Second tarsal
84402	Wide	85666	Third tarsal
84403	Margin	85667	Fourth tarsal
84404	Sclerotic	85668	Fifth tarsal
84405	Non-Sclerotic	84917	Dimensions
84406	Cortex	84918	Height ___cm
84407	Intact	84919	Transversely ___cm
84408	Destruction	84920	AP (anteroposteriorly) ___cm
84409	Endosteal Scalloping	84921	Pattern
84410	Expansion	84922	Geographic
84411	Thickening	84923	Moth-eaten
84412	Thinning	84924	Permeative
84413	Soft Tissue Mass	84925	Zone Of Transition
84414	Suspected	84926	Narrow
84415	Seen	84927	Wide
84416	Periosteal Reaction	84928	Margin
84417	Thick	84929	Sclerotic
84418	Thin	84930	Non-Sclerotic
84419	Uniform	84931	Cortex
84420	Irregular	84932	Intact
84421	Dense	84933	Destruction
84422	Amorphous	84934	Endosteal Scalloping
84423	Wavy	84935	Expansion
84424	Lamellated	84936	Thickening
84425	Sunburst	84937	Thinning
84426	Spiculated	84938	Soft Tissue Mass
84427	Codman Triangle	84939	Suspected
84428	Matrix	84940	Seen
84429	Osteoid	84941	Periosteal Reaction
84430	Chondral	84942	Thick
84431	Septation	84943	Thin
84432	Trabecular	84944	Uniform
84433	Prominence	84945	Irregular
84434	Thickening	84946	Dense
84435	Sequestrum	84947	Amorphous
84436	Ground Glass Appearence	84948	Wavy
84908	Sclerotic Lesion	84949	Lamellated
84909	Location	84950	Sunburst
84910	Superior	84951	Spiculated

X-RAY, CONT.

84952	Codman Triangle	84993	Suspected
84953	Matrix	84994	Seen
84954	Osteoid	84995	Periosteal Reaction
84955	Chondral	84996	Thick
84956	Septation	84997	Thin
84957	Trabecular	84998	Uniform
84958	Prominence	84999	Irregular
84959	Thickening	85000	Dense
84960	Sequestrum	85001	Amorphous
84961	Ground Glass Appearence	85002	Wavy
84962	Mixed Lytic / Sclerotic Lesion	85003	Lamellated
84963	Location	85004	Sunburst
84964	Superior	85005	Spiculated
84965	Inferior	85006	Codman Triangle
84966	Medial	85007	Matrix
84967	Lateral	85008	Osteoid
84968	Anterior	85009	Chondral
84969	Posterior	85010	Septation
84970	Central	85011	Trabecular
85669	Right	85012	Prominence
85670	First tarsal	85013	Thickening
85671	Second tarsal	85014	Sequestrum
85672	Third tarsal	85015	Ground Glass Appearence
85673	Fourth tarsal	13887	**Foot**
85674	Fifth tarsal	102874	Views
85675	Left	28378	Anteroposterior And Lateral Views
85676	First tarsal	28379	Three Or More Views
85677	Second tarsal	27074	Right Foot
85678	Third tarsal	27075	Left Foot
85679	Fourth tarsal	27076	Both Feet
85680	Fifth tarsal	102875	No Radiographic Evidence Of Any
84971	Dimensions		Osteoarticular Abnormality
84972	Height ___ cm	80292	Fracture
84973	Transversely ___ cm	80293	Open
84974	AP (anteroposteriorly) ___ cm	80294	Closed
84975	Pattern	80295	Acute
84976	Geographic	80296	Old
84977	Moth-eaten	80297	Stress
84978	Permeative	80298	Complete
84979	Zone Of Transition	80299	Incomplete
84980	Narrow	80300	Pathologic
84981	Wide	80301	Pediatric
84982	Margin	80302	Torus
84983	Sclerotic	80303	Greenstick
84984	Non-Sclerotic	80304	Salter Type I
84985	Cortex	80305	Salter Type II
84986	Intact	80306	Salter Type III
84987	Destruction	80307	Salter Type IV
84988	Endosteal Scalloping	80308	Intra-articular
84989	Expansion	80309	Extra-articular
84990	Thickening	80310	Comminuted
84991	Thinning	80311	Minimally
84992	Soft Tissue Mass	80312	Moderately

X-RAY, CONT.

80313	Severely	80862	Right First Metatarsophalangeal Joint
80314	Simple		
80315	Displaced	80863	Right Second Metatarsophalangeal Joint
80318	Non-displaced		
80326	Pattern	80864	Right Third Metatarsophalangeal Joint
80319	Angulated		
80320	Spiral	80865	Right Fourth Metatarsophalangeal Joint
80321	Oblique		
80322	Transverse	80866	Right Fifth Metatarsophalangeal Joint
80323	Butterfly Component		
80324	Complex	80867	Chopart, Left Foot
80325	Avulsion	80868	Lisfranc, Left Foot
80327	Location	80869	Left First Metatarsophalangeal Joint
80328	Proximal	80870	Left Second Metatarsophalangeal Joint
80329	Middle		
80330	Medial	80871	Left Third Metatarsophalangeal Joint
80331	Lateral	80872	Left Fourth Metatarsophalangeal Joint
80332	Anterior		
80333	Posterior	80873	Left Fifth Metatarsophalangeal Joint
80334	Section	17965	Osteopenia
80335	Metaphyseal	101243	Juxta-articular
80336	Diaphyseal	101244	Diffuse
80337	Epiphyseal	102157	1st Tarsal-Metatarsal Joint
80640	Right Calcaneous	102160	Base
80641	Right Navicular	102161	2nd Tarsal-Metatarsal Joint
80642	Right Cuboid	102162	Base
80643	Right First Cuneiform	102164	3rd Tarsal-Metatarsal Joint
80644	Right Second Cuneiform	102165	Base
80645	Right Third Cuneiform	102166	4th Tarsal-Metatarsal Joint
80646	Right First Metatarsal	102167	Base
80647	Right Second Metatarsal	102169	5th Tarsal-Metatarsal Joint
80648	Right Third Metatarsal	102170	Base
80649	Right Fourth Metatarsal	102171	Intertarsal Joints
80650	Right Fifth Metatarsal	102175	Calcaneus
80651	Left Calcaneous	102176	Talus
80652	Left Navicular	102177	Cuboid
80653	Left Cuboid	102178	Navicular
80654	Left First Cuneiform	102179	Medial Cuneiform
80655	Left Second Cuneiform	102180	Middle Cuneiform
80656	Left Third Cuneiform	102181	Lateral Cuneiform
80657	Left First Metatarsal	102182	Subtalar Joint
80658	Left Second Metatarsal	102183	Posterior Facet
80659	Left Third Metatarsal	102184	Medial Facet
80660	Left Fourth Metatarsal	102185	Anterior Facet
80661	Left Fifth Metatarsal	102186	Tibiotalar Joint
80786	Dislocation	102187	Talar Dome
80787	Partial	102188	Medial Malleolus
80788	Complete	102189	Distal Fibula
80789	Acute	17966	Soft Tissue Swelling
80790	Old	101245	Periarticular
80791	Recurrent	101246	Diffuse
80860	Chopart, Right Foot	101247	Fusiform
80861	Lisfranc, Right Foot	102193	1st Tarsal-Metatarsal Joint

X-RAY, CONT.

102194	Base	102249	Distal Fibula
102195	2nd Tarsal-Metatarsal Joint	101242	Proliferative Changes
102196	Base	101250	Sclerosis
102197	3rd Tarsal-Metatarsal Joint	101348	Lateral
102198	Base	101349	Medial
102199	4th Tarsal-Metatarsal Joint	101350	Anterior
102200	Base	101351	Posterior
102201	5th Tarsal-Metatarsal Joint	101251	Osteophytes
102202	Base	101252	Large
102203	Intertarsal Joints	101254	Small
102204	Calcaneus	101320	Lateral
102205	Talus	101321	Medial
102206	Cuboid	101322	Anterior
102207	Navicular	101487	Posterior
102208	Medial Cuneiform	101257	Periosteal Reaction
102209	Middle Cuneiform	101258	Amorphous
102210	Lateral Cuneiform	101259	Solid
102211	Subtalar Joint	101492	Lateral
102212	Posterior Facet	101493	Medial
102213	Medial Facet	101494	Anterior
102215	Anterior Facet	101495	Posterior
102216	Tibiotalar Joint	101269	Bony Proliferation
102217	Talar Dome	101345	At the Achilles Tendon Insertion
102218	Medial Malleolus		on the Calcaneus
102219	Distal Fibula	101346	At the Plantar Fascia Insertion on
17964	Joint Space Narrowing		the Calcaneus
101248	Uniform	102253	1st Tarsal-Metatarsal Joint
101249	Non-Uniform	102254	Base
102224	1st Tarsal-Metatarsal Joint	102255	2nd Tarsal-Metatarsal Joint
102225	Base	102256	Base
102226	2nd Tarsal-Metatarsal Joint	102258	3rd Tarsal-Metatarsal Joint
102227	Base	102259	Base
102228	3rd Tarsal-Metatarsal Joint	102260	4th Tarsal-Metatarsal Joint
102229	Base	102261	Base
102230	4th Tarsal-Metatarsal Joint	102262	5th Tarsal-Metatarsal Joint
102231	Base	102263	Base
102232	5th Tarsal-Metatarsal Joint	102264	Intertarsal Joints
102233	Base	102265	Calcaneus
102234	Intertarsal Joints	102266	Talus
102235	Calcaneus	102267	Cuboid
102236	Talus	102268	Navicular
102237	Cuboid	102269	Medial Cuneiform
102238	Navicular	102270	Middle Cuneiform
102239	Medial Cuneiform	102271	Lateral Cuneiform
102240	Middle Cuneiform	102273	Subtalar Joint
102241	Lateral Cuneiform	102274	Posterior Facet
102242	Subtalar Joint	102275	Medial Facet
102243	Posterior Facet	102276	Anterior Facet
102244	Medial Facet	102277	Tibiotalar Joint
102245	Anterior Facet	102278	Talar Dome
102246	Tibiotalar Joint	102279	Medial Malleolus
102247	Talar Dome	102280	Distal Fibula
102248	Medial Malleolus	101264	Bony Ankylosis

X-RAY, CONT.

102285	1st Tarsal-Metatarsal Joint		102365	Tibiotalar Joint
102286	Base		102366	Talar Dome
102287	2nd Tarsal-Metatarsal Joint		102367	Medial Malleolus
102288	Base		102368	Distal Fibula
102289	3rd Tarsal-Metatarsal Joint		17967	Erosions
102290	Base		101278	Marginal
102291	4th Tarsal-Metatarsal Joint		101279	Central
102292	Base		101290	Lateral
102293	5th Tarsal-Metatarsal Joint		101291	Medial
102294	Base		101292	Anterior
102295	Intertarsal Joints		101293	Posterior
102296	Calcaneus		101280	Overhanging Edge
102297	Talus		101294	Lateral
102298	Cuboid		101295	Medial
102299	Navicular		101296	Anterior
102300	Medial Cuneiform		101297	Posterior
102301	Middle Cuneiform		102314	1st Tarsal-Metatarsal Joint
102302	Lateral Cuneiform		102315	Base
102303	Subtalar Joint		102316	2nd Tarsal-Metatarsal Joint
102304	Posterior Facet		102317	Base
102305	Medial Facet		102318	3rd Tarsal-Metatarsal Joint
102306	Anterior Facet		102319	Base
102307	Tibiotalar Joint		102320	4th Tarsal-Metatarsal Joint
102308	Talar Dome		102321	Base
102309	Medial Malleolus		102322	5th Tarsal-Metatarsal Joint
102310	Distal Fibula		102323	Base
17968	Subchondral Cysts		102324	Intertarsal Joints
101334	Lateral		102325	Calcaneus
101336	Medial		102326	Talus
101337	Anterior		102327	Cuboid
101338	Posterior		102328	Navicular
102343	1st Tarsal-Metatarsal Joint		102329	Medial Cuneiform
102344	Base		102330	Middle Cuneiform
102345	2nd Tarsal-Metatarsal Joint		102331	Lateral Cuneiform
102346	Base		102332	Subtalar Joint
102347	3rd Tarsal-Metatarsal Joint		102333	Posterior Facet
102348	Base		102334	Medial Facet
102349	4th Tarsal-Metatarsal Joint		102335	Anterior Facet
102350	Base		102336	Tibiotalar Joint
102351	5th Tarsal-Metatarsal Joint		102337	Talar Dome
102352	Base		102338	Medial Malleolus
102353	Intertarsal Joints		102339	Distal Fibula
102354	Calcaneus		101281	Soft Tissue Calcification
102355	Talus		101298	Lateral
102356	Cuboid		101299	Medial
102357	Navicular		101300	Anterior
102358	Medial Cuneiform		101301	Posterior
102359	Middle Cuneiform		102380	1st Tarsal-Metatarsal Joint
102360	Lateral Cuneiform		102381	Base
102361	Subtalar Joint		102382	2nd Tarsal-Metatarsal Joint
102362	Posterior Facet		102383	Base
102363	Medial Facet		102384	3rd Tarsal-Metatarsal Joint
102364	Anterior Facet		102385	Base

X-RAY, CONT.

102386	4th Tarsal-Metatarsal Joint	101286	Neuropathic Joint Appearance
102387	Base	101308	Subluxation
102388	5th Tarsal-Metatarsal Joint	101310	Dislocation
102389	Base	101311	Debris
102390	Intertarsal Joints	101313	Destruction
102391	Calcaneus	101314	Increased Density
102392	Talus	102432	1st Tarsal-Metatarsal Joint
102393	Cuboid	102433	Base
102394	Navicular	102434	2nd Tarsal-Metatarsal Joint
102395	Medial Cuneiform	102435	Base
102396	Middle Cuneiform	102436	3rd Tarsal-Metatarsal Joint
102397	Lateral Cuneiform	102437	Base
102398	Subtalar Joint	102438	4th Tarsal-Metatarsal Joint
102399	Posterior Facet	102439	Base
102400	Medial Facet	102440	5th Tarsal-Metatarsal Joint
102401	Anterior Facet	102441	Base
102402	Tibiotalar Joint	102442	Intertarsal Joints
102403	Talar Dome	102443	Calcaneus
102404	Medial Malleolus	102444	Talus
102405	Distal Fibula	102445	Cuboid
101283	Deformity	102446	Navicular
101285	Dislocation	102447	Medial Cuneiform
101284	Subluxation	102448	Middle Cuneiform
101302	Lateral	102449	Lateral Cuneiform
101304	Medial	102450	Subtalar Joint
101305	Anterior	102451	Posterior Facet
101306	Posterior	102452	Medial Facet
102406	1st Tarsal-Metatarsal Joint	102453	Anterior Facet
102407	Base	102454	Tibiotalar Joint
102408	2nd Tarsal-Metatarsal Joint	102455	Talar Dome
102409	Base	102456	Medial Malleolus
102410	3rd Tarsal-Metatarsal Joint	102457	Distal Fibula
102411	Base	101287	Distribution
102412	4th Tarsal-Metatarsal Joint	101288	Bilaterally Symmetrical
102413	Base	101289	Bilaterally Assymmetrical
102414	5th Tarsal-Metatarsal Joint	101342	Ray
102415	Base	102152	1st Digit
102416	Intertarsal Joints	102153	2nd Digit
102417	Calcaneus	102154	3rd Digit
102418	Talus	102155	4th Digit
102419	Cuboid	102156	5th Digit
102420	Navicular	102458	1st Tarsal-Metatarsal Joint
102421	Medial Cuneiform	102459	Base
102422	Middle Cuneiform	102460	2nd Tarsal-Metatarsal Joint
102423	Lateral Cuneiform	102461	Base
102424	Subtalar Joint	102462	3rd Tarsal-Metatarsal Joint
102425	Posterior Facet	102463	Base
102426	Medial Facet	102464	4th Tarsal-Metatarsal Joint
102427	Anterior Facet	102465	Base
102428	Tibiotalar Joint	102466	5th Tarsal-Metatarsal Joint
102429	Talar Dome	102467	Base
102430	Medial Malleolus	102468	Intertarsal Joints
102431	Distal Fibula	102469	Calcaneus

MEDCIN - TESTS

X-RAY, CONT.

102470	Talus
102471	Cuboid
102472	Navicular
102473	Medial Cuneiform
102474	Middle Cuneiform
102475	Lateral Cuneiform
102476	Subtalar Joint
102477	Posterior Facet
102478	Medial Facet
102479	Anterior Facet
102480	Tibiotalar Joint
102481	Talar Dome
102482	Medial Malleolus
102483	Distal Fibula
17970	Chondrocalcinosis
17971	Periosteal Bone Resorption
17972	Periosteal New Bone Formation
17951	"Pencil-in-Cup" Deformity
17953	Whittling of Phalangeal Tufts
83519	Lytic Lesion
83520	Septated
83521	Non-Septated
83522	Dimensions
83523	Height ___ cm
83524	Transverse ___ cm
83525	AP ___ cm
83526	Location
83527	Cortical
83528	Medullary
83529	Central
83530	Eccentric
83531	Epiphyseal
83532	Proximal
83533	Distal
83534	Metaphyseal
83535	Proximal
83536	Distal
83537	Diaphyseal
83948	Right
83949	First Metatarsal
83950	Second Metatarsal
83951	Third Metatarsal
83952	Fourth Metatarsal
83953	Fifth Metatarsal
83954	Left
83955	First Metatarsal
83956	Second Metatarsal
83945	Third Metatarsal
83958	Fourth Metatarsal
83959	Fifth Metatarsal
86758	Pattern
86759	Geographic
86760	Moth-eaten
86761	Permeative
86762	Zone Of Transition
86763	Narrow
86764	Wide
86765	Margin
86766	Sclerotic
86767	Non-Sclerotic
86768	Cortex
86769	Intact
86770	Destruction
86771	Endosteal Scalloping
86772	Expansion
86773	Thickening
86774	Thinning
86775	Superior
86776	Inferior
86777	Medial
86778	Lateral
86779	Anterior
86780	Posterior
86781	Periosteal Reaction
86782	Thick
86783	Thin
86784	Uniform
86785	Irregular
86786	Dense
86787	Amorphous
86788	Wavy
86789	Lamellated
86790	Sunburst
86791	Spiculated
86792	Codman Triangle
86793	Matrix
86794	Osteoid
86795	Chondral
86796	Soft Tissue Mass
86797	Suspected
86798	Seen
86799	Superior
86800	Inferior
86801	Medial
86802	Lateral
86803	Anterior
86804	Trabecular
86805	Prominence
86806	Thickening
86807	Sequestrum
86808	Ground Glass Appearence
83538	Sclerotic Lesion
83539	Septated
83540	Non-Septated
83541	Dimensions
83542	Height ___ cm

X-RAY, CONT.

83543	Transverse ___ cm	86734	Irregular
83544	AP ___ cm	86735	Dense
83545	Location	86736	Amorphous
83546	Cortical	86737	Wavy
83547	Medullary	86738	Lamellated
83548	Central	86739	Sunburst
83549	Eccentric	86740	Spiculated
83550	Epiphyseal	86741	Codman Triangle
83551	Proximal	86742	Matrix
83552	Distal	86743	Osteoid
83553	Metaphyseal	86744	Chondral
83554	Proximal	86745	Soft Tissue Mass
83555	Distal	86746	Suspected
83556	Diaphyseal	86747	Seen
83936	Right	86748	Superior
83937	First Metatarsal	86749	Inferior
83938	Second Metatarsal	86750	Medial
83939	Third Metatarsal	86751	Lateral
83940	Fourth Metatarsal	86752	Anterior
83941	Fifth Metatarsal	86753	Trabecular
83942	Left	86754	Prominence
83943	First Metatarsal	86755	Thickening
83944	Second Metatarsal	86756	Sequestrum
83957	Third Metatarsal	86757	Ground Glass Appearence
83946	Fourth Metatarsal	83177	Mixed Lytic / Sclerotic Lesion
83947	Fifth Metatarsal	83178	Septated
86707	Pattern	83179	Non-Septated
86708	Geographic	83180	Dimensions
86709	Moth-eaten	83181	Height ___ cm
86710	Permeative	83182	Transverse ___ cm
86711	Zone Of Transition	83183	AP ___ cm
86712	Narrow	83184	Location
86713	Wide	83185	Cortical
86714	Margin	83186	Medullary
86715	Sclerotic	83187	Central
86716	Non-Sclerotic	83188	Eccentric
86717	Cortex	83189	Epiphyseal
86718	Intact	83190	Proximal
86719	Destruction	83191	Distal
86720	Endosteal Scalloping	83192	Metaphyseal
86721	Expansion	83193	Proximal
86722	Thickening	83194	Distal
86723	Thinning	83195	Diaphyseal
86724	Superior	83926	Right
86725	Inferior	83931	First Metatarsal
86726	Medial	83932	Second Metatarsal
86727	Lateral	83933	Third Metatarsal
86728	Anterior	83934	Fourth Metatarsal
86729	Posterior	83935	Fifth Metatarsal
86730	Periosteal Reaction	83924	Left
86731	Thick	83925	First Metatarsal
86732	Thin	83927	Second Metatarsal
86733	Uniform	83928	Third Metatarsal

X-RAY, CONT.

83929	Fourth Metatarsal	28377	**Toes**
83930	Fifth Metatarsal	102904	Views
86656	Pattern	28380	Of The Right Foot
86657	Geographic	28381	Of The Left Foot
86658	Moth-eaten	28382	Of Both Feet
86659	Permeative	102876	No Radiographic Evidence Of Any
86660	Zone Of Transition		Osteoarticular Abnormality
86661	Narrow	80338	Fracture
86662	Wide	80339	Open
86663	Margin	80340	Closed
86664	Sclerotic	80341	Acute
86665	Non-Sclerotic	80342	Old
86666	Cortex	80343	Stress
86667	Intact	80344	Complete
86668	Destruction	80345	Incomplete
86669	Endosteal Scalloping	80346	Pathologic
86670	Expansion	80347	Pediatric
86671	Thickening	80348	Torus
86672	Thinning	80349	Greenstick
86673	Superior	80350	Salter Type I
86674	Inferior	80351	Salter Type II
86675	Medial	80352	Salter Type III
86676	Lateral	80353	Salter Type IV
86677	Anterior	80354	Intra-articular
86678	Posterior	80355	Extra-articular
86679	Periosteal Reaction	80356	Comminuted
86680	Thick	80357	Minimally
86681	Thin	80358	Moderately
86682	Uniform	80359	Severely
86683	Irregular	80360	Simple
86684	Dense	80361	Displaced
86685	Amorphous	80364	Non-displaced
86686	Wavy	80372	Pattern
86687	Lamellated	80365	Angulated
86688	Sunburst	80366	Spiral
86689	Spiculated	80367	Oblique
86690	Codman Triangle	80368	Transverse
86691	Matrix	80369	Butterfly Component
86692	Osteoid	80370	Complex
86693	Chondral	80371	Avulsion
86694	Soft Tissue Mass	80373	Location
86695	Suspected	80374	Proximal
86696	Seen	80375	Middle
86697	Superior	80376	Medial
86698	Inferior	80377	Lateral
86699	Medial	80378	Anterior
86700	Lateral	80379	Posterior
86701	Anterior	80380	Section
86702	Trabecular	80381	Metaphyseal
86703	Prominence	80382	Diaphyseal
86704	Thickening	80383	Epiphyseal
86705	Sequestrum	80662	Right Great Toe
86706	Ground Glass Appearence	80663	Proximal Phalanx

X-RAY, CONT.

80664	Distal Phalanx		80885	Right Fourth Toe Joint
80665	Right Second Toe		80886	MTP
80666	Proximal Phalanx		80887	PIP
80667	Middle Phalanx		80888	DIP
80668	Distal Phalanx		80889	Right Little Toe Joint
80669	Right Middle Toe		80890	MTP
80670	Proximal Phalanx		80891	PIP
80671	Middle Phalanx		80892	DIP
80672	Distal Phalanx		80893	Left Great Toe
80673	Right Fourth Toe		80894	MTP
80674	Proximal Phalanx		80895	IP
80675	Middle Phalanx		80896	Left Second Toe Joint
80676	Distal Phalanx		80897	MTP
80677	Right Little Toe		80898	PIP
80678	Proximal Phalanx		80899	DIP
80679	Middle Phalanx		80900	Left Third Toe Joint
80680	Distal Phalanx		80901	MTP
80681	Left Great Toe		80902	PIP
80682	Proximal Phalanx		80903	DIP
80683	Distal Phalanx		80904	Left Fourth Toe Joint
80684	Left Second Toe		80905	MTP
80685	Proximal Phalanx		80906	PIP
80686	Middle Phalanx		80907	DIP
80687	Distal Phalanx		80908	Left Little Toe Joint
80688	Left Middle Toe		80909	MTP
80689	Proximal Phalanx		80910	PIP
80690	Middle Phalanx		80911	DIP
80691	Distal Phalanx		101499	Bony Ankylosis
80692	Left Fourth Toe		101500	Subchondral Cysts
80693	Proximal Phalanx		101501	Lateral
80694	Middle Phalanx		101502	Medial
80695	Distal Phalanx		101503	Anterior
80696	Left Little Toe		101504	Posterior
80697	Proximal Phalanx		101439	Osteopenia
80698	Middle Phalanx		101906	Right
80699	Distal Phalanx		101907	Left
80792	Dislocation		101440	Juxta-articular
80793	Partial		101441	Diffuse
80794	Complete		101442	1st Interphalangeal Joint
80795	Acute		101443	Proximal End
80796	Old		101444	Distal End
80797	Recurrent		101445	2nd Distal Interphalangeal Joint
80874	Right Great Toe		101446	Proximal End
80875	MTP		101447	Distal End
80876	IP		101448	3rd Distal Interphalangeal Joint
80877	Right Second Toe Joint		101449	Proximal End
80878	MTP		101450	Distal End
80879	PIP		101451	4th Distal Interphalangeal Joint
80880	DIP		101452	Proximal End
80881	Right Third Toe Joint		101453	Distal End
80882	MTP		101454	5th Distal Interphalangeal Joint
80883	PIP		101455	Proximal End
80884	DIP		101456	Distal End

101457	2nd Proximal Interphalangeal Joint
101458	Proximal End
101459	Distal End
101460	3rd Proximal Interphalangeal Joint
101461	Proximal End
101462	Distal End
101463	4th Proximal Interphalangeal Joint
101464	Proximal End
101465	Distal End
101466	5th Proximal Interphalangeal Joint
101467	Proximal End
101468	Distal End
101517	1st Metatarsal Phalangeal Joint
101518	Proximal End
101519	Metatarsal Head
101534	2nd Metatarsal Phalangeal Joint
101535	Proximal End
101537	Metatarsal Head
101538	3rd Metatarsal Phalangeal Joint
101539	Proximal End
101540	Metatarsal Head
101541	4th Metatarsal Phalangeal Joint
101542	Proximal End
101543	Metatarsal Head
101546	5th Metatarsal Phalangeal Joint
101547	Proximal End
101548	Metatarsal Head
101469	Soft Tissue Swelling
101909	Right
101910	Left
101470	Periarticular
101471	Diffuse
101472	Fusiform
101382	1st Interphalangeal Joint
101389	Proximal End
101390	Distal End
101391	2nd Distal Interphalangeal Joint
101392	Proximal End
101393	Distal End
101399	3rd Distal Interphalangeal Joint
101400	Proximal End
101401	Distal End
101404	4th Distal Interphalangeal Joint
101405	Proximal End
101406	Distal End
101409	5th Distal Interphalangeal Joint
101410	Proximal End
101412	Distal End
101417	2nd Proximal Interphalangeal Joint
101418	Proximal End
101420	Distal End
101428	3rd Proximal Interphalangeal Joint
101429	Proximal End
101430	Distal End
101433	4th Proximal Interphalangeal Joint
101434	Proximal End
101435	Distal End
101436	5th Proximal Interphalangeal Joint
101437	Proximal End
101438	Distal End
101563	1st Metatarsal Phalangeal Joint
101564	Proximal End
101565	Metatarsal Head
101566	2nd Metatarsal Phalangeal Joint
101567	Proximal End
101568	Metatarsal Head
101569	3rd Metatarsal Phalangeal Joint
101570	Proximal End
101571	Metatarsal Head
101572	4th Metatarsal Phalangeal Joint
101573	Proximal End
101574	Metatarsal Head
101575	5th Metatarsal Phalangeal Joint
101576	Proximal End
101577	Metatarsal Head
101473	Joint Space Narrowing
101911	Right
101912	Left
101474	Uniform
101475	Non-Uniform
101590	1st Interphalangeal Joint
101591	Proximal End
101592	Distal End
101594	2nd Distal Interphalangeal Joint
101595	Proximal End
101596	Distal End
101597	3rd Distal Interphalangeal Joint
101598	Proximal End
101599	Distal End
101600	4th Distal Interphalangeal Joint
101601	Proximal End
101602	Distal End
101603	5th Distal Interphalangeal Joint
101604	Proximal End
101606	Distal End
101607	2nd Proximal Interphalangeal Joint
101608	Proximal End
101609	Distal End
101610	3rd Proximal Interphalangeal Joint
101611	Proximal End
101613	Distal End
101614	4th Proximal Interphalangeal Joint
101615	Proximal End
101616	Distal End
101617	5th Proximal Interphalangeal Joint
101618	Proximal End

X-RAY, CONT.

101619	Distal End	101667	Proximal End
101620	1st Metatarsal Phalangeal Joint	101668	Metatarsal Head
101621	Proximal End	101669	2nd Metatarsal Phalangeal Joint
101623	Metatarsal Head	101670	Proximal End
101624	2nd Metatarsal Phalangeal Joint	101671	Metatarsal Head
101625	Proximal End	101672	3rd Metatarsal Phalangeal Joint
101626	Metatarsal Head	101673	Proximal End
101627	3rd Metatarsal Phalangeal Joint	101674	Metatarsal Head
101628	Proximal End	101675	4th Metatarsal Phalangeal Joint
101629	Metatarsal Head	101676	Proximal End
101630	4th Metatarsal Phalangeal Joint	101677	Metatarsal Head
101631	Proximal End	101678	5th Metatarsal Phalangeal Joint
101632	Metatarsal Head	101679	Proximal End
101633	5th Metatarsal Phalangeal Joint	101680	Metatarsal Head
101634	Proximal End	101482	Osteophytes
101635	Metatarsal Head	101485	Lateral
101476	Proliferative Changes	101505	Medial
101914	Right	101486	Anterior
101915	Left	101488	Posterior
101477	Sclerosis	101685	1st Interphalangeal Joint
101478	Lateral	101686	Proximal End
101479	Medial	101687	Distal End
101480	Anterior	101688	2nd Distal Interphalangeal Joint
101481	Posterior	101689	Proximal End
101639	1st Interphalangeal Joint	101690	Distal End
101640	Proximal End	101691	3rd Distal Interphalangeal Joint
101641	Distal End	101692	Proximal End
101642	2nd Distal Interphalangeal Joint	101693	Distal End
101643	Proximal End	101694	4th Distal Interphalangeal Joint
101644	Distal End	101695	Proximal End
101645	3rd Distal Interphalangeal Joint	101696	Distal End
101646	Proximal End	101697	5th Distal Interphalangeal Joint
101647	Distal End	101698	Proximal End
101648	4th Distal Interphalangeal Joint	101699	Distal End
101649	Proximal End	101700	2nd Proximal Interphalangeal
101650	Distal End		Joint
101651	5th Distal Interphalangeal Joint	101701	Proximal End
101652	Proximal End	101702	Distal End
101653	Distal End	101703	3rd Proximal Interphalangeal Joint
101654	2nd Proximal Interphalangeal	101704	Proximal End
	Joint	101705	Distal End
101655	Proximal End	101706	4th Proximal Interphalangeal Joint
101656	Distal End	101707	Proximal End
101657	3rd Proximal Interphalangeal Joint	101708	Distal End
101658	Proximal End	101709	5th Proximal Interphalangeal Joint
101659	Distal End	101710	Proximal End
101660	4th Proximal Interphalangeal Joint	101711	Distal End
101661	Proximal End	101712	1st Metatarsal Phalangeal Joint
101662	Distal End	101713	Proximal End
101663	5th Proximal Interphalangeal Joint	101714	Metatarsal Head
101664	Proximal End	101715	2nd Metatarsal Phalangeal Joint
101665	Distal End	101716	Proximal End
101666	1st Metatarsal Phalangeal Joint	101717	Metatarsal Head

X-RAY, CONT.

101718	3rd Metatarsal Phalangeal Joint	101813	Metatarsal Head
101719	Proximal End	101814	5th Metatarsal Phalangeal Joint
101720	Metatarsal Head	101815	Proximal End
101721	4th Metatarsal Phalangeal Joint	101816	Metatarsal Head
101722	Proximal End	101491	Solid
101723	Metatarsal Head	101324	Lateral
101724	5th Metatarsal Phalangeal Joint	101326	Medial
101725	Proximal End	101327	Anterior
101726	Metatarsal Head	101329	Posterior
101507	Periosteal Reaction	101817	1st Interphalangeal Joint
101490	Amorphous	101818	Proximal End
101775	1st Interphalangeal Joint	101819	Distal End
101776	Proximal End	101820	2nd Distal Interphalangeal Joint
101777	Distal End	101821	Proximal End
101778	2nd Distal Interphalangeal Joint	101822	Distal End
101779	Proximal End	101823	3rd Distal Interphalangeal Joint
101780	Distal End	101824	Proximal End
101781	3rd Distal Interphalangeal Joint	101825	Distal End
101782	Proximal End	101826	4th Distal Interphalangeal Joint
101783	Distal End	101827	Proximal End
101784	4th Distal Interphalangeal Joint	101828	Distal End
101785	Proximal End	101829	5th Distal Interphalangeal Joint
101786	Distal End	101830	Proximal End
101787	5th Distal Interphalangeal Joint	101831	Distal End
101788	Proximal End	101832	2nd Proximal Interphalangeal Joint
101789	Distal End		
101790	2nd Proximal Interphalangeal Joint	101833	Proximal End
		101834	Distal End
101791	Proximal End	101835	3rd Proximal Interphalangeal Joint
101792	Distal End		
101793	3rd Proximal Interphalangeal Joint	101836	Proximal End
		101837	Distal End
101794	Proximal End	101838	4th Proximal Interphalangeal Joint
101795	Distal End		
101796	4th Proximal Interphalangeal Joint	101839	Proximal End
		101840	Distal End
101797	Proximal End	101841	5th Proximal Interphalangeal Joint
101798	Distal End		
101799	5th Proximal Interphalangeal Joint	101842	Proximal End
		101843	Distal End
101800	Proximal End	101844	1st Metatarsal Phalangeal Joint
101801	Distal End	101845	Proximal End
101802	1st Metatarsal Phalangeal Joint	101846	Metatarsal Head
101803	Proximal End	101847	2nd Metatarsal Phalangeal Joint
101804	Metatarsal Head	101848	Proximal End
101805	2nd Metatarsal Phalangeal Joint	101849	Metatarsal Head
101806	Proximal End	101850	3rd Metatarsal Phalangeal Joint
101807	Metatarsal Head	101851	Proximal End
101808	3rd Metatarsal Phalangeal Joint	101852	Metatarsal Head
101809	Proximal End	101853	4th Metatarsal Phalangeal Joint
101810	Metatarsal Head	101854	Proximal End
101811	4th Metatarsal Phalangeal Joint	101855	Metatarsal Head
101812	Proximal End	101856	5th Metatarsal Phalangeal Joint

X-RAY, CONT.

101857	Proximal End	101970	Metatarsal Head
101858	Metatarsal Head	101971	3rd Metatarsal Phalangeal Joint
101496	Bony Proliferation	101972	Proximal End
101497	At the Achilles Tendon Insertion on the Calcaneous	101973	Metatarsal Head
		101974	4th Metatarsal Phalangeal Joint
101498	At the Plantar Fascia Insertion on the Calcaneous	101975	Proximal End
		101976	Metatarsal Head
101863	Erosions	101977	5th Metatarsal Phalangeal Joint
101917	Right	101978	Proximal End
101918	Left	101979	Metatarsal Head
101932	Marginal	101877	Soft Tissue Calcification
101933	Central	101921	Right
101934	Lateral	101922	Left
101935	Medial	101878	Lateral
101936	Anterior	101879	Medial
101937	Posterior	101880	Anterior
101872	Overhanging Edge	101881	Posterior
101873	Lateral	101980	1st Interphalangeal Joint
101874	Medial	101981	Proximal End
101875	Anterior	101982	Distal End
101876	Posterior	101983	2nd Distal Interphalangeal Joint
101938	1st Interphalangeal Joint	101984	Proximal End
101939	Proximal End	101985	Distal End
101940	Distal End	101986	3rd Distal Interphalangeal Joint
101941	2nd Distal Interphalangeal Joint	101987	Proximal End
101942	Proximal End	101988	Distal End
101943	Distal End	101989	4th Distal Interphalangeal Joint
101944	3rd Distal Interphalangeal Joint	101990	Proximal End
101945	Proximal End	101991	Distal End
101946	Distal End	101992	5th Distal Interphalangeal Joint
101947	4th Distal Interphalangeal Joint	101993	Proximal End
101948	Proximal End	101994	Distal End
101949	Distal End	101995	2nd Proximal Interphalangeal Joint
101950	5th Distal Interphalangeal Joint	101996	Proximal End
101951	Proximal End	101997	Distal End
101952	Distal End	101998	3rd Proximal Interphalangeal Joint
101953	2nd Proximal Interphalangeal Joint	101999	Proximal End
101954	Proximal End	102000	Distal End
101955	Distal End	102001	4th Proximal Interphalangeal Joint
101956	3rd Proximal Interphalangeal Joint	102002	Proximal End
101957	Proximal End	102003	Distal End
101958	Distal End	102004	5th Proximal Interphalangeal Joint
101959	4th Proximal Interphalangeal Joint	102005	Proximal End
101960	Proximal End	102006	Distal End
101961	Distal End	102007	1st Metatarsal Phalangeal Joint
101962	5th Proximal Interphalangeal Joint	102008	Proximal End
101963	Proximal End	102009	Metatarsal Head
101964	Distal End	102010	2nd Metatarsal Phalangeal Joint
101965	1st Metatarsal Phalangeal Joint	102011	Proximal End
101966	Proximal End	102012	Metatarsal Head
101967	Metatarsal Head	102013	3rd Metatarsal Phalangeal Joint
101968	2nd Metatarsal Phalangeal Joint	102014	Proximal End
101969	Proximal End	102015	Metatarsal Head

X-RAY, CONT.

102016	4th Metatarsal Phalangeal Joint	102060	Metatarsal Head
102017	Proximal End	102061	5th Metatarsal Phalangeal Joint
102018	Metatarsal Head	102062	Proximal End
102019	5th Metatarsal Phalangeal Joint	102063	Metatarsal Head
102020	Proximal End	101889	Neuropathic Joint Appearance
102021	Metatarsal Head	101927	Right
101882	Deformity	101928	Left
101923	Right	101890	Subluxation
101924	Left	101891	Dislocation
101883	Dislocation	101892	Debris
101884	Subluxation	101893	Destruction
101885	Lateral	101894	Increased Density
101886	Medial	102064	1st Interphalangeal Joint
101887	Anterior	102104	Proximal End
101888	Posterior	102105	Distal End
102022	1st Interphalangeal Joint	102065	2nd Distal Interphalangeal Joint
102023	Proximal End	102066	Proximal End
102024	Distal End	102067	Distal End
102025	2nd Distal Interphalangeal Joint	102068	3rd Distal Interphalangeal Joint
102026	Proximal End	102069	Proximal End
102027	Distal End	102070	Distal End
102028	3rd Distal Interphalangeal Joint	102071	4th Distal Interphalangeal Joint
102029	Proximal End	102072	Proximal End
102030	Distal End	102073	Distal End
102031	4th Distal Interphalangeal Joint	102074	5th Distal Interphalangeal Joint
102032	Proximal End	102075	Proximal End
102033	Distal End	102076	Distal End
102034	5th Distal Interphalangeal Joint	102077	2nd Proximal Interphalangeal Joint
102035	Proximal End	102078	Proximal End
102036	Distal End	102079	Distal End
102037	2nd Proximal Interphalangeal Joint	102080	3rd Proximal Interphalangeal Joint
102038	Proximal End	102081	Proximal End
102039	Distal End	102082	Distal End
102040	3rd Proximal Interphalangeal Joint	102083	4th Proximal Interphalangeal Joint
102041	Proximal End	102084	Proximal End
102042	Distal End	102085	Distal End
102043	4th Proximal Interphalangeal Joint	102086	5th Proximal Interphalangeal Joint
102044	Proximal End	102087	Proximal End
102045	Distal End	102088	Distal End
102046	5th Proximal Interphalangeal Joint	102089	1st Metatarsal Phalangeal Joint
102047	Proximal End	102090	Proximal End
102048	Distal End	102091	Metatarsal Head
102049	1st Metatarsal Phalangeal Joint	102092	2nd Metatarsal Phalangeal Joint
102050	Proximal End	102093	Proximal End
102051	Metatarsal Head	102094	Metatarsal Head
102052	2nd Metatarsal Phalangeal Joint	102095	3rd Metatarsal Phalangeal Joint
102053	Proximal End	102096	Proximal End
102054	Metatarsal Head	102097	Metatarsal Head
102055	3rd Metatarsal Phalangeal Joint	102098	4th Metatarsal Phalangeal Joint
102056	Proximal End	102099	Proximal End
102057	Metatarsal Head	102100	Metatarsal Head
102058	4th Metatarsal Phalangeal Joint	102101	5th Metatarsal Phalangeal Joint
102059	Proximal End	102102	Proximal End

X-Ray, cont.

102103	Metatarsal Head	102147	Metatarsal Head
101895	Distribution	83559	Lytic Lesion
101929	Right	83560	Septated
101930	Left	83561	Non-Septated
101896	Bilateral Symmetric	83562	Dimensions
101897	Bilateral Assymmetric	83563	Height ___ cm
101898	Ray	83564	Transverse ___ cm
101899	1st Digit	83565	AP ___ cm
102148	2nd Digit	83566	Location
102149	3rd Digit	83567	Cortical
102150	4th Digit	83568	Medullary
102151	5th Digit	83569	Central
102106	1st Interphalangeal Joint	83570	Eccentric
102107	Proximal End	83571	Epiphyseal
102108	Distal End	83572	Proximal
102109	2nd Distal Interphalangeal Joint	83573	Distal
102110	Proximal End	83574	Metaphyseal
102111	Distal End	83575	Proximal
102112	3rd Distal Interphalangeal Joint	83576	Distal
102113	Proximal End	83577	Diaphyseal
102114	Distal End	83891	Proximal Phalanx
102115	4th Distal Interphalangeal Joint	83892	Right Great Toe
102116	Proximal End	83893	Right Second Toe
102117	Distal End	83894	Right Third Toe
102118	5th Distal Interphalangeal Joint	83895	Right Fourth Toe
102119	Proximal End	83896	Right Little toe
102120	Distal End	83897	Left Great Toe
102121	2nd Proximal Interphalangeal Joint	83898	Left Second Toe
102122	Proximal End	83899	Left Third Toe
102123	Distal End	83900	Left Fourth Toe
102124	3rd Proximal Interphalangeal Joint	83901	Left Little toe
102125	Proximal End	83902	Middle Phalanx
102126	Distal End	83904	Right Second Toe
102127	4th Proximal Interphalangeal Joint	83905	Right Third Toe
102128	Proximal End	83906	Right Fourth Toe
102129	Distal End	83907	Right Little toe
102130	5th Proximal Interphalangeal Joint	83909	Left Second Toe
102131	Proximal End	83910	Left Third Toe
102132	Distal End	83911	Left Fourth Toe
102133	1st Metatarsal Phalangeal Joint	83912	Left Little toe
102134	Proximal End	83913	Distal Phalanx
102135	Metatarsal Head	83914	Right Great Toe
102136	2nd Metatarsal Phalangeal Joint	83915	Right Second Toe
102137	Proximal End	83916	Right Third Toe
102138	Metatarsal Head	83917	Right Fourth Toe
102139	3rd Metatarsal Phalangeal Joint	83918	Right Little toe
102140	Proximal End	83919	Left Great Toe
102141	Metatarsal Head	83920	Left Second Toe
102142	4th Metatarsal Phalangeal Joint	83921	Left Third Toe
102143	Proximal End	83922	Left Fourth Toe
102144	Metatarsal Head	83923	Left Little toe
102145	5th Metatarsal Phalangeal Joint	86911	Pattern
102146	Proximal End	86912	Geographic

X-RAY, CONT.

86913	Moth-eaten	83582	Height ___cm
86914	Permeative	83583	Transverse ___ cm
86915	Zone Of Transition	83584	AP ___cm
86916	Narrow	83585	Location
86917	Wide	83586	Cortical
86918	Margin	83587	Medullary
86919	Sclerotic	83588	Central
86920	Non-Sclerotic	83589	Eccentric
86921	Cortex	83590	Epiphyseal
86922	Intact	83591	Proximal
86923	Destruction	83592	Distal
86924	Endosteal Scalloping	83593	Metaphyseal
86925	Expansion	83594	Proximal
86926	Thickening	83595	Distal
86927	Thinning	83596	Diaphyseal
86928	Superior	83858	Proximal Phalanx
86929	Inferior	83859	Right Great Toe
86930	Medial	83860	Right Second Toe
86931	Lateral	83861	Right Third Toe
86932	Anterior	83862	Right Fourth Toe
86933	Posterior	83863	Right Little toe
86934	Periosteal Reaction	83864	Left Great Toe
86935	Thick	83865	Left Second Toe
86936	Thin	83866	Left Third Toe
86937	Uniform	83867	Left Fourth Toe
86938	Irregular	83868	Left Little toe
86939	Dense	83869	Middle Phalanx
86940	Amorphous	83871	Right Second Toe
86941	Wavy	83872	Right Third Toe
86942	Lamellated	83873	Right Fourth Toe
86943	Sunburst	83874	Right Little toe
86944	Spiculated	83876	Left Second Toe
86945	Codman Triangle	83877	Left Third Toe
86946	Matrix	83878	Left Fourth Toe
86947	Osteoid	83879	Left Little toe
86948	Chondral	83880	Distal Phalanx
86949	Soft Tissue Mass	83881	Right Great Toe
86950	Suspected	83882	Right Second Toe
86951	Seen	83883	Right Third Toe
86952	Superior	83884	Right Fourth Toe
86953	Inferior	83885	Right Little toe
86954	Medial	83886	Left Great Toe
86955	Lateral	83887	Left Second Toe
86956	Anterior	83888	Left Third Toe
86957	Trabecular	83889	Left Fourth Toe
86958	Prominence	83890	Left Little toe
86959	Thickening	86860	Pattern
86960	Sequestrum	86861	Geographic
86961	Ground Glass Appeerence	86862	Moth-eaten
83578	Sclerotic Lesion	86863	Permeative
83579	Septated	86864	Zone Of Transition
83580	Non-Septated	86865	Narrow
83581	Dimensions	86866	Wide

X-RAY, CONT.

86867	Margin		83205	Medullary
86868	Sclerotic		83206	Central
86869	Non-Sclerotic		83207	Eccentric
86870	Cortex		83208	Epiphyseal
86871	Intact		83209	Proximal
86872	Destruction		83210	Distal
86873	Endosteal Scalloping		83211	Metaphyseal
86874	Expansion		83212	Proximal
86875	Thickening		83213	Distal
86876	Thinning		83214	Diaphyseal
86877	Superior		83768	Proximal Phalanx
86878	Inferior		83769	Right Great Toe
86879	Medial		83770	Right Second Toe
86880	Lateral		83771	Right Third Toe
86881	Anterior		83772	Right Fourth Toe
86882	Posterior		83773	Right Little toe
86883	Periosteal Reaction		83810	Left Great Toe
86884	Thick		83811	Left Second Toe
86885	Thin		83812	Left Third Toe
86886	Uniform		83813	Left Fourth Toe
86887	Irregular		83814	Left Little toe
86888	Dense		83779	Middle Phalanx
86889	Amorphous		83817	Right Second Toe
86890	Wavy		83818	Right Third Toe
86891	Lamellated		83819	Right Fourth Toe
86892	Sunburst		83820	Right Little toe
86893	Spiculated		83822	Left Second Toe
86894	Codman Triangle		83823	Left Third Toe
86895	Matrix		83824	Left Fourth Toe
86896	Osteoid		83825	Left Little toe
86897	Chondral		83809	Distal Phalanx
86898	Soft Tissue Mass		83827	Right Great Toe
86899	Suspected		83828	Right Second Toe
86900	Seen		83829	Right Third Toe
86901	Superior		83830	Right Fourth Toe
86902	Inferior		83831	Right Little toe
86903	Medial		83832	Left Great Toe
86904	Lateral		83833	Left Second Toe
86905	Anterior		83834	Left Third Toe
86906	Trabecular		83835	Left Fourth Toe
86907	Prominence		83836	Left Little toe
86908	Thickening		86809	Pattern
86909	Sequestrum		86810	Geographic
86910	Ground Glass Appearence		86811	Moth-eaten
83196	Mixed Lytic / Sclerotic Lesion		86812	Permeative
83197	Septated		86813	Zone Of Transition
83198	Non-Septated		86814	Narrow
83199	Dimensions		86815	Wide
83200	Height ___ cm		86816	Margin
83201	Transverse ___ cm		86817	Sclerotic
83202	AP ___ cm		86818	Non-Sclerotic
83203	Location		86819	Cortex
83204	Cortical		86820	Intact

X-RAY, CONT.

86821	Destruction	13900	Sclerotic Lesion
86822	Endosteal Scalloping	13901	Bone Island
86823	Expansion	13902	Bone Enlargement
86824	Thickening	13903	Stippled Epiphyses
86825	Thinning	13904	Calcifications
86826	Superior	13905	Joint Space
86827	Inferior	13906	Tendon
86828	Medial	13907	Muscle
86829	Lateral	13908	Bursal
86830	Anterior	13909	Vascular
86831	Posterior	13910	Scoliosis
86832	Periosteal Reaction	13911	Joint Space Narrowing
86833	Thick	13912	Aseptic Necrosis
86834	Thin	13913	Bone Metastases
86835	Uniform	13914	Osteolytic
86836	Irregular	13915	Osteoblastic
86837	Dense	13916	Soft Tissue
86838	Amorphous	13917	Calcifications
86839	Wavy	13918	Gas
86840	Lamellated	13919	Mammogram
86841	Sunburst	22676	Screening
86842	Spiculated	22677	Unilateral
86843	Codman Triangle	22678	Bilateral
86844	Matrix	22679	Stereotactic Biopsy Localization
86845	Osteoid	22680	Preoperative Wire Localization
86846	Chondral	13920	Mass - Not Suggestive of Malignancy
86847	Soft Tissue Mass		___cm
86848	Suspected	26218	Abnormal
86849	Seen	13921	Mass - Suggestive of Malignancy
86850	Superior		___cm
86851	Inferior	13922	Gastrointestinal Radiography
86852	Medial	13923	**Abdominal Flat Plate**
86853	Lateral	22658	With Oblique And Coned Views
86854	Anterior	22659	With Decubitus And / Or Erect Views
86855	Trabecular	22660	With Decubitus, Erect Views And
86856	Prominence		CXR
86857	Thickening	13924	Mass ___ cm
86858	Sequestrum	13925	RUQ
86859	Ground Glass Appearence	13926	LUQ
13888	Findings At Sites Not Elsewhere	13927	Epigastrium
	Classified	13928	RLQ
13889	Fracture	13929	LLQ
13890	Recent	13930	Flank
13891	Old	13931	Suprapubic
21019	Multiple, in various stages of healing	13932	Solitary
13892	Bone Density Decreased	13933	Multiple
13893	Periarticular	13934	Cystic
13894	Bone Density Increased	13935	Calcified
13895	Periosteal Elevation	13936	Hepatomegaly
13896	Cystic Bone Lesion	13937	Hepatic Calcification
13897	Lytic Bone Lesion	13938	Splenomegaly
13898	Solitary	13939	Splenic Calcification
13899	Multiple		

13940	Biliary Calcification	13990	Hypotensive Lower Esophageal
13941	Adrenal Calcification		Sphincter
13942	Pneumobilia	13991	Diffuse Esophageal Spasm
13943	Hydrops of Gallbladder	13992	Tertiary Contractions
13944	Calcified Gallbladder	13993	Reflux
13945	Abdominal Aortic Aneurysm	13994	Esophageal Ulcer
13946	Calcified	13995	Esophageal Extrinsic Compression
13947	Pancreatic Mass ___ cm	13996	Hiatal Hernia
13948	Calcified	13997	Sliding
13949	Non-Calcified	13998	Paraesophageal
13950	Pancreatic Calcifications	13999	Tracheo-esophageal Fistula
13951	Gastric Dilation	14000	Esophageal Foreign Body
13952	Gastric Outlet Obstruction	14001	Surgical Clips
13953	Bezoar	14002	Esophageal Obstruction
13954	Sentinel Loop	14003	Esophageal Varices
13955	Small Bowel Obstruction	14004	Esophageal Rupture
13956	Ileus	14005	Esophageal Perforation
13957	Small Bowel Wall Thickened	14006	Esophageal Mass ___ cm
13958	Ascites	14007	Benign Neoplasm
13959	Thumbprinting	14008	Malignant Neoplasm
13960	Large Bowel	14009	Esophageal Web
13961	Small Bowel	14010	Esophageal Stricture
13962	Volvulus	14011	Mid-Esophageal
13963	Cecal	14012	Esophageal Mucosal Irritation
13964	Sigmoid	14013	Shaggy Exudate
13965	Gastric	14014	Esophageal / Schatzki's Ring
13966	Megacolon	14015	Esophageal Post-Surgical Change
13967	Gas Absent in Rectum	14016	Colonic Interposition
13968	Bowel Filled With Stool	14017	Nasogastric Tube in Place
13969	Retained Barium	14018	Gastric Diverticula
13970	Air in Bowel Wall	14019	Juxtapyloric
13971	Intraluminal Foreign Body	14020	Juxtacardiac
13972	Intraluminal Calcified Material	14021	Perforated
18596	Misplaced IUD	14022	Gastric Motility
13973	Surgical Hardware	14023	Delayed Emptying
13974	Lumen Occluded	14024	Gastric Ulcer
13975	Large Bowel	14025	Antrum Benign
13976	Small Bowel	14026	Antrum Malignant
13977	Calcified Fibroid	14027	Antrum Perforated
13978	**Abdominal Upright**	14028	Fundus Benign
13979	Demonstrating Free Air	14029	Fundus Malignant
13980	Air Fluid Levels Present	14030	Fundus Perforated
13981	**Upper GI Series - Barium Swallow**	14031	Gastric Extrinsic Compression
14102	With Air Contrast	14032	Gastro-colic Fistula
13982	Esophageal Diverticula	14033	Gastric Dilation
13983	Zenker's	19110	Gastroptosis
13984	Epiphrenic	19111	Hourglass Stricture
13985	Perforated	14034	Gastric Perforation
13986	Esophageal Motility Disorder	14035	Gastric Volvulus
13987	Achalasia	14036	Gastric Varices
13988	Nutcracker Esophagus	14037	Gastric Foreign Body
13989	Hypertensive Lower Esophageal	14038	Surgical Clips
	Sphincter	14039	Gastric Outlet Obstruction

22569	Elongated Pyloric Canal	14089	Which Looked Like A Benign Neoplasm ___cm
14040	Bezoar		
14041	Gastric Mass ___cm	14090	Which Looked Like A Malignant Neoplasm ___cm
14042	Benign Neoplasm ___cm		
14043	Malignant Neoplasm ___cm	14091	Extrinsic Compression
14044	Infiltrative Malignant Neoplasm ___cm	14092	Mucosal Inflammation
		14093	With Ischemia
14045	Hypertrophy of Gastric Folds	14094	Dilation
14046	Gastric Post-Surgical Change	14095	With A Malabsorptive Pattern
14047	Partial Gastrectomy	14096	Malrotation
14048	Total Gastrectomy	14097	Foreign Body
14049	Gastroduodenostomy - Billroth I	14098	Surgical Clips
14050	Gastrojejunostomy - Billroth II	14099	Post-Surgical Change
14051	Gastroenterostomy	14100	Small Bowel Resection
14053	Duodenal Diverticula	14101	Small Bowel (Cantor) Tube in Place
14054	Perforated	14103	**Barium Enema**
14055	Duodenal Ulcer	14104	Rectum
14056	Perforated	14105	Polyp, Solitary
14057	Deformed Duodenal Bulb	14106	Polyp, Multiple
14058	Duodenal-biliary Fistula	14107	Intraluminal Mass Lesion ___cm
14059	Duodenal Irritability	14108	Constricting Mass Lesion ___cm
14060	Duodenal Scarring	14109	Extrinsic Compression
14061	Duodenal Perforation	14110	Stricture
14062	Duodenal Mass ___cm	14111	Ulceration, Solitary
14063	Benign Neoplasm ___cm	14112	Ulceration, Multiple
14064	Malignant Neoplasm ___cm	14113	Fistulae
14065	Duodenal Foreign Body	14114	Perforation
14066	Surgical Clips	14115	Foreign Body
14067	Widening of Duodenal Sweep	14116	Surgical Clips
14068	Duodenal Post-Surgical Change	14117	Absence
14069	Plication of Ulcer	14118	Sigmoid Colon
14070	Pyloroplasty	14119	Polyp, Solitary
14071	Dedicated Small Bowel Series	14120	Polyp, Multiple
29064	Diverticula	14121	Intraluminal Mass Lesion ___cm
14072	Single	14122	Constricting Mass Lesion ___cm
18331	Below Ligament of Treitz	14123	Extrinsic Compression
14073	Multiple	14124	Stricture
14074	Perforated	14125	Ulceration, Solitary
14075	Rapid Transit Time	14126	Ulceration, Multiple
14076	Dilated Loops	14127	Fistulae
14077	Air Fluid Levels	14128	Perforation
29065	Ulcer	14129	Diverticula
14078	Single	14130	Volvulus
14079	Multiple	14131	Intussusception
14080	Perforated	14132	Thumbprinting
14081	Entero-entero Fistula	14133	Dilation
14082	Entero-colic Fistula	14134	Foreign Body
14083	Entero-cutaneous Fistula	14135	Surgical Clips
14084	Entero-vesicle Fistula	14136	Absence
14085	Enterovaginal Fistula	14137	Descending Colon
14086	Perforation	14138	Polyp, Solitary
14087	Obstruction	14139	Polyp, Multiple
14088	Mass ___cm	14140	Intraluminal Mass Lesion ___cm

14141	Constricting Mass Lesion ___ cm	14191	Extrinsic Compression
14142	Extrinsic Compression	14192	Stricture
14143	Stricture	14193	Ulceration, Solitary
14144	Ulceration, Solitary	14194	Ulceration, Multiple
14145	Ulceration, Multiple	14195	Fistulae
14146	Fistulae	14196	Perforation
14147	Perforation	14197	Diverticula
14148	Diverticula	18667	Intussusception
18664	Intussusception	14198	Thumbprinting
14149	Thumbprinting	14199	Dilation
14150	Dilation	14200	Foreign Body
14151	Foreign Body	14201	Surgical Clips
14152	Surgical Clips	14202	Ascending Colon
14153	Absence	14203	Polyp, Solitary
14154	Splenic Flexure	14204	Polyp, Multiple
14155	Polyp, Solitary	14205	Intraluminal Mass Lesion ___ cm
14156	Polyp, Multiple	14206	Constricting Mass Lesion ___ cm
14157	Intraluminal Mass Lesion ___ cm	14207	Extrinsic Compression
14158	Constricting Mass Lesion ___ cm	14208	Stricture
14159	Extrinsic Compression	14209	Ulceration, Solitary
14160	Stricture	14210	Ulceration, Multiple
14161	Ulceration, Solitary	14211	Fistulae
14162	Ulceration, Multiple	14212	Perforation
14163	Fistulae	14213	Diverticula
14164	Perforation	18668	Intussusception
14165	Diverticula	14214	Thumbprinting
18665	Intussusception	14215	Dilation
14166	Thumbprinting	14216	Foreign Body
14167	Dilation	14217	Surgical Clips
14168	Foreign Body	14218	Absence
14169	Surgical Clips	14219	Cecum
14170	Transverse Colon	14220	Polyp, Solitary
14171	Polyp, Solitary	14221	Polyp, Multiple
14172	Polyp, Multiple	14222	Intraluminal Mass Lesion ___ cm
14173	Intraluminal Mass Lesion ___ cm	14223	Constricting Mass Lesion ___ cm
14174	Constricting Mass Lesion ___ cm	14224	Extrinsic Compression
14175	Extrinsic Compression	14225	Stricture
14176	Stricture	14226	Ulceration, Solitary
14177	Ulceration, Solitary	14227	Ulceration, Multiple
14178	Ulceration, Multiple	14228	Fistulae
14179	Fistulae	14229	Perforation
14180	Perforation	14230	Diverticula
14181	Diverticula	14231	Volvulus
18666	Intussusception	14232	Intussusception
14182	Thumbprinting	14233	Thumbprinting
14183	Dilation	14234	Dilation
14184	Foreign Body	14235	Foreign Body
14185	Surgical Clips	14236	Surgical Clips
14186	Hepatic Flexure	14237	Absence
14187	Polyp, Solitary	14238	Absence of Colon
14188	Polyp, Multiple	14239	Appendix
14189	Intraluminal Mass Lesion ___ cm	14240	Solitary Mass Lesion ___ cm
14190	Constricting Mass Lesion ___ cm	14241	Extrinsic Compression

14242	Fistulae	18930	Multiple
14243	Perforation	18931	Not Well Visualized
14244	Foreign Body	18932	Intra-Hepatic Duct
14245	Surgical Clips	18933	Dilated
14246	Absence	18934	Focal
14247	Terminal Ileum	18935	Diffuse
14248	Polyp, Solitary	18936	Cysts
14249	Polyp, Multiple	18937	Single
14250	Intraluminal Mass Lesion ___ cm	18938	Multiple
14251	Constricting Mass Lesion ___ cm	18939	Not Well Visualized
14252	Extrinsic Compression	18940	Gallbladder
14253	Stricture	18941	Not Well Visualized
14254	Ulceration, Solitary	18942	Dilated
14255	Ulceration, Multiple	18943	Soft Tissue Mass ___ cm
14256	Fistulae	18944	Wall Thickened
14257	Perforation	14265	Cineradiography
14258	Diverticula	14266	Cineesophagram
14259	Thumbprinting	14267	**Oral Cholecystogram**
14260	Dilatation	18952	Calculi
14261	Foreign Body	18953	Solitary
14262	Surgical Clips	18954	Radiopaque
14263	with Air Contrast	18955	Radiolucent
14264	**ERCP**	18956	Multiple
22661	With Biliary Catheterization	18957	Radiopaque
18903	Pancreas	18958	Radiolucent
18904	Mass ___ cm	18959	Sludge
18905	Body	18960	Polyp
18906	Tail	18961	Wall Thickened
18907	Uncinate	18962	Soft Tissue Mass ___ cm
18908	Diffuse Enlargement	18963	Septated
18909	Cyst	18964	Non-Visualized Gallbladder
18910	Head	14268	**IV Cholangiography**
18911	Body	18900	Calculi
18912	Tail	18901	Solitary
18913	Uncinate	18902	Multiple
18914	Calcification	14269	**Percutaneous Transhepatic**
18915	Focal		**Cholangiography**
18916	Diffuse	19398	Injection Procedure
18917	Pancreatic Duct	18974	Common Bile Duct
18918	Dilated	18975	Dilated
18919	Calculi	18976	Focal
18920	Small Ducts Poorly Filled	18977	Diffuse
18921	Pancreas Divisum	18978	Containing Soft Tissue Mass
18922	Aberrant Attachment of Duct of	18979	Cysts
	Santorini	18980	Single
18923	Common Bile Duct	18981	Multiple
18924	Dilated	18982	Not Well Visualized
18925	Focal	18983	Intra-Hepatic Duct
18926	Diffuse	18984	Dilated
18927	Containing Soft Tissue Mass	18985	Focal
	___ cm	18986	Diffuse
18928	Cysts	18987	Cysts
18929	Single	18988	Single

18989	Multiple		14312	Multiple Ureter Calculi
18990	Not Well Visualized		14313	In The Right Ureter Only
18991	Gallbladder		14314	In The Left Ureter Only
18992	Not Well Visualized		14315	In Both Ureters
18993	Dilated		14316	Solitary Bladder Calculus
18994	Soft Tissue Mass		14317	Multiple Bladder Calculi
18995	Wall Thickened		14318	**Intravenous Pyelogram (IVP)**
13655	Pneumoencephalography		14319	Absent Kidney
13656	Suprasellar Extension		14320	On The Right Only
13657	Empty Sella		14321	On The Left Only
21434	Sialography		14322	Bilaterally
14270	**Renal**		14323	Nonvisualization of Kidney
14271	**Kidneys, Ureter and Bladder (KUB)**		14324	On The Right Only
14272	Absent Kidney		14325	On The Left Only
14273	On The Right Only		14326	Bilaterally
14274	On The Left Only		14327	Delayed Visualization of Kidney
14275	Bilaterally		14328	On The Right Only
14276	Small Kidney		14329	On The Left Only
14277	On The Right Only		14330	Bilaterally
14278	On The Left Only		14331	Large Kidney
14279	Bilaterally		14332	On The Right Only
14280	Large Kidney		14333	On The Left Only
14281	On The Right Only		14334	Bilaterally
14282	On The Left Only		14335	Small Kidney
14283	Bilaterally		14336	On The Right Only
14284	Ectopic Kidney		14337	On The Left Only
14285	On The Right Only		14338	Bilaterally
14286	On The Left Only		14339	Extrinsic Compression of Kidney
14287	Bilaterally		14340	From Above
14288	Fusion of Kidneys		14341	From Below
14289	Renal Calcification		14342	Right Kidney Only
14290	Solitary Renal Cyst		14343	Left Kidney Only
14291	On The Right Only		14344	Both Kidneys
14292	On The Left Only		14345	Fusion of Kidneys
14293	Bilaterally		14346	Ectopic Kidney
14294	Multiple Renal Cysts		14347	Kidney Mass Lesion
14295	On The Right Only		24763	Solitary ___ cm
14296	On The Left Only		14348	On The Right Only
14297	Bilaterally		14349	On The Left Only
14298	Enlarged Bladder		14350	In Both Kidneys
14299	Calculi		24764	Multiple ___ cm
14300	Solitary Kidney Calculus		14351	On The Right Only
14301	Right Kidney Only		14352	On The Left
14302	Left Kidney Only		14353	In Both Kidneys
14303	Both Kidneys		14354	Calcified ___ cm
14304	Multiple Kidney Calculi		14355	Kidney Cyst
14305	In The Right Kidney Only		24765	Solitary
14306	In The Left Kidney Only		14356	On The Right Only
14307	In Both Kidneys		14357	On The Left Only
14308	Solitary Ureter Calculus		14358	Bilaterally
14309	In The Right Ureter Only		24766	Multiple
14310	In The Left Ureter Only		14359	On The Left Only
14311	In Both Ureters		14360	On The Right

14361	Bilaterally	14414	Multiple
14362	Calcification of Wall	14415	Calcification of Wall
14363	Papillary Necrosis	14416	Bladder Polyp
14364	On The Right Only	14417	Solitary
14365	On The Left Only	14418	Multiple
14366	Bilaterally	14419	Extravasation
14367	Nephrocalcinosis	24767	Of The Kidney
14368	On The Right Only	14420	On The Right Only
14369	On The Left Only	14421	On The Left Only
14370	Bilaterally	14422	Bilaterally
14371	Obstructive Pattern	24768	Of The Ureter
14372	On The Right Only	14423	On The Right Only
14373	On The Left Only	14424	On The Left Only
14374	Bilaterally	14425	Bilaterally
14375	Dilated Terminal Collecting Ducts	14426	Of The Bladder
14376	Filling Defect	14427	**Retrograde Pyelogram**
14377	Calculi	14428	Obstructive Pattern
14378	Solitary Kidney Calculus	14429	On The Right Only
14379	On The Right Only	14430	On The Left Only
14380	On The Left Only	14431	Bilaterally
14381	In Both Kidneys	14432	Displacement of Ureters
14382	Multiple Kidney Calculi	14433	On The Right Only
14383	Right Only	14434	On The Left Only
14384	Left Only	14435	Bilaterally
14385	In Both Kidneys	14436	Fused Kidneys
14386	Solitary Ureter Calculus	14437	Small Kidney
14387	On The Right Only	14438	On The Right Only
14388	On The Left Only	14439	On The Left Only
14389	Bilaterally	14440	Bilaterally
14390	Multiple Ureter Calculi	14441	Enlarged Kidney
14391	In The Right Ureter Only	14442	On The Right Only
14392	In The Left Ureter Only	14443	On The Left Only
14393	In Both Ureters	14444	Bilaterally
14394	Solitary Bladder Calculus	14445	Kidney Mass Lesion ___ cm
14395	Multiple Bladder Calculi	24769	Solitary
14396	Solitary Urethral Calculus	14446	Solitary, Right Only
14397	Multiple Urethral Calculi	14447	Solitary, Left Only
14398	Ureter Displacement	14448	In Both Kidneys
14399	On The Right Only	24770	Multiple
14400	On The Left Only	14449	Right Kidney Only
14401	Bilaterally	14450	Left Kidney Only
14402	Enlarged Bladder	14451	Both Kidneys
14403	Extrinsic Compression of Bladder	14452	Calcified
14404	From Above	14453	Kidney Cyst
14405	From Below	24771	Solitary
14406	To The Right	14454	On The Right Only
14407	To The Left	14455	On The Left Only
14408	Bladder Mass ___ cm	14456	Both Kidneys
14409	Solitary	24772	Multiple
14410	Multiple	14457	Right Kidney Only
14411	Calcified	14458	Left Kidney Only
14412	Bladder Cyst	14459	Both Kidneys
14413	Solitary	14460	Calcification of Wall

14461	Filling Defect	29330	With nuclear scan
14462	Papillary Necrosis	14504	Bladder
14463	On The Right Only	14505	Enlarged
14464	On The Left Only	14506	Small
14465	Bilaterally	14507	Delayed Emptying
14466	Nephrocalcinosis	14508	Extravasation
14467	Extrinsic Compression of Kidney	14509	Urethra
14468	From Above	14510	Extravasation
14469	From Below	14511	Anomaly
14470	On The Right Only	14512	Extrinsic Compression
14471	On The Left Only	21435	Hysterosalpingography
14472	Bilaterally	14513	Tomogram
14473	Ectopic Kidney	14514	Base of Skull
14474	On The Right Only	14515	Bone Erosion
14475	On The Left Only	14516	Mediastinum
14476	Bilaterally	14517	Pulmonary
14477	Absent Kidney	14518	Spine
14478	On The Right Only	14519	Bone Erosion
14479	On The Left Only	14520	Renal
14480	Bilaterally	19231	Computer Enhanced
14481	Kidney Calculi	19232	Cardiac
24773	Solitary	19233	Coronary
14482	On The Right Only	19235	Calcification
14483	On The Left Only	19234	Valvular
14484	Both Kidneys	14522	Digital Fluoroscopy
24774	Multiple	14523	Carotid
14485	On The Right Only	14524	Vertebral
14486	On The Left Only	14525	Aorta
14487	Both Kidneys	14526	Thoracic
14488	Ureter Calculi	14527	Abdominal
24775	Solitary	14528	Iliac
14489	On The Right Only	14529	Extremities
14490	On The Left Only	14530	Upper
14491	Both Ureters	14531	Lower
24776	Multiple	14814	**CT Scan**
14492	On The Right Only	14815	**Head**
14493	On The Left Only	28521	With Contrast
14494	Both Ureters	28522	First Without, Then With Contrast
14495	Extravasation of Kidney	14816	Ventricles
14496	On The Right Only	14817	Enlarged
14497	On The Left Only	14818	Right Lateral only
14498	Bilaterally	14819	Left Lateral only
14499	Extravasation of Ureter	14820	Both Laterals
14500	On The Right Only	14821	Both Laterals, 3rd
14501	On The Left Only	14822	Both Laterals, 3rd and 4th
14502	Bilaterally	14823	Small
19383	Antegrade Pyelogram	14824	Compressed
19384	Injection Of Contrast Material	14825	Shifted
19439	Ureterography	14826	Non-Visualization
19440	Injection Of Contrast Material	14827	Cortical Sulci
	Through Ureterostomy	14828	Basal Cisterns
19441	Injection To Visualize Ileal Conduit	14829	Suprasellar
14503	Voiding Cystourethrogram	14830	Atrophy

CT SCAN, CONT.

14831	Cerebral (Widened Sulci)	14884	Intrasellar
14832	Diffuse	14885	Subdural
14833	Frontal	14886	Right
14834	Temporal	14887	Left
14835	Cerebellar	14888	Bilateral
14836	Midline (Vermis)	14889	White Matter only
14837	Hemispheric	14890	Mass Lesion ___ cm
14838	Generalized	14891	Single
14839	Pontine	14892	Multiple
14840	Decreased Density	14893	Frontal
14841	Single	14894	Right
14842	Multiple	14895	Left
14843	Frontal	14896	Midline
14844	Right	14897	Temporal
14845	Left	14898	Right
14846	Midline	14899	Left
14847	Temporal	14900	Parietal
14848	Right	14901	Right
14849	Left	14902	Left
14850	Parietal	14903	Midline
14851	Right	14904	Occipital
14852	Left	14905	Right
14853	Midline	14906	Left
14854	Occipital	14907	Basal Ganglia
14855	Right only	14908	Right
14856	Left only	14909	Left
14857	Bilateral	14910	Thalamus
14858	Basal Ganglia	14911	Right
14859	Right	14912	Left
14860	Left	14913	Hypothalamus
14861	Internal Capsule	14914	Pineal
14862	Right	14915	Midbrain
14863	Left	14916	Right
14864	Thalamus	14917	Left
14865	Right	14918	Tectum
14866	Left	14919	Pons
14867	Hypothalamus	14920	Right
14868	Pineal	14921	Left
14869	Midbrain	14922	Medulla
14870	Right	14923	Right
14871	Left	14924	Left
14872	Tectum	14925	Cerebellum
14873	Pons	14926	Right
14874	Right	14927	Left
14875	Left	14928	Midline
14876	Medulla	14929	Intraventricular
14877	Right	14930	Right Lateral
14878	Left	14931	Left Lateral
14879	Cerebellum	14932	Third
14880	Right	14933	Fourth
14881	Left	14934	Cerebellopontine Angle
14882	Midline	14935	Right
14883	Suprasellar	14936	Left

CT SCAN, CONT.

14937	Suprasellar	14990	Left
14938	Intrasellar	14991	Suprasellar
14939	Parasellar (Cavernous Sinus)	14992	Intrasellar
14940	Sphenoid Ridge	14993	Parasellar (Cavernous Sinus)
14941	Petrous Apex	14994	Sphenoid Ridge
14942	Clivus	14995	Petrous Apex
14943	Foramen Magnum	14996	Clivus
14944	Contrast Enhancing Lesion	14997	Foramen Magnum
14945	Single	14998	Contrast Enhancement
14946	Multiple	14999	Meninges
14947	Frontal	15000	Cortical
14948	Right	15001	Basal
14949	Left	15002	Tentorium
14950	Midline	15003	Choroid Plexus
14951	Temporal	15004	Cavernous Sinus
14952	Right	15005	Right
14953	Left	15006	Left
14954	Parietal	15007	Bilateral
14955	Right	15008	Middle Cerebral Artery
14956	Left	15009	Right
14957	Midline	15010	Left
14958	Occipital	15011	Bilateral
14959	Right	15012	Basilar Artery
14960	Left	15013	Calcification
14961	Basal Ganglia	15014	Midline
14962	Right	15015	Symmetrical
14963	Left	15016	Asymmetrical
14964	Thalamus	15017	Cortical
14965	Right	15018	Right
14966	Left	15019	Left
14967	Hypothalamus	15020	Periventricular
14968	Pineal	15021	Frontal
14969	Midbrain	15022	Right
14970	Right	15023	Left
14971	Left	15024	Midline
14972	Tectum	15025	Temporal
14973	Pons	15026	Right
14974	Right	15027	Left
14975	Left	15028	Parietal
14976	Medulla	15029	Right
14977	Right	15030	Left
14978	Left	15031	Midline
14979	Cerebellum	15032	Occipital
14980	Right	15033	Right
14981	Left	15034	Left
14982	Midline	15035	Basal Ganglia
14983	Intraventricular	15036	Right
14984	Right Lateral	15037	Left
14985	Left Lateral	15038	Thalamus
14986	Third	15039	Right
14987	Fourth	15040	Left
14988	Cerebellopontine Angle	15041	Hypothalamus
14989	Right	15042	Pineal

CT SCAN, CONT.

15043	Midbrain		15096		Left
15044		Right	15097		Subarachnoid
15045		Left	29039	Foreign Body	
15046		Tectum	29040		Frontal
15047	Pons		29046		Right
15048		Right	29047		Left
15049		Left	29041		Temporal
15050	Medulla		29048		Right
15051		Right	29053		Left
15052		Left	29042		Parietal
15053	Suprasellar		29049		Right
15054	Intrasellar		29054		Left
15055	Hemorrhage		29043		Occipital
15056		Frontal	29050		Right
15057		Right	29055		Left
15058		Left	29044		Basal Ganglia
15059		Temporal	29051		Right
15060		Right	29056		Left
15061		Left	29045		Posterior Fossa
15062		Parietal	29052		Right
15063		Right	29057		Left
15064		Left	29024	Skull	
15065		Occipital	29023		Fracture
15066		Right	29025		Frontal
15067		Left	29031		Right
15068		Basal Ganglia	29032		Left
15069		Right	29026		Temporal
15070		Left	29033		Right
15071		Thalamus	29034		Left
15072		Right	29027		Parietal
15073		Left	29035		Right
15074		Hypothalamus	29036		Left
15075		Midbrain	29028		Occipital
15076		Right	29037		Right
15077		Left	29038		Left
15078		Pons	29029		Sphenoid
15079		Medulla	29030		Nasal
15080		Cerebellum	20847		Mastoid
15081		Right	20848		Air Cells Obscured
15082		Left	20849		Sclerotic
15083		Midline	15098	**Orbits**	
15084		Intrasellar	22656		With Contrast
15085		Intraventricular	22657		Without, Then With Contrast
15086		Right Lateral	15099		Mass ___ cm
15087		Left Lateral	15100		Bone Erosion
15088		Third	22690	**Sella**	
15089		Fourth	22691		With Contrast
15090		All Four	22692		Without, Then With Contrast
15091		Epidural	22693	**Posterior Fossa**	
15092		Right	22694		With Contrast
15093		Left	22695		Without, Then With Contrast
15094		Subdural	15101	**Base of Skull**	
15095		Right	22696		With Contrast

CT SCAN, CONT.

22697	Without, Then With Contrast		15120	**Cervical Spine**
15102	Mass ___cm		28526	With Contrast
15103	Orbital Apex		28527	First Without, Then With Contrast
15104	Orbital Roof		15147	Osteophytes
15105	Lateral Orbital Wall		15148	Disc Herniation
15106	Medial Orbital Wall		15149	Erosion
15107	Parasellar		15150	Vertebral Body
15108	Middle Fossa Floor		15151	Pedicle
15109	Petrous Apex		15152	Lamina
15110	Posterior Fossa Floor		15153	Spinous Process
15111	Bone Erosion		15154	Paraspinal Mass ___cm
15112	Orbital Apex		15155	Intradural Extramedullary Mass ___cm
15113	Orbital Roof		15156	Epidural Mass ___cm
15114	Lateral Orbital Wall		15157	Spina Bifida
15115	Medial Orbital Wall		15158	Canal Stenosis
15116	Parasellar		15159	Cord Enlargement
15117	Middle Fossa Floor		15160	Intramedullary Mass ___cm
15118	Petrous Apex		15161	Cyst
15119	Posterior Fossa Floor		15162	Diastematomyelia
22698	**Outer, Middle and Inner Ear**		15163	Arnold Chiari Malformation
22699	With Contrast		15164	**Thorax**
22700	Without, Then With Contrast		22640	Without Contrast
19135	**Neck**		22641	With Contrast
22701	With Contrast		22642	Without, Then With Contrast
22702	Without, Then With Contrast		15165	Lung
15121	Thyroid		18027	Hilar Lymphadenopathy
15122	Enlargement		18126	Unilaterally
15123	Focal		15252	On The Right Only
15124	Diffuse		15253	On The Left Only
15125	Mass ___cm		15254	Bilaterally
15126	Solitary ___cm		18272	Symmetrical
15127	Multiple ___cm		18273	Asymmetrical
15128	Cyst		15166	Pulmonary Nodule (<6cm.)
15129	Solitary		18128	Solitary
15130	Multiple		15167	On The Right Only
15131	Absent		15168	On The Left Only
15132	Surgical Change		15169	Calcified
15133	Parathyroid		18165	Fat Density
15134	Enlargement		18129	Multiple
15135	Solitary		15170	On The Right Only
15136	Multiple		15171	On The Left Only
15137	Ectopic Gland		15172	Bilaterally
15138	Lymph Node Enlargement		15173	Calcified
15139	Diffuse		18151	Calcified "Buckshot" Pattern
15140	Solitary		18152	Mass Lesion ___cm
15141	Larynx		18153	Apical
15142	Mass ___cm		18154	Hilar
15143	Post-Surgical Change		18155	Peripheral
15144	Vocal Cord Mass Lesion ___cm		18156	Pleural Based
15145	Branchial Cleft Cyst		18157	Basal
15146	Hypopharyngeal Mass ___cm		18164	Fat Density
19136	Parapharyngeal Mass ___cm		15181	Cavitary Lesion
19137	Nasopharyngeal Mass ___cm		15182	Thin Wall

CT SCAN, CONT.

15183	Thick Wall	15201	Absence of One Lung
18030	Central	15202	Surgical Change
18031	Eccentric	15203	Pleura
15184	Multiple	15204	Pleural Effusion
15185	Partially Filled With An Air	15205	On The Right Only
	Meniscus	15206	On The Left Only
15174	Bulla(e)	15207	Bilaterally
18215	Upper Lobe	15208	Pleural Mass ___ cm
18216	Lower Lobe	15209	On The Right Only
18130	Solitary	15210	On The Left Only
15175	On The Right Only	15211	Bilaterally
15176	On The Left Only	15212	Pleural Thickening
18131	Multiple	15213	Diffuse
15178	On The Right Only	15214	Focal
15179	On The Left Only	15215	Pleural Calcification
15180	Bilaterally	15216	Bronchopleural Fistula
18214	Cyst(s)	15217	On The Right Only
15186	Bronchiectasis	15218	On The Left Only
15187	On The Right Only	15219	Bilaterally
15188	On The Left Only	15220	Post-Surgical Change
15189	Bilaterally	15221	Pericardium
15190	Hyperinflation	15222	Thickened
15191	Pneumothorax	15223	Diffuse
15192	On The Right Only	15224	Asymmetric
15193	On The Left Only	15225	Pericardial Effusion
15194	Bilaterally	15226	Post-Surgical Change
15195	Atelectasis	15227	Chest Wall
15196	On The Right Only	15228	Mass ___ cm
15197	On The Left Only	15229	On The Right Only
15198	Bilaterally	15230	On The Left Only
15199	Infiltrate	15231	Bilaterally
18132	Unilaterally	15232	Calcified
18133	Bilaterally	15233	Diaphragm
18135	Apical predominance	15234	Elevated
18134	Basilar predominance	15235	On The Right Only
18136	Perihilar predominance	15236	On The Left Only
18137	Peripheral predominance	15237	Bilaterally
15200	Interstitial	15238	Mass ___ cm
18138	Nodular	15239	On The Right Only
18139	Reticular	15240	On The Left Only
18140	Reticular-Nodular	15241	Bilaterally
18141	Honeycomb Pattern	15242	Calcified
18142	Scarring	15243	Hernia
18143	Apical	15244	Post-Surgical Change
18144	Basilar	15245	Mediastinum
18145	Peripheral	15246	Mass ___ cm
18146	Alveolar	15248	Anterior
18147	Lobar / localized	18160	Middle
18148	Diffuse / patchy	15249	Posterior
18033	Air Bronchogram	15247	Superior
18149	Miliary	15250	Containing Calcium
18274	Hilar Calcification	15251	Lymph Node Enlargement
18150	Pulmonary Calcification	18127	Unilaterally

CT SCAN, CONT.

15255	On The Right Only		15296	Vertebral Body
15256	On The Left Only		15297	Pedicle
15257	Bilaterally		15298	Lamina
18267	Symmetric		15299	Spinous Process
18268	Asymmetric		15300	Paraspinal Mass ___ cm
18269	Containing Calcium		15301	Intradural Extramedullary Mass ___ cm
18260	Widening		15302	Epidural Mass ___ cm
15258	Pneumomediastinum		15303	Spina Bifida
18271	Air Containing Structure		15304	Cord Enlargement
15259	Substernal Thyroid		15305	Intramedullary Mass ___ cm
15260	Thymus Gland Enlargement		15306	Cyst
15261	Heart		15307	Diastematomyelia
15262	Myxoma		**15308**	**Abdomen**
15263	Left Atrial		22643	Without Contrast
15264	Cardiac Enlargement		22644	With Contrast
15265	Valvular Calcification		22645	Without, Then With Contrast
15266	Mitral		15309	Adrenal Glands
15267	Aortic		15310	Diffuse Enlargement
15268	Post-Surgical Change		15311	On The Right Only
15269	Arteries		15312	On The Left Only
15270	Aortic Aneurysm		15313	Bilaterally
15271	Calcified Aorta		15314	Not Visualized
15272	Calcified Coronary Artery		15315	On The Right Only
15273	Pulmonary Artery Enlargement		15316	On The Left Only
15274	Post-Surgical Change		15317	Bilaterally
18125	**Thoracic Spine**		15318	Atrophy
22148	Injection Of Contrast Material		15319	On The Right Only
28528	With Contrast		15320	On The Left Only
28529	First Without, Then With Contrast		15321	Bilaterally
15275	Osteophytes		15322	Focal Mass Lesion ___ cm
15276	Disc Herniation		24777	Solitary
15277	Erosion		15323	On The Right Only
15278	Vertebral Body		15324	On The Left Only
15279	Pedicle		15325	Bilaterally
15280	Lamina		24778	Multiple
15281	Spinous Process		15326	On The Right Only
15282	Paraspinal Mass ___ cm		15327	On The Left Only
15283	Intradural Extramedullary Mass ___ cm		15328	Bilaterally
15284	Epidural Mass ___ cm		15329	Cyst
15285	Spina Bifida		24779	Solitary
15286	Canal Stenosis		15330	On The Right Only
15287	Cord Enlargement		15331	On The Left Only
15288	Intramedullary Mass ___ cm		15332	Bilaterally
15289	Cyst		24780	Multiple
15290	Diastematomyelia		15333	On The Right Only
15291	**Lumbar Spine**		15334	On The Left Only
22147	Injection Of Contrast Material		15335	Bilaterally
28530	With Contrast		15336	Calcification
28531	First Without, Then With Contrast		15337	On The Right Only
15292	Canal Stenosis		15338	On The Left Only
15293	Osteophytes		15339	Bilaterally
15294	Disc Herniation		15340	Pancreas
15295	Erosion		15341	Mass ___ cm

CT SCAN, CONT.

15342	Head
15343	Body
15344	Tail
15345	Uncinate
15346	Diffuse Enlargement
15347	Pancreatic Phlegmon
15348	Atrophy
15349	Focal
15350	Diffuse
15351	Cyst
15352	Head
15353	Body
15354	Tail
15355	Uncinate
15356	Calcification
15357	Focal
15358	Diffuse
15359	Not Well Visualized
15360	Pancreatic Duct
15361	"Chain-of-Lakes" Appearance
15362	Dilated
15363	Calculi
15364	Liver
15365	Mass Lesion ___ cm
15366	Solitary ___ cm
15367	Multiple ___ cm
15368	Satellites ___ cm
15369	Calcified ___ cm
15370	Cyst
15371	Solitary
15372	Multiple
15373	Multilocular
15374	Satellites
15375	Calcified Wall
15376	Diffuse Enlargement
15377	Fatty Infiltration
15378	Focal Enlargement
15379	Fatty Infiltration
15380	Right Lobe
15381	Left Lobe
15382	Caudate
15383	Quadrate
18945	Fibrotic Changes
18946	Regenerating Nodules
18947	Shrunken Liver
15384	Calcifications
15385	Diffuse
15386	Focal
15387	Density (HU)
15388	Common Bile Duct
15389	Dilated
15390	Focal
15391	Diffuse

15392	Containing Soft Tissue Mass
15393	Calculi
15394	Not Well Visualized
15395	Intra-Hepatic Duct
15396	Dilated
15397	Focal
15398	Diffuse
15399	Calculi
15400	Not Well Visualized
15401	Gallbladder
15402	Not Well Visualized
15403	Calculi
15404	Dilated
15405	Soft Tissue Mass
15406	Wall Thickened
15407	Spleen
15408	Enlarged
15409	Wandering
15410	Polysplenia
15411	Absence
15412	Mass Lesion ___ cm
15413	Focal ___ cm
15414	Solitary ___ cm
15415	Multiple ___ cm
15416	Cyst
15417	Focal
15418	Solitary
15419	Multiple
15420	Calcified Wall
15421	Calcification
15422	Diffuse
15423	Focal
15424	Hematoma
15425	Atrophy
15426	Kidney
81938	Dimensions
81936	Right Kidney Long Axis ___ cm
81939	Right Kidney Short Axis ___ cm
81937	Left Kidney Long Axis ___ cm
81940	Left Kidney Short Axis ___ cm
15427	Enlarged
15428	On The Right Only
15429	On The Left Only
15430	Bilaterally
81941	Small
81942	On The Right Only
81943	On The Left Only
81944	Bilaterally
15431	Mass ___ cm
15432	On The Right Only
15433	On The Left Only
15434	Bilaterally
15435	Renal Pelvis

CT SCAN, CONT.

15436	Calcified		15484	On The Left Only
15437	Cyst		15485	Bilaterally
24781	Solitary		15486	Inferior Vena Cava
15438	On The Right Only		15487	Thrombosis
15439	On The Left Only		15488	Calcified
15440	Bilaterally		15489	Soft Tissue Mass
24782	Multiple		15490	Hemorrhage
15441	On The Right Only		15491	Abdominal Wall and Peritoneal Cavity
15442	On The Left Only		15492	Herniation of Bowel
15443	Bilaterally		24786	Inguinal
15444	Calcified Wall		15493	On The Right Only
15445	Calculi		15494	On The Left Only
24783	Solitary		15495	Bilaterally
15446	On The Right Only		24787	Femoral
15447	On The Left Only		15496	On The Right Only
15448	Bilaterally		15497	On The Left Only
24784	Multiple		15498	Ventral
15449	On The Right Only		15499	Hiatal
15450	On The Left Only		15500	Umbilical
15451	Bilaterally		15501	Intraperitoneal Fluid
15452	Nephrocalcinosis		15502	Loculated
15453	On The Right Only		15503	Anterior Abdominal Wall Hematoma
15454	On The Left Only		15504	Anterior Abdominal Wall Mass
15455	Bilaterally			___cm
15456	Obstructive Pattern		15505	Solitary
15457	On The Right Only		15506	Multiple
15458	On The Left Only		15507	Calcified
15459	Bilaterally		15508	Intraperitoneal Cyst
15460	Absence		15509	Solitary
15461	On The Right Only		15510	Multiple
15462	On The Left Only		15511	Calcified Wall
15463	Fused		15512	Peritoneal Mass ___cm
15464	Ptosis		15513	Solitary
15465	On The Right Only		15514	Multiple
15466	On The Left Only		15515	Calcified
15467	Bilaterally		15516	Intraabdominal Pregnancy
15468	Found in Pelvis		15517	Alimentary Tract
15469	Extravasation		15518	Intraluminal Mass Lesion ___cm
15470	On The Right Only		24788	Gastric ___cm
15471	On The Left Only		15519	Single ___cm
15472	Bilaterally		15520	Multiple ___cm
15473	Retroperitoneum		24789	Duodenal ___cm
15474	Lymph Nodes		15521	Single ___cm
15475	Enlarged		15522	Multiple ___cm
15476	Calcified		24790	Jejunal ___cm
15477	Abdominal Aorta		15523	Single ___cm
15478	Fusiform Dilatation		15524	Multiple ___cm
15479	Saccular Dilation		24791	Ileal ___cm
15480	Calcified Wall		15525	Single ___cm
15481	Thrombosis		15526	Multiple ___cm
15482	Renal Artery		24792	Cecal ___cm
24785	Dilation		15527	Single ___cm
15483	On The Right Only		15528	Multiple ___cm

CT SCAN, CONT.

24793	Appendiceal ___cm	
15529	Single ___cm	
15530	Multiple ___cm	
24794	Ascending Colon ___cm	
15531	Single ___cm	
15532	Multiple ___cm	
24795	Transverse Colon ___cm	
15533	Single ___cm	
15534	Multiple ___cm	
24796	Descending Colon ___cm	
15535	Single ___cm	
15536	Multiple ___cm	
24797	Sigmoid Colon ___cm	
15537	Single ___cm	
15538	Multiple ___cm	
24798	Rectum ___cm	
15539	Single ___cm	
15540	Multiple ___cm	
15541	Calcified ___cm	
15542	Dilation	
15543	Gastric	
15544	Small Intestinal	
15545	Colonic	
15546	Diverticula	
15547	Gastric	
15548	Small Intestinal	
15549	Colonic	
15550	Malrotation	
15551	Gastric	
15552	Small Intestinal	
15553	Colonic	
15554	Wall Thickened	
15555	Gastric	
15556	Duodenal	
15557	Jejunal	
15558	Ileal	
15559	Cecal	
15560	Appendiceal	
15561	Ascending Colon	
15562	Transverse Colon	
15563	Descending Colon	
15564	Sigmoid Colon	
15565	Rectum	
15566	Intussusception	
15567	Post-Surgical Changes	
15568	Stomach Partly Absent	
15569	Stomach Totally Absent	
15570	Small Bowel Partly Resected	
15571	Ascending Colon Absent	
15572	Descending Colon Absent	
15573	Sigmoid Colon Absent	
15574	Rectum Absent	
15575	Entire Colon Absent	
15576	Foreign Bodies	
15577	Surgical Hardware	
15578	Clips	
15579	**Pelvis**	
15580	Soft Tissue Mass	
15581	Bone Erosion	
15582	Bladder	
15583	Enlarged	
15584	Obstructive Pattern	
15585	Mass ___cm	
15586	Solitary ___cm	
15587	Multiple ___cm	
15588	Polyp	
15589	Solitary	
15590	Multiple	
15591	Wall Thickened	
15592	Focal	
15593	Diffuse	
15594	Calculi	
15595	Solitary	
15596	Multiple	
15597	Extravasation	
15598	Post-Surgical Changes	
15599	Prostate	
15600	Enlarged	
15601	Mass ___cm	
15602	Calcification	
15603	Seminal Vesicles	
15604	Enlarged	
15605	On The Right Only	
15606	On The Left Only	
15607	Bilaterally	
15608	Undescended Testicle	
15609	On The Right Only	
15610	On The Left Only	
15611	Bilaterally	
15612	Mass Present ___cm	
15613	Uterus	
15614	Enlarged	
15615	Atrophied	
15616	Calcification	
15617	Absence	
15618	Mass Lesion ___cm	
15619	Solitary ___cm	
15620	Multiple ___cm	
15621	Calcified ___cm	
15622	Bicornate	
15623	Fetus	
15624	Ovaries	
15625	Enlargement	
15626	On The Right Only	
15627	On The Left Only	
15628	Bilaterally	

CT SCAN, CONT.

15629	Atrophied	
15630	On The Right Only	
15631	On The Left Only	
15632	Bilaterally	
15633	Absence	
15634	On The Right Only	
15635	On The Left Only	
15636	Bilaterally	
15637	Mass ___ cm	
15638	On The Right Only	
15639	On The Left Only	
15640	Bilaterally	
15641	Calcified	
15642	Cystic lesion	
15643	On The Right Only	
15644	On The Left Only	
15645	Bilaterally	
15646	Calcified	
15647	Fallopian Tubes	
15648	Absence	
15649	On The Right Only	
15650	On The Left Only	
15651	Bilaterally	
15652	Mass ___ cm	
15653	On The Right Only	
15654	On The Left Only	
15655	Bilaterally	
15656	Intraabdominal Pregnancy	
15657	Lymph Nodes	
15658	Enlarged	
15659	Calcified	
15660	Iliac Artery	
15661	On The Right Only	
15662	On The Left Only	
15663	Bilaterally	
15664	Thrombosis	
15665	Calcified	
15666	Iliac Vein	
15667	On The Right Only	
15668	On The Left Only	
15669	Bilaterally	
15670	Thrombosis	
15671	Calcified	
15672	Rectum	
15673	Intraluminal Mass Lesion ___ cm	
15674	Solitary ___ cm	
15675	Multiple ___ cm	
15676	Wall Thickened	
15677	Foreign Bodies	
15678	Surgical Hardware	
15679	Clips	
19356	**Cine-CT**	
19357	Cardiac	

22618	**MRI**	
15684	**Head**	
15906	Without Contrast	
22647	With Contrast	
22648	Without, Then With Contrast	
15683	T1 Weighted (IR)	
15685	Ventricles	
15686	Enlarged	
15687	Right Lateral only	
15688	Left Lateral only	
15689	Both Laterals	
15690	Both Laterals, 3rd	
15691	Both Laterals, 3rd and 4th	
15692	Small	
15693	Compressed	
15694	Shifted	
15695	Non-Visualization	
15696	Cortical Sulci	
15697	Basal Cisterns	
15698	Suprasellar	
15699	Atrophy	
15700	Cerebral (Widened Sulci)	
15701	Diffuse	
15702	Frontal	
15703	Temporal	
15704	Cerebellar	
15705	Midline (Vermis)	
15706	Hemispheric	
15707	Generalized	
15708	Pontine	
15709	Increased Signal Intensity (decreased T1)	
15710	Single Location	
15711	Multiple Locations	
15712	Frontal	
15713	On The Right	
15714	On The Left	
15715	At The Midline	
15716	Temporal	
15717	On The Right	
15718	On The Left	
15719	Parietal	
15720	On The Right	
15721	On The Left	
15722	Midline	
15723	Occipital	
15724	On The Right	
15725	On The Left	
15726	Basal Ganglia	
15727	On The Right	
15728	On The Left	
15729	Internal Capsule	
15730	On The Right	

MRI, CONT.

15731	On The Left	15783	On The Left
15732	Thalamus	15784	Parietal
15733	On The Right	15785	On The Right
15734	On The Left	15786	On The Left
15735	Hypothalamus	15787	Midline
15736	Pineal	15788	Occipital
15737	Midbrain	15789	On The Right
15738	On The Right	15790	On The Left
15739	On The Left	15791	Basal Ganglia
15740	Tectum	15792	On The Right
15741	Pons	15793	On The Left
15742	On The Right	15794	Internal Capsule
15743	On The Left	15795	On The Right
15744	Medulla	15796	On The Left
15745	On The Right	15797	Thalamus
15746	On The Left	15798	On The Right
15747	Cerebellum	15799	On The Left
15748	On The Right	15800	Hypothalamus
15749	On The Left	15801	Pineal
15750	Midline	15802	Midbrain
15751	Intraventricular	15803	On The Right
15752	Right Lateral	15804	On The Left
15753	Left Lateral	15805	Tectum
15754	Third	15806	Pons
15755	Fourth	15807	On The Right
15756	Cerebellopontine Angle	15808	On The Left
15757	On The Right	15809	Medulla
15758	On The Left	15810	On The Right
15759	Periventricular	15811	On The Left
15760	Suprasellar	15812	Cerebellum
15761	Intrasellar	15813	On The Right
15762	Parasellar (Cavernous Sinus)	15814	On The Left
15763	Sphenoid Ridge	15815	Midline
15764	Petrous Apex	15816	Intraventricular
15765	Clivus	15817	Right Lateral
15766	Foramen Magnum	15818	Left Lateral
15767	Subarachnoid	15819	Third
15768	Epidural	15820	Fourth
15769	On The Left Only	15821	Cerebellopontine Angle
15770	On The Right	15822	On The Right
15771	Subdural	15823	On The Left
15772	On The Right	15824	Periventricular
15773	On The Left	15825	Suprasellar
15774	Decreased Signal Intensity (prolonged T1)	15826	Intrasellar
		15827	Parasellar (Cavernous Sinus)
15775	Single Location	15828	Sphenoid Ridge
15776	Multiple Locations	15829	Petrous Apex
15777	Frontal	15830	Clivus
15778	On The Right	15831	Foramen Magnum
15779	On The Left	15832	Subarachnoid
15780	Midline	15833	Epidural
15781	Temporal	15834	On The Right
15782	On The Right	15835	On The Left

MRI, CONT.

15836	Subdural
15837	On The Right
15838	On The Left
15839	Mass Effect ___ cm
15840	Single Location
15841	Multiple Locations
15842	Frontal
15843	On The Right
15844	On The Left
15845	Midline
15846	Temporal
15847	On The Right
15848	On The Left
15849	Parietal
15850	On The Right
15851	On The Left
15852	Midline
15853	Occipital
15854	On The Right
15855	On The Left
15856	Basal Ganglia
15857	On The Right
15858	On The Left
15859	Internal Capsule
15860	On The Right
15861	On The Left
15862	Thalamus
15863	On The Right
15864	On The Left
15865	Hypothalamus
15866	Pineal
15867	Midbrain
15868	On The Right
15869	On The Left
15870	Tectum
15871	Pons
15872	On The Right
15873	On The Left
15874	Medulla
15875	On The Right
15876	On The Left
15877	Cerebellum
15878	On The Right
15879	On The Left
15880	Midline
15881	Intraventricular
15882	Right Lateral
15883	Left Lateral
15884	Third
15885	Fourth
15886	Cerebellopontine Angle
15887	On The Right
15888	On The Left

15889	Periventricular
15890	Suprasellar
15891	Intrasellar
15892	Parasellar (Cavernous Sinus)
15893	Sphenoid Ridge
15894	Petrous Apex
15895	Clivus
15896	Foramen Magnum
15897	Subarachnoid
15898	Epidural
15899	On The Right
15900	On The Left
15901	Subdural
15902	On The Right
15903	On The Left
15905	T2 Weighted (SE)
15907	Ventricles
15908	Enlarged
15909	Right Lateral only
15910	Left Lateral only
15911	Both Laterals
15912	Both Laterals, 3rd
15913	Both Laterals, 3rd and 4th
15914	Small
15915	Compressed
15916	Shifted
15917	Non-Visualization
15918	Cortical Sulci
15919	Basal Cisterns
15920	Suprasellar
15921	Atrophy
15922	Cerebral (Widened Sulci)
15923	Diffuse
15924	Frontal
15925	Temporal
15926	Cerebellar
15927	Midline (Vermis)
15928	Hemispheric
15929	Generalized
15930	Pontine
15931	Increased Signal Intensity (prolonged T2)
15932	Single Location
15933	Multiple Locations
15934	Frontal
15935	On The Right
15936	On The Left
15937	Midline
15938	Temporal
15939	On The Right
15940	On The Left
15941	Parietal
15942	On The Right

MRI, CONT.

15943	On The Left
15944	Midline
15945	Occipital
15946	On The Right
15947	On The Left
15948	Basal Ganglia
15949	On The Right
15950	On The Left
15951	Internal Capsule
15952	On The Right
15953	On The Left
15954	Thalamus
15955	On The Right
15956	On The Left
15957	Hypothalamus
15958	Pineal
15959	Midbrain
15960	On The Right
15961	On The Left
15962	Tectum
15963	Pons
15964	On The Right
15965	On The Left
15966	Medulla
15967	On The Right
15968	On The Left
15969	Cerebellum
15970	On The Right
15971	On The Left
15972	Midline
15973	Intraventricular
15974	Right Lateral
15975	Left Lateral
15976	Third
15977	Fourth
15978	Cerebellopontine Angle
15979	On The Right
15980	On The Left
15981	Periventricular
15982	Suprasellar
15983	Intrasellar
15984	Parasellar (Cavernous Sinus)
15985	Sphenoid Ridge
15986	Petrous Apex
15987	Clivus
15988	Foramen Magnum
15989	Subarachnoid
15990	Epidural
15991	On The Right
15992	On The Left
15993	Subdural
15994	On The Right
15995	On The Left

15996	Decreased Signal Intensity (shortened T2)
15997	Single Location
15998	Multiple Locations
15999	Frontal
16000	On The Right
16001	On The Left
16002	Midline
16003	Temporal
16004	On The Right
16005	On The Left
16006	Parietal
16007	On The Right
16008	On The Left
16009	Midline
16010	Occipital
16011	On The Right
16012	On The Left
16013	Basal Ganglia
16014	On The Right
16015	On The Left
16016	Internal Capsule
16017	On The Right
16018	On The Left
16019	Thalamus
16020	On The Right
16021	On The Left
16022	Hypothalamus
16023	Pineal
16024	Midbrain
16025	On The Right
16026	On The Left
16027	Tectum
16028	Pons
16029	On The Right
16030	On The Left
16031	Medulla
16032	On The Right
16033	On The Left
16034	Cerebellum
16035	On The Right
16036	On The Left
16037	Midline
16038	Intraventricular
16039	Right Lateral
16040	Left Lateral
16041	Third
16042	Fourth
16043	Cerebellopontine Angle
16044	On The Right
16045	On The Left
16046	Periventricular
16047	Suprasellar

MRI, CONT.

16048	Intrasellar	16101	On The Left
16049	Parasellar (Cavernous Sinus)	16102	Midline
16050	Sphenoid Ridge	16103	Intraventricular
16051	Petrous Apex	16104	Right Lateral
16052	Clivus	16105	Left Lateral
16053	Foramen Magnum	16106	Third
16054	Subarachnoid	16107	Fourth
16055	Epidural	16108	Cerebellopontine Angle
16056	On The Right	16109	On The Right
16057	On The Left	16110	On The Left
16058	Subdural	16111	Periventricular
16059	On The Right	16112	Suprasellar
16060	On The Left	16113	Intrasellar
16061	Mass Effect	16114	Parasellar (Cavernous Sinus)
16062	Single Location	16115	Sphenoid Ridge
16063	Multiple Locations	16116	Petrous Apex
16064	Frontal	16117	Clivus
16065	On The Right	16118	Foramen Magnum
16066	On The Left	16119	Subarachnoid
16067	Midline	16120	Epidural
16068	Temporal	16121	On The Right
16069	On The Right	16122	On The Left
16070	On The Left	16123	Subdural
16071	Parietal	16124	On The Right
16072	On The Right	16125	On The Left
16073	On The Left	22649	**Orbits, Face And Neck**
16074	Midline	16126	With Contrast
16075	Occipital	15904	Orbits
16076	On The Right	19358	**Thorax**
16077	On The Left	19359	With Contrast
16078	Basal Ganglia	29381	**Cardiac**
16079	On The Right	29383	For Morphology
16080	On The Left	29382	With Contrast
16081	Internal Capsule	29384	For Function
16082	On The Right	29386	Of Multiple Chambers
16083	On The Left	29387	Of A Single Chamber
16084	Thalamus	29385	For Flow Velocity
16085	On The Right	22634	**Spine**
16086	On The Left	22635	Cervical
16087	Hypothalamus	22650	With Contrast
16088	Pineal	22651	Without, Then With Contrast
16089	Midbrain	22636	Thoracic
16090	On The Right	22652	With Contrast
16091	On The Left	22653	Without, Then With Contrast
16092	Tectum	22637	Lumbar
16093	Pons	22654	With Contrast
16094	On The Right	22655	Without, Then With Contrast
16095	On The Left	18669	**Abdomen**
16096	Medulla	18670	Adrenal Gland
16097	On The Right	18671	Diffuse Enlargement
16098	On The Left	18672	On The Right
16099	Cerebellum	18673	On The Left
16100	On The Right	18674	Bilaterally

MRI, CONT.

18675	Not Visualized		18724	Multilocular
18676	On The Right		18725	Satellites
18677	On The Left		18726	Diffuse Enlargement
18678	Bilaterally		18727	Fatty Infiltration
18679	Atrophy		18728	Focal Enlargement
18680	On The Right		18729	Fatty Infiltration
18681	On The Left		18730	Right Lobe
18682	Bilaterally		18731	Left Lobe
18683	Focal Mass Lesion		18732	Caudate
24799	Solitary		18733	Quadrate
18684	On The Right Only		18948	Fibrotic Changes
18685	On The Left Only		18949	Regenerating Nodules
18686	Bilaterally		18950	Shrunken Liver
24800	Multiple		18734	Increased Iron
18687	On The Right Only			Common Bile Duct
18688	On The Left Only		18735	
18689	Bilaterally		18736	Dilated
18690	Cyst		18737	Focal
24801	Solitary		18738	Diffuse
18691	On The Right Only		18739	Containing Soft Tissue Mass
18692	On The Left Only		18740	Not Well Visualized
18693	Bilaterally		18741	Intra-Hepatic Duct
24802	Multiple		18742	Dilated
18694	On The Right Only		18743	Focal
18695	On The Left Only		18744	Diffuse
18696	Bilaterally		18745	Not Well Visualized
18697	Pancreas		18746	Gallbladder
18698	Mass		18747	Not Well Visualized
18699	Head		18748	Dilated
18700	Body		18749	Soft Tissue Mass
18701	Tail		18750	Wall Thickened
18702	Uncinate		18951	Septated
18703	Diffuse Enlargement		18751	Spleen
18704	Pancreatic Phlegmon		18752	Enlarged
18705	Atrophy		18753	Wandering
18706	Focal		18754	Polysplenia
18707	Diffuse		18755	Absence
18708	Cyst		18756	Mass Lesion
18709	Head		18757	Focal
18710	Body		18758	Solitary
18711	Tail		18759	Multiple
18712	Uncinate		18760	Cyst
18713	Not Well Visualized		18761	Focal
18714	Pancreatic Duct		18762	Solitary
18715	Dilated		18763	Multiple
18716	Liver		18765	Hematoma
18717	Mass Lesion		18766	Atrophy
18718	Solitary		18767	Kidney
18719	Multiple		18768	Enlargement
18720	Satellites		18769	On The Right Only
18721	Cyst		18770	On The Left Only
18722	Solitary		18771	Bilaterally
18723	Multiple		18772	Mass
			18773	On The Right Only

MRI, CONT.

18774	On The Left Only	18822	On The Left Only
18775	Bilaterally	18823	Ventral
18776	Renal Pelvis	18824	Hiatal
18777	Cyst	18825	Umbilical
24803	Solitary	18826	Intraperitoneal Fluid
18778	On The Right Only	18827	Loculated
18779	On The Left Only	18828	Anterior Abdominal Wall Hematoma
18780	Bilaterally	18829	Anterior Abdominal Wall Mass
24804	Multiple	18830	Solitary
18781	On The Right Only	18831	Multiple
18782	On The Left Only	18832	Intraperitoneal Cyst
18783	Bilaterally	18833	Solitary
18784	Obstructive Pattern	18834	Multiple
18785	On The Right Only	18835	Peritoneal Mass
18786	On The Left Only	18836	Solitary
18787	Bilaterally	18837	Multiple
18788	Absence	18838	Intraabdominal Pregnancy
18789	On The Right Only	18839	Alimentary Tract
18790	On The Left Only	18840	Intraluminal Mass Lesion
18791	Fused	24808	Gastric
18792	Ptosis	18841	Single
18793	On The Right Only	18842	Multiple
18794	On The Left Only	24809	Duodenal
18795	Bilaterally	18843	Single
18796	Found in Pelvis	18844	Multiple
18797	Extravasation	24810	Jejunal
18798	On The Right Only	18845	Single
18799	On The Left Only	18846	Multiple
18800	Bilaterally	24811	Ileal
18801	Retroperitoneum	18847	Single
18802	Lymph Nodes	18848	Multiple
18803	Enlarged	24812	Cecal
18804	Abdominal Aorta	18849	Single
18805	Fusiform Dilation	18850	Multiple
18806	Saccular Dilation	24813	Appendiceal
18807	Thrombosis	18851	Single
18808	Renal Artery	18852	Multiple
24805	Dilation	24814	Ascending Colon
18809	On The Right Only	18853	Single
18810	On The Left Only	18854	Multiple
18811	Bilaterally	24815	Transverse Colon
18812	Inferior Vena Cava	18855	Single
18813	Thrombosis	18856	Multiple
18814	Soft Tissue Mass	24816	Descending Colon
18815	Hemorrhage	18857	Single
18816	Abdominal Wall and Peritoneal Cavity	18858	Multiple
18817	Herniation of Bowel	24817	Sigmoid Colon
24806	Inguinal	18859	Single
18818	On The Right Only	18860	Multiple
18819	On The Left Only	24818	Rectum
18820	Bilaterally	18861	Single
24807	Femoral	18862	Multiple
18821	On The Right Only	18863	Dilation

MRI, CONT.

18864	Gastric	18054	Neck and Chest I-131
18865	Small Intestinal	18055	Ectopic uptake
18866	Colonic	16137	Heart
18867	Diverticula	16186	Lung
18868	Gastric	18319	Perfusion
18869	Small Intestinal	18320	V/Q
18870	Colonic	29448	Angiography
18871	Malrotation	29449	Flow Imaging
18872	Gastric	18427	Lower Extremity
18873	Small Intestinal	18428	Unilateral
18874	Colonic	18429	Bilateral
18875	Wall Thickened	16251	Fibrinogen I-125
18876	Gastric	16187	Adrenal (Iodocholesterol)
18877	Duodenal	16188	Uptake
18878	Jejunal	16189	On The Right Only
18879	Ileal	16190	On The Left Only
18880	Cecal	16191	Bilaterally
18881	Appendiceal	16192	Post Dexamethasone Uptake
18882	Ascending Colon	16193	On The Right Only
18883	Transverse Colon	16194	On The Left Only
18884	Descending Colon	16195	Bilaterally
18885	Sigmoid Colon	16196	Adrenal MIBG (Labelled Catecholamine Precursor)
18886	Rectum		
18887	Intussusception	16197	Liver
18888	Post-Surgical Changes	16198	Technetium
18889	Stomach Partly Absent	16199	Hepatomegaly
18890	Stomach Totally Absent	16200	Poor Uptake
18891	Small Bowel Partly Resected	16201	Filling Defect
18892	Ascending Colon Absent	16202	Single
18893	Descending Colon Absent	16203	Multiple
18894	Sigmoid Colon Absent	16204	HIDA
18895	Rectum Absent	16205	Renal
18896	Entire Colon Absent	16206	Kidney
18897	Foreign Bodies	16207	Enlarged
18898	Surgical Hardware	16208	On The Right Only
18899	Clips	16209	On The Left Only
19236	Cardiac Magnetic Resonance Spectroscopy	16210	Bilaterally
18997	Bone Mass Studies	16211	Small
18998	Single-Photon Absorptiometry	16212	On The Right Only
18999	Dual-Photon Absorptiometry	16213	On The Left Only
19000	Dual-Energy X-ray Absorptiometry	16214	Bilaterally
19001	Quantitative Computed Tomography	16215	Absent
16127	**Isotopic Scans**	16216	On The Right Only
16128	Brain	16217	On The Left Only
16129	Salivary Gland	16218	Bilaterally
16130	Thyroid	16219	Delayed Function
18056	Diffuse Enlargement	16220	On The Right Only
16131	Single Hot Nodule	16221	On The Left Only
16132	Cold Nodule	16222	Bilaterally
16133	Inhomogeneous ("Multinodular")	16223	Ectopic
16134	Substernal	16224	On The Right Only
16135	Absent	16225	On The Left Only
16136	Ectopic	16226	Bilaterally

16227	Mass Lesion	22665	Unilateral
16228	On The Right Only	22666	Nonselective
16229	On The Left Only	23115	Main Artery
16230	Bilaterally	23116	Right Branch
16231	Extravasation	23117	Left Branch
16232	On The Right Only	16271	Genito-Urinary
16233	On The Left Only	16272	Carotid
16234	Bilaterally	29782	External
16235	Obstructive Pattern	29783	Unilateral
16236	On The Right Only	29787	Bilateral
16237	On The Left Only	29784	Internal
16238	Bilaterally	29788	Unilateral
16239	Bladder	29789	Bilateral
16240	Enlarged	29785	Cerebral
16241	Small	29790	Unilateral
16242	Mass Lesion	22662	Bilateral
16243	Extravasation	29786	Cervical
16244	Spleen	29791	Unilateral
16245	Salivary Gland	29792	Bilateral
16246	Bone	16273	Vertebral
16247	Bone Marrow	16274	Spinal
16248	Meckel	16275	Arteriovenous Malformation
16249	Gallium	16276	Tumor Blush
16250	131 I-19 Iodocholestrol	29781	Brachial
81346	Nuclear Thyroid Studies	16277	Cerebral
12801	Iodine Radioactive Uptake (24 hr.)	29780	Cervical
12802	After Perchlorate (As % of baseline)	18386	Arterial Narrowing
12803	<2%	18387	Internal Carotid
22498	Technetium Uptake (24 hr.)	18388	External Carotid
16252	Myelography	18389	Vertebral
22146	Injection Of Contrast Material	18390	Basilar
16253	Filling Defect	18391	Carotid Siphon
16254	Intradural	18392	Anterior Cerebral
18034	Intramedullary	18393	Middle Cerebral
18035	Extramedullary	18394	Posterior Cerebral
16255	Extradural	16278	Vessels Occluded
16256	Root Sleeve	18381	Bilateral Carotids but anastomotic vessel network seen
16257	Diverticula		
16258	Along Roots	16279	Beaded Vessels
16259	Blockage	16280	Vessels Malformed
16260	Expanded Spinal Cord	16281	Arteriovenous
18036	Cisternal Myelogram	16282	Arteriovenous Fistula
16261	**Angiography**	16283	Vessels Shifted
16267	Aorta	16284	Tumor Blush
16268	Thoracic	16285	Aneurysm
29778	By Serialography	16286	Ophthalmic Artery
16269	Abdominal	16287	On The Right
29779	And Bilateral Ileofemoral Artery	16288	On The Left
16270	Iliac	16289	Internal Carotid
16266	Pulmonary	16290	On The Right
29390	Injection Procedure	16291	On The Left
29391	Imaging Supervision And Report	16292	Anterior Communicating Artery
22664	Bilateral	16293	Anterior Cerebral Artery

16294	On The Right		16346	On The Right Only
16295	On The Left		16347	On The Left Only
16296	Middle Cerebral Artery		16348	Bilaterally
16297	On The Right		16349	Fusion of Kidneys
16298	On The Left		16350	Ectopic Kidney
16299	Posterior Communicating Artery		16351	Kidney Mass Lesion
16300	On The Right		16352	Solitary
16301	On The Left		16353	On The Right Only
16302	Posterior Cerebral Artery		16354	On The Left Only
16303	On The Right		16355	Bilaterally
16304	On The Left		16356	Multiple
16305	Basilar Tip		16357	On The Right Only
16306	Basilar Artery		16358	On The Left Only
16307	Cerebellar Artery		16359	Bilaterally
16308	On The Right		16360	Tumor Blush
16309	On The Left		16361	Calcified
16310	Vertebral Artery		16362	Kidney Cyst
16311	On The Right		16363	Solitary
16312	On The Left		16364	On The Right Only
16313	Parathyroid		16365	On The Left Only
16314	Abdominal		16366	Bilaterally
16315	Celiac		16367	Multiple
16316	Pancreas		16368	On The Right Only
16317	Vessel Displacement		16369	On The Left Only
16318	Tumor Blush		16370	Bilaterally
16319	Vessel Sheathing		16371	Calcification of Wall
16320	Superior Mesenteric		16372	Papillary Necrosis
16321	Inferior Mesenteric		16373	On The Right Only
16322	Renal		16374	On The Left Only
22663	Bilateral		16375	Bilaterally
16323	Absent Kidney		16376	Nephrocalcinosis
16324	On The Right Only		16377	On The Right Only
16325	On The Left Only		16378	On The Left Only
16326	Bilaterally		16379	Bilaterally
16327	Nonvisualization of Kidney		16380	Obstructive Pattern
16328	On The Right Only		16381	On The Right Only
16329	On The Left Only		16382	On The Left Only
16330	Bilaterally		16383	Bilaterally
16331	Delayed Visualization of Kidney		16384	Renal Artery Stenosis
16332	On The Right Only		16385	On The Right Only
16333	On The Left Only		16386	On The Left Only
16334	Bilaterally		16387	Bilaterally
16335	Large Kidney		16388	Renal Artery Dilation
16336	On The Right Only		16389	On The Right Only
16337	On The Left Only		16390	On The Left Only
16338	Bilaterally		16391	Bilaterally
16339	Small Kidney		16392	Renal Artery Anomaly
16340	On The Right Only		16393	Solitary Kidney Calculus
16341	On The Left Only		16394	On The Right Only
16342	Bilaterally		16395	On The Left Only
16343	Extrinsic Compression of Kidney		16396	Bilaterally
16344	From Above		16397	Multiple Kidney Calculi
16345	From Below		16398	On The Right Only

16399	On The Left Only	22704	Procedures
16400	Bilaterally	19187	Left Heart Catheterization
16401	Extravasation of Kidney	19188	Percutaneous
16402	On The Right Only	19189	Cutdown
16403	On The Left Only	19190	By Left Ventricular Puncture
16404	Bilaterally	19186	Right Heart Catheterization
16405	Extremities	19191	With Transseptal Left Heart Catheterization
16406	Lower		
16407	Upper	19192	Through Existing Defect
16408	Venography	19193	Combined Right & Left Heart Catheterization
28329	Injection Of Contrast Material		
16409	Orbital	19194	With Retrograde Left Heart Catheterization
16410	Non-Visualization of Cavernous Sinus		
		19195	Combined Transseptal & Retrograde Left Heart Catheterization
16411	Lower Extremities		
22667	Bilaterally	19196	With Left Ventricular Puncture
16412	Upper Extremities	16262	Angiography
16413	Inferior Vena Cava	22712	Contrast Material Used
16414	Superior Vena Cava	22713	Renografin-60
16415	Hepatic	22714	Renografin-76
28545	With Hemodynamic Evaluation	22715	Hypaque-76
16416	Hepatoportal	22716	Angiovist-370
28546	With Hemodynamic Evaluation	22717	Iohexol
16417	Splenoportal	22718	Contrast A
19395	Injection Of Dye	22719	Contrast B
16418	Renal	22720	Hexabrix
16419	Lymphangiography	22721	Isovue
19442	Injection Procedure	22722	Conray
22668	Extremities	16263	Coronary
22669	Unilateral	27218	repeat study
22670	Right Arm	27320	post op study
22671	Left Arm	19180	Left Heart Ventriculography
22672	Right Leg	22731	Biplane
22673	Left Leg	22732	Monoplane
22674	Both Arms	22063	Echo-Guided
22675	Both Legs	22064	Fluoroscopic
27096	Intra-Coronary Angioscopy	22065	Pigtail Catheter Inserted
22705	**Cardiac Catheterization**	22066	Pigtail Catheter Removed
82685	Indications	19181	Aortography
82686	CHF	19184	Right Heart Ventriculography
82687	Cardiogenic Shock	22733	Biplane
82688	Valvular Heart Disease	22734	Monoplane
82689	For Diagnosis Of Heart Disease Of Unknown Etiology	23120	Digital Subtraction (DSA)
		24878	Premedication
82690	Cardiac Arrhythmia	24880	Diazepam
82691	Cardiac Arrest	24879	Demerol
82692	Ischemic Heart Disease	24881	Atropine
82693	Endocarditis	24882	Thorazine
82694	Cardiomyopathy	24883	Phenergan
82695	Percardial Disease	24884	Curare
82696	Congenital Heart Disease	24885	Flaxedil
82697	For Follow-Up	24886	Pavulon
82698	Prosthetic Valve Dysfunction	24887	Ketamine

CARDIAC CATHETERIZATION, CONT.

24888	Droperidol	23073	The Right Brachial Artery
24889	Fentanyl	26783	Catheter Size
25046	An Anesthetic	23088	Percutaneous
25047	A Local Anesthetic	23102	Cutdown
25048	A General Anesthetic	23074	The Left Axillary Artery
23055	With Amyl Nitrite Provocation	26784	Catheter Size
23056	With Infusion	23089	Percutaneous
23058	Of Atropine	23103	Cutdown
27097	Of Diazepam	23075	The Right Axillary Artery
27098	Of Digoxin	26785	Catheter Size
27099	Of Ergonovine	23090	Percutaneous
27219	Negative Response	23104	Cutdown
27220	Positive Response	23076	The Left Axillary Vein
27221	Equivocal Response	26786	Catheter Size
27100	Of Fentanyl	23091	Percutaneous
27101	Of Hydralazine	23105	Cutdown
23057	Of Isuprel	23077	The Right Axillary Vein
27102	Of Ketamine	26787	Catheter Size
27103	Of Ketanserin	23092	Percutaneous
27104	Of Lidocaine	23106	Cutdown
27105	Of Midazolam	23078	The Left Femoral Artery
27106	Of Nifedipine	26788	Catheter Size
27107	Of Nitroglycerin	23093	Percutaneous
27108	Of Persantine	23107	Cutdown
23060	Of Priscoline	23079	The Right Femoral Artery
23059	Of Prostoglandin	26789	Catheter Size
27109	Of Streptokinase	23094	Percutaneous
27110	Of tPA	23108	Cutdown
27111	Of Verapamil	23080	The Left Femoral Vein
27112	Of Nitroprusside	26790	Catheter Size
27113	Of Dobutamine	23095	Percutaneous
27114	Of Adenosine	23109	Cutdown
27115	Of Methergine	23081	The Right Femoral Vein
27094	Thrombolytic Infusion	26791	Catheter Size
23061	With Oxygen Inhalation	23096	Percutaneous
23062	With Catheter Tip Pressures	23110	Cutdown
28081	With Catheter Tip Ultrasound	23082	The Left Jugular Vein
23063	With Catheter Tip Phono	26792	Catheter Size
23064	Coronary Sinus Flow Measurements	23097	Percutaneous
23065	Thermodilution Flow Studies	23111	Cutdown
23068	With Exercise	23083	The Right Jugular Vein
23069	Supine	26793	Catheter Size
23070	Upright	23098	Percutaneous
23071	Isometric	23112	Cutdown
23066	Cardiac Pacing Studies	23084	The Left Basilic Vein
23067	With Intracardiac ECG	26794	Catheter Size
27093	Special Laboratory Drug Protocol	23099	Percutaneous
23049	Coexistent Conditions	23113	Cutdown
22706	Insertion Sites	23085	The Right Basilic Vein
23072	The Left Brachial Artery	26795	Catheter Size
26782	Catheter Size	23100	Percutaneous
23087	Percutaneous	23114	Cutdown
23101	Cutdown		

CARDIAC CATHETERIZATION, CONT.

23086	Transthoracic Left Ventricular Puncture		26856	End Diastolic
12663	Hemodynamics		26857	Right Coronary Artery
12670	Intracardiac & Intra-arterial Pressures		26858	Peak Systolic
26827	Aortic Root		26859	Mean Systolic
26828	Peak Systolic		27147	Mean
26829	Mean Systolic		26860	Mean Diastolic
26830	C-Wave		26861	End Diastolic
27160	Mean		26862	Subclavian Artery
26831	Mean Diastolic		26863	Peak Systolic
26832	Early Diastolic		26864	Mean Systolic
26833	Mid Diastolic		27148	Mean
26834	End Diastolic		26865	Mean Diastolic
26835	Ascending Aorta		26866	End Diastolic
12671	Systole		25286	Brachial Artery
25267	Peak		25287	Systolic Pressure
25268	Mean		25288	Diastolic Pressure
25269	C-Wave		25289	Mean Pressure
27161	Mean		25290	Femoral Artery
12672	Diastole		25291	Systolic Pressure
25270	Mean		25292	Diastolic Pressure
25271	End		25293	Mean Pressure
25272	Mid		26867	Blalock
25273	Early		26868	Main
26837	Aortic Arch		26869	Peak Systolic
26838	Peak Systolic		26870	Mean Systolic
26839	Mean Systolic		27149	Mean
27143	Mean		26871	Mean Diastolic
26840	Mean Diastolic		26872	End Diastolic
26841	End Diastolic		26873	Left
26842	Aortic Conduit		26874	Peak Systolic
26843	Peak Systolic		26875	Mean Systolic
26844	Mean Systolic		27150	Mean
27144	Mean		26876	Mean Diastolic
26845	Mean Diastolic		26877	End Diastolic
26846	End Diastolic		26878	Right
26847	Descending Aorta		26879	Peak Systolic
26848	Peak Systolic		26880	Mean Systolic
26849	Mean Systolic		27151	Mean
27145	Mean		26881	Mean Diastolic
26850	Mean Diastolic		26882	End Diastolic
26851	End Diastolic		26883	Collateral
81045	Abdominal Aorta		27023	Main
81046	Peak Systolic		26884	Peak Systolic
81047	Mean Systolic		26885	Mean Systolic
81048	Mean		27152	Mean
81049	Mean Diastolic		26886	Mean Diastolic
81050	End Diastolic		26887	End Diastolic
26852	Left Coronary Artery		27024	Upper
26853	Peak Systolic		27025	Peak Systolic
26854	Mean Systolic		27026	Mean Systolic
27146	Mean		27153	Mean
26855	Mean Diastolic		27027	Mean Diastolic
			27028	End Diastolic

CARDIAC CATHETERIZATION, CONT.

27029	Lower		26912	End Diastolic
27030	Peak Systolic		26913	Right
27031	Mean Systolic		26914	Peak Systolic
27154	Mean		26915	Mean Systolic
27032	Mean Diastolic		26916	Mean Diastolic
27033	End Diastolic		26917	End Diastolic
27034	Left		26918	Inferior Vena Cava
27035	Peak Systolic		26919	Above Diaphragm
27036	Mean Systolic		26920	Systolic
27155	Mean		26921	Diastolic
27037	Mean Diastolic		26922	Mean
27038	End Diastolic		26923	Below Diaphragm
27039	Right		26924	Systolic
27040	Peak Systolic		26925	Diastolic
27041	Mean Systolic		26926	Mean
27156	Mean		26927	Pulmonary Vein
27042	Mean Diastolic		27011	Systolic
27043	End Diastolic		27012	Diastolic
26888	Brachiocephalic Vein		27013	Mean
27014	Main		26928	Left Atrium
26889	Systolic		27162	Systolic
26890	Diastolic		26930	Peak Systolic
26891	Mean		26931	Mean Systolic
27015	Left		26932	C-Wave
27016	Systolic		12673	Mean
27017	Diastolic		25274	A-Wave
27018	Mean		25275	V-Wave
27019	Right		27163	Diastolic
27020	Systolic		26933	Mid Diastolic
27021	Diastolic		26934	End Diastolic
27022	Mean		26999	Gradient
26892	Superior Vena Cava		27000	Peak
26893	Main		27001	Mean
26894	Peak Systolic		12674	Right Atrium
26895	Mean Systolic		27164	Systolic
26896	Mean Diastolic		26935	Peak Systolic
26897	End Diastolic		26936	Mean Systolic
25294	Gradient		26937	C-Wave
25295	Mean Pressure		26929	Mean
26898	Upper		25276	A-Wave
26899	Peak Systolic		25277	V-Wave
26900	Mean Systolic		12675	Prominent V wave
26901	Mean Diastolic		27165	Diastolic
26902	End Diastolic		26938	Mid Diastolic
26903	Lower		26939	End Diastolic
26904	Peak Systolic		26940	Coronary Sinus
26905	Mean Systolic		26941	Systolic
26906	Mean Diastolic		26942	Diastolic
26907	End Diastolic		26943	Mean
26908	Left		12676	Pulmonary Artery
26909	Peak Systolic		19185	Flow-directed Catheter Placement
26910	Mean Systolic		12677	Systole
26911	Mean Diastolic		26944	Peak

CARDIAC CATHETERIZATION, CONT.

26945	Mean		26969	Mean
12678	Diastole		26970	Gradient
26946	Mean		26971	Post Amyl Nitrite
26947	End		27159	Mean
12679	Mean		26972	Diastole
12680	Pulmonary Wedge		26973	Mid
26948	Peak Systolic		26974	End
26949	Mean Systolic		26975	Mean
26950	Mid Diastolic		12686	Right Ventricle Systole
26951	End Diastolic		22727	Peak Pressure
26952	Mean Diastolic		22728	Mean Pressure
12681	Mean		12687	Right Ventricle Diastole
25278	A-Wave		22729	End Pressure
12682	A waves increased		22730	Mean Pressure
25279	V-Wave		12696	Intercavitary (LV-RV Diastolic)
12683	V waves increased		12688	Equalized Pressures
26953	Balloon		26976	RVOT
26954	Peak Systolic		26977	Main
26955	Mean Systolic		26978	Peak Systolic
27157	Mean		26979	Mean Systolic
26956	Mid Diastolic		26980	Mean Diastolic
26957	End Diastolic		26981	End Diastolic
26958	Mean Diastolic		26982	Upper
26959	Right Artery		26983	Peak Systolic
26960	Peak Systolic		26984	Mean Systolic
26961	Mean Systolic		26985	Mean Diastolic
27158	Mean		26986	End Diastolic
26962	Mid Diastolic		26987	Mid
26963	End Diastolic		26988	Peak Systolic
26964	Mean Diastolic		26989	Mean Systolic
28205	Left Artery		26990	Mean Diastolic
28206	Peak Systolic		26991	End Diastolic
28207	Mean Systolic		26992	Lower
28208	Mean		26993	Peak Systolic
28209	Mid Diastolic		26994	Mean Systolic
28210	End Diastolic		26995	Mean Diastolic
28211	Mean Diastolic		26996	End Diastolic
26836	Left Ventricle		12689	Gradient
12684	Systole		12690	Aortic Valve (Systolic)
22723	Peak Pressure		12692	Valvular
22724	Mean Pressure		24819	Peak Systolic
12695	Intracavitary Gradient		24820	Mean
26997	Peak		12694	Supravalvular
26998	Mean		24830	Peak Systolic
23167	Gradient Post-intervention		24831	Mean
23168	Post Amyl Nitrite		12693	Subvalvular (LVOT)
12685	Diastole		24373	Peak Systolic
26965	Mid Pressure		24374	Mean
22725	End Pressure		12691	Mitral Valve (Diastolic)
22726	Mean Pressure		25280	Maximum Instantaneous
26966	Common Ventricle			Gradient (DFP)
26967	Systole		25281	Mean Gradient (DFP)
26968	Peak		25001	Pulmonary Valve (Systolic)

CARDIAC CATHETERIZATION, CONT.

25003	Valvular		28334	Cardiac Stroke Work Index (gm-m/m2)
24310	Peak Systolic		12665	LV Ejection Fraction (%)
24311	Mean		24635	Regular Beat
25004	Supravalvular		24634	Post Ectopic Beat
25282	Peak Systolic		24636	Questionable Beat
25283	Mean		24178	RV Ejection Fraction (SV/EDV)
25005	Subvalvular		12705	Systemic Vascular Resistance (d-sec/cm5)
24354	Peak Systolic			
24355	Mean		12706	Pulmonary Vascular Resistance (d-sec/cm5)
25002	Tricuspid Valve (Diastolic)			
25284	Maximum Instantaneous Gradient (DFP)		25303	Total (No Wedge)
			25304	RP/RS Resistance Ratio
25285	Mean Gradient (DFP)		25305	Differential Pulmonary Arteriolar Resistance
12697	Intravenous Pressures			
12698	Central		12707	Systolic Time Intervals
12699	Peripheral (cm H2O)		12708	PEP Index
12700	Antecubital		12709	LVET Index
25049	Volume Measurements		12710	PEP/LVET Index
25050	LVESV		25491	Diastolic Filling Period
25296	Index		25306	Valve Areas
25051	LVEDV		25307	Aortic (Modified)
25297	Index		25308	Aortic (Gorlin)
25052	LVSV		25309	Mitral (Modified)
25298	Index		25310	Mitral (Gorlin)
25483	RVESV		24589	Assessment
25484	Index		24590	Systemic Hypertension
25485	RVEDV		24591	Systemic Hypotension
25486	Index		24592	Pulmonary Hypertension
25487	RVSV		24593	"V" Wave
25488	Index		24594	Consistent With Tricuspid Regurgitation
25299	Regurgitant Index			
25300	Stroke Work Value		24595	Consistent With Mitral Regurgitation
12664	Cardiac Output (l/min)			
25301	Index (l/min/m2)		24596	Pressure Relationships
25302	Stroke Volume Index (ml/beat/m2)		24597	Constrictive Disease
22707	Thermodilution Curves		24598	Restrictive Disease
22708	Arteriovenous O2 Saturation Gradient		16265	Left Heart Findings
			24103	Dilation
12701	Dye-Dilution Curves (Brachial Sampling)		24104	Hypertrophy of the left ventricle
			24587	Hypoplasia Of The Left Ventricle
29392	Subsequent Measurement		24108	Contractility Of The Left Ventricle
12702	Inferior Vena Cava Injection		24109	Global
12703	Right Ventricular Injection		24110	Hyperkinesia
12704	Pulmonary Artery Injection		24111	Hypokinesia
12666	Hydrogen Appearance Time		24112	Regional
12667	Shortened at Level of Right Atrium		24113	Anterobasal
			24114	Hyperkinesia
12668	Shortened at Level of Right Ventricle		24115	Hypokinesia
			24116	Akinesia
12669	Shortened at Level of Pulmonary Artery		24117	Dyskinesia
			24118	Anterolateral
22709	Increased		24126	Hyperkinesia
22710	Decreased		24133	Hypokinesia

CARDIAC CATHETERIZATION, CONT.

24141	Akinesia	24172	Diaphragmatic
24149	Dyskinesia	24173	Posterobasal
24119	Apical	24174	Basal Septal
24156	Hyperkinesia	24175	Apical Septal
24134	Hypokinesia	24176	Posterolateral
24142	Akinesia	24177	Lateral
18057	Dyskinesia	24832	Mass ___cm
24120	Diaphragmatic	24833	Anterobasal ___cm
24127	Hyperkinesia	24834	Anterolateral ___cm
24135	Hypokinesia	24835	Apical ___cm
24143	Akinesia	24836	Diaphragmatic ___cm
24150	Dyskinesia	24837	Posterobasal ___cm
24121	Posterobasal	24838	Basal Septal ___cm
24128	Hyperkinesia	24839	Apical Septal ___cm
24136	Hypokinesia	24840	Posterolateral___cm
24144	Akinesia	24841	Lateral ___cm
24151	Dyskinesia	24349	LVOT
24122	Basal Septal	24105	Hypertrophy
24129	Hyperkinesia	24368	Atresia
24137	Hypokinesia	24369	Obstruction
24145	Akinesia	24370	Peak Systolic Gradient
24152	Dyskinesia	24371	Mean Gradient
24123	Apical Septal	24372	Subaortic Obstruction
24130	Hyperkinesia	24599	Aortic Valve
24138	Hypokinesia	24679	Cusps
24146	Akinesia	24680	Unicuspid With Single Commissure
24153	Dyskinesia		
24124	Posterolateral	24681	Bicuspid
24131	Hyperkinesia	24731	Deformed Tricuspid
24139	Hypokinesia	24682	Quadracuspid
24147	Akinesia	24683	Atresia
24154	Dyskinesia	24248	Regurgitation
24125	Lateral	24249	Native Valve
24132	Hyperkinesia	24250	Prosthetic Valve
24140	Hypokinesia	24251	Periprosthetic Valve
24148	Akinesia	24684	Stenosis
24155	Dyskinesia	24829	Supravalvular
24157	Aneurysm	24729	Prosthetic Aortic Valve
29271	Anterior	24824	Type
24158	Anterobasal	24821	St. Jude
24159	Anterolateral	24822	Starr Edwards
24160	Apical	24823	Bjork-Shiley
24161	Diaphragmatic	24825	Function
24162	Posterobasal	24726	Aortic Root
24163	Basal Septal	19182	Regurgitation
24164	Apical Septal	24732	Fistula
24165	Posterolateral	24733	Sinus To Right Ventricle
24166	Lateral	24734	Sinus To Right Atrium
24167	False Aneurysm	24735	Sinus To Left Atrium
18059	Thrombus Formation	24600	Mitral Valve
24168	Anterobasal	24106	Regurgitation
24169	Anterolateral	24637	Catheter Induced
24170	Apical	24644	Absent

CARDIAC CATHETERIZATION, CONT.

24646	Prolapse	24539	Intact
24648	Cleft Anterior Leaflet	24540	Defect
24649	Complete	24541	Patent Foramen Ovale
24650	Partial	24542	Ostium Secundum
24647	Parachute Valve	24549	Ostium Primum
24642	Atresia	24543	Sinus Venosus
24643	Dysplasia	24544	Coronary Sinus
24645	Stenosis	24545	Common Atrium
24601	Left AV Valve	24546	Aneurysm Of Fossa Ovalis
24652	Overriding	24547	Atrioventricular Canal
24651	Straddling	24548	Partial
24638	Atresia	24550	Intermediate
24639	Imperforate Membrane	24551	Complete
24640	Dysplasia	24552	Type A
24653	Ebstein Anomaly	24553	Type B
24107	Regurgitation	24554	Type C
24641	Stenosis	24555	Atrioventricular Valve Incompetence
24654	Prosthetic Left AV Valve	24556	Cor Triatriatum
24655	Type	24557	Left Atrial Supravalvular Mitral Ring
24656	St. Jude		
24657	Starr Edwards	24558	Cor Triatriatum Dexter
24658	Bjork-Shiley	24854	Mass ___ cm
24659	Function	24538	Ventricular Septum
24559	Left Atrium	24569	Intact
24852	Mass ___ cm	24570	Defect
24563	Juxtaposed Atrial Appendages	24571	Aneurysm Of Membranous Septum
24560	Giant Atrium		
24561	Aneurysm Of Atrial Appendage	24572	Membranous
24562	Double Outlet	24573	Supracristal
24685	Congenital Findings Of Functional Left Ventricle	24574	Outlet Infundibular
		24575	Inlet Sub-tricuspid (AV Canal Type)
24686	Morphology		
24687	Left Ventricular	24576	Left Ventricle To The Right Atrium
24688	Right Ventricular		
24689	Anatomy	24577	Single Muscular
24690	Left Ventricular	24578	Multiple Muscular (<4)
24691	Right Ventricular	24579	Fenestrated
24692	Inlet	24580	Sub-Pulmonary
24693	Double	24581	Sub-Aortic
24694	Common	24582	Non-committed
24695	Single	24583	Doubly committed
24696	No Rudimentary Chambers	24584	Postoperative
24697	Hypoplastic Subpulmonary Right Ventricle	24585	Restrictive
		24586	Restricted Outflow Tract
24698	Hypoplastic Subaortic Right Ventricle	24855	Mass ___ cm
		16264	Right Heart Findings
24699	Hypoplastic Double Outlet Right Ventricle	18049	Ventricular Dilation
		24179	Hypertrophy of the right ventricle
24700	Anomalous Muscle Bundle	24588	Hypoplasia Of The Right Ventricle
24701	Hypoplasia	24183	Contractility Of The Right Ventricle
24702	Diverticulum	24184	Global
22751	Septa	24185	Hyperkinesia
24537	Atrial Septum	24186	Hypokinesia

CARDIAC CATHETERIZATION, CONT.

24187	Regional		24240	Apical Septal
24188	Anterobasal		24241	Posterolateral
24189	Hyperkinesia		24242	Lateral
24190	Hypokinesia		24243	False Aneurysm
24191	Akinesia		24725	Right Atrium To Right Ventricle
24192	Dyskinesia			Conduit
24193	Anterolateral		24366	Peak Systolic Gradient
24194	Hyperkinesia		24367	Mean Gradient
24195	Hypokinesia		24365	Stenosis
24196	Akinesia		24842	Mass ___cm
24197	Dyskinesia		24843	Anterobasal ___cm
24198	Apical		24844	Anterolateral ___cm
24199	Hyperkinesia		24845	Apical ___cm
24200	Hypokinesia		24846	Diaphragmatic ___cm
24201	Akinesia		24847	Posterobasal ___cm
24202	Dyskinesia		24848	Basal Septal ___cm
24203	Diaphragmatic		24849	Apical Septal ___cm
24204	Hyperkinesia		24850	Posterolateral ___cm
24205	Hypokinesia		24851	Lateral ___cm
24206	Akinesia		24348	RVOT
24207	Dyskinesia		24180	Hypertrophy
24208	Posterobasal		24351	Peak Systolic Gradient
24209	Hyperkinesia		24352	Mean Gradient
24210	Hypokinesia		24350	Obstruction
24211	Akinesia		24727	Subpulmonary Membrane
24212	Dyskinesia		24353	Obstruction
24223	Posterolateral		24728	Conduit
24224	Hyperkinesia		24357	Peak Systolic Gradient
24225	Hypokinesia		24358	Mean Gradient
24226	Akinesia		24356	Stenosis
24227	Dyskinesia		24757	Prominent Conal Branch
24228	Lateral		24308	Pulmonary Valve
24229	Hyperkinesia		24313	Absent
24230	Hypokinesia		24309	Stenosis
24231	Akinesia		24312	Regurgitation
24232	Dyskinesia		24603	Tricuspid Valve
24213	Basal Septal		24181	Regurgitation
24214	Hyperkinesia		24665	Absent
24215	Hypokinesia		24668	Prolapse
24216	Akinesia		24670	Cleft
24217	Dyskinesia		24669	Parachute Valve
24218	Apical Septal		24664	Atresia
24219	Hyperkinesia		24666	Dysplasia
24220	Hypokinesia		24667	Stenosis
24221	Akinesia		24604	Right AV Valve
24222	Dyskinesia		24672	Overriding
24233	Aneurysm		24671	Straddling
24234	Anterobasal		24660	Atresia
24235	Anterolateral		24661	Imperforate Membrane
24236	Apical		24662	Dysplasia
24237	Diaphragmatic		24673	Ebstein Anomaly
24238	Posterobasal		24182	Regurgitation
24239	Basal Septal		24663	Stenosis

CARDIAC CATHETERIZATION, CONT.

24674	Prosthetic Right AV Valve	24254	Sinus Of Valsalva Aneurysm
24675	Type	24257	Arteriovenous Fistula
24676	St. Jude	24258	Of Aortic Arch
24677	Bjork-Shiley	24260	Rupture
24678	Function	24259	Generalized Arteriopathy
24564	Right Atrium	24261	Aortic Arch
24565	Juxtaposed Atrial Appendages	24262	Anomalies
24566	Giant Atrium	24263	Aortic Branches
24567	Aneurysm Of Atrial Appendage	24264	Double Aortic Arch
24568	Double Outlet	24265	Both Patent
24853	Mass ___ cm	24266	One Atretic
24703	Congenital Findings Of Functional Right Ventricle	24267	Cervical Arch
		24269	Right Arch
24704	Morphology	24268	Left Arch
24705	Right Ventricular	24272	Interruption Of Arch
24706	Left Ventricular	24273	Between The Brachiocephalic Trunk And The Left Carotid Artery
24707	Anatomy		
24708	Right Ventricular		
24709	Left Ventricular	24274	At The Left Carotid
24710	Inlet	24275	Between The Left Carotid And Subclavian Arteries
24711	Double		
24712	Common	24276	Distal To The Left Subclavian Artery
24713	Single		
24714	No Rudimentary Chambers	24277	Coarctation
24715	Hypoplastic Subpulmonary Left Ventricle	24278	Peak Systolic Gradient
		24279	Mean Gradient
24716	Hypoplastic Subaortic Left Ventricle	24280	Pseudocoarctation
		24283	Truncus Arteriosus
24717	Hypoplastic Double Outlet Left Ventricle	24346	Main Pulmonary Artery From Truncus
24718	Anomalous Muscle Bundle	24347	Right And Left Pulmonary Artery Separate From Truncus
24720	Hypoplasia		
24721	Diverticulum	24284	Bilateral Conus
22752	Arteriographic Findings Of The Great Arteries	24736	Aortic Conduit
		24286	Peak Systolic Gradient
24244	Aorta	24287	Mean Gradient
24245	Dilation	24285	Stenosis
24246	Root And Sinuses	24737	Aortic To Pulmonary Outflow Tract Septal Defect
24247	Ascending Aorta		
24252	Dissection	24738	Aortic To Left Ventricular Tunnel
24826	From The Ascending Aorta Through The Arch And The Descending Aorta	24288	Systemic
		24289	Persistent Left Ductus Arteriosus
		24290	Persistent Right Ductus Arteriosus
24827	Through The Aortic Arch	24291	Persistent Bilateral Ductus Arteriosus
24828	Descending From The Left Subclavian Artery		
		24292	Aneurysm Of Ductus Arteriosus
24253	Aneurysm	24293	The Right Subclavian Artery Arose From The Descending Aorta
24255	Ascending		
24256	Aortic Arch	24294	The Left Subclavian Artery Arose From The Descending Aorta
24281	Descending		
24282	Abdominal	24295	The Right Subclavian Artery Was Isolated From The Aorta
24270	Hypoplasia		
24271	Tubular, Of The Aortic Arch		

CARDIAC CATHETERIZATION, CONT.

24296	The Left Subclavian Artery Was Isolated From The Aorta	24344	Pulmonary A-V Fistula
24297	Systemic-Pulmonary Collateral	24345	Direct Communication From PA To Left Atrium
24298	Congenital	22753	Great Veins
24299	Acquired	24425	Pulmonary Veins
24300	Arteriovenous Fistula	24426	Connections
24301	Hepatic	24442	Total APVC
24302	Hypertension	24443	To Right SVC
24303	Arterial Occlusion	24444	To Left SVC
24304	Femoral	24445	To Azygous Vein
24305	Pulmonary Artery	24446	To Hemiazygous Vein
24328	Normal Pressure And Resistance	24447	To Brachiocephalic Vein
24306	Stenosis	24448	To The Coronary Sinus
24314	Supravalvular	24449	To The Right Atrium
24315	Peak Systolic Gradient	24450	To The Left Atrium
24316	Mean Gradient	24722	Situs Ambiguous
24317	The Left Branch	24723	Situs Inversus
24319	Peak Systolic Gradient	24451	Infradiaphragmatic to IVC
24321	Mean Gradient	24452	Infradiaphragmatic To Portal Vein
24318	The Right Branch	24453	Mixed Drainage
24320	Peak Systolic Gradient	24454	Hemi APVC
24322	Mean Gradient	24455	Right Pulmonary Veins To The Azygous Vein
24323	Peripheral Artery System		
24324	Peak Systolic Gradient	24456	Right Pulmonary Veins To The Coronary Sinus
24325	Mean Gradient		
24739	Pulmonary Outflow Conduit	24457	Right Pulmonary Veins To The Inferior Vena Cava
24359	Stenosis		
24360	Peak Systolic Gradient	24458	Right Pulmonary Veins To The Right Atrium
24361	Mean Gradient		
24740	Right Atrium To Pulmonary Artery Conduit	24459	Right Pulmonary Veins To The Right Superior Vena Cava
24362	Stenosis	24460	Left Pulmonary Veins To The Left Superior Vena Cava
24363	Peak Systolic Gradient		
24364	Mean Gradient	24461	Left Pulmonary Veins To The Coronary Sinus
24326	Hypertension		
24327	An Embolus	24462	Left Pulmonary Veins To Hemi-azygous Vein
24341	Idiopathic Dilation		
24337	Aneurysm	24463	Left Pulmonary Veins To The Right Superior Vena Cava
24338	Of The Right Pulmonary Artery		
24339	Of The Left Pulmonary Artery	24464	Partial APVC
24340	Hypoplasia	24466	Right Pulmonary Veins To The Azygous Vein
24307	Atresia		
24329	Nonconfluent Arteries	24486	The Upper Region
24330	Incomplete Central Artery Distribution	24496	The Middle Region
		24511	The Lower Region
24331	Anomalous Origin	24475	Right Pulmonary Veins To Hemi-azygous Vein
24332	RPA From The Ascending Aorta		
24333	LPA From The Ascending Aorta	24487	The Upper Region
24334	RPA From The Descending Aorta	24497	The Middle Region
24335	LPA From The Descending Aorta	24512	The Lower Region
24336	Vascular Sling	24467	Right Pulmonary Veins To The Coronary Sinus
24342	Left PA Supplied By Ductus		
24343	Right PA Supplied By Ductus		

CARDIAC CATHETERIZATION, CONT.

27304	The Upper Region	24474	Left Pulmonary Veins To The
27305	The Middle Region		Right Superior Vena Cava
27306	The Lower Region	24494	The Upper Region
24468	Right Pulmonary Veins To The	24509	The Middle Region
	Inferior Vena Cava	24524	The Lower Region
24482	The Upper Region	24480	Left Pulmonary Veins To The
24499	The Middle Region		Brachiocephalic Vein
24514	The Lower Region	24495	The Upper Region
24469	Right Pulmonary Veins To The	24510	The Middle Region
	Right Atrium	24525	The Lower Region
24483	The Upper Region	24465	Abnormality Of Otherwise Normal
24500	The Middle Region		Pulmonary Vein
24515	The Lower Region	24427	Thrombosis
24470	Right Pulmonary Veins To The	24428	Veno-occlusive Disease
	Right Superior Vena Cava	24429	Occlusion
24484	The Upper Region	24430	Stenosis
24501	The Middle Region	24431	Systemic
24516	The Lower Region	24432	Connections
24476	Right Pulmonary Veins To The	24526	Left SVC To Right Atrium Via
	Left Superior Vena Cava		Coronary Sinus
24485	The Upper Region	24527	Left SVC Directly To The Left
24502	The Middle Region		Atrium
24517	The Lower Region	24528	Left SVC To Left Atrium Via
24477	Left Pulmonary Veins To The		Coronary Sinus
	Azygous Vein	24529	Coronary Sinus To The Left
24488	The Upper Region		Atrium, No Accessory SVC
24503	The Middle Region	24530	Unroofed Coronary Sinus
24518	The Lower Region	24531	Absent Right Superior Vena Cava
24473	Left Pulmonary Veins To	24532	Azygous Vein Continuation To
	Hemi-azygous Vein		Right SVC, Interrupted IVC
24489	The Upper Region	24533	Azygous Vein Continuation To
24504	The Middle Region		Coronary Sinus, Interrupted IVC
24519	The Lower Region	24534	Hemi-azygous Vein Continuation
24472	Left Pulmonary Veins To The		To Left SVC, Interrupted IVC
	Coronary Sinus	24535	Inferior Vena Cava Connected To
27307	The Upper Region		The Left Atrium
27308	The Middle Region	24536	Accessory Right Superior Vena
27309	The Lower Region		Cava, Situs Inversus
24478	Left Pulmonary Veins To The	24433	Inferior Vena Cava
	Inferior Vena Cava	24434	Abnormalities
24491	The Upper Region	24435	Obstruction
24506	The Middle Region	24436	Superior Vena Cava
24521	The Lower Region	24437	Abnormalities
24479	Left Pulmonary Veins To The	24438	Obstruction
	Right Atrium	24439	Femoral Vein
24492	The Upper Region	24440	Abnormalities
24507	The Middle Region	24441	Obstruction
24522	The Lower Region	22748	Coronary Arteries
24471	Left Pulmonary Veins To The	22742	Native Arteries
	Left Superior Vena Cava	19202	Ergonovine Provocation
24493	The Upper Region	22743	Dominance
24508	The Middle Region	22744	Left
24523	The Lower Region	22745	Right

CARDIAC CATHETERIZATION, CONT.

22746	Balanced	22786	Aneurysm
22747	Undetermined	22787	Discrete
27116	Coronaries Not Done. Both Not	22788	Diffuse
	Injected	22789	Multiple
22755	Left Coronary Artery System	24752	Dissection
22757	Not Injected	27125	Not Visible
22756	Left Main Artery	27126	Poorly Visualized
22758	Stenosis	22790	Dist LAD
24747	Ostial Stenosis	22820	Stenosis
24748	Ostial Membrane	22842	Single Discrete
22759	Single Discrete	23420	Single Discrete, Concentric
23416	Single Discrete, Concentric	23448	Single Discrete, Eccentric
	Morphology	22865	Multiple Discrete
23417	Single Discrete, Eccentric	22888	Diffuse
	Morphology	22911	Tubular
22760	Multiple Discrete	22934	Calcific
22761	Diffuse	22957	Aneurysm
22762	Tubular	22980	Discrete
22763	Calcific	23003	Diffuse
102898	Thrombotic	23026	Multiple
102899	Length ___ mm	24753	Dissection
22764	Aneurysm	27127	Not Visible
22765	Discrete	27128	Poorly Visualized
22766	Diffuse	27117	Left Anterior Descending Artery
22767	Multiple		Branches
24749	Dissection	22791	Diag-1
27119	Not Visible	22821	Stenosis
27121	Poorly Visualized	22843	Single Discrete
22768	Prox LAD	23421	Single Discrete, Concentric
22769	Stenosis	23449	Single Discrete, Eccentric
22770	Single Discrete	22866	Multiple Discrete
23418	Single Discrete, Concentric	22889	Diffuse
23446	Single Discrete, Eccentric	22912	Tubular
22771	Multiple Discrete	22935	Calcific
22772	Diffuse	22958	Aneurysm
22773	Tubular	22981	Discrete
22774	Calcific	23004	Diffuse
22775	Aneurysm	23027	Multiple
22776	Discrete	27131	Not Visible
22777	Diffuse	27132	Poorly Visualized
22778	Multiple	22792	Diag-2
24751	Dissection	22822	Stenosis
27122	Not Visible	22844	Single Discrete
27124	Poorly Visualized	23422	Single Discrete, Concentric
22779	Mid LAD	23450	Single Discrete, Eccentric
22780	Stenosis	22867	Multiple Discrete
22781	Single Discrete	22890	Diffuse
23419	Single Discrete, Concentric	22913	Tubular
23447	Single Discrete, Eccentric	22936	Calcific
22782	Multiple Discrete	22959	Aneurysm
22783	Diffuse	22982	Discrete
22784	Tubular	23005	Diffuse
22785	Calcific	23028	Multiple

CARDIAC CATHETERIZATION, CONT.

27133	Not Visible	23454	Single Discrete, Eccentric
27134	Poorly Visualized	22871	Multiple Discrete
22793	Septal-1	22894	Diffuse
22823	Stenosis	22917	Tubular
22845	Single Discrete	22940	Calcific
23423	Single Discrete, Concentric	22963	Aneurysm
23451	Single Discrete, Eccentric	22986	Discrete
22868	Multiple Discrete	23009	Diffuse
22891	Diffuse	23032	Multiple
22914	Tubular	24755	Dissection
22937	Calcific	27137	Not Visible
22960	Aneurysm	27138	Poorly Visualized
22983	Discrete	27118	Circumflex Artery Branches
23006	Diffuse	22797	OM-1
23029	Multiple	22827	Stenosis
27129	Not Visible	22849	Single Discrete
27130	Poorly Visualized	23427	Single Discrete, Concentric
22794	Intermedius	23455	Single Discrete, Eccentric
22824	Stenosis	22872	Multiple Discrete
22846	Single Discrete	22895	Diffuse
23424	Single Discrete, Concentric	22918	Tubular
23452	Single Discrete, Eccentric	22941	Calcific
22869	Multiple Discrete	22964	Aneurysm
22892	Diffuse	22987	Discrete
22915	Tubular	23010	Diffuse
22938	Calcific	23033	Multiple
22961	Aneurysm	27139	Not Visible
22984	Discrete	27140	Poorly Visualized
23007	Diffuse	22798	OM-2
23030	Multiple	22828	Stenosis
24756	Dissection	22850	Single Discrete
27180	Not Visible	23428	Single Discrete, Concentric
27181	Poorly Visualized	23456	Single Discrete, Eccentric
22795	Prox Circ	22873	Multiple Discrete
22825	Stenosis	22896	Diffuse
22847	Single Discrete	22919	Tubular
23425	Single Discrete, Concentric	22942	Calcific
23453	Single Discrete, Eccentric	22965	Aneurysm
22870	Multiple Discrete	22988	Discrete
22893	Diffuse	23011	Diffuse
22916	Tubular	23034	Multiple
22939	Calcific	27141	Not Visible
22962	Aneurysm	27142	Poorly Visualized
22985	Discrete	22799	OM-3
23008	Diffuse	22829	Stenosis
23031	Multiple	22851	Single Discrete
24754	Dissection	23429	Single Discrete, Concentric
27135	Not Visible	23457	Single Discrete, Eccentric
27136	Poorly Visualized	22874	Multiple Discrete
22796	Dist Circ	22897	Diffuse
22826	Stenosis	22920	Tubular
22848	Single Discrete	22943	Calcific
23426	Single Discrete, Concentric	22966	Aneurysm

CARDIAC CATHETERIZATION, CONT.

22989	Discrete	23433	Single Discrete, Concentric
23012	Diffuse	23461	Single Discrete, Eccentric
23035	Multiple	22877	Multiple Discrete
27166	Not Visible	22900	Diffuse
27167	Poorly Visualized	22923	Tubular
22800	L AV Groove	22946	Calcific
22830	Stenosis	22969	Aneurysm
22852	Single Discrete	22992	Discrete
23430	Single Discrete, Concentric	23015	Diffuse
23458	Single Discrete, Eccentric	23038	Multiple
22875	Multiple Discrete	27176	Not Visible
22898	Diffuse	27177	Poorly Visualized
22921	Tubular	22803	L Postlat-3
22944	Calcific	22833	Stenosis
22967	Aneurysm	22855	Single Discrete
22990	Discrete	23434	Single Discrete, Concentric
23013	Diffuse	23462	Single Discrete, Eccentric
23036	Multiple	22878	Multiple Discrete
27168	Not Visible	22901	Diffuse
27169	Poorly Visualized	22924	Tubular
23121	L Postlat Seg	22947	Calcific
23122	Stenosis	22970	Aneurysm
23123	Single Discrete	22993	Discrete
23431	Single Discrete, Concentric	23016	Diffuse
23459	Single Discrete, Eccentric	23039	Multiple
23124	Multiple Discrete	27178	Not Visible
23125	Diffuse	27179	Poorly Visualized
23126	Tubular	22804	Right Coronary Artery System
23127	Calcific	22805	Not Injected
23128	Aneurysm	22806	Proximal RCA
23129	Discrete	22834	Stenosis
23131	Diffuse	24745	Ostial Stenosis
23130	Multiple	24746	Ostial Membrane
27172	Not Visible	22856	Single Discrete
27173	Poorly Visualized	23435	Single Discrete, Concentric
22801	L Postlat-1	23463	Single Discrete, Eccentric
22831	Stenosis	22879	Multiple Discrete
22853	Single Discrete	22902	Diffuse
23432	Single Discrete, Concentric	22925	Tubular
23460	Single Discrete, Eccentric	22948	Calcific
22876	Multiple Discrete	22971	Aneurysm
22899	Diffuse	22994	Discrete
22922	Tubular	23017	Diffuse
22945	Calcific	23040	Multiple
22968	Aneurysm	24750	Dissection
22991	Discrete	27182	Not Visible
23014	Diffuse	27183	Poorly Visualized
23037	Multiple	24758	Prominent Right Ventricular
27174	Not Visible		Branch
27175	Poorly Visualized	22807	Mid-RCA
22802	L Postlat-2	22835	Stenosis
22832	Stenosis	22857	Single Discrete
22854	Single Discrete	23436	Single Discrete, Concentric

CARDIAC CATHETERIZATION, CONT.

23464	Single Discrete, Eccentric	22812	R Posterolat Seg
22880	Multiple Discrete	22838	Stenosis
22903	Diffuse	22861	Single Discrete
22926	Tubular	23440	Single Discrete, Concentric
22949	Calcific	23468	Single Discrete, Eccentric
22972	Aneurysm	22884	Multiple Discrete
22995	Discrete	22907	Diffuse
23018	Diffuse	22930	Tubular
23041	Multiple	22953	Calcific
27184	Not Visible	22976	Aneurysm
27185	Poorly Visualized	22999	Discrete
22808	Distal RCA	23022	Diffuse
22836	Stenosis	23045	Multiple
22858	Single Discrete	27190	Not Visible
23437	Single Discrete, Concentric	27191	Poorly Visualized
23465	Single Discrete, Eccentric	22813	R Posterolat-1
22881	Multiple Discrete	22839	Stenosis
22904	Diffuse	22862	Single Discrete
22927	Tubular	23441	Single Discrete, Concentric
22950	Calcific	23469	Single Discrete, Eccentric
22973	Aneurysm	22885	Multiple Discrete
22996	Discrete	22908	Diffuse
23019	Diffuse	22931	Tubular
23042	Multiple	22954	Calcific
27186	Not Visible	22977	Aneurysm
27187	Poorly Visualized	23000	Discrete
22809	AMV-1	23023	Diffuse
22837	Stenosis	23046	Multiple
22859	Single Discrete	27192	Not Visible
23438	Single Discrete, Concentric	27193	Poorly Visualized
23466	Single Discrete, Eccentric	22814	R Posterolat-2
22882	Multiple Discrete	22840	Stenosis
22905	Diffuse	22863	Single Discrete
22928	Tubular	23442	Single Discrete, Concentric
22951	Calcific	23470	Single Discrete, Eccentric
22974	Aneurysm	22886	Multiple Discrete
22997	Discrete	22909	Diffuse
23020	Diffuse	22932	Tubular
23043	Multiple	22955	Calcific
22810	AMV-2	22978	Aneurysm
22811	was not visualized	23001	Discrete
23486	Stenosis	23024	Diffuse
22860	Single Discrete	23047	Multiple
23439	Single Discrete, Concentric	27194	Not Visible
23467	Single Discrete, Eccentric	27195	Poorly Visualized
22883	Multiple Discrete	22815	R Posterolat-3
22906	Diffuse	22841	Stenosis
22929	Tubular	22864	Single Discrete
22952	Calcific	23443	Single Discrete, Concentric
22975	Aneurysm	23471	Single Discrete, Eccentric
22998	Discrete	22887	Multiple Discrete
23021	Diffuse	22910	Diffuse
23044	Multiple	22933	Tubular

CARDIAC CATHETERIZATION, CONT.

22956	Calcific	23178	Prox Circ
22979	Aneurysm	23179	Dist Circ
23002	Discrete	23180	OM-1
23025	Diffuse	23181	OM-2
23048	Multiple	23182	OM-3
27196	Not Visible	23183	L AV Groove
27197	Poorly Visualized	23184	L Postlat Seg
22816	Posterior Descending Arteries	23185	L Postlat-1
23132	Left PDA	23186	L Postlat-2
23134	Stenosis	23187	L Postlat-3
23135	Single Discrete	23188	Proximal RCA
23444	Single Discrete, Concentric	23189	Middle RCA
23472	Single Discrete, Eccentric	23190	Distal RCA
23136	Multiple Discrete	23191	AMV-1
23137	Diffuse	23192	AMV-2
23138	Tubular	23193	R Posterolat Seg
23139	Calcific	23194	R Posterolat-1
23140	Aneurysm	23195	R Posterolat-2
23141	Discrete	23196	R Posterolat-3
23142	Diffuse	23197	Left PDA
23143	Multiple	23198	Right PDA
27170	Not Visible	23350	Y Graft
27171	Poorly Visualized	23344	Sequential
23133	Right PDA	23356	Obstruction
23144	Stenosis	23357	Single Discrete
23145	Single Discrete	23474	Single Discrete, Concentric
23445	Single Discrete, Concentric	23475	Single Discrete, Eccentric
23473	Single Discrete, Eccentric	23358	Multiple Discrete
23146	Multiple Discrete	23359	Diffuse
23147	Diffuse	23360	Tubular
23148	Tubular	23361	Calcific
23149	Calcific	23362	Aneurysm
23150	Aneurysm	23363	Discrete
23151	Discrete	23364	Diffuse
23152	Diffuse	23365	Multiple
23153	Multiple	23158	RIMA
27188	Not Visible	23199	Insertion Sites Visualized
27189	Poorly Visualized	23204	Left Main
22817	Congenital Abnormalities	23209	Prox LAD
22818	Left	23214	Mid LAD
22819	Right	23219	Dist LAD
19183	CABG	23224	Diag-1
23154	Origin	23229	Diag-2
23157	LIMA	23234	Septal-1
23169	Insertion Sites Visualized	23239	Intermed Branch
23170	Left Main	23244	Prox Circ
23171	Prox LAD	23249	Dist Circ
23172	Mid LAD	23254	OM-1
23173	Dist LAD	23259	OM-2
23174	Diag-1	23264	OM-3
23175	Diag-2	23269	L AV Groove
23176	Septal-1	23274	L Postlat Seg
23177	Intermed Branch	23279	L Postlat-1

CARDIAC CATHETERIZATION, CONT.

23284	L Postlat-2	23330	R Posterolat-3
23289	Proximal RCA	23335	Left PDA
23294	Middle RCA	23340	Right PDA
23299	Distal RCA	23352	Y Graft
23304	AMV-1	23346	Sequential
23309	AMV-2	23367	Obstruction
23314	R Posterolat Seg	23372	Single Discrete
23319	R Posterolat-1	23477	Single Discrete, Concentric
23324	R Posterolat-2	23482	Single Discrete, Eccentric
23329	R Posterolat-3	23377	Multiple Discrete
23334	Left PDA	23382	Diffuse
23339	Right PDA	23387	Tubular
23351	Y Graft	23392	Calcific
23345	Sequential	23397	Aneurysm
23366	Obstruction	23402	Discrete
23371	Single Discrete	23407	Diffuse
23476	Single Discrete, Concentric	23412	Multiple
23481	Single Discrete, Eccentric	23161	SVG-2
23376	Multiple Discrete	23201	Insertion Sites Visualized
23381	Diffuse	23206	Left Main
23386	Tubular	23211	Prox LAD
23391	Calcific	23216	Mid LAD
23396	Aneurysm	23221	Dist LAD
23401	Discrete	23226	Diag-1
23406	Diffuse	23231	Diag-2
23411	Multiple	23236	Septal-1
23160	SVG-1	23241	Intermed Branch
23200	Insertion Sites Visualized	23246	Prox Circ
23205	Left Main	23251	Dist Circ
23210	Prox LAD	23256	OM-1
23215	Mid LAD	23261	OM-2
23220	Dist LAD	23266	OM-3
23225	Diag-1	23271	L AV Groove
23230	Diag-2	23276	L Postlat Seg
23235	Septal-1	23281	L Postlat-1
23240	Intermed Branch	23286	L Postlat-2
23245	Prox Circ	23291	Proximal RCA
23250	Dist Circ	23296	Middle RCA
23255	OM-1	23301	Distal RCA
23260	OM-2	23306	AMV-1
23265	OM-3	23311	AMV-2
23270	L AV Groove	23316	R Posterolat Seg
23275	L Postlat Seg	23321	R Posterolat-1
23280	L Postlat-1	23326	R Posterolat-2
23285	L Postlat-2	23331	R Posterolat-3
23290	Proximal RCA	23336	Left PDA
23295	Middle RCA	23341	Right PDA
23300	Distal RCA	23353	Y Graft
23305	AMV-1	23347	Sequential
23310	AMV-2	23368	Obstruction
23315	R Posterolat Seg	23373	Single Discrete
23320	R Posterolat-1	23478	Single Discrete, Concentric
23325	R Posterolat-2	23483	Single Discrete, Eccentric

CARDIAC CATHETERIZATION, CONT.

23378	Multiple Discrete	23203	Insertion Sites Visualized
23383	Diffuse	23208	Left Main
23388	Tubular	23213	Prox LAD
23393	Calcific	23218	Mid LAD
23398	Aneurysm	23223	Dist LAD
23403	Discrete	23228	Diag-1
23408	Diffuse	23233	Diag-2
23413	Multiple	23238	Septal-1
23162	SVG-3	23243	Intermed Branch
23202	Insertion Sites Visualized	23248	Prox Circ
23207	Left Main	23253	Dist Circ
23212	Prox LAD	23258	OM-1
23217	Mid LAD	23263	OM-2
23222	Dist LAD	23268	OM-3
23227	Diag-1	23273	L AV Groove
23232	Diag-2	23278	L Postlat Seg
23237	Septal-1	23283	L Postlat-1
23242	Intermed Branch	23288	L Postlat-2
23247	Prox Circ	23293	Proximal RCA
23252	Dist Circ	23298	Middle RCA
23257	OM-1	23303	Distal RCA
23262	OM-2	23308	AMV-1
23267	OM-3	23313	AMV-2
23272	L AV Groove	23318	R Posterolat Seg
23277	L Postlat Seg	23323	R Posterolat-1
23282	L Postlat-1	23328	R Posterolat-2
23287	L Postlat-2	23333	R Posterolat-3
23292	Proximal RCA	23338	Left PDA
23297	Middle RCA	23343	Right PDA
23302	Distal RCA	23355	Y Graft
23307	AMV-1	23349	Sequential
23312	AMV-2	23370	Obstruction
23317	R Posterolat Seg	23375	Single Discrete
23322	R Posterolat-1	23480	Single Discrete, Concentric
23327	R Posterolat-2	23485	Single Discrete, Eccentric
23332	R Posterolat-3	23380	Multiple Discrete
23337	Left PDA	23385	Diffuse
23342	Right PDA	23390	Tubular
23354	Y Graft	23395	Calcific
23348	Sequential	23400	Aneurysm
23369	Obstruction	23405	Discrete
23374	Single Discrete	23410	Diffuse
23479	Single Discrete, Concentric	23415	Multiple
23484	Single Discrete, Eccentric	27222	Y-Graft
23379	Multiple Discrete	27223	Obstruction
23384	Diffuse	27224	Single Discrete
23389	Tubular	27225	Single Discrete, Concentric
23394	Calcific	27226	Single Discrete, Eccentric
23399	Aneurysm	27227	Multiple Discrete
23404	Discrete	27228	Diffuse
23409	Diffuse	27229	Tubular
23414	Multiple	27230	Calcific
23163	SVG-4	27231	Aneurysm

CARDIAC CATHETERIZATION, CONT.

27232	Discrete	23494	Single Discrete
27233	Diffuse	23500	Single Discrete, Concentric
27234	Multiple	23506	Single Discrete, Eccentric
27271	Sequential Graft	23512	Multiple Discrete
27272	Obstruction	23518	Diffuse
27273	Single Discrete	23524	Tubular
27274	Single Discrete, Concentric	23530	Calcific
27275	Single Discrete, Eccentric	23536	Aneurysm
27276	Multiple Discrete	23542	Discrete
27277	Diffuse	23548	Diffuse
27278	Tubular	23554	Multiple
27279	Calcific	23567	Flow
27280	Aneurysm	23572	TIMI Score
27281	Discrete	23577	Antegrade
27282	Diffuse	23582	Retrograde
27283	Multiple	23587	Decreased
27284	Sequential IMA Graft	23592	Present
27285	Obstruction	23597	Absent
27286	Single Discrete	23602	Uncertain
27287	Single Discrete, Concentric	22750	SGV-1
27288	Single Discrete, Eccentric	23489	Obstruction
27289	Multiple Discrete	23495	Single Discrete
27290	Diffuse	23501	Single Discrete, Concentric
27291	Tubular	23507	Single Discrete, Eccentric
27292	Calcific	23513	Multiple Discrete
27293	Aneurysm	23519	Diffuse
27294	Discrete	23525	Tubular
27295	Diffuse	23531	Calcific
27296	Multiple	23537	Aneurysm
23155	Body	23543	Discrete
22749	LIMA	23549	Diffuse
23487	Obstruction	23555	Multiple
23493	Single Discrete	23568	Flow
23499	Single Discrete, Concentric	23573	TIMI Score
23505	Single Discrete, Eccentric	23578	Antegrade
23511	Multiple Discrete	23583	Retrograde
23517	Diffuse	23588	Decreased
23523	Tubular	23593	Present
23529	Calcific	23598	Absent
23535	Aneurysm	23603	Uncertain
23541	Discrete	23164	SVG-2
23547	Diffuse	23490	Obstruction
23553	Multiple	23496	Single Discrete
23559	Flow	23502	Single Discrete, Concentric
23560	TIMI Score	23508	Single Discrete, Eccentric
23561	Antegrade	23514	Multiple Discrete
23562	Retrograde	23520	Diffuse
23566	Decreased	23526	Tubular
23563	Present	23532	Calcific
23564	Absent	23538	Aneurysm
23565	Uncertain	23544	Discrete
23159	RIMA	23550	Diffuse
23488	Obstruction	23556	Multiple

CARDIAC CATHETERIZATION, CONT.

23569	Flow	27247	Absent
23574	TIMI Score	27248	Uncertain
23579	Antegrade	27249	Retrograde Flow
23584	Retrograde	27250	Decreased
23589	Decreased	27251	Absent
23594	Present	27252	Uncertain
23599	Absent	27253	Sequential Graft
23604	Uncertain	27254	Antegrade Flow
23165	SVG-3	27255	Decreased
23491	Obstruction	27256	Absent
23497	Single Discrete	27257	Uncertain
23503	Single Discrete, Concentric	27258	Retrograde Flow
23509	Single Discrete, Eccentric	27259	Decreased
23515	Multiple Discrete	27260	Absent
23521	Diffuse	27261	Uncertain
23527	Tubular	27262	Sequential IMA Graft
23533	Calcific	27263	Antegrade Flow
23539	Aneurysm	27264	Decreased
23545	Discrete	27265	Absent
23551	Diffuse	27266	Uncertain
23557	Multiple	27267	Retrograde Flow
23570	Flow	27268	Decreased
23575	TIMI Score	27269	Absent
23580	Antegrade	27270	Uncertain
23585	Retrograde	23156	Insertion Sites
23590	Decreased	23607	Left Main
23595	Present	23677	Side-To-Side
23600	Absent	23636	Graft Termination
23605	Uncertain	23678	Direct
23166	SVG-4	23679	Branch
23492	Obstruction	23665	Obstruction
23498	Single Discrete	23666	Single Discrete
23504	Single Discrete, Concentric	23667	Single Discrete, Concentric
23510	Single Discrete, Eccentric	23668	Single Discrete, Eccentric
23516	Multiple Discrete	23669	Multiple Discrete
23522	Diffuse	23670	Diffuse
23528	Tubular	23671	Tubular
23534	Calcific	23672	Calcific
23540	Aneurysm	23673	Aneurysm
23546	Discrete	23674	Discrete
23552	Diffuse	23675	Diffuse
23558	Multiple	23676	Multiple
23571	Flow	23608	Prox LAD
23576	TIMI Score	23680	Side-To-Side
23581	Antegrade	23637	Graft Termination
23586	Retrograde	23707	Direct
23591	Decreased	23736	Branch
23596	Present	23761	Obstruction
23601	Absent	23789	Single Discrete
23606	Uncertain	23817	Single Discrete, Concentric
27244	Y Graft	23836	Single Discrete, Eccentric
27245	Antegrade Flow	23864	Multiple Discrete
27246	Decreased	23892	Diffuse

CARDIAC CATHETERIZATION, CONT.

23920	Tubular	23961	Aneurysm
23939	Calcific	23991	Discrete
23958	Aneurysm	24019	Diffuse
23988	Discrete	24047	Multiple
24016	Diffuse	23612	Diag-2
24044	Multiple	23684	Side-To-Side
23609	Mid LAD	23641	Graft Termination
23681	Side-To-Side	23711	Direct
23638	Graft Termination	23740	Branch
23708	Direct	23765	Obstruction
23737	Branch	23793	Single Discrete
23762	Obstruction	23821	Single Discrete, Concentric
23790	Single Discrete	23840	Single Discrete, Eccentric
23818	Single Discrete, Concentric	23868	Multiple Discrete
23837	Single Discrete, Eccentric	23896	Diffuse
23865	Multiple Discrete	23924	Tubular
23893	Diffuse	23943	Calcific
23921	Tubular	23962	Aneurysm
23940	Calcific	23992	Discrete
23959	Aneurysm	24020	Diffuse
23989	Discrete	24048	Multiple
24017	Diffuse	23613	Septal-1
24045	Multiple	23685	Side-To-Side
23610	Dist LAD	23642	Graft Termination
23682	Side-To-Side	23712	Direct
23639	Graft Termination	23741	Branch
23709	Direct	23766	Obstruction
23738	Branch	23794	Single Discrete
23763	Obstruction	23822	Single Discrete, Concentric
23791	Single Discrete	23841	Single Discrete, Eccentric
23819	Single Discrete, Concentric	23869	Multiple Discrete
23838	Single Discrete, Eccentric	23897	Diffuse
23866	Multiple Discrete	23925	Tubular
23894	Diffuse	23944	Calcific
23922	Tubular	23963	Aneurysm
23941	Calcific	23993	Discrete
23960	Aneurysm	24021	Diffuse
23990	Discrete	24049	Multiple
24018	Diffuse	23614	Intermed Branch
24046	Multiple	23686	Side-To-Side
23611	Diag-1	23643	Graft Termination
23683	Side-To-Side	23713	Direct
23640	Graft Termination	23742	Branch
23710	Direct	23767	Obstruction
23739	Branch	23795	Single Discrete
23764	Obstruction	23823	Single Discrete, Concentric
23792	Single Discrete	23842	Single Discrete, Eccentric
23820	Single Discrete, Concentric	23870	Multiple Discrete
23839	Single Discrete, Eccentric	23898	Diffuse
23867	Multiple Discrete	23926	Tubular
23895	Diffuse	23945	Calcific
23923	Tubular	23964	Aneurysm
23942	Calcific	23994	Discrete

CARDIAC CATHETERIZATION, CONT.

24022	Diffuse	23618	OM-2
24050	Multiple	24102	Side-To-Side
23615	Prox Circ	23647	Graft Termination
23687	Side-To-Side	23717	Direct
23644	Graft Termination	23746	Branch
23714	Direct	23771	Obstruction
23743	Branch	23799	Single Discrete
23768	Obstruction	24074	Single Discrete, Concentric
23796	Single Discrete	23846	Single Discrete, Eccentric
23824	Single Discrete, Concentric	23874	Multiple Discrete
23843	Single Discrete, Eccentric	23902	Diffuse
23871	Multiple Discrete	24083	Tubular
23899	Diffuse	24095	Calcific
23927	Tubular	23968	Aneurysm
23946	Calcific	23998	Discrete
23965	Aneurysm	24026	Diffuse
23995	Discrete	24054	Multiple
24023	Diffuse	23619	OM-3
24051	Multiple	23690	Side-To-Side
23616	Dist Circ	23648	Graft Termination
23688	Side-To-Side	23718	Direct
23645	Graft Termination	23747	Branch
23715	Direct	23772	Obstruction
23744	Branch	23800	Single Discrete
23769	Obstruction	24075	Single Discrete, Concentric
23797	Single Discrete	23847	Single Discrete, Eccentric
24072	Single Discrete, Concentric	23875	Multiple Discrete
23844	Single Discrete, Eccentric	23903	Diffuse
23872	Multiple Discrete	24084	Tubular
23900	Diffuse	24096	Calcific
24081	Tubular	23969	Aneurysm
24093	Calcific	23999	Discrete
23966	Aneurysm	24027	Diffuse
23996	Discrete	24055	Multiple
24024	Diffuse	23620	L AV Groove
24052	Multiple	23691	Side-To-Side
23617	OM-1	23649	Graft Termination
23689	Side-To-Side	23719	Direct
23646	Graft Termination	23748	Branch
23716	Direct	23773	Obstruction
23745	Branch	23801	Single Discrete
23770	Obstruction	24076	Single Discrete, Concentric
23798	Single Discrete	23848	Single Discrete, Eccentric
24073	Single Discrete, Concentric	23876	Multiple Discrete
23845	Single Discrete, Eccentric	23904	Diffuse
23873	Multiple Discrete	24085	Tubular
23901	Diffuse	24097	Calcific
24082	Tubular	23970	Aneurysm
24094	Calcific	24000	Discrete
23967	Aneurysm	24028	Diffuse
23997	Discrete	24056	Multiple
24025	Diffuse	23621	L Postlat Seg
24053	Multiple	23692	Side-To-Side

CARDIAC CATHETERIZATION, CONT.

23650	Graft Termination	23752	Branch
23720	Direct	23777	Obstruction
23749	Branch	23805	Single Discrete
23774	Obstruction	24080	Single Discrete, Concentric
23802	Single Discrete	23852	Single Discrete, Eccentric
24077	Single Discrete, Concentric	23880	Multiple Discrete
23849	Single Discrete, Eccentric	23908	Diffuse
23877	Multiple Discrete	24089	Tubular
23905	Diffuse	24101	Calcific
24086	Tubular	23974	Aneurysm
24098	Calcific	24004	Discrete
23971	Aneurysm	24032	Diffuse
24001	Discrete	24060	Multiple
24029	Diffuse	23625	Proximal RCA
24057	Multiple	23696	Side-To-Side
23622	L Postlat-1	23654	Graft Termination
23693	Side-To-Side	23724	Direct
23651	Graft Termination	23753	Branch
23721	Direct	23778	Obstruction
23750	Branch	23806	Single Discrete
23775	Obstruction	23825	Single Discrete, Concentric
23803	Single Discrete	23853	Single Discrete, Eccentric
24078	Single Discrete, Concentric	23881	Multiple Discrete
23850	Single Discrete, Eccentric	23909	Diffuse
23878	Multiple Discrete	23928	Tubular
23906	Diffuse	23947	Calcific
24087	Tubular	23977	Aneurysm
24099	Calcific	24005	Discrete
23972	Aneurysm	24033	Diffuse
24002	Discrete	24061	Multiple
24030	Diffuse	23626	Middle RCA
24058	Multiple	23697	Side-To-Side
23623	L Postlat-2	23655	Graft Termination
23694	Side-To-Side	23725	Direct
23652	Graft Termination	23754	Branch
23722	Direct	23779	Obstruction
23751	Branch	23807	Single Discrete
23776	Obstruction	23826	Single Discrete, Concentric
23804	Single Discrete	23854	Single Discrete, Eccentric
24079	Single Discrete, Concentric	23882	Multiple Discrete
23851	Single Discrete, Eccentric	23910	Diffuse
23879	Multiple Discrete	23929	Tubular
23907	Diffuse	23948	Calcific
24088	Tubular	23978	Aneurysm
24100	Calcific	24006	Discrete
23973	Aneurysm	24034	Diffuse
24003	Discrete	24062	Multiple
24031	Diffuse	23627	Distal RCA
24059	Multiple	23698	Side-To-Side
23624	L Postlat-3	23656	Graft Termination
23695	Side-To-Side	23726	Direct
23653	Graft Termination	23755	Branch
23723	Direct	23780	Obstruction

CARDIAC CATHETERIZATION, CONT.

23808	Single Discrete	23858	Single Discrete, Eccentric
23827	Single Discrete, Concentric	23886	Multiple Discrete
23855	Single Discrete, Eccentric	23914	Diffuse
23883	Multiple Discrete	23933	Tubular
23911	Diffuse	23952	Calcific
23930	Tubular	23982	Aneurysm
23949	Calcific	24010	Discrete
23979	Aneurysm	24038	Diffuse
24007	Discrete	24066	Multiple
24035	Diffuse	23631	R Posterolat-1
24063	Multiple	23702	Side-To-Side
23628	AMV-1	23660	Graft Termination
23699	Side-To-Side	23731	Direct
23657	Graft Termination	23759	Branch
23727	Direct	23784	Obstruction
23756	Branch	23812	Single Discrete
23781	Obstruction	23831	Single Discrete, Concentric
23809	Single Discrete	23859	Single Discrete, Eccentric
23828	Single Discrete, Concentric	23887	Multiple Discrete
23856	Single Discrete, Eccentric	23915	Diffuse
23884	Multiple Discrete	23934	Tubular
23912	Diffuse	23953	Calcific
23931	Tubular	23983	Aneurysm
23950	Calcific	24011	Discrete
23980	Aneurysm	24039	Diffuse
24008	Discrete	24067	Multiple
24036	Diffuse	23632	R Posterolat-2
24064	Multiple	23703	Side-To-Side
23629	AMV-2	23661	Graft Termination
23700	Side-To-Side	23732	Direct
23658	Graft Termination	23760	Branch
23728	Direct	23785	Obstruction
23757	Branch	23813	Single Discrete
23782	Obstruction	23832	Single Discrete, Concentric
23810	Single Discrete	23860	Single Discrete, Eccentric
23829	Single Discrete, Concentric	23888	Multiple Discrete
23857	Single Discrete, Eccentric	23916	Diffuse
23885	Multiple Discrete	23935	Tubular
23913	Diffuse	23954	Calcific
23932	Tubular	23984	Aneurysm
23951	Calcific	24012	Discrete
23981	Aneurysm	24040	Diffuse
24009	Discrete	24068	Multiple
24037	Diffuse	23633	R Posterolat-3
24065	Multiple	23704	Side-To-Side
23630	R Posterolat Seg	23662	Graft Termination
23701	Side-To-Side	23733	Direct
23659	Graft Termination	24090	Branch
23730	Direct	23786	Obstruction
23758	Branch	23814	Single Discrete
23783	Obstruction	23833	Single Discrete, Concentric
23811	Single Discrete	23861	Single Discrete, Eccentric
23830	Single Discrete, Concentric	23889	Multiple Discrete

23917	Diffuse	27210	not visualized - status uncertain
23936	Tubular	27211	SVG-3
23955	Calcific	27213	appears abnormal
23985	Aneurysm	27214	not visualized - status uncertain
24013	Discrete	27215	SVG-4
24041	Diffuse	27216	appears abnormal
24069	Multiple	27217	not visualized - status uncertain
23634	Left PDA	27235	Y Graft
23705	Side-To-Side	27236	appears abnormal
23663	Graft Termination	27237	not visualized - status uncertain
23734	Direct	27238	Sequential Graft
24091	Branch	27239	appears abnormal
23787	Obstruction	27240	not visualized - status uncertain
23815	Single Discrete	27241	Sequential IMA
23834	Single Discrete, Concentric	27242	appears abnormal
23862	Single Discrete, Eccentric	27243	not visualized - status uncertain
23890	Multiple Discrete	27313	Internal Mammary Bypass Graft
23918	Diffuse	27314	Endarterectomy
23937	Tubular	27315	Implantation
23956	Calcific	27310	Myocardium
23986	Aneurysm	27311	Foreign Body
24014	Discrete	27312	Removal Using Cath Technique
24042	Diffuse	24724	Congenital Anomalies
24070	Multiple	24856	An Absent Left Coronary Artery
23635	Right PDA	24857	An Absent Right Coronary Artery
23706	Side-To-Side	24858	An Anomalous Coronary Origin
23664	Graft Termination	24859	Of The Left Coronary Artery
23735	Direct		From The Pulmonary Artery
24092	Branch	24860	Of The Right Coronary Artery
23788	Obstruction		From The Pulmonary Artery
23816	Single Discrete	24861	Of Both Coronary Arteries From
23835	Single Discrete, Concentric		The Pulmonary Artery
23863	Single Discrete, Eccentric	24862	Of The Right Coronary Artery
23891	Multiple Discrete		From The Left Coronary Artery
23919	Diffuse	24863	Of The Left Coronary Artery
23938	Tubular		From The Right Coronary Artery
23957	Calcific	24864	Of The Left Circumflex Artery
23987	Aneurysm		From The Right Coronary Artery
24015	Discrete	24865	Of The Left Anterior Descending
24043	Diffuse		Artery From The Right Coronary
24071	Multiple		Artery
27198	Graft Status	24866	An Accessory Left Anterior
27199	LIMA		Descending Artery From The Right
27200	appears abnormal		Coronary Artery
27201	not visualized - status uncertain	24867	With A Prominent Conal Branch
27202	RIMA	24868	With A Prominent RV Branch
27203	appears abnormal	24869	A Double Orifice Left Coronary
27204	not visualized - status uncertain		Artery
27205	SVG-1	24870	A Double Orifice Right Coronary
27206	appears abnormal		Artery
27207	not visualized - status uncertain	24871	A Coronary Fistula
27208	SVG-2	24872	An Aneurysm
27209	appears abnormal	24873	Anomalies Of The Coronary Veins

CARDIAC CATHETERIZATION, CONT.

27316	Revascularization	24399	Right Ventricle Superior To The Left Ventricle
27317	Endarterectomy		
27318	Prosthetic Bypass Graft	24400	Right Ventricle Inferior To The Left Ventricle
27319	Piggy-Back Homograft		
22754	Shunts	24401	Valves
25311	Systemic Flow (No Shunt) (l/min)	24402	Aortic Valve Was Anterior To The Pulmonary Valve
25312	Index (l/min/m2)		
25313	Systemic Flow (Shunt) (l/min)	24403	Aortic Valve Was Posterior To The Pulmonary Valve
25314	Index (l/min/m2)		
25315	Pulmonary Flow	24404	Aortic Valve Was To The Right Of The Pulmonary Valve
25316	Index		
25317	Effective Pulmonary Flow	24405	Aortic Valve Was To The Left Of The Pulmonary Valve
25318	Index		
25319	QP/QS Ratio	24378	Cardia
25320	Left To Right (Content) (%)	24424	Levocardia, Normal Cardiac Apex
25321	Right To Left (Content Difference) (%)	24406	Dextrocardia
25322	Left To Right (Forward Triangle) (%)	24407	Mesocardia
25323	Right To Left (Forward Triangle) (%)	24408	Ambiguous Cardiac Apex
25324	Left To Right (Carter) (%)	24409	Ectopic Cordis
24741	Left To Right	24379	Viscera
24742	Right To Left	24410	Inversus
24744	Both Right To Left And Left To Right	24411	Ambiguous
24743	Systemic Arterial Desaturation	24412	Liver Was To The Right
24375	Situs	24413	Liver Was To The Left
24376	Atria	24414	Liver Was Midline
24380	Inversus	24415	Stomach Was On The Right
24381	Ambiguous	24416	Stomach Was On The Left
24382	Bilateral Right Appendages	24417	Stomach Was Midline
24383	Bilateral Left Appendages	24418	Asplenia
24384	Pulmonary Veins On The Left	24419	Polysplenia
24385	Pulmonary Veins On The Right	24420	Bronchial Anatomy Solitus
24386	Bilateral Pulmonary Veins	24421	Bronchial Anatomy Inversus
24387	Superior Vena Cava Drains To The Left Atrium	24422	Bilateral "Right" Bronchi
		24423	Bilateral "Left" Bronchi
24388	Superior Vena Cava Drains To The Right Atrium	23050	Complications
		25006	Arrhythmias
24389	Bilateral Superior Vena Cava Veins	25007	Ventricular Fibrillation
		25008	Supraventricular Tachycardia
24390	Inferior Vena Cava Drains To The Left Atrium	25009	Prolonged Ventricular Tachycardia
		25010	Heart Block
24391	Inferior Vena Cava Drains To The Right Atrium	25042	With Low Blood Pressure
		25011	Bradycardia
24392	Bilateral Inferior Vena Cava Veins	25012	With Low Blood Pressure
		25013	With Low Blood Pressure Causing Termination Of The Procedure
24393	Hepatic Veins Were On The Left		
24394	Hepatic Veins Were On The Right	25014	Low Blood Pressure Requiring Treatment
24395	Bilateral Hepatic Veins		
24377	Ventricles	82703	Contrast Reaction
24396	Ambiguous	82704	Anaphylactic
24397	Right Ventricle To The Right Of The Left Ventricle (D-Loop)	25036	Thrombophlebitis
		25044	Arterial Flow Abnormality
24398	Right Ventricle To The Left Of The Left Ventricle (L-Loop)	25015	Lost Pulse
		25016	Requiring Exploration

CARDIAC CATHETERIZATION, CONT.

25017	With Symptomatic Ischemia
25018	With Limb Ischemia
25019	Major Blood Loss
25043	False Aneurysm Requiring Exploration
25020	Hypoxic Episode
25021	Coronary Ischemia
25022	Pulmonary Edema
25023	Myocardial Infarction
82701	Transmural
82702	Transmyocardial
25024	Dissection Of Major Artery
25025	Thromboemboli
25026	Pulmonary Emboli
25027	Cerebral emboli
25028	Cerebral thrombus
25029	Perforation Of The Heart
25030	During Injection Of Contrast
25031	With Resulting Hemopericardium
25032	With Resulting Cardiac Tamponade
25033	With Mediastinal Bleeding
25034	With Resulting Hemothorax
25035	Pneumothorax
25037	Infection
25038	Local
25039	Sepsis
25040	Endocarditis
82699	PTCA Required
82700	CABG Required
25045	Cardiac Arrest
25041	Death
23051	Broken Catheter
23052	Broken Guide
23053	Catheter Knot
23054	Incomplete Study
27321	Drug Intervention
28298	Dacryocystography
28299	Injection Of Contrast Medium
13079	Plethysmography
19260	Total Body
19261	Tracing Only
19262	Interpretation Only
18414	Ocular
18415	Impedance, Lower Extremity
29396	Thermography
29397	Cephalic
29398	Peripheral
89045	Other Imaging Studies
22539	Sinogram
22540	Injection Of Contrast Material
18037	Discography
22216	Cervical
22217	Injection Of Contrast Material

22220	Radiological Supervision And Interpretation
22218	Lumbar
22219	Injection Of Contrast Material
22221	Radiological Supervision And Interpretation
19489	Transglottic Catheterization
19490	Tracheal Constrast Instillation
19491	With Catheterization
19492	Transtracheal Injection For Bronchography
13101	Bronchography
22589	Unilateral
22590	Bilateral
19493	Catheterization With Bronchial Brush Biopsy
82218	**Pathology**
22183	Percutaneous Aspiration
22184	Spinal Cord Cyst
22185	Spinal Syrinx
13050	Cytology
13051	Cervical Pap Smear
28600	Overread By Physician
28601	With Hormonal Indices
29285	Vaginal Pap Smear
29286	Overread By Physician
29287	With Hormonal Indices
13052	Gynecologic (Tzanck Smear)
13053	Sputum For Malignant Cells
13054	Gastric For Malignant Cells
13055	Colonic For Malignant Cells
13056	Pulmonary Artery Blood for Fetal Products
18549	Pulmonary Microvascular
13057	Urine
19354	Defective p53 Gene
13058	Wound
16459	**Biopsy**
22681	CT-Guidance
28548	Transcatheter
28549	With Radiologic Supervision And Interpretation
28547	Eye
82272	Site
22689	Eyelid
82918	Right Upper
82919	Nasal Aspect
82920	Temporal Aspect
82921	Right Lower
82922	Nasal Aspect
82923	Temporal Aspect
82924	Left Upper
82925	Nasal Aspect

BIOPSY, CONT.

82926	Temporal Aspect		82297	Histology
82927	Left Lower		82934	Benign
82928	Nasal Aspect		82402	Apocrine Adenoma
82929	Temporal Aspect		82308	Fuchs Adenoma
82284	Lacrimal Duct		82342	Pleomorphic Adenoma
82380	Right		82403	Sebaceous Adenoma
82381	Left		82302	Angiomatosis Retinae
82382	Bilaterally		82300	Astrocytoma
82279	Lacrimal Gland		82391	Benign Hereditary Intraepithelial
82365	Right			Dyskeratosis
82366	Left		82416	Benign Lymphoepithelial lesion
82367	Bilaterally		82353	Fibromatosis
82290	Orbit		82306	Glioneuroma
82347	Left		82311	Hemangioma
82348	Right		82346	Capillary Hemangioma
82291	Bilaterally		82303	Cavernous Hemangioma
28293	Extraocular Muscle		82388	Lymphoid Hyperplasia
82280	Conjunctival		82411	Atypical Lymphoid Hyperplasia
82368	Right		82410	Reactive Lymphoid Hyperplasia
82369	Left		82390	Pseudocarcinomatous Hyperplasia
82419	Bilaterally		82917	Premalignant
22620	Cornea		82392	Actinic Keratosis
82371	Right		82409	Melanoma
82372	Left		82406	Congenital Epithelial Melanosis
82373	Bilaterally		82935	Malignant
82275	Iris		82399	Adenocarcinoma
82287	Right		82404	Sebaceous Adenocarcinoma
82288	Left		82345	Adenocarcinoma Arising De
82289	Bilaterally			Novo
82276	Crystalline Lens		82397	Basal Cell Carcinoma
82292	Right		82395	Squamous Cell Carcinoma
82293	Left		82344	Adenoid Cystic Carcinoma
82294	Bilaterally		82343	Pleomorphic Carcinoma
82274	Ciliary Body		82394	Carcinoma in Situ
82273	Right		82351	Hemangiopericytoma
82285	Left		82352	Fibrous Histiocytoma
82286	Bilaterally		82355	Leimyoma
82383	Uveal Tract		82340	Mesectodermal Leiomyoma
82384	Right		82358	Lipoma
82385	Left		82350	Lymphangioma
82386	Bilaterally		82307	Medulloepithelioma
82283	Choroid		82398	Mucoepidermoid
82377	Right		82417	Lymphoma
82378	Left		82304	Malignant Lymphoma
82379	Bilaterally		82413	Leukemia
82282	Retina		82407	Primary Acquired Melanosis
82374	Right		82408	Secondary Acquired Melanosis
82375	Left		82405	Nevus
82376	Bilaterally		82309	Melanocytic Nevi
82277	Sclera		82362	Isolated Neurofibroma
82295	Right		82361	Diffuse Neurofibroma
82364	Left		82360	Plexiform Neurofibroma
82296	Bileterally		82310	Choroidal Osteoma

BIOPSY, CONT.

82370	Squamous cell papilloma	82749	Adenoid Cystic Carcinoma
82414	Plasmacytoma	82750	Carcinoma In Pleomorphic
82363	Schwannoma		Adenoma
82354	Fibrosarcoma	82751	Malignant Myoepithelioma
82356	Leimyosarcoma	82752	Epithelial-myoepithelial Carcinoma
82359	Liposarcoma	82753	Clear Cell Carcinoma
82357	Rhabdomyosarcoma	82754	Carcinoid Tumour
82341	Jeuvenile Xanthogranuloma	82755	Atypical Carcinoid Tumour
86145	Differentiation	82756	Small Cell Carcinoma
82312	Well Differentiated	82757	Lymphoepithclial Carcinoma
82313	Poorly Differentiated	82758	Fibroma
28296	Nasal Cavity Neoplasm	82759	Aggressive Fibromatosis
82314	Site	82760	Angiofibroma
82315	Right	82761	Myxoma
82420	Naris	82762	Fibrous Histiocytoma
82421	Cartilage	82763	Leiomyoma
82422	Mucosa	82764	Haemangioma
82423	Septum	82765	Haemangiopericytoma
82424	Turbinate	82766	Neurilemmoma
82316	Left	82767	Paraganglioma
82317	Naris	82768	Fibrosarcoma
82318	Cartilage	82769	Malignant Fibrous Histiocytoma
82319	Mucosa	82770	Leiomyosarcoma
82320	Septum	82771	Rhabdomyosarcoma
82321	Turbinate	82772	Angiosarcoma
82322	Showed	82773	Malignant Haemangiopericytoma
82324	Verrucous Carcinoma	82774	Malignant Nerve Sheath Tumour
82729	Sinonasal Papilloma	82775	Malignant Paraganglioma
82325	Spindle Cell Carcinoma	82776	Ewing Sarcoma
82326	Adenosquamous Carcinoma	28297	Nasopharyngeal Neoplasm
82327	Adenoid Cystic Carcinoma	82777	Location
82328	Adenocarcinoma	82425	Superior Wall
82329	Mucoepidermoid Carcinoma	82426	Posterior Wall
82330	Kaposi's Sarcoma	82427	Lateral Wall
82331	Anaplastic Carcinoma	82428	Anterior Wall
82332	Leiomyosarcoma	82778	Showed
82333	Carcinosarcoma	82779	Papilloma
82334	Melanoma	82780	Pleomorphic Adenoma
82335	Carcinoid Tumour	82781	Oncocytoma
82730	Exophytic papilloma	82782	Basal Cell Adenoma
82731	Inverted papilloma	82783	Ectopic Pituitary Adenoma
82732	Columnar Cell papilloma	82784	Nasopharyngeal Carcinoma
82733	Pleomorphic Adenoma	82785	Squamous Cell Carcinoma
82739	Myoepithelioma	82786	Differentiated Non-Keratinizing
82740	Oncocytoma		Carcinoma
82741	Basal Cell Adenoma	82787	Adenocarcinoma
82742	Sinonasal Carcinoma	82788	Papillary Adenocarcinoma
82743	Squamous Cell Carcinoma	82789	Mucoepidermoid Carcinoma
82744	Cylindrical Cell Carcinoma	82790	Adenoid Cystic Carcinoma
82745	Papillary Adenocarcinoma	82791	Angiofiroma
82746	Intestinal-type Adenocarcinoma	82792	Haemangioma
82747	Acinic cell carcinoma	82793	Haemangiopericytoma
82748	Mucoepidermoid Carcinoma	82794	Neurilemmoma

BIOPSY, CONT.

82795	Neurofibroma	82857	Papillary Cystadenoma
82797	Paraganglioma	82858	Mucinous Cystadenoma
82799	Fibrosarcoma	82860	Acinic Cell Carcinoma
82800	Rhabdomyosarcoma	82861	Mucoepidermoid Carcinoma
82801	Angiosarcoma	82864	Adenoid Cystic Carcinoma
82802	Kaposisarcoma	82865	Polymorphous Low Grade
82804	Malignant Haemangiopericytoma		Adenocarcinoma
82805	Malignant Nerve Sheath Tumour	82866	Epithelial-Myoepithelial Carcinoma
82807	Synovial Sarcoma	82867	Basal Cell Adenocarcinoma
82429	Sinus Neoplasm	16463	Brain
82430	Location	82445	Location
82431	Maxillary	82446	Right Optic Tract
82432	Ethmoid	82474	Glioblastoma Multiformi
82433	Frontal	82502	Anaplastic Astrocytoma
82434	Sphenoid	82503	Astrocytoma
82435	Oropharyngeal Neoplasm	82504	Oligodendroglioma
82436	Tonsil	82447	Left Optic tract
82437	Tonsillar Fossa	82475	Glioblastoma Multiformi
82439	Tonsillar Pillars	82505	Anaplastic Astrocytoma
82438	Vallecula	82506	Astrocytoma
82440	Anterior Aspect of the Epiglottis	82507	Oligodendroglioma
82441	Lateral Wall	82449	Right Optic Nerve
82442	Posterior Wall	82476	Glioblastoma Multiformi
82443	Branchial Cleft	82508	Anaplastic Astrocytoma
82444	Lip Neoplasm	82509	Astrocytoma
82810	Vermillion Border Upper Lip	82586	Pilocytic Astrocytoma
82812	Vermillion Border Lower Lip	82510	Oligodendroglioma
82814	Outer Aspect Lower Lip	82448	Left Optic Nerve
82813	Inner Aspect Lower Lip	82477	Glioblastoma Multiformi
82817	Tongue Neoplasm	82511	Anaplastic Astrocytoma
82818	Location	82512	Astrocytoma
82819	Base	82587	Pilocytic Astrocytoma
82821	Dorsal Surface	82513	Oligodendroglioma
82822	Tip And Lateral Border	82450	Optic Chiasm
82823	Ventral Surface	82478	Glioblastoma Multiformi
82825	Anterior Two-Thirds	82514	Anaplastic Astrocytoma
82826	Junctional Zone	82515	Astrocytoma
82827	Lingual Tonsil Neoplasm	82588	Pilocytic Astrocytoma
82830	Parotid Neoplasm	82516	Oligodendroglioma
82832	Salivary Gland Neoplasm	82589	Hypothalamus
82833	Showed	82590	Glioblastoma Multiformi
82836	Pleomorphic Adenoma	82591	Anaplastic Astrocytoma
82837	Myoepithelioma	82592	Astrocytoma
82840	Basal Cell Adenoma	82593	Oligodendroglioma
82842	Adenolymphoma	82594	Pilocytic Astrocytoma
82843	Oncocytoma	82639	Primary CNS Lymphoma
82845	Canalicular Adenoma	82451	Anterior Corpus Callosum
82847	Sebaceous Adenoma	82479	Glioblastoma Multiformi
82849	Ductal Papilloma	82517	Anaplastic Astrocytoma
82851	Inverted Ductal Papilloma	82518	Astrocytoma
82852	Intraductal Papilloma	82519	Oligodendroglioma
82853	Sialadenoma Papilliferum	82640	Primary CNS Lymphoma
82855	Cystadenoma	82452	Medior Corpus Callosum

BIOPSY, CONT.

82480	Glioblastoma Multiformi	82631	Hemangioblastoma
82520	Anaplastic Astrocytoma	82647	Primary CNS Lymphoma
82521	Astrocytoma	82670	Pleiomorphic Xanthoastrocytoma
82522	Oligodendroglioma	82679	Ganglioglioma
82641	Primary CNS Lymphoma	82459	Right Parietal
82453	Posterior Callosum	82487	Glioblastoma Multiformi
82481	Glioblastoma Multiformi	82541	Anaplastic Astrocytoma
82523	Anaplastic Astrocytoma	82542	Astrocytoma
82524	Astrocytoma	82606	Ependymoma
82525	Oligodendroglioma	82543	Oligodendroglioma
82642	Primary CNS Lymphoma	82632	Hemangioblastoma
82454	Multifocal	82648	Primary CNS Lymphoma
82482	Glioblastoma Multiformi	82671	Pleiomorphic Xanthoastrocytoma
82526	Anaplastic Astrocytoma	82680	Ganglioglioma
82527	Astrocytoma	82460	Left Parietal
82528	Oligodendroglioma	82488	Glioblastoma Multiformi
82643	Primary CNS Lymphoma	82544	Anaplastic Astrocytoma
82456	Right Frontal	82545	Astrocytoma
82483	Glioblastoma Multiformi	82607	Ependymoma
82529	Anaplastic Astrocytoma	82546	Oligodendroglioma
82530	Astrocytoma	82633	Hemangioblastoma
82602	Ependymoma	82649	Primary CNS Lymphoma
82531	Oligodendroglioma	82672	Pleiomorphic Xanthoastrocytoma
82628	Hemangioblastoma	82681	Ganglioglioma
82644	Primary CNS Lymphoma	82461	Right Occipital
82667	Pleiomorphic Xanthoastrocytoma	82489	Glioblastoma Multiformi
82676	Ganglioglioma	82547	Anaplastic Astrocytoma
82455	Left Frontal	82548	Astrocytoma
82484	Glioblastoma Multiformi	82608	Ependymoma
82532	Anaplastic Astrocytoma	82549	Oligodendroglioma
82533	Astrocytoma	82634	Hemangioblastoma
82603	Ependymoma	82650	Primary CNS Lymphoma
82534	Oligodendroglioma	82673	Pleiomorphic Xanthoastrocytoma
82629	Hemangioblastoma	82682	Ganglioglioma
82645	Primary CNS Lymphoma	82462	Left Occipital
82668	Pleiomorphic Xanthoastrocytoma	82490	Glioblastoma Multiformi
82677	Ganglioglioma	82550	Anaplastic Astrocytoma
82457	Right Temporal	82551	Astrocytoma
82485	Glioblastoma Multiformi	82609	Ependymoma
82535	Anaplastic Astrocytoma	82552	Oligodendroglioma
82536	Astrocytoma	82635	Hemangioblastoma
82604	Ependymoma	82651	Primary CNS Lymphoma
82537	Oligodendroglioma	82674	Pleiomorphic Xanthoastrocytoma
82630	Hemangioblastoma	82683	Ganglioglioma
82646	Primary CNS Lymphoma	82463	Right Thalamic
82669	Pleiomorphic Xanthoastrocytoma	82491	Glioblastoma Multiformi
82678	Ganglioglioma	82553	Anaplastic Astrocytoma
82458	Left Temporal	82554	Astrocytoma
82486	Glioblastoma Multiformi	82555	Oligodendroglioma
82538	Anaplastic Astrocytoma	82652	Primary CNS Lymphoma
82539	Astrocytoma	82464	Left Thalamic
82605	Ependymoma	82492	Glioblastoma Multiformi
82540	Oligodendroglioma	82556	Anaplastic Astrocytoma

BIOPSY, CONT.

82557	Astrocytoma	82597	Pilocytic Astrocytoma
82558	Oligodendroglioma	82612	Ependymoma
82653	Primary CNS Lymphoma	82579	Oligodendroglioma
82465	Right Midbrain	82636	Hemangioblastoma
82493	Glioblastoma Multiformi	82660	Primary CNS Lymphoma
82559	Anaplastic Astrocytoma	82472	Thoratic Spinal Cord
82560	Astrocytoma	82500	Glioblastoma Multiformi
82561	Oligodendroglioma	82580	Anaplastic Astrocytoma
82654	Primary CNS Lymphoma	82581	Astrocytoma
82466	Left Midbrain	82598	Pilocytic Astrocytoma
82494	Glioblastoma Multiformi	82613	Ependymoma
82562	Anaplastic Astrocytoma	82582	Oligodendroglioma
82563	Astrocytoma	82637	Hemangioblastoma
82564	Oligodendroglioma	82661	Primary CNS Lymphoma
82655	Primary CNS Lymphoma	82473	Lumbar Spinal Cord
82467	Pons	82501	Glioblastoma Multiformi
82495	Glioblastoma Multiformi	82583	Anaplastic Astrocytoma
82565	Anaplastic Astrocytoma	82584	Astrocytoma
82566	Astrocytoma	82599	Pilocytic Astrocytoma
82567	Oligodendroglioma	82622	Ependymoma
82656	Primary CNS Lymphoma	82585	Oligodendroglioma
82468	Medulla	82638	Hemangioblastoma
82496	Glioblastoma Multiformi	82662	Primary CNS Lymphoma
82568	Anaplastic Astrocytoma	82600	Cerebal Hemisphere
82569	Astrocytoma	82601	Pilocytic Arinocytoma
82570	Oligodendroglioma	82615	Intraventricular
82657	Primary CNS Lymphoma	82616	Right Lateral Ventrical
82469	Right Cerebellum	82621	Ependymoma
82497	Glioblastoma Multiformi	82617	Left Lateral Ventrical
82571	Anaplastic Astrocytoma	82614	Ependymoma
82572	Astrocytoma	82618	3rd Ventricle
82595	Pilocytic Astrocytoma	82623	Ependymoma
82610	Ependymoma	82619	4th Ventricle
82573	Oligodendroglioma	82624	Ependymoma
82626	Hemangioblastoma	82620	Brainstem
82658	Primary CNS Lymphoma	82625	Ependymoma
82664	Medulloblastoma	82675	Pleiomorphic Xanthoastrocytoma
82663	Midline Cerebellum	82684	Ganglioglioma
82665	Medulloblastoma	22211	Transoral Approach To Skull Base
82470	Left Cerebellum	22212	Transoral Approach To Brain Stem
82498	Glioblastoma Multiformi	22213	Transoral Approach To Upper Spinal
82574	Anaplastic Astrocytoma		Cord
82575	Astrocytoma	22181	Stereotactic
82596	Pilocytic Astrocytoma	22182	CT-Guided
82611	Ependymoma	22210	Tumor Pathology
82576	Oligodendroglioma	17906	Astrocytoma
82627	Hemangioblastoma	17907	Anaplastic (Malignant) Astrocytoma
82659	Primary CNS Lymphoma	17908	Glioblastoma Multiforme
82666	Medulloblastoma	17909	Gliosarcoma
82471	Cervical Spinal Cord	16464	Globoid Cells
82499	Glioblastoma Multiformi	17910	Oligodendroglioma
82577	Anaplastic Astrocytoma	17911	Anaplastic (Malignant)
82578	Astrocytoma		Oligodendroglioma

BIOPSY, CONT.

17912	Ependymoma	39983	Polyposis Coli
17913	Anaplastic (Malignant) Ependymoma	39984	Familial
17914	Mixed Glioma	39985	Congenital
17915	Mixed Malignant Glioma	39986	Retention
17916	Brain Stem Glioma	39987	Hyperplastic Polyp
17917	Cystic Cerebellar Astrocytoma	39988	Gardner's Syndrome
17918	Hypothalamic Glioma	39989	Sigmoid Polyps
17919	Optic Nerve Glioma	39990	Adenomatous Polyp
17920	Calcification	39991	Turcot's syndrome
17921	Tumor Infiltration of Meninges	82912	Malignant
17922	Gemistocytic Component	39956	Mucinous Adenocarcinoma
17923	Lymphocytic Infiltration	39957	Signet-ring Cell Carcinoma
17924	"Sarcomatous" Component	39958	Squamous Cell Carcinoma
17925	Giant Cells	39959	Adenosquamous Carcinoma
18377	Spongiform Encephalopathy	39960	Small Cell Carcinoma
16465	angiostrongylus cantonensis	39961	Undifferentiated Carcinoma
82882	Large Intestine Neoplasm	39962	Leiomyosarcoma
82883	Location	39963	Carcinoid Tumour
82884	Cecum	39964	Mixed Carcinoid-
82885	Ileocecal Valve		Adenocarcinoma
82886	Ileocecal Junction	39965	Kaposi's Sarcoma
39972	Adenocarcinoma	39966	Lymphoma
82887	Ascending Colon	39967	Adenocarcinoma
39973	Adenocarcinoma	39975	Duke's A
82888	Hepatic Flexure	39976	Duke's B
39968	Adenocarcinoma	39977	Duke's B1
82889	Splenic Flexure	39978	Duke's B2
39974	Adenocarcinoma	39979	Duke's C
82890	Transverse Colon	39980	Duke's C1
39969	Adenocarcinoma	39981	Duke's C2
82891	Descending Colon	39982	Duke's D
39970	Adenocarcinoma	16471	Temporal Artery
82892	Sigmoid Colon	16472	Thrombosis
39971	Adenocarcinoma	16473	Inflammatory Infiltrates
82893	Overlapping Lesion	16474	Giant Cells
82894	Showed	16475	Elastic Lamina
82914	Benign	16476	Fragmented
82895	Lipoma	16477	Absent
82896	Lipomatosis	16478	Thickened Intima
82897	Adenoma	18046	By Fibrous Tissue
82898	Tubular Adenoma	18047	By Granulomatous Tissue
82899	Tubulovillous Adenoma	16460	Artery
82900	Villous Adenoma	16461	Nerve
82901	Adenomatosis	16462	Metachromatic Material
82902	Leiomyoma	16487	Fat
82903	Hemangioma	16489	Lymph Node
82904	Lymphangioma	19416	Needle
82905	Neurilemmoma	19417	Superficial
82906	Neurofibroma	19418	Deep Node
82907	Neurofibromatosis	19419	Excisional
39953	Granular Cell Tumour	19420	Superficial
39954	Ganglioneuroma	19421	Deep
39955	Ganglioneuromatosis	19429	Staging Lymphadenectomy

BIOPSY, CONT.

19430	Retroperitoneal	82976		Anaplastic Thyroid Carcinoma
19431	Para-aortic	82978		Recurrence After Ablation
19432	Pelvic	82979		Lymphoma
16490	Cervical	82980		Metastasis To Thyroid
19422	Superficial	16503	Soft Tissue Of The Neck	
19423	Deep	29061	Soft Tissue Of The Shoulder	
19424	With Excision Of Scalene Fat Pad	29062	Superficial	
19425	With Dissection Of Jugular Nodes	29063	Deep	
16491	fungi	22735	Soft Tissue Of The Thorax	
18163	Supraclavicular	22736	Soft Tissue Of The Back	
16492	Axillary	22737	Superficial	
19427	Superficial	22738	Deep	
19428	Deep	22739	Soft Tissue Of The Flank	
19426	Internal Mammary	22740	Superficial	
16494	Mediastinal	22741	Deep	
16495	Mesenteric	24605	Soft Tissue Of The Upper Arm	
16493	Inguinal	24606	Superficial	
18405	Reed-Sternberg Cells	24607	Deep	
18406	Epstein-Barr Virus DNA	24608	Soft Tissue Of The Elbow	
16510	Lip	24610	Deep	
16511	Minor Salivary Glands	24611	Soft Tissue Of The Forearm	
19443	Vestibule Of Mouth	24609	Superficial	
19444	Tongue	24612	Deep	
19445	Anterior Two-thirds	24613	Soft Tissue Of The Wrist	
19446	Posterior One-third	24614	Superficial	
19447	Floor Of Mouth	24615	Deep	
16508	Gingival	24616	Soft Tissue Of The Pelvis	
16552	Intranasal	24617	Superficial	
16551	Pharyngeal	24618	Deep	
16509	Laryngeal	24619	Soft Tissue Of The Hip	
16496	Thyroid	24620	Superficial	
82954	Showed	24621	Deep	
16497	Benign	24622	Soft Tissue Of The Thigh	
16498	Follicular Adenoma	24623	Superficial	
82956	Thyroid Adenoma	24624	Deep	
82957	Malignant	24625	Soft Tissue Of The Knee	
16499	Follicular Thyroid Carcinoma	24626	Superficial	
16501	Metastatic To Lung	24627	Deep	
82958	Metastatic To Bone	24628	Soft Tissue Of The Lower Leg	
82959	Papillary Thyroid Carcinoma	24629	Superficial	
82961	Metastatic To Regional Lymph Nodes	24630	Deep	
		24631	Soft Tissue Of The Ankle	
82962	Cervical	24632	Superficial	
82964	Supraclavicular	24633	Deep	
82965	Mediastinal	16504	Breast	
82966	Medullary Thyroid Carcinoma	16505	Estrogen Receptor Assay	
82968	Familial	18546	Progesterone Receptor Assay	
82970	Recurrence	18547	Immuno-Staining For Haptoglobin-Related Protein	
82971	Metastatic To Regional Lymph Nodes			
		16506	Skin	
82972	Cervical	16507	Snip	
82974	Supraclavicular	22688	Each Additional Lesion	
82975	Mediastinal	18382	Collagen Assay	

BIOPSY, CONT.

18383	Defiency - Type I	45372	Thoracolumbar
18384	Defiency - Type II	45373	Combined Extra-Intradural
18385	Defiency - Type III	22144	Spinal Cord
19084	Area of Alopecia	22215	Percutaneous Needle
19085	Catagen Hairs	22145	Stereotactic
19086	Keratin Plugs	19275	Perineal
19087	Dilated Follicular Infundibula	19274	Vulvar
19088	Trichomalacia	16526	Vaginal
29436	Nail	19276	Extensive
29437	Bed	16525	Cervical
29438	Plate	16528	Endometrial, Without Cervical Dilation
29439	Matrix	16527	Ovarian
29440	Hyponychium	16529	Esophageal
29441	Proximal Folds	16530	Stomach
29442	Lateral Folds	19292	By Laparotomy
16512	Lung	18595	CLO-test
16513	percutaneous	16534	Small Intestine
16514	transbronchial	16535	Duodenal
16515	mycobacterium avium-intracellulare	16536	Jejunal
16516	pneumocystis carinii	16537	anisakis marina
16517	Endobronchial brush biopsy	16538	angiostrongylus costaricensis
16518	pneumocystis carinii	16539	Large Intestine
16519	mycobacterium avium-intracellulare	19360	Peroral Intestinal Biopsy
16554	Pleural	19361	By Capsule
19496	Open	19362	By Tube
16555	mycobacterium	16531	Spleen
16556	mycobacterium tuberculosis	16532	Liver
16520	Open Lung	19396	Percutaneous Needle
19494	Major	19397	Wedge
16521	dirofilaria	18208	Iron (ug/ 100 mg. dry wt.)
16522	mycobacterium avium-intracellulare	16533	Bile Duct
16523	pneumocystis carinii	16540	Rectal
16524	Mediastinum	19371	Surgical Biopsy Of Anorectal Wall
16553	Pericardial	19401	Pancreatic
19197	Endomyocardial	19402	Surgical
23119	Left Ventricular	19403	Percutaneous Needle
22072	Right Ventricular	19405	Abdominal / Peritoneal
22073	Echo-Guided	19406	Needle Biopsy Of Mass
22074	Fluoroscopic Guidance	19407	Retroperitoneal
22225	Intraspinal Laminectomy	19408	Needle Biopsy Of Mass
45359	Extradural	16542	Renal
45360	Cervical	19372	Open
45361	Thoracic	16543	Light Microscopy
45362	Lumbar	16544	Immunofluorescence Microscopy
45363	Sacral	16545	Electron Microscopy
45364	Intradural	16546	Ureter
45365	Extramedullary, Cervical	16547	Renal Cyst Aspiration
45366	Extramedullary, Thoracic	19382	Culture
45367	Extramedullary, Lumbar	16548	Cytology
45368	Sacral	16549	Cyst Fluid Lipid Analysis
45369	Intramedullary	18060	Adrenal
45370	Cervical	18061	CT directed aspiration for
45371	Thoracic		cytology/culture

BIOPSY, CONT.

18062	Open		16917	plasmodium malariae
18340	Silver stain		16918	plasmodium ovale
18341	cryptococcus neoformans		16919	plasmodium vivax
18342	Culture		16920	wuchereria bancrofti
18343	cryptococcus neoformans		16921	Wet mount smear
16550	Prostate		16922	borrelia
16557	Testicular		81208	Buffy Coat Smear
16541	Bladder		16996	Histoplasma capsulatum
19463	Urethra		16924	streptococcus pneumoniae
16480	Muscle		16925	trypanosoma cruzi
22523	Superficial		16926	Gram stain
22524	Deep		16927	(-) Bacilli
22525	Percutaneous Needle		82705	(+) Bacilli
16481	Inflammation		16928	(+) Cocci
16482	Fiber Necrosis		82706	(-) Cocci
16483	Fiber Atrophy		16929	Giemsa stain
16484	Abnormal Fibers		16930	borrelia
16485	Basophilic Rim		16931	trypanosoma gambiense
16486	Vasculitis		16932	trypanosoma rhodesiense
16479	Joint		16933	wuchereria bancrofti
16467	Bone		16934	wuchereria malayai
22526	Trocar		18322	TRAP stain
22527	Superficial		16935	Wright stain
22528	Deep		16936	spirillum minus
22529	Needle		16937	Culture
22530	Superficial		16938	bacteria
22531	Deep		82796	gram (-)
22532	Excisional		82798	using EMB
22533	Superficial		82803	using an MAC agar
22534	Deep		82806	gram (+)
22535	Vertebral Body, Open		82808	using a CNA agar
22536	Thoracic		82809	using a PEA agar
22537	Lumbar		16939	acinetobacter
22538	Cervical		82874	aeromonas
16468	Decreased Matrix (Osteoporosis)		82875	using a CIN agar
16469	Decreased Mineralization		18335	avium intracellulare
16470	Osteitis Fibrosa Cystica		16940	bacillus antracis
16488	Bone Marrow		16941	bacteroides
18329	Fine needle aspirate biopsy		82811	using a kanamycin-vancomycin
18210	Excision For Pathology			caked blood agar
18211	Gallbladder		16942	bacteroides fragilis
18212	Cryptosporidia		82723	using a BBE agar
19302	**Microbiology**		16943	bacteroides melaninogenicus
16907	**Blood**		16944	bartonella bacilliformis
16908	Smear For Parasites		82838	bordetella
16909	bartonella bacilliformis		82839	using a Regan-Lowe medium
16910	histoplasma capsulatum		16945	bordetella pertussis
16911	acanthocheilonema perstans		82724	using a Bordet-Yengou agar
16912	mansonella ozzardi		82834	bordetella parapertussis
16913	trypanosoma cruzi		82835	using a Bordet-Yengou agar
16914	Thick smear		82828	borellia
16915	loa loa		82831	using a Kelly medium
16916	plasmodium falciparum			

MICROBIOLOGY, CONT.

16947	brucella	82881	using an XLD agar
82841	campylobacter	16971	spirillum minus
82844	using a campylobacter selective	16972	staphylococcus
	medium	16973	staphylococcus epidermidis
16946	clostridium botulinum		(albus)
82846	clostridium difficile	16974	staphylococcus aureus
82848	using a CCPA agar	18396	penicillin-resistant
16948	clostridium perfringens	18397	methicillin-resistant
16949	clostridium welchii	82824	using a mannitol salt agar
82850	coxynebacterium diptheriae	16999	spirillum minus
82854	using a Tinsdale agar	16975	streptobacillus monilliformis
16950	enterobacter	16976	streptococcus
82856	enterococci	16977	streptococcus faecalis
82859	using a bile-esculin agar		(Enterococcus)
16952	escherichia coli	16978	streptococcus pneumoniae
82815	using a sorbitol-MacConkey	16979	streptococcus Group A Beta
	agar		Hemolytic
16955	eikenella corrodens	16980	streptococcus viridans
16951	francisella tularensis	82870	vibrio
16953	hemophilus influenzae	82871	using a TCBS agar
82725	using a chocolate agar	82872	yersinia
16954	klebsiella pneumoniae	82873	using a CIN agar
82862	legionella	16981	yersinia enterocolitica
82863	using a BCYE agar	16982	yersinia pestis
16991	leptospira	16983	yersinia pseudotuberculosis
82816	using a Fletcher medium	16984	fungi
16992	leptospira canicola	16990	actinomyces israelii
16993	leptospira icterohemorrhagiae	16985	aspergillus
16994	leptospira pomona	82712	blastomyces dermatidis
16956	listeria monocytogenes	16986	candida
16957	mycobacterium	16987	cryptococcus neoformans
16958	neisseria gonorrhoeae	82713	fusarium
82820	using a Thayer-Martin agar	16988	histoplasma capsulatum
16959	neisseria meningitidis	29329	virus
82868	nocardia	16998	Inoculation
82869	using a BCYE agar	16989	colorado tick virus
16960	proteus	82718	cytomegalovirus
16961	pseudomonas	82721	enterovirus
16962	pseudomonas aeruginosa	82707	parasites
16963	pseudomonas mallei	16995	leishmania donovani
16964	pseudomonas pseudomallei	18568	Peripheral Blood Mononuclear Cells
16965	salmonella	18569	Culture
16966	chloraesuis	18570	HIV-1
16967	enteriditis	18571	HIV-2
16968	paratyphus	17000	**Serum**
16969	typhi	17003	Culture
18338	typhimurium	82720	adenovirus
82876	using selenite broth	29283	ebola virus
82877	using an HE agar	17004	rift valley
82878	using an XLD agar	17005	togavirus B: Dengue
16970	serratia	17006	togavirus B: West Nile fever
82879	shigella	82719	varicella zoster virus
82880	using an HE agar	17007	Sabin-Feldman dye test

MICROBIOLOGY, CONT.

17008	toxoplasma gondii		83253	babesia microti
12461	VDRL		82708	coxiella burnetii
28607	RPR		83272	ehrlichia phagocytophila
17009	Complement fixation		83286	ehrlichia chaffensis
17010	blastomyces dermatitidis		17059	legionella pneumophilia
17011	coccidioides immitis		17060	legionella micdadei ("Pittsburgh
17012	coxiella burnetii			pneumonia agent")
17013	histoplasma capsulatum		17061	toxoplasma gondii
17014	paracoccidioides brasilensis		17062	trichinella spiralis
17015	pseudomonas pseudomallei		17063	trypanosoma gambiense
17016	foot & mouth virus		17064	trypanosoma rhodesiense
17017	leishmania donovani		17065	wuchereria bancrofti
17018	influenza		17066	Fluorescent specific antiserum
22081	parainfluenza		17067	legionella pneumophilia
17019	mycoplasma pneumoniae		17068	chlamydia trachomatis
17020	mumps		19677	Fluorescent Immunoassay
17021	togavirus B: Dengue		19678	rubella
17022	varicella		17069	Fluorescent treponemal antibody (FTA)
17023	atypical organism		28608	Treponema Pallidum MHA
17024	chlamydia trachomatis		28609	Treponema Pallidum Immobilization
17025	mycoplasma pneumoniae		17071	Immunofluorescence
17026	pseudomonas mallei		17072	campylobacter jejuni (Vibrio fetus)
17027	rickettsiae akari		19522	Enzyme Immunoassay
17028	rickettsiae australis		28599	Multiple Step Method
17029	pseudomonas pseudomallei		18354	borrelia burgdorferi
17030	rickettsiae conori		101028	chlamydia trachomatis
17031	rickettsiae prowazeki		19675	rubella
17032	rickettsiae mooseri		19523	streptococcal antigen
17033	rickettsiae rickettsii		17073	Direct agglutination
17034	streptococcus		82184	Titre 1:___
17035	rickettsiae tsutsugamushi		17074	brucella
17036	fasciola hepatica		17075	francisella tularensis
17037	strongyloides stercoralis		17076	spirillum minus
17038	loa loa		19521	streptococcus Group A Beta Hemolytic
17039	toxoplasma gondii		17077	pseudomonas pseudomallei
17040	schistosoma		17078	streptobacillus monilliformis
17041	trichinella spiralis		17079	toxoplasma gondii
17042	trypanosoma cruzi		17080	trypanosoma gambiense
17044	trypanosoma gambiense		17081	pseudomonas pseudomallei
17045	trypanosoma rhodesiense		17082	trypanosoma rhodesiense
17046	wuchereria bancrofti		17083	leptospira
17047	wuchereria malayai		12399	Monospot
17048	Neutralization test		17084	Indirect hemagglutination
17050	polio		17085	entamoeba histolytica
17051	rabies virus		17086	plasmodium falciparum
17052	Fluorescent antibody		17091	trypanosoma cruzi
82161	Titre 1:___		17092	wuchereria bancrofti
17053	leishmania		17093	wuchereria malayai
17054	mycobacterium tuberculosis		17094	Hemagglutination
17055	trypanosoma cruzi		17096	fasciola hepatica
17056	wuchereria bancrofti		17097	pseudomonas pseudomallei
17057	wuchereria malayai		17098	pseudomonas pseudomallei
17058	Indirect fluorescent antibody		17099	yersinia enterocolitica

MICROBIOLOGY, CONT.

17095	reovirus	17136	streptococcus Group A Beta
17087	plasmodium malariae		Hemolytic
17088	plasmodium ovale	81518	Hepatitis Markers
17089	plasmodium vivax	12361	Hepatitis A Markers
17090	toxoplasma gondii	12362	A Antibody
17100	Hemagglutination inhibition	12363	IgM
17101	bacillus antracis	12364	IgG
17102	coxsackie	12345	Hepatitis B Markers
17103	influenza	12346	B Core Antibody
22080	parainfluenza	82163	IgM
17104	measles (Rubeola)	82164	IgM + IgG
17105	rubella	12347	B Core Antigen
17106	togavirus B: Dengue	12348	B Surface Antibody
17107	togavirus A: Eastern equine	12349	B Surface Antigen
	encephalitis	82165	Be Antibody
17108	togavirus A: Western equine	82166	Be Antigen
	encephalitis	18509	Hepatitis C Markers
17109	togavirus B: Japanese B	18510	C Antibodies
17110	togavirus B: St. Louis encephalitis	82167	Immunoblot
17111	trypanosoma cruzi	82168	Polymerase Chain Reaction
17112	Latex agglutination	18440	Hepatitis D
83325	cytomegalovirus	81517	Hepatitis E Markers
19676	rubella	12350	E Antibody
82722	streptococcal antigen	12351	E Antigen
17113	Cold agglutinins	12244	Viral Antibody
82141	Titre 1:___	12245	Cytomegalovirus
17114	cytomegalovirus	12246	Epstein-Barr
17115	togavirus B: Yellow fever	83826	IgA VCA
17116	mycoplasma pneumoniae	83837	IgG VCA
17117	Immunodiffusion	83815	IgM VCA
82173	Gel Diffusion	83838	IgG-EA/D
17118	aspergillus	83839	IgA-EA/D
17119	aspergillus fumigatus	83840	IgG-EA/R
17120	coccidioides immitis	83841	Anti-EBNA
17121	leishmania	12247	herpes simplex
17122	rickettsiae rickettsii	17070	ELISA
17123	Counterimmunoelectrophoresis	18409	HIV-1
17124	chlamydia trachomatis	18410	HIV-2
17125	C-Reactive protein	18583	HTLV-I
17126	streptococcus Group A Beta Hemolytic	18584	HTLV-II
17127	Anti-deoxyribonucleotidase B	18563	Recombinant ELISA
17128	Antihyaluronidase	83518	HCV
17129	streptococcus Group A Beta Hemolytic	18565	HIV-1
17130	Anti-DNAse-B	18566	HIV-2
17131	streptococcus Group A Beta	18585	HTLV-I
	Hemolytic	18586	HTLV-II
17132	Antistreptokinase	18352	Immunoblot (Western blot)
17133	Antistreptozyme	18564	HIV-1
19520	streptococcus Group A Beta	12248	HIV-2
	Hemolytic	18587	HTLV-I
17134	Antistreptolysin O titers	18588	HTLV-II
82036	screen	83557	Parvo B
17135	streptococcus	12249	mycoplasma pneumonia

MICROBIOLOGY, CONT.

12250	parainfluenza	17156	rift valley
12251	rubella	17157	rabies virus
12252	rubeola	17158	rubella
29282	ebola virus	17159	togavirus A: Chikungunya
12253	Antigen	17160	togavirus A: Eastern equine encephalitis
12255	Cryptococcal		
83358	Hemophilus influenzae	17161	echovirus
83326	Streptococcus pneumoniae	17162	togavirus A: Sindbis
12256	Weil-Felix	17163	togavirus A: Venezuelan equine encephalitis
12257	OX-2		
12258	OX-19	17164	togavirus A: Western equine encephalitis
12259	OX-K		
12260	Widal	17165	Epstein-Barr virus
18336	P24	17166	togavirus B: Japanese B
18337	Polymerase Chain Reaction	17167	togavirus B: St. Louis encephalitis
84438	Bacteria	17168	togavirus B: West Nile fever
83397	Borrelia burgdorferi	17169	togavirus B: Yellow fever
29288	GC/chlamydia DNA	17170	varicella
29294	(+) For Chlamydia	17171	variola
29295	(+) For N. Gonorrhoeae	17172	toxoplasma gondii
83479	Mycobacterium tuberculosis	17173	chlamydia psittaci
84439	Viruses	17174	paragonimus
83436	Cytomegalovirus	17175	**Sputum**
83437	Epstein-Barr	17178	Smear
83438	Hepatitis C	17179	blastomyces dermatitidis
83477	Herpes simplex	17180	paracoccidioides brasilensis
82171	HIV Antigen	17181	paragonimus
18567	HIV-1 DNA	17182	Wet mount smear
83478	JCV	18370	Charcot-Leyden crystals
84440	Parasites	18371	Curschman's spirals
17137	Acute & convalescent titers (1:X)	17183	phycomycetes (Mucor)
17138	streptococcus	17184	strongyloides stercoralis
17139	yersinia pestis	101059	Acridine Orange stain
17140	virus	101060	bacteria
17141	adenovirus	101061	fungi
17142	bunyavirus	17185	Gram stain
19089	uukuvirus	17190	(+) Bacilli
19090	nairovirus	82726	(-) Bacilli
19091	phlebovirus	17192	(-) Encapsulated organism
19092	hantaan virus	17193	(-) Pleomorphic organism
17143	coxsackie	17194	(+) Cocci
17144	coxsackie A	17195	(+) Cocci in clusters
17145	coxsackie B	17196	(+) Cocci lancet-shaped in pairs
17146	cytomegalovirus	17197	(+) Cocci in chains
17147	herpes simplex type I	17191	(-) Cocci
17148	herpes simplex type II	17186	bacteria
17149	influenza	17189	mixed flora
17150	measles (Rubeola)	17187	mycobacterium
17151	mumps	17177	yersinia pestis
17152	Orf	17188	fungi
17153	pseudomonas mallei	17198	Hyphae
17154	pseudomonas pseudomallei	17199	White Cells
17155	polio	17200	Polynuclear Neutrophils

MICROBIOLOGY, CONT.

17201	Mononuclear Cells		17233	streptococcus pneumoniae
17202	Macrophages		17234	streptococcus viridans
17203	Intraleukocytic organisms		17235	yersinia pestis
101054	Calcofluor White stain		17236	fungi
101055	acanthamoeba		17237	aspergillus
101056	pneumocystis		17238	blastomyces dermatitidis
17204	Ziehl-Neelsen stain		17239	coccidioides immitis
17206	actinomyces israelii		17240	cryptococcus neoformans
83558	cryptosporidium oocysts		17241	histoplasma capsulatum
83607	legionella micdadei		17242	pseudallescheria boydii
17176	mycobacterium tuberculosis		17243	phycomycetes (Mucor)
17205	nocardia		17244	paracoccidioides brasilensis
17210	pneumocystis carinii		17248	Endobronchial brush biopsy specimen
83597	rhodococcus		17249	bacteria
17207	KOH stain		17250	mycobacterium
17208	Methylene blue stain		17251	fungi
17209	Methenamine silver stain		17252	phycomycetes (Mucor)
101057	Toluidine Blue-O stain		17253	pneumocystis carinii
101058	pneumocystis carinii		17254	mycobacterium avium-intracellulare
18351	Gram-Weigert		17255	Transtracheal aspiration
18350	pneumocystis carinii		17256	bacteria
83598	Periodic Acid Schiff Stain		17257	mycobacterium
17211	Culture		17258	fungi
17212	bacteria		101126	Sputum and Bronchial aspiration
17213	acinetobacter		101132	pneumocystis carinii
17245	actinomyces israelii		101161	parasite
17214	bacteroides fragilis		101127	pulmonary amebiasis
82908	using a BBE agar		101128	ascariasis
17247	eikenella corrodens		101129	strongyloidiasis
17215	enterobacter		101130	hookworm larvae
17216	escherichia coli		101131	cryptosporidium
82909	using a sorbitol-MacConkey agar		17259	Direct fluorescent antibody
17217	fusobacterium		17260	legionella pneumophilia
17218	klebsiella		19079	Immunofluorescence
17219	klebsiella pneumoniae		19081	Human herpesvirus 6 (HHV-6)
17220	mycobacterium		17261	Indirect hemagglutination
17246	mycobacterium avium-intracellulare		17262	paracoccidioides brasilensis
17221	mycobacterium tuberculosis		17263	**Urine**
17222	mycobacterium kansasii		17265	Smear
17223	neisseria meningitidis		17266	schistosoma haemotobium
17224	nocardia		17267	Wet mount smear
82910	using a BCYE agar		17268	onchocerca volvulus
17225	pasturella multocida		17269	trichomonas vaginalis
17226	francisella tularensis		17270	Gram stain
17227	proteus		17271	(-) Bacilli
17228	pseudomonas		17272	(-) Bacilli
17229	serratia		17273	(+) Bacilli
17230	staphylococcus aureus		17274	(-) Cocci bacteria
18398	penicillin-resistant		17275	(+) Cocci bacteria
18399	methicillin-resistant		17276	Culture
82911	using a mannitol salt agar		17277	bacteria
17231	streptococcus pyogenes		82734	escherichia coli
17232	streptococcus		17283	leptospira canicola

MICROBIOLOGY, CONT.

17284	leptospira icterohemorrhagiae	17575	leptospira pomona
17285	leptospira pomona	17543	listeria monocytogenes
17278	mycobacterium tuberculosis	17544	mycobacterium tuberculosis
82735	proteus	17545	neisseria gonorrhoeae
17279	salmonella	17546	neisseria meningitidis
17280	salmonella typhi	17567	nocardia
17281	streptococcus faecalis	17548	proteus
	(Enterococcus)	17549	pseudomonas
83599	providencia	17550	pseudomonas aeruginosa
82727	virus	17551	staphylococcus
17264	cytomegalovirus	17553	staphylococcus aureus
82728	fungi	17552	staphylococcus epidermidis
17282	cryptococcus neoformans		(albus)
17286	Antibody-coated bacteria	17555	streptococcus
29328	direct fluorescent antibody	17556	streptococcus faecalis
29327	legionella pneumophilia		(Enterococcus)
17514	**Cerebral Spinal Fluid**	17557	streptococcus pneumoniae
17515	Smear	17558	streptococcus Group A Beta
17516	toxoplasma gondii		Hemolytic
17517	trypanosoma gambiense	17554	streptococcus pyogenes
17518	trypanosoma rhodesiense	17559	streptococcus viridans
17519	Wet mount smear	17560	fungi
17520	naegleria	17561	aspergillus
17521	Gram stain	17562	candida albicans
17522	bacteria	17563	coccidioides immitis
17523	(-) Bacilli	17564	cryptococcus neoformans
17524	(+) Bacilli	17565	histoplasma capsulatum
17525	(-) Cocci	17566	phycomycetes (Mucor)
17526	(+) Cocci	17568	sporotrichum schencki
17527	neisseria meningitidis	17569	virus
17528	(+) Cocci in clusters	22186	herpes simplex type I
17529	(+) Cocci lancet-shaped in pairs	22187	herpes simplex type II
17530	India ink	17570	polio
17531	fungi	17571	togavirus A
17532	cryptococcus neoformans	17572	togavirus B
17533	Ziehl-Neelsen stain	17576	lassa virus
17534	bacteria	17577	mokola virus
17535	mycobacterium tuberculosis	17578	Complement fixation
17536	KOH stain	17579	coccidioides immitis
17537	coccidioides immitis	17580	measles (Rubeola)
17538	Methylene blue stain	17581	Neutralization test
28610	Rapid Bacterial Antigen Identification Kit - CSF	17582	rabies virus
		18368	Fluorescent treponemal antibody
82709	escheria coli (K1)	17583	Direct agglutination
28612	hemophilus influenzae	82185	Titre 1:___
82710	niesseria meningitidis	17584	leptospira
82711	streptococcus pneumoniae	17585	Hemagglutination inhibition
17539	Culture	17586	rubella
17540	bacteria	17587	Latex agglutination
17541	hemophilus influenzae	17588	cryptococcus neoformans
17542	klebsiella pneumoniae	17589	Acute & convalescent titers
17573	leptospira canicola	17590	togavirus A: Venezuelan equine
17574	leptospira icterohemorrhagiae		encephalitis

MICROBIOLOGY, CONT.

17591	Subdural	17630	bacteria
17592	Culture	17631	Nasopharyngeal
17593	bacteroides	17632	Gram stain
17594	escherichia coli	17633	(-) Bacilli
17595	proteus	17634	Methylene blue stain
17596	pseudomonas	17635	corynebacterium diphtheriae
17597	staphylococcus aureus	17636	pseudomonas pseudomallei
17598	streptococcus faecalis (Enterococcus)	17637	Culture
17599	streptococcus viridans	17638	bordetella pertussis
17600	Brain	17639	corynebacterium diphtheriae
17601	Biopsy	17640	klebsiella ozenae
17602	mokola virus	17641	neisseria meningitidis
17603	Conjunctiva	17642	pseudomonas aeruginosa
17604	Giemsa stain	17643	streptococcus Group A Beta Hemolytic
17605	Culture	17644	phycomycetes (Mucor)
17606	bacteria	17645	virus
17607	adenovirus	17646	adenovirus
17608	newcastle disease	17647	coxsackie
17609	chlamydia trachomatis	17648	influenza
22622	Cornea	82715	type A
22624	Smear	82716	type B
22623	Culture	82717	type C
17610	Ear	17649	respiratory syncytial virus
18348	Gram-Weigert	17650	rhinovirus
17611	Culture	19504	coronavirus
17612	bacteria	19505	parainfluenza
20846	bacteroides	17651	Pharynx
20843	hemophilus influenzae	17652	Methylene blue stain
20844	moraxella	17653	corynebacterium diphtheriae
17613	pseudomonas aeruginosa	17654	Culture
17614	staphylococcus aureus	17655	bacteria
20841	streptococcus pneumoniae	17656	corynebacterium diphtheriae
20842	streptococcus pyogenes	17657	hemophilus influenzae
20845	virus	17658	mycobacterium tuberculosis
18345	Biopsy	17659	neisseria gonorrhoeae
18346	Lesion	17660	serratia
17615	Sinus	17661	streptococcus
18349	Gram-Weigert	17662	streptococcus Group A Beta Hemolytic
17616	Culture	17663	virus
17617	bacteria	17664	influenza
17618	phycomycetes (Mucor)	17665	respiratory syncytial virus
18347	Biopsy	17666	rabies virus
17619	Oral	17667	Esophageal
17620	Culture	17668	Smear
17621	phycomycetes (Mucor)	17669	herpes simplex type I
17622	Biopsy	17670	Gram stain
17623	phycomycetes (Mucor)	17671	KOH stain
17624	Gingival	17672	Culture
17625	Culture	17673	bacteria
17626	mycobacterium tuberculosis	17674	fungi
17627	Buccal Mucosa	17675	candida albicans
17628	Salivary Duct	17676	Gastric
17629	Culture	17677	Culture

MICROBIOLOGY, CONT.

17678	clostridium botulinum
18594	Helicobacter pylori
17679	Lymph nodes
17680	Gram stain
17681	(-) Bacilli
17682	Ziehl-Neelsen stain
17683	mycobacterium tuberculosis
17684	Giemsa stain
17685	wuchereria bancrofti
17686	wuchereria malayai
17687	Culture
17688	bacteria
17689	mycobacterium
17690	mycobacterium avium
17691	mycobacterium tuberculosis
17692	mycobacterium kansasii
17693	mycobacterium scrofulaceum
17694	yersinia pestis
17695	chlamydia trachomatis
17696	leishmania donovani
17697	Biopsy
17698	toxoplasma gondii
17699	Fluorescent antibody
17700	mycobacterium tuberculosis
17701	Pleural Fluid
17702	Smear
17703	paragonimus
17704	Gram stain
17705	bacteria
17706	Giemsa stain
17707	wuchereria bancrofti
17708	wuchereria malayai
17709	Sudan III stain
17710	Culture
17711	bacteria
17712	bacteroides fragilis
17713	fusobacterium
17714	mycobacterium
17715	mycobacterium tuberculosis
17716	streptococcus
22076	streptococcus Group A Beta Hemolytic
17717	fungi
17718	actinomyces israelii
22077	staphylococcus
22078	hemophilus influenzae
22075	streptococcus pneumoniae
17719	Neutralization test
17720	bacteria
17721	mycobacterium
17722	fungi
17723	Direct fluorescent antibody
17724	legionella pneumophilia
17725	Lung
17726	Ziehl-Neelsen stain
17727	legionella micdadei ("Pittsburgh pneumonia agent")
17728	Dieterle Stain
17729	legionella pneumophilia
17730	Biopsy
17731	cryptococcus neoformans
81861	silica
17732	Fluorescent antibody
17733	legionella pneumophilia
17734	Peritoneal Fluid
17735	Gram stain
17736	bacteria
17737	Ziehl-Neelsen stain
17738	bacteria
17739	Giemsa stain
17740	wuchereria bancrofti
17741	wuchereria malayai
17742	Culture
17743	bacteria
17744	mycobacterium
17745	mycobacterium tuberculosis
17746	candida albicans
17747	Hemagglutination inhibition
17748	bacteria
17749	Pericardial Fluid
17750	Wet mount smear
17751	echinococcus granulosus
17752	entamoeba histolytica
17753	Gram stain
17754	(+) Cocci in clusters
17755	(+) Cocci lancet-shaped in pairs
17756	Culture
17757	bacteria
17758	brucella abortus
17759	mycobacterium tuberculosis
17761	streptococcus Group A Beta Hemolytic
17760	staphylococcus aureus
17762	Mediastinal Fluid
17763	Muscle
17764	Biopsy
83697	cysticerus of Taenia solium
83714	diphyllobothrium latum
17765	trichinella spiralis
17766	Joint Fluid
17767	Gram stain
17768	bacteria
17769	fungi
17770	(-) Cocci
17771	neisseria
17772	Ziehl-Neelsen stain
17773	Methylene blue stain
17774	Giemsa stain

MICROBIOLOGY, CONT.

17775	wuchereria bancrofti		17821	Culture
17776	wuchereria malayai		17822	bacteria
17777	Culture		17826	chlamydia trachomatis
17778	bacteria		17823	listeria monocytogenes
83731	borrelia burgdorferi		17824	neisseria gonorrhoeae
17779	mycobacterium tuberculosis		17825	neisseria gonorrhoeae PPNG
17780	neisseria gonorrhoeae		83842	virus
17781	spirillum minus		29289	herpes simplex type II
17782	streptobacillus monilliformis		29297	human papilloma virus
17783	fungi		17287	Urethral
17784	Bursae		17288	Smear
17785	Gram stain		17289	chlamydia trachomatis
17786	bacteria		17290	Wet mount smear
17787	Culture		17291	trichomonas vaginalis
17788	bacteria		17292	Gram stain
17789	Bone		17294	(-) Cocci
17790	Gram stain		17295	neisseria gonorrhoeae
17791	bacteria		17293	bacteria
17792	Culture		17296	Giemsa stain
17793	bacteria		17297	trichomonas vaginalis
17794	mycobacterium tuberculosis		17298	Culture
17795	actinomyces israelii		17299	bacteria
17796	Bone Marrow		17300	neisseria gonorrhoeae
83732	Giemsa stain		17301	neisseria gonorrhoeae PPNG
83766	histoplasma capsulatum		82736	direct fluorescent antibody
83767	Ziehl-Neelsen stain		82737	chlamydia trachomatis
83806	mycobacterium tuberculosis		17302	Skin test
83807	methenamine silver stain		17303	Vaginal Discharge
83808	histoplasma capsulatum		17304	Vaginal
17799	Culture		17305	Wet mount smear
17800	brucella		17306	candida
17801	mycobacterium tuberculosis		82738	clue cells
17802	salmonella typhi		17307	glitter cells
17803	histoplasma capsulatum		17308	trichomonas vaginalis
17804	leishmania donovani		17309	KOH stain
18366	Immunofluorescence		17310	candida albicans
18367	Epstein-Barr virus		17311	Giemsa stain
17805	Small Intestine Fluid		17312	trichomonas vaginalis
17806	Wet mount smear		17313	Culture
17807	strongyloides stercoralis		17314	bacteria
17808	Giemsa stain		17315	bacteroides fragilis
17809	entamoeba histolytica		18209	chlamydia trachomatis
17810	Culture		17316	clostridium perfringens
17811	bacteria		83600	gardnerella vaginalis
17812	mycobacterium tuberculosis		83601	mobiluncus
17813	streptococcus viridans		17317	neisseria gonorrhoeae
17814	Aspiration		17318	nisseria gonorrhoeae PPNG
17815	strongyloides stercoralis		17319	staphylococcus aureus
17816	Cervical		17320	streptococcus faecalis (Enterococcus)
17817	Wet mount smear		17321	streptococcus Group A Beta Hemolytic
17818	trichomonas vaginalis		17322	candida albicans
17819	Gram stain		29290	herpes simplex type II
17820	(-) Cocci		17323	Direct agglutination

MICROBIOLOGY, CONT.

17324	candida albicans	22294	bacteria
29293	Vulvar	17367	clostridium botulinum
29292	Culture	17368	neisseria gonorrhoeae
29291	herpes simplex type II	17369	salmonella chloraesuis
17325	Small Bowel	17370	salmonella enteriditis
17326	Ziehl-Neelsen stain	17371	salmonella typhimurium
17327	avium-intracellulare	17372	salmonella paratyphus
17328	Stool	17373	salmonella typhi
17329	Smear	17374	shigella
17330	vibrio cholerae	17375	staphylococcus aureus
18332	ancylostoma ceylanicum	17376	campylobacter jejuni (Vibrio fetus)
17331	ancylostoma duodenale	17377	vibrio cholerae
17332	ascaris lumbricoides	17378	vibrio parahemolyticus
17333	balantidium coli	17380	yersinia enterocolitica
18067	blastocystis hominis	17379	virus
17334	capillaria phillippinensis	17381	coxsackie
17335	chilomastix mesnili	17382	polio
17336	clonorchis sinensis	17383	Scotch tape test
18068	cryptosporidia	17384	taenia saginata
17337	diphyllobothrium latum	17385	Complement fixation
17338	endolimax nana	17386	rotavirus
17339	entamoeba coli	17387	Fluorescent antibody
17340	entamoeba histolytica	17388	rotavirus
17341	fasciola hepatica	17389	ELISA
17342	fasciolopsis buski	17390	rotavirus
17343	giardia lamblia	17391	Immunofluorescence
18333	Heterophyes heterophyes	17392	taenia solium
17344	hymenolepsis diminuta	17393	Rectal
17345	hymenolepsis nana	17394	Smear
17346	iodamoeba buetschlii	17395	neisseria gonorrhoeae
18334	Metagonimus yakagawa	17396	entamoeba histolytica
17347	necator americanus	17397	Culture
17348	opisthocerciasis	17398	neisseria gonorrhoeae
17349	opisthocerciasis felineus	17399	shigella
17350	opisthocerciasis viverini	17400	reovirus
17351	paragonimus	17401	Biopsy
17352	schistosoma	17402	balantidium coli
17354	schistosoma haemotobium	83611	cryptosporidium
17355	schistosoma Japonicum	83614	entamoeba histolytica
17356	schistosoma mansoni	83625	schistosoma japonicum
17357	schistosoma mekongi	83624	schistosoma mansoni
17358	strongyloides stercoralis	17403	Scotch tape test
17359	taenia saginata	17404	enterobius vermicularis
17360	taenia solium	17405	Complement fixation
17361	trichuris trichiura	17406	rotavirus
17362	trichomonas hominis	17407	Fluorescent antibody
17363	trichostrongylus	17408	rotavirus
17364	Thick smear	17409	ELISA
17365	trichostrongylus	83637	chlamydia trachomatis
83602	Trichrome stain	83643	Respiratory Syncytial Virus
83603	Lugol's Iodine stain	17410	rotavirus
83605	Iron Hematoxylin stain	17411	Skin
17366	Culture	17412	parasites

MICROBIOLOGY, CONT.

17413	Culture	17459	blastomyces dermatitidis
17414	bacteria	17460	candida albicans
17415	streptococcus	17461	monosporium apiospermum
17416	Aspiration	17462	pseudallescheria boydii
17417	bacteria	17463	sporotrichum schencki
17418	streptococcus Group A Beta Hemolytic	17464	coxsackie A
17419	Biopsy	17465	herpes simplex type I
17420	dipetalonema streptocerca	17466	variola
81841	Fibroblast Culture	17467	actinomyces israelii
17421	Skin lesion	17468	chlamydia trachomatis
17423	ancylostoma braziliens	17469	leishmania tropica
83660	leishmania	17470	Biopsy
83661	mycobacterium marinum	18339	cryptococcus neoformans
83670	pseudomonas	17471	diphyllobothrium manson
83671	sporothrix schenckii	17472	gnathostoma spinigerum
83680	treponema pallidium	17473	Abscess
17422	yersinia pestis	17474	Gram stain
17424	Smear	17475	bacteria
17425	blastomyces dermatitidis	17476	Ziehl-Neelsen stain
17426	monosporium apiospermum	17477	mycobacterium tuberculosis
17427	leishmania braziliensis	17478	Giemsa stain
17428	leishmania peruviana	17479	entamoeba histolytica
17429	leishmania tropica	17480	Culture
17430	loa loa	17481	bacteria
17431	Gram stain	17482	mycobacterium tuberculosis
17432	clostridium	17483	fungi
17433	hemophilus ducreyi	17484	Ulcer
17434	pseudomonas mallei	17485	Methylene blue stain
17435	streptococcus Group A Beta Hemolytic	17486	corynebacterium diphtheriae
17436	KOH stain	17487	Culture
17437	candida albicans	17488	corynebacterium diphtheriae
17438	malassezia furfur	17489	Biopsy
17439	Giemsa stain	17490	histoplasma capsulatum
17440	multinucleated Giant Cells	17491	Wound
17441	Culture	17492	Smear
17442	bacteria	17493	draculculus medinensis
17443	bacillus antracis	17494	Gram stain
17444	bartonella bacilliformis	17495	bacteria
17445	clostridium	17496	staphylococcus
17446	hemophilus ducreyi	17497	streptococcus
17447	mycobacterium marinum	17498	actinomyces israelii
17448	neisseria gonorrhoeae	17499	(-) Bacilli
17449	neisseria meningitidis	17500	(-) Cocci
17450	nocardia	17501	Ziehl-Neelsen stain
17451	pseudomonas mallei	17502	mycobacterium tuberculosis
17452	staphylococcus	17503	actinomyces israelii
17453	staphylococcus aureus	17504	Culture
17454	streptococcus pyogenes	17505	bacteria
17455	streptococcus	17506	clostridium perfringens
17456	streptococcus Group A Beta Hemolytic	17507	clostridium tetani
		17508	pasturella multocida
17457	yersinia pestis	17509	staphylococcus aureus
17458	fungi	17510	streptococcus Group A Beta Hemolytic

MICROBIOLOGY, CONT.

17511	histoplasma capsulatum		17832	toxocara canis
17512	phycomycetes (Mucor)		17833	toxocara cati
17513	actinomyces israelii		83855	toxoplasma gondii
84441	Rapid Streptococcus Group Identification (Kit)		29331	User Finding:

28611	streptococcus Group A Beta Hemolytic
86962	streptococcus Group B
86963	streptococcus Group C
86964	streptococcus Group D
86965	streptococcus Group E
86966	streptococcus Group F
86967	streptococcus Group G
17827	Food Substances
17828	Culture
101080	bacteria
83845	bacillus cereus
83843	brucella
83846	campylobacter jejuni
17829	clostridium botulinum
83844	clostridium perfringens
83847	escherichia coli
83848	listeria
83849	salmonella
83850	staphylococcus aureus
83851	vibrio cholerae
83852	vibrio parahemolyticus
83853	vibrio vulnificus
83854	yersina enterocolitica
101083	fungi
101084	amanitotoxin
101085	parasite
101086	cryptosporidiosis
101087	giardiasis
101088	trichenellosis
101089	virus
101102	Hepatitis A
101103	Norwalk and Parvo-like
29332	Culture Result
29333	no growth at 24 hours
29334	no growth at 48 hours
29335	no growth at 7 days
29336	less than 10,000 colonies
29337	less than 50,000 colonies
29338	less than 100,000 colonies
29339	more than 100,000 colonies
29340	mixed flora
29341	mixed skin flora
17830	Pets
83856	bartonella henselae
17835	colorado tick virus
17836	o'nyong-nyong
83857	pasteurella multocida
17831	reovirus

Part V
DIAGNOSES, SYNDROMES, AND CONDITIONS

39448	Diagnoses, Syndromes And Conditions	36760		Senile
34847	**Normal Examination**	36761		Mechanical
34845	Normal Routine Annual History And Physical	36762		Spastic
		36763		Cicatricial
34846	Normal Annual Health Maintenance Checkup	36764	Lagophthalmos	
		36765		Paralytic
34848	Normal Annual "Physical"	36766		Mechanical
34849	Normal Pre-Employment Screening Examination	36767		Cicatricial
		36768	Ptosis	
30719	**Ophthalmology**	36769		Paralytic
90108	Refractive Disorders	36770		Myogenic
30749	Refractive Error	36771		Mechanical
34053	Hypermetropia	36772		Blepharochalasis
36608	Myopia	36773	Abnormal Innervation Syndrome	
30751	Astigmatism	36775	Disorders Of The Lacrimal System	
36609	Regular	36783	Dacryoadenitis	
36610	Irregular	36784		Acute
36623	Diplopia	36785		Chronic
36624	Polyopia	36786		Chronic Enlargement Of The Lacrimal Gland
36611	Anisometropia			
36612	Aniseikonia	36787	Lacrimal Cysts	
36613	Presbyopia	36788	Lacrimal Atrophy	
36617	Transient Change	36789		Primary
30757	Eyestrain	36790		Secondary
90104	Eyelids; Lacrimal Sac, Duct, Gland	36791	Dry Eye Syndrome	
35584	Foreign Body - Lacrimal Punctum	36792	Dislocation Of Lacrimal Gland	
39753	Right	36793	Epiphora	
39754	Left	36794		Due To Excess Lacrimation
39756	Both	36795		Due To Insufficient Drainage
30735	Sty (Hordeolum Externum)	30759	Dacryocystitis	
39762	Right Eye	36796		Acute
39763	Left Eye	36797		Chronic
39764	Both Eyes	36798		Phlegmonous
36746	Hordeolum Internum	36799	Lacrimal Canaliculitis	
36747	Eyelid Abscess	36800		Acute
39765	Right Eye	36801		Chronic
39766	Left Eye	36803	Lacrimal Mucocele	
39767	Both Eyes	36804	Eversion Of Lacrimal Punctum	
30736	Chalazion	36805	Lacrimal Stenosis	
36748	Dermatitis Of Eyelid	36806		Lacrimal Punctum
36749	Eczematous	36807		Lacrimal Canaliculi
36750	Contact, Allergic	36808		Lacrimal Sac
36753	Infective	30734	Tear Duct Occlusion	
36751	Xeroderma Of Eyelid	36802		Neonatal
36752	Discoid Lupus Erythematosus Of Eyelid	39768		Right Eye
36754	Parasitic Infestation Of Eyelid	39769		Left Eye
30733	Entropion	39771		Both Eyes
36755	Senile	30758	Lacrimal Calculus	
36756	Mechanical	39772		Right Eye
36757	Spastic	39773		Left Eye
36758	Cicatricial	39774		Both Eyes
36759	Trichiasis Of Eyelid	36809	Lacrimal Fistula	
30761	Ectropion	39775		Right Eye

OPHTHALMOLOGY, CONT.

39776	Left Eye		36724	Contact
39777	Both Eyes		39539	Right Eye
34059	Blepharitis		39540	Left Eye
30760	Chronic Marginal		39541	Both Eyes
36744	Ulcerative		35583	Foreign Body - Conjunctival Sac
36745	Squamous		39750	Right
36810	Lacrimal Passage Granuloma		39751	Left
39778	Right Eye		39752	Both
39779	Left Eye		36352	Conjunctival Degeneration
39780	Both Eyes		36735	Xerosis
90094	Conjunctiva		36736	Concretions
30991	Conjunctivitis		36737	Pigmentations
34056	Acute		36738	Argyrosis
36714	Serous		36733	Pinguecula
36715	Follicular		36734	Pseudopterygium
38354	Vernal		39800	Right Eye
36716	Pseudomembranous		39801	Left Eye
36717	Atopic		39802	Both Eyes
30992	Hemophilus Bordetella Pertussis		36353	Conjunctival Deposits
30999	Koch Weeks Bacillus		39803	Right Eye
36725	Rosacea		39804	Left Eye
34057	Chronic		39805	Both Eyes
36718	Simple		36739	Conjunctival Granuloma
36719	Follicular		39806	Right Eye
36720	Vernal		39807	Left Eye
36721	Chronic Allergic		39808	Both Eyes
38554	Giant Papillary		36740	Conjunctival Adhesions
36722	Parasitic		36741	Localized
36726	In Mucocutaneous Disease		36742	Extensive
30993	Keratoconjunctivitis		39809	Right Eye
36677	Phlyctenular		39810	Left Eye
36678	Vernal		39812	Both Eyes
36679	Sicca		36743	Conjunctival Scarring
36680	Exposure		39813	Right Eye
36681	Neurotrophic		39815	Left Eye
36224	Tuberculous		39817	Both Eyes
30994	Meningococcus		90095	Cornea
30995	Acute Hemorrhagic		34054	Keratitis
30996	Inclusion		30738	Superficial
30997	Epidemic Kerato		36671	Punctate
30998	Gonococcal		36672	Macular
31000	Hemophilus Parainfluenzae		36673	Filamentary
31001	Neonatal		36674	Photokeratitis
38549	Chemical		36675	Snow Blindness
39533	Right Eye		36676	Welders' Keratitis
39534	Left Eye		30739	Interstitial
39535	Both Eyes		36682	Diffuse
38550	Subconjunctival Hemorrage		36683	Cogan's Syndrome
39537	Right Eye		36684	Sclerosing
39536	Left Eye		36685	Corneal Abscess
39538	Both Eyes		36222	Tuberculous
36351	Blepharoconjunctivitis		39542	Right Eye
36723	Angular		39543	Left Eye

OPHTHALMOLOGY, CONT.

39544	Both Eyes
34055	Corneal Degeneration
36693	Senile
36694	Recurrent Erosion
36695	Keratomalacia
36696	Nodular
36697	Salzmann's Nodular Dystrophy
36698	Peripheral
36699	Marginal
39619	Right Eye
39617	Left Eye
39618	Both Eyes
30744	Corneal Foreign Body
39620	Right Eye
39621	Left Eye
39622	Both Eyes
30730	Bullous Keratopathy
38462	Corneal Scar
39781	Right Eye
39782	Left Eye
39784	Both Eyes
36347	Corneal Neovascularization
36686	Localized
36687	Pannus
36688	Deep
36689	Ghost Vessels
39785	Right Eye
39786	Left Eye
39787	Both Eyes
36348	Corneal Edema
36690	Idiopathic
36691	Secondary
36692	Contact Lens-Induced
39788	Right Eye
39789	Left Eye
39790	Both Eyes
36349	Corneal Dystrophy
36700	Juvenile Epithelial
36701	Anterior
36702	Granular
36703	Lattice
36704	Macular
36705	Stromal
36706	Endothelial
36707	Posterior
39791	Right Eye
39792	Left Eye
39793	Both Eyes
36350	Corneal Deformity
36710	Ectasia
36711	Descemetocele
36712	Staphyloma
39794	Right Eye

39795	Left Eye
39796	Both Eyes
36713	Contact Lens-Induced Corneal Disorder
38555	Poorly-Fitting Contact Lens
31116	Corneal Ulcer
36663	Marginal
36664	Ring
36665	Central
36666	Hypopyon
36667	Serpiginous
36668	Mycotic
36669	Perforated
36670	Mooren's
31117	Pseudomonas
31118	Proteus
39797	Right Eye
39798	Left Eye
39799	Both Eyes
34058	Pterygium
36727	Peripheral
36728	Stationary
36729	Progressive
36730	Central
36731	Double
36732	Recurrent
30740	Keratoconus
36708	Stable Condition
36709	Acute Hydrops
90101	Anterior Chamber
36518	Hyphema
90098	Iris / Uveal Tract
34039	Sympathetic Uveitis
32477	Sympathetic Ophthalmia
30741	Iridocyclitis
34040	Acute
36511	Primary
36512	Recurrent
36513	Secondary
36514	Infectious
36515	Noninfectious
34041	Chronic
34042	Fuchs' Heterochromic Cyclitis
36516	Glaucomatocyclitic Crises
36517	Lens-Induced
34043	Vogt-Kayanagi Syndrome
36223	Tuberculous
39548	Right Eye
39549	Left Eye
39550	Both Eyes
31159	Iritis
38552	Traumatic
39551	Right Eye
39552	Left Eye

OPHTHALMOLOGY, CONT.

39553	Both Eyes	38465	Anterior Dislocation Of Lens
36519	Rubeosis Iridis	39737	Right Eye
36520	Iris Atrophy	39739	Left Eye
36521	Essential	39741	Both Eyes
36522	Progressive	30745	Cataract
39556	Right Eye	34050	Presenile
39557	Left Eye	36575	Anterior Subcapsular Polar
39559	Both Eyes	36576	Posterior Subcapsular Polar
38547	Aniridia	36577	Cortical
36523	Iridoschisis	36578	Lamellar
36524	Pigmentary Iris Degeneration	36579	Zonular
36525	Acquired Heterochromia	36580	Nuclear
36526	Pigment Dispersion Syndrome	36581	Combined Forms
36527	Translucency	34051	Senile
39589	Right Eye	36582	Pseudoexfoliation Of Lens Capsule
39590	Left Eye	36583	Immature
39591	Both Eyes	36584	Anterior Subcapsular Polar
36528	Degeneration Of Pupillary Margin	36585	Posterior Subcapsular Polar
36529	Atrophy Of The Sphincter	36586	Cortical
36530	Ectropion Of The Pigment Epithelium	36587	Nuclear
36534	Anterior Uveal Cysts	36588	Total
36535	Idiopathic	36589	Hypermature
36536	Implantation	36590	Combined Forms
36537	Exudative	34052	Traumatic
36538	Pars Plana	36591	Localized
36539	Primary	36592	Total
36540	Exudative	36593	Partially Resolved
39592	Right Eye	36594	Secondary To Ocular Disorders
39594	Left Eye	36595	Glaucomatous Flecks
39596	Both Eyes	36596	In Inflammatory Disorders
34049	Adhesions Of Iris	36597	With Neovascularization
36541	Posterior Synechiae	36598	In Degenerative Disorders
36544	Iris Bombe	36599	Secondary To Systemic Disorders
36545	Pupillary Occlusion	36600	Diabetic
36546	Iridodialysis	36601	Tetanic
36548	Ectopic Pupil	36602	Myotonic
90102	Crystalline Lens	36603	Toxic
30743	Congenital Ectopic Lens	36604	Radiation-Induced
38463	Aphakia	36345	After-Cataract
38467	Pseudophakia	36605	Not Obscuring Vision
38651	Anterior Chamber	36606	Obscuring Vision
38652	Posterior Chamber	36607	Soemmering's Ring
38653	Iris Fixated	90096	Vitreous
38654	Subluxation	34037	Endophthalmitis
38655	Anterior Dislocation	34038	Acute
38656	Posterior Dislocation	36423	Chronic
39725	Right Eye	36427	Parasitic
39726	Left Eye	36424	Panophthalmitis
39727	Both Eyes	36425	Vitreous Abscess
38464	Subluxation Of Lens	36426	Panuveitis
39729	Right Eye	36428	Ophthalmia Nodosa
39731	Left Eye	39545	Right Eye
39734	Both Eyes	39546	Left Eye

OPHTHALMOLOGY, CONT.

39547	Both Eyes		39611	Left Eye
36782	Vitreous Disorders		39612	Both Eyes
30726	Vitreous Hemorrhage		34048	Choroidal Detachment
39714	Right Eye		36509	Serous
39716	Left Eye		36510	Hemorrhagic
39718	Both Eyes		39613	Right Eye
38324	Vitreous Floaters		39614	Left Eye
39719	Right Eye		39615	Both Eyes
39721	Left Eye		30742	Retrolental Fibroplasia
39723	Both Eyes		38387	Retinopathy Of Prematurity
30722	Posterior Vitreous Detachment		30720	Macular Degeneration
38285	Post-Surgical Cataract Fragments In Eye		36459	Nonexudative
90097	Retina / Choroid		36460	Exudative
30415	Color Blindness		36461	Cystoid
36637	Protan Defect		36462	Macular Cyst
36638	Deutan Defect		36463	Macular Hole
36639	Tritan Defect		36464	Macular Pseudohole
36641	Acquired		36465	Toxic Maculopathy
36640	Achromatopsia		36466	Drusen
39524	Right Eye		39627	Right Eye
39525	Left Eye		39628	Left Eye
39526	Both Eyes		39629	Both Eyes
36642	Night Blindness		38566	Ischemic Maculopathy
36643	Congenital		30721	Central Serous Retinopathy
36644	Acquired		38580	Serous Detachment Of Retinal Pigment Epithelium
36645	Abnormal Dark Adaptation Curve			
39527	Right Eye		38581	Hemorrhagic Detachment Of Retinal Pigment Epithelium
39528	Left Eye			
39529	Both Eyes		38471	Retinal Hemorrhage
34046	Choroidal Degeneration		38582	Retinal Edema
36494	Senile Atrophy		38470	Radiation Retinopathy
36495	Diffuse Secondary Atrophy		38560	Sickle Cell Retinopathy
36496	Angioid Streaks		30724	Retinal Detachment
36497	Hereditary Choroidal Dystrophy		36321	With Retinal Defect
36498	Circumpapillary		36322	Partial
36499	Partial		36323	With Single Defect
36500	Total		36324	With Multiple Defects
36501	Central		36325	With Giant Tear
36502	Partial		36326	With Retinal Dialysis
36503	Total		36327	Old
36504	Choroideremia		36328	Total
36505	Diffuse Sclerosis		36329	Old
36506	Generalized Gyrate Atrophy		36330	Without Retinal Defect (Serous)
39604	Right Eye		36338	Traction Detachment
39605	Left Eye		38664	With ____ Grade PVR
39606	Both Eyes		39630	Right Eye
36507	Choroidal Hemorrhage		39631	Left Eye
36508	Expulsive		39632	Both Eyes
39607	Right Eye		36331	Retinoschisis
39608	Left Eye		36332	Flat
39609	Both Eyes		36333	Bullous
34047	Choroidal Rupture		39683	Right Eye
39610	Right Eye		39684	Left Eye

OPHTHALMOLOGY, CONT.

39685	Both Eyes	36491	Pigment Epitheliopathy
38469	Macular Puckering	36492	Pars Planitis
36334	Retinal Cysts	36221	Tuberculous
36335	Primary	39702	Right Eye
36336	Secondary	39704	Left Eye
36337	Pseudocyst	39706	Both Eyes
39686	Right Eye	36493	Solar Retinopathy
39687	Left Eye	38567	Retinal Scar
39688	Both Eyes	39709	Right Eye
36451	Retinal Defects Without Detachment	39711	Left Eye
30723	Retinal Tear	39712	Both Eyes
36452	Round Hole Of Retina	38591	Congenital Hypertrophy Of The Retinal
36453	Horseshoe Tear		Pigment Epithelium
36454	Multiple Defects	38466	Posterior Dislocation Of Lens
39692	Right Eye	39742	Right Eye
39694	Left Eye	39743	Left Eye
39695	Both Eyes	39744	Both Eyes
36455	Hypertensive Retinopathy	30728	Central Serous Choroidopathy
38563	Talc Retinopathy	30750	Malignant Myopia
38558	Retinal Telangiectasia	90114	Sclera
38561	Retinal Neovascularization	36894	Scleral Disorders
38559	Coats' Syndrome	36895	Scleritis
34044	Peripheral Retinal Degeneration	36896	Nodular
36467	Paving Stone	36897	Anterior
36468	Microcystoid	36899	Posterior
36469	Lattice	36904	Sclerotenonitis
36470	Senile Reticular	36898	Brawny
36471	Secondary Pigmentary	36900	Episcleritis Periodica Fugax
36472	Secondary Vitroretinal	36901	Scleromalacia Perforans
39696	Right Eye	36902	Scleroperikeratitis
39699	Left Eye	36903	Scleral Abscess
39700	Both Eyes	36905	Scleral Ectasia
34045	Hereditary Retinal Dystrophy	36906	Staphyloma Posticum
36473	Juvenile Retinoschisis	90105	Optic Nerve
36474	Albipunctate	30727	Foster Kennedy Syndrome
30731	Retinitis Pigmentosa	30732	Ophthalmoplegia
36475	Progressive Cone Dystrophy	36346	Disorder Of Accomodation
36476	Stagardt's Disease	36614	Paresis
36477	Fundus Flavimaculatus	36615	Total Internal Ophthalmoplegia
36478	Vitelliform Dystrophy	36616	Spasm
36479	Hyaline Dystrophy	36618	Drug-Induced
36480	Pseudoinflammatory Foveal Dystrophy	36619	Toxic
36481	Hereditary Drusen	36781	Disorders Of Gaze
30725	Chorioretinitis	36890	Conjugate Gaze Palsy
36482	Focal	36891	Spasm Of Conjugate Gaze
36483	Juxtapapillary	36892	Convergence Palsy
36484	Posterior Pole	36893	Convergence Spasm
36485	Peripheral	30756	Adie's Tonic Pupil
36486	Disseminated	36835	Optic Atrophy
36487	Posterior Pole	36836	Primary
36488	Peripheral	36837	Postinflammatory
36489	Generalized	36838	Associated With Retinal Dystrophy
36490	Metastatic	36839	Glaucomatous

OPHTHALMOLOGY, CONT.

38564	Pseudopapilledema		36570	With Uveitis
38568	Optic Disc Drusen		36571	With Intraocular Tumors
38565	Myleinated Optic Nerve Fibers		36572	With Trauma
36840	Optic Papillitis		36573	With Increased Episcleral Venous Pressure
36843	Hemorrhage In Optic Nerve Sheath		36342	Combined Mechanism
90099	Glaucoma / Intraocular Pressure		36343	Primary
36531	Miotic Cysts Of The Pupillary Margin		36344	Secondary
36532	Degenerative Changes Of The Chamber Angle		36574	Hypersecretion
36533	Degenerative Changes Of The Ciliary Body		36436	Absolute
			38468	Post-Iridotomy Condition
36542	Anterior Synechiae		90115	Orbit
36543	Goniosynechiae		36774	Disorders Of The Orbit
39597	Right Eye		36811	Inflammation Of The Orbit
39598	Left Eye		36812	Acute
39599	Both Eyes		36813	Chronic
36547	Recession Of Chamber Angle		30762	Orbital Periostitis
36429	Ocular Siderosis		30763	Orbital Granuloma
36430	Ocular Chalcosis		30764	Orbital Cellulitis
36431	Hypotony Of Eye		38391	Periorbital Cellulitis
36432	Primary		30765	Orbital Abscess
36433	Secondary		30766	Periorbital Abscess
39601	Right Eye		36814	Orbital Osteomyelitis
39602	Left Eye		36815	Tenonitis
39603	Both Eyes		36816	Orbital Myositis
36434	Blind Hypotensive Eye		36817	Orbital Parasitic Infestation
36435	Phthisis Bulbi		36818	Orbital Hemorrhage
36339	Preglaucoma		36819	Orbital Edema
36549	Open Angle With Borderline Findings		36820	Orbital Deformity
36550	Anatomical Narrow Angle		36821	Due To Bone Disease
36551	Steroid Responders		36822	Associated With Craniofacial Deformities
36552	Ocular Hypertension		36823	Post-Traumatic
30746	Glaucoma		36825	Hypertelorism Of Orbit
36340	Open-Angle		37675	Craniosynostosis
36553	Low Tension		36824	Exostosis Of Orbit
36554	Residual Stage		36826	Orbital Atrophy
30747	Primary		36827	Enlargement Of Orbit
35596	Secondary		38551	Exophthalmos
36555	Pigmentary		36828	Enophthalmos
36556	Corticosteroid-Induced		36829	Due To Atrophy Of Orbital Tissue
36557	Glaucomatous Stage		36830	Post-Traumatic
36558	Residual Stage		36832	Orbital Cyst
36566	Lens-Induced		36833	Orbital Encephalocele
36567	Phacolytic		36834	Extraocular Myopathy
36568	Pseudoexfoliation		90109	Motility Disorders
36341	Angle-Closure		30752	Amblyopia
30748	Primary		36620	Strabismic
36559	Intermittent		36621	Deprivation
36560	Acute		36622	Refractive
36561	Chronic		36625	Binocular Vision Disorder
36562	Residual Stage		36626	Suppression
35595	Secondary			
36569	With Pupillary Block			

OPHTHALMOLOGY, CONT.

36627	Simultaneous Perception Without Fusion
36628	Fusion With Defective Stereopsis
36629	Abnormal Retinal Correspondence
30753	Strabismus
30754	Non-Paralytic
36778	Esotropia
36844	Monocular
36845	With A Pattern
36846	With V Pattern
36847	With X Pattern
36848	With Y Pattern
36849	Intermittent
36850	Alternating
36851	With A Pattern
36852	With V Pattern
36853	With X Pattern
36854	With Y Pattern
36855	Intermittent
36779	Exotropia
36856	Monocular
36857	With A Pattern
36858	With V Pattern
36859	With X Pattern
36860	With Y Pattern
36861	Intermittent
36862	Alternating
36863	With A Pattern
36864	With V Pattern
36865	With X Pattern
36866	With Y Pattern
36867	Intermittent
36876	Cyclophoria
36877	Vertical
36878	Alternating
36780	Hypertropia
36868	Constant
36869	Intermittent
36870	Hypotropia
36871	Cyclotropia
36872	Monofixation Syndrome
36873	Heterophoria
36874	Esophoria
36875	Exophoria
30755	Paralytic
36879	Third Nerve Palsy
36880	Partial
36881	Total
36882	Fourth Nerve Palsy
36883	Sixth Nerve Palsy
36884	External Ophthalmoplegia
36885	Total Ophthalmoplegia
36777	Mechanical

36886	Brown's Tendon Sheath Syndrome
36887	Due To Other Musculofascial Disorders
36888	Limited Duction
36889	Duane's Syndrome
38557	Pseudoesotropia
90103	Eye Trauma
36318	Intraocular Foreign Body
37777	Magnetic
36319	Retained, Magnetic
36437	Anterior Chamber
36438	Iris
36439	Ciliary Body
36440	Lens
36441	Vitreous
36442	Posterior Wall
38636	Orbit
36443	Multiple Sites
36320	Retained, Nonmagnetic
36444	Anterior Chamber
36445	Iris
36446	Ciliary Body
36447	Lens
36448	Vitreous
36449	Posterior Wall
38637	Orbit
36450	Multiple Sites
36831	Retained, Old, Following Penetrating Wound
39623	Right Eye
39625	Left Eye
39626	Both Eyes
30729	Foreign Body - Eye
39745	Right Eye
39746	Left Eye
39748	Both Eyes
35736	Traumatic Blindness
39758	Right Eye
39760	Left Eye
39761	Both Eyes
38562	Eye Trauma
90100	Degree Of Visual Impairment; Field Defects
36646	Visual Impairment
36647	In One Eye
36648	Profound
36649	Moderate Or Severe
36650	In Both Eyes
36651	Profound
36652	Total Impairment In Both Eyes
36653	Better Eye: Near-Total
36654	Better Eye: Near-Total; Lesser Eye: Total

OPHTHALMOLOGY, CONT.

36655	Near-Total Impairment In Both Eyes	31227	Acute Serous
		37520	Allergic
36656	Better Eye: Profound Impairment	34062	Acute Mucoid
36657	Better Eye: Profound Impairment; Lesser Eye: Total	37521	Allergic
		34064	Acute Suppurative
36658	Better Eye: Profound Impairment; Lesser Eye: Near-Total	37530	With Spontaneous Rupture Of Ear Drum
36659	Profound Impairment In Both Eyes	37519	Acute Sanguinous
		37522	Allergic
36660	Moderate Or Severe In Better Eye; Lesser: Profound	34061	Chronic Serous
		37523	Chronic Mucoid
36661	Moderate Or Severe In Both Eyes	31228	Chronic Suppurative
36662	Legally Blind (USA Definition)	37531	Tubotympanic
39530	Right Eye	37532	Atticoantral
39531	Left Eye	31373	Tonsillitis
39532	Both Eyes	34114	Chronic
36630	Visual Field Defect	31301	Peritonsillar Abscess
36631	Central Scotoma	31284	Pharyngitis
36632	Centrocecal	31285	Adenovirus
36633	Paracentral	31286	Streptococcus, Group A: B Hemolytic
36634	Enlarged Blind Spot Syndrome		
36635	Sector Defect	38389	Chronic
36636	Generalized Contraction	38390	Recurrent
38667	**Otorhinolaryngology**	30950	Acute Lymphonodular (Coxsackie Virus)
31349	Sinusitis		
31350	Acute	31287	Gonococcus
34095	Maxillary	31288	Hemophilus Influenzae
34096	Frontal	34106	Chronic
34097	Ethmoidal	31317	Retropharyngeal Abscess
34098	Sphenoidal	34060	Acquired Stenosis Of External Ear Canal
34099	Pansinusitis		
31351	Chronic	34072	Labyrinthine Fistula
34109	Maxillary	37578	Round Window
34110	Frontal	37579	Oval Window
34111	Ethmoidal	37580	Semicircular Canal
34112	Sphenoidal	37581	Combined Sites
34113	Pansinusitis	34073	Labyrinthine Dysfunction
31071	Common Cold	37582	Hyperactive
31224	Otitis Externa	37588	Unilateral
31225	Malignant	37583	Bilateral
37508	Infective	37584	Hypoactive
37509	Chronic	37589	Unilateral
37510	Mycotic	37585	Bilateral
37517	Acute Swimmer's Ear	37586	Total Loss Of Reactivity
37511	Acute	37590	Unilateral
37512	Actinic	37587	Bilateral
37513	Chemical	30774	Otosclerosis
37514	Contact	37591	Oval Window, Nonobliterative
37515	Exzematoid	37592	Oval Window, Obliterative
37516	Reactive	37593	Cochlear
34963	Cerumen Impaction	37594	Otic Capsule
31226	Otitis Media	37595	Round Window
37518	Acute Nonsuppurative	30775	Foreign Body - Ear

OTORHINOLARYNGOLOGY, CONT.

31352	Submastoid Abscess		30783	Post Zero Gravity State
31180	Mastoiditis		30784	Congenital Deafness
34065	Acute		30785	Presbycusis
37533	Subperiosteal Mastoid Abscess		37596	Transient Ischemic Deafness
34066	Chronic		34076	Hearing Loss
37536	Postmastoidectomy Complications		34074	Conductive
37537	Mucosal Cyst		37598	External Ear
37538	Recurrent Cholesteatoma		37599	Tympanic Membrane
37539	Chronic Granulations		37600	Middle Ear
37540	Postauricular Fistula		37601	Inner Ear
37549	Tympanosclerosis		37602	Combined Sites
37550	Involving Membrane Only		34075	Sensorineural
37551	Involving Membrane And Ear Ossicles		37603	Sensory
			37604	Neural
37552	Involving Membrane, Ear Ossicles And Middle Ear		37605	Central
			37606	Combined Types
37556	Abnormality Of Middle Ear		34077	Mixed Conductive And Sensorineural
37557	Ankylosis Of Malleus			
37558	Ankylosis Of Ear Ossicles, Except Malleus		37607	Deaf Mutism
			30786	Tympanic Membrane Rupture
37559	Discontinuity Of Ear Ossicles		37542	Central
37560	Dislocation Of Ear Ossicles		37543	Attic
37561	Partial Loss Of Ear Ossicles		37544	Marginal
37562	Necrosis Of Ear Ossicles		37545	Multiple
37567	Cholesterin Granuloma		37546	Total
37568	Foreign Body Of Middle Ear		37547	Atrophic Flaccid Tympanic Membrane
31505	Cholesteatoma		37548	Atrophic Nonflaccid Tympanic Membrane
37563	Of Attic			
37564	Of Middle Ear		30787	Acoustic Trauma (Explosive)
37565	Of Middle Ear And Mastoid		30788	Noise-Induced Hearing Loss
37566	Diffuse Cholesteatosis		37597	Sudden Hearing Loss Of Unknown Etiology
34068	Myringitis			
34069	Acute		37529	Patulous Eustachian Tube
34070	Chronic		30789	Eustachian Tube Block
37541	Bullous		37526	Osseous
34071	Adhesive Otitis		37527	Intrinsic
37553	Drum Head To Incus		37528	Extrinsic
37554	Drum Head To Stapes		38479	Eustachian Tube Dysfunction
37555	Drum Head To Promontorium		34063	Eustachian Salpingitis
31229	Otitic Barotrauma		37524	Acute
30776	Polyp - External Auditory Meatus		37525	Chronic
30777	Labyrinthitis		30790	Rhinitis
37573	Suppurative		30791	Allergic
37574	Serous		39929	Pollen
37575	Viral		39931	Trees
37576	Toxic		39932	Grasses
37577	Circumscribed		39933	Ragweed
30778	Motion Sickness		39934	Animals
38062	Suffocation		39935	Cats
30779	Space Adaptation Syndrome		39936	Dogs
30780	Acute Space Motion Sickness		39937	Dust Mite
30781	Malaise		39938	Feathers
30782	Frank Sickness		39930	Kapok

OTORHINOLARYNGOLOGY, CONT.

30792	Medicamentosa
30793	Sicca
30794	Vasomotor
34107	Chronic
38388	Purulent
30795	Foreign Body - Nose
34104	Deviated Nasal Septum (Acquired)
30796	Cancrum Oris
31160	Ludwig's Angina
31161	Laryngitis
31162	Hemophilus Influenzae
36208	Tuberculous
34115	Chronic
34100	Acute Tracheitis
34101	With Obstruction
31163	Acute Laryngotracheitis
31164	With Obstruction
34116	Chronic Laryngotracheitis
31090	Epiglottitis
31091	With Obstruction
34102	Croup
34103	Acute Laryngopharyngitis
34117	Laryngeal Spasm
30797	Laryngeal Ulcer
30798	Oral Foreign Body
30799	Lingual Myositis
30800	Leukoplakia
30801	Foreign Body - Pharyngeal
33808	Foreign Body - Laryngeal
35585	Foreign Body - Tracheal
30802	Foreign Bodies - Bronchial
32884	Broncholithiasis
33801	Tracheal Perforation
33802	Iatrogenic
33803	Traumatic
33804	Pharyngeal Perforation
33805	Iatrogenic
33806	Traumatic
33807	Diverticular
30804	Vocal Cord Paralysis
30805	Glossitis
30806	Atrophic
30807	Stomatitis
30808	Alveolar Abscess
34158	Alveolitis Of Jaw
34159	Exostosis Of Jaw
30809	Aphthous Ulcer
30810	Pharyngeal Pouch
30811	Laryngocele
30812	Salivary Calculus
34160	Salivary Gland Abscess
31253	Suppurative Parotitis

30767	Temporomandibular Joint-Pain Dysfunction Syndrome
30813	Ill-Fitting Dentures
30814	Caries
30815	Dental Abscess
34151	With Sinus
30816	Unerupted 3rd Molar
30817	Impacted Tooth
34155	Acquired Absence Of Teeth
34156	Atrophy Of Edentulous Alveolar Ridge
34157	Retained Dental Root
34154	Gum And Periodontal Disease
30818	Gum Papilloma
30819	Gingivitis
30820	Acute
30821	Chronic
34152	Gingival Recession
34148	Pulpitis
34149	Acute
34150	Chronic
30822	Periodontitis
34145	Acute
34146	Acute Apical Of Pulpul Origin
34147	Chronic
34153	Periodontosis
30823	Pyorrhea Alveolaris

38666	**Cardiology**
35990	Normal Heart
39913	Conduction System
33193	ECG Normal Variant
35851	Rhythm Disorder
33185	Sinus Tachycardia
33471	Normal Response To Vigorous Exercise
33397	Sinus Bradycardia
33194	Enhanced Vagal Tone
36100	Sinoatrial Node Dysfunction
33407	Sick Sinus Syndrome
33393	Sinus Arrhythmia
33391	Sinoatrial Arrest
33392	Sinoatrial Block
33191	Supraventricular Tachycardia
33192	With Aberrant Conduction
33409	Paroxysmal Supraventricular Tachycardia
33176	Atrial Premature Complex
33177	With Block
33169	Wandering Atrial Pacemaker
33168	Automatic Atrial Tachycardia
33183	Paroxysmal Atrial Tachycardia
33184	With Block
33232	Atrial Tachycardia With Block
33179	Multifocal Atrial Tachycardia

CARDIOLOGY, CONT.

33166	Atrial Flutter
33167	With Block
33165	Atrial Fibrillation
33175	Bigeminal Rhythm
33174	Trigeminal Rhythm
33171	A-V Junctional Beats
33172	A-V Junctional Tachycardia
33173	With Block
33178	Ectopic Junctional Beats
33182	Ectopic Ventricular Beats
33240	Bundle Branch Block
33241	Complete Right
33242	Incomplete Right
33243	Complete Left
33244	Incomplete Left
33245	Left Anterior Hemiblock
33246	Left Posterior Hemiblock
33247	Bifasicular
33248	Trifascicular
33249	Intraventricular Conduction Delay
33234	A-V Block
33235	First Degree
33236	Second Degree
33237	Second Degree: Mobitz Type I
33238	Second Degree: Mobitz Type II
33239	Third Degree
33451	Complete Heart Block
33189	Ventricular Tachycardia
33190	Torsades De Pointes (Polymorphic)
33188	Cardiac Arrest
33186	Ventricular Fibrillation
33187	Asystole
33759	Electromechanical Dissociation
33170	Austin-Flint Murmur
33453	Stokes-Adams
33250	HIS Extra Systole
90004	Lenegre's Disease
33251	Lev's Disease
33252	Retrograde Concealed Conduction
33286	Hyperkinetic Heart Syndrome
33760	Pacemaker-Mediated Tachycardia
38068	During Procedure
33181	Prolonged QT Interval Syndrome
33408	Ventriculophasic Sinus Arrythmia
33435	Wolff-Parkinson-White Syndrome
33310	Lown-Ganong-Levine Syndrome
33287	Holt-Oram Syndrome
38225	Polydactyly - Syndactyly Syndrome
33398	Digitalis Effect
33180	Pacemaker Failure
38284	Implantable Automatic Defibrillator Malfunction
33164	A-V Dissociation

39914	Coronary Arteries
35988	Coronary Artery Disease
38160	Coronary Artery Spasm
38162	Coronary Collateral Circulation
37499	Coronary Arteriosclerosis
33228	Asymptomatic
37498	Calcific
33337	Anterolateral
33220	Beta-Blocker Withdrawal (Rebound Angina)
33221	Arteriosclerosis Obliterans
36038	Atypical Chest Pain
33706	Induced CPK Elevation
33215	Angina Pectoris
38678	Class I (Marked Exertion)
38679	Class II (Moderate Exertion)
38680	Class III (Mild Exertion)
38312	Class IV (At Rest)
33216	Crescendo
33217	Decubitus
33218	Prinzmetal's
33219	Unstable
38320	Atypical
33333	Myocardial Ischemia
33334	Anterior Wall
33335	Anteroseptal
38478	Septal
33336	Lateral
33338	Anteroapical
33339	Inferior Wall
38474	Inferoapical Wall
38475	Inferolateral Wall
38476	Inferoseptal Wall
38648	Infero-Septal-Apical
33340	Posterior Wall
38473	Apical Wall
33341	Subendocardial
38368	Silent
34083	Chronic Diffuse
33331	Papillary Muscle Dysfunction
38255	Hibernating Myocardium
33317	Acute Myocardial Infarction
35874	Left Ventricle
33318	Anterior Wall
35870	Anterobasal
33322	Anteroapical
33321	Anterolateral
35871	Antero-Lateral-Apical
33319	Anteroseptal
35872	Antero-Septal-Apical
33320	Lateral Wall
35873	Septal Wall
33323	Inferior Wall

CARDIOLOGY, CONT.

35875	Inferobasal	36042	Regional	
35876	Inferoapical	33468	Coronary Artery Stenosis	
35877	Inferolateral	33470	Left Main	
35878	Infero-Lateral-Apical	33469	Multi-Vessel	
35879	Inferoseptal	38241	3-Vessel	
38647	Infero-Septal-Apical	38242	Proximal	
33324	Posterior Wall	38243	Distal	
35880	Posteroapical	38244	2-Vessel	
35881	Posterolateral	38245	Proximal	
35885	Apical	38246	Distal	
35886	Apicoseptal	38247	Single Vessel	
38352	Apicolateral	38248	Coronary Bypass Graft Stenosis	
35869	Right Ventricle	38303	Autologous	
36039	Silent	38304	Nonautologous	
33325	Non-Q-Wave (Subendocardial)	38221	Ostial Stenosis	
35882	Papillary Muscle	38222	Coronary Ostial Membrane	
35883	Antero-Lateral	33441	Coronary Artery Embolism	
35884	Postero-Medial	33442	Coronary Artery Thrombosis	
33326	Atrial	37503	Traumatic Coronary Injury	
35908	Extension	38219	Multiple Coronary Aneurysms	
35887	Expansion	38220	Coronary Ectasia	
33327	Arrhythmias	39916	Myocardium	
33328	Cardiac Rupture	33263	Cardiomyopathy	
33329	Dressler's Syndrome	35909	Dilated	
33330	Septal Perforation	35910	Ischemic	
33332	Cardiogenic Shock	33265	Alcoholic	
38351	Prior Myocardial Infarction	38477	Postpartum	
38330	Anterior Wall	33264	Congestive	
38331	Anterobasal	35911	Diffuse	
38332	Anteroapical	35912	Segmental	
38333	Anterolateral	35913	Anterior	
38334	Antero-Lateral-Apical	35914	Inferior	
38335	Anteroseptal	35915	Lateral	
38336	Antero-Septal-Apical	35916	Apical	
38337	Lateral Wall	35917	Septal	
38338	Septal Wall	35918	Multiple Sites	
38339	Inferior Wall	35919	Non-Dilated	
38340	Inferobasal	33266	Restrictive	
38341	Inferoapical	35926	Infiltrative	
38342	Inferolateral	35927	Secondary To Amyloidosis	
38343	Infero-Lateral-Apical	35928	Secondary To Hemochromatosis	
38344	Inferoseptal	35929	Secondary To Sarcoidosis	
38649	Infero-Septal-Apical	33281	Endomyocardial Fibrosis	
38345	Posterior Wall	33279	Endocardial Fibroelastosis	
38353	Posteroapical	37465	Left Atrial	
38347	Posterolateral	37466	Right Atrial	
38348	Apical	37467	Left Ventricular	
38349	Apicoseptal	37468	Right Ventricular	
38346	Apicolateral	37469	Atrial Septal	
38350	Right Ventricle	37470	Ventricular Septal	
34082	Healed Previous Myocardial Infarction	37471	Venous	
36040	Cardiac Wall Motion Dysfunction	35920	Hypertrophic	
36041	Global	35921	Non-Obstructive	

CARDIOLOGY, CONT.

35922	Obstructive	33345		'Parachute' Mitral Valve
35923	Mid-Septal Variant	36031		Late Systolic
35924	Apical Variant	36032		Diastolic
35925	Myectomy / Myotomy Visualized	33348		Prolapsing Mitral Valve Leaflet Syndrome
33267	Obliterative			
35810	Familial Hypertrophic	33342		Mitral Annular Calcification
35930	Right Ventricular	36028		Mitral Sclerosis
33268	Congestive Heart Failure	33346		Mitral Stenosis
33269	Right-Sided	36034		Rheumatic
33270	Left-Sided	36033		Silent
33271	Combined	33745		With Pulmonary Fibrosis
36043	Cardiomegaly	36035		Cleft Mitral Valve
34081	Hypertensive Heart Disease	33375		Pulmonary Valve Insufficiency
33230	Athlete's Heart	33370		Pulmonary Valve Stenosis
33231	Physical Conditioning	33374		Congenital
33316	Myocardial Contusion	33373		Infundibular
38161	Myocardial Bridge	38254		Subpulmonic Obstruction
37266	Laceration Of Heart	38233		Pulmonary Artery Stenosis
37267	With Penetration Of Heart Chambers	38234		Supravalvular
37268	With Open Wound Into Thorax	38230		Main
37306	Gunshot Wound Of The Heart	38231		Left
35837	Myocardial Degeneration	38232		Right
30909	Chagas Disease	33371		Branch
30910	Acute	36095		Peripheral
30911	Chronic	33372		Pulmonary Vein Stenosis
33440	Marantic Endocarditis	38235		Left Superior
33349	Acute Myocarditis	38236		Left Inferior
37628	Idiopathic Myocarditis	38237		Right Superior
39915	Heart Valves	38238		Right Inferior
35999	Valvular Heart Disease	38239		Peripheral
39908	Primary	33421		Tricuspid Regurgitation
39909	Secondary	33422		Tricuspid Stenosis
36037	Multiple Valves	36036		Straddling Tricuspid Valve
33472	Functional Murmur	34079		Combined Mitral And Aortic Valvular Disease
33254	Aortic Regurgitation			
36027	Aortic Sclerosis	33257		Idiopathic Hypertrophic Subaortic Stenosis
33399	Aortic Stenosis			
33400	Calcific	37432		Prosthetic Valve Functioning Normally
33401	Congenital Subaortic Stenosis	37433		Aortic
33405	Congenital Valvular	37434		Mitral
33402	Congenital Supravalvular	37435		Pulmonary
33403	Congenital Discrete Subvalvular	37436		Tricuspid
36018	Discrete Subaortic Membrane	35989		Prosthetic Valve Malfunction
33404	Bicuspid Valve	37437		Aortic
36029	Unicuspid Valve	37438		Mitral
36030	Quadracuspid Valve	37439		Pulmonary
36058	Williams Syndrome	37440		Tricuspid
33406	Post-Operative Aortic Valve State	35991		Bacterial Endocarditis
33343	Mitral Regurgitation	31321		Acute
34549	Congenital	31322		Group A Strep
33344	Rupture Of Papillary Muscle	31323		Fungal
36044	Rupture Of Chordae	31324		Staph Aureus
36045	Papillary Muscle Dysfunction	31325		Subacute

CARDIOLOGY, CONT.

31326	Enterococcus	33205	Ventricular Aneurysm
31327	Fungal	36047	Left
31328	Serratia	36048	Right
31329	Staph Epidermidis	36088	Septal Wall
31330	Staph Aureus	36089	Atrial Aneurysm
31331	Strep Viridans	36090	Septal Wall
35992	Aortic	36091	Appendage
36023	Aortic Root Abscess	33206	Ventricular Pseudoaneurysm
35993	Mitral	39918	Pericardium
35994	Pulmonary	33456	Cardiac Tamponade
35995	Tricuspid	33353	Pericarditis
30901	Prosthetic Valve	35931	Constrictive
30902	Staphylococcus Aureus Coagulase Positive	35935	Acute
		33358	Subacute
30903	Pseudomonas	33362	Chronic
30904	Staphylococcus Epidermidis Coagulase Negative	35932	Restrictive
		35933	Effusive
30905	Staph Epidermidis	33360	Acute
30906	Enterococcus	33357	Subacute Effusive-Constrictive
36024	On Catheter	33359	Chronic
36025	Pacing	35934	Fibrinous
36026	Monitoring	33361	Acute
36046	Valvular Vegetation	35936	Subacute
31305	Rheumatic Fever	35937	Chronic
31306	Acute Rheumatic Carditis	33356	Chronic Adhesive
31307	Extracardiac	33355	Uremic
31308	Chronic Rheumatic Myocarditis	37501	Purulent
31309	Chronic Rheumatic Carditis	33354	Coxsackie Group B Virus
34078	Rheumatic Aortic Stenosis	33465	Pericardial Effusion
35985	Rheumatic Heart Disease	37500	Hemopericardium
33285	Graham-Steell Murmur	33047	Pericardial Cyst
39917	Heart Chambers	38215	Pericardial Disease
33427	Left Ventricular Hypertrophy	38216	Absent Pericardium
33428	Concentric	38217	Pericardial Defect
33429	Asymmetrical Septal Hypertrophy	38218	Pericardial Tumor
33430	Right Ventricular Hypertrophy	33288	Hypertension
33431	Combined Ventricular Hypertrophy	33291	Essential
33432	Right Atrial Enlargement	33293	Systolic
33433	Left Atrial Enlargement	33290	Diastolic
33434	Bi-Atrial Enlargement	34080	Benign
38317	Right Ventricular Enlargement	33289	Accelerated
38318	Left Ventricular Enlargement	33292	Malignant
36072	Ventricular Thrombosis	38503	Iatrogenic
36073	Left	39910	Secondary
36074	Right	39911	Benign
37472	Septal	39912	Malignant
33455	Atrial Thrombosis	33363	Pulmonary Hypertension
36075	Left	33364	Primary
36076	Left Appendage	33365	Veno-Occlusive Disease
37473	Septal	33366	Plexogenic Arteriopathy
36077	Right	33367	Secondary
36078	Right Appendage	35814	Persistent Of The Newborn
37502	Myocardial Foreign Body	35836	Congenital Heart Disease

CARDIOLOGY, CONT.

33452	Congenital Heart Block	35907	Double Outlet Of Left Ventricle
33162	Congenital Heart Defect	37497	Double Outlet From Outlet Chamber
33415	Tetralogy Of Fallot	38170	Abnormal Left Ventricle
36053	Left To Right Shunt	36056	Common Inlet Ventricle
36054	Right To Left Shunt	38197	LV Type
33223	Atrial Septal Defect	38198	No Rudimentary Chambers
33224	Ostium Secundum	38199	Hypoplastic Sub Pulmonary RV
33225	Ostium Primum	38200	Hypoplastic Sub Aortic RV
33226	Sinus Venosus	38201	Hypoplastic Double Outlet RV
35945	Coronary Sinus	38202	RV Type
35946	Fenestrated	38203	No Rudimentary Chambers
35947	Restrictive	38204	Hypoplastic LV Present
35948	Residual / Recurrent	38205	Undifferentiated
35949	Common Atrium	37453	Double Inlet Ventricle
35898	Aortic Atresia	38174	LV Type
35902	Subaortic Atresia	38177	No Rudimentary Chambers
33466	Truncus Arteriosis	38178	Hypoplastic Sub Pulmonary RV
35899	Mitral Atresia	38179	Hypoplastic Sub Aortic RV
36055	Absent Pulmonary Valve Syndrome	38180	Hypoplastic Double Outlet RV
33369	Pulmonary Atresia	38181	RV Type
35903	Subpulmonary Atresia	38182	No Rudimentary Chambers
35900	Left A-V Valve Atresia	38183	Hypoplastic LV Present
33413	Tricuspid Atresia	38184	Undifferentiated
35892	With Pulmonary Atresia (Type I-A)	38188	Single Inlet Ventricle
35893	With Pulmonary Stenosis (Type I-B)	38186	LV Type
35894	Without Pulmonary Stenosis (Type I-C)	38189	No Rudimentary Chambers
		38190	Hypoplastic Sub Pulmonary RV
35895	With Transposed Great Arteries And Pulmonary Atresia (Type II-A)	38191	Hypoplastic Sub Aortic RV
		38192	Hypoplastic Double Outlet RV
35896	With Transposed Great Arteries And Pulmonary Stenosis (Type II-B)	38193	RV Type
		38194	No Rudimentary Chambers
35897	With Transposed Great Arteries But No Pulmonary Stenosis (Type II-C)	38195	Hypoplastic LV Present
		38196	Undifferentiated
35901	Right A-V Valve Atresia	37454	Common Atrioventricular Inlet
35904	Double Inlet A-V Valve Atresia	35982	Morphologic Left Ventricular Hypertrophy
33278	Endocardial Cushion Defect		
33262	Hypoplastic Left Heart Syndrome	35983	Morphologic Right Ventricular Hypertrophy
38159	Hypoplastic Valve		
35950	Atrioventricular Canal	35984	Hypertrophied Common Ventricle
35954	Partial	37457	Single Outlet Heart
35955	Complete	37455	Absence Of One Atrioventricular Connection
35956	Type A		
35957	Type B	37456	Criss-Cross Atrioventricular Relationship
35958	Type C		
35959	Univentricular Heart	37452	Atrioventricular Ambiguous
35960	Type A-I	37448	Atrioventricular Concordance
35961	Type A-II	37449	Atrioventricular Discordance
35962	Type A-III	37450	Ventriculo-Great Artery Concordance
35963	Obstructed Outlet Foramen	37451	Ventriculo-Great Artery Discordance
35964	Non-Obstructed Outlet	33426	Ventricular Septal Defect
35965	Type A-IV	35967	Inflow Muscular
35966	Type C	35968	Trabecular Muscular
35906	Double Outlet Of Right Ventricle	35969	Outflow Muscular

CARDIOLOGY, CONT.

35970	Paramembranous Muscular	33444	Aberrant Right Subclavian Artery
35971	Supracristal	33445	Double Aortic Arch
35972	Paramembranous Restrictive	33446	Right Sided Aortic Arch
35973	Outflow Restrictive	37654	Dextraposition Of Aorta
35974	Malalignment Inflow	37655	Overriding Aorta
35975	Malalignment Outflow	33277	Ebstein's Anomaly
35976	Multiple	35905	Criss-Cross Heart
35977	Residual	35986	Shone's Anomaly
35978	Recurrent	38323	Cardiac Neoplasm
36059	Cor Biloculare	33299	Benign
36057	Paradoxical Emboli	38206	Unspecified
33283	Ellis-van Creveld	38207	Left Atrial
38229	Gargoyle Syndrome	38208	Right Atrial
33275	Cor Triatriatum	38209	Left Ventricular
37445	Ectopic Cordis	38210	Right Ventricular
33276	Dextrocardia	38212	Atrial Septal
37446	Levocardia	38213	Ventricular Septal
37447	Mesocardia	38211	Venous
33280	Uhl's Anomaly (RV Hypoplasia)	35888	Myxoma
33272	Noonan's Syndrome	33300	Left Atrial
36123	Orthodeoxia	35889	Right Atrial
33273	Coarctation Of The Aorta	35890	Left Ventricular
38314	Hypoplastic Aortic Arch	35891	Right Ventricular
36060	Interrupted Aortic Arch	37463	Atrial Septal
36019	Congenital Absence Of Pericardium	37464	Ventricular Septal
33274	Congenital Pulmonary Vein Stenosis	37481	Venous
33351	Patent Foramen Ovale	33301	Lipoma
33352	Patent Ductus Arteriosus	35944	Myocardial Fibroma
33227	Aorticopulmonary Septal Defect	37474	Left Atrial
36092	Anomalous Pulmonary Venous Return	37475	Right Atrial
33255	Partial	37476	Left Ventricular
33412	Total	37477	Right Ventricular
37441	Right Ventricular Outflow Tract Anomaly	37478	Atrial Septal
		37479	Ventricular Septal
37442	Left Ventricular Outflow Tract Anomaly	37480	Venous
		35951	Papilloma
33376	Partial Transposition Of The Pulmonary Veins	35952	Multiple Intracardiac
		37482	Hamartoma
37443	Congenital Anomaly Of Coronary Artery	37483	Left Atrial
		37484	Right Atrial
33256	Anomalous Pulmonary Origin Of Coronary Artery	37485	Left Ventricular
		37486	Right Ventricular
33767	Anomalous Origin Of Left Coronary Artery From Right Cusp	37487	Atrial Septal
		37488	Ventricular Septal
33378	Complete Transposition Of The Great Arteries	37489	Venous
		33303	Rhabdomyoma
33379	Corrected	37490	Left Atrial
38171	Complete Transposition Of The Great Vessels	37491	Right Atrial
		37492	Left Ventricular
38172	Levorotation	37493	Right Ventricular
38173	Dextrorotation	37494	Atrial Septal
34886	Coronary Artery Arising From Left Aortic Sinus Of Valsalva	37495	Ventricular Septal
		37496	Venous

CARDIOLOGY, CONT.

35953	Multiple	33380	Raynaud's Disease
33302	Papillary Fibroelastoma	33383	Raynaud's Phenomenon
33304	Malignant	34824	Vibration White Finger
33305	Angiosarcoma	33411	Thromboangiitis Obliterans (Buerger's Disease)
33306	Rhabdomyosarcoma		
33307	Mesothelioma	33282	Erythromelalgia
33308	Fibrosarcoma	33385	Rubenstein-Taybi Syndrome
38886	Location	33436	Avascular Necrosis
38887	Endocardium	33437	Carotid Cavernous Sinus Fistula
38888	Epicardium	33438	Carotid Sinus Syndrome
38889	Myocardium	33439	Carotid Stenosis
38890	Pericardium	33347	Subclavian Stenosis
38891	Right Ventricle	38315	Brachiocephalic Stenosis
38892	Left Ventricle	34720	Basilar Artery Stenosis
38893	Right Atrium	33195	Vertebral Artery Stenosis
38894	Left Atrium	33309	Leriche Syndrome
38895	Overlapping Lesion Of Heart, Mediastinum, And Pleura	33447	Inferior Vena Cava Syndrome
		33448	Renal Infarction
35979	Heart Disease Secondary To Carcinoid Tumor	33450	Hypersensitivity Angiitis
		33163	Acrocyanosis
39920	Vasculature	33311	Livedo Reticularis
33454	Subclavian Steal Syndrome	37090	Atrophie Blanche
38490	Vertebrobasilar Artery Syndrome	33386	Omphalitis
38321	Intermittent Claudication	36066	Aortic Artery Thrombosis
33229	Atherosclerosis	36067	Ascending
38290	Aorta	36068	Aortic Arch
38291	Extremities	36069	Descending
38292	With Intermittent Claudication	36070	Abdominal
38293	With Rest Pain	36071	Pulmonary Artery Thrombosis
38294	With Ulcerations	36119	Main
38295	With Gangrene	36120	Saddle
38296	Of A Bypass Graft Of The Extremities	36121	Right
		36122	Left
38297	Autologous	33449	Vena Caval Thrombosis
38298	Nonautologous	36064	Inferior
38163	Atherosclerotic Ulcers	36065	Superior
35852	Acute Ischemia	33384	Femoral Vein Thrombosis
35853	Upper Limb	33387	Portal Vein Thrombosis
35854	Lower Limb	33388	Renal Vein Thrombosis
38319	Pulmonary Artery Enlargement	33390	Veno-Occlusive Disease
38214	Venous Thrombosis	33394	Scalenus Anticus Syndrome
36101	Thrombus On Catheter	33832	Pulmonary Arteriovenous Fistula
36102	Vegetation On Catheter	33410	Takayasu's Disease
38065	Dialysis Catheter - Mechanical Complication	33831	Pulmonary Vein Varicosity
		33315	Monckeberg's Arteriosclerosis
33841	Pulmonary Artery Dilation	33395	Shock
33892	Azygos / Hemiazygos Venous Dilation	33396	Hemorrhagic
33368	Postphlebitis Syndrome	38504	Postoperative
33259	Coronary Arteriovenous Fistula	33294	Renal Artery Stenosis
33258	Pulmonary Coronary Fistula	33295	Renal Artery Hyperplasia
33381	Chilblains (Pernio)	33296	Renal Arterial Occlusion
37151	Erythrocyanosis	33816	Renal Artery Aneurysm
33382	Thoracic Outlet Syndrome	33297	Celiac Artery Compression Syndrome

CARDIOLOGY, CONT.

33457	Arterial Embolism	38307	Brachial Artery Aneurysm
33458	Upper Extremity	38308	Radial Artery Aneurysm
34088	Iliac Artery	38309	Ulnar Artery Aneurysm
33459	Femoral Artery	33211	Iliac Artery Aneurysm
33460	Popliteal Artery	34086	Femoral Artery Aneurysm
33462	Cavernous Sinus Thrombosis	34087	Popliteal Artery Aneurysm
38583	Ophthalmic Artery Occlusion	36051	Coronary Artery Aneurysm
33463	Central Retinal Artery Occlusion	33212	Subclavian Artery Aneurysm
38612	Septic Embolus	36052	Pulmonary Artery Aneurysm
38611	Of Retina / Choroid	33213	Acute Arterial Occlusion
36456	Retinal Arterial Branch Occlusion	33214	Aortitis
33464	Retinal Vein Occlusion	33222	Aortic Sinus Aneurysm
36457	Central	38240	With Fistula
36458	Venous Tributary	33233	Anterior Tibial Compartment Syndrome
38587	Partial		
38586	Normal Variant Of Retinal Venous Circulation	33253	Arteriovenous Fistula
		38064	Mechanical Complication
38588	Post-Laser Retinal Condition	33260	Capillary Leak Syndrome
33467	Eisenmenger Syndrome	33261	Cavernous Hemangioma
33473	Inferior Vena Cava Obstruction	35855	Deep Venous Insufficiency
38316	Mesenteric Artery Stenosis	33791	Chronic Venous Insufficiency
33474	Mesenteric Vein Thrombosis	33423	Varicose Veins
33913	Mesenteric Vasculitis	33424	Primary
33475	Aneurysm Sinus Of Valsalva	33425	Secondary
33476	Rupture	34094	With Ulcer And Inflammation
33477	Splenic Vein Thrombosis	33312	Lymphedema
33196	Dissection	33313	Milroy's Disease
36017	Of The Aorta	33314	Postmastectomy Syndrome
33197	Type I	33478	Blood Vessel Injury
33198	Type II	33479	Carotid Artery
33199	Descending Aorta - Type III	33480	Internal Jugular Vein
38289	Abdominal Aorta	33481	External Jugular Vein
37504	Of A Coronary Artery	33482	Thoracic Aorta
37505	On The Right Only	33483	Superior Vena Cava
37506	On The Left Only	33484	Pulmonary Artery
37507	Bilaterally	33485	Pulmonary Vein
33200	Carotid Artery	33486	Abdominal Aorta
33201	Vertebral Artery	33487	Inferior Vena Cava
36049	Aortic Aneurysm	38066	Umbrella Device, Vena Cava - Mechanical Complication
35856	Thoracic Aorta		
36050	Aortic Root	33488	Gastric Artery
33207	Ascending	33489	Hepatic Artery
33210	Aortic Arch	33490	Splenic Artery
33209	Descending	33491	Superior Mesenteric Artery
33208	Abdominal Aorta	33492	Inferior Mesenteric Artery
38301	Thoracoabdominal Aorta	33493	Superior Mesenteric Vein
33787	Ruptured Aortic Aneurysm	33494	Inferior Mesenteric Vein
38299	Thoracic	33495	Portal Vein
33204	Ascending	33496	Splenic Vein
38300	Descending	33497	Renal Artery
33203	Abdominal	33498	Renal Vein
38302	Thoracoabdominal	33499	Hypogastric Artery
38306	Axillary Artery Aneurysm	33500	Hypogastric Vein

CARDIOLOGY, CONT.

33501	Iliac Artery
33502	Iliac Vein
33503	Uterine Artery
33504	Uterine Vein
33505	Ovarian Artery
33506	Ovarian Vein
33507	Axillary Artery
33508	Axillary Vein
33509	Brachial Blood Vessel
33510	Radial Blood Vessel
33511	Ulnar Blood Vessel
33512	Palmar Artery
33513	Digital Blood Vessel
33514	Common Femoral Artery
33515	Superficial Femoral Artery
33516	Femoral Veins
33517	Saphenous Veins
33518	Popliteal Artery
33519	Popliteal Vein
33520	Tibial Vessels
33521	Deep Plantar Blood Vessel
33414	Trench Foot
33416	Thrombophlebitis
33417	Of Lower Extremity Superficial Vessels
34089	Femoropopliteal Vein
34090	Saphenous Vein
33418	Of Lower Extremity Deep Vessels
34091	Femoral Vein
34092	Popliteal Vein
34093	Tibial Vein
37629	Of Superficial Veins Of Upper Extremities
37630	Of Deep Veins Of Upper Extremities
33419	Migratory
33389	Budd-Chiari Syndrome
31731	Trousseau's Syndrome
33420	Peri-Menstrual Edema
39921	Other Conditions
35996	Cardiac Neurosis
33202	Aneurysm, NOS
35997	Post-Operative Heart Disease
35998	Valvular
36000	Congenital
36113	Heart Transplant Candidate
36114	Heart Transplant Donor
36115	Heart Transplant Recipient
38023	Heart Valve Transplant Recipient
36116	Lung Transplant Candidate
36117	Lung Transplant Donor
36118	Lung Transplant Recipient
37444	Postoperative Cardiac Repair
33161	Heart Disease

32874	**Pulmonary Medicine**
35857	Reactive Airway Disease
32881	Asthma
34127	Extrinsic
34128	Intrinsic
33783	Exercise-Induced
32882	Occupational
33784	Baker's
32887	Byssinosis
32883	Diisocyanates
34827	Laboratory Worker's
34825	Western Red Cedar
33071	Status Asthmaticus
32889	Tungsten Carbide Obstructive Airway Syndrome
32875	Amniotic Fluid Embolism
34345	Puerperal Pulmonary Embolism
35544	Obstetrical Septic Embolism
32876	Adult Respiratory Distress Syndrome
34823	Post
32890	Acute Bronchitis
32877	Acute Respiratory Failure
36016	Chronic Respiratory Failure
32878	Acute Ventilatory Failure
35754	Respiratory Arrest
32879	Acute Berylliosis
35757	Pulmonary Hypoplasia
32885	Bronchiolitis
32886	Bronchopulmonary Sequestration
34122	Chronic Obstructive Pulmonary Disease
32891	Chronic Bronchitis
34873	Acute Exacerbation
34123	Simple
34124	Mucopurulent
34125	Diffuse Obstructive
34826	Asthmatic
32998	Emphysema
33002	Hereditary (Alpha 1-Antitrypsin Deficiency)
34126	Bleb Emphysema
33001	Subcutaneous Emphysema
30986	Influenza
30987	Type A
30988	Type B
30989	Type C
30990	Parainfluenza
90252	Haemophilus Influenzae Type B
31256	Mycoplasma Pneumonia (Primary Atypical)
31257	Bacterial Pneumonia
31259	Pneumococcal (Streptococcus Pneumoniae)

PULMONARY MEDICINE, CONT.

90250	Drug Resistant	32917	Chronic Berylliosis
31260	Streptococcal Group A	32918	Diatomaceous Earth Disease
35224	Salmonella	32919	Rare Earth
31264	Staphylococcal	32920	Fuller's Earth
31267	Geriatric Presentation	32921	Antimony
31265	Gram Negative	32922	Tin (Stannosis)
31261	Klebsiella	32923	Kaolinosis
31262	Pseudomonas	32924	Bakelite
31263	Hemophilus Influenzae	32925	Mica
34821	Acinetobacter	32926	Nepheline
31266	Neisseria Meningiditis	32927	Mullite
31268	Legionnaire's Disease	32928	Carbon / Graphite
31258	Pittsburgh Pneumonia Agent (L. micdadei)	32929	Thesaurosis
		32930	Tungsten Carbide
31270	Viral Pneumonia	32931	Titanium Dust
34119	Respiratory Syncytial Virus	32932	Zirconium
34118	Adenovirus	32933	Sillimanite
34120	Parainfluenza Virus	32934	Inhalation Of Noxious Gases
33900	Varicella	32935	HCl Gas
31271	Fungal Pneumonia	32936	Nitric Oxide
31272	Cryptococcal	32937	Nitrous Oxide
31273	Pulmonary Mucormycosis (Zygomycosis)	32938	Picric Acid
		32939	Ammonia
32880	Aspiration Pneumonia	32940	Bromine
34121	Bronchopneumonia	32941	Carbon Tetrachloride
32892	Chylothorax	32942	Hydrogen Sulfide
32893	Pseudo-Chylothorax	32943	Paraquat
32894	Cor Pulmonale	32944	Formaldehyde
32895	Chronic Obstructive	32945	Kerosene
32896	Chronic Mountain Sickness	32946	Methane
32897	Dung Lung	32947	Chlorine
32898	Ondine's Curse	32948	Diesel Emissions
33869	Benign Asbestos Pleural Effusion	32949	Excessive Heat
33870	Asbestos Pleural Plaques	32950	Polytetrafluoroethylene
32899	Pneumoconiosis	32951	Polyvinyl Chloride
32900	Shaver's Disease (Bauxite)	32952	Sulphur Dioxide
32901	Cement	32953	Smoke
32902	Fibrous Erionite	32954	Nitrogen Dioxide
32903	Aluminum Lung	32955	Ozone
32904	Aluminum Fibrosis	32956	Osmium Bronchitis
32905	Hematite	32957	Trimelitic Anhydride Pneumonitis
32906	Mixed Dust	32958	Phosgenes
32907	Polyvinyl Chloride	32959	Hydrogen Fluoride Gas
32908	Shale	32960	Pneumonitis
32909	Coal Workers' (Uncomplicated)	32961	Inhalation Of Metal Fumes
32910	Coal Workers' (Complicated)	32962	Barium
32911	Talc	32963	Cadmium
32912	Baritosis	32964	Copper
32913	Siderosis (Arc Welder's Disease)	32965	Iron
32914	Silver Polisher's Lung	32966	Magnesium
32915	Asbestosis	32967	Mercury
32916	Silicosis	32968	Manganese
35009	Fulminant Silicosis	32969	Nickel

PULMONARY MEDICINE, CONT.

32970	Silver		33747	Post Pulmonary Infarction
32971	Selenium		33880	Mediastinal Lipomatosis
32972	Vanadium		31220	Infectious Mediastinitis
32973	Zinc		37269	Contusion Of Lung
32974	Hypersensitivity Pneumonitis		37271	With Open Wound Into Thorax
32975	"Air-Conditioning"		37270	Laceration Of Lung
32976	Furrier's Lung		37272	With Open Wound Into Thorax
32977	Fish Meal Worker's Lung		37308	Gunshot Wound Of The Lung
32978	Cheese Worker's Lung		32490	Crushed Chest
32979	Suberosis		33748	Post Chest Trauma
32980	Wood Dust		33842	Mediastinal Hematoma
32981	Sequoiosis		33897	Post Mediastinal Hematoma
32982	Maple Bark Disease		38069	Post-Operative Hematoma
32983	Detergent Worker's Lung		33896	Post Thoracic Surgery
32984	Pituitary Snuff Taker's Lung		34141	Post Tracheostomy
32985	Wood Pulp Worker's Lung		34142	Hemorrhage
32986	Bagassosis		34143	Obstruction
32987	Bird Fancier's Disease		34144	Sepsis
32988	Mushroom Grower's Disease		33749	Post Pulmonary Resection
32989	Maltworker's Lung		33873	Post Cardiac Surgery
32990	Farmer's Lung		33017	Hydrothorax
32991	Coffee Workers' Lung		34129	Postinflammatory Pulmonary Fibrosis
32992	"Doghouse Disease"		33019	Diffuse Interstitial Fibrosis
32993	Wheat Weevil Disease		33020	Idiopathic Pulmonary Fibrosis
32994	Animal Handler's Lung		33021	Usual Interstitial Pneumonia
32995	Paint Refinisher's Disease			(Carrington-Liebow)
32996	Plastic Worker's Lung		33022	Desquamative Interstitial Pneumonia
32997	Tungsten Carbide		33027	Idiopathic Pulmonary Hemosiderosis
31269	Chronic Eosinophilic Pneumonia		33023	Lymphoid Interstitial Pneumonia
33004	Eosinophilic Pulmonary Reactions		33061	Pulmonary Alveolar Proteinosis
33003	Alpha 1-Antitrypsin Deficiency		33024	Bronchiolitis Obliterans
33005	Diaphragmatic Displacement		33025	Giant Cell Interstitial Pneumonia
33006	Diaphragmatic Eventration		33026	Lymphoplasmacytic Interstitial
33007	Diaphragmatic Congenital Absence			Pneumonia
33008	Diaphragmatic Rupture		33028	Kartagener's Syndrome
33009	Fat Embolism		33029	Lipoid Pneumonia
33010	Fibrosing Mediastinitis		33030	Loeffler's Syndrome
33011	Drug Induced Hypersens. Lung Disease		33888	Hemangioma
			33889	Mediastinal Gasteroenteric Cyst
33012	Pulmonary Edema: Non-Cardiac		33890	Mediastinal Neurenteric Cyst
33013	Pulmonary Edema: Acute Cardiac		33062	Pickwickian Syndrome
33018	Hyperventilation Syndrome		33063	PIE Syndrome
31174	Lung Abscess		33064	Pleuritis
33746	Post Pneumonia State		33065	Pleural Effusion
33871	Post Empyema State		36013	Right-Sided
33823	Post Lung Abscess		36014	Left-Sided
33824	Post Septic Embolism		36015	Bilateral
33826	Post Tuberculosis State		33066	Pulmonary Embolism
33825	Post Histoplasmosis		33067	Multiple
37975	Non-Hodgkin's Lymphoma		33068	Septic
33895	Hodgkin's Disease - Post Treatment		38488	Iatrogenic
33827	Post Coccidioidomycosis		33877	Pulmonary Infarction
33828	Post Chicken Pox		38489	Iatrogenic

PULMONARY MEDICINE, CONT.

33443	Air Emboli		38485	Vibrio Parahaemolyticus
33069	Radiation Pneumonitis		38486	Vibrio Vulnificus
33898	Radiation Pulmonary Fibrosis		31119	Gastroenteritis
33899	Post Mediastinal Radiation		31120	Pseudomonas
33070	Sleep Apnea		31121	Staphylococcus Aureus
33072	Superior Vena Cava Syndrome		36193	Enteropathogenic E. Coli
33073	Weingarten's Syndrome		36194	Enteroinvasive E. Coli
33074	Respiratory Acidosis		36195	Enterohemorrhagic E. Coli
33075	Respiratory Alkalosis		90253	Serotype O157:H7
33076	Pneumothorax		31122	Clostridia
33077	Secondary		34132	Cytomegalovirus
33078	Tension		31128	Toxigenic E. Coli
33079	Spontaneous		31123	Campylobacter
33080	Traumatic		31129	Yersinia Enterocolitica
37262	With Open Wound Into Thorax		36196	Gram-Negative Enteritis
38274	Iatrogenic		35227	Viral
36206	Tuberculous		31125	Enterovirus
31092	Empyema		31126	Reovirus
31093	Group A Streptococcus		31127	Rotavirus
31094	Pneumococcus		36197	Adenovirus
31095	Klebsiella Pneumoniae		36198	Norwalk Virus
31096	Anaerobic		36199	Small Round Virus
31097	Fusobacterium		36200	Calcivirus
31098	Staphylococcus		36201	Astrovirus
31099	Tuberculous		36202	Torovirus
31100	Bacteroides		31124	Vibrio Parahemolyticus
33083	Pyopneumothorax		31130	Shigellosis (Bacillary Dysentery)
33014	Hemothorax		36185	Shigella Dysenteriae
33015	Traumatic		36186	Shigella Flexneri
37263	With Open Wound Into Thorax		36187	Shigella Boydii
33872	Post Hemothorax		36188	Shigella Sonnei
37264	Pneumohemothorax		31131	Giardiasis
37265	With Open Wound Into Thorax		34133	Isosporiasis
33016	Fibrothorax		31132	Cryptosporidiosis
33000	Mediastinal Emphysema		31133	Chronic
32999	Interstitial Emphysema		36192	Protozoal Intestinal Disease
33789	Pneumopericardium		90241	Esophagus
33081	Bronchiectasis		30002	Achalasia
36205	Tuberculous		30003	Cricopharyngeal Achalasia
33082	Decompression Sickness		30084	Diffuse Esophageal Spasm
33084	Tracheal Stenosis		30081	Dysphagia Lusoria
33085	Bronchial Stenosis		30091	Iatrogenic Dysphagia
33086	Atelectasis		30086	Esophagitis
33829	Round		30087	Acute
33876	Right Middle Lobe Syndrome		30088	Chronic Reflux
34165	**Gastroenterology**		30089	Corrosive
90242	Gastrointestinal Infections		30090	Radiation
33942	Food Poisoning		38250	Esophageal Reflux
38483	Bacterial		30036	Acute Variceal Hemorrhage
30941	Botulism		30096	Esophageal Ulcer
38484	Clostridium		30097	Drug Induced
35225	Clostridium Perfringens		35518	Acute, With Hemorrhage
33941	Staphylococcal			

GASTROENTEROLOGY, CONT.

35519	Acute, With Perforation		37634	Due To H. Pylori
35520	Chronic, With Hemorrhage		30006	Hemorrhagic
35521	Chronic, With Perforation		30007	Hypertrophic
30100	Esophageal Varices		30008	Alcoholic
35067	With Hemorrhage		30009	Phlegmonous
38249	Esophageal Hemorrhage		35513	Chronic Atrophic
38251	Esophageal Leukoplakia		30010	Fundal Gland
30103	Barrett's Esophagus		30011	Chronic Antral
30217	Post-Nissen Repair		35522	Radiation
30101	Lower Esophageal Ring		35515	Achlorhydria
30102	Esophageal Web		30170	Hypersecretory Gastropathy
30092	Esophageal Stricture		30134	Gastric Varices
30181	Kelly-Patterson (Plummer-Vinson)		35068	With Hemorrhage
	Syndrome		30128	Gastric Eosinophilic Granuloma
30076	Esophageal Diverticulum		30202	Postgastrectomy Syndrome
30077	Pulsion		30203	Gastritis
30078	Traction		30204	Malabsorption
30079	Perforated		30205	Afferent Loop Obstruction
30075	Zenker's Diverticulum		30206	Jejunogastric Intussusception
33810	Perforated		30207	Retained Antrum
30074	Epiphrenic Diverticula		30208	Retroanastamotic Herniation
30083	Esophageal Foreign Body		30209	Dumping Syndrome
30085	Esophageal Perforation		30210	Late Postprandial
30094	Iatrogenic Esophageal Perforation		30211	Anemia
30082	Boerhaave's Syndrome		30191	Menetrier's Disease
30093	Mallory-Weiss Syndrome		30139	Antral Web
35863	Gastrointestinal Bleeding		34976	Gastric Perforation
30292	Upper Tract		30073	Gastric Diverticula
30143	Hiatal Hernia		33811	Perforated
30144	Paraesophageal		30105	Stomach Laceration
30145	Sliding		30080	Gastrointestinal Duplication
30146	Diaphragmatic Hernia		33878	Gastroenteric Cyst
35561	Gangrenous		30212	Postvagotomy Syndrome
35565	With Obstruction		30221	Peptic Ulcer
33843	Foramen Of Morgagni		30227	Gastric
33844	Foramen Of Bochdalek		34161	Acute, With Hemorrhage
90244	Gastrum And Duodenum		34162	Acute, With Perforation
35514	Persistent Vomiting (Nongravida)		34163	Chronic, With Hemorrhage
30136	Gastric Volvulus		35501	Chronic, With Perforation
30135	Volvulus		30228	Antral
30012	Acute Gastric Dilation		33925	Pre-Pyloric
30025	Gastric Outlet Obstruction		30225	Pyloric Channel
35557	Gastroptosis		30229	Gastrojejunal
35558	Gastric Hourglass Stricture		35509	Acute, With Hemorrhage
30166	Pyloric Stenosis		35510	Acute, With Perforation
30167	Adult Hypertrophic		35511	Chronic, With Hemorrhage
30168	Congenital		35512	Chronic, With Perforation
34942	Pylorospasm		30222	Duodenal
30104	Foreign Body - Stomach		30223	Acute, With Hemorrhage
30037	Bezoars		34164	Acute, With Perforation
33882	Hair Ball (Trichobezoar)		30224	Chronic, With Hemorrhage
30004	Gastritis		35502	Chronic, With Perforation
30005	Acute Erosive		30226	Zollinger-Ellison Syndrome

GASTROENTEROLOGY, CONT.

30230	Drug Induced	30286	Crohn's Disease Of The Appendix
30231	Stress Induced	30287	Diffuse Granulomatous Jejunoileitis
30232	Perforated	30288	Crohn's (Granulomatous) Colitis
30233	Hemorrhage	30194	Nongranulomatous Ulcerative Jejunoileitis
33927	Duodenitis		
35516	Acute	34131	Foreign Body - Small Intestine
35517	Chronic	30129	Gallstone Ileus
30070	Duodenal Diverticulosis	30293	Ileus
33814	Perforated	38024	Post Ileostomy
30140	Duodenal Web	38493	Enterostomy Complication
30017	Meconium Obstruction	38494	Infection
90243	Jejunum And Ileum	30106	Small Intestine Laceration
30239	Radiation Enteritis	37273	Duodenal
30240	Small Bowel Bacterial Overgrowth	37274	With Open Wound Into Cavity
30040	Malabsorption Syndrome	37305	Gunshot Wound Of Small Intestine
30041	Malnutrition (Insufficient/Improper)	30279	Post Small Intestine Resection
30182	Lactase Deficiency Syndrome	34135	Intestinal Pseudopolyps
30183	Primary	30034	Appendicitis
30184	Secondary	35559	With Generalized Peritonitis
30099	Eosinophilic Enteritis	35560	Chronic
30192	Nontropical (Celiac) Sprue	33924	Gangrenous
30193	Collagenous Sprue	36177	Amebic
30291	Tropical Sprue	30033	Appendiceal Abscess
30259	Whipple's Disease	37340	Laceration Of The Appendix
30071	Multiple Jejunal Diverticulosis	37341	Gunshot Wound Of The Appendix
33813	Perforated	90245	Colon And Rectum
30072	Meckel's Diverticulosis	30185	Megacolon
33812	Perforated	30186	Aganglionic (Hirschsprung's Disease)
30043	Chronic Arterial Insufficiency Of Bowel	30187	Acute Toxic
30014	Acute Bowel Ischemia / Infarction	30188	Chronic Idiopathic (Psychogenic)
35573	Duodenal Varices	30189	Acquired
35574	With Hemorrhage	34559	Colonic Stricture
30015	Chronic Intestinal Pseudo-Obstruction	34170	Atony Of Colon
30195	Pneumatosis Cystoides Intestinalis	30018	Ogilvie's Syndrome
30179	Intussusception	30171	Antibiotic Associated Colitis
34134	Intestinal Malrotation	30172	Radiation Colitis
35845	Congenital Volvulus	30173	Ischemic Colitis
30022	Small Bowel Stricture	30174	Acute Fulminating
30023	Stenosis Of Small Intestine	30175	Subacute
30013	Acute Mesenteric Lymphadenitis	30176	Ulcerative Colitis
30016	Acute Intestinal Obstruction	38275	Enterocolitis
35844	Infantile Colic	38276	Ileocolitis
30241	Intramural Small Intestinal Hemorrhage	38277	Left-Sided
		38278	Pancolitis
30200	Blind Loop Syndrome	38280	Pseudopolyposis Of The Colon
30201	Short Bowel Syndrome	30213	Post-Ureterosigmoidostomy Syndrome
30275	Peutz-Jeghers Syndrome	30214	Protein Losing Enteropathy
30281	Regional Enteritis (Crohn's Ileitis)	30019	Colon Obstruction
30282	Crohn's Disease Of The Esophagus	30044	Chronic Constipation
30283	Crohn's Disease Of The Stomach	34973	Foreign Body - Colon
30284	Crohn's Disease Of The Duodenum	34136	Fecal Artifact
30285	Crohn's Disease Of The Jejunum	30098	Stercoral Ulcer

GASTROENTEROLOGY, CONT.

30021	Stenosis Of Large Intestine		34173	With Acute Cholecystitis
30069	Diverticulosis		34175	With Chronic Cholecystitis
30061	Colonic Diverticulosis		37636	With Obstruction
33815	Perforated		30064	Acalculous Cholecystitis
30067	Diverticulitis		33863	Cryptosporidial Cholecystitis
30068	With Abscess		30062	Acute Cholecystitis
30178	Spicy / Hot Food Syndrome		37635	With Obstruction
30280	Irritable Bowel Syndrome		33923	Gangrenous
35572	Functional Diarrhea		30063	Chronic Cholecystitis
30137	Sigmoid Volvulus		30197	Postcholecystectomy Syndrome
30138	Cecal Volvulus		33875	Post Cholecystectomy
30196	Pneumatosis Cystoides Coli		30169	Hydrops Gallbladder
30060	Colonic Angiodysplasia		30095	Empyema Gallbladder
30265	Colonic Arteriovenous Malformation		30294	Gallbladder Rupture
30290	Colonic Perforation		37300	Gallbladder Hematoma (Traumatic)
34171	Colostomy / Enterostomy Malfunction		37301	Laceration Of Gallbladder
34561	Iatrogenic		37302	Gunshot Wound Of Gallbladder
38491	Colostomy Complication		30050	Adenomyosis Of The Gallbladder
38492	Infection		34177	Gallbladder Obstruction
34139	Post Colectomy		34178	Cholesterolosis Of Gallbladder
30107	Large Intestine Laceration		30049	Choledocholithiasis
37275	Ascending		34174	With Acute Cholecystitis
37276	Transverse		34176	With Chronic Cholecystitis
37277	Descending		30126	Common Bile Duct Stricture
37278	Sigmoid		37296	Laceration Of The Common Bile Duct
37279	Multiple Sites		30065	Ascending Cholangitis
37280	With Open Wound Into Cavity		30066	Pericholangitis
37304	Gunshot Wound Of Large Intestine		30219	Primary Sclerosing Cholangitis
31318	Proctitis		30220	Secondary Sclerosing Cholangitis
31319	Gonococcal		30038	Biliary Atresia
34979	Syphilitic		37668	Biliary Atresia, Congenital
30177	Ulcerative Proctitis		30039	Biliary Dyskinesia
38279	Ulcerative Proctosigmoiditis		30125	Extrahepatic Bile Duct Stricture
30262	Rectal Prolapse		30127	Extrahepatic Biliary Obstruction
30263	Rectal Ulcer		35581	Choledochal Cyst
31316	Rectal Abscess		35580	Spasm Of Sphincter Of Oddi
30264	Rectal Stricture		90247	Liver
34138	Rectal Trauma		30151	Hepatitis
30045	Fecal Impaction		30152	Type A ("Infectious")
34977	Rectal Perforation		36278	With Hepatic Coma
30123	Foreign Body - Rectal		30153	Type B ("Serum")
30215	Proctalgia Fugax		36279	With Hepatic Coma
30141	Hemorrhoids		36280	With Hepatitis Delta
30142	Thrombosed		30155	Type C (Non-A, Non-B)
37631	Internal With Complication		36281	With Hepatic Coma
37632	External With Complication		38272	Chronic
30026	Anal Fissure		38273	With Hepatic Coma
30027	Anal Stricture		30154	Delta
35586	Anal Foreign Body		36282	With Hepatic Coma
30028	Anal Ulcer		36142	Type E
90246	Gallbladder And Biliary Tree		36283	With Hepatic Coma
30261	Gallbladder Disease		34872	Cytomegalovirus
30048	Cholelithiasis		34870	Epstein-Barr

GASTROENTEROLOGY, CONT.

30156	Toxic / Drug Induced		37284	Hepatic Hematoma
30157	Subacute Active		37285	With Open Wound Into Cavity
30158	Chronic Active		30199	Postoperative Jaundice
30159	Lupoid		36104	Liver Transplant Candidate
30160	Chronic Persistent		36105	Liver Transplant Donor
30161	Fulminant		36106	Liver Transplant Recipient
30162	Granulomatous		30059	Polychlorinated Biphenol Adsorption
30163	Alcoholic Hepatitis		90248	Pancreas
33944	Syphilitic Hepatitis		30029	Acute Pancreatitis
33862	Chlamydial Perihepatitis		36284	Mumps
31148	Gonococcal Perihepatitis		30030	Chronic Pancreatitis
30051	Fatty Liver		35582	Pancreatic Steatorrhea
34172	Alcoholic		33864	Pancreatic Phlegmon
31175	Liver Abscess		34980	Pancreas Divisum
31176	Bacterial		30032	Macroamylasemia
30052	Cirrhosis		30270	Pancreatic Insufficiency
30053	Alcoholic (Laennec's)		30269	Pancreatic B Islet Cell Hyperplasia
30054	Postnecrotic		37609	Glucagonoma
30055	Primary Biliary		31255	Pancreatic Abscess
30056	Secondary Biliary		30031	Pancreatic Pseudocyst
30057	Cardiac		35523	Pancreatic Laceration
30058	Rare Types		37334	Head
35577	Portal Pyemia		37335	Body
36913	Cholestasis In The Newborn		37336	Tail
30277	Portal Hypertension		37337	Multiple Sites
30278	Idiopathic		37338	With Open Wound Into Cavity
35578	Chronic Passive Hepatic Congestion		37339	Gunshot Wound Of The Pancreas
30035	Ascites		36107	Pancreas Transplant Candidate
30236	Rotor Syndrome		36108	Pancreas Transplant Donor
30164	Gilbert's Syndrome		36109	Pancreas Transplant Recipient
30046	Dubin-Johnson Syndrome		30133	Gaucher's Disease (Adult)
30266	Drug Induced Cholestasis		90249	Peritoneal Cavity
30124	Benign Familial Recurrent Cholestasis		30147	Umbilical Hernia
30218	Benign Intrahepatic Cholestasis		35566	Gangrenous
30130	Glucuronyl Transferase Deficiency		35567	With Obstruction
30131	Type I (Crigler-Najjar)		30148	Inguinal Hernia
30132	Type II		38593	On The Right
30165	Recurrent Jaundice Of Pregnancy		38594	Recurrent
30234	Reye's Syndrome		38595	On The Left
30242	Hepatic Cyst		38596	Recurrent
30243	Hepatic Infarct		38597	Bilateral
30244	Hepatic Rupture		38598	Recurrent
30245	Hepatic Fibrosis		34166	With Obstruction
30246	Congenital		34167	Gangrenous
30247	Hepatic Artery Aneurysm		30149	Ventral Hernia
30248	Hepatic Subcapsular Hematoma		33817	With Obstruction
30249	Peliosis Hepatis		35562	Gangrenous
30250	Hepatic Arteriovenous Malformation		33914	Incisional Hernia
30108	Hepatic Laceration		35563	Gangrenous
37281	With Open Wound Into The Cavity		35564	With Obstruction
37303	Gunshot Wound Of The Liver		30150	Femoral Hernia
37282	Hepatic Contusion		38599	On The Right
37283	With Open Wound Into Cavity		38600	Recurrent

GASTROENTEROLOGY, CONT.

38601	On The Left	35071	Pancreaticocutaneous
38602	Recurrent	30295	Aorticoduodenal
38603	Bilateral	34186	Urethroperineal
38604	Recurrent	34187	Urethrorectal
34168	With Obstruction	34188	Urethroscrotal
34169	Gangrenous	34189	Urethrovaginal
33915	Obturator Hernia	34190	Urethrovesicovaginal
33916	Spigelian Hernia	30118	Intestinoureteral
30001	Abdominal Abscess	30119	Rectovaginal
31298	Peritonitis	35185	Vaginoperineal
33922	Bacterial	34137	Rectocutaneous
33917	Spontaneous	30120	Rectovesical
33920	Candida	35781	Rectourethral
33919	Gonococcal	30121	Small Bowel
33918	Pneumococcal	30260	Liver, Stomach Or Bowel Disease, NOS
31299	Tuberculous	30627	**Nephrology**
35714	Meconium	30630	Absence Of One Kidney
33921	Starch	34767	Kidney Injury
30190	Mesenteric Lipodystrophy	34768	With Open Wound Into Cavity
30235	Retractile Mesenteritis (Weber-Christian)	37287	Hematoma Of Kidney
		37288	Laceration Of Kidney
30289	Perforated Viscus	37289	With Open Wound Into Cavity
30296	Abdominal Trauma	30703	Kidney Rupture
37298	Peritoneal Hematoma (Nontraumatic)	34814	Traumatic Anuria
37299	Peritoneal Hematoma (Traumatic)	30631	Acute Glomerulonephritis
30238	Retroperitoneal Hematoma (Nontraumatic)	30632	Chronic Membrano-Proliferative (Hypocomplementemic)
37297	Retroperitoneal Hematoma (Traumatic)	30633	Focal Sclerosing
33874	Post Abdominal Surgery	30634	Minimal Change (Nil Disease)
30297	Abdominal Adhesions	30635	Idiopathic Membranous
35568	Intestinal	30636	Berger's Disease
35569	Small Bowel	30637	Proliferative
35570	Colonic	30638	Acute Poststreptococcal
35571	Peritoneal	30639	Rapidly Progressive
31276	Retroperitoneal Abscess	30640	Chronic Glomerulonephritis
30237	Retroperitoneal Fibrosis	30629	Interstitial Nephritis
30110	Fistulae	31313	Renal Abscess
38071	Persistent Postoperative	31279	Perinephric Abscess
30111	In-ANO	31280	Tuberculous
30112	Cholecystoenteric	31281	Pyelonephritis
30113	Cholecystoduodenocolic	31282	Acute Bacterial
35579	Choledochoduodenal	31283	Chronic
33928	Entero-Entero	34179	Pyeloureteritis Cystica
33929	Entero-Colic	30718	Hydronephrosis
30114	Enterocutaneous	30641	Acute Tubular Necrosis
30115	Enterovesical	35755	Renal Insufficiency
34560	Colo-Vesical	36096	Renal Failure
35070	Colocutaneous	30642	Acute
35069	Colovaginal	30643	Hepato-Renal Syndrome
34130	Enterovaginal	30644	With Cortical Necrosis
30122	Tracheo-Esophageal	35538	Following Childbirth
30116	Gastrocolic	30645	Chronic
30117	Gastrojejunocolic	30646	Uremia

GASTROENTEROLOGY, CONT.

36110	Renal Transplant Candidate	30696	Gouty
36111	Renal Transplant Donor	30697	Acute Urate
36112	Renal Transplant Recipient	30698	Sarcoid
30648	Renal Transplant Rejection	30699	Hypokalemic
30649	Alport's Syndrome	34876	Analgesic
30653	Crossed Ectopia	30628	**Urology**
30654	Cystinuria	30920	Cystitis
36139	Glycinuria	34181	Acute
30656	Renal Tubular Acidosis	34182	Chronic
30657	Proximal (Type II)	34183	Chronic Interstitial
30658	Distal (Type I)	34184	Follicular
30659	Segmental Hypoplasia	31394	Urinary Tract Infection
30660	Renal Colic	36011	Pediatric Presentation
30661	Nephrolithiasis	31395	Geriatric Presentation
30662	Idiopathic With Hyperuricosuria	31389	Urethritis
30663	Idiopathic Hypercalcuria - Hyperabsorption	31390	Chlamydia Trachomitis
		31391	Gonococcus
30664	Idiopathic Hypercalcuria - Hyperexcretion	31392	Treponema Pallidum
		31393	Ureaplasma Urealyticum ('T Mycoplasma')
30665	Triple Phosphate		
38025	Post Cystostomy	37290	Bladder Hematoma
30668	Medullary Cystic Disease	37291	Laceration Of Bladder
30669	Medullary Sponge Kidney	30704	Ruptured Bladder
30670	Myoglobinuria	37292	Gunshot Wound Of Bladder
34822	Cocaine-Associated Rhabdomyolysis	30650	Neurogenic Bladder
30671	Nephrotic Syndrome	30651	Bladder Outlet Obstruction
37681	Proteinuria	34185	Diverticulum Of Bladder
37682	Bence-Jones Proteinuria	34180	With Calculus
30672	Orthostatic Proteinuria	30710	Bladder Calculus
30673	Papillary Necrosis	30652	Bladder Foreign Body
30674	Nephrosclerosis	37679	Urge Incontinence
30675	Benign	30680	Stress Incontinence
30676	Malignant	37680	Male Stress Incontinence
30677	Simple Renal Cyst	34243	Female Stress Incontinence
30678	Polycystic Kidney	38609	Pollakiuria
36916	Autosomal Dominant	30705	Congenital Ureteral Obstruction
36917	Autosomal Recessive	34769	Ureter Injury
30679	Benign Postural Proteinuria	37294	Ureteral Laceration
30681	Radiation Nephritis	30706	Ureteral Stricture
30683	Horseshoe Kidney	35768	Ureteral Obstruction
30684	Unilateral Renal Dysplasia	30707	Vesicoureteral Reflux
30685	Unilateral Fused Kidneys	30708	Urethral Stricture
30686	Unilateral Hypoplasia Of The Kidney	35770	Urethral Obstruction
30688	Fanconi's Syndrome	34192	Urethral Caruncle
30689	Balkan Nephropathy	34833	Urethral Abscess
30690	Nephropathy	30709	Urethral Foreign Body
30691	Diabetic	37293	Urethral Laceration
30692	Amyloid	34191	Urethral Diverticulum
34894	HIV-Associated	34193	Urethral Prolapse
30693	Multiple Myeloma	30711	Ureteral Stone
30694	Sickle Cell	30712	Urethral Stone
30695	Hypercalcemic	34194	Urinary Obstruction
34877	Lead	34195	Essential Hematuria

GASTROENTEROLOGY, CONT.

34203	Organic Impotence	30606	Ovarian Torsion
35587	Foreign Body - Penis	35186	Ovarian Atrophy (Acquired)
31439	Prostatitis	36267	Oophoritis
31440	Acute Bacterial	36268	Tuberculous
31441	Gonococcal	90001	Fallopian Tubes
31442	Chronic Bacterial	30615	Fallopian Tube Block
30666	Benign Prostatic Hypertrophy	35187	Torsion Of Fallopian Tube
34196	Calculus Of Prostate	35769	Rupture Of Fallopian Tube
30667	Post Prostatectomy	35188	Laceration Of Broad Ligament
38027	Post Ureterostomy		(Masters-Allen Syndrome)
30713	Meatal Stenosis	30614	Congenital Anomaly Of Fallopian
35833	Phimosis		Tube
34200	Priapism	31386	Salpingitis
34201	Balanoposthitis	34206	Acute
34202	Balanitis Xerotica Obliterans	31387	Gonococcal
30714	Spermatic Cord Torsion	34207	Chronic
35834	Torsion Of Epididymis	31388	Gonococcal
34204	Seminal Vesiculitis	36218	Tuberculous
30715	Spermatocele	34230	Uterus
30716	Hydrocele Of Male Genital Organs	34244	Perimenopausal Menorrhagia
30717	Scrotal Hernia	30594	Menopause
35576	Scrotal Varices	34245	Postmenopausal Bleeding
31101	Epididymitis	35205	Post-Artificial Menopause State
31102	Tuberculous	34410	Climacteric Arthritis
30687	Gential Ulcers - Male	30607	Ruptured Endometrioma
31141	Chancroid	30610	Endometriosis
31143	Lymphogranuloma Venereum	34215	Ovarian
31145	Granuloma Inguinale	34216	Fallopian Tube
31146	Gonorrhea	34214	Uterine
31147	PPNG	34217	Pelvic Peritoneum
30682	Testicular Feminization	34218	Rectovaginal Septum And Vagina
38669	**Gynecology**	34219	Intestinal
39997	Breast Disorders	35181	In Scar
35160	Breast Atrophy	30612	Endometrial Polyps
33094	Fat Necrosis Of The Breast	35190	Non-Puerperal Uterine Hypertrophy
33091	Mammary Duct Ectasia	35761	Endometrial Hyperplasia
33092	Mondor's Disease	34226	Benign Cystic
33093	Fibrocystic Disease	35762	Adenomatous
33159	Breast Abscess	35763	Atypical Adenomatous
33095	Mastitis	34227	Hematometra
34599	Neonatal Infective	34228	Uterine Adhesions
35720	Neonatal Noninfective	30595	Asherman's Syndrome
33160	Chronic Cystic Mastitis	30616	Congenital Anomaly Of Uterus
33121	Sucrosuria		Leading To Infertility
33146	Submammary Abscess	30617	Endometritis
35161	Nonpuerperal Galactorrhea	30618	Gonococcal
33148	Mastodynia	30619	Tuberculous
33145	Breast Cyst	35165	Acute
33147	Galactocele	35166	Subacute
34850	Normal Pelvic Exam	35167	Chronic
90000	Ovaries	35168	Endomyometritis
30605	Anovulatory Bleeding	35169	Acute
34211	Peritubal / Tubo-Ovarian Adhesions		

GYNECOLOGY, CONT.

35170	Subacute
35171	Chronic
35172	Myometritis
35173	Acute
35174	Subacute
35175	Chronic
35176	Pyometra
35177	Acute
35178	Subacute
35179	Chronic
35180	Nabothian Cyst
34241	Mittelschmerz
34240	Dysmenorrhea
34242	Pelvic Congestion Syndrome
30620	Vicarious Menstruation
35268	Amenorrhea
35269	Primary
35270	Secondary
35201	Pubertal Menorrhagia
35202	Ovulatory Bleeding
35203	Metrorrhagia
35204	Postcoital Bleeding
30621	Misplaced IUD
34982	Retained IUD During Pregnancy
35325	Congenital Abnormality Of Uterus
34984	Didelphic
35326	Unicornuate
35327	Bicornuate
35328	Septate
35329	Arcuate
30622	Retroversion Of Uterus
34225	Chronic Uterine Subinvolution
34229	Chronic Uterine Inversion
30623	Uterine Prolapse
34844	Uterine Foreign Body
30624	Uterine Perforation
30625	Uterine Rupture
34220	Uterovaginal Prolapse
34221	Incomplete
34222	Complete
90003	Cervix
30613	Cervical Erosion
34231	Dysplasia Of Cervix (Uteri)
34232	Leukoplakia Of Cervix (Uteri)
35189	Old Laceration Of Cervix
34233	Cervical Stenosis / Stricture
35780	Cervical Foreign Body
31382	Cervicitis
31383	Gonococcus
31384	Chlamydia Trachomitis
31385	Chronic Cystic
34235	Vaginal Disorder
30591	Bartholin Gland Cyst

30592	Gonococcus
34236	Vaginal Dysplasia
34237	Vaginal Leukoplakia
34238	Vaginal Stricture
38253	Vaginal Adhesions (Postoperative)
35191	Tight Hymenal Ring (Perforate)
35192	Old Vaginal Laceration
35193	Noninfective Leukorrhea
34239	Vaginal Polyp
30593	Vaginal Foreign Body
35182	Vaginal Wall Prolapse
31397	Vaginitis
31398	Candida Albicans
31399	Gonococcus
31400	Nonspecific
31401	Trichomonas Vaginitis
34247	Postmenopausal Atrophic
35183	Post-Hysterectomy Vaginal Vault Prolapse
35122	Vaginal Hematoma (Non-Puerperal)
35184	Old Perineal Laceration
34834	Vaginal Enterocele
34208	Parametritis
34209	Acute
34210	Chronic
35162	Female Pelvic Peritonitis
35163	Acute
35164	Chronic
31139	Genital Ulcers - Female
31140	Chancroid - Female
31142	Lymphogranuloma Venereum - Female
31144	Granuloma Inguinale - Female
35764	Cystocele
35765	Cystourethrocele
35766	Rectocele
35767	Urethrocele
34248	Hematocele, Genital
34249	Broad Ligament
34250	Fallopian Tube
34251	Uterine
34252	Vaginal
34253	Vulvar
34254	Hydrocele Of Canal Of Nuck
39996	External Genitalia
35196	Clitoral Hypertrophy (Non-Endocrine)
35197	Labial Hypertrophy
38326	Vulvovaginitis
35195	Vulvar Atrophy
35194	Vulvar Dystrophy
34212	Vulvar Abscess
34213	Vulvar Ulceration
38327	Candida Albicans

GYNECOLOGY, CONT.

38328	Gonococcus
38329	Trichomonas Vaginitis
35575	Vulvar Varices
35199	Vulvar Hematoma
35200	Vulvar Polyp
35198	Old Vulvar Laceration
31396	Bartholin's Gland Abscess
34246	Female Infertility
38670	**Obstetrics**
34579	Maternal Condition Affecting Fetus / Newborn
37677	Cocaine
38283	Diethylstilbestrol
34580	Hypertension
35698	Diabetes Mellitus
34581	Renal Disease
34582	Urinary Tract Infection
34583	Infectious Disease
35615	Nutritional Disorders
35616	Maternal Injury
35617	Maternal Surgery
34584	Noxious Influences Via Placenta Or Breast Milk
36103	Collagen Vascular Disease
34585	Pregnancy Complication Affecting Fetus / Newborn
34586	Incompetent Cervix
34587	Premature Rupture Of Membranes
34588	Polyhydramnios
34589	Ectopic Pregnancy
34590	Multiple Pregnancy
35618	Placenta Previa Affecting Fetus / Newborn
35619	Placental Abruption Affecting Fetus / Newborn
34591	Placental Dysfunction Affecting Fetus / Newborn
35620	Placental Transfusion Syndromes Affecting Fetus / Newborn
35621	Prolapsed Cord Affecting Fetus / Newborn
35622	Nuchal Cord Affecting Fetus / Newborn
35623	Knot In Cord Affecting Fetus / Newborn
35624	Vasa Previa Affecting Fetus / Newborn
35625	Umbilical Cord Thrombosis Affecting Fetus / Newborn
35626	Short Umbilical Cord Affecting Fetus / Newborn
35627	Chorioamnionitis Affecting Fetus / Newborn

34594	Labor / Delivery Complications
	Affected Fetus / Newborn
34592	Caesarean Delivery
34593	Abnormal Uterine Contractions
35631	Intrauterine Growth Retardation
35628	Small For Gestational Age At Delivery
35629	Malnourished
35630	Intrauterine Malnutrition
30596	Pregnancy
34286	Normal Delivery
34297	Caesarean Delivery
34267	Complication - Hypertension
34268	Essential
34269	Secondary To Renal Disease
34270	Transient
34263	With Hemorrhage Before 23rd Gestational Week
34264	Threatened Abortion
32392	Hyperemesis Gravidarum
34271	With Metabolic Disturbance
33907	Mild
35292	In 2nd Half Of Pregnancy
30598	Hydatidiform Mole (Molar)
34981	Invasive (Non-Metastatic GTD)
35206	Blighted Ovum
30599	Toxemia
30600	Ectopic
34256	Abdominal
34257	Tubal
34258	Ovarian
34983	Cervical
34234	Cervical Incompetence
34272	Threatened Premature Labor
34273	Early Onset Of Delivery
34274	Prolonged
34278	Complications
34279	Diabetes Mellitus
34280	Thyroid Dysfunction
34281	Anemia
34282	Drug Dependence
34283	Mental Disorder
35298	Cardiovascular Disorders
35297	Congenital Cardiovascular Disorders
34284	Back, Pelvis Or Lower Limb Disorder
34285	Abnormal Glucose Tolerance
35293	Renal Disease
35294	Peripheral Neuropathy
35295	Asymptomatic Bacteriuria
35296	Genitourinary Tract Infection
35299	Infectious Disease

OBSTETRICS, CONT.

35300	Syphilis	35286	Postabortal Shock
35301	Gonorrhea	35287	Postabortal Embolism
35302	Tuberculosis	34255	Missed Abortion
35303	Malaria	34277	Habitual Aborter (Gravid)
35304	Rubella	35123	Habitual Aborter (Non-Gravid)
35305	Toxoplasmosis	30601	Preeclampsia
35306	Herpes Simplex	35290	Severe
35307	Cytomegalovirus	30602	Eclampsia
34276	Excessive Weight Gain In Pregnancy	35291	Superimposed On Chronic Hypertension
34261	Abortion	30603	Pseudocyesis
35271	With Complications	34287	Multiple Gestation
35272	Pelvic Infection	34288	Twins
35273	Hemorrhage	34289	Triplets
30604	Spontaneous	34943	Quadruplets
35274	Complicated By Pelvic Infection	34290	Malpresentation Of Fetus
35275	Complicated By Pelvic Hemorrhage	34291	Breech
37637	Complicated By Damage To Pelvic Organs Or Tissues	37678	Before Labour
		35308	Frank
37638	Complicated By Shock	35309	Complete
34259	Elective	35310	Incomplete
35276	Complicated By Pelvic Infection	35311	Successful Version
35277	Complicated By Pelvic Hemorrhage	35312	Transverse Presentation
		35313	Oblique Presentation
37639	Complicated By Damage To Pelvic Organs Or Tissues	35314	Face Presentation
		35315	Brow Presentation
37640	Complicated By Renal Failure	35316	High Head At Term
37641	Complicated By Shock	35317	In Multiple Gestation
37642	Complicated By Embolism	35318	Prolapsed Arm
34260	Self-Induced	34292	Disproportion
35278	Complicated By Pelvic Infection	34293	Contracted Pelvis
35279	Complicated By Pelvic Hemorrhage	35319	Inlet Contracture Of Pelvis
		35320	Outlet Contracture Of Pelvis
37643	Complicated By Damage To Pelvic Organs Or Tissue	34294	Fetopelvic
		34295	Unusually Large Fetus
37644	Complicated By Renal Failure	35321	Fetal Hydrocephaly
37645	Complicated By Shock	34296	Congenital Abnormality Of Uterus (Obstetric)
37646	Complicated By Embolism		
34262	Failed Attempted Abortion	34985	Unicornuate
35280	Complicated By Pelvic Infection	34986	Bicornuate
35281	Complicated By Pelvic Hemorrhage	34987	Septate
37647	Complicated By Damage To Pelvic Organs Or Tissues	34988	Arcuate
		35322	Uterine Neoplasms (Obstetric)
37648	Complicated By Renal Failure	35330	Dehiscence Of Uterine Scar
37649	Complicated By Shock	35331	Retroversion Of Uterus (Obstetric)
37650	Complicated By Embolism	35756	Sacculation Of Gravid Uterus
31456	Septic Abortion	35332	Uterine Prolapse (Obstetric)
31457	Postabortal Sepsis	35333	Cervical Incompetence (Obstetric)
35282	Delayed Postabortal Hemorrhage	34298	Congenital Abnormality Of Gravid Cervix
35283	Postabortal Pelvic / Abdominal Organ Damage		
		35334	Vaginal Stricture (Obstetric)
35284	Postabortal Renal Failure	35335	Vaginal Neoplasm (Obstetric)
35285	Postabortal Metabolic Disorder	35336	Vulvar Abnormality (Obstetric)

OBSTETRICS, CONT.

35337	Vulvar Neoplasm (Obstetric)		35355	Shoulder Dystocia
34299	Fetal Abnormality Affecting Care Of Mother		35356	Interlocked Twins
			30608	Placenta Abruptio
35338	CNS		35289	Antepartum Hemorrhage Due To Coagulation Defects
35339	Chromosomal			
35340	Hereditary Disease			Placenta Previa
35345	Fetal Damage Affecting Care Of Mother		30609	
			34266	Without Hemorrhage
35341	Viral		34265	With Hemorrhage
35342	From Toxoplasmosis		34318	Failed Trial Of Labor
35343	From Drug		35357	Failed Forceps / Vacuum Delivery
35344	From Radiation		34319	Uterine Inertia
34300	Fetal-Maternal Hemorrhage Affecting Care Of Mother		34320	Primary
			34321	Secondary
35346	Rh Isoimmunization Affecting Care Of Mother		34322	Precipitate Labor
			35524	Hypertonic Uterine Contractions
35347	ABO Isoimmunization Affecting Care Of Mother		34323	Prolonged Labor
			35525	First Stage
34301	Fetal Distress Affecting Care Of Mother		35526	Second Stage
			35527	Delayed Second Delivery In Multiple Pregnancy
33908	Intrauterine Fetal Death Affecting Care Of Mother		34324	Umbilical Cord Complication
			35012	Prolapse
34302	Poor Fetal Growth Affecting Care Of Mother		35108	Nuchal Cord With Compression
			35109	Knot In Cord With Compression
34303	Excessive Fetal Growth Affecting Care Of Mother		35013	Cord Entanglement
			35014	With Compression
34304	Placental Infarct Affecting Care Of Mother		35015	Short Cord
			35016	Vasa Previa
34305	Lithopedian Affecting Care Of Mother		35017	Vascular Lesion(s)
34275	Papyraceous Fetus		35750	Rupture
34306	Polyhydramnios		34325	Perineal Laceration During Delivery
34308	Premature Rupture Of Membranes		34326	First-Degree
34307	Oligohydramnios		34327	Second-Degree
34309	Delayed Delivery After Spontaneous Rupture Of Membranes		34328	Third-Degree
			35018	Fourth-Degree
35348	Delayed Delivery After Artificial Rupture Of Membranes		35528	Obstetrical Vulvar / Perineal Hematoma
34310	Infection Of Amniotic Cavity		35529	Prelabor Uterine Rupture
35349	Amnion Nodosum		35530	Uterine Rupture During Or After Labor
35758	Amniotic Band Syndrome		35019	Uterine Inversion During Delivery
34311	Failed Mechanical Induction		35020	Cervical Laceration During Delivery
34312	Failed Medical Induction		35021	Vaginal Laceration During Delivery
35350	Maternal Pyrexia During Labor		35531	Obstetrical Pelvic Organ Damage
35351	Maternal Sepsis During Labor		35022	Pelvic Hematoma During Delivery
34313	Grand Multiparity		34329	Obstetrical Injury Of Pelvic Joints / Ligaments
35352	Elderly Primigravida			
35353	Deep Transverse Arrest During Labor		34330	Postpartum Hemorrhage
35354	Persistent Occiput Posterior Position During Labor		34331	Third-Stage
			34332	Delayed / Secondary
34314	Obstructed Labor		35532	Postpartum Coagulation Defects
34315	Due To Malposition Of Fetus		35533	Retained Intact Placenta Without Hemorrhage
34316	By Bony Pelvis			
34317	By Abnormal Pelvic Soft Tissue			

Obstetrics, cont.

34333	Retained Partial Placenta / Membranes Without Hemorrhage	37660	Unilateral, Complete
		37661	Unilateral, Incomplete
34334	Complication From Anesthesia / Sedation During Parturition	37662	Bilateral, Complete
		37663	Bilateral, Incomplete
35534	Pulmonary	30403	Cleft Palate
35535	Cardiac	37656	Unilateral, Complete
35536	CNS	37657	Unilateral, Incomplete
34336	Maternal Distress	37658	Bilateral, Complete
34335	Obstetric Shock	37659	Bilateral, Incomplete
35537	Maternal Hypotension Syndrome	34551	Cleft Palate With Cleft Lip
35539	Obstetrical Surgical Complications	37664	Unilateral, Complete
34337	Forceps / Vacuum Extractor Delivery	37665	Unilateral, Incomplete
34338	Breech Extraction	37666	Bilateral, Complete
34339	Parturition Complication	37667	Bilateral, Incomplete
31300	Puerperal Sepsis	34552	Tongue Tie
35540	Varicose Leg Veins In Pregnancy / Puerperium	34553	Congenital Absence Of Uvula
		35842	Persistent Omphalomesenteric Duct
35541	Obstetrical Vulvar Varicosities	30024	Atresia Of Small Intestine
34340	Venous Complication In Pregnancy / Puerperium	36126	Duodenum
		36127	Ileum
34341	Superficial Thrombophlebitis	36128	Jejunum
34343	Antepartum Deep-Vein Thrombophlebitis	30020	Atresia Of Large Intestine
		35843	Patent Urachus
34342	Postpartum Deep-Vein Thrombophlebitis	30404	Club-Foot
		30405	Congenital Dislocation Of Hip
35542	Puerperal Hemorrhoids	30406	Unilateral
34344	Puerperal Pyrexia	30407	Bilateral
35545	Obstetrical Cerebrovascular Disorders	30397	Congenital Rubella
35546	Disruption Of Uterine Incision After Cesarean	33856	Fetal Alcohol Syndrome
		35812	Fetal Hydantoin Syndrome
35547	Obstetrical Perineal Breakdown	38226	Thalidomide Syndrome
35548	Obstetrical Surgical Wound Complications	30399	Congenital Cytomegalovirus Infection
		36020	Congenital Herpes Simplex Infection
35549	Placental Polyp	30400	Congenital Toxoplasmosis
35550	Puerperal Infections Of Nipple	35682	Tetanus Neonatorum
35551	Puerperal Breast Abscess	35683	Neonatal Omphalitis
34346	Puerperal Mastitis	35684	Neonatal Candidiasis
34347	Purulent	34600	Fetal Blood Loss
34348	Nonpurulent	34601	Umbilical Hemorrhage After Birth
35552	Retraction Of Nipple In Puerperium	34602	Neonatal Gastrointestinal Hemorrhage
35553	Cracked Nipple In Puerperium	35685	Neonatal Adrenal Hemorrhage
35554	Breast Engorgement In Puerperium	35686	Neonatal Cutaneous Hemorrhage
34349	Agalactia	30626	Rh Incompatibility (Erythroblastosis Fetalis)
35555	Suppressed Lactation		
35556	Puerperal Galactorrhea	35687	Isoimmunized Hydrops Fetalis
30396	**Pediatrics**	35688	Isoimmunized Kernicterus Of The Newborn
34538	Agenesis Of Brain		
35749	Anencephaly	35689	Isoimmunized Anemia Of The Newborn
36912	Cranial Meningocele		
34539	Diastematomyelia	35716	Non-Isoimmunized Anemia Of The Newborn
34540	Hydromyelia		
34550	Cleft Nose	35690	Perinatal Jaundice
30402	Cleft Lip	35691	From Hereditary Anemias

PEDIATRICS, CONT.

35692	From Exogenous Agents / Events	30413	Chediak-Higashi Disease (Oculocutaneous Albinism)
35693	With Preterm Delivery		
35694	From Conjugated Hyperbilirubinemia	30414	Seminiferous Tubule Dysgenesis
		30418	Trisomy
38252	From Breast Milk	35835	5p
35695	From Hepatocellular Damage	30419	13
35813	Neonatal Hyperbilirubinemia	30420	18
35700	Neonatal Hematological Disorders	30421	Down Syndrome (Trisomy 21 - Mongolism)
35701	Hemorrhagic		
35702	Transient Thrombocytopenia	38661	Translocation
35703	DIC	38223	Trisomic Abnormality (Not Downs)
35704	Polycythemia	38662	Cri-Du-Chat Syndrome
35705	Congenital Anemia	38663	Antimongolism Syndrome
35706	Anemia Of Prematurity	30422	Triple X Syndrome
35707	Neutropenia	30423	Klinefelter's Syndrome (XXY)
35743	Neonatal Digestive Disorders	30424	XYY Syndrome
35709	Intestinal Obstruction From Inspissated Milk	37676	Sex Chromosome Mosaicism
		30425	Turner's Syndrome (XO)
35710	Swallowed Maternal Blood Syndrome	30416	Laurence-Moon-Biedl Syndrome
		38657	Weill-Marchesani Syndrome
35711	Transitory Ileus Of Newborn	30417	Prader-Willi Syndrome
35712	Necrotizing Enterocolitis	36129	Cornelia De Lange
35713	Intestinal Perforation	36130	Smith-Lemli-Opitz
35717	Sclerema Neonatorum	33881	Hermaphroditism
35718	Hypothermia Of Newborn	34554	Congenital Absence Of Ovaries
35719	Hyperthermia Of Newborn	30426	Congenital Absence Of Uterus (Mullerian Dysgenesis Syndromes
35715	Congenital Hydrocele		
30401	Congenital Nystagmus	34557	Embryonic Fallopian Tube Cyst
34030	Growth Hormone Deficiency (Pituitary Dwarfism)	33857	Congenital Absence Of Thyroid Gland
		30427	Bloom's Syndrome
37615	Dwarfism	30428	Congenital Absence Of Intrinsic Factor
31958	Werner's Syndrome (Adult Progeria)	30429	Congenital Abnormal Intrinsic Factor
30409	Marfan's Syndrome	30430	Situs Inversus
38282	Fragile X Syndrome	34578	Conjoined Twins
38228	Delange Syndrome	34595	Extreme Immaturity At Birth
30410	Cystic Fibrosis	34596	Preterm Infant
34541	Congenital Anophthalmos	35632	Macrosomic Infant
34542	Congenital Cryptophthalmos	35633	Exceptionally Large (>10 Lbs.)
34543	Congenital Microphthalmos	35634	Post-Term Infant (AGA)
38613	Congenital Nanophthalmos	34874	Low Apgar Score
30411	Congenital Glaucoma	35635	Birth Trauma
36563	With Chamber Angle Anomalies	35637	Cerebral Hemorrhage
36564	With Anomalies Of Iris	35638	Scalp Injury
36565	With Systemic Syndromes	36907	Caput Succedaneum
34544	Congenital Cataract	36908	Chignon
34545	Congenital Aphakia	36909	Massive Epicranial Subaponeurotic Hemorrhage
34546	Congenital Ptosis		
34547	Congenital Eyelid Deformity	36910	Skull Injury
34548	Congenital Ear Deformity	36911	Cephalohematoma
35981	Connective Tissue Defect	35639	Fracture Of Clavicle
38548	Oculocutaneous Albinism	35640	Fracture Of Long Bones
30412	Hermansky-Pudlak (Oculocutaneous Albinism)	35641	Skull Fracture
		34597	Spinal Injury

PEDIATRICS, CONT.

35642	Facial Nerve Injury	33530	Beriberi (Thiamine)
35643	Eye Damage	33531	Formiminotransferase Deficiency
35644	Testicular Hematoma	33532	Alcaptonuria
35645	Vulvar Hematoma	33533	Glucose Phosphate Isomerase Deficiency
35646	Scalpel Wound		
35647	Fetal Hypoxia	33534	Hereditary Nadh-Methemoglobin Reductase Deficiency
35648	Death From Asphyxia Or Anoxia		
35649	During Labor	33536	Arginnosuccinic Aciduria
35650	Liveborn Infant - Fetal Distress Before Labor	33537	Lesch-Nyhan Syndrome (HGPRT Deficiency)
35651	Liveborn Infant - Fetal Distress During Labor	33538	Cystinosis
		33539	Maple Syrup Disease
35653	Mild / Moderate Birth Asphyxia	33543	Cysthathioninuria
35652	Severe Birth Asphyxia	33540	Carnosinemia
34598	Respiratory Distress Syndrome Of Newborn	33535	Histidinemia
		33559	Hyperammonemia
35654	Respiratory Conditions Of Fetus Or Newborn	36140	Transient In The Newborn
		33560	Carbamyl Phosphate Synthetase Deficiency
35655	Congenital Pneumonia		
35656	Massive Aspiration Syndrome	33561	Ornithine Transcarbamylase Deficiency
35657	Interstitial Emphysema		
35658	Pulmonary Hemorrhage	36134	Arginosuccinic Acidemia
35659	Primary Atelectasis	36135	Argininemia
35660	Secondary Atelectasis	33542	Citrullinemia
35661	Transient Tachypnea	36131	Argininosuccinic Aciduria
35662	Bronchopulmonary Dysplasia	36138	N-Acetylglutamate Synthetase Deficiency
35663	Interstitial Pulmonary Fibrosis		
35664	Wilson-Mikity Syndrome	36133	Hyperornithinemia
34603	Convulsions In Newborn	36136	Gyrate Atrophy Of The Choroid
34604	CNS Dysfunction In Newborn	36137	HHH Syndrome
35722	Neonatal Drug Reaction	33541	Propionic Acidemia
35723	Neonatal Drug Withdrawal Syndrome	30963	Familial Mediterranean Fever
35724	Amphetamine	33544	Orotic Aciduria
35725	Cocaine	33545	Fructose Intolerance
35726	Opioids	33546	Galactosemia
35727	Sedatives	36141	In The Newborn
35721	Neonatal Feeding Problems	33547	Hyperglycinemia
34605	Perinatal Fetal Death Due To Termination Of Pregnancy	33548	Glycogen Storage Disease
		33549	Von Gierke's Disease (GSD Type I)
34606	Stillbirth	33550	Pompe's Disease (GSD Type II)
34820	Sudden Infant Death Syndrome	33551	Forbes' Disease (GSD Type III)
38671	**Metabolic Disorders**	33552	Andersen's Disease (GSD Type IV)
33522	Nutritional Amblyopia	33553	Mc Ardle's Disease (GSD Type V)
33523	Ariboflavinosis	33554	Hers' Disease (GSD Type VI)
31790	Amyloidosis	33555	Liver Phosphorylase Kinase Deficiency (GSD Type Via)
31791	Primary		
31792	Secondary	33556	Phosphofructokinase Deficiency (GSD Type VII)
33524	Homocystinuria		
33525	Fabry's Disease	33557	Glycogen Synthetase Deficiency (GSD Type O)
33526	Hyperprolinemia		
33527	Type I	33558	Hyper-B-Alaninemia
33528	Type II	33562	Hydroxyprolinemia
33529	Dihydrofolate Reductase Deficiency	33563	Isovaleric Acidemia

METABOLIC DISORDERS, CONT.

33564	Familial Lipoprotein Lipase Deficiency	33592	Pseudo-Hurler's (GM1 Gangliosidosis)
33855	Familial Apolipoprotein C-II Deficiency	36915	Cerebrohepatorenal Syndrome (Zellweger Syndrome)
33565	Abetalipoproteinemia (Bassen-Kornzweig)	36918	Beckwith Syndrome
		33593	Hyperoxaluria
33566	Tangier Disease (Familial HDL Deficiency)	33594	Type I
		33595	Type II
38632	Fish-Eye Disease (Familial HDL Deficiency)	33596	Porphyria
		33597	Porphyria Cutanea Tarda (PCT)
38633	APO A-I Deficiency	33598	Erythropoietic Uroporphyria (CEP)
33567	Lecithin Cholesterol Acyltransferase (LCAT) Deficiency	33599	Hereditary Coproporphyria (HCP)
		33600	Acute Intermittent Porphyria (AP)
38634	Heterozygous	33601	Erythropoietic Protoporphyria (PP)
38635	Homozygous	33602	Porphyria Variegata (VP)
33568	Cholesterol Ester Storage Disease	33603	Pseudohyponatremia
33284	Familial Hypercholesterolemia	33604	Renal Glycosuria
38627	Heterozygous	33605	Pseudohyperkalemia
38628	Homozygous	33606	Hypersarcosinemia
33852	Familial Combined Hyperlipidemia	33607	Sulfituria
33854	Familial Hypertriglyceridemia	33608	Tyrosinosis
38631	Familial Defective Apoliprotein B-100	33609	Tyrosinemia
30578	Familial Hypobetalipoproteinemia	33610	Hypervalinemia
38630	Familial Abetalipoproteinemia	33611	Xanthinuria
33853	Familial Dysbetalipoproteinemia	33612	Hyperlysinemia
33571	Hyperlipoproteinemia	33613	Periodic
33572	Type I	33614	Persistent
33573	Type II-A	33620	Hartnup Disease
33574	Type II-B	33621	Carotenemia
33575	Type III	33622	Hypervitaminosis A
33576	Type IV	33623	Hypervitaminosis D
33577	Type V	33624	Pellagra
31733	Waldenstrom's Macroglobulinemia	33625	Rickets
31812	Benign Monoclonal Hypergammaglobulinemia	33626	Scurvy
		33627	Vitamin K Deficiency
33570	Wolman's Disease	33628	Menkes' Kinky Hair Disease
36914	Alpha 1-Antitrypsin Deficiency	33629	Methylmalonic Aciduria
33578	Mucopolysaccharidoses	33630	Vitamin B12 - Responsive
33579	B Mercaptolactate Cysteine Disulfiduria	33631	Vitamin B12 - Unresponsive
		33632	Vitamin A Deficiency
33580	Type 1H (Hurler)	33633	Pyridoxine (Vitamin B6) Deficiency
33581	Type 1S (Scheie)	33634	Zinc Deficiency
33582	Type II: Hunter Syndrome	33635	Acrodermatitis Enteropathica
33583	Type III: Sanfilippo Syndromes	33636	Kwashiorkor
33584	Type A (MPS IIIA)	33637	Marasmus
33585	Type B (MPS IIIB)	33638	Hypoxia
33586	Type IV: Morquio Syndrome	38501	Cerebral, Iatrogenic
33587	Type VI: Maroteaux:Lamy Syndrome	33639	Fluid Overload
		33640	Hyponatremia
33588	Mild	33641	Hypernatremia
33589	Classic	33642	Hyperkalemia
33590	Type VII: B Glucuronidase Deficiency	33643	Hemolysis, In Vitro
		33644	Hypokalemia
33591	Mcardle-Schmid-Pearson Disease	33645	Hypercalcemia

METABOLIC DISORDERS, CONT.

33646	Familial Hypocalcuric (FHH)
32487	Hereditary Hyperphosphatasia
32489	Hypophosphatemic Rickets
33647	Hypophosphatemia
33648	Riboflavin (Vitamin B2) Deficiency
34031	Localized Adiposity
33649	Obesity
33821	Exogenous
33822	Secondary
38487	Morbid
33650	Hypocalcemia
33651	Neonatal
33652	Hypomagnesemia
33653	Neonatal
33654	Hypermagnesemia
33655	Compression Arthralgia
33656	Malignant Hyperthermia
34883	Food Toxicity
34884	Cyclamates
33657	Allergic Drug Reaction
33758	Penicillin
35828	Immunization Reaction
35829	Pertussis
33658	Drug Fever
33659	Drug Toxicity
33660	Antabuse
33661	Acetaminophen
33662	Aspirin
33663	Anticholinesterase
33664	Antihypertensives
34819	Azidothymidine
33887	HMG-COA Reductase Inhibitors
33665	Oral Hypoglycemics
33666	Anticholinergics
33667	Adrenocorticosteroids
38472	Topical Ocular Corticosteroids
33668	Anabolic Steroids
33669	Chloramphenicol
34947	Penicillins
33671	Aminoglycosides
33672	Anesthetic
33673	ARA-A (Adenine Arabinoside)
33674	Interleukin-2
33675	Antimetabolites
33676	Antiarrhythmics
33677	Amiodarone
34893	Encainide
34892	Flecanide
33678	Procainamide
33679	Quinidine
33680	Anticoagulants
38546	Antihistamines
33681	Beta Adrenergic Blocking Agents

33682	Cardiac Glycosides
38322	Cardiac
33683	Chemotherapeutics
35980	Adriamycin
33741	Bleomycin
33739	Busulfan
33684	Cyclophosphamide
33740	Methotrexate
38544	5-Fluorouracil
38556	Contact Lens Solution
33685	Cyclosporin-A Supression
33686	Diltiazem
33687	Dopamine
33688	Dilantin
33689	Diuretics
33690	Estrogen
33691	Ergot Alkaloids
33692	Flagyl
33693	Haloperidol
33694	Levodopa
33695	Lithium
33696	Minor Tranquilizer
33697	Nifedipine
33742	Nitrofurantoin
33698	Nitroglycerine
35760	Nonsteroidals
33699	Oral Contraceptives
33670	Penicillamine
33700	Phenothiazine
33701	Quinine
33702	Spironolactone
34880	Sulfonamides
34882	Tetracycline
33703	Theophylline
34881	Thiazides
33704	Outdated Tetracycline
33705	Verapamil
38589	Warfarin
34878	Toxicity To Radiographic Contrast Material

38672 Endocrinology

30433	Congenital Adrenal Hyperplasia
30434	C 21 Hydroxylase Deficiency (Salt Losing)
30435	C 21 Hydroxylase Deficiency (Non Salt Losing)
30436	C 11 Hydroxalase Deficiency
30437	C 17 Hydroxylase Deficiency
30438	C 18 Hydroxalase Deficiency
30439	3B OL Dehydrogenase Deficiency
30440	Bilateral Adrenal Hyperplasia
30562	Adrenal Crisis
30563	Adrenal Hemorrhage

ENDOCRINOLOGY, CONT.

37295	Adrenal Hematoma (Traumatic)		30470	Reifenstein's (Androgen Insensitivity) Syndrome
30431	Primary Adrenal Insufficiency ("Addison's Disease")		30471	Osteomalacia
30432	Primary Adrenal Insufficiency (Not Autoimmune)		38480	Hypotension
			38311	Orthostatic
35006	Secondary Adrenal Insufficiency		30476	Idiopathic
30441	Aldosteronism		38310	Chronic
30442	Primary - Aldosterone Producing Adenoma		38481	Iatrogenic
			30477	Hypoinsulinism
30443	Primary - Due To Bilateral Adrenal Hyperplasia		30478	Insulin Lipodystrophy
			30479	Diabetes Mellitus
30550	Primary - Idiopathic Hyperplasia		30480	Type II (Insulin Independent - 'Adult Onset')
30551	Bartter's Syndrome		30481	Type I (Insulin Dependent - 'Juvenile Onset')
30444	Secondary			
30575	Hypoaldosteronism		33909	Gestational
30576	With Low Renin Activity		35697	Neonatal
30577	Primary Selective		30482	Under Control
30446	Licorice Toxicity		35007	Poorly Controlled
30445	Male Infertility		30483	Diabetic Ketoacidosis
34197	Azoospermia		35214	With Coma
34198	Oligospermia		30484	Hyperglycemic Hyperosmolar Nonketotic State
34199	Iatrogenic			
30447	Dysfunctional Uterine Bleeding		37608	Secondary To Pancreatectomy
30448	Galactorrhea With Normal Prolactins		30485	Nonproliferative Diabetic Retinopathy
30449	Hypoglycemia			
30450	Tumor Associated (Non-Islet Cell)		30486	Proliferative Diabetic Retinopathy
30451	Reactive		30487	Diabetic Peripheral Neuropathy
30452	Neonatal		33846	Diabetic Amyotrophy / Mononeuritis Multiplex
30565	Alimentary			
35830	Neonatal Tetany		30488	Diabetic Autonomic Neuropathy
35778	Impaired Glucose Tolerance		30489	Diabetic Ophthalmoplegia
30453	Inadequate Luteal Phase		30490	Diabetic Gastropathy
30454	Milk-Alkali Syndrome		34949	Diabetic Foot Ulcer
30455	Multiple Endocrine Neoplasia		37896	Diabetic Hypoglycemia
30456	Type I		33119	Seip-Lawrence Syndrome
30457	Type II		30491	Hyperinsulinism (Exogenous)
30458	Type III		35215	With Coma
35211	C-Cell Hyperplasia		30268	Nesidioblastosis
33849	Polyendocrine Failure Sydnrome		30492	Diabetes Insipidus - Central
30459	Hyperparathyroidism		30493	Nephrogenic Diabetes Insipidus
30460	Ectopic (Pseudohyperparathyroidism)		30494	Gigantism
			30495	Empty Sella Syndrome
30461	Familial		30496	Acromegaly, Inactive
30462	Primary - Adenoma		30497	Hypopituitarism
30463	Primary - Hyperplasia		30498	Iatrogenic
30464	Secondary		30500	Sheehan's Syndrome (Postpartum Necrosis)
30465	Nodular Hyperplasia			
30466	Albright's Syndrome		30501	Lymphocytic (Granulomatous) Hypophysitis
30468	Hyperthecosis			
30469	Polycystic Ovary (Stein-Leventhal Syndrome)		36164	Pituitary Abscess
			36165	Tuberculous
34915	Luteoma Of Pregnancy		30502	Pituitary Neoplasm

ENDOCRINOLOGY, CONT.

30503	Acth Producing ("Basophilic") Adenoma (Cushing's Disease)	33795	With Hyperthyroidism
30504	Non-Secretory ("Chromophobe") Adenoma	30538	Thyroiditis
		30540	Pyogenic
30505	Growth Hormone Producing ("Eosinophilic") Adenoma	30541	Riedel's
		30542	Subacute
30506	Prolactinoma	30543	Post-Partum
30507	TSH Producing Adenoma - Inappropriate TSH	30544	Substernal Thyroid
		30545	Goiter
30508	Carcinoma	30546	Simple
30509	Pituicytoma	30547	Familial (Dyshormonogenic)
30510	Granular Cell Tumor	30548	Endemic Iodine Deficient
32386	Sotos Syndrome	31675	Thyroid Cyst
31513	Forbes-Albright Syndrome	35213	With Hemorrhage
31504	Carcinoid Syndrome	30549	Thyroglossal Cyst
30511	Nelson's Syndrome	31681	Parathyroid Cyst
30512	Hypoparathyroidism	30555	Inappropriate Tsh Syndrome - Pituitary Resistance To Thyroid
30513	Idiopathic		
30514	Postoperative	30556	Generalized Resistance To Thyroid Hormone
30515	Postoperative, Transient		
30516	Pseudo	30559	Increased Thyroid Binding Globulin
30517	Pseudo-Pseudo	30560	Decreased Thyroid Binding Globulin
30518	"Pseudo-Pseudo-Pseudo"	37893	Nontoxic Nodular Goiter
30519	Pseudo With Bone/Kidney Variance	34991	Thyroid Nodule, Solitary
30520	'Hungry Bone' Syndrome	30557	Nontoxic Multinodular Goiter
30524	Hypothyroidism	30558	Nontoxic Autonomous Nodule
30525	Primary	31672	Thyroid Neoplasm
30526	Postsurgical	38682	Benign
30527	Post Radio-Iodine Therapy	38683	Follicular Adenoma
30528	Secondary	31674	Thyroid Adenoma, NOS
30529	Myxedema Coma	38681	Malignant
30530	Myxedema	31676	Follicular Thyroid Carcinoma
30531	Postablative	38757	Metastatic To Lung
36012	Congenital	38759	Metastatic To Bone
30523	Cretinism (Hypothyroid)	31678	Papillary Thyroid Carcinoma
30532	Hyperthyroidism	38712	Metastatic To Regional Lymph Nodes
37894	Thyrotoxicosis With Or Without Goiter		
		38713	Cervical
30521	Graves' Disease (Diffuse Toxic Goiter)	38715	Supraclavicular
		38716	Mediastinal
30522	Graves' Ophthalmopathy	31677	Medullary Thyroid Carcinoma
30553	Toxic Thyroid Adenoma	35212	Familial
34029	Toxic Unilateral Goiter	33794	Recurrence
30552	Toxic Multinodular Goiter	38775	Metastatic To Regional Lymph Nodes
30533	Thyroid Crisis (Storm)		
30534	Exogenous, Iatrogenic	38776	Cervical
35699	Transient Neonatal	38777	Supraclavicular
30535	Apathetic	38778	Mediastinal
30554	Iodine Induced Thyrotoxicosis (Iod-Basedow)	31673	Anaplastic Thyroid Carcinoma
		33793	Recurrence After Ablation (Differentiated)
30536	Exogenous (Thyrotoxicosis Factitia)		
		31679	Lymphoma
30537	Treated / Under Control	31680	Metastasis To Thyroid
30539	Hashimoto's Thyroiditis	31622	Parathyroid Neoplasm

ENDOCRINOLOGY, CONT.

31623	Carcinoma	37127	Venenata
30564	Adrenal Adenoma	37128	Cosmetica
30566	ACTH Producing Pituitary Hyperplasia	37129	Pomade
	(Cushing's Disease)	37130	Detergicans
30567	Cushing's Syndrome	37131	Mechanica
30568	Due To Ectopic ACTH	37132	Excoriated
30569	Iatrogenic	36125	Conglobata
30570	Due To Adrenal Adenoma	37119	Fulminans
30571	Due To Adrenal Carcinoma	37120	Keloidalis
30572	Due To Adrenal Macronodular	37124	Tropical
	Hyperplasia	37125	Aestivalis
31468	Adrenal Rest Tumor	37122	Neonatal
30561	Adrenocortical Carcinoma	36124	Infantile
30573	Hemochromatosis	37123	Childhood
33859	Primary	34396	Varioliformis
33860	Carrier State	37049	Acrodermatitis Continua
33861	Secondary	37077	Acrokeratoelastoidosis Of Costa
30574	Hyperuricemia Asymptomatic	33088	Actinic Keratosis
30579	Lactic Acidosis	36998	Actinic Reticuloid
30580	Metabolic Acidosis	33114	Adiposis Dolorosa (Dercum's Disease)
30581	Metabolic Alkalosis	33154	Alopecia Areata
35267	Mixed Acid-Base Balance Disorder	37105	Ophiasis
30582	Froehlich's Syndrome	33089	Alopecia Mucinosa
30583	Testicular Failure	33155	Alopecia Totalis
30584	Primary (Hypergonadotrophic	37086	Anetoderma
	Hypogonadism)	37087	Jadassohn
35217	Iatrogenic	37088	Schweninger-Buzzi
30585	Secondary (Hypogonadotrophic	37181	Angioma Serpiginosum
	Hypogonadism)	33090	Arsenical Keratoses
37612	Postirradiation	34390	Atrophoderma
37613	Postsurgical	37095	Atrophoderma Vermiculata
37669	Undescended Testicle	33096	Basal-Cell Nevus Syndrome
30700	Hypogonadism	33143	Blue Rubber-Bleb Nevus Syndrome
30701	Prepubertal	33151	Breast Nipple Eczema
30702	Postpubertal	33149	Breast Nipple Keratosis
37670	Hypospadias/Epispadias	37116	Bromhidrosis
30586	Ovarian Failure	37183	Calcinosis Cutis
30587	Primary (Hypergonadotrophic	37184	Circumscripta
	Hypogonadism)	37185	Universalis
35216	Iatrogenic	37186	Dystrophic
37611	Postsurgical Ovarian Failure	37187	Metastatic
30588	Secondary (Hypogonadotrophic	37188	Calciphylaxis
	Hypogonadism)	37065	Callus
30589	Precocious Puberty	37111	Canities Segmentata Sideropenica
37614	Delayed Puberty	36163	Chloracne
30590	Inappropriate ADH Syndrome	37117	Chromhidrosis
	(SIADH)	33110	Chronic Cutaneous Ulcers
34350	**Dermatology**	33111	Venous Stasis
90180	Non-Infectious	33112	Arterial Insufficiency
33087	Acanthosis Nigricans	33113	Decubitus
33153	Acne	34400	Nondecubitus Of Lower Limbs
34397	Vulgaris	37135	Neurotrophic
37126	Premenstrual		

DERMATOLOGY, CONT.

37145	Cutaneous Diphtheria
37146	Necrobiosis Lipoidica Diabeticorum
37149	Meleney's
37153	Post-Traumatic
37154	Chemical-Induced
37155	Factitious
37137	Tropical
37138	Septic Desert Ulcer
37139	Mycotic
37140	Frambesia
37141	Buruli
37142	Leishmania
37143	Of Kaposi's Sarcoma
37144	Desert Sore
37091	Colloid Degeneration
37189	Colloid Milium
37094	Confluent And Reticulate Papillomatosis
33125	Contact Dermatitis
34372	Due To Detergents
34374	Due To Oils / Greases
34375	Due To Solvents
34376	Due To Skin Contact With Medications
34377	Due To Chemical Products
34378	Due To Food Touching Skin
34379	Due To Plants
37003	Due To Jewelry
37004	Due To Furs
38392	Due To Metal
38393	Due To Animals
34387	Corns
37063	Hard
37064	Soft
35808	Coumarin-Induced Skin Necrosis
33109	Cowden's Syndrome
37037	Cutaneous Lupus Erythematosis
37038	Chronic
33152	Discoid
37033	Localized
37034	Widespread
37043	With Systemic Involvement
37036	Verrucous
37039	Palmoplantar Erosive Discoid
37040	Chillblain
37035	Panniculitis
37041	With Discoid Lupus Erythematosis
37042	With Systemic Lupus Erythematosis
37032	Subacute
37044	Papulosquamous
37045	Annular
37046	Acute
37099	Darier's Disease Of The Nails

34380	Dermatitis Due To Consumed Food
33136	Dermatitis Factitia
33098	Dermatitis Herpetiformis
34381	Dermatitis Medicamentosa
37150	Drug-Induced Cutaneous Ulcers
33099	Eczematoid Dermatitis
37082	Elastosis Perforans Serpiginosa
37177	Ephelides
31103	Erysipelas
33138	Erythema Multiforme
37027	Minor
37026	Stevens-Johnson Syndrome
33140	Erythema Nodosum
35831	Erythema Toxicum Of The Newborn
34853	Erythroderma
37018	Familial Benign Chronic Pemphigus
37078	Focal Acral Hyperkeratosis
37107	Folliculitis Decalvans
37190	Foreign Body Granulomas Of The Skin
34395	Fox-Fordyce Disease
33157	Frostbite
37118	Granulosis Rubra Nasi
38227	Hallerman Streiff Syndrome
37074	Hereditary Palmoplantar Keratoderma
31151	Hidradenitis Suppurativa
36996	Hydroa Aestivale
33100	Hypertrichosis Lanuginosa
33101	Ichthyosis
33102	Vulgaris
31157	Impetigo
37012	Impetigo Herpetiformis
37097	Ingrowing Nail
33133	With Infection
37073	Keratoderma Climactericum
37085	Keratosis Blennorrhagica
38385	Keratosis Pilaris
37071	Keratosis Punctata Of The Palmar Creases
37076	Keratosis Punctata Of The Palmar Creases
37083	Kyrle's Disease
37104	Laugier-Hunziker Syndrome
37172	Lentigo
37173	Simplex
37174	Senilis
34385	Lichen Nitidus
33117	Lichen Planus
37070	Lichen Sclerosus Et Atrophicus
33118	Lichen Simplex Chronicus
37051	Lichen Striatus
37152	Lupus Pernio
37081	Mal De Meleda

DERMATOLOGY, CONT.

33144	Malignant Atrophic Papulosis (Degos Disease)	36991	Berloque
37102	Median Nail Dystrophy	36992	Dermatitis Bullosa Striata Pratensis
37058	Melanotic Prurigo Of Pierini And Borda	36993	Phytophotodermatitis
37176	Melasma	36990	Phototoxicity Due To Systemic Sensitizer
37005	Miliaria	36988	Photoallergic Contact Dermatitis
37006	Crystallina	36989	Photoallergy Due To Systemic Sensitizer
34393	Heat Rash		
37007	Pustulosa	36994	In Tattoo
37008	Profunda	37180	Pigmented Purpuric Lichenoid Dermatitis
37010	Tropical Anhidrotic Asthenia	31274	Pilonidal Cyst
37011	Occlusion	31275	With Abscess
37052	Morbus Moniliformis	36984	Pityriasis Alba
34386	Morphea	33141	Pityriasis Rosea
37066	Guttate	34392	Pityriasis Rubra Pilaris
37067	Generalized	36995	Polymorphous Light Eruption
37068	Pansclerotic, Of Children	34394	Pompholyx
37069	Linear Scleroderma	37072	Porokeratosis Palmaris Et Plantaris Disseminata
37175	Moynahan's Syndrome		
33103	Multiple Lentigines Syndrome	37009	Postmiliarial Hypohidrosis
37075	Mutatilating Keratoderma Of Vohwinkel	34965	Primary Vitiligo
30655	Nail-Patella Syndrome	37178	Progressive Pigmentary Dermatosis
33105	Necrolytic Migratory Erythema	37059	Prurigo Mitis
37061	Neurtoic Excoriation	36985	Prurigo Nodularis
37115	Neutrophilic Eccrine Hidradenitis	37060	Prurigo Polycythemica Of Kocsard
33104	Nodular Fat Necrosis	37057	Prurigo Simplex
34443	Of The Neck	37053	Pruritus Ani
33135	Nummular Eczematous Dermatitis	37055	Pruritus Scroti
37080	Olmstead Syndrome	37054	Pruritus Vulvae
33106	Pachydermoperiostosis	37108	Pseudopelade
37079	Papillon-Lefevre Syndrome	33107	Psoriasis
37056	Papular Urticaria	37048	Palmoplantar Pustular
37050	Parapsoriasis	36982	Bacterid
34384	Pemphigoid	31819	Psoriatic Arthropathy
37019	Bullous	37098	Psoriatic Nails
37020	Localized	37179	Purpura Annularis Telangiectodes
37021	Childhood	33137	Pyoderma Gangrenosum
37022	Cicatricial	34370	Pyogenic Granuloma
37023	Brunsting-Perry	37101	Racquet Nails
37024	Herpes Gestationis	37000	Radiation Dermatitis
33158	Pemphigus	37001	Non-Solar Ultraviolet
37013	Vulgaris	37002	X-Ray
37014	Vegetans	37084	Reactive Perforating Collagenosis
37015	Foliaceus	37031	Rhinophyma
37016	Brazilian	33127	Rosacea
37017	Erythematosus	34373	Sanitary Napkin Rash
34383	Malignant	34402	Scar
35747	Paraneoplastic	37182	Atrophic
37112	Perifolliculitis Capitis Abscedens Et Suffodiens	37092	Hypertrophic
		34389	Keloid
37030	Perioral Dermatitis	33108	Sebaceous Cyst
34855	Photodermatitis	37133	Pilar
36987	Phototoxic Contact Dermatitis	37134	Epidermal Inclusion

DERMATOLOGY, CONT.

34399	Seborrhea	36936	Wrist
37096	Seborrheic Keratosis	36937	Hand
38281	Inflamed	36938	Thumb
37089	Secondary Macular Atrophy	36939	Finger
33122	Senile Purpura	36925	Trunk
36999	Solar Elastosis	36926	Chest
34388	Striae Distensae	36927	Back
34382	Subcorneal Pustular Dermatosis	36928	Flank
33156	Sunburn	36929	Groin
37113	Sycosis Barbae	36930	Perineum
37114	Sycosis Lupoides	36940	Anorectal
37106	Telogen Effluvium	36931	Buttock
34854	Toxic Epidermal Necrolysis (TEN)	36941	Hip
37110	Trichorrhexis Invaginata	36942	Thigh
37109	Trichorrhexis Nodosa	36943	Popliteal Fossa
37100	Twenty Nail Dystropy	34355	Lower Leg
33123	Urticaria	36944	Ankle
34401	Allergic	34356	Foot
37156	Ingested Agent	36945	Plantar Surface
37157	Inhaled Agent	36946	Dorsal Surface
37158	Parenterally-Administered Agent	36947	Interdigital
37159	Invenomation	30907	Cellulitis
37160	Foreign Body	36976	Face
37161	Idiopathic	36977	Neck
31788	Cold	36978	Genital
37162	Heat	36979	Penile
36997	Solar	34359	Finger
37163	Dermatographic	34360	Toe
37165	Pressure-Induced	30908	Hemophilus Influenzae
37164	Vibratory	37148	Erythema Induratum
37166	Cholinergic	33139	Erythema Marginatum
37168	Exercise-Induced	33886	Erythema Nodosum Leprosum
37167	Adrenergic	36220	Erythema Nodosum Tuberculous
37170	Due To Chronic Infection	34391	Folliculitis
37171	Neoplasia-Related	37121	Gram-Negative
33124	Urticaria Pigmentosa	34351	Furuncle
33150	Varicocele	36948	Head
33142	Vogt-Koyanagi-Harada Disease	36949	Face
33097	Waardenburg Syndrome	36950	Scalp
37062	Winter Itch	36951	Ear
36919	Xerosis Cutis	36952	Neck
37103	Yellow Nail Syndrome	36953	Axilla
90181	Bacterial	36954	Shoulder
34354	Carbuncle	36955	Upper Arm
36921	Head	36956	Forearm
36920	Face	36957	Wrist
36923	Scalp	36958	Hand
36922	Ear	36959	Thumb
36924	Neck	36960	Finger
36932	Axilla	36961	Trunk
36933	Shoulder	36962	Chest
36934	Upper Arm	36963	Back
36935	Forearm	36964	Flank

DERMATOLOGY, CONT.

36965	Groin		30825	Infectious Arthritis
36966	Perineum		30826	Acute Bacterial
36967	Anorectal		30827	Gonococcal
36968	Buttock		30828	Chronic Tuberculous
36969	Hip		30829	Fungal
36970	Thigh		30830	Viral
36971	Popliteal Fossa		33757	Lyme
34352	Lower Leg		34828	Chronic
36972	Ankle		31818	Pseudogout
34353	Foot		33615	Gout
36973	Plantar Surface		33616	Primary
36974	Dorsal Surface		33617	Secondary
36975	Interdigital		33618	Acute
31291	Paronychia		33619	Chronic (Tophaceous)
34357	Finger		31841	Pprp Synthetase Excess
34358	Toe		34403	Chondrocalcinosis
31292	Fungal		38256	Due To Dicalcium Phosphate Crystals
31293	Staphylococcal		38257	Due To Pyrophosphate Crystals
36981	Perleche		31364	Sarcoidosis
37136	Pyoderma		31826	Uveoparotid Fever
34361	Skin Abscess		90210	Asymmetric Polyarticular Inflammation
34362	Face		31817	Juvenile Rheumatoid Arthritis
34363	Neck		33754	Systemic Onset (Still's Disease)
34364	Trunk		33755	Polyarticular
34365	Arm / Shoulder		35867	Rf Negative
34366	Wrist / Hand		35868	Rf Positive
34367	Buttock		33756	Pauciarticular
34368	Hip / Leg		35865	Type I
34369	Heel / Foot		35866	Type II
37029	Staphylococcal Scalded Skin Syndrome		35864	Monoarticular
37025	Toxic Erythema		34924	Adult Still's Disease
90182	Fungal		35858	Symmetric Polyarticular Inflammation
33115	Atopic Eczematous Dermatitis		31844	Rheumatoid Arthritis
33116	Barraquer-Simons Disease		31845	Felty's Syndrome
34371	Diaper Rash		33833	Necrobiotic Nodule
37047	Intertrigo		31837	Caplan's Syndrome
33134	Neurodermatitis		31835	Atlantoaxial Subluxation
36986	Nodular, Of The Scalp		31847	Systemic Lupus Erythematosus
34398	Seborrhea Capitis		31848	Drug Induced
33126	Seborrheic Dermatitis		31820	Arthritis Of Inflammatory Bowel Disease
36983	Of The Scalp		90212	Axial Polyarticular Inflammation
38495	Infantile		31789	Ankylosing Spondylitis
33120	Stasis Dermatitis		31821	Reiter's Syndrome
33128	Tinea Capitis		34409	Traumatic Arthropathy
38394	Tinea Corporis		37651	Charcot's Arthropathy
33129	Tinea Cruris		90228	Diabetic
33130	Tinea Imbricata		90229	Syringomyelic
33131	Tinea Pedis		90230	Syphilitic
33132	Tinea Versicolor		90219	Great Toe
90183	Parasitic		90220	Right
37093	Acrodermatitis Chronica Atrophicans		90221	Left
38673	**Rheumatology**		90216	Ankle
90211	Monoarticular Inflammation		90222	Right

RHEUMATOLOGY, CONT.

90223	Left	32485	Anserine
90217	Knee	32486	Subacromial
90224	Right	31840	Polymyalgia Rheumatica
90225	Left	35943	Fibromyalgia
90218	Hip	34465	Plantar Fascial Fibromatosis
90226	Right	34460	Ruptured Synovium
90227	Left	31843	Ruptured Baker's Cyst
34411	Transient Arthropathy	34467	Ruptured Muscle - Nontraumatic
34412	Unspecified Arthropathy	34468	Diastasis Of Muscle
31846	Osteoarthritis	34469	Muscle Spasm
34404	Localized	34470	Fasciitis
34406	Primary	38496	Necrotizing
34407	Secondary	90234	Connective Tissue Disorders
34405	Generalized	31793	Ehlers-Danlos Syndrome
34408	Kaschin-Beck Disease (Endemic Polyarthritis)	31794	Type I
		31795	Type II
34944	Osteoarthrosis	31796	Type III
31871	Xyphisternal Arthritis	31797	Type IV
31872	Tempromandibular Arthritis	31798	Type V
90214	Non-Articular Bone Disorders	31799	Type VI
30472	Osteoporosis	31800	Type VII
30473	Postmenopausal	33738	Type VIII
37653	Senile	31717	Polydysplastic Epidermolysis Bullosa
34477	Idiopathic	31801	Pseudoxanthoma Elasticum
30474	Disuse	31802	Cutis Laxa
30475	Drug-Induced	31803	Facialis
90213	Osteonecrosis	31811	Goodpasture's Syndrome
31232	Osteomyelitis	31823	Scleroderma
31233	Pseudomonas	36098	Crest Syndrome
31234	Hemophilus Influenzae	31838	Eosinophilic Fasciitis (Schulman's Syndrome)
31235	Mandibular		
31236	Proteus	31849	Mixed Connective Tissue Disease (MCTD)
31237	Salmonella		
31238	Staphylococcal	32478	Generalized Myositis Ossificans
36166	Tubercular	31824	Sjogren's Syndrome
31239	Vertebral	32479	Achondroplasia
34067	Petrositis	31825	Sicca Syndrome
37534	Acute	31842	Dupuytren's Contracture
37535	Chronic	32491	Fibrositis
32488	Osteogenesis Imperfecta	31221	Myositis
32492	Hyperostosis Frontalis Interna	34464	Infective
33765	Hyperostosis Generalisata With Pachydermia	31222	Clostridial Myositis
		31804	Polymyositis / Dermatomyositis:
33766	Hyperostosis Corticalis Generalisata	31805	Typical Polymyositis (Type I)
38422	Perichondritis	31806	Typical Dermatomyositis (Type II)
38423	Acute	31807	Typical Dermatomyositis With Malignancy (Type III)
38424	Chronic		
90231	Inflammatory Soft Tissue Disorders	31808	Childhood Dermatomyositis (Type IV)
32480	Bursitis	31809	Acute Myolysis (Type V)
32481	Trochanteric	31810	Polymyositis In Sjogren's Syndrome
32482	Olecranon	90232	Granulomatous Disorders
32483	Ischemic	31813	Histiocytoses (Histiocytosis X)
32484	Prepatellar	31814	Unifocal Eosinophilic Granuloma

Rheumatology, cont.

31815	Multifocal Eosinophilic Granuloma (Hand-Schuller-Christian)
31816	Letterer-Siwe Disease
31831	Wegener's Granulomatosis
33744	Talc Granulomatosis Of Drug Addicts
31832	Lymphomatoid Granulomatosis
90233	Vasculitides
31822	Behcet's Syndrome
34879	Acroosteolysis
33911	Necrotizing Vasculitis
31828	Hypersensitivity Vasculitis
31829	Polyarteritis Nodosa
34887	Microscopic
31827	Allergic Granulomatous Angiitis (Churg-Strauss)
31830	Temporal Arteritis
31834	Angioedema
33912	Rheumatoid Vasculitis
31870	Carotid Arteritis
39925	**Orthopedics**
32493	Fracture
32494	Skull
37705	Closed With Cerebral Laceration And Contusion
37706	Closed With Subarachnoid, Subdural, And Extradural Hemorrhage
37707	Closed With Other And Unspecified Intracranial Hemorrhage
37708	Closed With Intracranial Injury Of Unspecified Nature
37709	Open With Cerebral Laceration And Contusion
37710	Open With Subarachnoid, Subdural, And Extradural Hemorrhage
37711	Multiple Fractures
37712	Closed With Cerebral Laceration And Contusion
37713	Closed With Subarachnoid, Subdural, And Extradural Hemorrhage
37714	Open With Cerebral Laceration And Contusion
37715	Open With Subarachnoid, Subdural, And Extradural Hemorrhage
32495	Frontal / Parietal Bone
34608	Closed
32496	Closed With Cerebral Laceration And Contusion
37685	Closed With Subarachnoid, Subdural, And Extradural Hemorrhage
34609	Open
37686	Open Without Mention Of Intracranial Injury
37687	Open With Cerebral Laceration And Contusion
37688	Open With Subarachnoid, Subdural, And Extradural Hemorrhage
32497	Basilar
32498	Closed With Cerebral Laceration And Contusion
37689	Closed With Subarachnoid, Subdural, And Extradural Hemorrhage
37690	Open With Subarachnoid, Subdural, And Extradural Hemorrhage
32499	Nasal Bones - Closed
34610	Nasal Bones - Open
32500	Middle Cranial Fossa
32501	Mandibular / Lower Jaw - Closed
37691	Condylar Process
37692	Subcondylar
37693	Coronoid Process
37694	Ramus
37695	Angle Of Jaw
37696	Symphysis Of Body
37697	Alveolar Border Of Body
34611	Mandibular / Lower Jaw - Open
37698	Condylar Process
37699	Subcondylar
37700	Coronoid Process
37701	Ramus
37702	Angle Of Jaw
37703	Symphysis Of Body
37704	Alveolar Border Of Body
32502	Malar / Maxillary / Upper Jaw - Closed
34612	Malar / Maxillary / Upper Jaw - Open
32503	Orbital Floor (Blow-Out) - Closed
34613	Orbital Floor (Blow-Out) - Open
32504	Cervical Vertebral Body - Closed
34623	First
34617	Second
34624	Third
34625	Fourth
34618	Fifth
34619	Sixth
34626	Seventh

ORTHOPEDICS, CONT.

37191	Multiple	
35862	Compression	
34614	Cervical Vertebral Body - Open	
37897	Cervical Vertebral Body - Closed, With Spinal Cord Injury	
37905	C1-C4 Level	
37906	C1-C4 Level With Complete Lesion Of Cord	
37907	C1-C4 Level With Anterior Cord Syndrome	
37908	C1-C4 Level With Central Cord Syndrome	
37909	C5-C7 Level	
37910	C5-C7 Level With Complete Lesion Of Cord	
37911	C5-C7 Level With Anterior Cord Syndrome	
37912	C5-C7 Level With Central Cord Syndrome	
37898	Cervical Vertebral Body - Open, With Spinal Cord Injury	
37913	C1-C4 Level	
37914	C1-C4 Level With Complete Lesion Of Cord	
37915	C1-C4 Level With Anterior Cord Syndrome	
37916	C1-C4 Level With Central Cord Syndrome	
37917	C5-C7 Level	
37918	C5-C7 Level With Complete Lesion Of Cord	
37919	C5-C7 Level With Anterior Cord Syndrome	
37920	C5-C7 Level With Central Cord Syndrome	
32505	Thoracic Vertebral Body - Closed	
34615	Thoracic Vertebral Body - Open	
37899	Thoracic Vertebral Body - Closed, With Spinal Cord Injury	
37921	T1-T6 Level	
37922	T1-T6 Level With Complete Lesion Of Cord	
37923	T1-T6 Level With Anterior Cord Syndrome	
37924	T1-T6 Level With Central Cord Syndrome	
37925	T7-T12 Level	
37926	T7-T12 Level With Complete Lesion Of Cord	
37927	T7-T12 Level With Anterior Cord Syndrome	
37928	T7-T12 Level With Central Cord Syndrome	
37900	Thoracic Vertebral Body - Open, With Spinal Cord Injury	
37929	T1-T6 Level	
37930	T1-T6 Level With Complete Lesion Of Cord	
37931	T1-T6 Level With Anterior Cord Syndrome	
37932	T1-T6 Level With Central Cord Syndrome	
37933	T7-T12 Level	
37934	T7-T12 Level With Complete Lesion Of Cord	
37935	T7-T12 Level With Anterior Cord Syndrome	
37936	T7-T12 Level With Central Cord Syndrome	
32506	Lumbar Vertebral Body - Closed	
34616	Lumbar Vertebral Body - Open	
37901	Lumbar Vertebral Body - Closed, With Spinal Cord Injury	
37902	Lumbar Vertebral Body - Open, With Spinal Cord Injury	
37903	Sacrum / Coccyx - Closed, With Spinal Cord Injury	
37904	Sacrum / Coccyx - Open, With Spinal Cord Injury	
32507	Sacrum / Coccyx - Closed	
32508	With Complete Cauda Equina Lesion	
34620	Sacrum / Coccyx - Open	
32606	Rib(s) - Closed	
32607	Multiple	
34621	Rib(s) - Open	
34622	Multiple	
34627	Sternum - Closed	
34628	Sternum - Open	
32608	Flail Chest	
34629	Larynx And Trachea - Closed	
34630	Larynx And Trachea - Open	
32509	Pelvic	
32510	Acetabulum (Closed)	
37716	Acetabulum (Open)	
32511	Pubis (Closed)	
34631	Ilium	
34632	Ischium	
32512	Multiple, With Disruption Of Pelvic Circle	
32513	Of Clavicle	
34633	(Closed)	
34634	Sternal End	
34635	Shaft	
34636	Acromial End	
34637	(Open)	

34638	Sternal End	34681	Ulna Only
34639	Shaft	34682	Radius With Ulna
34640	Acromial End	34683	Shaft, Open
32514	Of Scapula	34684	Radius Only
34641	(Closed)	34685	Ulna Only
34642	Acromial Process	34686	Radius With Ulna
34643	Coracoid Process	34687	Distal End, Closed
34644	Glenoid Cavity / Neck Of Scapula	32524	Colles' Fracture
34645	(Open)	34688	Radius Only
34646	Acromial Process	34689	Ulna Only
34647	Coracoid Process	34690	Radius With Ulna
34648	Glenoid Cavity / Neck Of Scapula	34691	Distal End, Open
32515	Of Humerus	34692	Colles' Fracture
34649	Proximal End, Closed	34693	Radius Only
32516	Surgical Neck	34694	Ulna Only
34650	Anatomical Neck	34695	Radius With Ulna
34651	Greater Tuberosity	34696	Of Carpal Bone(s), Closed
34652	Proximal End, Open	32527	Navicular
34653	Surgical Neck	34697	Lunate Bone
34654	Anatomical Neck	34698	Triquetral Bone
34655	Greater Tuberosity	34699	Pisiform
32517	Shaft, Closed	34700	Trapezium Bone
32518	Shaft, Open	34701	Trapezoid Bone
34656	Distal End, Closed	34702	Capitate Bone
32519	Supracondylar	34703	Hamate Bone
34658	Lateral Condyle	34704	Of Carpal Bone(s), Open
32521	Medial Condyle	34705	Navicular
34660	Multiple	34706	Lunate Bone
34657	Distal End, Open	34707	Triquetral Bone
32520	Supracondylar	34708	Pisiform
34659	Lateral Condyle	34709	Trapezium Bone
32522	Medial Condyle	34710	Trapezoid Bone
34661	Multiple	34711	Capitate Bone
34662	Of Radius / Ulna	34712	Hamate Bone
34663	Proximal End, Closed	34713	Metacarpal Bone(s) (Closed)
34664	Olecranon Process	34714	Base Of Thumb
34665	Coronoid Process	34715	2nd To 5th
34666	Monteggia's Fracture	34716	Shaft
34667	Multiple	34717	Neck
32523	Head Of Radius	34718	Multiple
34668	Neck Of Radius	34719	Metacarpal Bone(s) (Open)
34670	Radius With Ulna	37192	Base Of Thumb
34671	Proximal End, Open	37193	2nd To 5th
34672	Olecranon Process	37194	Shaft
34673	Coronoid Process	37195	Neck
34674	Monteggia's Fracture	37196	Multiple
34675	Multiple	32525	Of Phalange(s) - Closed
34676	Head Of Radius	34721	Of Phalange(s) - Open
34677	Neck Of Radius	32526	Of Hand Bones, Multiple (Closed)
34669	Upper Radius NEC/NOS-Open	34722	Of Hand Bones, Multiple (Open)
34678	Radius With Ulna	34723	Involving Both Arms With Rib(s) Or
34679	Shaft, Closed		Sternum - Closed
34680	Radius Only	32528	Of Neck Of Femur - Closed

ORTHOPEDICS, CONT.

34724	Transcervical	37728	Cuneiform Bone (Foot)
34725	Transepiphyseal	32540	Metatarsal Bone(s)
34726	Midcervical	34751	Of Tarsal Bone(s) - Open
34727	Base Of Neck	37729	Astragalus
34728	Head Of Femur	37730	Navicular Bone (Foot)
34729	Pertrochanteric	37731	Cuboid
34730	Intertrochanteric	37732	Cuneiform Bone (Foot)
34731	Subtrochanteric	37733	Metatarsal Bone(s)
34732	Of Neck Of Femur - Open	32541	Of Phalange(s) (Foot) - Closed
34733	Transcervical	34752	Of Phalange(s) (Foot) - Open
34734	Transepiphyseal	32542	Pathologic
34735	Midcervical	38258	Of The Humerus
34736	Base Of Neck	38259	Of The Distal Radius And Ulna
34737	Pertrochanteric	38260	Of Vertebrae
34738	Intertrochanteric	38261	Of The Femur
34739	Subtrochanteric	38262	Of The Tibia
32529	Of Shaft Of Femur, Closed	38263	Of The Fibula
35987	Oblique Transverse	34480	Pseudarthrosis
32530	Of Shaft Of Femur, Open	32543	Dislocation
34740	Of Distal End Of Femur, Closed	32544	Temporomandibular
37717	Condyle, Femoral	37197	Open
37718	Epiphysis, Lower (Separation)	34454	Bone Spur
37719	Supracondylar Fracture Of Femur	32545	Of Shoulder
34741	Of Distal End Of Femur, Open	37198	Open
37720	Condyle, Femoral	32546	Of Elbow
37721	Epiphysis, Lower (Separation)	37199	Open
37722	Supracondylar Fracture Of Femur	32547	Of Wrist
32531	Of Patella - Closed	37200	Open
34742	Of Patella - Open	32548	Of Finger(s)
32532	Tibia, Closed	37201	Open
37937	Proximal	32549	Of Hip
37938	Shaft	38459	Right
34743	With Fibula	38460	Left
32533	Of Tibia, Open	38461	Bilateral
37939	Proximal	37202	Open
37940	Shaft	32550	Of Knee
32534	Of Fibula, Closed	34753	Bucket Handle Tear Of Medial Meniscus
32535	Of Fibula, Open	34754	Tear Of Lateral Cartilage
32536	Of Ankle (Closed)	34755	Tear Of Semilunar Cartilage
34745	Medial Malleolus	32551	Patella
34746	Lateral Malleolus	37206	Closed
34747	Bimalleolar	37734	Anterior Dislocation Of Tibia, Proximal End
34748	Trimalleolar	37735	Posterior Dislocation Of Tibia, Proximal End
32537	Of Ankle, Open		
37723	Medial Malleolus	37736	Medial Dislocation Of Tibia, Proximal End
37724	Lateral Malleolus		
37725	Bimalleolar	37737	Lateral Dislocation Of Tibia, Proximal End
37726	Trimalleolar		
32538	Of Heel - Closed	37205	Open
34750	Of Heel - Open	37738	Anterior Dislocation Of Tibia, Proximal End
34749	Of Tarsal Bone(s) - Closed		
32539	Navicular Bone (Foot)		
37727	Cuboid Bone		

ORTHOPEDICS, CONT.

37739	Posterior Dislocation Of Tibia, Proximal End	90206	Right
		90207	Left
37740	Medial Dislocation Of Tibia, Proximal End	90208	Bilateral
		32556	Sprain / Strain
37741	Lateral Dislocation Of Tibia, Proximal End	32557	Jaw
		32572	Neck
32552	Of Ankle	32558	Shoulder
37203	Open	34757	Acromioclavicular Joint
34756	Of Foot	37216	Acromioclavicular Ligament
37204	Open	37217	Coracoclavicular Ligament
32553	Cervical Vertebra	37218	Coracohumeral Ligament
37742	Closed	37219	Infraspinatus Muscle
37743	First	37220	Infraspinatus Tendon
37750	Second	32559	Rotator Cuff (Capsule)
37744	Third	37222	Subcapularis Muscle
37745	Fourth	32573	Supraspinatus Muscle
37746	Fifth	37221	Supraspinatus Tendon
37747	Sixth	37249	Right
37748	Seventh	37250	Left
37749	Multiple	37223	Upper Arm
37207	Open	32560	Elbow
37751	First	37225	Radiohumeral Joint
37752	Second	37226	Ulnohumeral Joint
37753	Third	37251	Right
37754	Fourth	37252	Left
37755	Fifth	37224	Forearm
37756	Sixth	37227	Radial Collateral Ligament
37757	Seventh	37228	Ulnar Collateral Ligament
37758	Multiple	32561	Wrist
32554	Lumbar Vertebra	37229	Carpal Joint
37208	Open	37230	Radiocarpal Joint
32555	Thoracic Vertebra	37231	Radiocarpal Ligament
37209	Open	37253	Right
37210	Coccyx	37254	Left
37211	Open	34758	Hand
37212	Sacrum	37232	Carpometacarpal Joint
37213	Open	37233	Metacarpophalangeal Joint
37214	Sternum	32562	Finger
37215	Open	32574	Pectoralis Minor
90193	Separation	37245	Sternum
32598	Shoulder	37246	Sternoclavicular Joint
90194	Right	37247	Sternoclavicular Ligament
90195	Left	37248	Chondrosternal Joint
90196	Bilateral	34764	Thoracic
90197	Elbow	34763	Lumbar
90198	Right	34761	Sacroiliac Region
90199	Left	34762	Lumbosacral Joint
90200	Bilateral	37241	Lumbosacral Ligament
90201	Hip	38176	Chronic Lumbosacral Strain
90202	Right	37242	Sacroiliac Ligament
90203	Left	37243	Sacrospinatus Ligament
90204	Bilateral	37244	Sacrotuberous Ligament
90205	Knee	32575	Lower Back

ORTHOPEDICS, CONT.

34765	Coccyx
32563	Hip
37234	Iliofemoral Ligament
37235	Ischiocapsular Ligament
32576	Thigh
32564	Knee
32565	Lateral Collateral Ligament
32566	Medial Collateral Ligament
32567	Cruciate Ligament
37310	Right
37311	Left
32568	Ankle
32569	Deltoid Ligament
37236	Calcaneofibular Ligament
37237	Tibiofibular Ligament
34759	Achilles Tendon
37312	Right
37313	Left
34760	Foot
37238	Tarsometatarsal Joint
37240	Tarsometatarsal Ligament
37239	Metatarsophalangeal Joint
32570	Toe
32620	Tendonitis
32621	Achilles
32622	Bicipital
32623	Patellar
32624	Posterior Tibial
32625	Rotator Cuff Tear
32626	Calcifying, Of Shoulder
32627	Supraspinatus
32628	Tricipital
32629	Tennis Elbow
34451	Adhesive Capsulitis Of Shoulder
34461	Tendon Rupture
34462	Rotator Cuff
32630	Bicipital
34463	Quadriceps
32631	Achilles
32633	Tenosynovitis
32634	Bicipital
34455	Trigger Finger (Acquired)
32635	De Quervain's
32618	Muscle Hematoma
32619	Neck Injury
34452	Medial Epicondylitis
32571	Unspecified Muscle Strain
34421	Intra-Articular Abnormality
34413	Internal Derangement Of Knee
33763	Meniscus Injury
34414	Old Bucket Handle Tear Of Medial Meniscus

34415	Anterior Horn Of Medial Meniscus
34416	Posterior Horn Of Medial Meniscus
34418	Lateral Meniscus
34417	Degeneration Of Internal Semilunar Cartilage
34419	Loose Body In Knee
34481	Chondromalacia
34420	Patellar Chondromalacia
34422	Articular Cartilage Disorder (Non-Genu)
32610	Intraarticular Bone Fragment (Non-Genu)
34423	Pathological Dislocation
34424	Recurrent Dislocation
34425	Contracture
34426	Ankylosis
34453	Calcaneal Spur
34555	Congenital Deformity
34556	Head
38224	Craniostosis
34571	Upper Limb
34575	Spine
34576	Lumbosacral Spondylolysis
34577	Spondylolisthesis
32604	Spina Bifida
35748	Absence Of Sacrum
38386	Hip
34572	Lower Limb
34573	Knee
34563	Foot
34564	Talipes Varus
34565	Talipes Equinovarus
34566	Metatarsus Primus Varus
34567	Metatarsus Varus
34568	Talipes Valgus
34570	Talipes Calcaneovalgus
34574	Toes
37671	Polydactyly Of Fingers
37672	Polydactyly Of Toes
37673	Syndactyly
37674	Cleft Hand
34482	Flat Foot
34569	Congenital
34485	Acquired Deformity
34486	Toe
34487	Hallux Valgus
34488	Hallux Varus
34489	Hallux Rigidus
34490	Hallux Malleus
34491	Claw Toe
34492	Forearm

ORTHOPEDICS, CONT.

34493	Cubitus Valgus		32612	Acute Chest Wall Trauma
34494	Cubitus Varus		32602	Arthrogryposis Multiplex Congenita
34495	Wrist		32600	Aseptic Necrosis
34496	Valgus		32601	Of Femoral Head
34497	Varus		34456	Bunion
34498	Wrist Drop		32613	Chest Wall Open Wound
34499	Claw Hand		37816	Chest Wall Open Wound, Complicated
34500	Club Hand		32599	Costochondritis (Tietze's Syndrome)
34502	Finger		31109	Felon
34503	Boutonniere		34459	Ganglion
34504	Swan-Neck		34458	Joint
34501	Mallet Finger		32636	Wrist
34505	Hip		34427	Hydrarthrosis
34506	Coxa Valga		32611	Intercostal Myositis
34507	Coxa Vara		32615	Intermittent Hydrarthrosis
34508	Knee		34466	Interstitial Myositis
34509	Genu Valgum		34475	Juvenile Osteochondrosis Of Foot
34510	Genu Varum		34472	Juvenile Osteochondrosis Of Spine
34511	Genu Recurvatum		34474	Juvenile Osteochondrosis Of Upper
34512	Ankle			Extremity
34513	Foot		32617	Legg-Perthe's Disease
34514	Equinovarus		32587	Melorheostosis
34515	Equinus		32603	Multiple Exostosis
34516	Cavus		32616	Osgood Schlatter Disease
34517	Cavovarus		34476	Osteochondritis Dissecans
34518	Claw Foot		33764	Osteomyelosclerosis
34519	Unequal Leg Length		32589	Osteopenia
38286	Tibial Torsion		32590	Osteopetrosis
38287	Medial		32588	Osteopoikilosis
38288	Lateral		32591	Paget's Disease
34529	Nose		32594	Pectus Excavatum
34530	Head		32592	Pigmented Villonodular Synovitis
34531	Neck		34946	Polyostotic Fibrous Dysplasia
34532	Chest		32593	Progressive Diaphyseal Dysplasia
34533	Ribs		32595	Pyknodysostosis
32614	Spondylolisthesis		32596	Relapsing Polychondritis
34535	Pelvis		32609	Rib Periostitis
34536	Cauliflower Ear		32597	Shoulder-Hand Syndrome
34537	Clavicle		34473	Slipped Upper Femoral Epiphysis
34483	Kyphosis (Acquired)		32605	Subluxation Atlas
34521	Adolescent Postural		38674	**Neurology**
34522	Radiation		90005	Disorders Of Consciousness
34523	Postlaminectomy		31875	Nerve Disorders
34484	Lordosis (Acquired)		31876	Neuromuscular Diseases
34524	Postlaminectomy		31877	Brain Death
32586	Kyphoscoliosis		31878	Cerebral Herniation
34520	Scoliosis		31879	Uncal
34562	Congenital		31880	Central
34525	Resolving Infantile Idiopathic		31881	Tonsillar
34526	Progressive Infantile Idiopathic		31882	Persistent Vegetative State
34527	Radiation		34035	Frontal Lobe Syndrome
34528	Thoracogenic		31883	Head Injury
90209	Other Disorders		37761	With Subarachnoid Hemorrhage

NEUROLOGY, CONT.

37762	With Subdural Hemorrhage	90007	CNS Infections
37763	With Extradural Hemorrhage	31192	Meningitis
37261	With Open Intracranial Wound	31193	Aseptic
37764	With Subarachnoid Hemorrhage	35668	Viral
37765	With Subdural Hemorrhage	31436	Mumps
37766	With Extradural Hemorrhage	31087	Lymphocytic Choriomeningitis
38396	With Dementia	31207	Coxsackie Group B Virus
31885	Concussion	31208	Echo Virus
37255	With No Loss Of Consciousness	36272	Adenovirus
37256	With Brief Loss Of Consciousness (Under 1 Hour)	31195	Bacterial
		31206	Meningococcal
37257	With Moderate Loss Of Consciousness (1-24 Hours)	31198	Pneumococcal
		31212	Streptococcus Pyogenes
37258	With Prolonged Loc (Over 24 Hr) And Return To Prev. Level	31210	Staph Aureus
		31204	Hemophilus Influenzae
37259	With Prolonged Loc (Over 24 Hr) Without Return To Prev. Level	31203	Gonococcal
		31199	Gram Negative
37260	With Loss Of Consciousness Of Unspecified Duration	36354	Aerobacter Aerogenes
		36355	Escherichia Coli
34034	Postconcussion Syndrome	36356	Friedlander Bacillus
31884	Cerebral Contusion	36357	Klebsiella Pneumoniae
37759	Cerebral Contusion With Open Intracranial Wound	36358	Proteus Morganii
		36359	Pseudomonas
37760	Cerebellar Contusion With Open Intracranial Wound	36360	Anaerobic
		36361	Bacteroides Fragilis
37309	Gunshot Wound Of The Brain	31213	Geriatric Presentation
32394	Vasovagal Syncope	31211	Staph Epidermidis (Albus)
36097	Presyncope Syndrome	31200	Listeria Monocytogenes
31986	Amnesia	35223	Salmonella
31987	Post-Traumatic	31205	Pasturella Multocida
31988	Transient Global	36362	Bacillus Pyocyaneus
90006	Headache Syndromes	31065	Leptospiral
31894	Tension Headache	31196	Tubercular
31887	Migraine Headache	31201	Fungal
36008	Classical	31197	Cryptococcal
36009	Common	31445	Coccidioidal
31888	Basilar Artery	36310	Parasitic
31889	Ophthalmoplegic	36311	Trypanosomiasis
36010	Hemiplegic	31209	Naegleria
31890	Abdominal	31194	Chemical
31891	Menstrual	31202	Eosinophilic
36003	Non-Migranous Vascular Headache	34036	Chronic
31893	Cluster Headache	35670	Meningeal Sarcoidosis
36005	Episodic	31214	Ventriculitis
36006	Primary Chronic	31215	Ependymitis
36007	Secondary Chronic	31216	Choroidal Plexitis
36411	Cerebral Edema	30879	Brain Abscess
36004	Chronic Paroxysmal Hemicrania	30880	Temporal Lobe
31892	Premenstrual Headache Syndrome	36210	Tuberculous
31895	Hangover	30881	Cerebellar
31896	Post-Lumbar Puncture Headache	30882	Frontal Lobe
31897	Lumbar Puncture Traumatic Tap	30883	Parietal Lobe
31898	Cerebrospinal Fluid Rhinorrhea	30884	Occipital Lobe

NEUROLOGY, CONT.

30885	Subdural Empyema		31899	Brain Tumor
30886	Epidural Empyema		31901	Glioblastoma Multiforme
31932	Intracranial Tuberculoma		34931	Anaplastic Astrocytoma
34932	Spinal Cord Tuberculoma		31902	Astrocytoma (Grades I & II)
36211	Tuberculous Abscess Of Spinal Cord		31900	Brain Stem Glioma
36212	Tuberculous Encephalitis		31948	Optic Nerve Glioma
36213	Tuberculous Myelitis		36776	Glioma Of The Optic Chiasm
30854	Viral Encephalitis		31941	Hypothalamic Neoplasm
30978	Herpes Simplex		31942	Ventromedial Nucleus
35669	Herpes Zoster		34995	Supraoptic Nucleus
36172	Mosquito-Borne		34996	Paraventricular Nucleus
30856	Eastern Equine		31943	Glioma
30857	Japanese		31912	Cerebellar Cystic Astrocytoma
30858	St. Louis		31903	Subependymal Giant Cell Astrocytoma
30855	California		31907	Oligodendroglioma
36273	La Crosse		34933	Anaplastic
36173	Tick-Borne		34993	Neurocytoma
36274	Russian Spring-Summer		34994	Anaplastic
36275	Louping Ill		31933	Ependymoma
36276	Central European		31904	Diffuse Histiocytic Lymphoma (RCS)
36277	Powassan		31905	Medulloblastoma
30859	Venezuelan Equine		31908	Neurofibroma - Trigeminal Nerve
30860	Western Equine		31909	Neurofibroma - Acoustic Nerve
31290	Progressive Multifocal Leukoencephalopathy		31910	Chordoma
			31911	Cerebellar Hemangioblastoma
31360	Subacute Sclerosing Panencephalitis (SSPE)		31913	Meningioma
			31914	Parasagittal
31296	Progressive Rubella Encephalitis		31915	Hemisphere Convexity
31380	Toxoplasma Meningoencephalitis		31916	Sphenoidal Ridge
31412	Encephalomyelitis		31917	Anterior Fossa Floor
31413	Postinfectious		31918	Middle Fossa Floor
31414	Postvaricella		31919	Posterior Fossa Floor
31415	Postmeasles		31920	Clivus
31416	Postmumps		31921	Foramen Magnum
34871	Epstein-Barr		31922	Tentorium
31417	Postvaccination		31923	Cerebellopontine Angle
31967	Acute Disseminated Encephalomyelitis		31924	Intraventricular
31968	Acute Necrotizing Hemorrhagic Leukoencephalitis		31925	Tuberculum Sellae
			31926	Falx
31022	Poliomyelitis		31927	Optic Nerve
36269	Paralytic		34997	Papillary
36270	Bulbar		34998	Malignant
36271	Nonparalytic		31514	Hemangiopericytoma
34471	Osteopathy		34999	Malignant
35779	Post-Polio Syndrome		31906	Meningeal Sarcoma
31421	Neurosyphilis		31929	Papilloma Of Choroid Plexus
31422	Meningeal		31930	Carcinoma Of Choroid Plexus
31425	Spinal		31931	Brain Metastasis
31424	Cerebral Meningovascular		31936	Craniopharyngioma
31426	Tabes		31937	Rathke's Pouch Cyst
31427	Paresis (GPI)		31938	Colloid Cyst Of Third Ventricle
31428	Optic Atrophy		31939	Germ Cell Tumor
90008	CNS Neoplasms		34936	Germinoma

NEUROLOGY, CONT.

34937	Non-Germinoma
31946	Teratoma (CNS)
34938	Embryonal Carcinoma
34939	Teratocarcinoma
34940	Choriocarcinoma
34941	Endodermal Sinus Tumor
31940	Pinealoma
35000	Pineoblastoma
35001	Pineocytoma
31944	Epidermoid Tumor (Cholesteatoma)
31945	Dermoid
31947	Lipoma (CNS)
31928	Carcinomatous Meningitis (Leptomeningeal Metastasis)
35666	Lymphomatous Meningitis (Leptomenigeal Metastasis)
35667	Leukemic Meningitis (Leptomenigeal Metastasis)
31949	Base Of Skull Metastasis
31950	Orbital Apex
31951	Parasellar
31952	Middle Fossa Floor
31953	Petrous Apex
31954	Posterior Fossa Floor
31934	Sphenoid Sinus Carcinoma
31935	Sphenoid Sinus Mucocele
31959	Paraganglioma (Chemodectoma)
31751	Glomus Jugulare Tumor
34935	Glomus Vagale Tumor
31752	Carotid Body Tumor
32216	Arachnoid Cyst
36410	Porencephalic Cyst
32217	Ependymal Cyst
90009	Neurocutaneous Disorders
31955	Von Hippel-Lindau - (Cerebelloretinal Hemangioblastomatosis)
31956	Neurofibromatosis Type I - (Von Recklinghausen's Disease)
34934	Neurofibromatosis Type II (Bilateral Acoustic)
31957	Tuberous Sclerosis (Bourneville's Disease)
31960	Sturge-Weber Disease (Encephalotrigeminal Syndrome)
33298	Klippel-Trenaunay-Weber Syndrome
33350	Hereditary Hemorrhagic Telangiectasia (Osler-Rendu-Weber)
32231	Ataxia-Telangiectasia (Louis-Bar Disease)
90010	Encephalopathies And Hydrocephalies
31962	Acute Hypoxic Encephalopathy
31963	Hypertensive Encephalopathy
31964	Hepatic Encephalopathy

31965	Acute Hypoglycemic Encephalopathy
30647	Uremic Encephalopathy
35671	Septic Encephalopathy
36312	Toxic Encephalopathy
36363	Lead
36364	Mercury
36365	Carbon Tetrachloride
36366	Hydroxyquinoline Derivatives
36367	Thallium
31961	Pseudotumor Cerebri
31969	Hydrocephalus
31970	Normal Pressure
31971	Increased Pressure
35672	Communicating
35673	Obstructive
36021	Congenital
36022	Hydranencephaly
31972	Aqueductal Stenosis
90011	Epilepsies
31974	Epilepsy
31975	Grand Mal
31980	Myoclonic
31978	Petit Mal
31976	Jacksonian
31979	Focal
36405	Visual
36406	Sensory
31977	Psychomotor
36407	Cursive
36408	Gelastic
31981	Petit Mal Status
31982	Grand Mal Status
36404	Infantile Spasms
36409	Epilepsia Partialis Continua
31983	Progressive Familial Myoclonic Epilepsy
31984	Mesial Temporal Sclerosis
31985	LaFora Body Disease
90012	Cerebral Degenerations, Extrapyramidal Disorders And Movement Disorders
31989	Alzheimer's Dementia
32693	Early Onset
38377	Uncomplicated
38378	With Delirium
38379	With Delusions
38380	With Depressed Mood
32688	Late Onset
32692	Uncomplicated
32689	With Delirium
32690	With Delusions
32691	With Depressed Mood
32694	Vascular Dementia
38381	Uncomplicated
38382	With Delirium

NEUROLOGY, CONT.

38383	With Delusions	36397	Diplegic
38384	With Depressed Mood	36398	Hemiplegic
31990	Pick's Disease	36399	Postnatal
38399	With Dementia	36400	Congenital
31991	Creutzfeldt-Jakob Disease	36401	Quadraplegic
38400	With Dementia	32258	Little's Disease
32228	Gerstmann-Straussler-Sheinker Syndrome	32012	Double Athetosis (Congenital Choreoathetosis)
35811	Fatal Familial Insomnia	36379	Athetoid Cerebral Palsy
33943	Kuru	32013	Kernicterus
30597	Chorea Gravidarum	32014	Ballismus / Hemiballismus
32015	Senile Chorea	32016	Familial (Benign Essential) Tremor
31310	Sydenham's Chorea	39995	Drug-Induced Essential Tremor
31992	Huntington's Chorea	32017	Senile Tremor
38398	With Dementia	32018	Spasmodic Torticollis
39993	Neuroleptic-Induced Acute Akathisia	31993	Acute Dystonic Reaction
31994	Tardive Dyskinesia	39992	Neuroleptic-Induced Acute Dystonia
39994	Neuroleptic-Induced	32019	Organic Writer's Cramp
35827	Restless Leg Syndrome	32020	Dystonia Musculorum Deformans
31995	Wilson's Disease	36378	Schwalbe-Ziehen-Oppenheim
31996	Hepatocerebral Degeneration (Non-Wilsonian)	32010	'Stiff Man' Syndrome
31997	Hallervorden-Spatz Disease	32021	Tolosa-Hunt Syndrome
31998	Jansky-Bielschowsky Disease	32041	Hemifacial Spasm
31999	Gaucher's Disease (Infantile)	38553	Blepharospasm
32000	Niemann-Pick Disease	36369	Akathesia
32001	Tay-Sachs Disease (Gm2 Gangliosidosis)	34439	Torticollis
33848	Tay-Sachs Carrier (Partial Hexosaminidase Deficiency)	35841	Congenital
33931	Sandhoff Disease	90014	Demyelinating Disorders
32002	Kufs' Disease (Ceroid Lipofuscinosis)	32022	Multiple Sclerosis
32003	Batten-Spielmayer-Vogt Disease	32023	Acute Transverse Myelitis
36371	Amaurotic (Familial) Idiocy	32024	Devic's Disease
36372	Alpers' Disease	32025	Optic Neuritis
36373	Infantile Necrotizing Encephalomyelopathy	32026	Retrobulbar Neuritis
36374	Leigh's Disease	32027	Central Pontine Myelinolysis
36375	Subacute Necrotizing Encephalopathy	32028	Schilder's Disease
36376	Rett's Syndrome	32029	Canavan's Disease (Van Bogaert-Bertrand-Canavan)
38371	Childhood Disintegrative Disorder	32033	Krabbe's Disease (Globoid Body Leukodystrophy)
32374	Fahr's Syndrome	32034	Pelizaeus-Merzbacher Disease ("Sudanophilic Leukodystrophy")
32004	Parkinson's Disease		
32005	Postencephalitic	32035	Hereditary (Leber's) Optic Atrophy
38397	With Dementia	32030	Metachromatic Leukodystrophy
32006	Pseudoparkinsonism	32031	Adrenoleukodystrophy
38626	Neuroleptic-Induced Parkinsonism	36370	Sulfatide Lipidosis
38660	Neuroleptic Malignant Syndrome	32032	Fibrinoid Leukodystrophy
32007	Juvenile Paralysis Agitans	32367	Marchiafava-Bignami
32008	Shy-Drager Syndrome	90091	Mitochondrial Disorders
32009	Progressive Supranuclear Palsy (Steele-Richardson-Olszewski)	36315	Mitochondrial Encephalopathy
		36314	Melas Syndrome
32011	Cerebral Palsy	36316	Merrf Syndrome
36402	Monoplegic	32349	Kearns-Sayre Syndrome
36403	Paraplegic	32346	Progressive Ophthalmoplegia

NEUROLOGY, CONT.

32347	Chronic External	32094	Subthalamic Nucleus (Hemichorea / Hemiballismus) - Left
90023	CNS Vascular Disorders		
32048	Amaurosis Fugax	32095	Pseudobulbar Palsy (Lacunar State)
32049	Transient Ischemic Attack (TIA)	36099	Multiple
32050	Stroke Syndrome	38502	Iatrogenic
32051	Internal Carotid Artery	32042	Dejerine-Roussy Syndrome
32052	- Right (Non-Dominant)	32096	Weber's Syndrome
32053	- Left (Dominant)	32097	- Right
32054	Middle Cerebral Artery	32098	- Left
32055	- Right (Non-Dominant)	32099	Claude's Syndrome
32056	- Left (Dominant)	32100	- Right
32057	Anterior Cerebral Artery	32101	- Left
32058	- Right (Non-Dominant)	32102	Benedikt's Syndrome
32059	- Left (Dominant)	32103	- Right
32060	Anterior Choroidal Artery	32104	- Left
32061	- Right (Non-Dominant)	32105	Nothnagel's Syndrome
32062	- Left (Dominant)	32106	Parinaud's Syndrome
32063	Posterior Cerebral Artery	32107	Millard-Gubler Syndrome
32064	- Right	32108	- Right
32065	- Left	32109	- Left
32066	Bilateral Occipital Infarct	32110	Raymond-Foville Syndrome
32067	Vertebral Artery	32111	- Right
32068	- Right	32112	- Left
32069	- Left	32113	Avellis Syndrome
32070	Posterior Inferior Cerebellar (Wallenberg's)	32114	- Right
		32115	- Left
32071	- Right	32116	Jackson's Syndrome
32072	- Left	32117	- Right
32073	Basilar Artery	32118	- Left
32074	Basilar Artery Occlusion	32119	Ophthalmic Artery Aneurysm
32075	Superior Cerebellar Artery	32120	- Right
32076	- Right	32121	- Left
32077	- Left	32122	Internal Carotid Artery Aneurysm
32078	Medial Medullary Syndrome	32123	- Right
32079	- Right	32124	- Left
32080	- Left	32125	Middle Cerebral Artery Aneurysm
32081	Anterior Inferior Cerebellar Artery	32126	- Right
32082	- Right	32127	- Left
32083	- Left	32128	Anterior Communicating Artery Aneurysm
32084	Lacunar		
32085	Basal Pons (Ataxic Hemiparesis) - Right	32129	Anterior Cerebral Artery Aneurysm
		32130	- Right
32086	Basal Pons (Ataxic Hemiparesis) - Left	32131	- Left
		32132	Posterior Communicating Artery Aneurysm
32087	Internal Capsule (Pure Motor) - Right		
		32133	- Right
32088	Internal Capsule (Pure Motor) - Left	32134	- Left
32089	Dysarthria - Clumsy Hand, Right	32135	Posterior Cerebral Artery Aneurysm
32090	Dysarthria - Clumsy Hand, Left	32136	- Right
32091	Thalamus (Pure Sensory) - Right	32137	- Left
32092	Thalamus (Pure Sensory) - Left	32138	Basilar Tip Aneurysm
32093	Subthalamic Nucleus (Hemichorea / Hemiballismus) - Right	32139	Basilar Artery Aneurysm
		32140	Superior Cerebellar Artery Aneurysm

NEUROLOGY, CONT.

32141	- Right	32187	Temporal - Right (Non-Dominant)
32142	- Left	32188	Temporal - Left (Dominant)
32143	Anterior Inferior Cerebellar Artery Aneurysm	32189	Parietal - Right (Non-Dominant)
		32190	Parietal - Left (Dominant)
32144	- Right	32191	Occipital - Right (Non-Dominant)
32145	- Left	32192	Occipital - Left (Dominant)
32146	Posterior Inferior Cerebellar Artery Aneurysm	32193	Basal Ganglia (Putaminal)
		32194	- Right (Non-Dominant)
32147	-Right	32195	- Left (Dominant)
32148	- Left	32196	Thalamic
32149	Vertebral Artery Aneurysm	32197	- Right (Non-Dominant)
32150	- Right	32198	- Left (Dominant)
32151	- Left	32199	Pontine
32152	Ruptured Cerebral Aneurysm	32200	Cerebellar
32153	Ophthalmic Artery - Right	32201	- Right
32154	Ophthalmic Artery - Left	32202	- Left
32155	Internal Carotid Artery - Right	32203	Locked-In Syndrome
32156	Internal Carotid Artery - Left	32204	Arteriovenous Malformation
32157	Middle Cerebral Artery - Right	32205	Cerebral
32158	Middle Cerebral Artery - Left	32206	Ruptured Cerebral
32159	Anterior Communicating Artery	32207	Brain Stem
32160	Anterior Cerebral Artery - Right	32208	Spinal
32161	Anterior Cerebral Artery - Left	32209	Aneurysm Of Vein Of Galen
32162	Posterior Communicating Artery - Right	32210	Foix-Alajouanine Syndrome
		32211	Acute Epidural Hemorrhage
32163	Posterior Communicating Artery - Left	32212	Subdural Hematoma
32164	Posterior Cerebral Artery - Right	32213	Acute
32165	Posterior Cerebral Artery - Left	35636	Traumatic Neonatal
32166	Basilar Tip	32214	Chronic
32167	Basilar Artery	32215	Subdural Hygroma
32168	Superior Cerebellar Artery - Right	34084	Cerebral Artery Thrombosis
32169	Superior Cerebellar Artery - Left	38305	Cerebral Embolism
32170	Anterior Inferior Cerebellar Artery - Right	32222	Cerebral Vasculitis
		34085	Moyamoya Disease
32171	Anterior Inferior Cerebellar Artery - Left	32223	Granulomatous Arteritis Of The Brain
		32218	Cerebral Vein Thrombosis
32172	Posterior Inferior Cerebellar Artery - Right	32219	Lateral Sinus
		32220	Superior Sagittal Sinus
32173	Posterior Inferior Cerebellar Artery - Left	32221	Cortical
		36393	Pseudobulbar Palsy
32174	Vertebral Artery - Right	90024	Cerebellar, Brainstem And Cranial Nerve Disorders
32175	Vertebral Artery - Left		
32176	Subarachnoid Hemorrhage	32224	Alcoholic Cerebellar Degeneration
32177	Neonatal	32225	Olivocerebellar Atrophy
32178	Pituitary Apoplexy	32226	Olivopontocerebellar Atrophy
32179	Intraventricular Hemorrhage	36377	Striatonigral Degeneration
32180	Neonatal	32229	Friedreich's Ataxia
32181	Intracerebral Hemorrhage	36380	Primary Cerebellar Degeneration
32182	Congophilic Angiopathy	36381	Cerebellar Ataxia
32183	Hypertensive Intracerebral Hemorrhage	36382	Marie's
32184	Lobar	36383	Sanger-Brown
32185	Frontal - Right (Non-Dominant)	36385	Sporadic
32186	Frontal - Left (Dominant)	32227	Familial

NEUROLOGY, CONT.

32368	Marinesco-Sjogren Syndrome
36384	Dyssynergia Cerebellaris Myoclonica
36386	Secondary Cerebellar Degeneration
36387	Due To Alcoholism
36388	Myxedema
36389	Paraneoplastic
32230	Miller - Fisher Syndrome
32234	Arnold-Chiari Malformation
32235	Klippel-Feil Deformity
32236	Platybasia
34809	Cranial Nerve Injury
37386	Olfactory Nerve
37387	Optic Nerve
37388	Oculomotor Nerve
37389	Trochlear Nerve
37390	Trigeminal Nerve
37391	Abducens Nerve
37392	Facial Nerve
37393	Acoustic Nerve
37394	Glossopharyngeal Nerve
37395	Vagus Nerve
37396	Accessory Nerve
37397	Hypoglossal Nerve
32232	Syringobulbia
30737	Ischemic Optic Neuropathy
36841	Nutritional Optic Neuropathy
36842	Toxic Optic Neuropathy
32036	Jacod's Syndrome
32037	Tic Douloureux
36412	Atypical Face Pain
32038	Glossopharyngeal Neuralgia
32046	Positional Vertigo Of Barany
32047	Vestibular Neuronitis
36413	Polyneuritis Cranialis
32311	Meniere's Disease
37569	Active Cochleovestibular
37570	Cochlear
37571	Vestibular
37572	Inactive
32340	Bell's Palsy
32341	Geniculate Ganglionitis
32370	Moebius' Syndrome
32371	Horner's Syndrome
32373	Collet-Sicard Syndrome
32376	Strachan's Syndrome
32377	Vernet's Syndrome
32378	Villaret's Syndrome
32379	Gradenigo's Syndrome
32385	Ramsay Hunt Syndrome (Geniculate Herpes)
90078	Spinal Disorders
32233	Syringomyelia
32237	Spinal Cord Injury

32238	Spinal Shock
34864	Cervical
37398	C1-C4 Level
37399	With Incomplete Lesion Of Cord
37400	With Complete Lesion Of Cord
37401	With Anterior Cord Syndrome
37402	With Central Cord Syndrome
37403	With Posterior Cord Syndrome
37404	C5-C7 Level
37405	With Incomplete Lesion Of Cord
37406	With Complete Lesion Of Cord
37407	With Anterior Cord Syndrome
37408	With Central Cord Syndrome
37409	With Posterior Cord Syndrome
34865	Thoracic
37410	T1-T6 Level
37411	With Incomplete Lesion Of Cord
37412	With Complete Lesion Of Cord
37413	With Anterior Cord Syndrome
37414	With Central Cord Syndrome
37415	With Posterior Cord Syndrome
37416	T7-T12 Level
37417	With Incomplete Lesion Of Cord
37418	With Complete Lesion Of Cord
37419	With Anterior Cord Syndrome
37420	With Central Cord Syndrome
37421	With Posterior Cord Syndrome
34866	Lumbar
34867	Cauda Equina
32239	Spinal Cord Tumor
32240	Foramen Magnum
32241	Cervical
32242	Thoracic
32243	Lumbar
31701	Conus Medullaris
32244	Cauda Equina
32245	Spinal Meningioma
33786	Vertebral Metastasis
32246	Spinal Epidural Metastases
32247	Brown-Sequard Syndrome
32248	Spinal Epidural Abscess
36368	Spinal Subdural Abscess
32249	Discitis
32250	Spinal Cord TIA
32251	Spinal Cord Infarction
32252	Spinal Hematoma
32253	Hematomyelia
36395	Subacute Necrotic Myelopathy
34428	Spinal Enthesopathy
34429	Sacroiliitis
32254	Cervical Spondylosis
34430	With Myelopathy
32255	Thoracic Spondylosis

NEUROLOGY, CONT.

32256	Lumbosacral Spondylosis	34810	Injury To Spinal Nerve Root
34431	Baastrup's Syndrome	35674	Cervical
32259	Familial Spastic Paraplegia	35675	Thoracic
32260	Subacute Combined Degeneration	35676	Lumbar
32261	Spinal Extramedullary Hematopoiesis	35677	Sacral
32262	Adhesive Arachnoiditis (Spinal)	35678	Brachial Plexus
31973	Dandy-Walker Syndrome	35679	Lumbosacral Plexus
32263	Meningomyelocele	34811	Injury To Cervical Sympathetic Nerve
32264	Cauda Equina Syndrome	32289	Peripheral Nerve Injury
32265	Lumbar Canal Stenosis	32290	Axillary Nerve
32266	Cervical Spine Stenosis	32291	Median Nerve
32267	Herniated Intervertebral Disc	32292	Ulnar Nerve
32268	(C5 - C6)	32293	Radial Nerve
32269	(C6 - C7)	34812	Digital Nerve
34830	Thoracic	32294	Sciatic Nerve
32270	(L3 - L4)	32295	Femoral Nerve
32271	(L4 - L5)	32296	Posterior Tibial Nerve
32272	(L5 - S1)	32297	Peroneal Nerve
37652	Schmorl's Nodes	34813	Multiple Nerves
34432	Intervertebral Disc Degeneration	37683	Abnormal Visually Evoked Potential
34433	Cervical	37684	Abnormal Electromyogram (EMG)
34434	Thoracic	32298	Peroneal Muscular Atrophy (Charcot-Marie-Tooth)
34435	Thoracolumbar		
34436	Lumbar	32299	Progressive Hypertrophic Polyneuropathy (Dejerine-Sottas)
34437	Lumbosacral		
34438	Postlaminectomy Syndrome	32300	Idiopathic Relapsing Polyneuropathy
36396	Drug-Induced Myelopathy	32301	Hereditary Sensory Neuropathy
32273	Radiation Myelopathy	36313	Subacute Sensory Neuropathy
32274	Radiation Plexopathy	32302	Guillain-Barre Syndrome
35861	Spinal Stenosis	32303	Levy-Roussy Syndrome
34447	Lumbago	32304	Refsum's Disease
34444	Klippel's Disease	32305	Familial Dysautonomia (Riley-Day Syndrome)
34448	Backache		
34449	Sacral Ankylosis	32308	Infantile Muscular Atrophy
34450	Spinal Ankylosis	32309	Werdnig Hoffman
35860	Spinal Joint Disease	36390	Adult Muscular Atrophy
90092	Disorders Of The Peripheral Nerves, Neuromuscular Junction, And Muscles	32257	Amyotrophic Lateral Sclerosis
		32306	Progressive Muscular Atrophy
32275	Polyneuropathy	32307	Kugelberg-Wellander
32276	Alcoholic	36391	Duchenne-Aran
32277	Amyloid	36392	Progressive Bulbar Palsy
32278	Arsenic	36394	Primary Lateral Sclerosis
32279	Cis-Platinum	32310	Oppenheim's Disease (Amyotonia Congenita)
37895	Diabetes		
32280	Diphtheric	32312	Nerve Palsy
32281	With Infectious Hepatitis	32313	Brachial Plexus
32282	Isoniazid	32314	Long Thoracic
32283	Lead	32315	Suprascapular
32284	Nitrofurantoin	32316	Axillary
32285	Porphyric	32317	Musculocutaneous
32286	Uremic	32318	Radial
32287	Vinblastine	32319	Median
32288	Vincristine	32320	Ulnar

NEUROLOGY, CONT.

36415	Tardy Ulnar Nerve
36416	Cubital Tunnel Syndrome
32321	Lateral Femoral Cutaneous
32322	Obturator
32323	Femoral
32324	Sciatic
32325	Common Peroneal
32326	Tibial
32327	Phrenic
32328	Brachial Plexus Palsy
32329	Upper (Erb-Duchenne)
32330	Lower (Dejerine-Klumpke)
32331	Lumbosacral Plexus Lesion
36414	Phantom Limb Syndrome
34440	Cervicalgia
34441	Barre-Lieou Syndrome
34442	Cervicobrachial Syndrome (Diffuse)
32332	Neuritis
35859	Cervical
32333	Brachial
32334	Sciatic
34445	Thoracic
34446	Lumbosacral
32335	Costoclavicular Syndrome
32336	Cervical Rib
32337	Carpal Tunnel Syndrome
32338	Tarsal Tunnel Syndrome
32339	Saturday Night Palsy
32342	Tick Paralysis
32343	Myasthenia Gravis
32344	Neonatal
32345	Eaton-Lambert Syndrome
32350	Progressive Muscular Dystrophy
32351	Duchenne
32352	Landouzy-Dejerine
32353	Limb Girdle
36422	Fascioscapulohumeral
32354	Becker
32348	Oculopharyngeal Muscular Dystrophy
32355	Periodic Paralysis Syndrome
32356	Hyperkalemic
32357	Normokalemic
32358	Hypokalemic
32359	Thyrotoxic
32360	Myotonic Dystrophy
32361	Congenital Myotonia
32362	Congenital Paramyotonia
32363	Chondrodystrophic Myotonia (Schwartz-Jampel Syndrome)
32364	Isaacs Syndrome
32365	Chronic Thyrotoxic Myopathy
36317	Toxic Myopathy

36417	Congenital Hereditary Muscular Dystrophy
32366	Benign Congenital Myopathy
36418	Central Core Disease
36419	Centronuclear Myopathy
36420	Myotubular Myopathy
36421	Nemaline Body Disease
32039	Neuralgia
32040	Postherpetic
32043	Causalgia
34992	Reflex Sympathetic Dystrophy
32044	Sudeck's Atrophy
32045	Mononeuritis Multiplex
90093	Other Disorders
32369	Mikulicz's Disease
32372	Morton's Neuroma
32375	Melkersson's Syndrome
35680	Tapia's Syndrome
32380	Foix's Syndrome
32381	Wernicke's Disease
36289	Polio Encephalopathy
36290	Nonalcoholic, Nutritional
36288	Korsakoff's Syndrome, Non-Alcoholic
32383	Immerslund's Syndrome
32384	Lowe's Syndrome
32387	Tarui's Disease
32388	Neuropathic Joint Disease
32389	Miner's Nystagmus
32390	Phenylketonuria
32391	Sinus Pericranii
32393	Ischemic Paralysis Of Upper Limb
32637	**Psychiatric Disorders**
90015	Childhood
32643	Attention-Deficit Disorder
90013	Primarily Inattentive Type
32642	With Hyperactivity
32644	With Hyperactivity, Residual State
32645	Solitary Aggressive Conduct Disorder
32646	Solitary Nonaggressive Conduct Disorder
32647	Group Type Aggressive Conduct Disorder
32648	Group Type Nonaggressive Conduct Disorder
32649	Disruptive Behavior Disorder
32650	Separation Anxiety Disorder Of Childhood
33845	School Phobia
32651	Avoidant Disorder Of Childhood Or Adolescence
32652	Overanxious Disorder

PSYCHIATRIC DISORDERS, CONT.

32653	Reactive Attachment Disorder Of Infancy Or Early Childhood
38373	Inhibited Type
38374	Disinhibited Type
32654	Introverted Disorder Of Childhood Or Adolescence
32655	Selective Mutism Of Childhood
32656	Oppositional Defiant Disorder Of Childhood
32657	Identity Disorder Of Childhood
32658	Anorexia Nervosa
38538	Restricting Type
38539	Binge-Eating And Purging Type
30042	Ketogenic Dieting
32659	Bulimia Nervosa
38540	Purging Type
38541	Non-Purging Type
32660	Pica
30267	Kleine-Levin Syndrome
32661	Rumination Disorder Of Infancy
32662	Atypical Eating Disorder
38372	Feeding Disorder Of Infancy / Early Childhood
32663	Transient Tic Disorder
35788	Single Episode
35789	Recurrent
32664	Chronic Motor Or Vocal Tic Disorder
32665	Tourette's Syndrome
32666	Atypical Tic Disorder
32667	Stereotypic Movement Disorder
38375	With Self-Injurious Behavior
32668	Stuttering
35106	Cluttering
32669	Functional Enuresis
32670	Functional Encopresis
32679	Specific Developmental Disorder
32680	Reading
32681	Arithmetic
35105	Expressive Writing
32682	Language
32683	Expressive
32684	Mixed Receptive-Expressive
32685	Phonological
35790	Coordination
32686	Mixed Specific
32687	Atypical Specific
35815	Pervasive Developmental Disorders
32673	Autistic Disorder (Infantile Autism, Full Syndrome Present)
32674	Autistic Disorder (Infantile Autism, Residual State)
32675	Autistic Disorder (Childhood Onset Pervasive Developmental)

32676	Full Syndrome Present
32677	Residual State
38370	Asperger's Disorder
32678	Atypical
32639	Mental Retardation
32640	With Other Behavioral Symptoms
32641	Without Other Behavioral Symptoms
35101	Mild
35102	Moderate
35103	Severe
35104	Profound
90016	Organic Disorders
35730	Delirium Of Known (Axis III) Etiology
35731	Delirium Of Unknown (Axis III) Etiology
35732	Dementia Of Known (Axis III) Etiology
35733	Dementia Of Unknown (Axis III) Etiology
35734	Amnestic Disorder Of Known (Axis III) Etiology
35735	Amnestic Disorder Of Unknown (Axis III) Etiology
35097	Psychotic Disorder Due To General Medical Condition, With Delusions
35098	Delusional Disorder Of Unknown (Axis III) Etiology
35099	Psychotic Disorder Due To General Medical Condition, With Hallucinations
35100	Hallucinosis Of Unknown (Axis III) Etiology
35092	Mood Disorder Due To General Medical Condition
35096	Mood Disorder Of Unknown (Axis III) Etiology
35095	Anxiety Disorder Due To General Medical Condition
38514	With Generalized Anxiety
38515	With Panic Attacks
38516	With Obsessive-Compulsive Symptoms
35094	Anxiety Disorder Of Unknown (Axis III) Etiology
38407	Personality Change Due To Axis III Etiology
38402	Labile Type
38403	Disinhibited Type
38408	Aggressive Type
38404	Apathetic Type
38405	Paranoid Type
38406	Combined Type

PSYCHIATRIC DISORDERS, CONT.

35091	Personality Disorder Of Known Axis III Etiology
36291	Explosive
32695	Personality Disorder Of Unknown (Axis III) Etiology
36292	Explosive
32696	Mental Disorder Of Known (Axis III) Etiology
35093	Mental Disorder Of Unknown (Axis III) Etiology
90017	Drug-Related Disorders
32396	Alcohol Disorders
32397	Intoxication
35219	Idiosyncratic
38410	Intoxication Delirium
32398	Withdrawal
32402	Withdrawal Delirium ("D. Tremens")
32399	Abuse
38411	Mood Disorder
38412	Anxiety Disorder
38413	Induced Sexual Dysfunction
38414	Sleep Disorder
32401	Dependence (Alcoholism)
35221	With Dementia
32400	Alcoholic Ketoacidosis
39907	Persistent Dementia
32382	Alcohol-Induced Persisting Amnestic Disorder
38409	Psychotic Disorder With Delusions
35220	Psychotic Disorder With Hallucinations
38415	Amphetamine-Related Disorders
32703	Dependence
32702	Abuse
38416	Intoxication
39883	With Delirium
35323	Withdrawal
35324	Amphetamine / Sympathomimetic Delirium
38418	Mood Disorder
38419	Anxiety Disorder
38420	Sexual Dysfunction
38421	Sleep Disorder
39882	Amphetamine-Induced Psychotic Disorders
35588	With Delusions
38417	Psychotic Disorder With Hallucinations
34888	Methamphetamine Abuse
34889	Methamphetamine Dependence
32466	MDMA ('Ecstasy')
34885	Fentanyl Analogues

38427	Caffeine-Related Disorders
38428	Intoxication
38429	Anxiety Disorder
38430	Sleep Disorder
38425	Cannabis-Related Disorders
32711	Dependence
32710	Abuse
38426	Intoxication
39880	With Delirium
39881	Anxiety Disorder
39878	Cannabis-Induced Psychotic Disorders
35592	With Delusions
39879	With Hallucinations
38431	Cocaine-Related Disorders
33850	Dependence
32701	Abuse
33790	Cardiovascular Effects
32395	Intoxication
35728	With Delirium
35681	Withdrawal
38440	Mood Disorder
39886	Anxiety Disorder
39887	Sexual Dysfunction
39888	Sleep Disorder
39884	Cocaine-Induced Psychotic Disorders
35589	With Delusions
39885	With Hallucinations
38432	Hallucinogen-Related Disorders
35792	Dependence
32709	Abuse
32467	LSD Hallucinosis / Abuse
35791	Persistent Perception Disorder
39890	Intoxication
39891	With Delirium
35784	Mood Disorder
39892	Anxiety Disorder
39889	Hallucinogen-Induced Psychotic Disorders
35591	With Delusions
35593	With Hallucinations
38433	Inhalant-Related Disorders
35786	Dependence
35594	Abuse
38437	Intoxication
39896	With Delirium
38441	Mood Disorder
39898	Anxiety Disorder
39897	Persistent Dementia
39893	Inhalant-Induced Psychotic Disorders
39894	With Delusions
39895	With Hallucinations
38434	Nicotine-Related Disorders
32712	Dependence

PSYCHIATRIC DISORDERS, CONT.

32456	Withdrawal	38444	Intoxication
38435	Opioid-Related Disorders	35739	Withdrawal
32700	Dependence	35738	Delirium
32699	Abuse	35737	Dementia
38438	Intoxication	35740	Amnestic Disorder
39901	With Delirium	35744	Delusional Disorder
32446	Withdrawal	35745	Hallucinosis
38442	Mood Disorder	35782	Mood Disorder
39902	Sleep Disorder	38456	Anxiety Disorder
39903	Sexual Dysfunction	38457	Sexual Dysfunction
39899	Opioid-Induced Psychotic Disorders	38458	Sleep Disorder
39877	With Delusions	33753	Drug-Seeking Behavior
39900	With Hallucinations	90018	Psychoses
38436	Phencyclidine-Related Disorders	35742	Schizophrenia
35787	Dependence	32717	Disorganized
32704	Abuse	32718	Subchronic (Episodic With No Interepisode Residual Symptoms)
38439	Intoxication		
35729	With Delirium	32719	Chronic (Episodic With Interepisode Residual Symptoms)
35785	Mood Disorder		
39906	Anxiety Disorder	32720	Subchronic With Acute Exacerbation (Episodic)
39904	Phencyclidine-Induced Psychotic Disorders		
		32721	Chronic With Acute Exacerbation (Episodic With Negative Sx)
35590	With Delusions		
39905	With Hallucinations	32722	In Remission
32706	Benzodiazepam Abuse	32723	Catatonic
32461	Benzodiazepam Withdrawal	32724	Subchronic (Episodic With No Interepisode Residual Symptoms)
32705	Benzodiazepam Dependence		
32697	Barbiturate Abuse	32725	Chronic (Episodic With Interepisode Residual Symptoms)
32453	Barbiturate Withdrawal		
32698	Barbiturate Dependence	32726	Subchronic With Acute Exacerbation (Episodic)
35089	Nitrous Oxide Abuse		
38443	Specified Sedative / Hypnotic / Anxiolytic Disorders	32727	Chronic With Acute Exacerbation (Episodic With Negative Sx)
32708	Dependence	32728	In Remission
38446	Abuse	32729	Paranoid
32707	Intoxication	32730	Subchronic (Episodic With No Interepisode Residual Symptoms)
35708	Withdrawal		
38447	With Perceptual Disturbances	32731	Chronic (Episodic With Interepisode Residual Symptoms)
38448	Intoxication Delirium		
38449	Withdrawal Delirium	32732	Subchronic With Acute Exacerbation (Episodic)
38450	Persistent Dementia		
35741	Amnestic Disorder	32733	Chronic With Acute Exacerbation (Episodic With Negative Sx)
38451	Delusions		
38452	Hallucinations	32734	In Remission
35783	Mood Disorder	35793	Stable
38453	Anxiety Disorder	32735	Undifferentiated
38454	Sexual Disturbances	32736	Subchronic (Episodic With No Interepisode Residual Symptoms)
38455	Sleep Disorder		
32713	Laxative Abuse	32737	Chronic (Episodic With Interepisode Residual Symptoms)
32714	Diuretic Abuse		
38445	Unspecified Substance Disorders	32738	Subchronic With Acute Exacerbation (Episodic)
32716	Dependence		
32715	Abuse		

PSYCHIATRIC DISORDERS, CONT.

32739	Chronic With Acute Exacerbation (Episodic With Negative Sx)	32764	Without Melancholia
32740	In Remission	32765	With Melancholia
32741	Residual	32766	With Psychotic Features
32742	Subchronic (Episodic With No Interepisode Residual Symptoms)	32767	In Remission
		32768	Major, Recurrent
32743	Chronic (Episodic With Interepisode Residual Symptoms)	32769	Without Melancholia
		32770	With Melancholia
32746	Childhood	32771	With Psychotic Features
35794	Late Onset	32772	In Remission
38658	Refractory	35816	Chronic
32744	Schizophreniform Disorder	38659	Refractory
35801	With Good Prognostic Features	35218	Postpartum Depression
35802	Without Good Prognostic Features	32749	Involutional Melancholia
32745	Schizoaffective Disorder	32773	Cyclothymic Disorder
35803	Bipolar	32774	Dysthymia (Depressive Neurosis)
35804	Depressive	36295	Primary
38401	Catatonic Disorder Due To Known Axis III Diagnosis	36296	Secondary
		36297	Early Onset
32747	Brief Psychotic Disorder	36298	Late Onset
38505	With Marked Stressor(s)	32775	Bipolar Affective Disorder NOS
38506	Without Marked Stressor(s)	32776	Depression NOS
38507	With Postpartum Onset	34869	Depression - Seasonal Pattern
32748	Atypical Psychosis	32779	Premenstrual Dysphoric Disorder
33796	Delusional (Paranoid) Disorder	90020	Personality Disorders
35795	Erotomanic	32847	Paranoid Personality Disorder
35796	Grandiose	32848	Schizoid Personality Disorder
35797	Jealous	32849	Schizotypal Personality Disorder
35798	Persecutory	32850	Histrionic Personality Disorder
35799	Somatic	32851	Narcissistic Personality Disorder
33797	Shared Psychotic Disorder	32852	Antisocial Personality Disorder
33798	Acute Paranoid Disorder	32853	Borderline Personality Disorder
33799	Atypical Paranoid Disorder	32854	Avoidant Personality Disorder
90019	Affective Disorders	32855	Dependent Personality Disorder
32750	Mixed Bipolar I Affective Disorder	32856	Obsessive Compulsive Personality Disorder
32751	Without Psychotic Features	32857	Passive Aggressive Personality Disorder
32752	With Psychotic Features		
32753	In Remission	32858	Personality Disorder NOS
32754	Manic Bipolar I Affective Disorder	90022	V-Code Dysfunctions
32755	Without Psychotic Features	38610	Failure To Thrive
32756	With Psychotic Features	33819	Child Neglect
32757	In Remission	32859	Child Abuser
32758	Depressed Bipolar I Affective Disorder	33847	Abused Child
32759	Without Melancholia	33820	Abused Spouse
32760	With Melancholia	33851	Spouse Abuser
32761	With Psychotic Features	32860	Malingering
32762	In Remission	32861	Borderline Intellectual Functioning
36294	Bipolar II Affective Disorder	32862	Adult Antisocial Behavior
38511	Bipolar Affective Disorder With Rapid Cycling	32863	Childhood / Adolescent Antisocial Behavior
36293	Seasonal Bipolar Affective Disorder	32864	Academic Problem
36309	Depression	32865	Occupational Problem
32763	Major, Single Episode	32866	Bereavement Without Complications

PSYCHIATRIC DISORDERS, CONT.

32867	Noncompliance With Medical Treatment	32794	Conversion Disorder (Hysterical Conversion)
32868	Phase Of Life Or Life Circumstance Problem	38517	With Motor Symptom / Deficit
		38518	With Sensory Symptom / Deficit
32869	Indigence	38519	With Seizures
32870	Marital Problem	38520	With Mixed Presentation
32871	Parent-Child Problem	32795	Pain Disorder Associated With Psychological Factors
32872	Other Specified Family Circumstances		
32873	Other Interpersonal Problem	38521	And A General Medical Condition
90021	Other Psychiatric Disorders	32796	Hypochondriasis
32777	Generalized Anxiety Disorder	35800	Body Dysmorphic Disorder
32778	Panic Disorder Without Agoraphobia	32797	Somatoform Disorder NOS
32780	Panic Disorder With Agoraphobia	32798	Chronic Pain Syndrome
32781	Agoraphobia Without History Of Panic Disorder	32799	Dissociative Amnesia
		32800	Dissociative Fugue
32782	Social Phobia	32801	Dissociative Identity Disorder
32783	Simple (Specific) Phobia	32802	Depersonalization Disorder
36001	Claustrophobia	32803	Dissociative Disorder, NOS
36002	Acrophobia	32804	Ego-Syntonic Homosexuality
34829	Bashful Kidney	32805	Ego-Dystonic Homosexuality
32784	Obsessive Compulsive Anxiety Disorder	32806	Transsexualism
		32807	Asexual
32785	Acute Post-Traumatic Stress Disorder	32808	Homosexual
38513	Chronic Post-Traumatic Stress Disorder	32809	Heterosexual
		36299	Gender Identity Disorder
32786	Delayed Post-Traumatic Stress Disorder	36300	Adolescent
		36301	Adult
38512	Acute Stress Disorder	38528	Sexually Attracted To Males
32787	Globus Hystericus	38529	Sexually Attracted To Females
32788	Suicide Risk	38530	Sexually Attracted To Both Sexes
32789	Suicide Attempt	38531	Sexually Attracted To Neither Sex
38138	Analgesics / Antipyretics / Antirheumatics	32810	Gender Identity Disorder Of Childhood
		32811	Gender Identity Disorder, NOS
38139	Barbiturates	36302	Sexual Disorder
38140	Tranquilizers / Psychotropic Agents	32812	Fetishism
38141	Corrosive / Caustic Substances	35107	Frotteurism
38142	Gas Distributed By Pipeline	32813	Transvestism
38143	Motor Vehicle Exhaust Gas	38537	Gender Dysphoric
38144	Hanging	32814	Zoophilia
38145	Suffocation By A Plastic Bag	32815	Pedophilia
38146	Handgun	38532	Sexually Attracted To Males
38147	Jumping / Lying Before Moving Object	38533	Sexually Attracted To Females
		38534	Sexually Attracted To Both Sexes
38148	Extremes Of Cold	38535	Limited To Incest
38149	Electrocution	38536	Only Attracted To Children (Exclusive)
38150	Crashing Of Motor Vehicle		
32790	Suicide Achieved	32816	Exhibitionism
32791	Anxiety Disorder NOS	32817	Voyeurism
32792	Psychogenic Water Drinking	32818	Sexual Masochism
31886	Psychogenic Unresponsiveness	32819	Sexual Sadism
32793	Somatization Disorder (Briquet's Syndrome)	32820	Paraphilia, NOS
		32821	Hypoactive Sexual Desire Disorder
		35817	Sexual Aversion Disorder

PSYCHIATRIC DISORDERS, CONT.

32822	Inhibited Sexual Excitement
34868	Psychogenic Impotence
35818	Female Sexual Arousal Disorder
35819	Male Erectile Disorder
32823	Female Orgasmic Disorder
32824	Male Orgasmic Disorder
32825	Premature Ejaculation
32826	Dyspareunia (Not Due To A Physical Condition)
32827	Vaginismus (Not Due To A Physical Condition)
32828	Sexual Dysfunction, NOS
38523	Female Hypoactive Sexual Desire Due To Physical Condition
38524	Male Hypoactive Sexual Desire Due To Physical Condition
38525	Male Erectile Disorder Due To Physical Condition
38526	Female Dyspareunia Due To A Physical Condition
38527	Male Dyspareunia Due To A Physical Condition
35820	Insomnia Related To Axis I/II Mental Disorder (Nonorganic)
35821	Insomnia Related Known Axis III Factor
35822	Primary Insomnia
35823	Hypersomnia Related To Axis I/II Mental Disorder (Nonorganic)
35824	Hypersomnia Related To Known Axis III Factor
35011	Primary Hypersomnia
38624	Parasomnia Related To Known Axis III Factor
38625	Mixed Type Sleep Disorder Due To Known Axis III Factor
35825	Circadian Rhythm Sleep Disorder
36303	Advanced
36304	Delayed
38542	Jet Lag Type
36305	Disorganized
36306	Frequently Changing
38622	Atypical Dyssomnia
35826	Nightmare Disorder
32672	Sleep Terror Disorder
32671	Sleepwalking Disorder
38621	Atypical Parasomnia
38623	REM Sleep Behavior Syndrome
33707	Factitious Fever
32829	Factitious Disorder With Psychological Symptoms
36307	Factitious Disorder With Physical Symptoms

32830	Munchausen's Syndrome
38522	Factitious Disorder With Psychological And Physical Symptoms
32831	Factitious Disorder, NOS
32832	Pathological Gambling
32833	Kleptomania
32834	Pyromania
33792	Sadistic Triad
32835	Intermittent Explosive Disorder
35072	Trichotillomania
32837	Impulse Control Disorder, NOS
32838	Adjustment Disorder With Depressed Mood
32839	Adjustment Disorder With Anxious Mood
32840	Adjustment Disorder With Mixed Emotional Features
32841	Adjustment Disorder With Disturbance Of Conduct
32842	Adjustment Disorder With Disturbance Of Emotions, Conduct
32843	Adjustment Disorder With Work (Or Academic) Inhibition
36308	Adjustment Disorder With Physical Complaints
32844	Adjustment Disorder With Withdrawal
35003	Adjustment Disorder With Denial Of Physical Disorder
32845	Adjustment Disorder, NOS
35665	Reaction To Chronic Stress
32846	Psychological Factors Affecting Physical Condition
32638	Requiring Hospitalization

30824 Infectious Disease

39998	See, Also: Affected System
90185	Viral
30926	Adenovirus
30831	Arbovirus:
30832	Fever, Malaise, Rash, Lymphadenopathy
30833	Dengue Fever
30834	West Nile Fever
30835	Fever, Malaise, Headache, Myalgia
30836	Bat Salivary Gland Virus
30837	Colorado Tick Fever
30839	Mayaro-Semliki Forest Virus Disease
30840	Phlebotomus Fever
30841	Rift Valley Fever
30842	Bunyamwera Group
30838	Bunyavirus
35090	Hantavirus
36174	With Renal Syndrome (HFRS)

INFECTIOUS DISEASE, CONT.

30843	Zika Virus	30981		Generalized
30844	Fever, Malaise, Rash, Arthralgia	30982		Traumatic Herpes
30845	Chikungunya	30970	Herpes Zoster	
30846	O'nyong-Nyong Fever	33938		With Ophthalmic Complications
30847	Ross River Virus	33939		With Otitis Externa
30848	Sindbis Virus	30985	Infectious Mononucleosis	
30849	Fever, Malaise, Hemorrhagic Signs	31172	Lassa Fever	
30850	Kyasanur Forest Disease	31419	Marburg Virus Disease	
30851	Congo-Crimean Hemorrhagic Fever	31181	Measles (Rubeola)	
30852	Omsk Hemorrhagic Fever	31420	Milker's Nodules	
30853	Yellow Fever	31429	Mokola Virus	
36175	Arenavirus Infection	31430	Mucormycosis	
36286	Argentine Fever	31431	Rhinocerebral	
36287	Bolivian Fever	31432	Gastrointestinal	
30932	Brill-Zinsser Disease	31433	Disseminated	
31407	Chickenpox	31434	Mumps	
30913	Cholera	31435	Orchitis	
36176	Vibrio Cholerae	31007	Murine (Endemic Flea-Borne) Typhus Fever	
36178	Vibrio Cholerae El Tor			
31408	Cowpox	31009	Newcastle Disease	
30946	Coxsackie Group A Virus Infections	31446	Orchitis	
30947	Diarrhea	31447	Gonococcal	
30948	Herpangina	31240	Pharyngoconjunctival Fever	
33940	Carditis	31023	Rabies	
30949	Hand, Foot & Mouth Disease	31025	Respiratory Syncytial Virus Infection	
30951	Tracheobronchitis	90235	Retrovirus Infections	
31018	Coxsackie Group B Virus Infections	90236	HTLV-I	
31019	Pleurodynia	90237	HTLV-II	
31410	Cytomegalovirus Colitis	90238	HTLV-III	
31409	Cytomegalovirus Disease	34816	HIV-1 Infection	
34815	Cytomegalovirus Retinitis	34925	Stage 0	
38325	Ebola Virus Hemorrhagic Fever	34926	Stage 1	
30953	Echo Virus	34927	Stage 2 (PGL)	
30954	Boston Exanthem	34928	Stage 3 (PGL)	
30955	Diarrhea	34929	Stage 4	
30956	Pneumonia	34930	Stage 5 (ARC)	
30957	Hemolytic / Uremic	31779	Acquired Immunodeficiency Syndrome (AIDS - HIV-1 Stage 6)	
30958	Myopericarditis			
30959	Neurologic	33883	Dementia	
30960	Pleurodynia	36264	Encephalopathy	
30961	Rash	36265	Oral Leukoplakia	
30962	Upper Respiratory	33884	Myelopathy	
31089	Encephalomyocarditis Viruses	33885	Polyneuropathy	
31086	Erythema Infectiousum	36266	Nephritis	
30971	Herpes Simplex	90239	HIV-2 Infection	
30972	Type I	90240	Lymphadenopathy-Associated Virus	
30973	Type II	31312	Roseola Infantum	
30974	Esophagitis	31182	Rubella	
30975	Eczema Herpeticum	31069	Smallpox (Variola)	
30976	Acute Gingivostomatitis	30966	Summer Grippe	
30977	Kerato Conjunctivitis	30914	Suppurative Cervicaladenitis	
30979	Chronic Perirectal	31070	Vaccinia	
30980	Rhinitis	31075	Verruca	

31402	Vesicular Stomatitis
31183	Viral Exanthem
38175	Viral Syndrome
34607	Viremia
31074	Warts
31076	Common
31077	Digital
31078	Flat
31079	Filiform
31080	Plantar
31138	Condylomata Acuminata
90184	Bacterial
30921	Actinomycosis
30922	Cervicofacial
36262	Cutaneous
30923	Pulmonary
36263	Madura Foot
30924	Abdominal
30925	Hematogenous
30927	Anthrax
36230	Cutaneous
36231	Pulmonary
36232	Gastrointestinal
36233	Septic
30872	Bacteremia
35847	Streptococcal
35848	Staphylococcal
35850	Salmonella
30935	Bartonellosis (Carrion's Disease)
30936	Oroya Fever
30937	Verruga Peruana
31084	Bejel (Treponema Pallidum)
30942	Boutonneuse Fever
30878	Brodie's Abscess - Staph
30943	Brucellosis
30944	Acute
30945	Chronic
36234	Brucella Melitensis
36235	Brucella Abortus
36236	Brucella Suis
36237	Brucella Canis
31218	Bubonic Plague
30888	Burns
34806	Of The Eye
37972	Of The Eyelids
37973	Chemical Burn
30889	Of The Face, Head, Or Neck
37342	First Degree
34859	Second Degree
30890	Third Degree
37344	Third, With Deep Necrosis Of Underlying Tissues
37345	With Loss Of A Body Part

30891	Of The Trunk
37343	First Degree
34860	Second Degree
30892	Third Degree
37346	Third, With Deep Necrosis Of Underlying Tissues
37347	With Loss Of A Body Part
30893	Of The Upper Limbs
37348	First Degree
34861	Second Degree
30894	Third Degree
37349	Third, With Deep Necrosis Of Underlying Tissues
37350	With Loss Of A Body Part
30895	Of The Wrists Or Hands
37351	First Degree
34862	Second Degree
30896	Third Degree
37352	Third, With Deep Necrosis Of Underlying Tissues
37353	With Loss Of A Body Part
30897	Of The Lower Limbs
37354	First Degree
34863	Second Degree
30898	Third Degree
37355	Third, With Deep Necrosis Of Underlying Tissues
37356	With Loss Of A Body Part
34807	Of Multiple Sites
37357	First Degree
37358	Second Degree
37359	Third Degree
37360	Third, With Deep Necrosis Of Underlying Tissues
37361	With Loss Of A Body Part
34808	Of Internal Organs
37362	Mouth
37363	Gums
37364	Tongue
37365	Pharynx
37366	Larynx
37367	Trachea
37368	Lung
37369	Esophagus
37370	Stomach
37371	Small Intestine
37372	Colon
37373	Rectum
37374	Vagina
37375	Uterus
37376	Involving Under 10% Of The Body Surface

INFECTIOUS DISEASE, CONT.

37377	Involving 10-19% Of The Body Surface	36254	Osteomyelitis
		36255	Urethritis
37378	Involving 20-29% Of The Body Surface	36256	Endometritis
		31344	Meningococcemia (Waterhouse - Friderichsen Syndrome)
37379	Involving 30-39% Of The Body Surface	31219	Molluscum Contagiosum
37380	Involving 40-49% Of The Body Surface	31016	Nocardiosis
		31448	Orf
37381	Involving 50-59% Of The Body Surface	31437	Parapharyngeal Space Abscess
		36145	Paratrachoma
37382	Involving 60-69% Of The Body Surface	31297	Paratyphoid Fever
		36179	Type A
37383	Involving 70-79% Of The Body Surface	36180	Type B
		36181	Type C
37384	Involving 80-89% Of The Body Surface	31252	Pasteurella Multocida
		31314	Perirectal Abscess
37385	Involving 90% Or More Of The Body Surface	31315	Anaerobic Streptococcal
		31438	Pertussis
30899	Pseudomonas	31082	Pinta (Treponema Carateum)
30900	Proteus	31027	Plague: Yersinia Pestis
34972	Campylobacter Colitis	36228	Pneumonic
31406	Cat Scratch Disease	31452	Pneumococcemia
30952	Diphtheria	31024	Psittacosis
31149	Disseminated Gonococcemia	36285	With Pneumonia
31459	Farcy	31040	Q Fever
30967	Gangrene	31304	Rat-Bite Fever (Spirillum Minus)
30968	Wet (Infected)	31311	Rhinoscleroma
30969	Dry (Ischemic)	36182	Salmonella Infection
33809	Gas	36183	Salmonella Arthritis
31458	Glanders	36184	Carrier State
30965	Granuloma Inguinale	31348	Salmonellosis
31037	Haverhill Fever	34817	Disseminated
34852	Jarisch-Herxheimer Reaction	31358	Scarlet Fever
31002	Leprosy	31359	Surgical
31003	Borderline	31340	Septic Shock (Endotoxic)
31004	Lepromatous	31341	Clostridial
31005	Tuberculoid	31342	Escherichia Coli
31064	Leptospirosis	31343	Klebsiella Pneumoniae
31066	Fort Bragg Fever	31345	Pseudomonas
31067	Myocarditis	31346	Staphylococcal
31068	Weil's Syndrome	30873	Septicemia
31085	Listeriosis	30874	Streptococcal
36238	Erysipelothrix Infection	30875	Staphylococcal
31006	Melioidosis (Pseudomonas Pseudomallei)	36257	Due To Bacteroides
36171	Meningococcal Infection	35849	Pneumococcal
31451	Acute	35222	Salmonella
31450	Chronic	30876	Gram-Negative
36248	Pericarditis	36258	Hemophilus Influenzae
36249	Endocarditis	36259	E. coli
36250	Myocarditis	36260	Pseudomonas
36251	Optic Neuritis	36261	Serratia
36252	Arthropathy	35759	Neonatal
36253	Sinusitis	30877	Geriatric Presentation

INFECTIOUS DISEASE, CONT.

31104	Staphylococcal Enterocolitis		33894	Chronic, Cavitary
31320	Subcutaneous Abscess		31444	Disseminated
31363	Subungal Abscess		33834	Cryptococcoma
31370	Suppurative Tenosynovitis, Staph		31411	Cryptococcosis
31042	Syphilis		31020	Dracunculiasis (Guinea Worm)
31043	Congenital		31241	Histoplasmoma
31044	Latent		31242	Histoplasmosis
31045	Primary		31243	Primary Infectious
31046	Anal		31244	Acute Pulmonary
31047	Secondary		31245	Chronic, Cavitary Pulmonary
31048	Late		31246	Progressive Disseminated
31049	Cardiovascular		31247	Ocular
31050	Aortic Valve		31248	Mucocutaneous (African)
33945	Pulmonary		31008	Mycetoma
31029	Tetanus		31249	Paragonimiasis
31365	Toxic Shock Syndrome		31250	Abdominal
90251	Streptococcal		31251	Cerebral
31028	Trachoma		31081	Phycomycosis
36143	Initial Stage		31021	Rhinosporidiosis
36144	Active		31036	Sporotrichosis
31031	Tularemia		90188	Mycobacterium
31032	Glandular		31051	Tuberculosis
31033	Pulmonary		36203	Primary
31034	Ulceroglandular		31057	Pulmonary
31035	Oculoglandular		33750	Post Primary
36229	Enteric		38313	Pericardial
31381	Typhoid Fever		31052	Gastrointestinal
31403	Wound Infection		31053	Latent
31404	Pseudomonas		31054	Miliary
31405	Clostridial		34948	Disseminated
31083	Yaws (Treponema Pertenue)		31055	Peritoneal
90187	Fungal		36204	Fibrosis
30928	Aspergillosis		31056	Pott's Disease
30929	Allergic Bronchopulmonary		31058	Pleural
33830	Mucoid Impaction		33800	Adrenal
30930	Aspergilloma		31059	Renal
30931	Pneumonia		36216	Bladder
30938	Blastomycosis		36217	Ureter
30939	North American		31060	Scrofula
30940	South American		36214	Hip
31010	Candidiasis		36215	Knee
31011	Esophagitis		36225	Thyroid Gland
33865	Pneumonia		36226	Splenic
31012	Systemic		36227	Esophageal
31013	Skin		36207	Tracheobronchial Adenopathy
31014	Oral Thrush		36219	Subcutaneous
31015	Vaginal		31061	Tuberculoma
38605	Endocarditis		36209	Meningeal
38606	Otitis Externa		33737	Chronic Tuberculous Cavity
38607	Meningitis		36168	Atypical Mycobacterial Infection
38608	Enteritis		31062	Pneumonia
33752	Coccidioidoma		36239	M. Avium Intracellulare
31443	Coccidioidomycosis		36240	M. Kansasii

INFECTIOUS DISEASE, CONT.

36241	M. Chelonei	31115	Foot & Mouth Disease
36242	M. Malmoense	31134	Gnathostomiasis
31063	Disseminated	33932	Heterophyiasis
36170	M. Xenopi	31152	Hookworm Disease (Ancylostomiasis)
36243	Cutaneous	31153	Hymenolepiasis
36244	M. Marinum	31154	Diminuta
36245	M. Ulcerans	31155	Nana
36246	M. Fortuitum	37461	Infestation By Fly Larvae
36247	M. Haemophilum	37460	Infestation By Maggots
36169	Scrofulaceum	37459	Infestation By Mites
31454	Tuberculous Gingivitis	37462	Infestation By Sand Fleas
90189	Rickettsia	31156	Intestinal Capillariasis
31026	Rickettsial Pox	31165	Leishmaniasis
31030	Trench Fever (Rickettsia Quintana)	31166	American Cutaneous
31038	Rocky Mountain Spotted Fever	31167	Uta
31039	Queensland Tick Typhus	31168	Espundia
31041	Scrub Typhus (Tsutsugamushi Disease)	31169	Kala-Azar
31460	South African Tick Fever	31170	Post Kala-Azar Dermal
30933	Epidemic (Louse Borne) Typhus Fever	31171	Old World Cutaneous
90190	Parasites	31173	Loiasis
30863	Amebiasis	31110	Lymphatic Filariasis
30864	Asymptomatic	31111	Bancroftian
36189	Acute	31112	Malayan
30865	Intestinal	31184	Malaria
36190	Cutaneous	31185	Plasmodium Vivax
30866	Pleuropulmonary	31186	Plasmodium Malariae
30867	Pericardial	31187	Plasmodium Ovale
35226	Amebic Nondysenteric Colitis	31188	Plasmodium Falciparum
30870	Amebic Liver Abscess	31189	Plasmodium Falciparum (Drug Resistant)
30868	Cerebral		
30869	Amebic Abscess (Non-Hepatic)	31190	Blackwater Fever
30862	Ameboma	31191	Cerebral
31135	Angiostrongyliasis	33933	Metagonimiasis
31136	Cantonensis	31230	Onchocerciasis
31137	Costaricensis	31231	Opisthorchiasis
30861	Anisakiasis	31461	Pediculosis Capitis
30871	Ascariasis	31462	Pediculosis Corporis
30934	Babesiosis	31463	Pediculosis Pubis
30887	Balantidiasis	31295	Pneumocystis Carinii
37458	Chiggers	34818	Extrapulmonary
30912	Clonorchiasis	31464	Ringworm
33935	Coenurosis	31339	Scabies
30918	Cutaneous Larva Migrans	31332	Schistosomiasis
30915	Cysticercosis	31333	Dermatitis ("Swimmer's Itch")
30916	Dipetalonemiasis	31334	Genitourinary (Haematobium)
30919	Diphyllobothrium Latum	31335	Intestinal (Mansoni)
33934	Dipylidiasis	31336	Asian (Japonicum/Mekongi)
31108	Dirofilariasis	31337	Katayama Fever
31088	Echinococciasis	31338	Portal Hypertension
31105	Enterobiasis (Pinworm)	30984	Septic Bursitis
31107	Fascioliasis	31347	Sparganosis
31106	Fasciolopsiasis	31114	Streptocerciasis
30964	Filariasis	31361	Strongyloidiasis

31362	Disseminated	30395	Thrombotic Thrombocytopenic Purpura
31372	Taeniasis Saginata	31836	Benign Hyperglobulinemic Purpura
31371	Taeniasis Solium	31839	Henoch-Schonlein Purpura
38590	Toxocariasis	30299	Pancytopenia
31375	Toxoplasmosis	34856	Leukopenia
31376	Congenital Chorioretinitis	34851	Granulocytopenia
31377	Chorioretinitis, Acquired	30301	Neutropenia
31378	Central Nervous System	37625	Cyclic
31379	Lymphadenopathic	37626	Drug-Induced
31366	Trichinosis	30302	Idiopathic Thrombocytopenic Purpura
31367	Trichomoniasis	30303	Acute
36191	Intestinal	30304	Chronic
31369	Trichostrongyliasis	30305	Methemoglobinemia
31368	Trichuriasis	30306	Myelofibrosis - Myeloid Metaplasia
31113	Tropical Eosinophilia (Amicrofilaremic Filariasis)	30307	Myeloproliferative Syndromes
		30308	Bernard-Soulier Syndrome
31374	Trypanosomiasis (African Sleeping Sickness)	35838	Coagulation Defects
		30309	Von Willebrand's Disease
31073	Vincent's Angina	37621	Acquired Coagulation Factor Deficiency
30917	Visceral Larva Migrans	37622	Due To Liver Disease
90191	Other Organisms	37623	Due To Vitamin K Deficiency
36980	Acute Lymphadenitis	30310	Clotting Factor Deficiency
33818	Blastocystis Hominis	30311	Factor I (Fibrinogen)
35746	Brazilian Purpuric Fever	30312	Factor II (Prothrombin)
34108	Chronic Nasopharyngitis	30313	Factor V
36167	DF-2 Infection	30314	Factor VII
35002	Eosinophilia-Myalgia Syndrome	30315	Factor VIII (Hemophilia)
31418	Fever Of Unknown Origin	34890	Carrier State For Hemophilia A (Factor VIII Deficiency)
38369	Human Granulocytic Ehrlichiosis		
31158	Kawasaki Disease	30316	Factor IX
31177	Lymphangiomyomatosis	34891	Carrier State For Hemophilia B (Factor IX Deficiency)
31178	Lymphangitis		
31179	Streptococcus	36162	Factor X
31223	Mansonelliasis Ozzardi	30317	Factor XI
31453	Meatitis	30318	Factor XII
31217	Midline Granuloma	30319	Factor XIII
31254	Ozena	35805	Antithrombin III Deficiency
31278	Pelvic Abscess	35806	Protein C Deficiency
31277	Pelvic Inflammatory Disease	35807	Protein S Deficiency
31289	Periostitis	30320	Anemia
31017	Petriellidiosis	30321	Hypochromic / Microcytic
31294	Psoas Abscess	30324	Sideroblastic
31303	Pylephlebitis	37620	Vitamin B6 Responsive
31455	Relapsing Fever	30325	Thalassemia
31302	Subphrenic Abscess	30322	Iron Deficiency
33891	Suppurative Spondylitis	30323	Secondary To Chronic Blood Loss
31449	Upper Respiratory Infection	30326	Macrocytic
31072	Vincent's Stomatitis	30327	Folic Acid Deficiciency
38675	**Hematology**	30328	Pernicious Anemia
39952	Blood Disorders	30329	Vitamin B12 Deficiency
30298	Thrombocytopenia	30330	Liver Disease
35809	Heparin-Induced	30331	Normochromic, Normocytic
37624	Drug-Induced		

HEMATOLOGY, CONT.

30332	Aplastic Anemia	30373	Stress Polycythemia (Gaisbock's
37618	Due To Infection		Syndrome)
37619	Due To Radiation	35938	Myelodysplastic Syndromes
30333	Of Chronic Disease	34857	Eosinophilia
30334	Endocrine Failure	30300	Essential Thrombocytosis
30335	Fanconi's Anemia	38585	Antiphospholipid Syndrome
30336	Hypothyroidism	30374	Sulfhemoglobinemia
30337	Myelophthisic	30375	Cryoglobulinemia
30338	Uremic	30376	Thromboasthenia
30339	Hemolytic	30377	Blood Transfusion Complications
30340	Congenital Heinz Body Hemolytic	30378	Extravascular
	Anemia	30379	Intravascular
30341	Hereditary Elliptocytosis	37944	Abo Incompatibity
30342	Hereditary Stomatocytosis	37945	Rh Incompatibilty
30343	Hereditary Spherocytosis	30380	Hypereosinophilic Syndromes
30344	Cryoglobulinemia	30381	Hemoglobin H Disease
30345	Drug Related Immune	30382	Alpha-Thalassemia Trait
30346	G6PD Deficiency	30383	Alpha-Thalassemia Silent Carrier
30347	Glucose Phosphate Isomerase	30384	B-Thalassemia
	Deficiency	30385	Heterozygous
30348	Hexokinase Deficiency	30386	Major Homozygous
30349	Uremic Syndrome	30387	Homozygous Intermedia
30350	Microangiopathic	30388	Disseminated Intravascular Coagulation
30351	Paroxysmal Cold Hemoglobinuria	30389	Congenital Fibrinogen Deficiency
37617	Hemoglobinuria From Exertion	33569	Transcobalamin II Deficiency
30352	Phosphoglycerate Kinase Deficiency	30390	Hemoglobin M Disease
30353	Paroxysmal Nocturnal	30391	Red Blood Cell Aplasia
	Hemoglobinuria	30392	Acquired
30354	Pyruvate Kinase Deficiency	30393	Congenital (Blackfan-Diamond)
30355	Sickle Beta-Thalassemia	30394	Drug Induced
30356	Sickle C Disease	38668	Splenic Disorders
30357	Sickle D Disease	30254	Hyposplenism
30358	Sickle Cell Crisis	36093	Asplenia
30359	Sickle Cell Anemia	30255	Hypersplenism
30360	Sickle Cell Trait	36094	Polysplenia
37616	Sickle Cell/Hb-C Disease	30256	Chronic Congestive Splenomegaly
30361	Triose Phosphate Isomerase	31353	Splenic Abscess
	Deficiency	31354	Bacteroides
30362	Spur Cell Anemia	31355	Enterobacteriaceae
30363	Warm Antibody Immunohemolytic	31356	Pseudomonas
30364	Cold Agglutinin Disease	31357	Serratia
30365	Homozygous Hemoglobin C Disease	30251	Splenic Cyst
30366	ABO Isoimmunization	30252	Splenic Artery Aneurysm
30367	Acute Posthemorrhagic	30253	Splenic Subcapsular Hematoma
30368	Refractory	30257	Splenic Infarct
35939	Sideroblastic	30258	Splenic Rupture
35940	With Excess Blasts	30109	Splenic Laceration
35941	With Transforming Blasts	37286	With Open Wound Into Cavity
30369	Post-Transfusion Rdw Elevation	34766	With Open Wound
30370	Familial Polycythemia	37307	Gunshot Wound Of The Spleen
30371	Secondary Polycythemia	30198	Postsplenectomy State
37627	Hypoxemic	38676	**Immunology**
30372	Polycythemia Vera	39923	Atopic Disorders

HEMATOLOGY, CONT.

31869	Hay Fever	39948	C1r
31866	Cosmetic Allergy	39949	C1s
31867	Drug Allergy	31855	C2
39926	Latex-Induced Dermatitis	31856	C3
39927	Latex-Induced Bronchospasm	31857	C4
31833	Anaphylaxis	31858	C5
38063	Adverse Food Reaction	31859	C5 Dysfunction
38264	Peanuts	31860	C6
37943	Shellfish	31861	C7
38268	Fish	31862	C8
38265	Fruits	33761	C9
38266	Vegetables	31863	C3b Inactivator Deficiency
38267	Nuts Or Seeds	39924	Other States/Disorders
38269	Food Additives	31782	Post-Bone Marrow Transplant
38270	Milk Products	31874	Graft-Versus-Host Disease (GVHD)
38271	Eggs	31864	C1 Inhibitor Deficiency ("Hereditary Angioedema")
39928	Latex		
39950	Bee Venom	34140	Sick Building Syndrome
39951	Wasp Venom	31868	Shellfish - Allergic Reaction
39922	Immunodeficiency	38072	Serum - Anaphylactic Shock
31781	Nezelof's Syndrome	31873	Serum Sickness
31785	Digeorge's Syndrome	34875	Drug-Induced
31865	Wiskott Aldrich Syndrome	**38665**	**Oncology**
31780	Severe Combined Immunodeficiency Disease	39999	See, Also, Affected System
		31465	Cancer, NOS
39939	Reticular Dysgenesis	34022	Eye Neoplasm
39940	Adenosine Deaminase Deficiency	38355	Benign
39941	Bare Lymphocyte Syndrome	90106	Histology
39942	Cd3 Deficiency	34026	Lacrimal Duct
39943	Interleukin-2 Deficiency	90118	Right
31783	Agammaglobulinemia	90120	Left
34033	Autosomal Recessive	31748	Lacrimal Gland
31784	X-Linked	90121	Right
34032	Swiss-Type	90124	Left
31786	Hypogammaglobulinemia	31747	Orbital
31787	Transient Of Infancy	31746	Hemangioma
34950	Common Variable	90146	Autonomic Nervous System
31850	Selective IgA Deficiency	90149	Right
31851	Selective IgM Deficiency	90150	Left
31852	Selective IgG Deficiency	90151	Connective Tissue
34951	Subclass G1	90152	Right
34952	Subclass G2	90153	Left
34953	Subclass G3	90155	Superior Rectus
34954	Subclass G4	90157	Right
30180	Intestinal Lymphangiectasia	90158	Left
39944	Phagocyte Deficiency	90159	Inferior Rectus
30408	Chronic Granulomatous Disease	90160	Right
39945	Leukocyte Adhesion Defect	90161	Left
39946	Hyperimmunoglobulin E Syndrome	90162	Medial Rectus
31853	Hereditary Serum Complement Deficiency	90163	Right
		90164	Left
31854	C1	90165	Lateral Rectus
39947	C1q	90166	Right

ONCOLOGY, CONT.

90167	Left	39854	Right	
90168	Superior Oblique	39855	Left	
90169	Right	39856	Superior Rectus	
90170	Left	39857	Right	
90171	Inferior Oblique	39858	Left	
90172	Right	39859	Inferior Rectus	
90173	Left	39860	Right	
90174	Peripheral Nerves	39861	Left	
90175	Right	39862	Medial Rectus	
90176	Left	39863	Right	
90177	Other Soft Tissue	39864	Left	
90178	Right	39865	Lateral Rectus	
90179	Left	39866	Right	
33981	Conjunctival	39867	Left	
34024	Cornea	39868	Superior Oblique	
38650	Dermoid	39869	Right	
90125	Right	39870	Left	
90126	Left	39871	Inferior Oblique	
38619	Iris	39872	Right	
90128	Right	39873	Left	
90129	Left	39874	Peripheral Nerves	
90131	Crystalline Lens	39875	Right	
90132	Right	39876	Left	
90133	Left	90111	Other Soft Tissue	
38618	Ciliary Body	90112	Right	
90134	Right	90113	Left	
90136	Left	38641	Metastatic	
90140	Uveal Tract	38361	Conjunctiva	
90141	Right	90117	Right	
90142	Left	90119	Left	
38356	Choroid	38642	Metastatic	
34025	Retina	38362	Cornea	
38367	Hemangioma	90122	Right	
38592	Melanocytoma	90123	Left	
90144	Right	38643	Metastatic	
90145	Left	38615	Iris	
38620	Sclera	90154	Right	
90143	Premalignant	90156	Left	
38357	Malignant	38639	Metastatic	
90107	Histology	38616	Crystalline Lens	
38584	Ocular Lymphoma	39821	Right	
38365	Lacrimal Duct	39822	Left	
90116	Right	38614	Ciliary Body	
90110	Left	39818	Right Eye	
38646	Metastatic	39819	Left Eye	
38360	Lacrimal Gland	38638	Metastatic	
90147	Right	39829	Uveal Tract	
90148	Left	39830	Right	
38359	Orbit	39831	Left	
39850	Autonomic Nervous System	38364	Choroid	
39851	Right	31749	Melanoma	
39852	Left	90127	Right	
39853	Connective Tissue	90130	Left	

ONCOLOGY, CONT.

38645	Metastatic		35409		Vallecula
38363	Retina		35411		Anterior Aspect Of Epiglottis
38366	Retinoblastoma		35413		Epiglottal Junctional Region
90135	Right		35415		Lateral Wall
90137	Left		35417		Posterior Wall
38644	Metastatic		35419		Branchial Cleft
38617	Sclera		35228	Lip Neoplasm	
90138	Right		35229		Vermilion Border Of Upper Lip
90139	Left		35230		Benign
38640	Metastatic		35231		Malignant
33948	Nasal Cavity Neoplasm		35232		Vermilion Border Of Lower Lip
33949	Malignant		35233		Benign
38809	Location		35234		Malignant
38810	Naris		35235		Inner Aspect Of Upper Lip
38811	Cartilage		35236		Benign
38812	Mucosa		35237		Malignant
38813	Septum		35238		Inner Aspect Of Lower Lip
38814	Turbinate		35239		Benign
31735	Nasal Polyps		35240		Malignant
31736	Nasopharyngeal Neoplasm		35244		Labial Commissure
31737	Benign		35245		Benign
35420	Superior Wall		35246		Malignant
35422	Posterior Wall		90316		Overlapping Lesion Of Lip
35424	Lateral Wall		33982	Tongue Neoplasm	
35426	Anterior Wall		33983		Benign
31738	Malignant		90192		Malignant
35421	Superior Wall		31727		Carcinoma
35423	Posterior Wall		31709		Leiomyosarcoma
35425	Lateral Wall		31710		Malignant Lymphoma
35427	Anterior Wall		31708		Squamous Cell Carcinoma
31721	Sinus Neoplasm		35247	Base	
38815	Location		35248		Benign
38816	Maxillary		35249		Malignant
38817	Ethmoid		90317		Dorsal Surface
38819	Frontal		90319		Posterior Third Of Tongue
38822	Sphenoid		90318		Posterior Tongue
38823	Overlapping Lesion		90320		Root Of Tongue
34105	Sinus Polyp		35250	Dorsal Surface	
35399	Oropharyngeal Neoplasm		35251		Benign
35400	Benign		35252		Malignant
35402	Tonsil		90321		Anterior 2/3 Of Tongue
35404	Tonsillar Fossa,		90322		Midline Of Tongue
35406	Tonsillar Pillars		90323		Anterior Of Tongue
35408	Vallecula		35253	Tip And Lateral Border	
35410	Anterior Aspect Of Epiglottis		35254		Benign
35412	Epiglottal Junctional Region		35255		Malignant
35414	Lateral Wall		35256	Ventral Surface	
35416	Posterior Wall		35257		Benign
35418	Branchial Cleft		35258		Malignant
35401	Malignant		90324		Anterior 2/3 Of Tongue
35403	Tonsil		90325		Frenulum Linguae
35405	Tonsillar Fossa		90326		Anterior Surface
35407	Tonsillar Pillars		35259		Anterior Two-Thirds

ONCOLOGY, CONT.

35260	Benign		35363	Benign
35261	Malignant		35364	Malignant
35262	Junctional Zone		35365	Gum Neoplasm
35263	Benign		35366	Benign
35264	Malignant		35367	Malignant
31729	Lingual Tonsil Neoplasm		35368	Benign Upper Gum
35265	Benign		35369	Malignant Upper Gum
35266	Malignant		35370	Benign Lower Gum
31745	Parotid Neoplasm		35371	Malignant Lower Gum
35358	Benign		35372	Neoplasm Of Floor Of Mouth
35359	Malignant		35373	Benign
31750	Salivary Gland Neoplasm		35375	Anterior Portion
33984	Benign		35377	Lateral Portion
39554	Pleomorphic Adenoma		35374	Malignant
39555	Myoepithelioma		31713	Squamous Cell Carcinoma
39558	Basal Cell Adenoma		35376	Anterior Portion
39560	Adenolymphoma		35378	Lateral Portion
39561	Oncocytoma		35379	Neoplasm Of Buccal Mucosa
39562	Canalicular Adenoma		35380	Benign
39563	Sebaceous Adenoma		35381	Malignant
39564	Ductal Papilloma		35382	Neoplasm Of Buccal Sulcus
39565	Inverted Ductal Papilloma		35383	Benign
39566	Intraductal Papilloma		35384	Malignant
39567	Sialadenoma Papilliferum		35385	Neoplasm Of Labial Sulcus
39568	Cystadenoma		35386	Benign
39569	Papillary Cystadenoma		35387	Malignant
39570	Mucinous Cystadenoma		35388	Neoplasm Of Hard Palate
35360	Malignant		35389	Benign
39571	Acinic Cell Carcinoma		35390	Malignant
39572	Mucoepidermoid Carcinoma		35391	Neoplasm Of Soft Palate
39573	Adenoid Cystic Carcinoma		35392	Benign
39574	Polymorphous Low Grade Adenocarcinoma		35393	Malignant
			31728	Carcinoma Of Palate
39575	Epithelial-Myoepithelial Carcinoma		35394	Neoplasm Of Uvula
			35395	Benign
39576	Basal Cell Adenocarcinoma		35396	Malignant
39577	Sebaceous Carcinoma		33946	Retromolar Area Neoplasm
39578	Papillary Cystadenocarcinoma		35397	Benign
39579	Mucinous Adenocarcinoma		35398	Malignant
39580	Oncocytic Carcinoma		30768	Epulis
39581	Salivary Duct Carcinoma		30769	Oral Mucocele
39582	Adenocarcinoma		31711	Oral Cancer
39583	Myoepithelioma		31712	Squamous Cell
39584	Carcinoma In Pleomorphic Adenoma		31726	Epithelioma
			35428	Hypopharyngeal Neoplasm
39585	Squamous Cell Carcinoma		35429	Benign
39586	Small Cell Carcinoma		31742	Malignant
39587	Undifferentiated Carcinoma		35430	Postcricoid Region, Benign
39588	Lymphoma		35431	Postcricoid Region, Malignant
39593	Submandibular Gland		35432	Pyriform Sinus, Benign
35361	Benign		33947	Pyriform Sinus, Malignant
35362	Malignant		35433	Aryepiglottic Fold, Benign
39595	Sublingual Gland		35434	Aryepiglottic Fold, Malignant

ONCOLOGY, CONT.

35435	Posterior Wall, Benign	38731	Upper Third Of Esophagus
35436	Posterior Wall, Malignant	38732	Middle Third Of Esophagus
31740	Pharyngeal Neoplasm	38734	Lower Third Of Esophagus
31741	Carcinoma	38802	Overlapping Lesion
35437	Waldeyer's Ring, Benign	38736	Cardioesophageal Junction
35438	Waldeyer's Ring, Malignant	38857	Metastatic To
90327	Location	38858	Regional Lymph Nodes
90328	Pharyngeal Wall	38860	Lung
90329	Lateral Wall	38859	Liver
90330	Posterior Wall	38861	Bone
90331	Retropharynx	31763	Gastric Neoplasm
90332	Throat	31766	Benign
31507	Esophageal Neoplasm	31767	Adenomatous Polyp
38727	Benign	31768	Diffuse Polyposis
38733	Squamous Cell Papilloma	33926	Lipoma
38737	Adenoma	31770	Hyperplastic Polyps
38738	Leiomyoma	31771	Leiomyoma
38740	Lipoma	38764	Adenoma
38742	Vascular Tumors	38765	Tubular Adenoma
38743	Neurogenic Tumors	38766	Villous Adenoma
38744	Granular Cell Tumor	38767	Tubulovillous Adenoma
35444	Cervical Esophagus	38768	Vascular Neoplasm
35446	Thoracic Esophagus	31769	Hemangioma
35448	Abdominal Esophagus	38769	Lymphangioma
35450	Upper Third Of Esophagus	38770	Glomus Tumor
35452	Middle Third Of Esophagus	38771	Neurogenic Neoplasm
35454	Lower Third Of Esophagus	38772	Neurilemmoma
38728	Malignant	38773	Neurofibroma
31510	Squamous Cell Carcinoma	38774	Granular Cell Neoplasm
38747	Verrucous Carcinoma	35456	Malignant
38749	Spindle Cell Carcinoma	31764	Adenocarcinoma
38751	Adenosquamous Carcinoma	39109	Papillary Adenocarcinoma
38753	Adenoid Cystic Carcinoma	39110	Tubular Adenocarcinoma
31508	Adenocarcinoma	39111	Mucinous Adenocarcinoma
38756	Mucoepidermoid Carcinoma	39112	Signet-Ring Cell Carcinoma
31511	Kaposi's Sarcoma	39113	Adenosquamous Carcinoma
38758	Anaplastic Carcinoma	39114	Squamous Cell Carcinoma
38760	Leiomyosarcoma	39115	Small Cell Carcinoma
38761	Carcinosarcoma	39116	Undifferentiated Carcinoma
38762	Melanoma	39117	Neurilemmoma
38763	Carcinoid Tumor	31772	Lymphoma
31509	Malignant Lymphoma	31773	Sarcoma
31512	Neurofibroma	31774	Leiomyosarcoma
35445	Cervical Esophagus	31775	Liposarcoma
35447	Thoracic Esophagus	31776	Kaposi's
35449	Abdominal Esophagus	31777	Carcinoid
35451	Upper Third Of Esophagus	39108	Mixed Carcinoid-
35453	Middle Third Of Esophagus		Adenocarcinoma
35455	Lower Third Of Esophagus	31765	Linitis Plastica
38717	Location	35462	Cardia
38718	Cervical Esophagus	35463	Pyloric
38729	Thoracic Esophagus	35464	Pyloric Antrum
38730	Abdominal Esophagus	35465	Fundal

ONCOLOGY, CONT.

35466	Body		39139	Mixed Carcinoid-
35467	Lesser Curvature			Adenocarcinoma
35468	Greater Curvature		31571	Kaposi's Sarcoma
38739	Location		31569	Leiomyosarcoma
38741	Cardia		31570	Lymphoma
38745	Fundus		31572	Intestinal Lymphoma
38746	Body			(Mediterranean Abdominal)
38748	Gastric Antrum		38782	Location
38750	Pylorus		38784	Duodenum
38752	Prepylorus		38783	Jejunum
38754	Lesser Curvature		38785	Ileum
38755	Greater Curvature		38786	Meckel's Diverticulum
38780	Anterior Wall		38803	Overlapping Lesion
38781	Posterior Wall		38837	Metastatic To
38779	Overlapping Lesion		38838	Regional Lymph Nodes
38827	Metastatic To		38839	Liver
38828	Regional Lymph Nodes		31573	Appendiceal Neoplasm
38829	Liver		31574	Carcinoid
38830	Lung		31575	Adenocarcinoma
30216	Gastric Pseudolymphoma		35469	Benign
35461	Small Intestine Neoplasm		35470	Malignant
31561	Benign		31548	Large Intestine Neoplasm
39118	Adenoma		39150	Benign
31562	Islet Cell Adenoma		34978	Lipoma
31564	Papillary Villous Adenoma		39154	Lipomatosis
39119	Tubular Adenoma		39158	Adenoma
39120	Tubular Adenoma		39160	Tubular Adenoma
39121	Villous Adenoma		39161	Tubulovillous Adenoma
39122	Tubulovillous Adenoma		31559	Villous Adenoma
39123	Adenomatosis		39170	Adenomatosis
39136	Mucinous Cystadenoma		39171	Leiomyoma
31563	Hemangioma		39172	Haemangioma
31565	Leiomyoma		39173	Lymphangioma
39124	Lipoma		39174	Neurilemmoma
39125	Lymphangioma		39175	Neurofibroma
39126	Neurilemmoma		39176	Neurofibromatosis
39127	Neurofibroma		39177	Granular Cell Tumour
39128	Neurofibromatosis		39178	Ganglioneuroma
39129	Gangliocytic Paraganglioma		39179	Ganglioneuromatosis
39130	Ganglioneuroma		39152	Malignant
39131	Ganglioneuromatosis		39180	Mucinous Adenocarcinoma
39132	Paraganglioma		39181	Signet-Ring Cell Carcinoma
31566	Malignant		39182	Squamous Cell Carcinoma
35457	Duodenum		39183	Adenosquamous Carcinoma
35458	Jejunum		39184	Small-Cell Carcinoma
35459	Ileum		39185	Undifferentiated Carcinoma
35460	Meckel's Diverticulum		39186	Leiomyosarcoma
31567	Adenocarcinoma		39187	Carcinoid Tumour
39133	Mucinous Adenocarcinoma		39188	Mixed Carcinoid-
39134	Signet-Ring Cell Carcinoma			Adenocarcinoma
39135	Undifferentiated Carcinoma		31560	Kaposi's Sarcoma
31568	Carcinoid Tumour		31558	Lymphoma
39137	Goblet Cell Carcinoid		31550	Adenocarcinoma

ONCOLOGY, CONT.

31551	Hepatic Flexure		38854	Regional Lymph Nodes
31552	Transverse Colon		38855	Liver
31553	Descending Colon		38856	Ovaries
31554	Sigmoid Colon		33985	Rectal Neoplasm
31555	Cecum		33986	Benign
31556	Ascending Colon		31720	Rectal Polyps
31557	Splenic Flexure		34975	Carcinoid
34955	Duke's A		39190	Malignant
34956	Duke's B		31718	Carcinoma
34959	B1		33930	Rectosigmoid Junction Carcinoma
34960	B2		35776	Metastatic To
34957	Duke's C		39636	Regional Lymph Nodes
34961	C1		39637	Liver
34962	C2		33987	Anal Neoplasm
34958	Duke's D		33988	Benign
39162	Polyps		39192	Malignant
30271	Polyposis Coli		31719	Carcinoma
30272	Familial		35487	Anal Canal
30273	Congenital		39193	Benign
30274	Retention ("Juvenile")		39198	Squamous Cell Papilloma
34974	Hyperplastic Polyp		35488	Malignant
30047	Gardner's Syndrome		39199	Squamous Cell Carcinoma
34558	Sigmoid Polyps		39200	Large Cell Keratinizing
31549	Adenomatous Polyp			Carcinoma
30276	Turcot's Syndrome		39201	Large Cell Non-Keratinizing
35471	Benign			Carcinoma
35475	Cecum		39202	Basaloid Carcinoma
35476	Ascending Colon		39203	Adenocarcinoma
35472	Hepatic Flexure		39204	Rectal-Type Adenocarcinoma
35473	Transverse Colon		39205	Adenocarcinoma Of Anal
35477	Splenic Flexure			Glands
35474	Descending Colon		39206	Small-Cell Carcinoma
35478	Sigmoid Colon		39207	Undifferentiated Carcinoma
35479	Malignant		39194	Anal Sphincter
35480	Cecum		35489	Benign
35481	Ascending Colon		35490	Malignant
35482	Hepatic Flexure		39195	Anal Margin
35483	Transverse Colon		39196	Benign
35484	Splenic Flexure		39409	Squamous Cell Papilloma
35485	Descending Colon		39410	Papillary Hidradenoma
35486	Sigmoid Colon		39197	Malignant
38787	Location		39411	Squamous Cell Carcinoma
38788	Cecum		39412	Verrucous Carcinoma
38789	Ileocecal Valve		39413	Basal Cell Carcinoma
38790	Ileocecal Junction		39414	Paget's Disease
38791	Ascending Colon		39415	Bowen's Disease
38792	Hepatic Flexure		38797	Location
38793	Transverse Colon		39191	Anal Margin
38794	Splenic Flexure		38798	Anal Canal
38795	Descending Colon		38799	Anal Sphincter
38796	Sigmoid Colon		38800	Cloacogenic Zone
38804	Overlapping Lesion		38805	Overlapping Lesion
38853	Metastatic To		31583	Liver Neoplasm

ONCOLOGY, CONT.

39416	Benign		39477	Lymphangioma
39418	Hepatocellular Adenoma		39478	Neurofibroma
39419	Biliary Papillomatosis		31642	Malignant
39420	Angiomyolipoma		39458	Carcinoma In Situ
39421	Lymphangioma		39459	Adenocarcinoma
39422	Lymphangiomatosis		39460	Papillary Adenocarcinoma
39424	Infantile Hemangioendothelioma		39461	Adenocarcinoma, Intestinal Type
31587	Hemangioma		39462	Mucinous Adenocarcinoma
31585	Hepatic Adenoma		39463	Clear Cell Adenocarcinoma
39446	Localized Fibrous Tumor		39464	Signet-Ring Cell Carcinoma
39447	Teratoma		39465	Adenosquamous Carcinoma
39417	Malignant		39466	Squamous Cell Carcinoma
31588	Hepatocellular Carcinoma		39467	Small Cell Carcinoma
36086	Hepatoblastoma		39468	Undifferentiated Carcinoma
39426	Combined Hepatocellular And Cholangiocarcinoma		39469	Carcinoid Tumor
39428	Undifferentiated Carcinoma		39470	Mixed Carcinoid-Adenocarcinoma
39429	Epithelioid Hemangioendothelioma		39479	Rhabdomyosarcoma
31589	Hemangioendothelioma		39480	Kaposi's Sarcoma
31586	Angiosarcoma		39481	Leiomyosarcoma
39434	Undifferentiated Sarcoma		39482	Fibrous Histiocytoma
39438	Rhabdomyosarcoma		39483	Angiosarcoma
31590	Lymphoma		39484	Carcinosarcoma
39442	Endodermal Sinus Tumor		39485	Melanoma
39443	Carcinosarcoma		39486	Lymphoma
39444	Kaposi's Sarcoma		39633	Metastatic To
39445	Rhabdoid Tumor		39634	Regional Lymph Nodes
33910	Focal Nodular Hyperplasia		39635	Liver
31584	Hepatic Metastases		35494	Extrahepatic Bile Duct Neoplasm
35491	Intrahepatic Bile Duct Neoplasm		35495	Benign
35492	Benign		39487	Adenoma
39440	Adenoma		39488	Tubular Adenoma
39441	Cystadenoma		39489	Papillary Adenoma
35493	Malignant		39490	Tubulopapillary Adenoma
31469	Intrahepatic Cholangiocarcinoma		39491	Cystadenoma
39439	Intrahepatic Bile Duct Cystadenocarcinoma		39492	Papillomatosis
			39493	Adenomatosis
39450	Gallbladder Neoplasm		39494	Paraganglioma
39449	Benign		39495	Granular Cell Tumor
39451	Adenoma		39496	Ganglioneurofibromatosis
39452	Tubular Adenoma		39497	Leiomyoma
39453	Papillary Adenoma		39498	Lipoma
39454	Tubulopapillary Adenoma		39499	Hemangioma
39455	Cystadenoma		39500	Lymphangioma
39456	Papillomatosis		39501	Neurofibroma
39457	Adenomatosis		35496	Malignant
39471	Paraganglioma		39502	Carcinoma In Situ
39472	Granular Cell Tumor		39503	Adenocarcinoma
39473	Ganglioneurofibromatosis		39504	Papillary Adenocarcinoma
39474	Leiomyoma		39505	Adenocarcinoma, Intestinal Type
39475	Lipoma		39506	Mucinous Adenocarcinoma
39476	Hemangioma		39507	Clear Cell Adenocarcinoma
			39508	Signet-Ring Cell Carcinoma

ONCOLOGY, CONT.

39509	Adenosquamous Carcinoma	38719	Intraductal Papillary-Mucinous
39510	Squamous Cell Carcinoma		Carcinoma
39512	Small Cell Carcinoma	38720	Noninvasive
39511	Undifferentiated Carcinoma	38721	Invasive
39513	Carcinoid Tumor	38722	Acinar Cell Carcinoma
39514	Mixed Carcinoid-	38723	Acinar Cell
	Adenocarcinoma		Cystadenocarcinoma
39515	Rhabdomyosarcoma	38724	Mixed Acinar-Endocrine
39516	Kaposi's Sarcoma		Carcinoma
39517	Leiomyosarcoma	38725	Solid-Pseudopapillary
39518	Fibrous Histiocytoma		Carcinoma
39519	Angiosarcoma	38726	Pancreatoblastoma
39520	Carcinosarcoma	31631	Microadenomatosis
39521	Melanoma	35207	Beta Cell Tumor
39522	Lymphoma	31632	Pancreatic Cholera (WDHA
31624	Pancreatic Neoplasm		Syndrome)
38684	Benign	35210	Islet Cell Tumor Secreting
38686	Serous Cystadenoma		V.I.P.
38687	Mucinous Cystadenoma	35208	Gastrinoma
38688	Intraductal Papillary-Mucinous	35209	Glucagonoma
	Adenoma	31634	Lymphoma
38689	Mature Teratoma	38706	Location
31625	Adenoma	38707	Head
38690	Uncertain Malignant Potential	38709	Body
38691	Mucinous Cystic Meoplasm	38710	Tail
	(Moderate Dysplasia)	38711	Duct
38692	Intraductal Papillary-Mucinous	38714	Islets Of Langerhans
	Neoplasm (Moderate Dysplasia)	38801	Overlapping Lesion
38693	Solid-Pseudopapillary Neoplasm	38831	Metastatic To
31630	Insulin Secreting Beta Cell	38832	Regional Lymph Nodes
	Tumors	38833	Liver
31633	Glucagonoma	38834	Peritoneal Surface
38685	Malignant	31666	Splenic Neoplasm
38694	Ductal Carcinoma In Situ	31667	Leiomyosarcoma
31626	Adenocarcinoma	31668	Fibrosarcoma
31627	Body	31669	Hemangioma
35497	Tail	31670	Lymphoma
35500	Ductal	31671	Lymphangioma
31629	Head	31641	Pseudomyxoma Peritonei
31628	Ampulla Of Vater	31636	Peritoneal Neoplasm
38695	Mucinous Noncystic Carcinoma	35503	Benign
38698	Signet-Ring Cell Carcinoma	35504	Malignant
38699	Adenosquamous Carcinoma	31637	Mesothelioma
38700	Anaplastic Carcinoma	35505	Mesentery
38701	Mixed Ductal-Endocrine	35506	Mesocolon
	Carcinoma	35507	Omentum
38702	Osteoclast-Like Giant Cell	35508	Rectouterine Pouch
	Neoplasm	31638	Metastases
38703	Serous Cystadenocarcinoma	31543	Retroperitoneal Neoplasm
38704	Mucinous Cystadenocarcinoma	35498	Benign
38705	Noninvasive	31546	Neuroma
38708	Invasive	35499	Malignant
		31544	Sarcoma

ONCOLOGY, CONT.

31545	Fibrosarcoma	
36079	Liposarcoma	
31743	Vocal Cord Polyp	
37633	Granuloma Of Vocal Cords	
33768	Tracheal Neoplasm	
33048	Carcinoma	
33769	Papillomatosis	
33770	Leiomyoma	
33771	Multiple	
31730	Tracheoepithelioma	
30803	Laryngeal Neoplasm	
33989	Benign	
35439	Of The Glottis	
35440	Of The Supraglottis	
35441	Of The Subglottis	
35442	Of The Laryngeal Cartilage	
31744	Malignant	
33950	Of The Glottis	
33951	Of The Supraglottis	
33952	Of The Subglottis	
35443	Of The Laryngeal Cartilage	
38835	Location	
38836	Glottis	
38840	Laryngeal Commissure	
38841	Vocal Cord	
38842	Supraglottis	
38843	Aryepiglottic Fold	
38844	Posterior Surface Of Epiglottis	
38845	False Cord	
38846	Subglottis	
38847	Laryngeal Cartilage	
38848	Arytenoid	
38849	Cricoid	
38850	Cuneiform	
38851	Thyroid	
38852	Overlapping Lesion	
31603	Pulmonary Artery Neoplasm	
31591	Lung Neoplasm	
31593	Bronchial Adenoma	
31595	Carcinoid	
33751	Hamartoma	
33773	Lipoma	
33837	Fibroma	
33838	Teratoma	
33774	Hemangioma	
33775	Endometriosis	
31596	Adenocarcinoma	
38806	Metastatic To	
38807	Brain	
38808	Bone	
31597	Oat Cell	
38818	Metastatic To	
38820	Brain	
38824	Kidneys	
38821	Bone	
31598	Pancoast Tumor	
31599	Squamous Cell	
38825	Metastatic To	
38826	Mediastinal Lymph Nodes	
33772	Large Cell	
31594	Bronchioalveolar Cell	
31600	Undifferentiated	
31592	Pulmonary Metastases	
33840	Hematogenous	
33743	Lymphangitic	
33785	Endobronchial	
33776	Chondroma	
33777	Hemangiopericytoma	
33778	Chemodectoma	
33835	Leiomyoma	
33779	Granular Cell Myoblastoma	
33780	Pulmonary Blastoma	
38865	Location	
38868	Right Lung And Bronchus	
38869	Main Stem Bronchus	
38881	Carina	
38882	Hilus	
38870	Upper Lobe	
38874	Middle Lobe	
38875	Lower Lobe	
38876	Left Lung And Bronchus	
38877	Main Stem Bronchus	
38884	Carina	
38885	Hilus	
38878	Upper Lobe	
38879	Lingula	
38880	Lower Lobe	
38883	Overlapping Lesion	
33781	Lymphoma Involving Lung	
31601	Kaposi's Sarcoma Of The Lung	
31602	Mesothelioma (Pleural)	
33867	Benign	
33868	Malignant	
33866	Traumatic Lung Cyst	
33836	Pulmonary Pseudotumor	
33839	Chest Wall Shadow Image	
31635	Pleural Neoplasm	
30771	Branchial Cyst	
30772	Branchial Fistula	
33031	Mediastinal Masses	
33032	Bronchogenic Cyst	
33033	Lipoma	
33034	Lymphoma	
33035	Mediastinal Masses - Anterior	
33036	Parathyroid Adenoma	
33037	Thyroid Adenoma	

ONCOLOGY, CONT.

33038	Carcinoma	90256	Mesenchymoma
33039	Dermoid Cyst	31500	Giant Cell Tumor
33040	Choriocarcinoma	90257	Leiomyosarcoma
33041	Mesenchymal Tumors	90258	Undifferentiated Sarcoma
33042	Seminoma	90259	Chordoma
33043	Thymoma	90260	Neurilemoma
33044	Teratomas	90261	Neurofibroma
33045	Thymic Cyst	90262	Adamantinoma
33046	Mediastinal Masses - Middle	31501	Reticulum Cell Sarcoma
33049	Metastases	31496	Metastases
33050	Mediastinal Masses - Posterior	33953	Skull
33051	Neuroblastoma	33954	Face
33052	Chromaffin Tumor	33960	Vertebral Column
33053	Ganglioneuroma	33955	Ribs, Sternum Or Clavicle
33054	Neurofibroma	33956	Scapula Or Long Bones Of Upper
33055	Pheochromocytoma		Limb
33056	Mediastinal Masses - Superior	33957	Short Bones Of Upper Limb
33057	Substernal Goiter	33958	Pelvic Bones, Sacrum Or Coccyx
33058	Lymphoma	33959	Long Bones Of Lower Limb
33060	Thymic Tumors	33999	Short Bones Of Lower Limb
31732	Thymoma	39682	Bone-Forming Neoplasms
33059	Superior Mediastinal Masses -	38896	Benign
	Parathyroid	31714	Osteoma
30773	Lymphangioma (Hygroma)	31494	Osteoid Osteoma
31506	Diaphragmatic Neoplasm	39697	Osteoblastoma
34478	Bone Cyst	39698	Malignant
34479	Solitary	39701	Aggressive Osteoblastoma
30770	Odontoma	39703	Osteosarcoma
31488	Bone Neoplasm	39705	Medullary Osteosarcoma
39770	Benign, NOS	39707	Conventional Central
39811	Fibrous Histiocytoma		Osteosarcoma
39814	Lipoma	39708	Telangiectatic Osteosarcoma
39816	Desmoplastic Fibroma	39713	Intraosseous Well-
31489	Aneurysmal Cyst		Differentiated Osteosarcoma
31491	Fibroma	39715	Round Cell Osteosarcoma
31492	Giant Cell Tumor	39717	Surface Osteosarcoma
33990	Skull	39720	Parosteal Osteosarcoma
31716	Osteoma Calvarium	39722	Periosteal Osteosarcoma
31703	Hemangioma	39724	High Grade Surface
33991	Face		Osteosarcoma
31715	Osteoma Of Nasal Sinus	31502	Osteogenic Sarcoma
33992	Vertebral Column	39691	Cartilage-Forming Neoplasms
33993	Ribs, Sternum Or Clavicle	39728	Benign
33994	Scapula Or Long Bones Of Upper	31490	Chondroma
	Limb	39732	Enchondroma
33995	Short Bones Of Upper Limb	39733	Periosteal Chondroma
33996	Pelvic Bones, Sacrum Or Coccyx	31493	Osteochondroma
33997	Long Bones Of Lower Limb	39735	Solitary Osteochondroma
33998	Short Bones Of Lower Limb	39736	Multiple Hereditary
31495	Malignant, NOS		Osteochondromas
31499	Fibrosarcoma	39738	Epiphyseal Chondroblastoma
90254	Fibrous Histiocytoma	39740	Chondromyxoid Fibroma
90255	Liposarcoma	39730	Malignant

ONCOLOGY, CONT.

31497	Chondrosarcoma	39054	T3
39747	Juxtacortical Chondrosarcoma	39055	T4
39749	Mesenchymal Chondrosarcoma	39056	T5
39755	Chondroblastoma	39057	T6
39757	Dedifferentiated	39058	T7
	Chondrosarcoma	39059	T8
39759	Clear Cell Chondrosarcoma	39060	T9
90263	Bone Marrow Neoplasm	39061	T10
90266	Malignant	39062	T11
31498	Ewing's Sarcoma	39063	T12
90264	Primitive Neuroectodermal	39064	L1
	Neoplasm	39065	L2
90265	Lymphoma	39066	L3
90267	Myeloma	39067	L4
90268	Vascular Bone Neoplasm	39068	L5
90269	Benign	39024	Intervertebral Disc
90271	Haemangioma	39069	Nucleus Pulposus
90272	Lymphangioma	39025	C1-2
90273	Glomangioma	39026	C2-3
90270	Malignant	39027	C3-4
90276	Angiosarcoma	39028	C4-5
90277	Haemangiopericytoma	39029	C5-6
90278	Indeterminate	39030	C6-7
90274	Haemangioendothelioma	39031	C7-T1
90275	Haemangiopericytoma	39032	T1-2
38897	Location	39033	T2-3
39000	Skull	39034	T3-4
39001	Facial Bones	39035	T4-5
39002	Frontal	39036	T5-6
39003	Nasal	39037	T6-7
39004	Ethmoid	39038	T7-8
39005	Zygomatic	39039	T8-9
39007	Malar	39040	T9-10
39006	Maxilla	39041	T10-11
39009	Occipital	39042	T11-12
39010	Orbital	39043	T12-L1
39011	Parietal	39044	L1-2
39012	Sphenoid	39045	L2-3
39013	Temporal	39046	L3-4
39008	Hyoid	39047	L4-5
39017	Mandible	39070	Ribs, Sternum, Clavicle
39018	Temporomandibular Joint	39071	Ribs
39019	Vertebral Column	39072	Right First Rib
39020	Vertebra	39073	Right Second Rib
39021	C1	39074	Right Third Rib
39022	C2	39075	Right Fourth Rib
39023	C3	39076	Right Fifth Rib
39048	C4	39077	Right Sixth Rib
39049	C5	39078	Right Seventh Rib
39050	C6	39079	Right Eighth Rib
39051	C7	39080	Right Ninth Rib
39052	T1	39081	Right Tenth Rib
39053	T2	39082	Right Eleventh Rib

ONCOLOGY, CONT.

39083	Right Twelfth Rib	39212	Fourth Rib
39084	Left First Rib	39213	Fifth Rib
39085	Left Second Rib	39214	Sixth Rib
39086	Left Third Rib	39215	Seventh Rib
39087	Left Fourth Rib	39216	Hip
39088	Left Fifth Rib	39217	Acetabulum
39089	Left Sixth Rib	39218	Right
39090	Left Seventh Rib	39219	Left
39091	Left Eighth Rib	39220	Joint
39092	Left Ninth Rib	39221	Right
39093	Left Tenth Rib	39222	Left
39094	Left Eleventh Rib	39223	Pelvic Bone
39095	Left Twelfth Rib	39224	Coccyx
39096	Costal Cartilage	39225	Ilium
39097	R1-2	39226	Innominate Bone
39098	R2-3	39227	Ischium
39099	R3-4	39228	Pubic Bone
39100	R4-5	39229	Symphysis Pubis
39101	R5-6	39230	Sacrum
39102	R6-7	39231	Sacroiliac Joint
39103	R7-8	39232	Right
39104	R8-9	39233	Left
39105	R9-10	39234	Overlapping Lesion Of Bones, Joints And Articular Cartilage
39106	R10-11		
39107	R11-12	38898	Long Bones Of Shoulder / Upper Limb
39138	L1-2		
39140	L2-3	38899	Acromioclavicular Joint
39141	L3-4	38900	Right
39142	L4-5	38901	Left
39143	L5-6	38902	Shoulder Bone
39144	L6-7	38903	Right
39145	L7-8	38904	Left
39146	L8-9	38905	Scapula
39147	L9-10	38906	Right
39148	L10-11	38907	Left
39149	L11-12	38908	Shoulder Girdle
39151	Costovertebral Joint	38909	Right
39153	First Rib	38910	Left
39155	Second Rib	38911	Shoulder Joint
39156	Third Rib	38912	Right
39157	Fourth Rib	38913	Left
39159	Fifth Rib	38914	Humerus
39163	Sixth Rib	38915	Right
39164	Seventh Rib	38916	Left
39165	Eighth Rib	38917	Elbow Joint
39166	Ninth Rib	38918	Right
39167	Tenth Rib	38919	Left
39168	Eleventh Rib	38920	Radius
39169	Twelfth Rib	38921	Right
39208	Sternocostal Joint	38922	Left
39209	First Rib	38923	Ulna
39210	Second Rib	38924	Right
39211	Third Rib	38925	Left

ONCOLOGY, CONT.

38926	Wrist		38979	Left
38927	Bone		38980	Foot
38928	Right		38981	Right
38929	Left		38982	Left
38930	Joint		38983	Toes
38931	Right		38984	Great Toe
38932	Left		38985	Right
38933	Hand		38986	Left
38934	Right		38987	2nd Toe
38935	Left		38988	Right
38936	Fingers		38989	Left
38937	Thumb		38990	Middle Toe
38938	Right		38991	Right
38939	Left		38992	Left
38940	Index Finger		38993	4th Toe
38941	Right		38994	Right
38942	Left		38995	Left
38943	Middle Finger		38996	Little Toe
38944	Right		38997	Right
38945	Left		38998	Left
38946	Ring Finger		38999	Overlapping Lesion Of Bones, Joints And Articular Cartilage
38947	Right			
38948	Left		39624	Cartilage
38949	Little Finger		34457	Synovial Cyst
38950	Right		31576	Joint Neoplasm
38951	Left		31577	Hemangioma
38952	Femur		31578	Lipoma
38953	Right		31579	Synovial Chondromatosis
38954	Left		31580	Synovioma
38955	Knee Joint		31581	Synovial Chondrosarcoma
38956	Right		34832	Jaw Cyst
38957	Left		31739	Jaw Sarcoma
38958	Semilunar Cartilage		33936	Connective Tissue Neoplasm
38959	Lateral Meniscus		34000	Benign
38960	Right		34001	Head, Face Or Neck
38961	Left		34002	Upper Limb, Including Shoulder
38962	Medial Meniscus		34003	Lower Limb, Including Hip
38963	Right		34004	Thorax
38964	Left		34005	Abdomen
38974	Patella		34006	Pelvis
38975	Right		33937	Malignant
38976	Left		33961	Head, Face Or Neck
38965	Tibia		33962	Upper Limb, Including Shoulder
38966	Right		33963	Lower Limb, Including Hip
38967	Left		33964	Thorax
38968	Fibula		33965	Abdomen
38969	Right		33966	Pelvis
38970	Left		31503	Bowen's Disease
38971	Tarsus		31704	Desmoid Tumor
38972	Right		36080	Angiosarcoma
38973	Left		31683	Rhabdomyosarcoma
38977	Heel		36085	Neuroblastoma
38978	Right		39014	Skin Neoplasm

ONCOLOGY, CONT.

34007	Benign	31662	Lentigo
31725	Subcutaneous Lipoma	31663	Metastatic
34008	Lip	31664	Nodular
34009	Eyelid	31665	Superficial Spreading
34010	Ear	31582	Kaposi's Sarcoma
34011	Face	39235	Location
34012	Scalp	39236	Eye
34013	Neck	39237	Eyelid
34014	Trunk	39238	Right Upper
34015	Upper Limb, Including Shoulder	39239	Right Lower
31722	Malignant	39240	Left Upper
31723	Basal Cell Carcinoma	39241	Left Lower
33967	Lip	39242	Canthus
33968	Eyelid	39243	Right Inner
33969	Ear	39244	Right Outer
31734	Auricular	39245	Left Inner
33970	Face	39246	Left Outer
33971	Scalp	39247	Meibomian Gland
33972	Neck	39248	Right
33979	Trunk	39249	Left
38862	Metastatic To	39250	External Ear
38863	Regional Lymph Nodes	39251	Pinna
38864	Lung From Inhaled	39258	Right
	Fragments	39259	Left
31724	Squamous Cell Carcinoma	39260	Right Concha
31707	Lip	39261	Left Concha
33974	Eyelid	39262	Right Helix
33975	Ear	39263	Left Helix
33976	Face	39264	Right Tragus
33977	Scalp	39265	Left Tragus
33978	Neck	39252	Earlobe
33980	Trunk	39253	Right
37147	Lower Extremities	39254	Left
38871	Metastatic To	39255	External Auditory Canal
38872	Regional Lymph Nodes	39256	Right
38873	Regional Nerve Axons	39257	Left
36146	Lip	39266	Ceruminal Gland
31661	Malignant Melanoma	39267	Right
36147	Eyelid	39268	Left
36148	Ear	39269	Face
36149	Forehead	39270	Forehead
36150	Eyebrow	39271	Eyebrow
36151	Temple	39272	Right
36152	Nose	39273	Left
36153	Cheek	39274	Temple
36154	Chin	39275	Right
36155	Scalp	39276	Left
36156	Neck	39277	Nose
36157	Trunk	39278	Columnella
36158	Shoulder	39279	Ala Nasi
36159	Upper Limb	39280	Cheek
36160	Hip	39281	Right
36161	Lower Limb	39282	Left

ONCOLOGY, CONT.

39283	Jaw	90034		Thumb
39284	Chin	90051		Right
39285	Head	90052		Left
39286	Scalp	90053		Lower Extremities
39287	Neck	90054		Hip
39288	Cervical Region	90065		Right
39289	Supraclavicular Region	90066		Left
39290	Trunk	90055		Thigh
39291	Infraclavicular Region	90064		Right
39292	Axilla	90067		Left
39293	Breast	90056		Knee
39294	Chest	90068		Right
39295	Chest Wall	90069		Left
39296	Thorax	90057		Popliteal Space
39297	Thoracic Wall	90070		Right
39298	Abdomen	90071		Left
39299	Umbilicus	90058		Leg
39300	Groin	90072		Right
39301	Inguinal Region	90073		Left
39302	Flank	90059		Calf
39303	Scapular Region	90074		Right
39304	Back	90075		Left
39305	Sacrococcygeal Region	90060		Ankle
39306	Buttock	90076		Right
39307	Gluteal Region	90077		Left
39308	Perineum	90061		Heel
39309	Perianal Skin	90079		Right
39310	Anus	90080		Left
90025	Upper Extremities	90062		Foot
90026	Shoulder	90081		Right
90035	Right	90082		Left
90036	Left	90083		Right Dorsal
90027	Arm	90084		Left Dorsal
90037	Right	90085		Right Plantar
90038	Left	90086		Left Plantar
90028	Elbow	90063		Toe
90039	Right	90087		Right
90040	Left	90088		Left
90029	Antecubital Space	90089		Right Nail Bed
90041	Right	90090		Left Nail Bed
90042	Left	31702	Extramammary Paget's Disease
90030	Forearm	31643	Breast Neoplasm
90043	Right	35124	Benign, Female
90044	Left	35125	Benign, Male
90031	Wrist	35126	Malignant, Female
90045	Right	35129	Nipple / Areola
90046	Left	35130	Central Portion
90032	Hand	35131	Upper-Inner Quadrant
90047	Right	35132	Lower-Inner Quadrant
90048	Left	35133	Upper-Outer Quadrant
90033	Palm	35134	Lower-Outer Quadrant
90049	Right	35135	Axillary Tail
90050	Left	35127	Malignant, Male Nipple / Areola

ONCOLOGY, CONT.

35128	Malignant, Male Breast Tissue	39346	Lower Breast
31644	Sclerosing Adenosis	39347	Right
31645	Intraductal Papilloma	39348	Left
31646	Papillary Cyst Adenoma	39349	Midline
31647	Adenocarcinoma	39350	Right
31648	Cystosarcoma Phylloides	39351	Left
31649	Adenofibrosarcoma	31607	Ovarian Neoplasm
31650	Fibroadenoma	34916	Benign Epithelial
31651	Fibrosarcoma	34917	Germinal Inclusional Cyst
31652	Hemangiosarcoma	34918	Serous Cystadenoma
31653	Lymphoma	34919	Mucinous Cystadenoma
31654	Nipple Epithelioma	34920	Cystadenofibroma
31655	Liposarcoma	34921	Endometrioid
31656	Neurosarcoma	34922	Brenner
31657	Scirrhous Carcinoma	31608	Adenocarcinoma (Epithelial)
31658	Paget's Disease	34895	Serous
31659	Fibroadenosis	34896	Mucinous
34205	Fibrosclerosis	34897	Endometroid
39311	Location	34898	Clear Cell
39312	Nipple	34899	Brenner
39313	Right	34900	Undifferentiated
39314	Left	34901	Carcinosarcoma
39315	Areola	34902	Stromal Cell
39316	Right	31609	Arrhenoblastoma (Sertoli-Leydig Cell)
39317	Left		
39318	Central Portion	34904	Sertoli
39319	Right Breast	31611	Granulosa Cell
39320	Left Breast	34903	Gynandroblastoma
39321	Upper Inner Quadrant	31612	Hilus Cell
39322	Right	31614	Theca Cell
39323	Left	31613	Lipoid Cell
39324	Upper Outer Quadrant	34905	Germ Cell
39325	Right	31616	Teratoma
39326	Left	31615	Struma Ovarii
39327	Lower Inner Quadrant	31619	Carcinoid Tumor
39328	Right	34923	Dermoid Cyst
39329	Left	34908	Teratocarcinoma
39330	Lower Outer Quadrant	31617	Choriocarcinoma
39331	Right	34906	Dysgerminoma
39332	Left	34907	Endodermal
39333	Axillary Tail	34909	Embryonal
39334	Right	34910	Mixed
39335	Left	34911	Gonadoblastoma
39336	Overlapping Lesion	34912	Mesenchymal
39337	Inner Breast	34913	Metastasis To Ovary
39338	Right	31618	Krukenberg
39339	Left	31610	Ovarian Fibroma
39340	Outer Breast	34224	Ovarian Cyst
39341	Right	31621	Ruptured
39342	Left	34223	Follicle
39343	Upper Breast	30467	Corpus Luteum
39344	Right	34914	Theca Lutein
39345	Left	31754	Meig's Syndrome

ONCOLOGY, CONT.

31620	Fallopian Tube Neoplasm		90288	Malignant
35087	Benign		31757	Sarcoma
35086	Adenocarcinoma		90294	Leiomyosarcoma
35772	Metastasis		90295	Epithelioid Leiomyosarcoma
39352	Right		90296	Myxoid Leiomyosarcoma
39353	Left		90309	Adenosarcoma
35143	Broad Ligament Neoplasm		90310	Homologous Adenosarcoma
35144	Benign		90311	Heterologous Adenosarcoma
35145	Malignant		90312	Carcinofibroma
35146	Parametrial Neoplasm		90313	Carcinosarcoma
35147	Benign		90314	Homologous Carcinosarcoma
35148	Malignant		90315	Heterologous Carcinosarcoma
39354	Uterine Ligament		31756	Endometrial Carcinoma
39355	Uterosacral Ligament		90299	Endometrioid Adenocarcinoma
35149	Round Ligament Neoplasm		90300	Secretory
35150	Benign		90301	Ciliated Cell
35151	Malignant		90303	Serous Adenocarcinoma
35088	Cervical Neoplasm		90302	Adenosquamous Carcinoma
35136	Benign		90304	Clear Cell Adenocarcinoma
30611	Polyps		90305	Mucinous Adenocarcinoma
31606	Cancer		90306	Squamous Cell Carcinoma
35137	Endocervical Canal		90307	Mixed Carcinoma
35138	Endocervical Gland		90308	Undifferentiated Carcinoma
35139	Exocervix		90293	High Grade Stromal Sarcoma
35140	Cervical Stump		35141	Corpus Fundus
35777	Metastasis		35142	Corpus Isthmus
39356	Location		90289	Uncertain Malignant Potential
39357	Endocervix		90290	Low Grade Endometrial Stromal
39358	Cervical Canal			Sarcoma
39359	Endocervical Canal		90291	Smooth Muscle Tumour
39360	Endocervical Gland		90292	Intravenous Leiomyomatosis
39361	Nabothian Gland		90297	Diffuse Leiomyomatosis
39362	Exocervix		35079	Leiomyomatous Degeneration
39363	Overlapping Lesion		35080	Carneous (Red)
34017	Uterine Neoplasm		35081	Hyaline
39600	Benign		35082	Cystic
31755	Leiomyoma		35083	Fatty
34016	Submucous		35084	Calcific
35073	Intramural		35085	Malignant (Sarcomatous)
35074	Subserous		35771	Metastasis
35075	Pedunculated		39364	Location
35076	Intraligamentous		39365	Isthmus
35077	Parasitic		39366	Endometrium
90279	Cellular Leiomyoma		39367	Endometrial Gland
90280	Epithelioid Leiomyoma		39368	Endometrial Stroma
90281	Bizarre Leiomyoma		39369	Myometrium
90298	Metastasizing Leiomyoma		39370	Fundus
90282	Lipoleiomyoma		39371	Overlapping Lesion
90283	Adenomatoid Tumour		34018	Vaginal Neoplasm
90284	Adenofibroma		34019	Benign
90285	Adenomyoma		31758	Cancer
90286	Atypical Polypoid Adenomyoma		35774	Metastasis
90287	Endometrial Stromal Nodule		39372	Location

ONCOLOGY, CONT.

39373	Vault
39374	Fornix
39375	Gartner's Duct
39376	Hymen
31682	Uterine ("Gestational")
	Choriocarcinoma (Metastatic GTD)
34989	Low Risk
34990	High Risk
34020	Vulvar Neoplasm
34021	Benign
35152	Labia Majora
35153	Bartholin's Gland
35154	Labia Minora
35155	Clitoris
31759	Cancer
35156	Labia Majora
35157	Bartholin's Gland
35158	Labia Minora
35159	Clitoris
35773	Metastatic
39377	Location
39378	Labium Majus
39379	Bartholin's Gland
39380	Skin
39381	Labium Minus
39382	Fourchette
39383	Mons Pubis
39384	Skin
39385	Clitoris
39386	Overlapping Lesion
31516	Penile Carcinoma
39387	Location
39388	Prepuce
39389	Glans Penis
39390	Corpus Cavernosum
39391	Right
39392	Left
39393	Skin
39394	Overlapping Lesion
31517	Penile Warts
31518	Testicular Neoplasm
31519	Teratoma
31520	Choriocarcinoma
31521	Interstitial Cell Tumor
31522	Seminoma
31523	Teratocarcinoma
31524	Fibroma
31525	Lipoma
31526	Adenoma
31527	Myxoma
31528	Embryonal Cell Carcinoma
39395	Location
39396	Descended Testis

39397	Right
39398	Left
39399	Bilaterally
39400	Undescended Testis
39401	Right
39402	Left
39403	Bilaterally
39404	Ectopic Testis
39405	Right
39406	Left
39407	Bilaterally
31660	Scrotal Carcinoma
39423	Skin
39425	Neoplasm Of Epididymis
39427	Neoplasm Of Spermatic Cord
39430	Neoplasm Of Seminal Vesicle
39431	Neoplasm Of Tunica Vaginalis
39432	Neoplasm Of Overlapping Lesion Of
	Male Genital Organs
34027	Prostatic Neoplasm
31640	Benign
31639	Adenocarcinoma
39015	Renal Neoplasm
31536	Benign
31537	Adenoma
31538	Renin Producing
31539	Fibrolipomyomas
31540	Angiomyolipoma
31541	Hemangioma
31542	Oncocytoma
31529	Malignant
31530	Juxtoglomerular Cell Tumor
31531	Wilm's Tumor (Nephroblastoma)
31532	Papillary Adenocarcinoma
31533	Papillary Transitional Cell
31534	Neuroblastoma
31535	Renal-Cell Carcinoma
39433	Location
39435	Parenchyma
39436	Right
39437	Left
39638	Metastatic To
39639	Regional Lymph Nodes
39640	Liver
39641	Lung
39642	Renal Pelvis Neoplasm
31547	Benign
34831	Malignant
39643	Location
39644	Renal Calyces
39645	Right
39646	Left
39647	Pelviureteric Junction

ONCOLOGY, CONT.

39648	Right
39649	Left
31760	Ureteral Carcinoma
34028	Bladder Neoplasm
31486	Benign
31487	Papilloma
39016	Malignant
31483	Carcinoma
31484	Solid
31485	Papillary
35775	Metastasis
39650	Location
39651	Trigone
39652	Dome
39653	Lateral Wall
39654	Anterior Wall
39655	Posterior Wall
39656	Bladder Neck
39657	Internal Urethral Orifice
39658	Ureteric Orifice
39659	Urachus
39660	Overlapping Lesion Of Bladder
31761	Urethral Carcinoma
39661	Location
39662	Cowper's Gland
39663	Prostatic Utricle
39664	Urethral Gland
39665	Paraurethral Neoplasm
31467	Pheochromocytoma
34858	Malignant
33782	Immunoblastic Lymphadenopathy
31466	Angioimmunoblastic Lymphadenopathy (AILD)
31778	Metastatic Cancer
31691	Hodgkin's Disease
31692	Lymphocyte Depleted
31693	Lymphocyte Predominant
31694	Mixed Cellularity
31695	Nodular Sclerosis
35839	Non-Hodgkin's Lymphoma
31684	Diffuse
31685	DM (Mixed Lymphocytic & Histiocytic)
31686	DLPD (Diffuse Lymphoma, Poorly Differentiated)
31687	DU (Undifferentiated)
31688	DLWD (Diffuse Lymphoma, Well Differentiated)
31689	DHL (Diffuse Histiocytic)
31690	Burkitt's
31696	Nodular
31697	NH (Nodular Histiocytic Lymphoma)

31698	NLPD (Nodular Lymphoma, Poorly Differentiated)
31699	NM (Nodular Mixed Cytologic Lymphoma)
31700	NLWD (Nodular Lymphoma, Well Differentiated)
36081	Lymphoma, NOS
36082	Acute
36083	Chronic
36084	In Remission
31515	Pseudolymphoma
31753	Histiocytic Medullary Reticulosis
31762	Mastocytosis
31470	Leukemia
36061	Acute
36062	Chronic
31471	Mast Cell (Mastocytosis)
31472	Erythroleukemia (Diguglielmo's Disease)
31473	Chronic Lymphocytic (CLL)
31474	Adult T-Cell
31475	Chronic Granulocytic (Myelogenous - CML)
35942	Chronic Myelomonocytic (CMML)
33858	Hairy-Cell
31476	Acute Myelogenous (AML)
31477	Acute Myelomonoblastic (AMML)
31478	Acute Lymphocytic (ALL)
31479	Megakaryocytic (Essential Thrombocythemia)
31480	Acute Undifferentiated
31481	Promyelocytic
31482	Eosinophilic
36063	In Remission
31604	Mycosis Fungoides Lymphoma
31605	Sezary Syndrome
31705	Multiple Myeloma
31706	Plasmacytoma
33893	Heavy Chain Disease
38677	**Environmental Disorders**
32403	Poisoning
32404	Acids
32405	Alkali
32406	Aniline
32407	Heavy Metals
32408	Antimony
32409	Arsenic
32410	Barium
32411	Bismuth
32412	Cadmium
32413	Copper
32414	Gold
32415	Lead

ENVIRONMENTAL DISORDERS, CONT.

32416	Mercury	38499	Silicone
32417	Manganese	38500	Tobacco
32418	Silver	32468	N-Hexamemethyl-N-Butyl Ketone
32419	Uranium	32464	Trichloroethylene
32420	Benzene	32460	Benzodiazepines
35004	Acute Toxicity	32462	Tricyclic Antidepressant
35005	Chronic Toxicity	32463	Belladonna / Atropine
35008	Toluene	32465	Amphetamine
32421	Boric Acid	32469	Phencyclidine (Angel Dust)
32422	Bromates / Chlorates	32470	Minor Tranquilizer
32423	Cantharidin	32471	Oxygen
32424	Carbon Monoxide	32472	Water
38059	Carbon Tetrachloride	32473	Glutethimide
32425	Cyanide	32474	Thallium
32426	Fluorides	32475	Ciguatera Poisoning
32427	Formaldehyde	37941	Scombroid Poisoning
38058	Fusel Oil	34770	Open Wound
32428	Glycols	34771	Ocular Adnexa
38060	Inorganic Lead Compounds	37767	Laceration Of Eyelid Skin And Periocular Area
32429	Iodine		
32430	Iron Salts	38543	Laceration Of Eyelid
32431	Isopropyl Alcohol	37768	Full-Thickness
32432	Magnesium	37769	Laceration Of Eyelid Involving Lacrimal Passages
32433	Methyl Alcohol		
32434	Monosodium Glutamate ("Chinese Restaurant Syndrome")	37770	Penetrating Wound Of Orbit
		37771	Penetrating Wound Of Orbit With Foreign Body
32435	Mushroom		
32436	Naphthalene / Mothballs	34772	Eyeball
32437	Nitrites	37776	Laceration Of Eye
32438	Organophosphate	37772	Ocular Laceration W/Out Prolapse Of Intraocular Tissue
32439	Paraquat		
32440	Petroleum Distillates	37773	Ocular Laceration With Prolapse/Exposure Of Intraocular Tissue
34966	Solvents		
34964	Pentachlorophenol		
32441	Phenol	37774	Rupture Of Eye With Partial Loss Of Intraocular Tissue
32442	Phosphorus		
32443	Salicylates	37775	Avulsion Of Eye
38061	Strychnine And Salts	34773	Ear
32444	Acetaminophen	37778	External Ear
32445	Opioid	37779	Auricle
32447	Sulfides	37780	Auditory Canal
32448	Ddt	37781	External Ear, Complicated
32449	Carbon Tetrachloride	34774	Head
32450	Tetrachloroethelene	37782	Scalp
32451	Paraldehyde	37783	Scalp, Complicated
32452	Barbiturate	34775	Face
32454	Bromides	37792	Forehead
32455	Strychnine	37793	Lip
32457	Caffeine	37794	Jaw
32458	Cannabis	37795	Face, Complicated
32459	Aflatoxin	37796	Cheek
38497	Asbestos	37797	Forehead
38498	Latex	37798	Lip

ENVIRONMENTAL DISORDERS, CONT.

37799	Jaw	37839	With Tendon Involvement
37784	Nose	34787	Finger(s)
37785	Nasal Septum	37840	Complicated
37786	Nasal Cavity	34788	With Tendon Involvement
37787	Nasal Sinus	37841	Upper Limb
37788	Nose, Complicated	37842	Complicated
37789	Nasal Septum	37843	With Tendon Involvement
37790	Nasal Cavity	37828	Abdominal Wall, Anterior
37791	Nasal Sinus	37829	Abdominal Wall, Anterior, Complicated
37800	Internal Structures Of Mouth		
37801	Gum (Alveolar Process)	37830	Abdominal Wall, Lateral
37802	Tooth (Broken)	37831	Abdominal Wall, Lateral, Complicated
37803	Tongue And Floor Of Mouth	34789	Hip / Thigh
37804	Palate	34790	Knee
34781	Internal Structures Of Mouth, Complicated	37852	Complicated
		37853	With Tendon Involvement
37805	Buccal Mucosa	34791	Leg
37806	Gum (Alveolar Process)	37854	Complicated
37807	Tooth (Broken)	37855	With Tendon Involvement
37808	Tongue And Floor Of Mouth	34792	Foot
37809	Palate	37856	Complicated
34776	Neck	37857	With Tendon Involvement
37810	Larynx	37858	Toe(s)
37811	Trachea	37859	Complicated
37812	Larynx, Complicated	37860	With Tendon Involvement
37813	Trachea, Complicated	37861	Lower Limb
37814	Thyroid Gland	37862	Complicated
37815	Thyroid Gland, Complicated	37863	With Tendon Involvement
37826	Breast	34780	Multiple
37827	Breast, Complicated	31150	Human Bites
34777	Back	38155	Injury Due To War
34778	Buttock	38156	Bullets
37825	External Genital Organs	38157	Accidental Explosion
37824	Penis	38158	Nuclear Weapons
37817	Penis, Complicated	37314	Gunshot Wound
37818	Scrotum And Testes	38126	Caused By Handgun
37819	Scrotum And Testes, Complicated	38127	Caused By Shotgun
37820	Vulva	38151	Due To Legal Intervention By Firearms
37821	Vulva, Complicated	37315	Ocular Adnexa
37822	Vagina	37316	Ear
37823	Vagina, Complicated	37317	Head
34782	Upper Arm	37318	Face
34783	Forearm	37319	Neck
37832	Complicated	37323	Shoulder Region
37833	With Tendon Involvement	37320	Back
34784	Elbow	37321	Buttock
37834	Complicated	37322	External Genital Organs
37835	With Tendon Involvement	37324	Upper Arm
34785	Wrist	37325	Forearm
37836	Complicated	37326	Elbow
37837	With Tendon Involvement	37327	Wrist
34786	Hand	37328	Hand
37838	Complicated	37329	Hip / Thigh

ENVIRONMENTAL DISORDERS, CONT.

37330	Knee
37331	Leg
37332	Foot
37333	Multiple
90333	Injury Due To Legal Intervention
38152	By Gas
90334	By Rubber Bullet(s)
90335	By Metal Bullet(s)
90336	By Grenade Fragments
90337	By A Piercing Instrument
38153	By Blunt Object
38154	By Other Specified Means
32577	Traumatic Amputation
32578	Of Thumb
32579	Of Finger(s)
32580	Of Arm And Hand
37848	Unilateral
37849	Complicated
37844	Below Elbow
37845	Complicated
37846	At Elbow Or Above
37847	Complicated
37850	Bilateral
37851	Bilateral, Complicated
32581	Of Toe(s)
37864	Complicated
32582	Of Foot
32583	Of Leg(s)
37865	Unilateral, Below Knee
37866	Complicated
37867	Unilateral, At/Above Knee
37868	Complicated
37869	Bilateral
37870	Complicated
34793	Late Effect Of Injury
37871	Internal, To Chest
37872	Internal, To Intra-Abdominal Organs
37873	Internal, To Other Internal Organs
37874	To Blood Vessel Of Head, Neck, & Extremities
37875	To Blood Vessel Of Thorax, Abdomen & Pelvis
37876	Foreign Body In Orifice
38070	Foreign Body Left During Procedure
37877	Certain Complications Of Trauma
37878	Late Effects Of Injuries To Skin & Subcutaneous Tissues
37879	Late Effect Of Contusion
37880	Late Effect Of Crushing
37881	Late Effect Of Burn Of Eye, Face, Head And Neck
37882	Late Effect Of Burn Of Wrist And Hand

37883	Late Effects Of Injuries To The Nervous System
37884	Cranial Nerve
37885	Spinal Cord
37886	Nerve Root(s), Spinal Plexus(es), Other Trunk Nerves
37887	Peripheral Nerve Of Shoulder Girdle & Upper Limb
37888	Peripheral Nerve Of Pelvic Girdle & Lower Limb
37889	Late Effect Of External Causes
37890	Toxic Effects Of Nonmedical Substances
37891	Radiation
37892	Complications Of Surgical And Medical Care
34794	Superficial Injury
34835	Face/Scalp
37974	Abrasion Of Face
37981	Infected
37976	Abrasion Of Scalp
37977	Infected
37978	Blister Of Face
37982	Infected
37979	Blister Of Scalp
37980	Infected
37983	Insect Bite, Nonvenomous, Of Face
37984	Infected
37985	Insect Bite, Nonvenomous, Of Scalp
37986	Infected
37987	Splinter Of Face
37988	Infected
37989	Splinter Of Scalp
37990	Infected
34836	Trunk
37991	Abrasion On Trunk
37992	Infected
37993	Blister On Trunk
37994	Infected
37995	Insect Bite, Nonvenomous, On Trunk
37996	Infected
37997	Splinter On Trunk
37998	Infected
34837	Shoulder And Upper Arm
37999	Abrasion Of Shoulder
38000	Infected
38001	Blister Of Shoulder
38002	Infected
38003	Insect Bite, Nonvenomous, Of Shoulder
38004	Infected
38005	Splinter Of Shoulder

ENVIRONMENTAL DISORDERS, CONT.

38006	Infected		38056	Superficial Laceration Of Cornea
34838	Forearm		38057	Conjunctival Injury
38007	Abrasion Of Forearm		34795	Contusion With Intact Skin Surface
38008	Infected		34796	Head / Neck
38009	Blister Of Forearm		37946	Face
38010	Infected		37947	Scalp
38011	Insect Bite, Nonvenomous, Of Forearm		34843	Eye / Adnexa (Black Eye)
38012	Infected		37948	Eyelids
38013	Splinter Of Forearm		37949	Orbital
38014	Infected		37952	Eyeball
34839	Hands		34797	Trunk
38015	Abrasion Of Hands		37950	Breast
38016	Infected		37951	Chest Wall
38017	Blister Of Hands		37953	Abdominal Wall
38018	Infected		34798	Back
38019	Insect Bite, Nonvenomous, Of Hand		37955	Genital Organs
38020	Infected		37954	Shoulder And Upper Arm
38021	Splinter Of Hand		34799	Shoulder
38022	Infected		37956	Elbow
34840	Fingers		37957	Hand
38026	Abrasion Of Fingers		37958	Finger
38028	Infected		34800	Hip And Thigh
38029	Blister Of Fingers		34801	Knee
38030	Infected		34802	Lower Leg
38031	Insect Bite, Nonvenomous, Of Fingers		34803	Ankle/Foot
38032	Infected		37959	Toe
38033	Splinter Of Fingers		34804	Multiple
38034	Infected		37960	Crush Injury
34841	Leg		37961	Face
38035	Abrasion Of Leg		37962	Neck
38036	Infected		37963	External Genitalia
38037	Blister Of Leg		37964	Shoulder And Upper Arm
38038	Infected		37965	Forearm
38039	Insect Bite, Nonvenomous, Of Leg		37966	Wrist And Hand
38040	Infected		37967	Finger
38041	Splinter Of Leg		37968	Hip And Thigh
38042	Infected		37969	Lower Leg
34842	Foot		37970	Foot
38043	Abrasion Of Foot		37971	Toe
38044	Infected		35023	Accident
38045	Blister Of Foot		35024	Train
38046	Infected		35025	Collision With Another Train
38047	Insect Bite, Nonvenomous, Of Foot		37422	Followed By Derailment
38048	Infected		35026	Collision With Another Object
38049	Splinter Of Foot		37423	A Fallen Tree On The Railway
38050	Infected		37424	A Rock On The Railway
38051	Eye/Adnexa		37425	The Platform
38052	Abrasion Of Eyelids/Periocular Area		37426	Gates
38053	Superficial Foreign Body		37427	A Streetcar
38054	Splinter		37428	A Nonmotor Vehicle
38055	Abrasion Of Cornea		35027	Derailment Without Antecedent Collision
			35028	Involving An Explosion Or Fire

ENVIRONMENTAL DISORDERS, CONT.

35029	A Fall In, On, Or From A Train	35111	Involving Suspended Cable Conveyances
35030	Hit By A Train	35112	Involving Ice Or Land Yacht
37429	Hit By An Object Falling In The Train	38122	Accident Caused By Explosion
37430	Injured By A Door Or Window	38123	Aerosol Can
37431	Train Hit By A Falling Object	38124	Fireworks
35031	Motor Vehicle Traffic	38125	Bomb
35032	Collision With Train	38128	Accident Caused By Electric Current
35033	Re-Entrant Collision With Another Motor Vehicle	38129	Domestic Wiring
		38130	Accident Caused By Exposure To Radiation
35034	Collision With Another Motor Vehicle On Road	38131	Infra-Red Heaters / Lamps
35035	Collision With A Non-Motor Vehicle On Road	38132	X-Rays / Electromagnetic Ionizing Radiation
35036	Collision With A Pedestrian	38133	Lasers
35037	Collision With A Stationary Or Moving Object	38113	Accident Caused By Machinery
		38114	Agricultural Machines
35038	Due To Loss Of Control Of Vehicle	38115	Mining / Earth-Drilling Machinery
35039	While Boarding Or Exiting A Vehicle	38116	Lifting Machinery / Appliances
		38117	Powered Lawn Mower
35040	Non-Traffic Motor Vehicle	38118	Powered Hand Tools
35041	Snowmobile	38119	Powered Household Appliances
35043	Off-Road Motor Vehicle	38120	Knives / Swords / Daggers
35042	Tractor	38121	Hand Tools
35044	Collision With Moving Object	35113	Accidental Poisoning Or Injury Occurred In
35045	Collision With Stationary Object		
35046	While Boarding / Alighting From	35114	The Home
38135	Late Effects Of Motor Vehicle Accident	35115	A Farm
		35116	A Mine Or Quarry
35047	Non-Motor Vehicle	35117	Industrial Premises
35048	Pedal Cycle	35118	A Recreation Area
35049	Animal-Drawn Vehicle	35119	A Street Or Highway
35050	Pony Cart	35120	A Public Building
35051	Animal Being Ridden	35121	A Residential Institution
35052	Foxhunting	38094	Accident Resulting From Conflagration In Private Dwelling
35053	Watercraft		
35054	Causing Submersion / Drowning	38095	Smoke And Fumes
35055	Causing Onboard Injury	38096	Injury Caused By Animals
35056	Submersion Or Drowning From Falling Overboard	38097	Dog Bite
		38098	Rat Bite
35057	Falling From Ladder / Down Stairs	35611	Shellfish
35058	Falling From One Level To Another	90338	Accidental Poisoning
35059	Machinery Injury	35597	Analgesic, Antipyretic, Antirheumatics
35060	Onboard Explosion Or Fire	35598	Barbiturates
35061	Aircraft	35599	Sedatives Or Hypnotics
35062	During Powered Takeoff Or Landing	35600	Tranquilizers
35063	Unpowered	35601	Psychotropic Agents
35064	Hang Glider	35602	CNS-Acting Medications
35065	Onboard Fall / Falling Off	35603	Antibiotics
35066	Spacecraft	35604	Alcohols
35110	Involving Powered Vehicle On Company Premises	35605	Cleaning Agents Or Paints
		35606	Petroleum Products
		35607	Agricultural Chemicals

ENVIRONMENTAL DISORDERS, CONT.

38083	Herbicides	37942	By Lightning
38084	Rodenticides	38137	Late Effects Of Accident - Natural / Environmental Factors
35608	Corrosives Or Caustics		
38086	Acids	35751	Sudden / Instantaneous Death
38088	Caustic Alkalis	35752	Unexplained Rapid Death
35609	Foods Or Plants	35753	Unattended Death
35610	Meat	35840	Ill-Defined Condition
35612	Fish (Finned)	33901	Unspecified Diagnosis
35613	Berries Or Seeds	38569	Patient Condition
35614	Mushrooms	38570	Good
38076	Synthetic Detergents/Shampoos	38571	Improved
38077	Soap Products	38579	Excellent
38079	Polishes	38572	Stable
38080	Paints And Varnishes	38573	Fair
38082	Lead Paint	38574	Seriously Ill
38108	Accidental Drowning	38575	Poor
38109	Bathtub	38576	Guarded
38110	Scuba Diving	38577	Terminal
38111	Struck Accidentally By Falling Object	38578	Expired
38112	Crushed By Human Stampede	35832	Free Text:
38136	Late Effects Of Accidental Fall	38395	User Finding:
32584	Diffuse Idiopathic Skeletal Hyperostosis (DISH)		
32585	Hypertrophic Pulmonary Osteoarthropathy		
33461	Dehydration (Na, H2O)		
35696	Neonatal		
38134	Overexertion / Strenuous Movements		
33762	Volume Depletion		
33708	Heat Stroke		
38105	Sunstroke		
34967	Heat Syncope		
34968	Heat Cramps		
34969	Heat Exhaustion		
34970	Anhydrotic		
34971	Due To Salt Depletion		
33709	Hypothermia		
38106	Exposure To Cold		
38107	Mountain Sickness		
33710	Narcolepsy		
33712	Bee Sting		
38103	Hornets / Wasps / Bees		
33711	Snake Bite		
38100	Venomous Snakes / Lizards		
38101	Spider Bite		
38102	Scorpion Sting		
38104	Venomous Marine Animals / Plants		
33713	Trauma		
33714	Hyperthermia - Non-Infectious		
33715	Saturday Night Fever		
35010	Radiation Sickness		
38545	Radiation Toxicity		
33736	Electrocution		

Part VI
THERAPY AND
MANAGEMENT

40000	**Therapy**
75223	**Physician Services And Protocols**
44459	Physician's Services
48277	Visit Status
48278	Patient Arrived
48280	Over One-half Hour Late
48279	Patient Did Not Show-up
48281	Visit Cancelled
48282	Due To Late Arrival Of Patient
48283	Due To Physician Being Delayed
48284	By Patient
48285	and Rescheduled
48286	By This Office
48287	and Rescheduled
48288	By Referral Source
48289	and Rescheduled
42435	Preventive Medicine Services
42436	New Patient Evaluation
42443	Infant Under 1 Year
42442	Early Childhood 1-4
49908	For School / Camp Physical
42441	Late Childhood 5-11
49909	For School / Camp Physical
42440	Adolescent 12-17
49910	For School / Camp Physical
42439	Adult 18-39
49911	For School / Camp Physical
42438	Adult 40-64
42437	Adult Over 64
42444	Established Patient Reevaluation
42445	Infant Under 1 Year
42446	Early Childhood 1-4
49912	For School / Camp Physical
42447	Late Childhood 5-11
49913	For School / Camp Physical
42448	Adolescent 12-17
49914	For School / Camp Physical
42449	Adult 18-39
49915	For School / Camp Physical
44977	Adult 40-64
44978	Adult Over 64
42451	Administration Pediatric Pneumogram
45767	Risk Factor Counseling
45768	Individual, 15 Minutes
45769	Individual, 30 Minutes
45770	Individual, 45 Minutes
45771	Individual, 60 Minutes
45772	Group, 30 Minutes
45773	Group, 60 Minutes
71073	Tobacco Use
71074	Alcohol Use
71075	Illicit Drug Use
71076	Inadequate Physicial Activity
71077	Unsafe Sexual Practices
71079	Violent Behavior / Firearm Use
71080	Smoking Near Bedding Or Upholstery
71096	Osteoporosis
71078	High Hot Water Temperature
45774	Administration Of Health Risk Questionnaire
42450	Administration Developmental Tests
72602	Unlisted Preventive Medicine Service
49916	Administrative Evaluation Services
49917	Basic Life / Disability Examination
49918	Work Related / Medical Disability Exam By Treating Physician
49919	Work / Medical Disability Exam, Not By Treating Physician
42339	Office Services - Primary Physician
42340	New Patient
42341	Focused H&P With Straightforward Decision Making
42342	Expanded H&P With Straightforward Decision Making
42343	Detailed H&P With Low Complexity Decision Making
42344	Comprehensive H&P With Moderate Complexity Decision Making
42345	Comprehensive H&P With High Complexity Decision Making
42346	Established Patient
42347	Minimal Service
42349	Focused H&P With Straightforward Decision Making
42350	Expanded H&P With Low Complexity Decision Making
42351	Detailed H&P With Moderate Complexity Decision Making
42352	Comprehensive H&P With High Complexity Decision Making
42353	Home Services - Primary Physician
42354	New Patient
42355	Focused H&P With Low Complexity Decision Making
42356	Expanded H&P With Moderate Complexity Decision Making
42357	Detailed H&P With High Complexity Decision Making
42359	Established Patient
42360	Focused H&P With Low Complexity Decision Making

E & M, CONT.

42361	Expanded H&P With Moderate Complexity Decision Making		45764	Detailed H&P With Low Complexity Decision Making
42362	Detailed H&P With High Complexity Decision Making		45765	Comprehensive H&P With Moderate Complexity Decison Making
42365	Hospital Services - Primary Physician		45766	Comprehensive H&P With High Complexity Decison Making
72532	Observation Care Discharge		42395	Inpatient Consultation
44979	Initial Observation Care		42396	Initial Service
42375	Detailed H&P With Low Complexity Decision Making		42397	Focused H&P With Straightforward Decision Making
42376	Comprehensive H&P With Moderate Complexity Decision Making		42398	Expanded H&P With Straightforward Decision Making
44980	Comprehensive H&P With High Complexity Decision Making		42399	Detailed H&P With Low Complexity Decision Making
42366	Initial Care		42400	Comprehensive H&P With Moderate Complexity Decison Making
42367	Detailed H&P With Low Complexity Decision Making		42401	Comprehensive H&P With High Complexity Decison Making
42368	Comprehensive H&P With Moderate Complexity Decision Making		42402	Follow-Up
42369	Comprehensive H&P With High Complexity Decision Making		42403	Focused H&P With Straightforward Decision Making
42371	Subsequent Care		42404	Focused H&P With Low Complexity Decison Making
42372	Focused H&P With Low Complexity Decision Making		42405	Expanded H&P With Moderate Complexity Decision Making
42373	Expanded H&P With Moderate Complexity Decision Making		42406	Detailed H&P With High Complexity Decision Making
42374	Detailed H&P With High Complexity Decision Making		42407	Confirmatory Consultation
42378	Hospital Discharge Day Management		42408	Focused H&P With Straightforward Decision Making
72533	More Than 30 Minutes		42409	Expanded H&P With Straightforward Decision Making
42379	ER Physician Services		42410	Detailed H&P With Low Complexity Decision Making
42382	Focused H&P With Straightforward Decision Making		42411	Comprehensive H&P With Moderate Complexity Decision Making
42383	Expanded H&P With Low Complexity Decision Making		42412	Comprehensive H&P With High Complexity Decision Making
42384	Expanded H&P With Moderate Complexity Decision Making		45778	Pathology Consultation
42385	Detailed H&P With Moderate Complexity Decision Making		45779	Limited
42386	Comprehensive H&P With High Complexity Decision Making		45780	Comprehensive With Review Of Medical Records
42394	Physician Direction of EMS Services		42509	Case Management
44981	Newborn Care		42510	Conference With Patient And/Or Family
42370	Initial H&P		42511	Half-Hour
72550	H&P When Assessed and Discharged On Same Day		42512	One Hour
44982	Outside Of Hospital		42513	Conference To Coordinate Interdisciplinary Care
42377	Subsequent Hospital Care		42514	Half-Hour
42112	Resuscitation		42515	One Hour
45761	Outpatient Consultation		42516	Telephone Call To Patient / Providers
45762	Focused H&P With Straightforward Decision Making		42517	Brief
45763	Expanded H&P With Straightforward Decision Making			

E & M, CONT.

42518	Intermediate	42746	Analysis Of Computerized Data
42519	Lengthy	42747	Special Review / Reporting Of Patient Status
72542	Care Plan Oversight Services		
72545	30-60 Minutes Per Month	72983	Unlisted Special Service Or Report
72547	Greater Than 60 Minutes Per Month	72537	Prolonged Physician Service With Direct Patient Contact
42751	Initial Critical Care Services		
42752	First Hour	42748	Prolonged Outpatient Physician Service
42753	Additional Half-Hour(s)		
42754	Follow-up Critical Care Services	42749	First Hour
48947	Patient Instructed To Call If Not Improved In (days)	42750	Each Additional 30 Minutes
		72534	Prolonged Inpatient Physician Service
42755	Neonatal Intensive Care	72535	First Hour
42756	Initial Care - Day Of Admission	72536	Each Additional 30 Minutes
42757	Subsequent Care Of Unstable Neonate For 1 Day	72538	Prolonged Physician Service Without Direct Patient Contact
42758	Subsequent Care Of Stable Neonate For 1 Day	72539	First Hour
		72540	Each Additional 30 Minutes
42452	Physician Supervised Infusion (Non-Chemo)	72541	Physician Stand-by Service Each 30 Minutes
42453	Initial Hour	42413	Physician Care In Nursing Facility
42454	Additional Hours	42414	Initial
42455	Physician Supervised Injection	42415	Detailed History With Low Complexity Decision Making
42456	Subcutaneous		
42457	Intramuscular	42416	Detailed History With Mod/High Complexity Decision Making
42458	Intra-arterial		
42459	Intravenous	42417	Comprehensive H&P With Mod-High Complexity Decision Making
42460	Intramuscular Antibiotic		
42461	Intravenous Allergy Medication	42418	Subsequent
42730	Special Physician-Supervised Services	42419	Focused H&P With Low Complexity Decision Making
42731	Specimen Handling / Transfer: Office To Lab	42420	Expanded H&P With Moderate Complexity Decision Making
42732	Specimen Handling / Transfer: Non-office To Lab	42421	Detailed H&P With Mod/High Complexity Decision Making
42733	Ordering / Handling / Fitting Patient Devices	44591	Flexible Fiberoptic Laryngoscopy
42734	Services Requested For After Office Hours	42423	Rest Home Visit
		42424	New Patient
42735	Services Requested For Between 10 PM And 8 AM	42425	Focused H&P With Low Complexity Decision Making
42736	Services Requested For Sundays Or Holidays	42426	Expanded H&P With Moderate Complexity Decision Making
42737	Outside Location Requested For Office-Type Services	42427	Detailed H&P With High Complexity Decision Making
42738	Office Services Provided On An Emergency Basis	42429	Established Patient
		42430	Focused H&P With Low Complexity Decision Making
42739	New Patient Visit With Starred (*) Surgical Procedure	42431	Expanded H&P With Moderate Complexity Decision Making
42740	Postoperative Visit, Without Charge	42432	Detailed H&P With High Complexity Decision Making
42741	Provision Of Special Supplies		
42742	Provision Of Educational Supplies	72604	Unlisted Evaluation and Management Service
42743	Group Educational Services		
42744	Medical Testimony	75222	Standard Therapies And Protocols
42745	Unusual Travel		

E & M, CONT.

41807	Active Rewarming		42070	Pump Infusion, More Than 8 Hours
42045	Allergen Desensitization		42072	Intra-arterial
42046	Supervision - Single Allergen Injection		42722	Push Technique
42047	Supervision - Multiple Allergenic Extract Injections		42723	By Infusion
42048	Injection and Supply Of Single Allergenic Extract		42724	Up To 1 Hour
			42725	Additional Infusion 1 To 7 Hours, Per Hour
42049	Injection and Supply Of Multiple Allergenic Extracts		42073	Pump Infusion, More Than 8 Hours
42050	Injection and Supply Of Stinging Insect Allergen		42074	Implantable Pump Refilling / Maintenance
45640	One Venom		42071	Portable Pump Refilling / Maintenance
45641	Two Venoms		40490	Intrathecal
45642	Three Venoms		42059	Via Reservoir
45643	Four Venoms		42060	Intracavitary
45644	Five Venoms		42726	Pleural Cavity
45645	Supervision and Supply Of Allergen		42727	Peritoneal Cavity
45646	One Antigen, One Dose Vials		42728	Provision Of Chemotherapy Agent
45647	Multiple Antigens, One Dose Vials		40066	Chest Physical Therapy
42052	One Or More Antigens, One Multiple Dose Vial		42326	Circadian System Adjustment By Light / Dark Exposure
45652	One Or More Antigens, Two Or More Multiple Dose Vials		42316	Cochlear Implant
42051	One Insect Allergen, Multiple Dose Vials		71062	Continue Current Therapy
			44694	Cool mist
45648	Two Insect Allergens, Multiple Dose Vials		40023	Cooling Blanket
			41804	Correct Malocclusion
45649	Three Insect Allergens, Multiple Dose Vials		40049	Decrease Joint Stress
			40019	Decreased Bathing Frequency
45650	Four Insect Allergens, Multiple Dose Vials		40027	Dentures
			48832	Dependence on Respirator
45651	Five Insect Allergens, Multiple Dose Vials		42526	Detoxification
			42527	Alcohol
42053	Supervision and Supply Of Insect Body Extract		42528	Drugs
			40029	Diet
42054	Rapid		41988	As Appropriate
42055	Insulin		40042	Weight Loss
42056	Penicillin		40028	Weight Gain
42057	Animal Serum		40041	Low Salt
40012	Arrange Treatment For Sexual Partner		40031	Low Fat
42212	Balloon Dilation of Prostate		40034	Low Cholesterol
40072	Bracing		41876	Diabetic
40060	Carotid Sinus Massage		40035	Controlled Carbohydrate
40073	Cervical Collar		40032	Lactose Free
42058	Chemotherapy Administration		40033	Gluten Free
42720	Subcutaneous Injection		40036	High Residue
42721	Intramuscular Injection		40030	Frequent Small Meals
42061	Intravenous Injection		40037	Polyunsaturated Fats
42066	Push Technique		40038	Liquid
42067	By Infusion		40039	High Protein
42068	Up To 1 Hour		40040	Low Protein
42069	Additional Infusion 1 To 7 Hours, Per Hour		40045	Low Copper
			74938	Doctor's Orders

E & M, cont.

74943	Restricted To Bed		74542	Fitting/Orientation/Checking Of
74944	Bedside Commode Permitted		74543	Repair/Modification Of
43951	Out Of Bed In A Chair		74545	Monaural
43952	Bathroom Privileges		74546	Air Conduction
43953	With Assistance		74547	Bone Conduction
43954	Ambulate As Tolerated		74548	In The Ear
40007	NPO		74595	Behind The Ear
74939	Except Medications		74597	Binaural
42113	Emetic Administration / Observation		74599	Body
40001	Enteric Precautions		74603	In The Ear
40002	Isolation		74607	Behind The Ear
74941	Respiratory		74608	Dispensing Fee
74942	Contact		74609	CROS
70197	Isolation Of All Body Fluids And Excretions		74610	In The Ear
			74611	Behind The Ear
42591	Ear Protector Attenuation Measurements		74612	Dispensing Fee
45869	Early Postnatal Feeding		74620	BICROS
42585	Electroacoustic Evaluation For Hearing Aid		74621	In The Ear
			74622	Behind The Ear
42586	Binaural		74623	Dispensing Fee
40052	Elevation of Extremity		74625	Bilateral
71053	Environmental Control Measures		74626	Dispensing Fee
41989	Electrostatic Dust Filter		74624	Miscellaneous
71054	Mattress / Pillow Covers		74627	Dispensing Fee
71055	HEPA Filters		40020	Heat
71056	Carpet Removal		42119	Heat Exchanger
71057	Drapery Removal		42759	Pump Assembly And Operation
71058	Removal Of Pets		42761	One Half-hour
71059	Frequent Vacuuming		42762	3/4-hour
71060	Humidity Control		42760	One Hour
40084	Fluid Balance		41997	Home Intervention
40016	Fluid Restriction		40091	Hydrostatic Dilation
40015	Fluids		40081	Hyperalimentation
44721	Gargle		42116	Hypothermia Induction
44722	Saltwater		42117	Regional
41844	Gastric Balloon		42118	Total Body
41980	Health Seminar		40018	Ice
41981	Smoking Cessation		40022	Ice Water Bath
41982	Drinking Cessation		40051	Immobilization
41983	Stress Management		74937	Instructions To Patient
41984	Prenatal Care		40024	Bed Rest
41985	Parent Effectiveness		40008	Abstinence From Alcohol
41986	AIDS Education		40009	Abstinence From Smoking
41987	Drugs Cessation		74940	Use A Condom During Sexual Intercourse
42589	Hearing Aid Check			
42590	Binaural		40011	Abstinence From Sexual Contact
42587	Hearing Aid Examination and Selection		40010	Terminate Exposure
42588	Binaural		40080	IV Hydration
74538	Hearing Services		73499	Leeches
74539	Hearing Screening		41839	Masters-Johnson Penis Squeeze Technique
74544	Conformity Evaluation			
74541	Hearing Aid		40076	MD Supervision of Hyperbaric Oxygen Session
74540	Assessment For			

E & M, CONT.

40092	Mechanical Dilation	45861	5% Dextrose In Water
40057	Medical Alert Badge	45862	10% Dextrose In Water
71061	Continue Current Medication	45863	15% Dextrose In Water
40043	Modify Drug Dosage	45864	20% Dextrose In Water
40044	Withdraw Offending Medication	45865	25% Dextrose In Water
40077	Medication Instruction	72107	50% Dextrose Injection IV
42120	Membrane Oxygenation	45866	Lactated Ringer's Solution
42763	Pump Assembly And Operation	45867	With 5% Dextrose
42764	One Half-hour	45868	With 10% Dextrose
42765	3/4-hour	41996	Parenting Evaluation
42766	One Hour	40006	**Patient Counseling**
40021	Moist Air	72300	Restraints
71518	Monitor Alarms	71092	Use Of Bicycle and Motorcycle
71519	Heart Rate		Helmets
71520	Blood Pressure	71093	Use Of Smoke Detectors
71521	Respiratory Rate	71097	Inquiry & Counseling
71522	Oxygen Content	71098	Contraceptive Practices
73963	Apnea	71100	Sexual Problems
73966	Pacemaker	71099	Family Functioning
73967	Includes Audible/Visible Check	71103	Distress Related To Retirement
	Systems	71104	Hearing Impairment
73969	Includes Digital/Visible Check	71101	Functional Status At Home
	Systems	71102	Symptoms Of TIA
70196	Notifiable Infectious Disease: Report To	41871	Patient Education
	National Epidemiologic Center	71095	Regular Dental Care
41862	Notify Authorities	41875	Dietary
44863	Observation	71084	Self-Examination
48853	Observation following accident at work	71085	Of Breasts
48854	Observation following motor vehicle	71086	Of Oral Cavity
	accident	71087	Of Skin
40079	Ommaya Reservoir Injection	71088	Of Testes
71045	Oral Appliances	42210	Back Care
71046	Tongue Retainer	71089	Need To Report Postmenopausal
71048	Snore Guard		Bleeding
71047	Mandibular Advancement Device	71090	Prevention Of Falls
48846	Other Physical Therapy	71094	Glaucoma Testing
40075	Oxygen	42018	Diabetes
71517	Via Nasal Cannula	41872	Blood Glucose Monitor
18364	Rate Of Supplemental Oxygen	73965	Home
71516	Fraction Of Inspired Air	72269	Voice Synthesized
40074	Oxygen Restriction	41873	Home Insulin Administration
41999	Parent Counseling	41874	Foot Care
41998	Parent Education	42020	Sexual Dysfunction
45856	Parenteral Fluids	42496	Dialysis
40062	Saline	42497	Completed Course Of Training
40063	Normal Saline	42498	Partial Completion Of Course, Per
72106	Half-Normal Saline		Session
40064	Hypertonic Saline	48831	Patient Requiring Intermittent Renal
45858	Dextrose		Dialysis
45857	5% Dextrose in Half-normal Saline	42021	Alcohol
45859	5% Dextrose in Third-normal Saline	42525	Drug Abstinence
45860	5% Dextrose in Quarter-normal	42019	HIV
	Saline	48951	Patient Goals

PATIENT COUNSELING, CONT.

48952	Decrease Weight By ___	72991	Community Reintegration Training - Per 15 Minutes
48953	Keep Fasting Blood Sugar Under ___		
48954	Decrease Cholesterol	42088	Infrared Treatment
48955	Begin Regular Exercise, Times Per Week	42089	Ultraviolet Treatment
		40065	Physical Therapy
48956	Increase Weight By ___	42090	___ Session Segments, 15 Minutes Each
48957	Test Blood Sugars and Bring in Results		
48958	Cut Smoking To	72987	Group Physical Therapy Session
42002	Personal Protective Equipment	42091	Exercises/ROM
42291	Head Gear	42092	Neuromuscular Re-education
42292	Face Shields	72984	Aquatic Therapy With Exercises
42004	Safety glasses	42093	Kinetic Training
42293	Shaded Lenses	42110	Physical Performance Testing
42013	Ear Muffs	42094	Gait Training
42014	Ear Plugs	42095	Electrical Stimulation
42295	Air-Purifiers	45653	Iontophoresis
42005	Mask	42096	Manual Traction
42294	Respirator	42097	Massage
42296	Cartridge - gas	42098	Contrast Baths
42297	Cartridge - chemical	42099	Ultrasound
42298	Cartridge - particulate	42101	Hubbard Tank
42299	Powered	72992	Wheelchair Training - Per 15 Minutes
42006	Air-Supply Respirator	42103	Manipulation By Physician, One Area
42003	Gloves	42104	Manipulation By Physician, Additional Area
42007	Rubber		
42008	Latex	72988	Soft Tissue Mobilization
42009	Leather	72989	Joint Mobilization
42010	Insulated	42105	Orthotics Training
42011	Cotton-lined	45658	Initial 30 Minutes
42012	Cushioned	45659	Additional 15 Minutes
42290	Puncture/Cut Resistant	42106	Prosthetic Use Training
42016	Coveralls	45660	Initial 30 Minutes
42017	Aprons	45661	Additional 15 Minutes
42300	Protective Suit	45666	Work Hardening / Conditioning
42301	Whole Body	45667	Initial 2 Hours
42302	Encapsulating	45668	Additional Hour
42303	Temperature Control Clothing	42111	Muscle Testing With Torque Curves
40090	Phlebotomy (Therapeutic)	40093	Pneumatic Dilation
44865	Phototherapy	42315	Prescribe Hearing Aid
42078	Physical Medicine	41841	Progressive Vaginal Dilation
42079	Cold Packs	40026	Proper Chewing of Food
42080	Hot Packs	40061	Rectal Digital Disimpaction
42081	Mechanical Traction	42529	Reduce Intake
42082	Electrical Stimulation (Unattended)	42530	Caffeine
42083	Vasopneumatic Device	40050	Reduce Strain
42084	Paraffin Bath	43336	Regular Exercise
42085	Microwave Treatment	43337	Institute Presribed Program
42086	Whirlpool Treatment	40082	Respirator
42087	Diathermy Treatment	40013	Screen Family
72986	Unlisted Therapy	41854	Self-Help Group
72985	Unlisted Modality	45781	Alcoholism-Related
72990	Self Care Training - Per 15 Minutes	41855	Alcoholics Anonymous
		45782	Al-Anon

PATIENT COUNSELING, CONT.

45783	Women For Sobriety		42134	Lifting
45784	Adult Children Of Alcoholics (ACOA)		42135	Not over 10 pounds
			42136	Not over 15 pounds
41856	Weight Watching		42137	Not over 20 pounds
45785	Weight Watchers		42138	Not over 25 pounds
45786	Over-Eaters Anonymous		42139	Not over 30 pounds
45787	Eating Disorders		42140	Not over 35 pounds
41857	Smoking Cessation		42141	Not over 40 pounds
41858	Narcotic-Use Cessation		42142	Not over 45 pounds
45789	Narcotics Anonymous (NA)		42143	Not over 50 pounds
41859	Gamblers Anonymous		42144	Not over 60 pounds
41979	Families of Severely Mentally Ill		42145	Sitting
45790	Alzheimer's Association		42146	Not over 10 minutes
45788	National Alliance for the Mentally Ill (NAMI)		42147	Not over 15 minutes
			42148	Not over 20 minutes
40069	Sleeping Posture		42149	Not over 30 minutes
48268	Status Of Employment Evaluation (Medical)		42150	Not over 45 minutes
			42151	Not over 60 minutes
48269	Pre-placement		42159	Should Stand Or Move As Needed
48270	Approved		42195	Limited Writing
48271	Not Approved		42196	No Writing
48272	Incomplete		42168	Should Keep Legs Elevated
48273	Promotion		42152	No Constant Standing
48274	Approved		42153	Limited Standing Only
48275	Not Approved		42154	Limited Walking Only
48276	Incomplete		42155	No Pushing Or Pulling
40085	Stomach Tube		42156	No Repeated Bending
40089	Gastric Intubation And Lavage		42157	Neck
72982	Gastric Intubation and Aspiration		42158	Back
40086	Nasogastric Suction		42162	Climbing
40088	Small Bowel (Cantor) Tube		42164	Avoid Stairs
72112	Levin Type		42165	A-Frame Type Ladders Only
40014	Take Pet to Vet		42166	No Ladders
40005	Treat Complications		42169	No Pole Gaffing
40004	Treat Predisposing Conditions		42167	No Poles
42576	Treat Secondary Symptoms		42279	Limited Shoulder Movement
40003	Treat Underlying Etiology		42163	No Reaching Above Shoulders
41806	Ultraviolet Light		42280	Limited Elbow Movement
40025	Wear Stockings		42281	Limited Wrist Movement
42131	**Work Restrictions**		42282	Limited Hand Movement
48267	Decision Pending Further Evaluation		42283	Limited Foot Movement
48262	Not Fit For Work		42170	Environmental
42208	Return To Work Requires Medical Dept. Clearance		42171	Must Work In Well Ventilated Area
			42180	Avoid High Noise Level
42132	Fit For Work		42328	Avoid Crowded, Overstimulating Conditions
48342	No Restrictions			
48343	With Restrictions		42179	No Working Alone
48344	Patient Not Returned to Service		42174	Must Avoid Prolonged Exposure To Cold
42201	All Restrictions Are Removed			
48266	Return To Work Requires Administrative Disposition		42175	Must Avoid Prolonged Exposure To Heat
42133	Physical		42176	Must Work Inside
42181	Sedentary Work Only		42324	Access To Fluids To Drink

WORK RESTRICTIONS, CONT.

42211	Close Proximity To Bathroom	42243	No Exposure To Plastics
42338	Private Bathroom Facilities	42244	acrylic resins
42177	No Working Underground	42245	epoxy resins
42178	No Working Aloft	42246	No Exposure To Chemical Vapors
42278	No Working At High Altitude	42247	formaldehyde
42172	No Dust Exposure	42248	halides
42260	asbestos	42249	No Exposure To Chemical Fumes
42269	animal	42250	polytetrafluoroethylene
42261	beryllium	42251	sulfides
42262	cadmium	42252	trimellitic anhydride
42263	cement	42253	No Exposure To Smoke
42264	coal	42254	No Exposure To Gases
42265	cotton	42255	carbon monoxide
42266	diatomaceous earth	42256	chlorine
42267	flour	42257	ozone
42268	grain	42258	No Exposure To Mists
42270	nickel	42259	No Exposure To Molds
42271	pentachlorophenol	42276	No Exposure To Fibers
42272	rare earth	42277	fiberglass
42273	silica	42320	No Exposure To Radiation
42274	vanadium	42182	Equipment
42275	wood	42183	Limited Typing
42173	No Exposure To Fumes	42184	No Typing
42213	No Exposure To Metals (Contact)	42185	Should Use Telephone Headset
42214	arsenic	42186	With Amplifier
42215	chromium	42187	Over-The-Head Type
42216	mercury	42188	Avoid Earpiece-Type Earphones
42217	nickel	42189	Avoid Using A Telephone Handset
42218	platinum	42190	Avoid Using A Telephone
42219	No Exposure To Metal Fumes	42191	Avoid Using Video Display Terminals
42220	cadmium		
42221	lead	42287	Must Use Anti-glare VDT Screen
42222	platinum	42161	Must Have Adjustable Keyboard Height
42223	vanadium		
42224	welding	42160	Must Have Ergonomic, Adjustable Chair
42225	zinc		
42226	No Exposure To Chemical Liquids	42192	No Driving Company Vehicle
42227	acids	42193	No Operating Dangerous Equipment
42228	alkalis	42194	No Operating High Voltage Equipment
42229	chromates		
42230	dyes	42288	Limit Use of Hand Tools
42231	epoxies	42284	No Operating Vibrating Equipment
42232	formaldehyde	42289	PPE
42233	gluteraldehyde	42304	No Head Gear
42235	isocyanates	42305	No Ear Plugs
42234	oils/greases	42306	No Respirator Use
42236	pesticides	42307	No Cartridge Respirator Use
42237	solvents	42309	No SCBA Respirator Use
42238	No Exposure To Chemical Powders	42308	No Glove Use
42239	detergents	42310	No Protective Suit Use
42240	phthalic anhydride	42197	Schedule
42241	salicylanilide	42198	No Overtime
42242	trimellitic anhydride	42199	Fixed Shift Only

WORK RESTRICTIONS, CONT.

42200	Half-Day Only
42286	Day Shift Only
42329	Flexible To Accommodate Therapy
42202	No Work Requiring Perfect Color Vision
42285	No Work Requiring Perfect Depth Perception
42321	No Work Requiring Normal Hearing
42203	Avoid Intensive Time-Measured Work
42204	Avoid Using Voice
42205	Avoid Using Affected Hand
42206	Avoid Using Affected Arm
42207	Avoid Customer Contact
42330	Requires Close Supervision
42209	Contact Medical Dept. For Patient-Specific Restrictions
44693	Services: (For Free Text For Billing For Services)
75131	**Office Services**
42531	Ophthalmological Services
42532	New Patient
42533	Initiation of Intermediate Level Care
42534	Initiation of Comprehensive Level Care
42535	Prior Patient
42536	Initiation of Intermediate Care
42537	Initiation of Comprehensive Level Care
42538	Exam Under Anesthesia
42539	Complete
42540	Limited
42541	Orthoptic / Pleoptic Training
42314	Contact Lenses
42542	Fitting and Supply of Therapeutic Lens
42543	Prescription And Fitting Services
42544	Bilateral Corneal Lenses (Not For Aphakia)
42545	Unilateral Corneal Lens For Aphakia
42546	Bilateral Corneal Lenses For Aphakia
42547	Corneoscleral Lens
42548	Prescription And Direction Of Fitting
42549	Bilateral Corneal Lenses (Not For Aphakia)
42550	Unilateral Corneal Lens For Aphakia
42551	Bilateral Corneal Lenses For Aphakia
42552	Corneoscleral Lens
42553	Modification of Lens
42554	Replacement of Lens
42555	Supply of Lenses (Not For Aphakia)
42556	Supply of Permanent Contact Lenses For Aphakia)
42557	Ocular Prosthetics (Artificial Eye)
42558	Prescription And Fitting
42559	Prescription And Direction Of Fitting
42571	Supply Of Artificial Eye
74503	Plastic
74504	Polishing/Resurfacing
74505	Enlargement
74506	Reduction
74507	Scleral Cover Shell
74508	Fabrication And Fitting
74509	Other Type
48864	Mechanical Complication Due To Ocular Lens Prosthesis
74510	Intraocular Lenses
74511	Anterior Chamber
74512	Iris Supported
74513	Posterior Chamber
74536	Processing, Preserving, Transporting Corneal Tissue
74537	Miscellaneous Vision Service
42560	Spectacle Services
42561	Fitting Monofocals (Not For Aphakia)
42562	Fitting Bifocals (Not For Aphakia)
42563	Fitting Multifocals (Not For Aphakia)
42564	Fitting Monofocals For Aphakia
42565	Fitting Multifocals For Aphakia
42566	Fitting Single Element System Low Vision Aid
42567	Fitting Complex Element System Low Vision Aid
42568	Temporary Prosthesis For Aphakia
42569	Repair And Refitting Glasses (Not For Aphakia)
42570	Repair And Refitting Prosthesis For Aphakia
42572	Supply Of Eyeglasses
74359	Frames
74360	Purchased
74361	Deluxe
42573	Supply Of Low Vision Aids
74498	Hand-Held, Non-Spectacle-Mounted Aids
74499	Single Lens Spectacle-Mounted
74500	Telescopic, Other Compound Lens System
42574	Supply Of Permanent Spectacles For Aphakia
42313	Eyeglasses Prescription

OFFICE SERVICES, CONT.

74300	Distance		74440	Aniseikonic
74389	Sphere		74441	Seg Width Over 28mm
74390	+/- 4.00, Per Lens		74442	Add Over 3.25d
74391	+/- 4.12-7.00d, Per Lens		74443	Speciality (By Report)
74392	+/- 7.12-20.00d, Per Lens		74305	Progressives
74393	Spherocylinder		74474	Single Vision
74394	With +/- 4.00d Sphere		74475	Bifocal
74395	0.12 To 2.00d Cylinder		74476	Other Type
74396	2.12 To 4.00d Cylinder		74303	Trifocals
74397	4.25 To 6.00d Cylinder		74445	Sphere
74398	Over 6.00d Cylinder		74446	+/- 4.00d, Per Lens
74399	With +/- 4.25-7.00d Sphere		74447	+/- 4.12-7.00d, Per Lens
74400	0.12 To 2.00d Cylinder		74448	+/- 7.12-20.00d, Per Lens
74401	2.12 To 4.00d Cylinder		74449	Spherocylinder
74402	4.25 To 6.00d Cylinder		74450	With +/- 4.00d Sphere
74403	Over 6.00d Cylinder		74451	0.12 To 2.00d Cylinder
74404	With +/- 7.25-12.00d Sphere		74452	2.12 To 4.00d Cylinder
74405	0.25 To 2.25d Cylinder		74453	4.25 To 6.00d Cylinder
74406	2.25 To 4.00d Cylinder		74454	Over 6.00d Cylinder
74407	4.25 To 6.00d Cylinder		74455	With +/- 4.25-7.00d Sphere
74408	With Over +/- 12.00d Sphere		74456	0.12 To 2.00d Cylinder
74414	Lenticular		74457	2.12 To 4.00d Cylinder
74410	Myodisc		74458	4.25 To 6.00d Cylinder
74411	Nonaspheric		74459	Over 6.00d Cylinder
74412	Aspheric		74460	With +/- 7.25-12.00d Sphere
74409	Aniseikonic		74461	0.25 To 2.25d Cylinder
74413	Not Otherwise Classified		74462	2.25 To 4.00d Cylinder
74301	Reading		74463	4.25 To 6.00d Cylinder
74302	Bifocals		74464	With Over +/- 12.00d Sphere
74416	Sphere		74465	Lenticular
74417	+/- 4.00d, Per Lens		74466	Myodisc
74418	+/- 4.12-7.00d, Per Lens		74467	Nonaspheric
74419	+/- 7.12-20.00d, Per Lens		74468	Aspheric
74420	Spherocylinder		74469	Aniseikonic
74421	With +/- 4.00d Sphere		74470	Seg Width Over 28mm
74422	0.12 To 2.00d Cylinder		74471	Add Over 3.25d
74423	2.12 To 4.00d Cylinder		74472	Speciality (By Report)
74424	4.25 To 6.00d Cylinder		75138	Prescription Less Than Manifest
74425	Over 6.00d Cylinder		75139	Right Lens
74426	With +/- 4.25-7.00d Sphere		75140	Left Lens
74427	0.12 To 2.00d Cylinder		75141	Both Lenses
74428	2.12 To 4.00d Cylinder		74921	Special Use Lenses
74429	4.25 To 6.00d Cylinder		74922	Industrial
74430	Over 6.00d Cylinder		74923	Carbon Arc Welding Or Furnace Operation (Shade 14)
74431	With +/- 7.25-12.00d Sphere		74924	Metallic Electric Arc Welding Over 250 Amperes (Shade 12)
74432	0.25 To 2.25d Cylinder			
74433	2.25 To 4.00d Cylinder		74925	Metal Arc Welding 75-250 Amperes (Shade 10)
74434	4.25 To 6.00d Cylinder			
74435	With Over +/- 12.00d Sphere		74926	Heavy Acetylene Cutting And Welding (Shade 8)
74436	Lenticular			
74437	Myodisc		74927	Acetylene Or Electrical Welding; Firebox Observation (Shade 6)
74438	Nonaspheric			
74439	Aspheric			

OFFICE SERVICES, CONT.

74928	Acetylene Burning, Brazing, Or Cutting (Shade 5)	74484	Spherical
74929	Light Brazing (Shade 3)	74485	Toric
74930	Laser Protection (Didymium)	74486	Bifocal
74931	X-Ray Protection	74487	Extended Wear
74932	Sunglasses	74318	Hard (PMMA)
74933	Neutral Gray (20-30%)	74489	Spherical
74934	Colored Green (30-70%)	74490	Toric
74935	Yellow (77%)	74491	Bifocal
74936	Brown Polaroid (21%)	74482	Color Vision Deficiency
74532	Photochromatic	74914	Aphakic
74915	Material	74913	Daily Wear
74917	Plastic	74320	Extended Wear
74920	High Index Plastic	74496	Other Types
74916	Polycarbonate	74304	Progressives
74918	Glass	74493	Scleral
74919	High Index Glass	74494	Gas Permeable
74514	Lens Additions	74495	Gas Impermeable
74515	Lens	44462	ENT - Upper Airway Services
74516	Balance	44463	Drain Nasal Abscess (internal approach)
74517	U-V	44464	Drain Nasal Hematoma (internal approach)
74518	Occluder		
74519	Oversize	44465	Drain Nasal Septum Abscess (internal approach)
74520	Progressive		
74521	Press-On	44466	Drain Nasal Septum Hematoma (internal approach)
74533	Special Base Curve		
74534	Prism	44467	Simple Excision Of Nasal Polyp
74535	Slab Off Prism	44472	Excision / Planing Of Rhinophyma
74522	Coating	44468	Simple Excision Of Dermoid Cyst (Subcutaneous)
74523	Anti-Reflective		
74524	Scratch Resistant	44478	Injection Into Turbinate
74525	Tint	44479	Displacement Therapy (Proetz Type)
74526	Plastic	44480	Insertion Of Nasal Septal Button
74527	Rose 1 Or 2	44481	Simple Removal Of Nasal Foreign Body
74528	Other Than Rose 1 Or 2		
74529	Glass	44499	Nasal Hemorrhage Control
74530	Rose 1 Or 2	44500	Simple, Anterior
74531	Other Than Rose 1 Or 2	44501	Complex, Anterior
74299	Contact Lens Prescription	44502	Posterior, Initial
74317	Soft	44503	Posterior, Subsequent
74312	Planned Replacement Lenses (Disposable)	44508	Lavage Of Maxillary Sinus
		44509	Lavage Of Sphenoid Sinus
74316	Daily / 1 Day	41598	Endotracheal Tube Insertion
74313	Daily / 1 Week	44818	Unsuccessful
74314	Daily / 2 Weeks	44567	Tube Change Prior To Mature Fistula
74315	Daily / 3 Months		
74308	Daily Wear Spherical	44568	Indirect Laryngoscopy
74309	Daily Wear Toric	44569	With Foreign Body Removal
74310	Daily Wear Bifocal/Multifocal	44570	With Removal Of Lesion
74306	Extended Wear Spherical	44571	With Vocal Cord Injection
74307	Extended Wear Toric	44603	Closed Laryngeal Fracture Repair
74311	Opaque	44604	With Manipulative Reduction
74319	Gas Permeable	44592	With Foreign Body Removal

OFFICE SERVICES, CONT.

44593	With Removal Of Lesion	41557	Psychiatric Therapy
70549	Simple Removal Of Intranasal Foreign Body	41846	Individual
		42462	Half Hour or Less
70550	Right Nostril	42463	Half Hour To One Hour
70551	By curette	45854	Interactive
70552	By irrigation	42499	Medical Psychoanalysis
70553	Left Nostril	42500	Family Medical Psychotherapy (Without Patient Present)
70554	By curette		
70555	By irrigation	42472	Counseling Family / Guardians
74628	Speech-Language Pathology Services	41851	Family (Conjoint)
74629	Repair/Modification Of	41853	Marital
74630	Augmentative Communicative System/Device	41847	Group (Interactive)
		45853	Group (Interview)
74631	Speech Screening	42464	Multiple-Family Group
74632	Language Screening	41848	Hypnosis
74633	Dysphagia Screening	42471	Environmental Intervention
42577	Special ENT Services	42473	Preparation of Psychiatric Status Report
42578	Examination Under General Anesthesia	48849	Examination Following Psychotherapy and Other Treatment for Mental Disorder
42579	Binocular Microscopy		
42580	Physician Evaluation of Speech/Hearing Problems	41849	Behavior Modification
		45855	Cognitive Therapy
42581	Physician Supervision of Speech/Hearing Therapy	41852	Sex
		42474	Electroconvulsive
42582	Individual	42475	Single Seizure
42583	Group	42476	Multiple Seizures, Per Day
42584	Nasopharyngoscopy With Endoscope	42477	Psychoactive Medication Management
48848	Speech Therapy	41850	In-Patient
44972	Cardiology Services	41863	Mandatory
44973	Patient Reassurance	42478	Biofeedback Therapy
44974	Patient Request	42479	By Electromyogram
44975	Evaluation Of Cardiac Transplant Donor	42480	In Conduction Disorder
		42481	In Blood Pressure Regulation
44976	Cardiac Evaluation Of Non-Cardiac Organ Donor	42482	Regulation of Skin Temperature
		42483	By Electroencephalogram
48948	Cerumen Removal	42484	By Electro-oculogram
48949	Right Ear	42030	Respiratory Therapy
70556	By irrigation	42031	Inhalation Treatment (Nonpressurized)
70557	Incomplete	42032	Intermittent Positive Pressure Breathing
70558	By curette	42033	Initiation
70559	Incomplete	42034	Continuation
48950	Left Ear	42035	Newborn
70560	By irrigation	42036	Continuous Positive Airway Pressure Ventilation
70561	Incomplete		
70562	By curette	42037	Sputum Mobilization / Induction
70563	Incomplete	42038	Initial
44864	Pediatric Services	42039	Continued
42465	Psychiatric Evaluation	42040	Chest Wall Manipulation
42466	Comprehensive Examination	42041	Initial
45852	Interactive	42042	Subsequent
42467	Review of Records and Reports	41558	Mechanical Ventilation
42469	Telephone Consultation	42026	Initiation
42470	Narcosynthesis	42027	Continuation
44428	Psychological Counseling	42028	Positive Endexpiratory Pressure

OFFICE SERVICES, CONT.

42029	Intermittent Mandatory Ventilation	75053	Grass Mix
71035	Inspiratory Pressure Support	75054	Individual Grasses
71034	Bilevel Positive Airway Pressure	75055	Timothy
75135	**Medications, Vaccines**	75056	Sweet Vernal
40096	Antidotes	75057	Rye
40097	Amyl Nitrate	75058	Red Top
40098	Calcium Chloride	75059	Kentucky Blue Grass
48521	Digoxin Immune Fab (Ovine)	75060	Meadow Fescue
40099	Liquid Petrolatum	75061	Orchard Grass
40100	Potassium Permanganate	75062	Velvet Grass
40101	Sodium Sulfate	75063	Bent Grass
40102	Sodium Thiosulfate	75064	Bermuda Grass
40103	Starch	75065	Johnson Grass
40104	Water	75066	Salt Grass
40105	Allergy and Immunological Preparations	75067	Bahia Grass
40106	Allergens	75068	Ragweed
40107	Allergenic Extracts	75069	Weed Mix
40108	Allergenic Extracts Alum-Precipitated	75070	Individual Weeds
		75071	Pigweed
40112	Stinging Insect Antigens-Combined	75072	Lamb's Quarter
		75073	Russian Thistle
74962	Drugs	75074	Fire Bush
74963	Penicillin G	75075	Wing Scale
74964	Pre-Penicillin	75076	Cocklebur
74965	Tree Mix	75077	Marshelder
74966	Individual Trees	75078	Sage
74967	Alder	75079	Mugwort
74968	American Beech	75080	Dock
74969	Red Birch	75081	Sheep Sorrel
74970	Cottonwood	75082	English Plantain
74971	American Elm	75083	Fungal Mix
74972	Shagbark Hickory	75084	Individual Fungi
75032	Maple Mix	75085	Alternaria
75033	Oak Mix (Red & White)	75086	Cladosporium
75034	Sycamore	75087	Aspergillus Fumigatus
75035	Black Walnut	75088	Epicoccum
75036	Sweet Gum	75089	Fusarium
75037	Mulberry (red)	75090	Penicillium (mixed)
75038	Cedar (red)	75091	Aspergillus
75039	Juniper	75092	Animals
75040	Pecan	75093	Cat
75041	Aspen	75094	Dog
75042	Black Willow	75095	Goat
75043	Boxelder	75096	Pig
75044	Cypress	75097	Monkey
75045	Olive	75098	Rabbit
75046	Poplar	75099	Guinea Pig
75047	Black Locust	75100	Rat
75048	Douglass Fir	75101	Mouse
75049	Red Spruce	75102	Gerbil
75050	Pine	75103	Hamster
75051	Hazelnut	75104	Sheep (Crude Wool)
75052	Privet	75105	Silk

MEDICATIONS AND VACCINES

75106	Cow	40127	Tetanus Immune Globulin
75107	Horse	72635	Injection
75108	Parakeet	40128	Hyperimmune Gamma Globulin
75109	Cockroach	40129	Immunomodulators
75110	Dust Mite	40130	Immunosuppressives
75111	Mixed Feathers	40131	Antithymocyte Globulin
75112	Pigeon	40132	Azothiaprin (Immuran)
75113	Insects	40133	Cyclosporin-A
75114	Aphid	44717	Muromonab-CD3 (Orthoclone OKT3)
75115	Black Fly		
75116	Caddis Fly	41905	Azidothymidine (AZT)
75117	Deer Fly	48701	Immunosupplement
75118	Horse Fly	48702	Pegademase
75119	May Fly	48769	Didanosine
75120	Ant Mix (Black & Red)	48805	Aldesleukin
75121	Mosquito Mix	75151	Interferon beta-1a
75122	Other	40134	Plant Sensitizers
75123	Latex	40135	Toxoids
75124	Kapok	40136	Diphtheria Antitoxin
75125	Pyrethrum	40137	Diphtheria + Tetanus Toxoids, Aluminum Hydroxide Adsorbed
75126	Cotton Seed		
75127	Acacia Gum	40139	Tetanus Toxoid, Al Hyd. Adsb.
75128	Carragheen Gum	40140	Tetanus Toxoid, Al. Phos. Adsb.
75129	Karaya Gum	40141	Tetanus Toxoid
75130	Tragacanth Gum	48855	Tetanus Toxoid - need for vaccination
40109	Poison Ivy Extract		
40110	Poison Ivy, Poison Oak and Sumac Extract Combined	40142	Vaccines
		48803	Polyvalent Vaccines
40111	Pseudomonas Polysaccharide	40144	DTP Vaccine
48714	Allergenic Control	48861	DTP - need for vaccination
48715	Histamine Phosphate	48863	DTP + Polio - need for vaccination
48716	Penicillin Allergen		
40113	Antiserum	48759	DTP-HbOC (Tetramune)
40114	Antivenin [Crotalidae] Polyvalent	44451	DT Vaccine
40115	Antivenin (Micrurus Fulvius)	44450	Td Vaccine
40116	Black Widow Spider Antivenin (Equine)	40152	Polio Virus Vaccine, Live Oral (Sabin)
40117	Botulism Antitoxin	44452	Polio Virus Vaccine, Inactivated (Salk)
40118	Rabies Anti-Serum		
40119	Biologicals, other	44425	Hepatitis A Vaccine
40120	Immuneglobulin	44453	Hemophilus Influenza Type B Vaccine
40121	Gamma Globulin		
40122	Globulin, Poliomyelitis Immune (Human)	71909	Hemophilus Influenza Type B + DTP Vaccine
48856	Poliomyelitis - need for vaccination	40147	Measles Vaccines
		48858	Measles - need for vaccination
48433	Globulin, Hepatitis B Immune (Human)	40149	Measles, Mumps and Rubella Vaccine, Live
40123	Mumps Immune Globulin (Human)	48862	MMR - need for vaccination
40124	Pertussis Immune Globulin (Human)	40146	Measles and Rubella Virus, Vaccine (Live)
40125	Rabies Immune Globulin (Human)		
40126	Rho D Immune Globulin (Human)	40148	Measles Virus Vaccine, Live, Attenuated
72677	Injection		

MEDICATIONS AND VACCINES

40150	Mumps Vaccine, Live	40196	Phenacetin
40155	Rubella and Mumps Virus Vaccine, Live	40167	Salicylates
		40168	Aminobenzoic Acid (Pabirin)
40156	Rubella Virus Vaccine, Live	40169	Aminobenzoic Preparations (Pabalate)
48859	Rubella - need for vaccination		
40157	Smallpox Vaccine	40170	Acetylsalicylic Acid (aspirin)
48857	Smallpox - need for vaccination	41895	Acetylsalicylic Acid - enteric coated (aspirin)
40145	Influenza Virus Vaccine		
44454	Whole Virus	41896	Acetylsalicylic Acid - suppositories (aspirin)
44455	Split Virus		
48860	Influenza - need for vaccination	41897	Acetylsalicylic Acid - buffered (Bufferin)
49943	Chickenpox Vaccine		
40143	Cholera Vaccine	41898	Acetylsalicylic Acid + AlOH3 + MgOH2
44436	Japanese Encephalitis Vaccine		
40151	Plague Vaccine	48692	Acetylsalicylic Acid + Sodium Bicarbonate + Citric Acid
40153	Rabies Vaccine		
40154	Rocky Mountain Spotted Fever Vaccine	40171	Choline Magnesium Trisalicylate
		40172	Choline Salicylate
40138	Staphylococcus Vaccine	40173	Magnesium Salicylate
40158	Typhoid Vaccine	40174	Potassium Salicylate (Pabalate)
40159	Vaccines (Live)	40175	Salicylamide
44445	Yellow Fever Vaccine	40176	Salicylsalicylic Acid
40160	Meningococcal Vaccine	40177	Sodium Acetylsalicylate
40161	Pneumococcal Vaccine	40178	Sodium Salicylate
44456	Anthrax Vaccine	72684	Injection
44458	BCG Vaccine, Live, Attenuated	48396	Sodium Thiosalicylate
42022	Antianemia	40179	Triethanolamine Salicylate
42023	epoetin (Epogen)	71921	Tramadol HCl (Ultram)
40162	Anti-Alcohol	40184	Local
40163	Disulfiram (Antabuse)	40185	Piperocaine HCl
40164	Analgesics	40186	Pitcher Plant Distillate (Sarapin)
40165	Acetaminophen	40187	Pramoxine HCl
48618	Acetaminophen + Diphenhydramine	40190	Narcotic
48628	Acetaminophen + Diphenhydramine HCl + Pseudoephedrine HCl	48696	Meperidine Hydrochloride + Promethazine Hydrochloride
48620	Acetaminophen + Aspirin + Caffeine	72653	Injection
48619	Acetaminophen + Caffeine	40191	Meperidine Hydrochloride (Demerol)
48626	Acetaminophen + Calcium Carbonate		
		72652	Injection
48623	Acetaminophen + Chlorpheniramine Maleate + Phenylpropanolamine HCl	40181	aspirin + codeine (Empirin with codeine)
		40189	acetaminophen + Codeine (Tylenol with codeine)
48627	Acetaminophen + Chlorpheniramine Maleate + Pseudoephedrine HCl		
		40180	Codeine
48621	Acetaminophen + Pamabrom + Pyridoxine	40182	Codeine Phosphate
		72599	Injection
48622	Acetaminophen + Pentazocine Hydrochloride	40183	Codeine Sulfate
		44698	Antitussives
48629	Acetaminophen + Pseudoephedrine HCl + Dextromethorphan Hydrobromide	44699	Hydromorphone (Dilaudid Cough Syrup)
		48653	Hydrocodone Polistirex + Chlorpheniramine Polistirex
48630	Acetaminophen + Pseudoephedrine HCl		

MEDICATIONS AND VACCINES

48651	Hydrocodone Bitartrate + Phenylpropanolamine HCl
44700	Hydrocodone
48646	Hydrocodone Bitartrate + Aspirin
40670	Hydrocodone Bitartrate
48624	Hydrocodone Bitartrate + Acetaminophen
40671	Hydrocodone Resin Complex
48649	Hydrocodone Bitartrate + Homatropine Methylbromide
44703	Hydrocodone + Guaifenesin
48642	Hydrocodone + Guaifenesin + Pseudoephedrine HCl
44701	Codeine Phosphate + Guaifenesin
48666	Codeine Phosphate + Guaifenesin + Pseudoephedrine HCl
44702	Codeine Phosphate + Calcium Iodide
48777	Codeine Phosphate + Pseudoephedrine HCl
44705	Codeine Phosphate + Iodinated Glycerol
44704	Codeine Phosphate + Promethazine HCl
40188	Morphine Sulfate
45848	Oxymorphone Hydrochloride
72657	Injection
48690	Opium + Belladonna
40192	Tincture of Opium
40193	Opiate Alkaloid Hydrochlorides (Pantopon injectable)
40195	Naloxone
41061	Levallorphan Tartrate (Lorfan)
40194	Opiate Antagonists/Agonists
71917	Nalmefene HCl
71918	Naltrexone HCl
40197	Synthetic Narcotics
40198	Alphaprodine Hydrochloride (Nisentil)
40200	Dihydrocodeine Bitartrate + Acetaminophen + Caffeine
48625	Dihydrocodeine Bitartrate + Aspirin + Caffeine
48398	Nalbuphine Hydrochloride
48670	Fentanyl Citrate + Droperidol
72641	Injection
40201	Fentanyl (Sublimaze, injectable)
44716	Sufentanil Citrate (Sufenta)
40202	Levorphanol Tartrate (Levo-Dromoran)
72645	Injection
40203	Oxycodone

41962	Oxycodone + Acetaminophen (Percocet)
48662	Oxycodone + Aspirin
40214	Pentazocine HCl (Talwin)
72687	Injection
40215	Pentazocine Lactate (Talwin)
48663	Propoxyphene HCl + Acetaminophen
40204	Propoxyphene HCl (Darvon)
48674	Propoxyphene HCl + Aspirin + Caffeine
40205	Propoxyphene Napsylate (Darvon-N)
41965	Propoxyphene Napsylate + Acetaminophen (Darvocet-N)
41060	Narcotic Detoxification agents
41062	Methadone Hydrochloride (Dolophine)
74284	Injection
41063	Naloxone Hydrochloride
40206	Topical
48806	Capsaicin
40207	Methyl Salicylate
40208	Phenylcarbinol
40209	Other
40210	Mefenamic Acid (Ponstel)
40211	Methotrimeprazine (Levoprome)
72646	Injection
40212	Orphenadrine Citrate
40213	Oxyphenbutazone
40216	Antiarthritics
40217	Anti-gout & Uricosuric agents
40218	Allopurinol (Zyloprim)
40219	Colchicine
72600	Injection
40220	Probenecid
48681	Probenecid + Colchicine
40221	Sulfinpyrazone
40222	Gold
40223	Aurothioglucose (Solganal)
72682	Injection
40224	Other
40225	Anesthetic
40226	General
40227	Halothane
40228	Ketamine Hydrochloride
40229	Methoxyflurane (Penthrane)
48411	Deslflurane
40230	Local Anesthetic
40231	Balsam Peru
40232	Benzyl Alcohol
40233	Bismuth Subgallate
40234	Bupivacaine Hydrochloride

MEDICATIONS AND VACCINES

40235	Chloroprocaine Hydrochloride		48576	Netilmicin Sulfate
72704	Injection		40340	Tobramycin Sulfate
40236	Cyclomethycaine (Surfacaine)		72691	Injection
40237	Dibucaine Hydrochloride		48667	Tobramycin + Dexamethasone
40238	Etidocaine Hydrochloride		44690	Azithromycin (Zithromax)
40239	Lidocaine Base (Xylocaine)		41918	Aztreonam
72648	Injection		40280	Cephaloridine
48672	Lidocaine + Prilocaine		40274	Bacitracin
40240	Mepivacaine Hydrochloride		40275	Capreomycin Sulfate
72583	Injection		45753	Cephalosporins
40241	Prilocaine HCl		44719	Cefaclor (Ceclor)
40242	Procaine HCl		48580	Cefadroxil Monohydrate
40243	Tetracaine HCl		40277	Cefazolin Sodium
40244	Regional Anesthetics		72584	Injection
40245	Topical		48581	Cefamandole Nafate
40246	Benzocaine		75161	Cefepime HCl
48656	Benzocaine + Butyl Aminobenzoate		48582	Cefmetazole Sodium
	+ Tetracaine HCl		44685	Cefixime (Suprax)
48413	Chloroethane		48583	Cefonicid Sodium
48412	Cocaine Hydrochloride		72586	Injection
40247	Dibucaine		48584	Cefoperazone Sodium
48414	Dichlorotetrafluoroethane + Ethyl		48585	Cefpodoxime Proxetil
	Chloride		41908	Cefotetan
40248	Diperodon Preparations		48586	Cefprozil
48409	Dyclonine Hydrochloride		41911	Cefotaxime
40249	Ethyl Aminobenzoate		41906	Cefoxitin
40250	Oxyquinoline Sulfate		41910	Ceftazidime
48418	Trichloromonofluoromethane		72085	Ceftibuten Dihydrate
40251	Anorexics		48588	Ceftizoxime Sodium
40252	Amphetamines		72594	Injection
40253	Amphetamine		41907	Ceftriaxone
40254	Benzphetamine Hydrochloride		41909	Cefuroxime
	(Didrex)		40278	Cephalexin
40255	Chlorphentermine Hydrochloride		40279	Cephaloglycin
40256	Clortermine Hydrochloride		40281	Cephalothin Sodium
44442	Dextroamphetamine Saccharate		72643	Injection
	(Obetrol)		40282	Cephapirin Sodium
40257	Methamphetamine Hydrochloride		72592	Injection
40258	Methanphetamine Preparations		40283	Cephradine
40259	Other		40284	Chloramphenicol
40260	Diethylpropion Hydrochloride		40285	Chloramphenicol Palmitate
40261	Fenfluramine Hydrochloride		40286	Chloramphenicol Sodium Succinate
40262	Mazindol (Sanorex)		72595	Injection
40263	Phendimetrazine Tartrate		40287	Chlortetracycline (Aureomycin)
40264	Phenmetrazine HCl (Preludin)		48419	Clarithromycin
40265	Phentermine HCl		40288	Clindamycin Hydrochloride Hydrate
40266	Phentermine Resin			(Cleocin HCl)
40267	Antimicrobials		40289	Clindamycin Palmitate
40268	Antibacterials			Hydrochloride (Cleocin)
45752	Aminoglycosides		40290	Clindamycin Phosphate (Cleocin)
40270	Amikacin Sulfate (Amikin)		40291	Colistimethate Sodium
40304	Gentamicin Sulfate (Garamycin)		72601	Injection
72632	Injection		40292	Colistin Sulfate

MEDICATIONS AND VACCINES

40293	Demeclocycline	72685	Injection
71754	Dirithromycin	40311	Nafcillin Sodium
40298	Erythromycin	40315	Oxacillin Sodium
40297	Erythromycin Estolate (Ilosone)	72671	Injection
40299	Erythromycin Enteric Coated	40330	Sodium Cloxacillin Monohydrate
	Tablets	45756	Carboxypenicillins
40300	Erythromycin Ethyl Succinate	40276	Carbenicillin Indanyl Sodium
40301	Erythromycin Gluceptate (Ilotycin)		(Geocillin)
72626	Injection	40295	Disodium Carbenicillin
40302	Erythromycin Lactobionate	40339	Ticarcillin Disodium
	Injectable (Erythrocin)	41915	Ticarcillin Disodium + Clavulonic
72627	Injection		Acid
40303	Erythromycin Stearate	45757	Ureidopenicillins
44718	Erythromycin + Sulfisoxazole	41917	Mezlocillin
48406	Furazolidone	41916	Piperacillin
40305	Gramicidin	48680	Polymyxin B Sulfate + Bacitracin
40306	Kanamycin Sulfate		Zinc + Neomycin Sulfate
40307	Lincomycin Hydrochloride	40325	Polymyxin B Sulfate
	Monohydrate	48669	Polymyxin B Sulfate + Neomycin
72649	Injection		Sulfate + Hydrocortisone
48420	Loracarbef	40326	Polymyxin Preparations
40308	Methacycline Hydrochloride	40327	Potassium Hetacillin
	(Rondomycin)	40328	Potassium Phenethicillin
75156	Meropenem	45758	Quinolones
40312	Neomycin	48447	Cinoxacin
40313	Neomycin Palmitate	41912	Ciprofloxacin
40314	Neomycin Sulfate	48451	Enoxacin
48679	Neomycin Sulfate + Polymyxin B	48450	Lomefloxacin Hydrochloride
	Sulfate	41913	Norfloxacin
48797	Neomycin Sulfate + Flucinolone	48449	Ofloxacin
	Acetonide	48727	Lomefloxacin HCl
40319	Penicillins	48422	Rifabutin
40318	Oral	40329	Silver Sulfadiazine
40346	Injectable	40331	Spectinomycin HCl
40320	Penicillin G, Benzathine	40332	Streptomycin Sulfate
40321	Penicillin G, Potassium	40345	Sulfonamides
72664	Injection	40269	Acetyl Sulfisoxazole (Gantrisin)
40322	Penicillin G, Procaine	40333	Sulfisoxazole
72661	Injection	40334	Sulfisoxazole Diolamine
40323	Penicillin G, Sodium	41534	Sulfamethoxazole
40324	Penicillin V Potassium .	41535	Sulfamethoxazole + Trimethoprim
45755	Aminopenicillins	48443	Sulfacetamide Sodium
40271	Amoxicillin (Polymox)	48444	Sulfacetamide Sodium +
41914	Amoxicillin + Clavulonic Acid		Prednisolone Acetate
	(Augmentin)	44746	Tetracyclines
40272	Ampicillin (Omnipen)	40335	Tetracycline
72554	Injection	72544	Injection
40273	Ampicillin Trihydrate	40336	Tetracycline HCl
41894	Ampicillin Sodium (Omnipen-N)	40337	Tetracycline Phosphate Complex
72555	Injection	40296	Doxycycline (Vibramycin)
45754	Semisynthetic Penicillins	40310	Minocycline Hydrochloride
40294	Dicloxacillin Sodium	40316	Oxytetracycline
40309	Methicillin Sodium	40317	Oxytetracycline HCl

MEDICATIONS AND VACCINES

72660	Injection
48783	Oxytetracycline HCl + Hydrocortisone Acetate
48784	Oxytetracycline HCl + Polymyxin B Sulfate
40338	Thienamycin
40341	Trimethoprim
48657	Trimethoprim Sulfate + Polymyxin B Sulfate
40342	Trisulfapyrimidines
40343	Troleandomycin
40344	Vancomycin
72697	Injection
40347	Antifungal
40348	Amphotericin B
41957	Miconazole (topical)
41899	Fluconazole
40349	Flucytosine
40350	Griseofulvin
48612	Itraconazole
40351	Ketoconazole (Nizoral)
41960	Oral (topical)
48807	Clotrimazole
41961	Nystatin
48541	Nystatin + Triamcinolone Acetonide
40352	Antiviral
40353	Acyclovir (Zovirax)
75158	Cidofovir
72100	Famciclovir
41919	Ganciclovir
41920	Ribavirin
40354	Adenine Arabinoside (Ara-A)
40355	Interferon
41877	Alpha
41878	Gamma
48740	Foscarnet Sodium
72631	Injection
72111	Indinavir Sulfate
75157	Nevirapine
72094	Ritonavir
72086	Saquinavir Mesylate
72109	Stavudine
71923	Valacyclovir HCl
40356	Anti TB
40357	Para-Aminosalicylic Acid
40358	Cycloserine
40359	Ethambutol Hydrochloride
40360	Ethionamide
40361	Isoniazid (INH)
40362	Rifampin
48676	Rifampin + Isoniazid

72108	Rifampin + Isoniazid + Pyrazinamide
40363	Viomycin Sulfate
40364	Pyrazinamide
72104	Folic Acid Inhibitors
72105	Trimetrexate Glucuronate
48760	Antileprosy
48761	Clofazimine
40365	Ophthalmologicals
40366	Sulfisoxazole Diolamine (Gantrisin)
40367	Polymyxin B-Bacitracin (Polysporin)
40368	Polymyxin B-Neomycin-Gramicidin (Neosporin)
40369	Antidiabetics
40370	Oral Hypoglycemics
72087	Acarbose
40371	Acetohexamide (Dymelor)
40372	Chlorpropamide (Diabinese)
72092	Glimepiride
41884	Glipizide (Glucotrol)
41883	Glyburide (Micronase)
71911	Metformin HCl
40373	Tolazamide (Tolinase)
40374	Tolbutamide (Orinase)
40375	Insulin preparations
40380	Insulin, Human (Humulin)
41936	regular (Humulin-R)
41937	NPH (Humulin-N)
41938	Lente (Humulin-L)
41939	Ultralente (Humulin-U)
41940	buffered regular for external insulin pump (Humulin-BR)
75155	Insulin Lispro
41941	Insulin, Mixed Beef-Pork (Iletin)
40377	Regular (Iletin I)
40376	NPH (Iletin I)
40378	PZI (Protamine, Zinc + Iletin I)
40381	Semilente (Semilente Iletin I)
40382	Lente (Lente Iletin I)
40383	Ultralente (Ultralente Iletin I)
40379	Insulin, Purified Pork
41943	Regular (Iletin II)
41942	NPH (Iletin II)
41944	PZI (Protamine, Zinc + Iletin II)
41945	Semilente
41946	Lente (Lente Iletin II)
41947	Insulin, Purified Beef
41948	Regular (Iletin II)
41949	NPH (Iletin II)
41950	PZI (Protamine, Zinc + Iletin II)
41951	Semilente
41952	Lente (Lente Iletin II)

MEDICATIONS AND VACCINES

41953	Ultralente
48473	Premixed Insulins
48475	Premixed Insulins Human Insulin
	Isophane Suspension + Human
	Insulin Injection
48476	Premixed Insulins Purified Pork
	Isophane Insulin Susp.+Purified
	Pork Insulin Inj
48477	Premixed Insulins NPH Human
	Insulin Isophane Susp.+Regular
	Human Insulin Inject
40384	Antidiuretics
40385	Lypressin (Diapid)
40386	Pitressin Tannate
44457	Desmopressin Acetate (DDAVP)
40387	Antiparasitic Agents
40388	Antimalarial
40403	Chloroquine Hydrochloride
72574	Injection
40404	Chloroquine Phosphate
40389	Hydroxychloroquine Sulfate
	(Plaquenil)
40390	Primaquine Phosphate
40391	Pyrimethamine (Daraprim)
40392	Quinine Sulfate
44446	Proguanil (Paludrine)
44447	Mefloquine
44448	Sulfadoxine + Pyrimethamine
	(Fansidar)
44449	Sulfalene + Pyrimethamine
	(Metakelfin)
40393	Antiprotozoan
48401	Atovaquone
40394	Quinacrine HCl (Atabrine)
40409	Metronidazole (Flagyl)
40395	Nifurtimox (Lampit)
40396	Pentamidine
42043	Aerosol (NebuPent)
40397	Pentavalent Antimony
40398	Suramin
40399	Antitoxoplasmosis
40401	Amebicides
40402	Carbarsone
40405	Dehydroemetine Dihydrochloride
40406	Diiodohydroxyquin (Diodoquin)
40407	Diloxanide Furoate (Furamide)
40408	Emetine HCl
40410	Paromomycin (Humatin)
40411	Anthelmintics
40412	Diethylcarbamazine
40413	Hexylresorcinol
40414	Mebendazole
40415	Metrifonate (Bilarcil)

40416	Piperazine Preparations (Antepar)
40417	Praziquantel
40418	Pyrantel Pamoate
40419	Pyrvinium Pamoate
40420	Niclosamide
40421	Niridazole
40422	Novarsenobenzol
40423	Tetrachlorethylene
40424	Thiabendazole
40425	Pediculicides
40426	Gamma Benzene Hexachloride
	(Kwell)
40427	Pyrethrins
40428	Scabicides
40429	Crotamiton (Eurax)
48808	Permethrin
40430	Trichomonacides
40432	Antihistamines
40433	d-Isoephedrine Sulfate
40434	Aminoacetic Acid (Corilin)
44709	Astemizole (Hismanal)
72096	Acrivastine + Pseudoephedrine HCl
40435	Azatadine Maleate +
	Pseudoephedrine Sulfate
40436	Brompheniramine Maleate
44710	Brompheniramine Maleate +
	Pseudoephedrine
48778	Brompheniramine Maleate +
	Pseudoephedrine +
	Dextromethorphan Hydrobromide
48779	Brompheniramine Maleate +
	Phenylpropanolamine HCl +
	Codeine Phosphate
40437	Carbinoxamine Maleate (Rondec)
72091	Cetirizine HCl
48430	Chlorpheniramine Maleate
72598	Injection
44819	Claritin
40438	Cyproheptadine Hydrochloride
	(Periactin)
40439	Dexbrompheniramine Maleate
40440	Dexchlorpheniramine Maleate
40441	Dimethindene Maleate
40442	Diphenhydramine Hydrochloride
40443	Diphenylpyraline Hydrochloride
75159	Fexofenadine HCl
44711	Clemastine Fumarate (Tavist)
41408	Hydroxyzine Hydrochloride
	(Atarax)
72701	Injection
41409	Hydroxyzine Pamoate (Vistaril)
72103	Levocabastine HCl

MEDICATIONS AND VACCINES

71753	Loratadine + pseudoephedrine sulfate	40468	Paramethasone Acetate
40444	Methapyrilene (Histadyl)	40469	Paramethasone Preparations
40445	Methapyrilene Fumarate	41886	Inhaled Steroids
40446	Methapyrilene Hydrochloride	41887	Beclomethasone nasal/oral inhalers
40447	Pyrrobutamine Phosphate	41460	Dipropionate
41967	Terfenadine	71049	Budesonide
44708	Terfenadine + Pseudoephedrine	41929	Flunisolide Nasal Inhaler
40448	Antihyperlipemics	71050	Fluticasone Propionate
40449	Cholestyramine	41930	Dexamethasone Nasal Inhaler (Decadron Respihaler)
40450	Clofibrate (Atromid-S)		
41864	Gemfibrozil	41888	Triamcinolone acetonide
40451	Colestipol Hydrochloride (Colestid)	40470	Intraarticular Steroids
40452	Probucol (Lorelco)	40471	Intrabursal Steroids
40453	Sitosterols (Cytellin)	40472	Other
40454	Dextrothyroxine (Choloxin)	40473	Fenoprofen Calcium (Nalfon)
44688	Anti-BPH	40474	Antipyretics
44689	Finasteride (Proscar)	40475	Antiseptics
40455	Anti-inflammatory	40476	Benzalkonium Chloride
40456	Enzymes	40477	Cetyl Dimethyl Ethyl Ammonium Bromine
40457	Non-steroidal		
48416	Flurbiprofen	40478	Chlorhexidine Gluconate
40166	Ibuprofen (non-prescription)	48610	Glutaraldehyde
40458	Ibuprofen	48455	Phenol
48603	Ketoprofen	48611	Tetrachlorosalicylanilide
48604	Diflunisal	40479	Anti-Thyroid Agents
72095	Diclofenac Potassium	40480	Iodine 131
48605	Diclofenac Sodium	41843	High dose (>50 mCi)
40459	Indomethacin (Indocin)	40481	Iodine Preparations (Lugols)
48575	Ketorolac Tromethamine	40482	Methimazole (Tapazole)
72642	Injection	40483	Propylthiouracil (PTU)
48606	Mesalamine	40484	Ipodate
40460	Naproxen	40485	Antivertigo
45940	Aleve (non-prescription; 200mg naproxen, 20mg Na)	40486	Buclizine Hydrochloride (Bucladin-S)
48607	Meclofenamate Sodium	40487	Diphenidol (Vontrol)
48394	Etodolac	40488	Meclizine Hydrochloride
41964	Sulindac (Clinoril)	40489	Cancer Chemotherapeutic agents
48397	Salsalate	40491	o,p'-DDD
40461	Phenylbutazone	40492	Actinomycin-D
48608	Nabumetone	48461	Altretamine
40462	Piroxican (Feldene)	40493	Asparaginase
48609	Oxaprozin	40494	5-Azacytidine
40463	Tolmetin Sodium (Tolectin)	40495	Azathioprine (Imuran)
40464	Steroids	71910	Bicalutamide
48472	Alclometasone Dipropionate	40496	Bleomycin Sulfate
40465	Betamethasone	40497	Busulfan (Myleran)
40466	Betamethasone Acetate	48464	Carboplatin
40467	Betamethasone Sodium Phosphate	40498	Carmustine
72591	Injection	48743	Mechlorethamine HCl
48520	Betamethasone Sodium Phosphate +Betamethasone Acetate	40499	Chlorambucil (Leukeran)
		42325	2-chlorodeoxyadenosine
72589	Injection	48465	Cisplatin

MEDICATIONS AND VACCINES

48468	Cladribine	40528	2-Amino-6-Mercaptopurine (Thioguanine)
72713	Injection		
40500	Cyclophosphamide (Cytoxan)	40529	Cis-Platinum
40501	Cytarabine	40530	Guanidine
40502	Cytosine Arabinoside	40531	32-Phosphorus
40503	Dacarbazine	40532	Streptozotocin
48457	Dactinomycin	42969	Colony-Stimulating Factors
45759	Daunorubicin (Cerubidine)	42970	Neupogen
40504	Diaziquone	40534	Cardio-Vascular Agents
75153	Docetaxel	40535	Anti-Anginal Preparations
40505	Doxorubicin HCl (Adriamycin)	40536	Dipyridamole
40506	Dromostanolone Preparations (Drolban)	72623	Injection
		40537	Erythrityl Tetranitrate
48460	Estramustine Phosphate Sodium	44691	Isosorbide Mononitrate (Ismo)
48428	Etoposide	40538	Isosorbide Dinitrate (Isordil)
40507	Floxuridine	40539	Magnesium Nicotinate
48469	Fludarabine Phosphate	40540	Nitrate & Nitrite Preparations
40508	5-Fluorouracil	40541	Nitroglycerin
48471	Flutamide	40542	Antihypertensives
75152	Gemcitabine HCl	40544	Clonidine Hydrochloride
40509	Hydroxyurea	48673	Clonidine Hydrochloride + Chlorthalidone
48470	Idarubicin Hydrochloride		
48462	Ifosfamide	40545	Cryptenamine Preparations
40510	Interleukin-2	40546	Cryptenamine Tannate
42127	Levamisole	40547	Deserpidine
40511	Lomustine	40548	Diazoxide
40512	Megestrol Acetate (Megace)	72637	Injection
40513	Melphalan (Alkeran)	48810	Guanabenz Acetate
74290	Injection	40549	Guanethidine Monosulfate (Esimil)
40514	6-Mercaptopurine (Purinethol)	40550	Guanethidine Sulfate (Ismelin)
40515	Methotrexate	48729	Guanadrel Sulfate
40516	Mithramycin	48809	Guanfacine HCl
40517	Mitomycin For Injection	40551	Hydralazine Hydrochloride
40518	Mitotane (Lysodren)	72572	Injection
48463	Mitoxantrone	41935	Hydralazine Hydrochloride + Hydrochlorothiazide (Apresazide)
74289	Injection		
40519	Nandrolone Phenpropionate Injection, N.F.	48658	Hydralazine Hydrochloride + Hydrochlorothiazide + Reserpine
72570	Injection	44820	Losartan potassium
48459	Pentostatin	48448	Mecamylamine HCl
40520	Pipobroman (Vercyte)	40552	Methyldopa (Aldomet)
48458	Plicamycin	41932	Methyldopa + Hydrochlorothiazide (Aldoril)
40521	Polyestradiol Phosphate		
40522	Procarbazine HCl	41933	Propranolol HCl + Hydorchlorothiazide
48467	Streptozocin		
44697	Taxol	48876	Methyldopa + Chlorothiazide
48466	Teniposide	41902	Minoxidil (Loniten)
40523	Testolactone	40553	Methyldopate HCl Injection
40524	Thioguanine	44686	Nicardipine HCl
40525	Thiotepa	40554	Paragyline HCl
40526	Vinblastine Sulfate	40555	Prazosin HCl
40527	Vincristine Sulfate	48774	Prazosin HCl + Polythiazide
		40557	Rauwolfia Preparations

MEDICATIONS AND VACCINES

40558	Rauwolfia Serpentina	72640	Injection
40559	Rescinnamine	48613	Betaxolol HCl
40560	Reserpine	48614	Bisoprolol Fumerate
48682	Reserpine + Chlorothiazide	48615	Bisoprolol Fumerate +
48683	Reserpine + Hydrochlorothiazide		Hydrochlorothiazide
40561	Sodium Nitroprusside	40579	Atenolol
40562	Syrosingopine	48661	Atenolol + Chlorthalidone
40563	Trimethaphan Camsylate	45440	Esmolol HCl (Brevibloc)
72575	Injection	48616	Carteolol HCl
41889	ACE Inhibitors	40580	Labetalol
48823	Benazepril HCl	40581	Metoprolol
41890	Captopril (Capoten)	41956	Metoprolol + Hydrochlorothiazide
44692	Captopril + Hctz (Capozide)		(Lopressor HCT)
48689	Lisinopril + Hydrochlorothiazide	48675	Nadolol + Bendroflumethiazide
41954	Lisinopril (Zestril)	40582	Nadolol
41900	Enalapril (Vasotec)	48617	Penbutolol Sulfate
41901	Enalapril + Hydrochlorothiazide	40583	Proctolol
	(Vaseretic)	40584	Pindolol
48824	Fosinopril Sodium	40585	Timolol
71922	Moexipril HCl	71752	Timolol Hemihydrate
44438	Quinapril (Accupril)	48691	Timolol Maleate +
48822	Ramipril		Hydrochlorothiazide
72528	Trandolapril	49808	Total Daily Dose
40564	Antiarrhythmics	41976	Beta-Adrenoceptor Partial Agonists
48813	Acebutolol HCl	41977	Xamoterol
48814	Adenosine	40586	Calcium Channel Blockers
72546	Injection	48818	Amlodipine Besylate
40565	Amiodarone	71913	Amlodipine Besylate + Benazepril
40566	Bretyllium Tosylate		HCl
40567	Disopyramide Phosphate (Norpace)	48819	Bepridil HCl
42126	Encainide (Enkaid)	40587	Diltiazem HCl
42125	Flecainide	44687	Felodipine (Plendil)
72093	Ibutilide Fumarate	48816	Isradipine
40568	Lidocaine Hydrochloride	40588	Nifedipine
44444	Mexiletine (Mexitil)	48817	Nimodipine
42327	Moricizine (Ethmozine)	72090	Nisoldipine
44443	Propafenone HCl (Rythmol)	40589	Verapamil
40569	Procainamide HCl	40590	Cardiac Glycosides
72670	Injection	40591	Acetyldigitoxin
40570	Quinidine	40592	Desianoside
40571	Quinidine Gluconate (Quinaglute)	40593	Digitalis Glycoside Preparations
40572	Quinidine Polygalacturonate	40594	Digitoxin
40573	Quinidine Sulfate	40595	Digoxin (Lanoxin)
48815	Sotalol HCl	72617	Injection
40574	Tocainide	40596	Gitalin
40575	Alpha Adrenergic Blocking Agents	40597	Lanatoside C (Cedilanid)
48811	Doxazosin Mesylate	40598	Ouabain (Strophanthin-G)
40576	Phenoxybenzamine HCl	40599	Diuretics
40577	Phentolamine (Regitine)	44714	Loop-Acting
48735	Metyrosine	40605	Furosemide (Lasix)
48812	Terazosin HCl	72644	Injection
40578	Beta Adrenergic Blocking agents	41882	Bumetanide
40556	Propranolol HCl	40604	Ethacrynic Acid

MEDICATIONS AND VACCINES

44713	Thiazides
40600	Bendroflumethiazide
40601	Benzthiazide
40602	Chlorothiazide
74283	Injection
40543	Chlorthalidone
40603	Cyclothiazide
40606	Hydrochlorothiazide
40607	Hydroflumethiazide
40610	Methyclothiazide
40612	Polythiazide
40617	Trichlormethiazide
48820	Amiloride HCl
41881	Amiloride + Hydrochlorothiazide
48821	Indapamide
40608	Mercaptomerin, Sodium (Thiomerin)
40609	Merethoxylline Procaine (Dicurin)
40611	Metolazone
40613	Quinethazone
40614	Spironolactone (Aldactone)
41966	Spironolactone + Hydrochlorothiazide
40615	Sterile Urea
41934	Hydrochlorothiazide + Triamterene (Dyazide)
44427	Hydrochlorothiazide + Triamterene (Maxzide)
72097	Torsemide
40616	Triamterene
40618	Mannitol
72651	Injection
40619	Hypertensives
40620	Levarteneol Bitartrate (Levophed)
40621	Metaraminol (Aramine)
72571	Injection
40622	Methoxamine Hydrochloride (Vasoxyl)
72699	Injection
40623	Vasodilators, Cerebral
40624	Isoxsuprine HCl
72698	Injection
40625	Papaverine HCl
72659	Injection
40626	Vasodilators, Coronary
40627	Aminophylline
72551	Injection
40628	Erythrityl Tetranitrate
40629	Isosorbide Dinitrate
40630	Vasodilators, General
40631	Cyclandelate
40632	Ethaverine HCl
40633	Nylidrin
40634	Theobromine

40635	Vasodilators, Peripheral
40636	Isoxsuprine Hydrochloride (Vasadilan)
40637	Nicotinyl Alcohol
40638	Nylidrin
40639	Theobromine Magnesium Oleate
40640	Tolazoline HCl (Priscoline)
72668	Injection
40641	Vasopressors
40646	Neosynephrine
40647	Norepinephrine
47702	Inotropes
40643	Dobutamine HCl
40645	Milrinone
74285	Injection
40642	Amrinone
49807	Vesnarinone
40644	Dopamine HCl
40648	Varicose Vein Sclerotics
40649	Morrhuate Sodium
40650	Sodium Tetradecyl Sulfate
41867	HMG-CoA Reductase Inhibitors
72102	fluvastatin (Lescol)
41868	lovastatin (Mevacor)
42575	pravastatin (Pravachol)
44437	simvastatin (Zocor)
40651	Chelating Agents
40652	Deferoxamine Mesylate
72605	Injection
40653	Dimercaprol (BAL)
72564	Injection
40654	Calcium Disodium Versenate
40655	D-Penicillamine
48825	Succimer
48522	Trientine Hydrochloride
41994	Cholesterol Solvents
41995	methyl tert-butyl ether (MTBE)
48703	Gall Stone Dissolution
48704	Ursodiol
40656	Cough & Cold Preparations
40657	Ammonium Chloride
40658	Benzonatate (Tessalon)
40659	Calcium Carbaspirin
40660	Calcium Iodide
40661	Caramiphen Edisylate (Tuss-Ornade)
40662	Carbetapentane Tannate (Rynatuss)
40663	Cetylpyridinium Chloride
40664	Chlorpheniramine Maleate
48776	Chlorpheniramine Maleate + Phenyltoloxamine Citrate + Phenylephrine HCl
40665	Chlorpheniramine + Pseudoephedrine (Co-Pyronil)

MEDICATIONS AND VACCINES

40666	Chlorpheniramine + Phenylpropanolamine	40689	Terpin Hydrate
40667	Chlorpheniramine Tannate	40690	Triprolidine HCl
40668	Dextromethorphan Hydrobromide	40691	Triprolidine Preparations
48688	Dextromethorphan Hydrobromide + Iodinated Glycerol	40692	Dermatologicals
		40693	Acne preparations
48693	Dextromethorphan Hydrobromide + Chloropheniramine Maleate + Phenylephrine HCl	40694	Acetone
		72084	Azelaic Acid
		40695	Benzoyl Peroxide
48697	Dextromethorphan Hydrobromide + Promethazine HCl	48659	Benzoyl Peroxide + Erythromycin
		40696	Chlordydroxyquinoline
40669	Guaifenesin	40697	Ethyl Alcohol
48636	Guaifenesin + Phenylephrine HCl	40698	Isotretinoin (Accutane)
48634	Guaifenesin + Pseudoephedrine	48544	Meclocycline Sulfosalicylate
48635	Guaifenesin + Pseudoephedrine HCl	40699	Polyoxyethylene Lauryl Ether (Benzagel)
48639	Guaifenesin + Phenylpropanolamine HCl	40700	Resorcinol
		40701	Resorcinol Monoacetate
48878	Guaifenesin + Phenylpropanolamine HCl + Phenylephrine HCl	40702	Salicylic Acid
		40703	Sulfated Oil Surfactants
48640	Guaifenesin + Dextromethorphan Hydrobromide	40704	Sulfur
		40705	Sulfur Preparations
40672	Hydromorphone Hydrochloride	40706	Sulfur, Colloidal
40673	Isopropamide Iodide (Ornade)	40707	Thymol
40674	Levopropoxyphene Napsylate (Novrad)	40708	Tretinoin (Retin-A)
		40709	Triethanolamine
40675	Methscopolamine Nitrate	40710	Antifungal
40676	Naphazoline HCl	40711	Acrisorcin (Akrinol)
40677	Pheniramine Maleate	48546	Ciclopirox Olamine
40678	Phenol (Chloraseptic)	48545	Clioquinol
40679	Phenylephrine Bitartrate	48550	Econazole Nitrate
40680	Phenylephrine HCl	40712	Haloprogin (Halotex)
48668	Phenylephrine HCl + Methscopolamine Nitrate + Chlorpheniramine Maleate	40713	Iodochlorhydroxyquin
		40714	Isopropyl Alcohol + Undecylenic Acid + Salicylic Acid
48677	Phenylephrine HCl + Naphazoline HCl + Pyrilamine Maleate	48547	Naftifine Hydrochloride
		41959	Nystatin (topical)
40681	Phenylephrine Tannate	48456	Sulconazole Nitrate
40682	Phenylpropanolamine Bitartrate	40715	Tannic Acid
40683	Phenylpropanolamine HCl	48551	Terbinafine Hydrochloride
40684	Phenyltoloxamine Resin Complex (Tussionex)	40716	Tolnaftate (Tinactin)
		48549	Oxiconazole Nitrate
40685	Pseudoephedrine HCl (Sudafed)	40717	Triacetin
48664	Pseudoephedrine HCl + Chlorpheniramine Maleate	40718	Undecylenate, Calcium
		40719	Undecylenate, Zinc
48678	Pseudoephedrine HCl + Chlorpheniramine Maleate + Dextromethorphan Hydrobromide	40720	Undecylenic Acid
		40721	Podophyllum
		40722	Antipruritics
40686	Pseudoephedrine + Triprolidine (Actifed)	40723	Calamine
		40724	Camphor
48877	Pseudoephedrine + Triprolidine + Codeine	40725	Dexpanthenol
		72110	Doxepin HCl
40687	Pyrilamine Maleate	48474	Fluticasone Propionate
40688	Pyrilamine Tannate (Rynatan)	40726	Ichthammol

MEDICATIONS AND VACCINES

40727	Menthol
40728	Methdilazine (Tacaryl)
40729	Vinylacetate Copolymers (Ivy-chex)
40730	Trimeprazine Tartrate (Temaril)
40731	Tripelennamine HCl
40732	Zirconium Oxide
40733	Antibacterial
40734	Entsufon Sodium (PhisoDerm)
40735	Hexachlorophene
40736	Mafenide Acetate (Sulfamylon)
48552	Mupirocin
40737	Nitrofurazone
40738	Povidone-Iodine (Betadine)
40739	Sodium Oxychlorosene (Clorpactin)
40740	Thimerosal
40741	Triclosan
48711	Tetrachlorosalicylanilide
40742	Anti-Psoriasis
40743	Allantoin
40744	Anthralin Preparations
72099	Calcipotriene
40745	Coal Tar
48553	Etretinate
40746	Tar Preparations
41971	Anti-Baldness
41972	Rogaine
40747	Astringents
40748	Witch Hazel
40749	Cleansing agents
48554	Eucerite
40750	Sodium Lauryl Sulfoacetate (Lowila)
40751	Mild Soaps (Dove)
48432	Nail Preparation
45751	Abrasives
40752	Debriding agents
40753	Carbamide Preparations
40754	Debrisan
40755	Desoxyribonuclease
40756	Enzymes
40757	Fibrinolysin
40758	Papain
48786	Papain + Urea
48787	Papain + Urea + Chlorophyllin Copper Complex
40759	Peroxide Preparations
40760	Streptokinase-Streptodornase (Varidase)
40761	Sutilains
48750	Topical Antineoplastics
48751	Fluorouracil
48755	Masoprocol
40762	Emollients
48827	Aloe Vera
71083	Ammonium Lactate (LAC-HYDRIN)
40763	Bismuth Subnitrate
40764	Cottonseed Oil Preparations (Lubath)
40765	Diisopropyl Sebacate
40766	Dimethisoquin Hydrochloride (Quotane)
48555	Essential Oils
40767	Isopropyl Myristate (Domol)
40768	Lanolin
40769	Methylbenzethonium Chloride
40770	Ointment Bases (Carmol)
40771	Hydrated Petrolatum
42015	Moisturizers
71082	Dimethicone (Moisturel)
48400	Moisturizers With Sunscreen
48403	Moisturizers With Ammonium Lactate
48404	Moisturizers With Lactic Acid
48826	Moisturizers
40772	Photodesensitizers
40773	Beta-carotene (Solatene)
40774	Repigmentation Agents
40775	Methoxsalen (Oxsoralen)
40776	Trioxsalen
72088	Retinoids
75160	Adapalene
72089	Tretinoin
40777	Skin Bleach
40778	Hydroquinone
48402	Monobenzone
40779	Topical Steroids
48528	Amcinonide
40780	Betamethasone Benzoate
40781	Betamethasone Dipropionate
40782	Betamethasone Valerate
48530	Clobetasol Propionate
40783	Desonide
48695	Desonide + Acetic Acid
40784	Desoximetasone
48529	Diflorasone Diacetate
48532	Fluocinonide
40785	Fluocinolone Acetonide (Synalar)
40786	Flumethasone Pivalate
40787	Fluoromethalone
40788	Flurandrenolide
48539	Fluticasone Propionate
40789	Halcinonide
48534	Halobetasol Propionate
40790	Hydrocortisone (Alcohol)

MEDICATIONS AND VACCINES

48602	Hydrocortisone Acetate + Pramoxine HCl
40791	Hydrocortisone Acetate
48537	Hydrocortisone Butyrate
48536	Hydrocortisone Valerate
48543	Mometasone Furoate
72098	Prednicarbate (Dermatop)
40792	Triamcinolone Acetonide
40793	Intralesional Steroids
40794	Shampoos
40795	Chloroxine
40796	Tar Shampoo
48556	Salicylic Acid
48828	Scalp Cleansing
40797	Selenium Sulfide (Selsun)
40798	Sulfur, Precipitated
40799	Zinc Pyrithione
40800	Sun Screens
40801	Benzophenones (Solbar)
40802	Cinoxate
40803	Digalloyl Trioleate
40804	Dioxybenzone
40805	Menthyl Anthranilate
40806	Padimate
40807	Para-Aminobenzoic Acid
40808	Red Petrolatum
40809	Salisobenzone
40810	Zinc Oxide
40811	Vesicants
40812	Canthardin Collodion
40813	Wart Therapeutic agents
40814	Cantharidin
48408	Podofilox
48399	Salicylic Acid
48410	Formaldehyde
40815	Lactic Acid (Duofilm)
40816	Wet Dressings
40817	Aluminum Acetate
40199	Aluminum Sulfate (Domeboro)
40818	Calcium Acetate (Domeboro)
40819	Chlorophyll Preparations
40820	Propionate Compounds
48754	Duoderm
48597	Wound Dressings
48598	Trypsin + Baslam Peru + Castor Oil
48599	Calcium-Sodium Alginate Fiber
48600	Polyurethane Membrane
48601	Zinc Oxide + Benzethonium Chloride
40821	Other
40822	Aluminum Chloride (Drysol)
48773	Aluminum Chlorhydroxide + Zinc Undecylenate + Formaldehyde

48728	Menthol
40823	Cod Liver Oil Concentrate
40824	Karaya Gum
40825	Melalenca Alternifolia Oil (Te-Tree Oint.)
40826	Diaminodiphenylsulfone (Dapsone)
48768	Nail Hardener
40827	Enzymes
40828	Collagenolytic
40829	Collagenase
40830	Digestants
40831	Amylolytic Enzyme
40832	Chymotrypsin
40833	Lactase (Lactaid)
40834	Pancreatic Preparations (Viokase)
40835	Pepsin
40836	Phenyltoloxamine Dihydrogen Citrate (Kutrase)
48724	Alglucerase
72549	Injection
48756	Alpha1-Proteinase Inhibitor (Human)
48764	Surfactants
48765	Colfosceril Palimate + Cetyl Alcohol + Tyloxapol
48766	Beractant
40837	Enzyme Inhibitors
48445	Hemin
40838	Trasylol
40839	Lipolytic
40840	Lipolytic Enzyme
40841	Lipolytic Preparations
40842	Fibrinolytic, Proteolytic
40843	Bromelains (Ananase)
40844	Fibrinolysin - d-RNAase (Elase)
40845	Proteolytic Preparations
40846	Trypsin - Chymotrypsin (Biozyme)
40847	Topical
40848	Hyaluronidase
72703	Injection
40849	Gastrointestinal Preparations
40850	Antacids
40851	Alginic Acid (Gaviscon)
44743	Aluminum-Containing
40852	Aluminum Hydroxide (Maalox)
40853	Al(OH)3 + Mg(OH)2 + Simethicone (Mylanta)
40854	Aluminum Hydroxide Gel, Dried (Mylanta)
40855	Aluminum Hydroxide Preparations (Amphojel)
40856	Bismuth Aluminate

MEDICATIONS AND VACCINES

40857	Calcium Carbonate + Magnesium Carbonate
72082	Calcium Carbonate + Magnesium Hydroxide
40858	Calcium Carbonate, Precipitated
40860	Dihydroxy Aluminum Aminoacetate (Robalate)
40861	Glycine (Titralac)
71916	Lansoprazole (Prevacid)
40862	Magaldrate (Riopan)
40863	Magnesium Carbonate
40864	Magnesium Hydroxide
48558	Magnesium Oxide
40865	Magnesium Trisilicate
41974	Misoprostol (Cytotec)
41973	Omeprazole (Losec)
40867	Simethicone
40868	Sodium Bicarbonate + Citric Acid + Potassium Bicarbonate
48557	Sodium Citrate
40869	Sucralfate (Carafate)
40870	Xanthine Oxidase Inhibitor (Zyloprim)
47654	Bismuth Subsalicylate (Pepto-Bismol)
41903	Histamine-2 Receptor Antagonists
40859	Cimetidine (Tagamet)
41904	Nizatidine (Axid)
41926	Famotidine (Pepcid)
40866	Ranitidine (Zantac)
41955	Metoclopramide (Reglan)
71081	Cisapride (Propulsid)
40871	Antidiarrheal
48559	Difenoxin Hydrochloride + Atropine Sulfate
40872	Diphenoxylate Hydrochloride (Lomotil)
40873	Kaolin (Donnagel)
40874	Lactobacillus Acidophilus
40875	Lactobacillus Bulgaricus
40876	Loperamide Hydrochloride (Imodium)
42317	Octreotide Acetate (Sandostatin)
40877	Opium Preparations
40878	Paregoric
40879	Pectin
40880	Antiflatulents
40881	Cellulase
40882	Cellulolytic Enzyme
48560	Charcoal + Simethicone
40883	Choline Bitartrate
40884	Enzymes, Digestive
40885	Ox Bile Extract
40886	Panthenol
48561	Simethicone
40887	Choleretics
40888	Dehydrocholic Acid (Hepahydrin)
40889	Emetics
40890	Apomorphine Hydrochloride
40891	Benzquinamide Hydrochloride (Emete-con)
72565	Injection
40892	Ipecac Preparation
40893	Enemas
40894	Bisacodyl (Dulcolax)
40895	Carbon Dioxide (Evac-Q-Kit)
48479	Hydrocortisone Retention
40896	Magnesium Citrate
42319	Mesalamine (Rowasa)
40897	Sodium Phosphate
40898	Sodium Phosphate, Dibasic
40899	Hemorrhoidal
40900	Benzocaine (Americaine)
40901	Dibucaine (Corticaine)
48564	Ephedrine Sulphate + Zinc Oxide
40902	Pramoxine HCl (ProctoFoam)
48563	Camphor + Ephedrine Sulphate + Zinc Oxide
48565	Shark Liver Oil + Live Yeast Cell Derivative
40903	Hydrocholeretics
40904	Laxatives
40905	Anthraquinone Preparations (Modane)
40906	Barley Malt Extract
48566	Calcium Polycarbophil
40907	Docusate Sodium (Dialose)
48671	Docusate Sodium + Phenolphthalein
40908	Casanthranol + Docusate Sodium
40909	Cascara Sagrada
40910	Castor Oil
40911	Cortex Rhamni Frangulae (Movicol)
40912	Danthron
40913	Dehydrocholic Acid
40914	Dioctyl Calcium Sulfosuccinate
40915	Dioctyl Sodium Sulfosuccinate
48567	Glycerin
40916	Gum Karaya
40917	Iron Bile Salts (Bilron)
48568	Lactulose
40918	Mineral Oil
40919	Phenolphthalein
40920	Plantago Seed (Konsyl)
40921	Psyllium Preparations
40922	Senna
40923	Senna Concentrates

MEDICATIONS AND VACCINES

48775	Senna Concentrate + Docusate Sodium
40924	Sodium Acid Pyrophosphate
48570	Sodium Bicarbonate + Potassium Bitartrate
48569	Sodium Phosphate
48829	Bowel Evacuants
48431	Polyethylene Glycol 3350
40925	Ulcerative Colitis agents
48421	Olsalazine Sodium
40926	Sulfasalazine
40927	Hematological Agents
40928	Anticoagulants
40932	Heparin Preparations
40933	Warfarin Sodium (Coumadin)
40929	Acenocoumarol (Sintrom)
40930	Anisindione (Miradon)
40931	Bishydroxycoumarin (Dicumarol)
40953	Thrombolytics
40954	Streptokinase
72686	Injection
43008	Anisoylated Plasminogen-Streptokinase Activator Complex
41869	Tissue Plasminogen Activator (Activase)
40955	Urokinase
44861	Antiplatelet
44862	Ticlopidine (Ticlid)
40934	Antifibrinolysis
40935	Aminocaproic Acid (Amicar)
40936	Microfibrillar Collagen (Avitene)
48424	Tranexamic Acid
40937	Heparin Antidote
40938	Protamine Sulfate
72673	Injection
48725	Hemorheologics
48726	Pentoxifylline
40939	Hemostatics
48571	Collagen
48572	Gelatin
40940	Thrombin
48573	Oxidized Regenerated Cellulose
40941	Leukocytic Promotional agents
48767	Sargramostim
72680	Injection
40942	Plasma Expanders
40943	Dextran-40
40944	Dextran-70
40945	Dextrans (Low Molecular Weight)
41831	Fresh Frozen Plasma
40946	Purified Plasma Fraction (PPF)
40947	Hetastarch
40948	Plasma Fractions, Human

40949	Albumin, Normal Serum
48436	Albumin + Globulin
40951	Factor VIII (AHF, AHG)
40950	Factor IX Complex (Human)
48452	Antithrombin III (Human)
44695	Plasma Fractions, Engineered
44696	Factor VIII (Recombinate)
40952	Protein Hydrolysate
48762	Other
48763	Pentastarch
48757	Antihemophilic Factors
48758	Kogenate
40956	Hormones
40990	Estrogens
40991	Chlorotrianisene
40992	Combined Estrogens
40993	Conjugated Estrogens (Premarin)
40994	Conjugated Estrogens for Injection (Premarin Intravenous)
71915	Conjugated Estrogens + Medroxyprogesterone Acetate
48771	Conjugated Estrogens + Meprobamate
48772	Conjugated Estrogens + Methyltestosterone
40995	Diethylstilbestrol Diphosphate
40996	Diethylstilbestrol
40997	Estradiol
40998	Estradiol Valerate
72610	Injection
40999	Estriol
41000	Estrogens, Conjugated (Equine)
72629	Injection
41001	Estrogens, Esterified
48795	Estrogens, Esterified + Methyltestosterone
41002	Estrogens, Esterified (Equine)
41003	Estrone
72628	Injection
41004	Piperazine Estrone Sulfate (Ogen)
48523	Polyestradiol Phosphate
48524	Quinestrol
41013	Progestrogens
41014	Dydrogesterone
41015	Medroxyprogesterone Acetate
72613	Injection
41016	Norethindrone Acetate
40971	Corticosteroids
40972	Cortisone Acetate
40973	Dexamethasone
40974	Dexamethasone Acetate
40975	Dexamethasone Sodium Phosphate

MEDICATIONS AND VACCINES

40976	Dexamethasone Sodium Phosphate Injection	41025		Dessicated
		48574		Pork
40977	Fludrocortisone Acetate	41027		Sodium Dextrothyroxine
40978	Hydrocortisone	41028		Sodium Levothyroxine
48542	Hydrocortisone Sodium Phosphate	41029		Sodium Liothyronine (Cytomel)
72636	Injection	41030		Sodium Levothyroxine (Synthroid, IV)
40979	Hydrocortisone Sodium Succinate			
72638	Injection	41031	Prostaglandins	
40980	Prednisolone	48527		Alprostadil
40981	Prednisolone Sodium Succinate	48526		Dinoprostone
40982	Prednisone	42318		Misoprostol (Cytotec)
71924	Rimexolone (Vexol)	40957	ACTH	
40983	Triamcinolone Diacetate	40958		Adrenocorticotropic Hormone
72693	Injection	40959	Anabolics	
40984	Triamcinolone Hexacetonide	40960		Methandrostenolone (Dianabol)
72694	Injection	40961		Methyltestosterone
40985	Triamcinolone	40962		Nandrolone Decanoate Injection N.F.
40986	Meprednisone (Betapar)			
40987	Methylprednisolone (Medrol)	40963		Oxymetholone
40988	Methylprednisolone Acetate	40964		Stanozolol
72611	Injection	40965	Androgens	
40989	Methylprednisolone Sodium Succinate	40966		Androgens (Formatrix)
		40967		Danazol (Danocrine)
48748	Keratolytics	40968		Fluoxymesterone
48749	Dichloroacetic Acid	71751		Testosterone
41005	Glucagon	40969	Corpus Luteum	
41006	Gonadotropin	40970		Chorionic Gonadotropin
48699	Luprolide Acetate	72596		Injection
48700	Nafarelin Acetate	41032	Other	
48830	Gonadorelin Acetate	48801		Protirelin
48721	Gonadorelin HCl	72674		Injection
72101	Menotropins	41033		Vasopressin
48720	Sermorelin Acetate	41034		Tamoxifen
48741	Goserelin Acetate Implant	72083		Anastrozole
48747	Histrelin Acetate	41035		Desmopressin Acetate
41007	Growth Hormones	41036		Bromocriptine Mesylate
48525	Somatrem	48802		Pentagastrin
41008	Somatropin	72662		Injection
41009	Mineralocorticoids	41037		Metyropone
41010	Desoxycorticosterone Acetate	41038		Aminoglutethimide
41011	Desoxycorticosterone Pivalate	41039	Ion Exchange Resins	
41012	Parathyroid	41040		Sodium Polystyrene Sulfonate (Kayexalate)
41026	Calcitonin			
72580	Injection	41041	Muscle Relaxants	
41017	Secretin	41042	Skeletal	
41018	Testosterones	48442		Atracurium Besylate
41019	Testosterone	48531		Baclofen
41020	Testosterone Cypionate	72559		Injection
41021	Testosterone Enanthate	41043		Carisoprodol
41022	Testosterone Propionate	48685		Carisoprodol + Aspirin
72689	Injection	48686		Carisoprodol + Aspirin + Codeine Phosphate
41023	Testosterone Methyl			
41024	Thyroid Preparations	41044		Chlorphenes in Carbamate

MEDICATIONS AND VACCINES

41045	Chlorzoxazone	41081	Methscopolamine Bromide (Pamine)
41046	Cyclobenzaprine Hydrochloride	41082	Mepenzolate Bromide (Cantil)
41047	Dantrolene Sodium	41083	Methixene Hydrochloride (Trest)
48441	Doxacurium Chloride	41084	Oxyphencyclimine HCl
41048	Metaxalone (Skelaxin)	41085	Oxyphenonium Bromide
41049	Methocarbamol (Robaxin)	41086	Pirenzipine
72678	Injection	41087	Propantheline Bromide
48781	Methocarbamol + Aspirin	41088	Scopolamine Hydrobromide
41050	Metocurine Iodide	41089	Scopolamine Preparations
72655	Injection	41090	Scopolamine Patch (Transderm V)
48438	Mivacurium Chloride	41091	Thiopropazate HCl
41051	Pancuronium Bromide Injection (Pavulon)	41092	Tridihexethyl Chloride
		74286	Injection
48533	Quinine Sulfate	41093	Anticonvulsants
41052	Succinylcholine Chloride	41098	Hydantoin Derivative (Dilantin)
72566	Injection	41963	Hydantoin Derivative (Dilantin) + Phenobarbital
41053	Tubocurarine Chloride		
48440	Vecuronium Bromide	41099	Mephenytoin (Mesantoin)
41054	Smooth	41094	Carbamazepine (Tegretol)
41055	Adiphenine Hydrochloride (Trasentine)	41095	Clonazepam (Clonopin)
		41096	Ethosuximide (Zarontin)
41056	Dioxyline Phosphate (Paveril)	41097	Ethotoin
41057	Ethaverine Hydrochloride	45938	Felbamate
48535	Papaverine Hydrochloride	45939	Gabapentin (Neurontin)
41058	Pentaerythritol Tetranitrate (Peritrate)	71912	Lamotrigine
		41100	Methsuximide (Celontin)
41059	Thiphenamil (Trocinate)	71919	Nefazodone HCl (Serzone)
48730	Neuromuscular Blockers	41101	Paramethadione
48731	Botulinum Toxin	41102	Phenacemide
48753	Ritodrine HCl	41103	Phensuximide
41064	Neurological Agents	41104	Phenytoin Sodium
71071	Anti-ALS agents	72618	Injection
71072	Riluzole	41105	Primidone
41065	Anticholinergics	41106	Trimethadione
41066	Anistropine Methylbromide (Valpin)	41107	Valproic Acid (Depakene)
41067	Atropine Derivatives	44439	Divalproex Sodium (Depakote)
41068	Atropine Nitrate, Methyl	41108	Antihyperammonia
41069	Atropine Sulfate	41109	Lactulose
72568	Injection	41110	Anticholinesterase
41071	Belladonna Extract	41111	Edrophonium Chloride (Tensilon)
41072	Belladonna Preparations	41112	Neostigmine Bromide (Prostigmin, tab.)
41073	Benztropine Mesylate		
72561	Injection	41113	Neostigmine Methylsulfate (Prostigmin, inj.)
41074	Biperiden (Akineton)		
72548	Injection	72672	Injection
41075	Clidinium Bromide (Quarzan)	41114	Physostigmine Salicylate
41076	Dicyclomine Hydrochloride (Bentyl)	41115	Pyridostigmine Bromide (Mestinon)
72562	Injection	41116	Antimigraine
41077	Diphemanil Methylsulfate	41117	Cyclizine Hydrochloride (Migral)
41078	Glycopyrrolate (Robinul)	41118	Dichloralphenazone
41079	Hexocyclium Methylsulfate	41119	Dihydroergotamine Mesylate (D.H.E.)
41080	Homatropine Methylbromide		
48538	Hyoscyamine Sulfate		

MEDICATIONS AND VACCINES

41120	Dihydroergotamine Methanesulfonate	48792	Butalbital + Aspirin + Caffeine + Codeine
41927	Ergotamine Tartrate (Ergomar)	48791	Butalbital + Aspirin + Caffeine
41928	Ergotamine Tartrate - Aerosol (Medihaler Ergotamine)	41149	Butalbital
		48655	Butalbital + Acetaminophen
41121	Ergotamine Tartrate + Caffeine (Cafergot)	48789	Butalbital + Acetaminophen + Caffeine
41122	Methysergide Maleate (Sansert)	48790	Butalbital + Acetaminophen + Caffeine + Codeine
43506	Sumatriptan (Imitrex)		
41123	Antinauseants	41150	Carbromal
41124	Buclizine Hydrochloride	41151	Mephobarbitol (Mebaral)
41125	Carbohydrates (Emetrol)	41152	Metharbital (Gemonil)
41126	Cyclizine Preparations (Marezine)	41153	Methohexital Sodium (Brevital)
41127	Dimenhydrinate (Dramamine)	41154	Pentobarbital
72622	Injection	41155	Phenobarbital
48660	Diphenhydramine HCl + Acetaminophen	48780	Phenobarbital + Belladonna
		41156	Phenobarbital Sodium
41128	Doxylamine Succinate (Benedictin)	72665	Injection
48434	Dronabinol	41157	Secobarbital Sodium
71750	Granisetron HCl	72681	Injection
48435	Perphenazine	45849	Amobarbital + Secobarbital
72695	Injection	45850	Amobarbital + Amphetamine Sulfate
41129	Phosphorated Carbohydrate Solution (Emetrol)	41159	Sodium Diethyl Barbiturate
		41160	Sodium Isobutylally Barbiturate
44684	Odansetron HCl (Zofran)	41161	Sodium Pentobarbital
41130	Prochlorperazine (Compazine)	72663	Injection
72603	Injection	41162	Sodium Phenylethylbarbiturate
41131	Thiethylperazine (Torecan)	41158	Sodium Butabarbital
41132	Trimethobenzamide HCl (Tigan)	41164	Thiamylal Sodium
72690	Injection	41165	Increasing dosage to counter decreased effect
45791	Anti-Alzheimer's drugs		
45792	Tacrine (Cognex)	41166	CNS Stimulants
41133	Anti-Parkinsonism drugs	41167	Caffeine and Sodium Benzoate
41134	Amantadine Hydrochloride	41958	Nicotine polacrilex (Nicorette gum)
41135	Carbidopa + L-dopa (Sinemet)	41975	Nicotine transdermal patch
41136	Cycrimine Hydrochloride	41168	Pentylenetetrazol
42130	Selegiline HCl	41170	Methylphenidate Hydrochloride (Ritalin)
41137	Levodopa		
41138	Orphenadrine HCl (Disipal)	41171	Pemoline (Cylert)
41139	Procyclidine HCl (Kemadrin)	41172	Organophosphate Anticholinesterase Antidote
48407	Pergolide Mesylate		
41140	Trihexyphenidyl HCl (Artane)	41173	Pralidoxime Chloride
41141	Bromocriptine	72675	Injection
41142	Barbiturates	41174	Parasympathomimetics
41143	Allobarbital (Dialog)	41175	Bethanechol Chloride (Myotonachol)
41144	Amobarbital (Amytal)		
72567	Injection	72576	Injection
41145	Amobarbital Sodium	41176	Deanol
41146	Aprobarbital	48540	Yohimbine Hydrochloride
41147	Barbiturate Preparations	41177	Sedatives
41148	Butabarbital	41178	Chloral Betaine
48793	Butalbital + Aspirin	41179	Chloral Hydrate

MEDICATIONS AND VACCINES

41070	Ergotamine + Belladonna + Phenobarbital (Bellergal)		41213	Ferrous Gluconate
			41214	Ferrous Sulfate
41180	Methaqualone (Quaalude)		41215	Ferrous Sulfate, Exsiccated
41181	Methaqualone Hydrochloride (Parest)		48633	Ferrous Sulfate + Vitamin C
			48631	Ferrous Sulfate + Folic Acid + Vitamin C
41182	Paraldehyde			
42646	Estazolam (ProSom)		48632	Ferrous Sulfate + Vitamin C + Vitamin B Complex
41183	Triazolam (Halcion)			
72531	Rohypnol (not approved for use in U.S.)		41216	Folic Acid
			41217	Intrinsic Factor Concentrate
41184	Sympathomimetics		41218	Iron & Ammonium Citrate
41185	Epinephrine		41219	Iron Choline Citrate (Ferrolip)
72543	Injection		41220	Iron Dextran Injection (Imferon)
41186	Isometheptane Mucate + Dichloralphenazone + Acetaminophen		41221	Iron Polysaccharide Complex
			48644	Iron Polysaccharide Complex + Folic Acid
41187	Nutritional		41222	Iron Preparations
41188	Absorbents		41223	Leucovorin, Calcium
41189	Activated Charcoal		72582	Injection
41190	Amino Acid preparations		41224	Infant Formulas
41191	L-Tryptophan		41225	Mineral Supplements
41192	Lysine		41226	Calcium
41193	Methionine		41227	Calcium & Calcium-Phosphorus Preparations
48737	Levocarnitine			
48738	Catecholamine Precursor		48736	Calcium Acetate
48739	L-Threonine		41228	Calcium (Oyster Shell)
41194	Protein & Calcium Preparations		41229	Calcium Glubionate
41195	Protein Hydrolysate		41230	Calcium Gluceptate
41196	Protein Preparations		41231	Calcium Gluconate
41197	Electrolytes		72577	Injection
41198	Salt Substitutes (Co-Salt)		41232	Calcium Glycerophosphate/ Calcium Lactate
41199	Sodium Chloride			
72683	Injection		72578	Injection
48596	Electrolyte Maintenance		41233	Calcium Lactate
41200	Fluorine preparations		41234	Calcium Pantothenate
41201	Sodium Fluoride		41235	Calcium-Protein Preparations
48798	Foods		41236	Copper Sulfate
41202	Specialized Foods		41237	Magnesium - Protein Complex
41203	Glucose (Dextrose)		41238	Magnesium Ascorbate
41204	High Nitrogen (Vivonex)		41239	Magnesium Gluconate
41205	High Protein		41240	Magnesium Oxide
41206	Medium Chain Triglycerides		41241	Magnesium Para Aminobenzoate
41207	Milk		41242	Magnesium Sulfate
41208	Yeast Preparations		41243	Manganese Chloride
41209	Hematinics		41244	Manganese Sulfate
41210	Ferric Pyrophosphate		41245	Phosphorus Preparations
41211	Ferrocholinate		41246	Zinc
41212	Ferrous Fumarate		41247	Zinc Sulfate
48637	Ferrous Fumarate + Vitamin C		41248	Zinc-Protein Complex
48638	Ferrous Fumarate + Folic Acid		41249	Parenteral Hyperalimentation
48641	Ferrous Fumarate + Intrinsic Factor		41250	Potassium preparations
48643	Ferrous Fumarate + Vitamin C + Vitamin B Complex		41251	Potassium Acetate
			41252	Potassium Bicarbonate

MEDICATIONS AND VACCINES

41253	Potassium Carbonate		41297	Vitamin B12
41254	Potassium Chloride		41298	Vitamin B2
41255	Potassium Citrate + Citric Acid		41299	Vitamin B6
41256	Potassium Gluconate + Potassium Chloride		41300	Vitamin C
			41301	Vitamin D
41257	Potassium Phosphate, Dibasic (Nutra-Phos-K)		41302	Vitamin D2 (Ergocalciferol)
			42121	D3 (Cholecalciferol)
41258	Potassium Phosphate, Monobasic (K-Phos)		42123	Calcifidiol (25 Hydroxy D3)
			42122	Calcitriol (1,25-Dihydroxy D3)
41259	Supplements, Dietary		72581	Injection
41260	Fatty Acids (Unsaturated)		41303	DHT (Dihydrotachysterol)
41261	Glucose Polymers		41304	Vitamin E
41262	Glutamic Acid		41305	Vitamin K
41263	Glutamic Acid Hydrochloride		41306	Vitamin K1
41265	Hydrochloric Acid Preparations		41307	Vitamin P
41264	Hesperidin Preparations		41308	Vitamins with Minerals
41266	Inositol		41309	Vitamins with Minerals, Therapeutic
41267	Liver Preparations		41870	Prenatal
41268	Liver, Dessicated		41310	Vitamins A & D
41269	Rutin		41311	Vitamins, Supplement
41270	Soybean Preparations		41312	Water-Soluble Vitamins
48437	Ubiquinone		41313	Vitamin B12 With Intrinsic Factor
41271	Vitamins		40533	Diphosphonate (EHDP)
41272	Bioflavonoids		48744	Etidronate Disodium
41273	Calciferol		72630	Injection
41274	Cocarboxylase		48742	Pamidronate Disodium
41275	Cyanocobalamin		72658	Injection
72702	Injection		71755	Aminobisphosphonate
41276	Dihydrotachysterol		71756	Alendronate sodium
41277	Ergocalciferol		41314	Ophthalmologicals
41278	Iodate Calcium		41315	Antiglaucoma agents
41279	Lecithin		48732	Methazolamide
41280	Menadiol Sodium Diphosphate (Synth. Vit. K)		41316	Acetazolamide (Diamox)
			44712	Dichlorphenamide (Daranide)
74288	Injection		41892	Pilocarpine (Pilocar)
48395	Multivitamins		41336	Timolol (Timoptic)
41281	Multivitamins with Fluoride		41317	Echothiphate Iodide
70564	Multivitamins with iron		41318	Epinephrine Bitartrate (Epitrate)
41282	Niacin		71920	Dorzolamide HCl (Trusopt)
41283	Niacinamide		75163	Latanoprost
41284	Nicotinic Acid		41893	Tetrahydrocannabinol
41285	Pantothenate, Calcium		41319	Antiherpes
41286	Para-Aminobenzoate, Potassium		41320	Idoxuridine (Stoxil)
41287	Phytonadione (AquaMEPHYTON)		48439	Trifluridine
41288	Potassium Sulfate		41321	Vidarabine
41289	Pyridoxine HCl		41322	Mydriatics
41290	Thiamine HCl		41323	Hydroxyamphetamine Hydrobromide
41291	Thiamine Mononitrate			
41292	Vitamin (Therapeutic)		41324	Phenylephrine HCl (Neo-Synephrine)
41293	Vitamin A			
41294	Vitamin B Complex		41325	Optic Opacities
41295	Vitamin B Complex with Vitamin C		41326	Anesthetic
41296	Vitamin B1		41327	Proparacaine HCl (Ophthaine)

MEDICATIONS AND VACCINES

41328	Anti-Inflammatory	41353	Isocarboxazid (Marplan)
41329	Prednisolone Acetate (Metimyd)	42336	Tranylcypromine Sulfate (Parnate)
72667	Injection	41356	Phenelzine Sulfate (Nardil)
41330	Prednisolone Sodium Phosphate	44434	Maprotiline HCl
	(Optimyd)	41411	Perphenazine + Amitriptyline HCl
72666	Injection	44440	Sertraline HCl (Zoloft)
41331	Dexamethasone Sodium Phosphate	41860	Trazodone HCl
	(Decadron)	44435	Trimipramine Maleate (Surmontil)
48687	Dexamethasone Sodium Phosphate +	41358	Antihypnotics
	Neomycin Sulfate	41359	Antimanic
41332	Other	41360	Lithium Carbonate
41333	Artificial Tears	44430	Lithium Citrate
48733	Tetrahydrozoline HCl + Glycerin	41394	Anxiolytics
41334	Chymotrypsin (Alpha Chymar)	41395	Benzodiazepines
41335	Silver Nitrate	41827	Alprazolam (Xanax)
41337	Otic Preparations	41396	Chlordiazepoxide
41338	Acetic Acid	72647	Injection
41339	Antipyrine + Benzocaine	41397	Chlordiazepoxide + Amitriptyline
41340	Boric Acid		HCl
44720	Cortisporin	41891	Chlordiazepoxide HCl + clidinium
41341	Glycerin Dehydrated		bromide (Librax)
41342	Parachlorometaxylenol (Orlex)	44432	Chlordiazepoxide HCl + estrogens
41343	Propylene Glycol		(Menrium)
41344	Triethanolamine Polypeptide Oleate-	41398	Clorazepate Dipotassium
	Condensate	41399	Clorazepate Monopotassium
41345	Hydrogen Peroxide		(Azene)
48734	Naphazoline HCl + Pheniramine	41400	Diazepam (Valium)
	Maleate	72696	Injection
41346	Psychotropic agents	41401	Lorazepam
41347	Antidepressants	72650	Injection
44433	Amoxapine (Asendin)	41403	Prazepam (Centrax)
41349	Benactyzine Hydrochloride +	44707	Short-Acting Benzodiazepines
	Meprobamate	44706	Midazolam (Versed)
42337	Bupropion (Wellbutrin)	41402	Oxazepam
41405	Desipramine Hydrochloride	45438	Benzodiazepine Antagonists
41350	Ergot Alkaloids (Hydrogenated)	45439	Flumazenil (Mazicon)
45936	Venlafaxine HCl	41861	Buspirone (BuSpar)
42335	Fluoxetine Hydrochloride (Prozac)	41404	Chlormezanone (Trancopal)
71914	Fluvoxamine maleate	41407	Droperidol
48446	Paroxetine Hydrochloride	72639	Injection
75162	Mirtazapine	41410	Meprobamate
44715	Tricyclics	48694	Meprobamate + Aspirin
41348	Amitriptyline Hydrochloride	41381	Hypnotics
72624	Injection	41382	Ethclorvynol (Placidyl)
41406	Doxepin Hydrochloride	41383	Ethinamate (Valmid)
41978	Clomipramine	41384	Flurazepam Hydrochloride
41351	Imipramine Hydrochloride		(Dalmane)
72692	Injection	41385	Glutethimide (Doriden)
41352	Imipramine Pamoate (Tofranil-	41386	Methyprylon
	PM)	48426	Propofol
41355	Nortriptyline HCl	48427	Quazepam
41357	Protriptyline HCl (Vivactil)	41387	Sodium Thiopental
41354	Monoamine - Oxidase Inhibitors	48429	Temazepam

MEDICATIONS AND VACCINES

41388	Triclofos Sodium	48577	Desogestrel + Ethinyl Estradiol
48425	Zolpidem Tartrate	41418	Ethinyl Estradiol
41389	Psychostimulants	41419	Ethynodial Diacetate
41390	Amphetamine Resin (Biphetamine)	48647	Ethynodial Diacetate + Ethinyl Estradiol
41391	Amphetamine Sulfate (Benzedrine)	48578	Levonorgestrel + Ethinyl Estradiol
41392	Dextroamphetamine Sulfate (Dexedrine)	41421	Mestranol Preparations
41393	Dextroamphetamine Tannate	41424	Norethindrone Preparations
41361	Antipsychotics	48648	Norethindrone + Ethinyl Estradiol
72210	Traditional	48650	Norethindrone + Mestranol
41362	Acetophenazine Maleate (Tindal)	48652	Norethindrone Acetate + Ethinyl Estradiol
41363	Butyrophenone		
41364	Chlorpromazine (Thorazine)	41425	Norethynodrel
41365	Chlorpromazine Hydrochloride	48579	Norgestimate + Ethinyl Estradiol
74287	Injection	41426	Norgestrel
41366	Chlorprothixene (Taractan)	48654	Norgestrel + Ethinyl Estradiol
41367	Fluphenazine Decanoate (Prolixin)	42627	Levenorgestrel Implants (Norplant)
		41422	Nonoxynol-9 (Delfen)
72669	Injection	41423	Nonyl Phenoxy Polyoxyethylene Ethanol
41368	Fluphenazine Enanthate		
41369	Fluphenazine Hydrochloride	41427	Octoxynol
41370	Haloperidol (Haldol)	41428	P-diisobutylphenoxypolyethoxyethanol (Ortho-gynol)
72633	Injection		
44429	Haloperidol Decanoate (Haldol)		
72634	Injection	41429	Vaginal Diaphragm & Apparatus
41371	Loxapine Hydrochloride (Loxitane)	41420	Intra-Uterine Devices
		42331	Copper-7
41372	Loxapine Succinate	42332	Progestasert
41373	Mesoridazine (Serentil)	42333	Dalkon Shield
41374	Molindone Hydrochloride	42323	Progesterone Inhibitors
41375	Phenothiazine Derivatives	42322	Mifepristone (RU 486)
44441	Pimozide (Orap)	41430	Fertility Agents
41376	Piperacetazine (Quide)	41431	Clomiphene Citrate (Clomid)
41377	Thioridazine	43333	Menotropins (Pergonal)
41378	Thiothixene	48587	Urofollitropin
72656	Injection	41432	Oxytocics
41379	Trifluoperazine HCl (Stelazine)	41433	Methylergonovine Maleate
41380	Triflupromazine (Vesprin)	72654	Injection
72700	Injection	41434	Oxytocin (Injection)
72211	Novel	41435	Oxytocin (Nasal Spray)
44431	Clozapine (Clozaril)	41436	Oxytocin Citrate-Oral
45937	Risperidone (Risperdal)	41437	Premenstrual Therapeutics
75212	Sertindole (Serlect)	41438	Pamabrom (Sunril)
75213	Olanzapine (Zyprexa)	41439	Uterine Contractants
72529	Anti-Obesity Agents	41440	Ergonovine Maleate
72530	Dexfenfluramine HCl	72625	Injection
41412	Reproductive System Agents	41441	Vaginal Preparations
41413	Antigonadotropin	41442	Aminacrine Hydrochloride (Vagilia)
41414	Contraceptives	41443	Aminacrine Preparations (Vagitrol)
41415	Cervical Caps (Rubber)	48589	Butoconazole Nitrate
41416	Condoms	48800	Conception Aid
41417	Dodecaethyleneglycol	41444	Candicidin
44742	Oral	41445	Chlordantoin

MEDICATIONS AND VACCINES

70370	clindamycin phosphate (Cleocin Cream)
41446	Clotrimazole
48794	Clotrimazole + Betamethasone Dipropionate
41447	Dienestrol
41448	Gentian Violet
70371	metronidazole gel (Metro-Gel)
41449	Miconazole Nitrate
41450	Nystatin
41451	Phenylmercuric Acetate
41452	Protozoacides
41453	Ricinoleic Acid
41454	Sodium Borate (Trichotine)
41455	Sulfathiazole + Sulfacetamide + Sulfabenzamide
41456	Sulfanilamide
48590	Terconazole
48799	Therapeutic Jelly
48591	Tioconazole
41457	Respiratory Agents
41458	Antiasthmatic
41461	Cromolyn Sodium
48453	Nedocromil Sodium
75154	Fluticasone propionate
41463	Ephedrine
41464	Ephedrine Hydrochloride
41465	Ephedrine Sulfate
48782	Ephedrine Sulfate + Theophylline + Hydroxyzine HCl
41466	Ephedrine Tannate
41467	Ethylnorepinephrine Hydrochloride
48684	Dyphylline + Guaifenesin
41468	Bronchodilators
41470	Albuterol
71051	Salmeterol (Serevent)
48592	Bitolterol Mesylate
41473	Isoetharine (Bronkosol)
41474	Isoproterenol Preparations (Isuprel)
41475	Metaproterenol Sulfate
71052	Formoterol
41885	Pirbuterol (Maxair)
41477	Protokylol HCl (Ventaire)
41478	Terbutaline Sulfate
72688	Injection
41931	Ipratropium Bromide (Atrovent)
41471	Epinephrine Bitartrate
41472	Epinephrine Racemic
41479	Theophylline
72679	Injection
48645	Theophylline + Guaifenesin
41480	Theophylline Calcium Salicylate
41481	Theophylline Monoethanolamine

41482	Theophylline Sodium Glycinate
48788	Theophylline Sodium Glycinate + Guaifenesin
41459	Aminophylline
41469	Choline Theophyllinate
48454	Oxtriphylline
41483	Xanthine Preparations
41476	Nebulizers (Norisodrin)
41484	Decongestants
41485	Chlorcyclizine Hydrochloride
41486	Oxymetazoline HCl
41487	Phenindamine Tartrate (Nolamine)
41488	Phenylephrine
41489	Phenyltoloxamine Citrate (Sinutab)
41490	Propylhexadrine
41491	Tetrahydrozoline HCl
41492	Thenyldiamine HCl
41493	Xylometazoline HCl (Otrivin)
41494	Expectorants
48593	Iodinated Glycerol
41495	Noscapine
48804	Phenylephrine Tannate + Chlorpheniramine Tannate + Pyrilamine Tannate
41496	Potassium Guaiacolsulfonate
41497	Potassium Iodide (SSKI)
41498	Promethazine HCl
48698	Phenylphrine HCl + Promethazine HCl
48770	Promethazine HCl + Phenylphrine HCl + Codeine
41499	Tripelennamine Preparations
41500	Inhalants
41501	Ammonia
41502	Saline
41503	Mucolytics
41504	Acetylcysteine (Mucomyst)
45935	Pulmozyme
41505	Respiratory Stimulants
41506	Doxapram Hydrochloride (Dopram)
41507	Nikethamide (Coramine)
41508	Sclerosing Agents
41509	Urological Agents
41510	Antienuresis Agents
41512	Antispasmodics
41513	Flavoxate Hydrochloride (Urispas)
41514	Hyoscyamine
41515	Hyoscyamine Sulfate
41516	Hyoscyamus Preparations
41517	Oxybutynin Chloride (Ditropan)
41518	Antibacterial
41519	Benzoic Acid
41520	Methenamine

MEDICATIONS AND VACCINES

41521	Methenamine Hippurate
41522	Methenamine Mandelate
41523	Methylene Blue
41524	Nalidixic Acid
41525	Nitrofurantoin
41526	Oxolinic Acid (Utibid)
48785	Oxytetracycline HCl + Sulfamethizole + Phenazopyridine HCl
41527	Phenazopyridine
41528	Phenazopyridine HCl
41529	Phenyl Salicylate
41530	Sulfacytine
41531	Sulfadiazine
41532	Sulfameter
41533	Sulfamethizole
41536	Urinary Acidifiers
41537	Potassium Acid Phosphate
41538	Sodium Acid Phosphate
41539	Sodium Phosphate, Monobasic
41540	Urinary Alkalinizing agents
41541	Sodium Citrate + Citric Acid
48594	Potassium Citrate + Sodium Citrate + Citric Acid
41542	Urinary Tract Analgesics
48752	Dimethyl Sulfoxide
72621	Injection
41543	Urological Irrigants
48705	Aminohippurate Sodium
48712	Anti-Hemorrhagic Cystitis Agents
48713	Mesna
48717	Contrast Agents
48718	Iohexol
48723	Gadolinium
48722	Gadopentetate Dimegumine
48745	Scanning Isotopes
48746	Gallium Nitrate
42024	**Administration Of Anesthesia**
42025	HEENT
42938	For Procedures On Skin Of Head
42939	For Repair Of Cleft Lip
72553	For Blepharoplasty
42940	For Electroconvulsive Therapy
42941	For Ear Procedures
42942	Otoscopy
42943	Tympanotomy
42944	For Eye Procedures
42945	Lens Surgery
42946	Corneal Transplant
42947	Vitrectomy
42948	Iridectomy
42949	Ophthalmoscopy
42950	For Procedures On Nose And Sinuses
42951	Radical Surgery
42952	Soft Tissue Biopsy
42953	For Oral Cavity Procedures
42954	Repair Of Cleft Palate
42955	Excision Of Retropharyngeal Tumor
42956	Radical Surgery
42957	For Procedures On Facial Bones
42958	Radical Surgery
43251	Jaw Reduction
42959	For Intracranial Procedures
42960	Subdural Taps
42961	Burr Holes
72556	Elevation Of Depressed Skull Fracture
42962	Vascular Procedures
42963	Procedures In Sitting Position
42964	Spinal Fluid Shunting Procedures
42965	Electrocoagulation Of Intracranial Nerve
42966	Neck
42967	For Procedures On Skin And Subcutaneous Tissue
42968	For Procedures On Deep Neck Structures
43009	Thyroid Aspiration Biopsy
43010	For Procedures On Major Neck Vessels
43011	Simple Ligation
43012	Thorax
43013	Procedures On Skin And Tissue Of Anterior Chest
43014	Reconstructive Procedures on Breast
43015	Radical Or Modified Radical Mastectomy
43016	With Internal Mammary Node Dissection
43017	For Elective Cardioversion
43018	Procedures On Skin And Tissue Of Upper Back
43019	Procedures On Clavicle And Scapula
43020	Radical Surgery
43021	Clavicular Biopsy
43022	For Partial Rib Resection
43023	For Thoracoplasty
43024	For Radical Procedures
43025	Intrathoracic
43026	For Procedures On Esophagus
43027	For Closed Chest Procedures
43028	Needle Biopsy Of Pleura
43029	Thoracentesis
43030	Mediastinoscopy
43031	For Transvenous Pacemaker Insertion
72560	For Access To Central Venous Circulation

ANESTHESIA

72563	For Transvenous Insertion Of Defibrillator	43077	Radical Hysterectomy
43032	For Thoracotomy Procedures	43078	Pelvic Exenteration
43033	Decortication	43079	Cesarean Section
43034	Pleurectomy	43080	Caesarean Hysterectomy
43035	Pulmonary Resection With Thoracoplasty	43081	Epidural For Labor - Caesarean Section
43036	Intrathoracic Repair Of Tracheal Or Bronchial Trauma	43082	For Extraperitoneal Procedures
43037	For Procedures On Heart And Great Vessels	43083	Renal
43038	Without Cardiopulmonary Bypass	43084	Total Cystectomy
43039	With Cardiopulmonary Bypass	72569	Radical Prostatectomy
43040	For Heart Or Heart/Lung Transplant	43085	Adrenalectomy
43041	Spine And Spinal Cord	43086	Renal Transplant (Recipient)
43042	Cervical	43087	Cystolithotomy
43043	Posterior Laminectomy In Sitting Position	43088	For Lithotripsy
43044	Thoracic	43089	With Water Bath
43045	Thoracolumbar Sympathectomy	43090	Without Water Bath
43046	Lumbar	43091	For Procedures On Major Vessels
43047	Lumbar Sympathectomy	43092	Inferior Vena Cava Ligation
43048	Chemonucleolysis	43093	Transvenous Umbrella Insertion
43049	Extensive Procedures	43094	Perineum
43050	Upper Abdomen	43095	For Biopsy / Procedures On Skin
43051	For Procedures On Anterior Wall	43096	Anorectal
43052	Percutaneous Liver Biopsy	43097	Radical Perineal Procedure
43053	For Procedures On Posterior Wall	43098	Vulvectomy
43054	For Upper Endoscopy	43099	Perineal Prostatectomy
43055	For Hernia Repairs	43100	For Transurethral Procedures
43056	Lumbar	43252	Cystoscopy
43057	Ventral (Incisional)	43101	Resection Of Bladder Tumor(s)
43060	Diaphragmatic (Transabdominal Repair)	43102	Resection Of Prostate
43058	Wound Dehiscence	43103	Post-resection Bleeding
43059	Omphalocele	72573	Removal of Ureteral Calculus
43061	For Procedures On Major Blood Vessels	43104	For Procedures On Male Genitalia
43062	For Intraperitoneal Procedures	43105	Seminal Vesicles
43063	Partial Hepatectomy	43106	Undescended Testis
43064	Pancreatectomy	43107	Radical Orchiectomy (Inguinal)
43065	Liver Transplant (Recipient)	43108	Radical Orchiectomy (Abdominal)
43066	Lower Abdomen	43109	Orchiopexy
43067	For Procedures On Anterior Wall	43110	Amputation Of Penis
43068	Panniculectomy	43111	With Inguinal Lymphadenectomy
43069	For Laparoscopic Procedures	43112	With Inguinal And Iliac Lymphadenectomy
43070	For Lower Endoscopy	43113	Insertion Of Penile Prosthesis (Perineal Approach)
43071	For Procedures On Posterior Wall	43114	For Vaginal Procedures
43072	For Hernia Repairs	43253	Cervical / Endometrial Biopsy
43073	Ventral / Incisional	43115	Colpotomy / Colpectomy / Colporrhaphy
43074	For Intraperitoneal Procedures	43116	Vaginal Hysterectomy
43075	Amniocentesis	43117	Vaginal Delivery
43076	Abdominoperineal Resection	43118	Cervical Cerclage
		43119	Culdoscopy
		43120	Hysteroscopy
		43121	For Labor - Vaginal Delivery (Continuous Epidural)

ANESTHESIA

43122	Pelvis
43123	For Procedures On Anterior Skin
43124	For Procedures On Posterior Skin
43125	For Procedures On Bony Pelvis
43126	For Body Cast Application Or Revision
43127	For Hind Quarter Amputation
43128	For Radical Pelvic Tumor Procedures (Not Amputation)
43129	For Closed Procedures On Symphysis Pubis Or Sacroiliac Joint
43130	For Open Procedures On Symphysis Pubis Or Sacroiliac Joint
43131	For Obturator Neurectomy
43132	Extrapelvic
43133	Intrapelvic
43134	Upper Leg
43135	For Closed Procedures Involving Hip Joint
43136	For Arthroscopic Procedures Of Hip Joint
43137	For Open Procedures Involving Hip Joint
43138	Hip Disarticulation
43139	Total Hip Replacement Or Revision
43140	For Closed Procedures Of Upper 2/3 of Femur
43141	For Open Procedures Of Upper 2/3 of Femur
43142	Amputation
43143	Radical Resection
43144	For Procedures On Skin
43145	For Procedures On Neuromuscular / Connective Tissue
43146	For Procedures On Veins
43147	For Procedures On Arteries
43148	Femoral Artery Ligation
43149	Femoral Artery Embolectomy
43150	Knee And Popliteal Area
43151	For Procedures On Skin
43152	For Procedures On Neuromuscular / Connective Tissue
43153	For Closed Procedures Of Lower 1/3 Of Femur
43154	For Open Procedures Of Lower 1/3 Of Femur
43155	For Closed Procedures On Knee Joint
43159	For Open Procedures On Knee Joint
43160	Total Knee Replacement
43161	Disarticulation At Knee
43156	For Arthroscopic Procedures Of Knee Joint
43162	For Knee Casting Procedures
43157	Closed Procedures Of Upper Ends Of Tibia, Fibula Or Patella
43158	Open Procedures Of Upper Ends Of Tibia, Fibula Or Patella
43163	For Procedures On Veins Of Knee And Popliteal Area
43164	Arteriovenous Fistula
43165	For Procedures On Arteries Of Knee And Popliteal Area
43166	Popliteal Thromboendarterectomy
43167	Excision Of Aneuyrsm
43168	Aneurysm Repair
43169	Lower Leg / Ankle / Foot
43254	For Procedures On Skin
43172	For Procedures On Neuromuscular / Connective Tissue
43177	Repair Of Ruptured Achilles Tendon
43178	Gastrocnemius Recession (Strayer Procedure)
43171	For Closed Procedures
43255	For Arthroscopic Procedures Of Joint
43173	For Open Procedures On Bones
43174	Radical Resection
43175	Osteotomy / Osteoplasty
43176	Total Ankle Replacement
43179	For Casting Procedures
43180	For Procedures On Veins
43181	Venous Thrombectomy
43182	For Procedures On Arteries
43183	Embolectomy
43184	Shoulder And Axilla
43170	For Procedures On Skin
43185	For Procedures On Neuromuscular / Connective Tissue
43186	For Closed Procedures
43192	For Arthroscopic Procedures Of Joint
43187	For Open Procedures On Bones
43188	Radical Resection
43189	Shoulder Disarticulation
43190	Forequarter Amputation
43191	Total Shoulder Replacement
43193	For Casting Procedures
43195	Shoulder Spica
43194	For Procedures On Veins
43196	For Procedures On Arteries
43197	Axillary-brachial Aneurysm Repair
43198	Bypass Graft
43199	Axillary-femoral
43200	Upper Arm And Elbow
43201	For Procedures On Skin
43202	For Procedures On Neuromuscular / Connective Tissue
43203	Open Tenotomy, Elbow To Shoulder

ANESTHESIA

43204	Tenoplasty, Elbow To Shoulder
43205	Tenodesis, Rupture Of Long Tendon Of Biceps
43206	For Closed Procedures
43213	For Arthroscopic Procedures Of Joint
43207	For Open Procedures On Bone Or Joint
43208	Osteotomy Of Humerus
43209	Repair Of Union Of Humerus
43210	Radical Procedures
43211	Excision Of Cyst Or Tumor
43212	Total Elbow Replacement
43214	For Procedures On Veins
43215	Repair
43216	For Procedures On Arteries
43217	Embolectomy
72579	For Repair of A-V Fistula
43218	Forearm / Wrist / Hand
43219	For Procedures On Skin
43220	For Procedures On Neuromuscular / Connective Tissue
43221	For Closed Procedures
43222	For Open Procedures On Bone Or Joint
43223	Total Wrist Replacement
43224	For Casting Procedures
43225	For Procedures On Veins
43226	Repair
43227	For Vascular Shunt Procedure
43228	For Procedures On Arteries
43229	Embolectomy
43230	For Radiological Procedures
43231	For Injection For Hysterosalpingography
43232	For Burr Hole(s) For Ventriculography
43233	For Injection For Pneumoencephalography
43234	For Injection For Myelography
43235	Lumbar
43236	Cervical
43237	Posterior Fossa
43238	For Injection For Discography
43239	Lumbar
43240	Cervical
43241	For Arteriogram (Needle)
43242	Carotid Or Vertebral
43243	Retrograde, Brachial Or Femoral
43244	For Cardiac Catheterization (Not Swan-Ganz)
43245	For Angioplasty
43246	For CT / MRI Scan
43247	For Ongoing Epidural / Intrathecal Drug Administration
43248	Regional IV Administration (Extremities)
43249	Physiological Support For Organ Harvesting
43250	Unlisted Procedure
72587	Patient Over Seventy
72588	Patient Under One Year
72590	Utilization Of Total Body Hypothermia
72593	Utilization Of Controlled Hypotension
72597	Under Emergency Conditions
75137	**Office And Lab Procedures**
72113	Dental Procedures
75215	Cleaning
75216	Filling
75217	Capping
75218	Root Canal
75219	Bridge Work
75220	Peridontal
42617	Cardiovascular Procedures
41805	Endocarditis Prophylaxis
42644	Physician Supervision Of Outpatient Cardiac Rehab Session
42645	With Continuous ECG Monitoring
40095	Elective Cardioversion
71237	Tilt Table Evaluation
48840	Adjustment of Cardiac Pacemaker
46021	Pacemaker Placement
42598	Temporary
42599	Transvenous
49573	Dual Chamber
42600	Transcutaneous
41607	Permanent
42592	Transvenous Electrode
42593	Atrial
42594	Ventricular
41828	Dual-chamber
42602	Subsequent Electrode Replacement
49576	Dual Chamber
42603	Subsequent Electrode Repositioning
42604	Insert Pulse Generator
42601	Replace Pulse Generator
49574	Dual Chamber
49575	Upgrade Single To Dual Chamber
42605	Repair Electrodes
49577	Dual Chamber
42606	Repair Electrodes And Replace Generator
42595	Epicardial Electrode
42596	By Thoracotomy
42597	By Xiphoid Approach
42614	Skin Pocket Revision / Relocation

OFFICE & LAB PROCEDURES, CONT.

71238	Electronic Analysis Of	46743	Distal RCA
	Antitachycardia Pacemaker	46744	AMV-1
42607	Remove Permanent Pacemaker	46745	AMV-2
49559	And Single Lead Transvenous	46746	R Posterolat Seg
	Electrode	46747	R Posterolat-1
49560	And Dual Lead Transvenous	46748	R Posterolat-2
	Electrodes	46749	R Posterolat-3
49564	And Transvenous Electrodes By	46750	Left PDA
	Thoracotomy	46751	Right PDA
49561	Remove Permanent Epicardial	46752	LIMA Graft
	Pacemaker By Thoracacotomy	46753	RIMA Graft
49562	Single Lead	46754	SVG-1
49563	Dual Lead	46755	SVG-2
41605	Cardiac Catheterization	46756	SVG-3
43259	Catheter Ablation	46757	SVG-4
43257	Arrhythmogenic Focus	46794	Initial Obstruction (%)
49597	For Ventricular Tachycardia	46795	Thrombus Visualized
43258	Arrhythmogenic Bypass Tracts	46796	Thrombolytic Agent
49598	For Ventricular Tachycardia	46807	Streptokinase
44744	Arrhythmogenic Bypass Tracts -	46808	TIMI Protocol Drugs
	RF - Fluoroscopic Guidance	46809	Urokinase
49599	For Ventricular Tachycardia	46810	tPA
44745	Arrhythmogenic Bypass Tracts -	46797	Outcome
	RF - Echocardiogram Guidance	46798	Successful
49600	For Ventricular Tachycardia	46799	Residual Stenosis
44899	His Ablation	38165	Unsuccessful
49596	Atrioventricular Node	46800	Flow Restoration Time
42624	Coronary Thrombolysis	46801	From Onset Of Drug Infusion
42625	Intracoronary Infusion	46802	From Onset Of Procedure
42626	Intravenous Infusion	74615	From Onset Of Symptoms
46016	Coronary Reperfusion	46803	Complications
46720	Culprit Lesion	46804	Hematoma
46721	Site	46805	Bleeding
46723	Left Main	46806	Stroke
46724	Prox LAD	46722	Non-culprit Lesion
46725	Mid LAD	46758	Site
46726	Dist LAD	46759	Left Main
46727	Diag-1	46760	Prox LAD
46728	Diag-2	46761	Mid LAD
46729	Septal-1	46762	Dist LAD
46730	Intermed Br	46763	Diag-1
46731	Prox Circ	46764	Diag-2
46732	Dist Circ	46765	Septal-1
46733	OM-1	46766	Intermed Br
46734	OM-2	46767	Prox Circ
46735	OM-3	46768	Dist Circ
46736	L AV Groove	46769	OM-1
46737	L Postlat Seg	46770	OM-2
46738	L Postlat-1	46771	OM-3
46739	L Postlat-2	46772	L AV Groove
46740	L Postlat-3	46773	L Postlat Seg
46741	Proximal RCA	46774	L Postlat-1
46742	Middle RCA	46775	L Postlat-2

OFFICE & LAB PROCEDURES, CONT.

46776	L Postlat-3	47721	Duration (sec)
46777	Proximal RCA	47798	Last Inflation Parameters
46778	Middle RCA	47799	Balloon Size (mm)
46779	Distal RCA	47800	Pressure (ATM)
46780	AMV-1	47801	Duration (sec)
46781	AMV-2	47802	Number of Inflations
46782	R Posterolat Seg	46054	Severity Of Stenosis
46783	R Posterolat-1	46055	Preprocedure
46784	R Posterolat-2	46056	Postprocedure
46785	R Posterolat-3	46057	Gradient
46786	Left PDA	46058	Preprocedure
46787	Right PDA	46061	Postprocedure
46788	LIMA Graft	46063	Assessment
46789	RIMA Graft	46064	Successful
46790	SVG-1	46065	Poor Distal Runoff
46791	SVG-2	46066	Lesion Could Not Be
46792	SVG-3		Crossed
46793	SVG-4	48980	Lesion Could Not Be Dilated
46811	Initial Obstruction (%)	46067	Intracoronary Thrombus
46812	Thrombus Visualized	46068	Complications
46813	Thrombolytic Agent	46069	Intimal Tear
46814	Streptokinase	46070	Dissection
46815	TIMI Protocol Drugs	46071	Perforation
46816	Urokinase	46072	Total Occlusion
46817	tPA	46073	Branch Vessel Occlusion
46818	Outcome	46074	Balloon Rupture
46819	Successful	46075	Catheter Transection
46820	Residual Stenosis	46025	Proximal Left Anterior
46821	Flow Restoration Time		Descending Artery
46822	From Onset Of Drug Infusion	46076	Lesion Classification
46823	From Onset Of Procedure	46104	High Probability of Success
46824	Complications		(>85%); Low Risk
46825	Hematoma	46132	Moderate Probability of
46826	Bleeding		Success (60-85%); Moderate
46827	Stroke		Risk
41610	Transluminal coronary angioplasty	46159	Low Probability of Success
	(PTCA)		(<60%); High Risk
44798	Emergency Procedure	47806	First Inflation Parameters
48868	Elective Procedure	47807	Balloon Size (mm)
75142	Same Day As Diagnostic	47808	Pressure (ATM)
	Catheterization	47809	Duration (sec)
46024	Left Main Artery	47810	Last Inflation Parameters
46053	Lesion Classification	47811	Balloon Size (mm)
46059	High Probability of Success	47812	Pressure (ATM)
	(>85%); Low Risk	47813	Duration (sec)
46060	Moderate Probability of	47814	Number of Inflations
	Success (60-85%); Moderate	46187	Severity Of Stenosis
	Risk	46215	Preprocedure
46062	Low Probability of Success	46243	Postprocedure
	(<60%); High Risk	46271	Gradient
47717	First Inflation Parameters	46299	Preprocedure
47719	Balloon Size (mm)	46327	Postprocedure
47720	Pressure (ATM)	46355	Assessment

OFFICE & LAB PROCEDURES, CONT.

46383	Successful	46674	Catheter Transection
46402	Poor Distal Runoff	46027	Distal Left Anterior Descending
46421	Lesion Could Not Be		Artery
	Crossed	46078	Lesion Classification
48981	Lesion Could Not Be Dilated	46106	High Probability of Success
46449	Intracoronary Thrombus		(>85%); Low Risk
46477	Complications	46134	Moderate Probability of
46505	Intimal Tear		Success (60-85%); Moderate
46533	Dissection		Risk
46561	Perforation	46161	Low Probability of Success
46589	Total Occlusion		(<60%); High Risk
46617	Branch Vessel Occlusion	47830	First Inflation Parameters
46645	Balloon Rupture	47831	Balloon Size (mm)
46673	Catheter Transection	47832	Pressure (ATM)
46026	Mid-Left Anterior Descending	47833	Duration (sec)
	Artery	47834	Last Inflation Parameters
46077	Lesion Classification	47835	Balloon Size (mm)
46105	High Probability of Success	47836	Pressure (ATM)
	(>85%); Low Risk	47837	Duration (sec)
46133	Moderate Probability of	47838	Number of Inflations
	Success (60-85%); Moderate	46189	Severity Of Stenosis
	Risk	46217	Preprocedure
46160	Low Probability of Success	46245	Postprocedure
	(<60%); High Risk	46273	Gradient
47818	First Inflation Parameters	46301	Preprocedure
47819	Balloon Size (mm)	46329	Postprocedure
47820	Pressure (ATM)	46357	Assessment
47821	Duration (sec)	46385	Successful
47822	Last Inflation Parameters	46404	Poor Distal Runoff
47823	Balloon Size (mm)	46423	Lesion Could Not Be
47824	Pressure (ATM)		Crossed
47825	Duration (sec)	48983	Lesion Could Not Be Dilated
47826	Number of Inflations	46451	Intracoronary Thrombus
46188	Severity Of Stenosis	46479	Complications
46216	Preprocedure	46507	Intimal Tear
46244	Postprocedure	46535	Dissection
46272	Gradient	46563	Perforation
46300	Preprocedure	46591	Total Occlusion
46328	Postprocedure	46619	Branch Vessel Occlusion
46356	Assessment	46647	Balloon Rupture
46384	Successful	46675	Catheter Transection
46403	Poor Distal Runoff	46028	First Diagonal Branch
46422	Lesion Could Not Be	46079	Lesion Classification
	Crossed	46107	High Probability of Success
48982	Lesion Could Not Be Dilated		(>85%); Low Risk
46450	Intracoronary Thrombus	46135	Moderate Probability of
46478	Complications		Success (60-85%); Moderate
46506	Intimal Tear		Risk
46534	Dissection	46162	Low Probability of Success
46562	Perforation		(<60%); High Risk
46590	Total Occlusion	47842	First Inflation Parameters
46618	Branch Vessel Occlusion	47843	Balloon Size (mm)
46646	Balloon Rupture	47844	Pressure (ATM)

OFFICE & LAB PROCEDURES, CONT.

47845	Duration (sec)	46406	Poor Distal Runoff
47846	Last Inflation Parameters	46425	Lesion Could Not Be
47847	Balloon Size (mm)		Crossed
47848	Pressure (ATM)	48985	Lesion Could Not Be Dilated
47849	Duration (sec)	46453	Intracoronary Thrombus
47850	Number of Inflations	46481	Complications
46190	Severity Of Stenosis	46509	Intimal Tear
46218	Preprocedure	46537	Dissection
46246	Postprocedure	46565	Perforation
46274	Gradient	46593	Total Occlusion
46302	Preprocedure	46621	Branch Vessel Occlusion
46330	Postprocedure	46649	Balloon Rupture
46358	Assessment	46677	Catheter Transection
46386	Successful	46030	First Anterior Septal Branch
46405	Poor Distal Runoff	46081	Lesion Classification
46424	Lesion Could Not Be	46109	High Probability of Success
	Crossed		(>85%); Low Risk
48984	Lesion Could Not Be Dilated	46137	Moderate Probability of
46452	Intracoronary Thrombus		Success (60-85%); Moderate
46480	Complications		Risk
46508	Intimal Tear	46164	Low Probability of Success
46536	Dissection		(<60%); High Risk
46564	Perforation	47866	First Inflation Parameters
46592	Total Occlusion	47867	Balloon Size (mm)
46620	Branch Vessel Occlusion	47868	Pressure (ATM)
46648	Balloon Rupture	47869	Duration (sec)
46676	Catheter Transection	47870	Last Inflation Parameters
46029	Second Diagonal Branch	47871	Balloon Size (mm)
46080	Lesion Classification	47872	Pressure (ATM)
46108	High Probability of Success	47873	Duration (sec)
	(>85%); Low Risk	47874	Number of Inflations
46136	Moderate Probability of	46192	Severity Of Stenosis
	Success (60-85%); Moderate	46220	Preprocedure
	Risk	46248	Postprocedure
46163	Low Probability of Success	46276	Gradient
	(<60%); High Risk	46304	Preprocedure
47854	First Inflation Parameters	46332	Postprocedure
47855	Balloon Size (mm)	46360	Assessment
47856	Pressure (ATM)	46388	Successful
47857	Duration (sec)	46407	Poor Distal Runoff
47858	Last Inflation Parameters	46426	Lesion Could Not Be
47859	Balloon Size (mm)		Crossed
47860	Pressure (ATM)	48986	Lesion Could Not Be Dilated
47861	Duration (sec)	46454	Intracoronary Thrombus
47862	Number of Inflations	46482	Complications
46191	Severity Of Stenosis	46510	Intimal Tear
46219	Preprocedure	46538	Dissection
46247	Postprocedure	46566	Perforation
46275	Gradient	46594	Total Occlusion
46303	Preprocedure	46622	Branch Vessel Occlusion
46331	Postprocedure	46650	Balloon Rupture
46359	Assessment	46678	Catheter Transection
46387	Successful	46031	Intermedius Branch

OFFICE & LAB PROCEDURES, CONT.

46082	Lesion Classification	47896	Pressure (ATM)
46110	High Probability of Success	47897	Duration (sec)
	(>85%); Low Risk	47898	Number of Inflations
46138	Moderate Probability of	46194	Severity Of Stenosis
	Success (60-85%); Moderate	46222	Preprocedure
	Risk	46250	Postprocedure
46165	Low Probability of Success	46278	Gradient
	(<60%); High Risk	46306	Preprocedure
47878	First Inflation Parameters	46334	Postprocedure
47879	Balloon Size (mm)	46362	Assessment
47880	Pressure (ATM)	46390	Successful
47881	Duration (sec)	46409	Poor Distal Runoff
47882	Last Inflation Parameters	46428	Lesion Could Not Be
47883	Balloon Size (mm)		Crossed
47884	Pressure (ATM)	48988	Lesion Could Not Be Dilated
47885	Duration (sec)	46456	Intracoronary Thrombus
47886	Number of Inflations	46484	Complications
46193	Severity Of Stenosis	46512	Intimal Tear
46221	Preprocedure	46540	Dissection
46249	Postprocedure	46568	Perforation
46277	Gradient	46596	Total Occlusion
46305	Preprocedure	46624	Branch Vessel Occlusion
46333	Postprocedure	46652	Balloon Rupture
46361	Assessment	46680	Catheter Transection
46389	Successful	46033	Distal Circumflex
46408	Poor Distal Runoff	46084	Lesion Classification
46427	Lesion Could Not Be	46112	High Probability of Success
	Crossed		(>85%); Low Risk
48987	Lesion Could Not Be Dilated	46140	Moderate Probability of
46455	Intracoronary Thrombus		Success (60-85%); Moderate
46483	Complications		Risk
46511	Intimal Tear	46167	Low Probability of Success
46539	Dissection		(<60%); High Risk
46567	Perforation	47902	First Inflation Parameters
46595	Total Occlusion	47903	Balloon Size (mm)
46623	Branch Vessel Occlusion	47904	Pressure (ATM)
46651	Balloon Rupture	47905	Duration (sec)
46679	Catheter Transection	47906	Last Inflation Parameters
46032	Proximal Circumflex	47907	Balloon Size (mm)
46083	Lesion Classification	47908	Pressure (ATM)
46111	High Probability of Success	47909	Duration (sec)
	(>85%); Low Risk	47910	Number of Inflations
46139	Moderate Probability of	46195	Severity Of Stenosis
	Success (60-85%); Moderate	46223	Preprocedure
	Risk	46251	Postprocedure
46166	Low Probability of Success	46279	Gradient
	(<60%); High Risk	46307	Preprocedure
47890	First Inflation Parameters	46335	Postprocedure
47891	Balloon Size (mm)	46363	Assessment
47892	Pressure (ATM)	46701	Successful
47893	Duration (sec)	46710	Poor Distal Runoff
47894	Last Inflation Parameters	46429	Lesion Could Not Be
47895	Balloon Size (mm)		Crossed

OFFICE & LAB PROCEDURES, CONT.

48989	Lesion Could Not Be Dilated	46142	Moderate Probability of Success (60-85%); Moderate Risk
46457	Intracoronary Thrombus		
46485	Complications		
46513	Intimal Tear	46169	Low Probability of Success (<60%); High Risk
46541	Dissection		
46569	Perforation	47926	First Inflation Parameters
46597	Total Occlusion	47927	Balloon Size (mm)
46625	Branch Vessel Occlusion	47928	Pressure (ATM)
46653	Balloon Rupture	47929	Duration (sec)
46681	Catheter Transection	47930	Last Inflation Parameters
46034	First Obtuse Marginal Branch	47931	Balloon Size (mm)
46085	Lesion Classification	47932	Pressure (ATM)
46113	High Probability of Success (>85%); Low Risk	47933	Duration (sec)
		47934	Number of Inflations
46141	Moderate Probability of Success (60-85%); Moderate Risk	46197	Severity Of Stenosis
		46225	Preprocedure
		46253	Postprocedure
46168	Low Probability of Success (<60%); High Risk	46281	Gradient
		46309	Preprocedure
47914	First Inflation Parameters	46337	Postprocedure
47915	Balloon Size (mm)	46365	Assessment
47916	Pressure (ATM)	46703	Successful
47917	Duration (sec)	46712	Poor Distal Runoff
47918	Last Inflation Parameters	46431	Lesion Could Not Be Crossed
47919	Balloon Size (mm)		
47920	Pressure (ATM)	48991	Lesion Could Not Be Dilated
47921	Duration (sec)	46459	Intracoronary Thrombus
47922	Number of Inflations	46487	Complications
46196	Severity Of Stenosis	46515	Intimal Tear
46224	Preprocedure	46543	Dissection
46252	Postprocedure	46571	Perforation
46280	Gradient	46599	Total Occlusion
46308	Preprocedure	46627	Branch Vessel Occlusion
46336	Postprocedure	46655	Balloon Rupture
46364	Assessment	46683	Catheter Transection
46702	Successful	46036	Third Obtuse Marginal Branch
46711	Poor Distal Runoff	46087	Lesion Classification
46430	Lesion Could Not Be Crossed	46115	High Probability of Success (>85%); Low Risk
48990	Lesion Could Not Be Dilated	46143	Moderate Probability of Success (60-85%); Moderate Risk
46458	Intracoronary Thrombus		
46486	Complications		
46514	Intimal Tear	46170	Low Probability of Success (<60%); High Risk
46542	Dissection		
46570	Perforation	47938	First Inflation Parameters
46598	Total Occlusion	47939	Balloon Size (mm)
46626	Branch Vessel Occlusion	47940	Pressure (ATM)
46654	Balloon Rupture	47941	Duration (sec)
46682	Catheter Transection	47942	Last Inflation Parameters
46035	Second Obtuse Marginal Branch	47943	Balloon Size (mm)
46086	Lesion Classification	47944	Pressure (ATM)
46114	High Probability of Success (>85%); Low Risk	47945	Duration (sec)
		47946	Number of Inflations

OFFICE & LAB PROCEDURES, CONT.

46198	Severity Of Stenosis
46226	Preprocedure
46254	Postprocedure
46282	Gradient
46310	Preprocedure
46338	Postprocedure
46366	Assessment
46704	Successful
46713	Poor Distal Runoff
46432	Lesion Could Not Be Crossed
48992	Lesion Could Not Be Dilated
46460	Intracoronary Thrombus
46488	Complications
46516	Intimal Tear
46544	Dissection
46572	Perforation
46600	Total Occlusion
46628	Branch Vessel Occlusion
46656	Balloon Rupture
46684	Catheter Transection
46037	Left Atrioventricular Groove Branch
46088	Lesion Classification
46116	High Probability of Success (>85%); Low Risk
46144	Moderate Probability of Success (60-85%); Moderate Risk
46171	Low Probability of Success (<60%); High Risk
47950	First Inflation Parameters
47951	Balloon Size (mm)
47952	Pressure (ATM)
47953	Duration (sec)
47954	Last Inflation Parameters
47955	Balloon Size (mm)
47956	Pressure (ATM)
47957	Duration (sec)
47958	Number of Inflations
46199	Severity Of Stenosis
46227	Preprocedure
46255	Postprocedure
46283	Gradient
46311	Preprocedure
46339	Postprocedure
46367	Assessment
46705	Successful
46714	Poor Distal Runoff
46433	Lesion Could Not Be Crossed
48993	Lesion Could Not Be Dilated
46461	Intracoronary Thrombus
46489	Complications
46517	Intimal Tear
46545	Dissection
46573	Perforation
46601	Total Occlusion
46629	Branch Vessel Occlusion
46657	Balloon Rupture
46685	Catheter Transection
46038	Left Posterolateral Segment
46089	Lesion Classification
46117	High Probability of Success (>85%); Low Risk
46145	Moderate Probability of Success (60-85%); Moderate Risk
46172	Low Probability of Success (<60%); High Risk
47962	First Inflation Parameters
47963	Balloon Size (mm)
47964	Pressure (ATM)
47965	Duration (sec)
47966	Last Inflation Parameters
47967	Balloon Size (mm)
47968	Pressure (ATM)
47969	Duration (sec)
47970	Number of Inflations
46200	Severity Of Stenosis
46228	Preprocedure
46256	Postprocedure
46284	Gradient
46312	Preprocedure
46340	Postprocedure
46368	Assessment
46706	Successful
46715	Poor Distal Runoff
46434	Lesion Could Not Be Crossed
48994	Lesion Could Not Be Dilated
46462	Intracoronary Thrombus
46490	Complications
46518	Intimal Tear
46546	Dissection
46574	Perforation
46602	Total Occlusion
46630	Branch Vessel Occlusion
46658	Balloon Rupture
46686	Catheter Transection
46039	First Left Posterolateral Branch
46090	Lesion Classification
46118	High Probability of Success (>85%); Low Risk

OFFICE & LAB PROCEDURES, CONT.

46146	Moderate Probability of Success (60-85%); Moderate Risk
46173	Low Probability of Success (<60%); High Risk
47974	First Inflation Parameters
47975	Balloon Size (mm)
47976	Pressure (ATM)
47977	Duration (sec)
47978	Last Inflation Parameters
47979	Balloon Size (mm)
47980	Pressure (ATM)
47981	Duration (sec)
47982	Number of Inflations
46201	Severity Of Stenosis
46229	Preprocedure
46257	Postprocedure
46285	Gradient
46313	Preprocedure
46341	Postprocedure
46369	Assessment
46707	Successful
46716	Poor Distal Runoff
46435	Lesion Could Not Be Crossed
48995	Lesion Could Not Be Dilated
46463	Intracoronary Thrombus
46491	Complications
46519	Intimal Tear
46547	Dissection
46575	Perforation
46603	Total Occlusion
46631	Branch Vessel Occlusion
46659	Balloon Rupture
46687	Catheter Transection
46040	Second Left Posterolateral Branch
46091	Lesion Classification
46119	High Probability of Success (>85%); Low Risk
46719	Moderate Probability of Success (60-85%); Moderate Risk
46174	Low Probability of Success (<60%); High Risk
47986	First Inflation Parameters
47987	Balloon Size (mm)
47988	Pressure (ATM)
47989	Duration (sec)
47990	Last Inflation Parameters
47991	Balloon Size (mm)
47992	Pressure (ATM)
47993	Duration (sec)
47994	Number of Inflations
46202	Severity Of Stenosis
46230	Preprocedure
46258	Postprocedure
46286	Gradient
46314	Preprocedure
46342	Postprocedure
46370	Assessment
46708	Successful
46717	Poor Distal Runoff
46436	Lesion Could Not Be Crossed
48996	Lesion Could Not Be Dilated
46464	Intracoronary Thrombus
46492	Complications
46520	Intimal Tear
46548	Dissection
46576	Perforation
46604	Total Occlusion
46632	Branch Vessel Occlusion
46660	Balloon Rupture
46688	Catheter Transection
46041	Third Left Posterolateral Branch
46092	Lesion Classification
46120	High Probability of Success (>85%); Low Risk
46147	Moderate Probability of Success (60-85%); Moderate Risk
46175	Low Probability of Success (<60%); High Risk
47998	First Inflation Parameters
47999	Balloon Size (mm)
48000	Pressure (ATM)
48001	Duration (sec)
48002	Last Inflation Parameters
48003	Balloon Size (mm)
48004	Pressure (ATM)
48005	Duration (sec)
48006	Number of Inflations
46203	Severity Of Stenosis
46231	Preprocedure
46259	Postprocedure
46287	Gradient
46315	Preprocedure
46343	Postprocedure
46371	Assessment
46709	Successful
46718	Poor Distal Runoff
46437	Lesion Could Not Be Crossed
48997	Lesion Could Not Be Dilated
46465	Intracoronary Thrombus
46493	Complications

OFFICE & LAB PROCEDURES, CONT.

46521	Intimal Tear	46177	Low Probability of Success
46549	Dissection		(<60%); High Risk
46577	Perforation	48022	First Inflation Parameters
46605	Total Occlusion	48023	Balloon Size (mm)
46633	Branch Vessel Occlusion	48024	Pressure (ATM)
46661	Balloon Rupture	48025	Duration (sec)
46689	Catheter Transection	48026	Last Inflation Parameters
46042	Proximal Right Coronary Artery	48027	Balloon Size (mm)
46093	Lesion Classification	48028	Pressure (ATM)
46121	High Probability of Success	48029	Duration (sec)
	(>85%); Low Risk	48030	Number of Inflations
46148	Moderate Probability of	46205	Severity Of Stenosis
	Success (60-85%); Moderate	46233	Preprocedure
	Risk	46261	Postprocedure
46176	Low Probability of Success	46289	Gradient
	(<60%); High Risk	46317	Preprocedure
48010	First Inflation Parameters	46345	Postprocedure
48011	Balloon Size (mm)	46373	Assessment
48012	Pressure (ATM)	46392	Successful
48013	Duration (sec)	46411	Poor Distal Runoff
48014	Last Inflation Parameters	46439	Lesion Could Not Be
48015	Balloon Size (mm)		Crossed
48016	Pressure (ATM)	48999	Lesion Could Not Be Dilated
48017	Duration (sec)	46467	Intracoronary Thrombus
48018	Number of Inflations	46495	Complications
46204	Severity Of Stenosis	46523	Intimal Tear
46232	Preprocedure	46551	Dissection
46260	Postprocedure	46579	Perforation
46288	Gradient	46607	Total Occlusion
46316	Preprocedure	46635	Branch Vessel Occlusion
46344	Postprocedure	46663	Balloon Rupture
46372	Assessment	46691	Catheter Transection
46391	Successful	46044	Distal Right Coronary Artery
46410	Poor Distal Runoff	46095	Lesion Classification
46438	Lesion Could Not Be	46123	High Probability of Success
	Crossed		(>85%); Low Risk
48998	Lesion Could Not Be Dilated	46150	Moderate Probability of
46466	Intracoronary Thrombus		Success (60-85%); Moderate
46494	Complications		Risk
46522	Intimal Tear	46178	Low Probability of Success
46550	Dissection		(<60%); High Risk
46578	Perforation	48034	First Inflation Parameters
46606	Total Occlusion	48035	Balloon Size (mm)
46634	Branch Vessel Occlusion	48036	Pressure (ATM)
46662	Balloon Rupture	48037	Duration (sec)
46690	Catheter Transection	48038	Last Inflation Parameters
46043	Mid-Right Coronary Artery	48039	Balloon Size (mm)
46094	Lesion Classification	48040	Pressure (ATM)
46122	High Probability of Success	48041	Duration (sec)
	(>85%); Low Risk	48042	Number of Inflations
46149	Moderate Probability of	46206	Severity Of Stenosis
	Success (60-85%); Moderate	46234	Preprocedure
	Risk	46262	Postprocedure

OFFICE & LAB PROCEDURES, CONT.

46290	Gradient	46609	Total Occlusion
46318	Preprocedure	46637	Branch Vessel Occlusion
46346	Postprocedure	46665	Balloon Rupture
46374	Assessment	46693	Catheter Transection
46393	Successful	46046	Second Acute Marginal Vessel
46412	Poor Distal Runoff	46097	Lesion Classification
46440	Lesion Could Not Be Crossed	46125	High Probability of Success (>85%); Low Risk
49000	Lesion Could Not Be Dilated	46152	Moderate Probability of Success (60-85%); Moderate Risk
46468	Intracoronary Thrombus		
46496	Complications		
46524	Intimal Tear	46180	Low Probability of Success (<60%); High Risk
46552	Dissection		
46580	Perforation	48058	First Inflation Parameters
46608	Total Occlusion	48059	Balloon Size (mm)
46636	Branch Vessel Occlusion	48060	Pressure (ATM)
46664	Balloon Rupture	48061	Duration (sec)
46692	Catheter Transection	48062	Last Inflation Parameters
46045	First Acute Marginal Vessel	48063	Balloon Size (mm)
46096	Lesion Classification	48064	Pressure (ATM)
46124	High Probability of Success (>85%); Low Risk	48065	Duration (sec)
		48066	Number of Inflations
46151	Moderate Probability of Success (60-85%); Moderate Risk	46208	Severity Of Stenosis
		46236	Preprocedure
		46264	Postprocedure
46179	Low Probability of Success (<60%); High Risk	46292	Gradient
		46320	Preprocedure
48046	First Inflation Parameters	46348	Postprocedure
48047	Balloon Size (mm)	46376	Assessment
48048	Pressure (ATM)	46395	Successful
48049	Duration (sec)	46414	Poor Distal Runoff
48050	Last Inflation Parameters	46442	Lesion Could Not Be Crossed
48051	Balloon Size (mm)		
48052	Pressure (ATM)	49002	Lesion Could Not Be Dilated
48053	Duration (sec)	46470	Intracoronary Thrombus
48054	Number of Inflations	46498	Complications
46207	Severity Of Stenosis	46526	Intimal Tear
46235	Preprocedure	46554	Dissection
46263	Postprocedure	46582	Perforation
46291	Gradient	46610	Total Occlusion
46319	Preprocedure	46638	Branch Vessel Occlusion
46347	Postprocedure	46666	Balloon Rupture
46375	Assessment	46694	Catheter Transection
46394	Successful	46047	Posterolateral Segment
46413	Poor Distal Runoff	46098	Lesion Classification
46441	Lesion Could Not Be Crossed	46126	High Probability of Success (>85%); Low Risk
49001	Lesion Could Not Be Dilated	46153	Moderate Probability of Success (60-85%); Moderate Risk
46469	Intracoronary Thrombus		
46497	Complications		
46525	Intimal Tear	46181	Low Probability of Success (<60%); High Risk
46553	Dissection		
46581	Perforation	48070	First Inflation Parameters

OFFICE & LAB PROCEDURES, CONT.

48071	Balloon Size (mm)	46378	Assessment
48072	Pressure (ATM)	46397	Successful
48073	Duration (sec)	46416	Poor Distal Runoff
48074	Last Inflation Parameters	46444	Lesion Could Not Be
48075	Balloon Size (mm)		Crossed
48076	Pressure (ATM)	49004	Lesion Could Not Be Dilated
48077	Duration (sec)	46472	Intracoronary Thrombus
48078	Number of Inflations	46500	Complications
46209	Severity Of Stenosis	46528	Intimal Tear
46237	Preprocedure	46556	Dissection
46265	Postprocedure	46584	Perforation
46293	Gradient	46612	Total Occlusion
46321	Preprocedure	46640	Branch Vessel Occlusion
46349	Postprocedure	46668	Balloon Rupture
46377	Assessment	46696	Catheter Transection
46396	Successful	46049	Second Right Posterolateral
46415	Poor Distal Runoff		Branch
46443	Lesion Could Not Be	46100	Lesion Classification
	Crossed	46128	High Probability of Success
49003	Lesion Could Not Be Dilated		(>85%); Low Risk
46471	Intracoronary Thrombus	46155	Moderate Probability of
46499	Complications		Success (60-85%); Moderate
46527	Intimal Tear		Risk
46555	Dissection	46183	Low Probability of Success
46583	Perforation		(<60%); High Risk
46611	Total Occlusion	48094	First Inflation Parameters
46639	Branch Vessel Occlusion	48095	Balloon Size (mm)
46667	Balloon Rupture	48096	Pressure (ATM)
46695	Catheter Transection	48097	Duration (sec)
46048	First Right Posterolateral Branch	48098	Last Inflation Parameters
46099	Lesion Classification	48099	Balloon Size (mm)
46127	High Probability of Success	48100	Pressure (ATM)
	(>85%); Low Risk	48101	Duration (sec)
46154	Moderate Probability of	48102	Number of Inflations
	Success (60-85%); Moderate	46211	Severity Of Stenosis
	Risk	46239	Preprocedure
46182	Low Probability of Success	46267	Postprocedure
	(<60%); High Risk	46295	Gradient
48082	First Inflation Parameters	46323	Preprocedure
48083	Balloon Size (mm)	46351	Postprocedure
48084	Pressure (ATM)	46379	Assessment
48085	Duration (sec)	46398	Successful
48086	Last Inflation Parameters	46417	Poor Distal Runoff
48087	Balloon Size (mm)	46445	Lesion Could Not Be
48088	Pressure (ATM)		Crossed
48089	Duration (sec)	49005	Lesion Could Not Be Dilated
48090	Number of Inflations	46473	Intracoronary Thrombus
46210	Severity Of Stenosis	46501	Complications
46238	Preprocedure	46529	Intimal Tear
46266	Postprocedure	46557	Dissection
46294	Gradient	46585	Perforation
46322	Preprocedure	46613	Total Occlusion
46350	Postprocedure	46641	Branch Vessel Occlusion

OFFICE & LAB PROCEDURES, CONT.

46669	Balloon Rupture
46697	Catheter Transection
46050	Third Right Posterolateral Branch
46101	Lesion Classification
46129	High Probability of Success (>85%); Low Risk
46156	Moderate Probability of Success (60-85%); Moderate Risk
46184	Low Probability of Success (<60%); High Risk
48106	First Inflation Parameters
48107	Balloon Size (mm)
48108	Pressure (ATM)
48109	Duration (sec)
48110	Last Inflation Parameters
48111	Balloon Size (mm)
48112	Pressure (ATM)
48113	Duration (sec)
48114	Number of Inflations
46212	Severity Of Stenosis
46240	Preprocedure
46268	Postprocedure
46296	Gradient
46324	Preprocedure
46352	Postprocedure
46380	Assessment
46399	Successful
46418	Poor Distal Runoff
46446	Lesion Could Not Be Crossed
49006	Lesion Could Not Be Dilated
46474	Intracoronary Thrombus
46502	Complications
46530	Intimal Tear
46558	Dissection
46586	Perforation
46614	Total Occlusion
46642	Branch Vessel Occlusion
46670	Balloon Rupture
46698	Catheter Transection
46051	Left Posterior Descending Artery
46102	Lesion Classification
46130	High Probability of Success (>85%); Low Risk
46157	Moderate Probability of Success (60-85%); Moderate Risk
46185	Low Probability of Success (<60%); High Risk
48118	First Inflation Parameters
48119	Balloon Size (mm)
48120	Pressure (ATM)
48121	Duration (sec)
48122	Last Inflation Parameters
48123	Balloon Size (mm)
48124	Pressure (ATM)
48125	Duration (sec)
48126	Number of Inflations
46213	Severity Of Stenosis
46241	Preprocedure
46269	Postprocedure
46297	Gradient
46325	Preprocedure
46353	Postprocedure
46381	Assessment
46400	Successful
46419	Poor Distal Runoff
46447	Lesion Could Not Be Crossed
49007	Lesion Could Not Be Dilated
46475	Intracoronary Thrombus
46503	Complications
46531	Intimal Tear
46559	Dissection
46587	Perforation
46615	Total Occlusion
46643	Branch Vessel Occlusion
46671	Balloon Rupture
46699	Catheter Transection
46052	Right Posterior Descending Artery
46103	Lesion Classification
46131	High Probability of Success (>85%); Low Risk
46158	Moderate Probability of Success (60-85%); Moderate Risk
46186	Low Probability of Success (<60%); High Risk
48130	First Inflation Parameters
48131	Balloon Size (mm)
48132	Pressure (ATM)
48133	Duration (sec)
48134	Last Inflation Parameters
48135	Balloon Size (mm)
48136	Pressure (ATM)
48137	Duration (sec)
48138	Number of Inflations
46214	Severity Of Stenosis
46242	Preprocedure
46270	Postprocedure
46298	Gradient
46326	Preprocedure
46354	Postprocedure
46382	Assessment
46401	Successful

OFFICE & LAB PROCEDURES, CONT.

46420	Poor Distal Runoff	47021	Lesion Classification
46448	Lesion Could Not Be Crossed	47028	High Probability of Success (>85%); Low Risk
49008	Lesion Could Not Be Dilated	47035	Moderate Probability of Success (60-85%); Moderate Risk
46476	Intracoronary Thrombus		
46504	Complications		
46532	Intimal Tear	47042	Low Probability of Success (<60%); High Risk
46560	Dissection		
46588	Perforation	48154	First Inflation Parameters
46616	Total Occlusion	48155	Balloon Size (mm)
46644	Branch Vessel Occlusion	48156	Pressure (ATM)
46672	Balloon Rupture	48157	Duration (sec)
46700	Catheter Transection	48158	Last Inflation Parameters
47008	Left Internal Mammary Graft	48159	Balloon Size (mm)
47020	Lesion Classification	48160	Pressure (ATM)
47027	High Probability of Success (>85%); Low Risk	48161	Duration (sec)
		48162	Number of Inflations
47034	Moderate Probability of Success (60-85%); Moderate Risk	47049	Severity Of Stenosis
		47056	Preprocedure
		47063	Postprocedure
47041	Low Probability of Success (<60%); High Risk	47070	Gradient
		47077	Preprocedure
48142	First Inflation Parameters	47084	Postprocedure
48143	Balloon Size (mm)	47091	Assessment
48144	Pressure (ATM)	47098	Successful
48145	Duration (sec)	47105	Poor Distal Runoff
48146	Last Inflation Parameters	47112	Lesion Could Not Be Crossed
48147	Balloon Size (mm)		
48148	Pressure (ATM)	49010	Lesion Could Not Be Dilated
48149	Duration (sec)	47119	Intracoronary Thrombus
48150	Number of Inflations	47126	Complications
47048	Severity Of Stenosis	47133	Intimal Tear
47055	Preprocedure	47140	Dissection
47062	Postprocedure	47147	Perforation
47069	Gradient	47154	Total Occlusion
47076	Preprocedure	47161	Branch Vessel Occlusion
47083	Postprocedure	47168	Balloon Rupture
47090	Assessment	47175	Catheter Transection
47097	Successful	47010	First Saphenous Vein Graft
47104	Poor Distal Runoff	47022	Lesion Classification
47111	Lesion Could Not Be Crossed	47029	High Probability of Success (>85%); Low Risk
49009	Lesion Could Not Be Dilated	47036	Moderate Probability of Success (60-85%); Moderate Risk
47118	Intracoronary Thrombus		
47125	Complications		
47132	Intimal Tear	47043	Low Probability of Success (<60%); High Risk
47139	Dissection		
47146	Perforation	48166	First Inflation Parameters
47153	Total Occlusion	48167	Balloon Size (mm)
47160	Branch Vessel Occlusion	48168	Pressure (ATM)
47167	Balloon Rupture	48169	Duration (sec)
47174	Catheter Transection	48170	Last Inflation Parameters
47009	Right Internal Mammary Graft	48171	Balloon Size (mm)

OFFICE & LAB PROCEDURES, CONT.

48172	Pressure (ATM)	49012	Lesion Could Not Be Dilated
48173	Duration (sec)	47121	Intracoronary Thrombus
48174	Number of Inflations	47128	Complications
47050	Severity Of Stenosis	47135	Intimal Tear
47057	Preprocedure	47142	Dissection
47064	Postprocedure	47149	Perforation
47071	Gradient	47156	Total Occlusion
47078	Preprocedure	47163	Branch Vessel Occlusion
47085	Postprocedure	47170	Balloon Rupture
47092	Assessment	47177	Catheter Transection
47099	Successful	47012	Third Saphenous Vein Graft
47106	Poor Distal Runoff	47024	Lesion Classification
47113	Lesion Could Not Be Crossed	47031	High Probability of Success (>85%); Low Risk
49011	Lesion Could Not Be Dilated	47038	Moderate Probability of Success (60-85%); Moderate Risk
47120	Intracoronary Thrombus		
47127	Complications		
47134	Intimal Tear	47045	Low Probability of Success (<60%); High Risk
47141	Dissection		
47148	Perforation	48190	First Inflation Parameters
47155	Total Occlusion	48191	Balloon Size (mm)
47162	Branch Vessel Occlusion	48192	Pressure (ATM)
47169	Balloon Rupture	48193	Duration (sec)
47176	Catheter Transection	48194	Last Inflation Parameters
47011	Second Saphenous Vein Graft	48195	Balloon Size (mm)
47023	Lesion Classification	48196	Pressure (ATM)
47030	High Probability of Success (>85%); Low Risk	48197	Duration (sec)
		48198	Number of Inflations
47037	Moderate Probability of Success (60-85%); Moderate Risk	47052	Severity Of Stenosis
		47059	Preprocedure
		47066	Postprocedure
47044	Low Probability of Success (<60%); High Risk	47073	Gradient
		47080	Preprocedure
48178	First Inflation Parameters	47087	Postprocedure
48179	Balloon Size (mm)	47094	Assessment
48180	Pressure (ATM)	47101	Successful
48181	Duration (sec)	47108	Poor Distal Runoff
48182	Last Inflation Parameters	47115	Lesion Could Not Be Crossed
48183	Balloon Size (mm)		
48184	Pressure (ATM)	49013	Lesion Could Not Be Dilated
48185	Duration (sec)	47122	Intracoronary Thrombus
48186	Number of Inflations	47129	Complications
47051	Severity Of Stenosis	47136	Intimal Tear
47058	Preprocedure	47143	Dissection
47065	Postprocedure	47150	Perforation
47072	Gradient	47157	Total Occlusion
47079	Preprocedure	47164	Branch Vessel Occlusion
47086	Postprocedure	47171	Balloon Rupture
47093	Assessment	47178	Catheter Transection
47100	Successful	47013	Fourth Saphenous Vein Graft
47107	Poor Distal Runoff	47025	Lesion Classification
47114	Lesion Could Not Be Crossed	47032	High Probability of Success (>85%); Low Risk

OFFICE & LAB PROCEDURES, CONT.

47039	Moderate Probability of Success (60-85%); Moderate Risk	47805	Severity of Stenosis
		47815	Preprocedure
		47816	Postprocedure
47046	Low Probability of Success (<60%); High Risk	47817	Gradient
		47827	Preprocedure
48202	First Inflation Parameters	47828	Postprocedure
48203	Balloon Size (mm)	47829	Assessment
48204	Pressure (ATM)	47839	Successful
48205	Duration (sec)	47840	Poor Distal Runoff
48206	Last Inflation Parameters	47841	Lesion Could Not Be Crossed
48207	Balloon Size (mm)		
48208	Pressure (ATM)	49015	Lesion Could Not Be Dilated
48209	Duration (sec)	47851	Intracoronary Thrombus
48210	Number of Inflations	47852	Complications
47053	Severity Of Stenosis	47853	Intimal Tear
47060	Preprocedure	47863	Dissection
47067	Postprocedure	47864	Perforation
47074	Gradient	47865	Total Occlusion
47081	Preprocedure	47875	Branch Vessel Occlusion
47088	Postprocedure	47876	Balloon Rupture
47095	Assessment	47877	Catheter Transection
47102	Successful	47887	Right Ventricular Outflow Tract
47109	Poor Distal Runoff	47888	Lesion Classification
47116	Lesion Could Not Be Crossed	47889	High Probability of Success (>85%); Low Risk
49014	Lesion Could Not Be Dilated	47899	Moderate Probability of Success (60-85%); Moderate Risk
47123	Intracoronary Thrombus		
47130	Complications	47900	Low Probability of Success (<60%); High Risk
47137	Intimal Tear		
47144	Dissection	47901	First Inflation Parameters
47151	Perforation	47911	Balloon Size
47158	Total Occlusion	47912	Pressure
47165	Branch Vessel Occlusion	47913	Duration
47172	Balloon Rupture	47923	Last Inflation Parameters
47179	Catheter Transection	47924	Balloon Size
47764	Truncus Arteriosus	47925	Pressure
47765	Lesion Classification	47935	Duration
47766	High Probability of Success (>85%); Low Risk	47936	Number of Inflations
		47937	Severity of Stenosis
47767	Moderate Probability of Success (60-85%); Moderate Risk	47947	Preprocedure
		47948	Postprocedure
47779	Low Probability of Success (<60%); High Risk	47949	Gradient
		47959	Preprocedure
47780	First Inflation Parameters	47960	Postprocedure
47781	Balloon Size	47961	Assessment
47782	Pressure	47971	Successful
47794	Duration	47972	Poor Distal Runoff
47795	Last Inflation Parameters	47973	Lesion Could Not Be Crossed
47796	Balloon Size		
47797	Pressure	49016	Lesion Could Not Be Dilated
47803	Duration	47983	Intracoronary Thrombus
47804	Number of Inflations	47984	Complications

OFFICE & LAB PROCEDURES, CONT.

47985	Intimal Tear	48164	Low Probability of Success
47995	Dissection		(<60%); High Risk
47996	Perforation	48165	First Inflation Parameters
47997	Total Occlusion	48175	Balloon Size
48007	Branch Vessel Occlusion	48176	Pressure
48008	Balloon Rupture	48177	Duration
48009	Catheter Transection	48187	Last Inflation Parameters
48019	Ascending Aorta	48188	Balloon Size
48020	Lesion Classification	48189	Pressure
48021	High Probability of Success	48199	Duration
	(>85%); Low Risk	48200	Number of Inflations
48031	Moderate Probability of	48201	Severity of Stenosis
	Success (60-85%); Moderate	48211	Preprocedure
	Risk	48212	Postprocedure
48032	Low Probability of Success	48213	Gradient
	(<60%); High Risk	48220	Preprocedure
48033	First Inflation Parameters	48221	Postprocedure
48043	Balloon Size	48228	Assessment
48044	Pressure	48229	Successful
48045	Duration	48236	Poor Distal Runoff
48055	Last Inflation Parameters	48237	Intracoronary Thrombus
48056	Balloon Size	48245	Complications
48057	Pressure	48246	Intimal Tear
48067	Duration	48249	Dissection
48068	Number of Inflations	48259	Perforation
48069	Severity of Stenosis	48260	Total Occlusion
48079	Preprocedure	48261	Branch Vessel Occlusion
48080	Postprocedure	48324	Balloon Rupture
48081	Gradient	48325	Catheter Transection
48091	Preprocedure	48326	A Left Blalock
48092	Postprocedure	48338	Lesion Classification
48093	Assessment	48339	High Probability of Success
48103	Successful		(>85%); Low Risk
48104	Poor Distal Runoff	48340	Moderate Probability of
48105	Lesion Could Not Be		Success (60-85%); Moderate
	Crossed		Risk
49017	Lesion Could Not Be Dilated	48341	Low Probability of Success
48115	Intracoronary Thrombus		(<60%); High Risk
48116	Complications	48885	First Inflation Parameters
48117	Intimal Tear	48886	Balloon Size
48127	Dissection	48887	Pressure
48128	Perforation	48888	Duration
48129	Total Occlusion	48889	Last Inflation Parameters
48139	Branch Vessel Occlusion	48890	Balloon Size
48140	Balloon Rupture	48891	Pressure
48141	Catheter Transection	48892	Duration
48151	A Main Blalock	48893	Number of Inflations
48152	Lesion Classification	48894	Severity of Stenosis
48153	High Probability of Success	48895	Preprocedure
	(>85%); Low Risk	48896	Postprocedure
48163	Moderate Probability of	48897	Gradient
	Success (60-85%); Moderate	48898	Preprocedure
	Risk	48899	Postprocedure

OFFICE & LAB PROCEDURES, CONT.

48900	Assessment	49037	Moderate Probability of
48901	Successful		Success (60-85%); Moderate
48902	Poor Distal Runoff		Risk
48903	Intracoronary Thrombus	49038	Low Probability of Success
48904	Complications		(<60%); High Risk
48905	Intimal Tear	49019	Bypass Graft
48906	Dissection	49020	Lesion Classification
48907	Perforation	49021	High Probability of Success
48908	Total Occlusion		(>85%); Low Risk
48909	Branch Vessel Occlusion	49022	Moderate Probability of
48910	Balloon Rupture		Success (60-85%); Moderate
48911	Catheter Transection		Risk
48912	A Right Blalock	49023	Low Probability of Success
48913	Lesion Classification		(<60%); High Risk
48914	High Probability of Success	49039	Severity of Stenosis
	(>85%); Low Risk	49040	Preprocedure
48915	Moderate Probability of	49041	Postprocedure
	Success (60-85%); Moderate	49042	Gradient
	Risk	49043	Preprocedure
48916	Low Probability of Success	49044	Postprocedure
	(<60%); High Risk	49050	Assessment
48917	First Inflation Parameters	49051	Successful
48918	Balloon Size	49052	Poor Distal Runoff
48919	Pressure	49054	Lesion Could Not Be
48920	Duration		Crossed
48921	Last Inflation Parameters	49055	Lesion Could Not Be Dilated
48922	Balloon Size	49053	Intracoronary Thrombus
48923	Pressure	49045	Complications
48924	Duration	49046	Intimal Tear
48925	Number of Inflations	49047	Dissection
48926	Severity of Stenosis	49048	Total Occlusion
48927	Preprocedure	49049	Branch Vessel Occlusion
48928	Postprocedure	49024	Bypass Graft #2
48929	Gradient	49025	Lesion Classification
48930	Preprocedure	49026	High Probability of Success
48931	Postprocedure		(>85%); Low Risk
48932	Assessment	49027	Moderate Probability of
48933	Successful		Success (60-85%); Moderate
48934	Poor Distal Runoff		Risk
48935	Intracoronary Thrombus	49028	Low Probability of Success
48936	Complications		(<60%); High Risk
48937	Intimal Tear	49029	Bypass Graft #3
48938	Dissection	49030	Lesion Classification
48939	Perforation	49031	High Probability of Success
48940	Total Occlusion		(>85%); Low Risk
48941	Branch Vessel Occlusion	49032	Moderate Probability of
48942	Balloon Rupture		Success (60-85%); Moderate
48943	Catheter Transection		Risk
49034	Vein Graft	49033	Low Probability of Success
49035	Lesion Classification		(<60%); High Risk
49036	High Probability of Success	42615	Each Additional Vessel
	(>85%); Low Risk	75143	Conclusions
		75144	Successful

OFFICE & LAB PROCEDURES, CONT.

38164	Unsuccessful	47006	Left Posterior Descending Artery
48871	Pulmonary Artery		
48872	Pulmonary Venous Obstruction	47007	Right Posterior Descending Artery
48979	Conduit Anastomosis		
48873	Systemic Venous Obstruction	47014	Left Internal Mammary Graft
48874	Aortic Coarctation	47015	Right Internal Mammary Graft
48875	Aortic Shunt		
46017	Stent Placement	47016	First Saphenous Vein Graft
46828	Number Of Stents Placed:	47017	Second Saphenous Vein Graft
46829	Stent 1		
46832	Location	47018	Third Saphenous Vein Graft
48879	Left Main Coronary Artery	47019	Fourth Saphenous Vein Graft
46980	Proximal Left Anterior Descending Artery	47722	Parameters
		47723	Size (mm)
46981	Mid-Left Anterior Descending Artery	47724	Inflation Pressure (ATM)
		47725	Duration (sec)
46982	Distal Left Anterior Descending Artery	47726	Lot ID
		47727	Type
46983	First Diagonal Branch	46833	Stenosis
46984	Second Diagonal Branch	46834	Predeployment
46985	First Anterior Septal Branch	46835	Postdeployment
46986	Intermedius Branch	46848	Gradient
46987	Proximal Circumflex	46849	Predeployment
46988	Distal Circumflex	46850	Postdeployment
46989	First Obtuse Marginal Branch	46836	Complications
		46837	Intimal Tear
46990	Second Obtuse Marginal Branch	46838	Dissection
		46839	Branch Vessel Occlusion
46991	Third Obtuse Marginal Branch	46840	Total Occlusion
		46841	Deployed In Wrong Segment
46992	Left Atrioventricular Groove Branch	46842	Assessment
		46843	Successful
46993	Left Posterolateral Segment	46844	Poor Distal Runoff
46994	First Left Posterolateral Branch	46845	Intracoronary Thrombus
		46846	Lesion Could Not Be Crossed
46995	Second Left Posterolateral Branch		
		46847	Stent Could Not Be Deployed
46996	Third Left Posterolateral Branch		
		46830	Stent 2
46997	Proximal Right Coronary Artery	47180	Location
		48880	Left Main Coronary Artery
46998	Mid-Right Coronary Artery	47182	Proximal Left Anterior Descending Artery
46999	Distal Right Coronary Artery		
47000	First Acute Marginal Vessel	47184	Mid-Left Anterior Descending Artery
47001	Second Acute Marginal Vessel		
		47186	Distal Left Anterior Descending Artery
47002	Posterolateral Segment		
47003	First Right Posterolateral Branch	47188	First Diagonal Branch
		47190	Second Diagonal Branch
47004	Second Right Posterolateral Branch	47192	First Anterior Septal Branch
		47194	Intermedius Branch
47005	Third Right Posterolateral Branch	47196	Proximal Circumflex
		47198	Distal Circumflex

OFFICE & LAB PROCEDURES, CONT.

47200	First Obtuse Marginal Branch	47262	Complications
		47264	Intimal Tear
47202	Second Obtuse Marginal Branch	47266	Dissection
		47268	Branch Vessel Occlusion
47204	Third Obtuse Marginal Branch	47270	Total Occlusion
		47272	Deployed In Wrong Segment
47206	Left Atrioventricular Groove Branch	47274	Assessment
		47276	Successful
47208	Left Posterolateral Segment	47278	Poor Distal Runoff
47210	First Left Posterolateral Branch	47280	Intracoronary Thrombus
		47282	Lesion Could Not Be Crossed
47212	Second Left Posterolateral Branch	47284	Stent Could Not Be Deployed
47214	Third Left Posterolateral Branch	46831	Stent 3
47216	Proximal Right Coronary Artery	47181	Location
		48881	Left Main Coronary Artery
47218	Mid-Right Coronary Artery	47183	Proximal Left Anterior Descending Artery
47220	Distal Right Coronary Artery		
47222	First Acute Marginal Vessel	47185	Mid-Left Anterior Descending Artery
47224	Second Acute Marginal Vessel	47187	Distal Left Anterior Descending Artery
47226	Posterolateral Segment		
47228	First Right Posterolateral Branch	47189	First Diagonal Branch
		47191	Second Diagonal Branch
47230	Second Right Posterolateral Branch	47193	First Anterior Septal Branch
		47195	Intermedius Branch
47232	Third Right Posterolateral Branch	47197	Proximal Circumflex
		47199	Distal Circumflex
47234	Left Posterior Descending Artery	47201	First Obtuse Marginal Branch
47236	Right Posterior Descending Artery	47203	Second Obtuse Marginal Branch
47238	Left Internal Mammary Graft	47205	Third Obtuse Marginal Branch
47240	Right Internal Mammary Graft	47207	Left Atrioventricular Groove Branch
47242	First Saphenous Vein Graft	47209	Left Posterolateral Segment
47244	Second Saphenous Vein Graft	47211	First Left Posterolateral Branch
47246	Third Saphenous Vein Graft	47213	Second Left Posterolateral Branch
47248	Fourth Saphenous Vein Graft		
47728	Parameters	47215	Third Left Posterolateral Branch
47729	Size (mm)		
47730	Inflation Pressure (ATM)	47217	Proximal Right Coronary Artery
47731	Duration (sec)		
47732	Lot ID	47219	Mid-Right Coronary Artery
47733	Type	47221	Distal Right Coronary Artery
47250	Stenosis	47223	First Acute Marginal Vessel
47252	Predeployment	47225	Second Acute Marginal Vessel
47254	Postdeployment		
47256	Gradient	47227	Posterolateral Segment
47258	Predeployment		
47260	Postdeployment		

OFFICE & LAB PROCEDURES, CONT.

47229	First Right Posterolateral Branch	47447	Atherectomy 1
47231	Second Right Posterolateral Branch	47450	Location
		48882	Left Main Coronary Artery
47233	Third Right Posterolateral Branch	47453	Proximal Left Anterior Descending Artery
47235	Left Posterior Descending Artery	47456	Mid-Left Anterior Descending Artery
47237	Right Posterior Descending Artery	47459	Distal Left Anterior Descending Artery
47239	Left Internal Mammary Graft	47462	First Diagonal Branch
47241	Right Internal Mammary Graft	47465	Second Diagonal Branch
		47468	First Anterior Septal Branch
47243	First Saphenous Vein Graft	47471	Intermedius Branch
47245	Second Saphenous Vein Graft	47474	Proximal Circumflex
		47477	Distal Circumflex
47247	Third Saphenous Vein Graft	47480	First Obtuse Marginal Branch
47249	Fourth Saphenous Vein Graft	47483	Second Obtuse Marginal Branch
47734	Parameters		
47735	Size (mm)	47486	Third Obtuse Marginal Branch
47736	Inflation Pressure (ATM)		
47737	Duration (sec)	47489	Left Atrioventricular Groove Branch
47738	Lot ID		
47739	Type	47492	Left Posterolateral Segment
47251	Stenosis	47495	First Left Posterolateral Branch
47253	Predeployment		
47255	Postdeployment	47498	Second Left Posterolateral Branch
47257	Gradient		
47259	Predeployment	47501	Third Left Posterolateral Branch
47261	Postdeployment		
47263	Complications	47504	Proximal Right Coronary Artery
47265	Intimal Tear		
47267	Dissection	47507	Mid-Right Coronary Artery
47269	Branch Vessel Occlusion	47510	Distal Right Coronary Artery
47271	Total Occlusion	47513	First Acute Marginal Vessel
47273	Deployed In Wrong Segment	47516	Second Acute Marginal Vessel
47275	Assessment		
47277	Successful	47519	Posterolateral Segment
47279	Poor Distal Runoff	47522	First Right Posterolateral Branch
47281	Intracoronary Thrombus		
47283	Lesion Could Not Be Crossed	47525	Second Right Posterolateral Branch
47285	Stent Could Not Be Deployed	47528	Third Right Posterolateral Branch
75149	Conclusions	47531	Left Posterior Descending Artery
75150	Successful		
38169	Unsuccessful	47534	Right Posterior Descending Artery
46018	Atherectomy		
48866	Device Used:	47537	Left Internal Mammary Graft
48867	Rotational	47540	Right Internal Mammary Graft
74613	Directional		
74614	Transluminal Extraction	47543	First Saphenous Vein Graft
47446	Number Performed:		

OFFICE & LAB PROCEDURES, CONT.

47546	Second Saphenous Vein Graft	47496	First Left Posterolateral Branch
47549	Third Saphenous Vein Graft	47499	Second Left Posterolateral
47552	Fourth Saphenous Vein Graft		Branch
47740	First Pass Parameters	47502	Third Left Posterolateral
48214	Blade Diameter		Branch
48215	Duration (sec)	47505	Proximal Right Coronary
48216	Last Pass Parameters		Artery
48217	Blade Diameter	47508	Mid-Right Coronary Artery
48218	Duration (sec)	47511	Distal Right Coronary Artery
48219	Number of Passes	47514	First Acute Marginal Vessel
47555	Stenosis	47517	Second Acute Marginal
47558	Preatherectomy		Vessel
47561	Postatherectomy	47520	Posterolateral Segment
47564	Gradient	47523	First Right Posterolateral
47567	Preatherectomy		Branch
47570	Postatherectomy	47526	Second Right Posterolateral
47573	Complications		Branch
47576	Intimal Tear	47529	Third Right Posterolateral
47579	Dissection		Branch
47582	Branch Vessel Occlusion	47532	Left Posterior Descending
47585	Total Occlusion		Artery
47588	Assessment	47535	Right Posterior Descending
47591	Successful		Artery
47594	Poor Distal Runoff	47538	Left Internal Mammary Graft
47597	Intracoronary Thrombus	47541	Right Internal Mammary
47600	Lesion Could Not Be		Graft
	Crossed	47544	First Saphenous Vein Graft
47603	Lesion Could Not Be Dilated	47547	Second Saphenous Vein
47448	Atherectomy 2		Graft
47451	Location	47550	Third Saphenous Vein Graft
48883	Left Main Coronary Artery	47553	Fourth Saphenous Vein Graft
47454	Proximal Left Anterior	47746	First Pass Parameters
	Descending Artery	48222	Blade Diameter
47457	Mid- Left Anterior	48223	Duration (sec)
	Descending Artery	48224	Last Pass Parameters
47460	Distal Left Anterior	48225	Blade Diameter
	Descending Artery	48226	Duration (sec)
47463	First Diagonal Branch	48227	Number of Passes
47466	Second Diagonal Branch	47556	Stenosis
47469	First Anterior Septal Branch	47559	Preatherectomy
47472	Intermedius Branch	47562	Postatherectomy
47475	Proximal Circumflex	47565	Gradient
47478	Distal Circumflex	47568	Preatherectomy
47481	First Obtuse Marginal	47571	Postatherectomy
	Branch	47574	Complications
47484	Second Obtuse Marginal	47577	Intimal Tear
	Branch	47580	Dissection
47487	Third Obtuse Marginal	47583	Branch Vessel Occlusion
	Branch	47586	Total Occlusion
47490	Left Atrioventricular Groove	47589	Assessment
	Branch	47592	Successful
47493	Left Posterolateral Segment	47595	Poor Distal Runoff

OFFICE & LAB PROCEDURES, CONT.

47598	Intracoronary Thrombus	47542	Right Internal Mammary Graft
47601	Lesion Could Not Be Crossed	47545	First Saphenous Vein Graft
47604	Lesion Could Not Be Dilated	47548	Second Saphenous Vein Graft
47449	Atherectomy 3	47551	Third Saphenous Vein Graft
47452	Location	47554	Fourth Saphenous Vein Graft
48884	Left Main Coronary Artery	47752	First Pass Parameters
47455	Proximal Left Anterior Descending Artery	48230	Blade Diameter
47458	Mid-Left Anterior Descending Artery	48231	Duration (sec)
		48232	Last Pass Parameters
47461	Distal Left Anterior Descending Artery	48233	Blade Diameter
		48234	Duration (sec)
47464	First Diagonal Branch	48235	Number of Passes
47467	Second Diagonal Branch	47557	Stenosis
47470	First Anterior Septal Branch	47560	Preatherectomy
47473	Intermedius Branch	47563	Postatherectomy
47476	Proximal Circumflex	47566	Gradient
47479	Distal Circumflex	47569	Preatherectomy
47482	First Obtuse Marginal Branch	47572	Postatherectomy
		47575	Complications
47485	Second Obtuse Marginal Branch	47578	Intimal Tear
		47581	Dissection
47488	Third Obtuse Marginal Branch	47584	Branch Vessel Occlusion
		47587	Total Occlusion
47491	Left Atrioventricular Groove Branch	47590	Assessment
		47593	Successful
47494	Left Posterolateral Segment	47596	Poor Distal Runoff
47497	First Left Posterolateral Branch	47599	Intracoronary Thrombus
		47602	Lesion Could Not Be Crossed
47500	Second Left Posterolateral Branch	47605	Lesion Could Not Be Dilated
		75145	Conclusions
47503	Third Left Posterolateral Branch	75146	Successful
		38166	Unsuccessful
47506	Proximal Right Coronary Artery	46019	Laser Angioplasty
		47286	Number Lased:
47509	Mid-Right Coronary Artery	47287	Lasering 1
47512	Distal Right Coronary Artery	47290	Location
47515	First Acute Marginal Vessel	48944	Left Main Coronary Artery
47518	Second Acute Marginal Vessel	47293	Proximal Left Anterior Descending Artery
47521	Posterolateral Segment	47296	Mid-Left Anterior Descending Artery
47524	First Right Posterolateral Branch	47299	Distal Left Anterior Descending Artery
47527	Second Right Posterolateral Branch	47302	First Diagonal Branch
		47305	Second Diagonal Branch
47530	Third Right Posterolateral Branch	47308	First Anterior Septal Branch
		47311	Intermedius Branch
47533	Left Posterior Descending Artery	47314	Proximal Circumflex
47536	Right Posterior Descending Artery	47317	Distal Circumflex
47539	Left Internal Mammary Graft		

OFFICE & LAB PROCEDURES, CONT.

47320	First Obtuse Marginal Branch	47404	Gradient
47323	Second Obtuse Marginal Branch	47407	Prelaser
		47410	Postlaser
47326	Third Obtuse Marginal Branch	47413	Complications
		47416	Intimal Tear
47329	Left Atrioventricular Groove Branch	47419	Dissection
		47422	Branch Vessel Occlusion
47332	Left Posterolateral Segment	47425	Total Occlusion
47335	First Left Posterolateral Branch	47428	Assessment
		47431	Successful
47338	Second Left Posterolateral Branch	47434	Poor Distal Runoff
		47437	Intracoronary Thrombus
47341	Third Left Posterolateral Branch	47440	Lesion Could Not Be Crossed
47344	Proximal Right Coronary Artery	47443	Lesion Could Not Be Lased
		47288	Lasering 2
47347	Mid-Right Coronary Artery	47291	Location
47350	Distal Right Coronary Artery	48945	Left Main Coronary Artery
47353	First Acute Marginal Vessel	47294	Proximal Left Anterior Descending Artery
47356	Second Acute Marginal Vessel	47297	Mid-Left Anterior Descending Artery
47359	Posterolateral Segment	47300	Distal Left Anterior Descending Artery
47362	First Right Posterolateral Branch	47303	First Diagonal Branch
47365	Second Right Posterolateral Branch	47306	Second Diagonal Branch
		47309	First Anterior Septal Branch
47368	Third Right Posterolateral Branch	47312	Intermedius Branch
		47315	Proximal Circumflex
47371	Left Posterior Descending Artery	47318	Distal Circumflex
		47321	First Obtuse Marginal Branch
47374	Right Posterior Descending Artery	47324	Second Obtuse Marginal Branch
47377	Left Internal Mammary Graft	47327	Third Obtuse Marginal Branch
47380	Right Internal Mammary Graft	47330	Left Atrioventricular Groove Branch
47383	First Saphenous Vein Graft	47333	Left Posterolateral Segment
47386	Second Saphenous Vein Graft	47336	First Left Posterolateral Branch
47389	Third Saphenous Vein Graft	47339	Second Left Posterolateral Branch
47392	Fourth Saphenous Vein Graft	47342	Third Left Posterolateral Branch
48238	First Pass Parameters		
48239	Duration (sec)		
48240	Number Of Bursts	47345	Proximal Right Coronary Artery
48247	Power (mjoules)		
48241	Last Pass Parameters	47348	Mid-Right Coronary Artery
48242	Duration (sec)	47351	Distal Right Coronary Artery
48243	Number Of Bursts	47354	First Acute Marginal Vessel
48248	Power (mjoules)	47357	Second Acute Marginal Vessel
48244	Number of Passes		
47395	Stenosis	47360	Posterolateral Segment
47398	Prelaser		
47401	Postlaser		

OFFICE & LAB PROCEDURES, CONT.

47363	First Right Posterolateral Branch	47301	Distal Left Anterior Descending Artery
47366	Second Right Posterolateral Branch	47304	First Diagonal Branch
		47307	Second Diagonal Branch
47369	Third Right Posterolateral Branch	47310	First Anterior Septal Branch
		47313	Intermedius Branch
47372	Left Posterior Descending Artery	47316	Proximal Circumflex
		47319	Distal Circumflex
47375	Right Posterior Descending Artery	47322	First Obtuse Marginal Branch
47378	Left Internal Mammary Graft	47325	Second Obtuse Marginal Branch
47381	Right Internal Mammary Graft	47328	Third Obtuse Marginal Branch
47384	First Saphenous Vein Graft		
47387	Second Saphenous Vein Graft	47331	Left Atrioventricular Groove Branch
47390	Third Saphenous Vein Graft	47334	Left Posterolateral Segment
47393	Fourth Saphenous Vein Graft	47337	First Left Posterolateral Branch
48250	First Pass Parameters		
48251	Duration (sec)	47340	Second Left Posterolateral Branch
48252	Number Of Bursts		
48253	Power (mjoules)	47343	Third Left Posterolateral Branch
48254	Last Pass Parameters		
48255	Duration (sec)	47346	Proximal Right Coronary Artery
48256	Number Of Bursts		
48257	Power (mjoules)	47349	Mid-Right Coronary Artery
48258	Number of Passes	47352	Distal Right Coronary Artery
47396	Stenosis	47355	First Acute Marginal Vessel
47399	Prelaser	47358	Second Acute Marginal Vessel
47402	Postlaser		
47405	Gradient	47361	Posterolateral Segment
47408	Prelaser	47364	First Right Posterolateral Branch
47411	Postlaser		
47414	Complications	47367	Second Right Posterolateral Branch
47417	Intimal Tear		
47420	Dissection	47370	Third Right Posterolateral Branch
47423	Branch Vessel Occlusion		
47426	Total Occlusion	47373	Left Posterior Descending Artery
47429	Assessment		
47432	Successful	47376	Right Posterior Descending Artery
47435	Poor Distal Runoff		
47438	Intracoronary Thrombus	47379	Left Internal Mammary Graft
47441	Lesion Could Not Be Crossed	47382	Right Internal Mammary Graft
47444	Lesion Could Not Be Lased	47385	First Saphenous Vein Graft
47289	Lasering 3	47388	Second Saphenous Vein Graft
47292	Location		
48946	Left Main Coronary Artery	47391	Third Saphenous Vein Graft
47295	Proximal Left Anterior Descending Artery	47394	Fourth Saphenous Vein Graft
		48315	First Pass Parameters
47298	Mid-Left Anterior Descending Artery	48316	Duration (sec)
		48317	Number Of Bursts
		48318	Power (mjoules)

OFFICE & LAB PROCEDURES, CONT.

48319	Last Pass Parameters	47768	First Inflation
48320	Duration (sec)	47769	Balloon Size (mm)
48321	Number Of Bursts	47770	Number Of Balloons
48322	Power (mjoules)	47771	Pressure (ATM)
48323	Number of Passes	47772	Duration (sec)
47397	Stenosis	47773	Last Inflation
47400	Prelaser	47774	Balloon Size (mm)
47403	Postlaser	47775	Number Of Balloons
47406	Gradient	47776	Pressure (ATM)
47409	Prelaser	47777	Duration (sec)
47412	Postlaser	47778	Number of Inflations
47415	Complications	48357	Severity of Stenosis
47418	Intimal Tear	48358	Preprocedure
47421	Dissection	48359	Postprocedure
47424	Branch Vessel Occlusion	48360	Gradient
47427	Total Occlusion	48361	Preprocedure
47430	Assessment	48362	Postprocedure
47433	Successful	48363	Assessment
47436	Poor Distal Runoff	48364	Successful
47439	Intracoronary Thrombus	48365	Lesion Could Not Be
47442	Lesion Could Not Be		Crossed
	Crossed	48366	Complications
47445	Lesion Could Not Be Lased	48367	Dissection
75147	Conclusions	48368	Perforation
75148	Successful	44802	Pulmonary
38167	Unsuccessful	47783	First Inflation
44799	Transluminal Valvular Angioplasty	47784	Balloon Size (mm)
44800	Aortic	47785	Number Of Balloons
47753	First Inflation	47786	Pressure (ATM)
47754	Balloon Size (mm)	47787	Duration (sec)
47755	Number Of Balloons	47788	Last Inflation
47756	Pressure (ATM)	47789	Balloon Size (mm)
47757	Duration (sec)	47790	Number Of Balloons
47758	Last Inflation	47791	Pressure (ATM)
47759	Balloon Size (mm)	47792	Duration (sec)
47760	Number Of Balloons	47793	Number of Inflations
47761	Pressure (ATM)	48369	Severity of Stenosis
47762	Duration (sec)	48370	Preprocedure
47763	Number of Inflations	48371	Postprocedure
48345	Severity of Stenosis	48372	Gradient
48346	Preprocedure	48373	Preprocedure
48347	Postprocedure	48374	Postprocedure
48348	Gradient	48375	Assessment
48349	Preprocedure	48376	Successful
48350	Postprocedure	48377	Lesion Could Not Be
48351	Assessment		Crossed
48352	Successful	48378	Complications
48353	Lesion Could Not Be	48379	Dissection
	Crossed	48380	Perforation
48354	Complications	44803	Tricuspid
48355	Dissection	48327	First Inflation
48356	Perforation	48328	Balloon Size (mm)
44801	Mitral	48329	Number Of Balloons

OFFICE & LAB PROCEDURES, CONT.

48330	Pressure (ATM)		43317	Revision
48331	Duration (sec)		43318	Removal
48332	Last Inflation		43262	Venipuncture (By Physician)
48333	Balloon Size (mm)		43263	On Child Under Age 3
48334	Number Of Balloons		43264	Deep Vein
48335	Pressure (ATM)		43265	Scalp Vein
48336	Duration (sec)		43286	Intravenous Catheter Placement
48337	Number of Inflations		43287	Superior Vena Cava
48381	Severity of Stenosis		49721	Inferior Vena Cava
48382	Preprocedure		49722	Renal
48383	Postprocedure		49723	Right
48384	Gradient		49724	Left
48385	Preprocedure		49725	Jugular
48386	Postprocedure		49726	Right
48387	Assessment		49727	Left
48388	Successful		49728	Axillary
48389	Lesion Could Not Be		49729	Right
	Crossed		49730	Left
48390	Complications		49731	Femoral
48391	Dissection		49732	Right
48392	Perforation		49733	Left
46020	Balloon Dilation		49734	Adrenal
48870	Non-Coronary Vessel		49735	Right
44853	Post-Operative Thrombolysis		49736	Left
44854	Acute Pre-Streptokinase		49737	Thyroid
44855	Post-Streptokinase		49738	Right
44856	Acute		49739	Left
44857	Chronic		49740	Petrosal Sinus
44858	PTCA		49741	Right
44859	Chronic		49742	Left
44860	tPA		49743	Right Heart
70369	Transmyocardial Revascularization		49744	Main Pulmonary Artery
41604	Pericardiocentesis		49745	Left Pulmonary Artery
43260	Subsequent		49746	Right Pulmonary Artery
44747	Fluid Volume		43266	Venous Cutdown
43302	Arterial Catheterization		43267	On Child Under Age 1
43303	Carotid		43268	Umbilical Vein Catheterization
43304	Vertebral		43269	Selective Venous Catheterization For
43305	Brachial Artery			Sampling
43306	Extremity Artery		49872	With Radiologic Supervision
43307	For Dialysis		41606	Percutaneous Central Venous Catheter
43308	Aortic - Translumbar			Placement
43309	Selective, Aortic Approach		42616	Infant or Newborn
43310	Placement		49747	Percutaneous Portal Vein Catheter
43311	Additional Placement - Thoracic			Placement
43312	Additional Placement - Cerebral		42619	Central Venous Catheter Placement By
43313	Additional Placement -			Cutdown
	Abdominal		42620	Infant or Newborn
43314	Indwelling Coronary		49748	Central Venous Catheter Repositioning
43261	Arterial Cannulation For			With Fluorscopic Guidance
	Chemotherapy		43276	Venous Sclerosing By Injection
43315	Intra-arterial Infusion Pump		43277	Single Vein
43316	Placement		43278	Multiple Veins - Same Leg

OFFICE & LAB PROCEDURES, CONT.

43279	Sclerosing Telangiectasia
43280	Limb / Trunk
43281	Face
43282	Venous Infusion Pump
43283	Insertion
43284	Revision
43285	Removal
49554	Venous Infusion Access Port
49555	Insertion
49556	Revision
49557	Removal
41809	Cardiopulmonary Resuscitation
41808	Internal Circulatory Assist Pump
42623	External Circulatory Assistance
49018	Left Heart Mechanical Device
44461	Pulmonary Procedures
42982	Digestive System Services
41636	Esophagoscopy (Rigid)
43007	Variceal Sclerotherapy
41645	Foreign Body Removal
43885	Proctosigmoidoscopy (Rigid)
43886	For Dilation
43887	For Foreign Body Removal
43888	For Removal Of Polyp Or Tumor
43892	By Electrocoagulation
43894	By Hot Biopsy
43893	By Laser Photocoagulation
43889	Multiple
43890	For Hemorrhage Control
43891	For Ablation Of Lesion(s)
43895	For Volvulus Decompression
43896	Sigmoidoscopy (Fiberoptic)
43897	For Foreign Body Removal
43898	For Polyp Removal
43899	For Hemorrhage Control
43900	For Ablation Of Lesion(s)
43901	By Electrocoagulation
43902	By Laser Photocoagulation
43903	By Hot Biopsy
43904	For Volvulus Decompression
41662	Complete Colonoscopy
43884	For Foreign Body Removal
43910	For Polyp Removal
43905	For Hemorrhage Control
43906	For Ablation Of Lesion(s)
43907	By Electrocoagulation
43908	By Laser Photocoagulation
43909	By Hot Biopsy
40087	Passage Of Sengstaken - Blakemore Tube For Varices
42983	Percutaneous Placement Of Gastrostomy Tube
42984	Change Of Gastrostomy Tube

45672	Musculoskeletal Procedures
45674	Incision Of Soft Tissue Abscess
45675	Superficial
45676	Deep
45685	Injection
45677	Sinus Tract
45686	Tendon Sheath
45687	Ligament
45688	Trigger Points
45689	Ganglion Cyst
45678	Foreign Body Removal
45679	Muscle
45680	Simple
45681	Deep
45682	Tendon Sheath
45683	Simple
45684	Deep
45690	Arthrocentesis
45691	Aspiration Of
45692	Small Joint
45695	Finger Joint
45696	Toe Joint
45693	Bursa Of Small Joint
45697	Bursa Of Finger
45698	Bursa Of Toe
45694	Ganglion Cyst Of Small Joint
45699	Ganglion Cyst Of Finger
45700	Ganglion Cyst of Toe
45701	Intermediate Joint
45702	Temporomandibular Joint
45703	Acromioclavicular Joint
45704	Wrist Joint
45705	Elbow Joint
45706	Ankle Joint
45707	Bursa Of Intermediate Joint
45708	Acromioclavicular Bursa
45709	Bursa Of Wrist
45710	Bursa Of Elbow
45711	Bursa Of Ankle
45712	Olecranon Bursa
45713	Ganglion Cyst Of Intermediate Joint
45714	Ganglion Cyst Of Wrist
45715	Major Joint
45716	Shoulder Joint
45717	Hip Joint
45718	Knee Joint
45719	Bursa Of Major Joint
45720	Subacromial Bursa
45721	Injection Of
45722	Small Joint
45723	Finger Joint
45724	Toe Joint

OFFICE & LAB PROCEDURES, CONT.

45725	Bursa Of Small Joint		45218	Spinal Anesthesia
45726	Bursa Of Finger		41833	Subarachnoid
45727	Bursa Of Toe		45219	Single
45728	Ganglion Cyst Of Small Joint		45220	Differential
45729	Ganglion Cyst Of Finger		45221	Continuous
45730	Ganglion Cyst of Toe		45222	Subdural
45731	Intermediate Joint		45223	Single
45733	Temporomandibular Joint		45224	Differential
45734	Acromioclavicular Joint		45225	Continuous
45735	Wrist Joint		41832	Epidural
45736	Elbow Joint		45226	Cervical
45737	Ankle Joint		45227	Thoracic
45738	Bursa Of Intermediate Joint		45228	Lumbar, Single
45732	Acromioclavicular Bursa		45229	Lumbar, Continuous
45739	Bursa Of Wrist		41834	Caudal
45740	Bursa Of Elbow		45230	Caudal, Single
45741	Bursa Of Ankle		45231	Caudal, Continuous
45742	Olecranon Bursa		45232	Injection Of Neurolytic Substance
45743	Ganglion Cyst Of Intermediate		45233	Subarachnoid
	Joint		45234	Epidural
45744	Ganglion Cyst Of Wrist		45235	Cervical
45745	Major Joint		45236	Thoracic
45746	Shoulder Joint		45237	Lumbar
45747	Hip Joint		45238	Caudal
45748	Knee Joint		45239	Injection For Chemonucleolysis Of
45749	Bursa Of Major Joint			Disk, With Discography
45750	Subacromial Bursa		41777	Chymopapain
45952	Aspiration		45240	Injection For Occlusion Of Spinal
45950	Bone Cyst			Arteriovenous Malformation
45953	Injection		41784	Nerve Block
45954	Bone Cyst		45441	Trigeminal
44866	Neurological Procedures		45442	Facial
45096	Transcatheter Occlusion		45443	Greater Occipital
45097	Intracranial		45444	Vagus
45098	For Tumor Destruction		45445	Phrenic
45099	To Achieve Hemostasis		45446	Spinal Accessory
45100	To Occlude A Vascular		45447	Cervical Plexus
	Malformation		45448	Brachial Plexus
45106	To Thrombose An Aneurysm		45449	Axillary
45101	Spinal Cord		45450	Suprascapular
45102	For Tumor Destruction		45451	Intercostal
45103	To Achieve Hemostasis		45452	Single Block
45104	To Occlude A Vascular		45453	Multiple Blocks
	Malformation		45454	Ilioinguinal
45105	To Thrombose Aneurysm		45455	Iliohypogastric
45107	Head (Non-CNS)		45456	Pudendal
45108	Neck		45457	Paracervical (uterine)
41758	Carotid Artery		45458	Paravertebral
41781	Spinal Tap		45459	Single Level
45214	For Drainage Of Fluid		45460	Thoracic
45215	Lumbar Injection		45461	Lumbar
45216	Of Blood		45462	Sacral
45217	Clot Patch		45463	Coccygeal

OFFICE & LAB PROCEDURES, CONT.

45464	Multiple Levels	71264		.6 to 1cm
45465	Paravertebral Facet Joint	72800		1.1 to 2cm
45466	Single Lumbar Level	72802		Over 2cm
45467	Additional Lumbar Level	71245	Ears	
45468	Sciatic	71265		Up To .5cm
45469	Chemical Sympathectomy	71266		.6 to 1cm
45470	Sphenopalatine Ganglion	71267		1.1 to 2cm
45471	Carotid Sinus	72805		Over 2cm
45472	Stellate Ganglion (Cervical)	71246	Scalp	
45473	Paravetebral	71268		Up To .5cm
45474	Thoracic	71269		.6 to 1cm
45475	Lumbar	71270		1.1 to 2cm
45476	Celiac Plexus	71271		Over 2cm
45902	Integumentary Procedures	71247	Neck	
45903	Acne Surgery	71272		Up To .5cm
72855	Facial Dermabrasion	71273		.6 to 1cm
45928	Paring / Curettage Of Benign	71274		1.1 to 2cm
	Hyperkeratotic Lesion	72809		Over 2cm
45929	Single Lesion	71248	Trunk	
45930	2-4	71276		Up To .5cm
45931	Over 4 Lesions	71277		.6 to 1cm
45932	Skin Tag Removal	71278		1.1 to 2cm
45933	Up To 15 Lesions	71279		Over 2cm
45934	Each Additional 10 Lesions	71249	Genitalia	
71069	Electrosurgical Skin Tags Destruction	71280		Up To .5cm
71070	An Additional 10 Lesions	71281		.6 to 1cm
72849	Intralesional Injections - Up To	72807		1.1 to 2cm
	Seven	71275		Over 2cm
72851	Intralesional Injections - More Than	71250	Arms	
	Seven	71282		Up To .5cm
71239	Shaving Of Lesion	71283		.6 to 1cm
71240	Face	71284		1.1 to 2cm
71254	Up To .5cm	71285		Over 2cm
71255	.6 to 1cm	71251	Hands	
71256	1.1 to 2cm	71286		Up To .5cm
72783	Over 2cm	71287		.6 to 1cm
71241	Eyelids	71288		1.1 to 2cm
71257	Up To .5cm	72812		Over 2cm
71258	.6 to 1cm	71252	Legs	
72789	1.1 to 2cm	71289		Up To .5cm
72792	Over 2cm	71290		.6 to 1cm
71242	Nose	71291		1.1 to 2cm
71259	Up To .5cm	71292		Over 2cm
71260	.6 to 1cm	71253	Feet	
72794	1.1 to 2cm	71293		Up To .5cm
72803	Over 2cm	71294		.6 to 1cm
71243	Lips	71295		1.1 to 2cm
71261	Up To .5cm	71296		Over 2cm
71262	.6 to 1cm	41746	Excision Of Lesion	
72797	1.1 to 2cm	71297	Face	
72796	Over 2cm	71312		Benign
71244	Mucous Membrane	71340		Up To .5cm
71263	Up To .5cm	71341		.6 to 1cm

OFFICE & LAB PROCEDURES, CONT.

71342	1.1 to 2cm		71383	.6 to 1cm
71343	2.1 to 3cm		71384	1.1 to 2cm
71356	3.1 to 4cm		71385	2.1 to 3cm
71357	Over 4cm		71386	3.1 to 4cm
71313	Malignant		71321	Malignant
71344	Up To .5cm		71387	Up To .5cm
71345	.6 to 1cm		71388	.6 to 1cm
71346	1.1 to 2cm		71389	1.1 to 2cm
71347	2.1 to 3cm		71390	2.1 to 3cm
71358	3.1 to 4cm		71391	3.1 to 4cm
71359	Over 4cm		71302	Ears
71298	Eyelids		71322	Benign
71314	Benign		71392	Up To .5cm
71348	Up To .5cm		71393	.6 to 1cm
71349	.6 to 1cm		71394	1.1 to 2cm
71350	1.1 to 2cm		71395	2.1 to 3cm
71360	2.1 to 3cm		71396	3.1 to 4cm
71361	3.1 to 4cm		71323	Malignant
71315	Malignant		71397	Up To .5cm
71351	Up To .5cm		71398	.6 to 1cm
71352	.6 to 1cm		71399	1.1 to 2cm
71353	1.1 to 2cm		71400	2.1 to 3cm
71362	2.1 to 3cm		71401	3.1 to 4cm
71363	3.1 to 4cm		71303	Scalp
71299	Nose		71324	Benign
71316	Benign		71402	Up To .5cm
71354	Up To .5cm		71403	.6 to 1cm
71355	.6 to 1cm		71404	1.1 to 2cm
71364	1.1 to 2cm		71405	2.1 to 3cm
71365	2.1 to 3cm		71406	3.1 to 4cm
71366	3.1 to 4cm		71407	Over 4cm
71317	Malignant		71325	Malignant
71367	Up To .5cm		71408	Up To .5cm
71368	.6 to 1cm		71409	.6 to 1cm
71369	1.1 to 2cm		71410	1.1 to 2cm
71370	2.1 to 3cm		71411	2.1 to 3cm
71371	3.1 to 4cm		71412	3.1 to 4cm
71300	Lips		71413	Over 4cm
71318	Benign		71304	Neck
71372	Up To .5cm		71326	Benign
71373	.6 to 1cm		71414	Up To .5cm
71374	1.1 to 2cm		71415	.6 to 1cm
71375	2.1 to 3cm		71416	1.1 to 2cm
71376	3.1 to 4cm		71417	2.1 to 3cm
71319	Malignant		71418	3.1 to 4cm
71377	Up To .5cm		71419	Over 4cm
71378	6 to 1cm		71327	Malignant
71379	1.1 to 2cm		71420	Up To .5cm
71380	2.1 to 3cm		71421	.6 to 1cm
71381	3.1 to 4cm		71422	1.1 to 2cm
71301	Mucous Membrane		71423	2.1 to 3cm
71320	Benign		71424	3.1 to 4cm
71382	Up To .5cm		71425	Over 4cm

OFFICE & LAB PROCEDURES, CONT.

71305	Trunk		71467	.6 to 1cm
71328	Benign		71468	1.1 to 2cm
71426	Up To .5cm		71469	2.1 to 3cm
71427	.6 to 1cm		71470	3.1 to 4cm
71428	1.1 to 2cm		71471	Over 4cm
71429	2.1 to 3cm		71310	Legs
71430	3.1 to 4cm		71336	Benign
71431	Over 4cm		71472	Up To .5cm
71329	Malignant		71473	.6 to 1cm
71432	Up To .5cm		71474	1.1 to 2cm
71433	.6 to 1cm		71475	2.1 to 3cm
71434	1.1 to 2cm		71476	3.1 to 4cm
71435	2.1 to 3cm		71477	Over 4cm
71436	3.1 to 4cm		71337	Malignant
71437	Over 4cm		71478	Up To .5cm
71306	Genitalia		71479	.6 to 1cm
71330	Benign		71480	1.1 to 2cm
71438	Up To .5cm		71481	2.1 to 3cm
71439	.6 to 1cm		71482	3.1 to 4cm
71440	1.1 to 2cm		71483	Over 4cm
71441	2.1 to 3cm		71311	Feet
71442	3.1 to 4cm		71338	Benign
71331	Malignant		71484	Up To .5cm
71443	Up To .5cm		71485	.6 to 1cm
71444	.6 to 1cm		71486	1.1 to 2cm
71445	1.1 to 2cm		71487	2.1 to 3cm
71446	2.1 to 3cm		71488	3.1 to 4cm
71447	3.1 to 4cm		71489	Over 4cm
71307	Arms		71339	Malignant
71332	Benign		71490	Up To .5cm
71448	Up To .5cm		71491	.6 to 1cm
71449	.6 to 1cm		71492	1.1 to 2cm
71450	1.1 to 2cm		71493	2.1 to 3cm
71451	2.1 to 3cm		71494	3.1 to 4cm
71452	3.1 to 4cm		71495	Over 4cm
71453	Over 4cm		71496	Excision For Hiradenitis
71333	Malignant		71497	Axillary
71454	Up To .5cm		71502	With Complex Repair
71455	.6 to 1cm		71498	Inguinal
71456	1.1 to 2cm		71503	With Complex Repair
71457	2.1 to 3cm		71499	Umbilical
71458	3.1 to 4cm		71504	With Complex Repair
71459	Over 4cm		71500	Perineal
71309	Hands		71505	With Complex Repair
71334	Benign		71501	Perianal
71460	Up To .5cm		71506	With Complex Repair
71461	.6 to 1cm		71063	Nails
71462	1.1 to 2cm		71507	Debridement
71463	2.1 to 3cm		71508	Manual
71464	3.1 to 4cm		71509	Each Additional
71465	Over 4cm		71510	With Electric Grinder
71335	Malignant		71511	Each Additional
71466	Up To .5cm		71065	Second Nail

OFFICE & LAB PROCEDURES, CONT.

71066	Additional Nails	70885	Axilla
71064	Evacuation Of Subungal Hematoma	70899	.1 to 2.5 cm
71067	Permanent Excision Of Nail And	70900	2.6 to 7.5 cm
	Matrix	70901	7.6 to 12.5 cm
71068	With Amputation Of Distal Tuft	70883	Trunk
72819	Repair of Nail Bed	70902	.1 to 2.5 cm
72820	Reconstruction of Nail Bed Using	70903	2.6 to 7.5 cm
	Graft	70904	7.6 to 12.5 cm
72822	Excision Of Ingrown Toe Nail	70905	12.6 to 20.0 cm
70879	Repair Of Superficial Wound	70906	20 to 30 cm
70880	Scalp	70907	over 30 cm
70887	.1 to 2.5 cm	70886	External Genitalia
70890	2.6 to 7.5 cm	70908	.1 to 2.5 cm
70888	7.6 to 12.5 cm	70909	2.6 to 7.5 cm
70889	12.6 to 20.0 cm	70884	Lower Extremities
70916	Face	70910	.1 to 2.5 cm
70922	.1 to 2.5 cm	70911	2.6 to 7.5 cm
70923	2.6 to 5.0 cm	70912	7.6 to 12.5 cm
70924	5.1 to 7.5 cm	70913	12.6 to 20.0 cm
70925	7.6 to 12.5 cm	70914	20 to 30 cm
70926	12.6 to 20.0 cm	70915	over 30 cm
70927	20 to 30 cm	70944	Closure Of Wound Dehiscence
70928	over 30 cm	70945	Layer Closure Of Wound
70917	Ears	70946	Scalp
70929	.1 to 2.5 cm	70961	.1 to 2.5 cm
70930	2.6 to 5.0 cm	70962	2.6 to 7.5 cm
70931	5.1 to 7.5 cm	70963	7.6 to 12.5 cm
70918	Eyelids	70964	12.6 to 20.0 cm
70932	.1 to 2.5 cm	70965	20 to 30 cm
70933	2.6 to 5.0 cm	71033	over 30 cm
70937	5.1 to 7.5 cm	70947	Face
70919	Nose	70966	.1 to 2.5 cm
70934	.1 to 2.5 cm	70967	2.6 to 5.0 cm
70935	2.6 to 5.0 cm	70968	5.1 to 7.5 cm
70936	5.1 to 7.5 cm	70969	7.6 to 12.5 cm
70920	Lips	70970	12.6 to 20.0 cm
70938	.1 to 2.5 cm	70971	20 to 30 cm
70939	2.6 to 5.0 cm	71032	over 30 cm
70940	5.1 to 7.5 cm	70948	Ears
70921	Mouth	70972	.1 to 2.5 cm
70941	.1 to 2.5 cm	70973	2.6 to 5.0 cm
70942	2.6 to 5.0 cm	70974	5.1 to 7.5 cm
70943	5.1 to 7.5 cm	70949	Eyelids
70881	Neck	70975	.1 to 2.5 cm
70891	.1 to 2.5 cm	70976	2.6 to 5.0 cm
70892	2.6 to 7.5 cm	70977	5.1 to 7.5 cm
70893	7.6 to 12.5 cm	70950	Nose
70894	12.6 to 20.0 cm	70978	.1 to 2.5 cm
70882	Upper Extremities	70979	2.6 to 5.0 cm
70895	.1 to 2.5 cm	70980	5.1 to 7.5 cm
70896	2.6 to 7.5 cm	70951	Lips
70897	7.6 to 12.5 cm	70981	.1 to 2.5 cm
70898	12.6 to 20.0 cm	70982	2.6 to 5.0 cm

OFFICE & LAB PROCEDURES, CONT.

70983	5.1 to 7.5 cm
70952	Mouth
70984	.1 to 2.5 cm
70985	2.6 to 5.0 cm
70986	5.1 to 7.5 cm
70953	Neck
70987	.1 to 2.5 cm
70988	2.6 to 7.5 cm
70989	7.6 to 12.5 cm
70990	12.6 to 20.0 cm
70991	20 to 30 cm
70992	Over 30 cm
70954	Axilla
70993	.1 to 2.5 cm
70994	2.6 to 7.5 cm
70995	7.6 to 12.5 cm
70996	12.6 to 20.0 cm
70997	20 to 30 cm
70955	Arms
70998	.1 to 2.5 cm
70999	2.6 to 7.5 cm
71000	7.6 to 12.5 cm
71001	12.6 to 20.0 cm
71002	20 to 30 cm
71003	Over 30 cm
70956	Hands
71004	.1 to 2.5 cm
71005	2.6 to 7.5 cm
71006	7.6 to 12.5 cm
71029	12.6 to 20.0 cm
71030	20 to 30 cm
71031	over 30 cm
70957	Trunk
71007	.1 to 2.5 cm
71008	2.6 to 7.5 cm
71009	7.6 to 12.5 cm
71010	12.6 to 20.0 cm
71011	20 to 30 cm
71012	Over 30 cm
70958	External Genitalia
71013	.1 to 2.5 cm
71014	2.6 to 7.5 cm
71015	7.6 to 12.5 cm
71028	12.6 to 20.0 cm
70959	Legs
71016	.1 to 2.5 cm
71017	2.6 to 7.5 cm
71018	7.6 to 12.5 cm
71019	12.6 to 20.0 cm
71020	20 to 30 cm
71021	Over 30 cm
70960	Feet
71022	.1 to 2.5 cm

71023	2.6 to 7.5 cm
71024	7.6 to 12.5 cm
71025	12.6 to 20.0 cm
71026	20 to 30 cm
71027	over 30 cm
71694	Complex Repair Of Wound
71695	Scalp
71710	1.1 to 2.5 cm
71711	2.6 to 7.5 cm
71712	over 7.5 cm
71696	Face
71713	1.1 to 2.5 cm
71714	2.6 to 7.5 cm
71715	over 7.5 cm
71697	Ears
71716	1.1 to 2.5 cm
71717	2.6 to 7.5 cm
71698	Eyelids
71718	1.1 to 2.5 cm
71719	2.6 to 7.5 cm
71699	Nose
71720	1.1 to 2.5 cm
71721	2.6 to 7.5 cm
71700	Lips
71722	1.1 to 2.5 cm
71723	2.6 to 7.5 cm
71701	Mouth
71724	1.1 to 2.5 cm
71725	2.6 to 7.5 cm
71702	Neck
71726	1.1 to 2.5 cm
71727	2.6 to 7.5 cm
71728	over 7.5 cm
71703	Axilla
71729	1.1 to 2.5 cm
71730	2.6 to 7.5 cm
71731	over 7.5 cm
71704	Arms
71732	1.1 to 2.5 cm
71733	2.6 to 7.5 cm
71734	over 7.5 cm
71705	Hands
71735	1.1 to 2.5 cm
71736	2.6 to 7.5 cm
71706	Trunk
71737	1.1 to 2.5 cm
71738	2.6 to 7.5 cm
71739	over 7.5 cm
71707	External Genitalia
71740	1.1 to 2.5 cm
71741	2.6 to 7.5 cm
71708	Legs
71742	1.1 to 2.5 cm

OFFICE & LAB PROCEDURES, CONT.

71743	2.6 to 7.5 cm
71744	over 7.5 cm
71709	Feet
71745	1.1 to 2.5 cm
71746	2.6 to 7.5 cm
71747	over 7.5 cm
71748	Secondary Closure Of Surgical Wound
71749	Secondary Closure Of Dehiscence
41747	Electrodessication & Curettage
70372	Destruction Of Flat Warts
70373	By Laser
70374	By Electrocautery
70375	By Cryosurgery
41748	Cryotherapy
48836	Elective Surgery Face-lift
48833	Elective Surgery Hair Transplant
48837	Elective Circumcision
43862	Urologic Services
41723	Urethral Catheterization
43864	Indwelling (Foley)
43863	Complicated
48865	Infection Due To Indwelling Urinary Catheter
41810	Dialysis
42492	End Stage Renal Disease Management (monthly)
42493	Patient Under 2 Years Old
45775	Patient 2-12 Years Old
45776	Patient 13-19 Years Old
42491	Patient Over 19 Years Old
45777	Related Daily Services For Less Than 1 Month
41811	Hemodialysis
42503	With Single Physician Evaluation
42504	With Repeated Physician Evaluations
41812	Peritoneal Dialysis
42505	With Single Physician Evaluation
42506	With Repeated Physician Evaluations
42494	Hemofiltration
42507	With Single Physician Evaluation
42508	With Repeated Physician Evaluations
42495	Hemoperfusion
42681	Gynecologic Services
42682	Vaginal Irrigation
42683	With Application of Medication
42684	Insertion Of Pessary
42685	Diaphragm Fitting With Instructions
42686	Placement Of Vaginal Hemostatic Agent or Pack (Non-OB)
42687	Insertion Of Intrauterine Device (IUD)

42688	Removal Of Intrauterine Device (IUD)
42689	Artificial Insemination
49860	Intracervical
49861	Intrauterine
42690	With Sperm Washing And Capacitation
42825	In Vitro Fertilization
42826	Oocyte Retrieval
42827	Culture & Fertilization of Oocytes
42828	Embryo Transfer
42829	Zygote Intrafallopian Transfer
42830	Gamete Intrafallopian Transfer
42691	Contrast Media Injection For Hysterosalpingography
49862	Transcervical Re-establishment Of Fallopian Tube Patency
42692	Hydrotubation Of Oviduct
42768	Pelvic Examination Under Anesthesia
42842	Obstetrical Services
42845	Antepartum Care Only
49863	4-6 Visits
49864	7 Or More Visits
42846	Comprehensive Antepartum, Vaginal Delivery And PP Care
42923	Comprehensive Antepartum, Cesarean Section And PP Care
42847	Vaginal Delivery And Postpartum Care
49865	Cesarean Section
42924	And Postpartum Care
42848	Postpartum Care Only
42849	External Cephalic Version
42844	Insertion Of Cervical Dilator
42843	Placement Of Internal Fetal Monitor
42850	Hospital Delivery Of Placenta Following Home Birth
42926	Medically Induced Abortion
49870	By Amniotic Fluid Injection(s)
49871	By Vaginal Suppositories
41559	**Surgery**
41571	Eyes
45793	Globe
45794	Evisceration
73640	Right
73641	Left
45795	Without Implant
45796	With Implant
73642	With Removal of Corneal Epithelium
73643	With Removal of Entire Cornea
73644	Without Signs of Orbital Infection
45797	Enucleation
73645	Right
73646	Left

SURGERY, CONT.

45798	Without Implant	45825	Nonmagnetic Technique
45799	With Implant	45826	Repair Of Laceration
73647	Hydroxyapetite	45827	Closure Of Conjunctiva
73648	Silicone	73733	Right
45800	Without Muscle Attachment	73734	Left
45801	With Muscle Attachment	73735	Bilateral
45802	Exenteration Of Orbit	45828	By Mobilization And
73649	Right		Rearrangement
73650	Left	45829	With Hospitalization
45803	With Removal Of Bone	45830	Closure Of Nonperforating
45804	With Muscle Graft		Corneal Laceration
49799	With Myocutaneous Flap	73758	Right
73651	With Clean Tumor Margins	73759	Left
45805	Modification Of Ocular Implant	73760	Bilateral
73652	Of The Right Eye	45831	Closure Of Perforating Corneal
73653	Of The Left Eye		Laceration
73654	With Implant Exchange	45832	Not Involving Uveal Tissue
45806	Insertion Of Ocular Implant	45833	With Repair Of Uveal Tissue
73655	Into The Right Globe	45834	With Application Of Tissue
73656	Into The Left Globe		Glue
45807	Subsequent To Evisceration	45835	Closure Of Perforating Scleral
73657	Into The Right Orbit		Laceration
73658	Into The Left Orbit	73761	Right
45808	Subsequent To Enucleation	73762	Left
73659	Hydroxyapetite	73763	Bilateral
73660	Silicone	45836	Not Involving Uveal Tissue
45809	Without Muscle Attachment	45837	With Repair Of Uveal Tissue
45810	With Muscle Attachment	45838	With Application Of Tissue
45811	Reinsertion Of Ocular Implant		Glue
73661	Into The Right Orbit	45839	Repair Of Extraocular Muscle
73662	Into The Left Orbit		Laceration
45812	With Conjunctival Graft	73764	Right
45813	With Reinforcement Using	73765	Left
	Foreign Material	73766	Bilateral
45814	With Muscle Attachment	45840	Repair Of Tendon Laceration
45815	Removal Of Ocular Implant	73767	Right
73663	From The Right Orbit	73768	Left
73664	From The Left Orbit	73769	Bilateral
45816	Removal Of Foreign Body	45841	Repair Of Tenon's Capsule
45817	From Conjuctiva	73770	Right
73665	Right Eye	73771	Left
73666	Left Eye	73772	Bilateral
45818	Superficial	45842	Cornea
45819	Embedded	45843	Excision Of Lesion
45820	From The Cornea	73736	Right
73667	Right Eye	73737	Left
73668	Left Eye	45844	Excision Of Pterygium
45821	Utilizing A Slit Lamp	73773	Right
45822	Intraocular	73774	Left
45823	From Posterior Segment	45846	With Graft
73669	Right Eye	73671	With Topical Mitomycin
73670	Left Eye	45845	Transposition Of Pterygium
45824	Magnetic Technique	73775	Right

SURGERY, CONT.

73776	Left	73801	Left
45847	With Graft	49797	With Excimer Laser Keratectomy
49218	Removal Of Epithelium	49235	Correction Of Surgically Induced
73738	Right Cornea		Astigmatism
73739	Left Cornea	73802	Right
49219	With Chemocauterization	73803	Left
49220	With Application Of Chelating	73804	Bilateral
	Agent	49236	By Relaxing Incision
49221	Destruction Of Lesion	49237	By Wedge Resection
73777	Right	73672	By Excimer Laser
73778	Left	49238	Anterior Chamber
49222	By Cryotherapy	49239	Paracentesis
49223	By Photocoagulation	73805	Right
49224	By Thermocauterization	73806	Left
49225	Multiple Punctures	49240	With Release Of Aqueous
73779	Right	49243	With Discission Of Anterior
73780	Left		Hyaloid Membrane
41574	Transplant	49244	And Air Injection
73781	Right	49245	With Removal Of Blood
73782	Left	49246	And Irrigation
49226	Lamellar	49247	And Air Injection
49227	Penetrating	73673	With Inadvertent Lens Capsule
49798	Phakic		Rupture
49228	(In Aphakia)	49248	Goniotomy
49229	(In Pseudophakia)	73807	Right
49230	Keratomileusis	73808	Left
73783	Right	73809	Bilateral
73784	Left	49249	Trabeculotomy Ab Externo
49231	Keratophakia	73810	Right
73785	Right	73811	Left
73786	Left	73812	Bilateral
49232	Keratoprosthesis	49250	Laser Trabeculoplasty
73787	Right	73740	Right Eye
73788	Left	73742	Superior Half
49233	Epikeratoplasty	73743	Inferior Half
73789	Right	73744	Nasal Half
73790	Left	73745	Temporal Half
49234	Radial Keratotomy	73741	Left Eye
73791	Right	73746	Superior Half
73792	Left	73747	Inferior Half
73793	Bilateral	73748	Nasal Half
49794	Excimer Laser Photorefractive	73749	Temporal Half
	Keratectomy	49251	Severing Lesions Of The Anterior
73794	Right		Segment
73795	Left	73813	Right
73796	Bilateral	73814	Left
49795	Excimer Laser Phototherapeutic	49252	By Laser
	Keratectomy	49253	By Incision
73797	Right	49255	With Air Injection
73798	Left	49256	With Fluid Injection
73799	Bilateral	49254	Goniosynechiae
49796	Automated Lamellar Keratectomy	49257	Anterior Synechiae
73800	Right	49258	Posterior Synechiae

SURGERY, CONT.

49259	Corneovitreal	73843	Right
49260	Removal Of Epithelial Downgrowth	73844	Left
73815	Right	73845	At ___ o'clock
73816	Left	49276	Revision Of Aqueous Shunt To Extraocular Reservoir
49261	Removal Of Implanted Material	73846	Right
73817	Right	73847	Left
73818	Left	73848	At ___ o'clock
49262	Removal Of A Blood Clot	49277	Repair Of Scleral Staphyloma
73819	Right	73849	Right
73820	Left	73850	Left
49263	Injection Of Medication	73851	From ___ o'clock
73821	Right	73852	To ___ o'clock
73822	Left	49278	With Graft
49264	Anterior Sclera	49279	Repair / Revision Of Operative Wound Of Anterior Segment
49265	Excision Of Lesion		
73823	Right	73853	Right
73824	Superior Half	73854	Left
73825	Inferior Half	73855	From ___ o'clock
73826	Nasal Half	73856	To ___ o'clock
73827	Temporal Half	49280	Iris
73828	Left	49282	Iridotomy
73829	Superior Half	73857	Right
73830	Inferior Half	73858	Left
73831	Nasal Half	73859	At ___ o'clock
73832	Temporal Half	49283	By Stab Incision
49266	Fistulization For Glaucoma	49285	With Transfixion
73833	Right	49284	By Laser
73834	Superior Half	73676	Argon
73835	Inferior Half	73677	YAG
73836	Nasal Half	73678	Dye
73837	Temporal Half	41573	Iridectomy
73838	Left	73860	Right
73839	Superior Half	73861	Left
73840	Inferior Half	73862	At ___ o'clock
73841	Nasal Half	49286	With Corneal Section
73842	Temporal Half	49287	With Corneoscleral Section
49267	By Trephination Including Iridectomy	49288	For Removal Of Lesion
		49289	With Cyclectomy
49268	By Thermocauterization Including Iridectomy	49290	Peripheral, For Glaucoma
		49291	Sector, For Glaucoma
49269	By Sclerectomy By Punch, Including Iridectomy	49292	Optical
		49297	By Laser
49270	By Sclerectomy By Scissors, Including Iridectomy	49293	Repair
		73863	Right
49271	By Iridencleisis	73864	Left
49272	By Iridotasis	73865	From ___ o'clock
49273	By Trabeculectomy Ab Externo	73866	To ___ o'clock
73674	From ___ o'clock	49295	Suture, With Retrieval Through Small Incision
73675	To ___ o'clock		
49274	In The Presence Of Previous Scarring	49298	Iridoplasty By Photocoagulation
		73867	Right
49275	Aqueous Shunt To Extraocular Reservoir	73868	Left

SURGERY, CONT.

73869	From ___ o'clock	49316	By Phacofragmentation With Aspiration
73870	To ___ o'clock		
49299	Destruction Of Cyst	49317	By Pars Plana Approach
73871	Right	49318	With Vitrectomy
73872	Left	73680	Partial
73873	At ___ o'clock	73681	Total
49300	Destruction Of Lesion	73679	For Dislocated Lens
73874	Right	73682	With Vitreous Hemorrhage
73875	Left	73683	With Retinal Detachment
73876	At ___ o'clock	49319	Intracapsular
49281	Ciliary Body	49320	For Dislocated Lens
49294	Repair	73684	For Subluxated Lens
73877	Right	41572	Extracapsular
73878	Left	49322	Intracapsular Cataract Extraction With Insertion Of Prosthesis
73879	From ___ o'clock		
73880	To ___ o'clock	73897	Right
49296	Suture, With Retrieval Through Small Incision	73898	Left
		73899	With Vitreous Loss
49301	Destruction	49323	Extracapsular Cataract Extraction With Insertion Of Prosthesis
73881	Right		
73882	Left	73900	Right
73883	From ___ o'clock	73901	Left
73884	To ___ o'clock	73902	With Vitreous Loss
49302	By Diathermy	49324	Insertion Of Intraocular Prosthesis, Cataract Previously Removed
49303	By Cyclophotocoagulation		
49304	By Cryotherapy	73903	Right
49305	By Cyclodialysis	73904	Left
49306	Destruction Of Cyst	73905	With Vitreous Present
73885	Right	73906	Into the Anterior Chamber
73886	Left	73907	Into the Posterior Chamber
73887	At ___ o'clock	49312	Repositioning Of Intraocular Prosthesis By Incision
49307	Destruction Of Lesion		
73888	Right	73911	Right
73889	Left	73912	Left
73890	At ___ o'clock	73913	With Vitreous Present
49308	Lens	49325	Exchange Of Intraocular Lens
49309	Discission Of Secondary Membranous Cataract	73915	Right
		73916	Left
73891	Right	73917	With Vitreous Present
73892	Left	73918	Into the Anterior Chamber
49310	By Stab Incision	73919	Into the Posterior Chamber
49311	By Laser	49326	Vitreous
49313	Removal Of Secondary Membranous Cataract With Corneo-Scleral Section	73920	Right
		73922	Left
		49327	Partial Removal Of Vitreous By Anterior Approach
73893	Right		
73894	Left	49328	Subtotal Removal Of Vitreous By Anterior Approach With Mechanical Vitrectomy
49321	With Iridectomy		
49314	Removal Of Lens Material		
73895	Right	49330	Aspiration / Release Of Subretinal Fluid By Pars Plana Approach
73896	Left		
49315	By Aspiration	49331	Aspiration / Release Of Choroidal Fluid By Pars Plana Approach

SURGERY, CONT.

49332	Intravitreal Injection Of A Pharmacologic Agent	49347	With Scleral Buckling
		71523	With Implant
73923	Vancomycin	71524	With Lincoff Balloon
73925	Amikacin	49348	With Vitrectomy
73926	Amphotericin	49349	By Injection Of ___cc Gas
73927	Gancyclovir	73706	___% SF6
73928	Cidovivir	73707	___% C2F6
73929	Gentamycin	73708	___% C3F8
73930	Ceftriaxone	49350	In Presence Of Previous Repair
49333	Discission Of Vitreous By Pars Plana Approach	49351	Release Of Encircling Band
		49907	Release Of Encircling Buckle
49334	Severing By Laser Surgery	49352	Removal Of Implanted Material
49335	Of Vitreous Strands	49353	Extraocular
49336	Of Vitreous Face Adhesions	49354	Intraocular
49337	Of Vitreous Membranes	49355	Prophylaxis Of Detachment
49338	Of Vitreous Opacities	49356	By Cryotherapy
49339	Mechanical Vitrectomy By Pars Plana Approach	49357	By Diatherapy
		49358	By Laser
49340	With Epiretinal Membrane Stripping	49359	By Xenon Arc
		49360	Localized Lesion Destruction
49341	With Focal Endolaser Photocoagulation	73709	Choroidal Neovascularization
		73710	Diabetic Macula Edema
49342	With Endolaser Panretinal Photocoagulation	73711	Macula Edema From Vein Occlusion
73685	With Air-Fluid Exchange	73712	Central Serous Retinopathy
73686	With Intraocular Gas Tamponade	49361	By Cryotherapy
73687	___% SF6	49362	By Diatherapy
73688	___% C2F6	49363	By Laser
73689	___% C3F8	49364	By Xenon Arc
73690	With ___centistroke Silicone Oil Tamponade	49365	By Implantation Of Radiation Source
49343	Retina	49366	Destruction Of Extensive / Progressive Retinopathy
41575	Repair Of Detachment		
73696	Rhegmatogenous	73713	From Proliferative Diabetic Retinopathy
73701	With Retinal Break(s)		
73702	Superior	73714	From Neovascularization Due To Vein Occlusion
73703	Inferior		
73704	Nasal	73715	Due To Rubeosis
73705	Temporal	49367	By Cryotherapy
73697	Traction	49368	By Diatherapy
73699	With ___grade PVR	49369	By Laser
73698	Combined Rhegmatogenous And Traction	49370	By Xenon Arc
		49371	Sclera
73700	With ___grade PVR	73932	Right
73691	From ___o'clock	73933	Left
73692	To ___o'clock	73934	From ___ o'clock
73693	Right Eye	73935	To ___ o'clock
73694	Left Eye	49372	Reinforcement
73695	With Macular Detachment	49373	With Graft
49344	By Cryotherapy	49374	Extraocular Muscles
49345	By Diatherapy	49378	Strabismus
41576	By Laser	49379	By ___mm Recession
49346	By Xenon Arc	49380	Of One Horizontal Muscle

SURGERY, CONT.

73716	___mm Right Medial Rectus	74262	Left Inferior Rectus
73717	___mm Right Lateral Rectus	74263	Left Inferior Oblique
73718	___mm Left Medial Rectus	49390	Of The Superior Oblique Muscle
73719	___mm Left Lateral Rectus		
49381	Of Two Horizontal Muscles	74265	Right Eye
73937	___mm Right Medial Rectus	74266	Left Eye
73938	___mm Right Lateral Rectus	74267	Bilateral
73939	___mm Left Medial Rectus	49396	By Posterior Fixation Suture
73940	___mm Left Lateral Rectus	49391	For A Patient With Previous Eye Surgery Not Involving The Extraocular Muscles
49382	Of One Vertical Muscle		
74227	Right Superior Rectus		
74228	Right Inferior Rectus	49392	For A Patient With Scarring From A Prior Ocular Injury
74229	Right Inferior Oblique		
74230	Left Superior Rectus	49393	For A Patient With Scarring From Prior Strabismus Surgery
74231	Left Inferior Rectus		
74232	Left Inferior Oblique	49394	For A Patient With Scarring From Prior Retinal Detachment Surgery
49383	Of Two Or More Vertical Muscles		
		49395	For A Patient With A Restrictive Myopathy
74233	Right Superior Rectus		
74234	Right Inferior Rectus	49398	With Placement Of Adjustable Suture(s)
74235	Right Inferior Oblique		
74236	Left Superior Rectus	49397	With Exploration / Repair Of Detached Extraocular Muscle(s)
74237	Left Inferior Rectus		
74238	Left Inferior Oblique	49399	Release Of Extensive Scar Tissue Without Detaching Extraocular Muscle
49384	Of The Superior Oblique Muscle		
74211	Right	49400	Chemodenervation Of Extraocular Muscle
74212	Left		
74213	Bilateral	74214	Right Medial Rectus
49385	By Resection	74215	Right Lateral Rectus
49386	Of One Horizontal Muscle	74216	Right Superior Rectus
74239	___mm Right Medial Rectus	74217	Right Inferior Rectus
74240	___mm Right Lateral Rectus	74218	Right Superior Oblique
74241	___mm Left Medial Rectus	74219	Right Inferior Oblique
74242	___mm Left Lateral Rectus	74220	Left Medial Rectus
49387	Of Two Horizontal Muscles	74221	Left Lateral Rectus
74246	___mm Right Medial Rectus	74222	Left Superior Rectus
74247	___mm Right Lateral Rectus	74223	Left Inferior Rectus
74248	___mm Left Medial Rectus	74224	Left Superior Oblique
74250	___mm Left Lateral Rectus	74225	Left Inferior Oblique
49388	Of One Vertical Muscle	49375	Orbit
74251	Right Superior Rectus	49401	Orbitotomy
74252	Right Inferior Rectus	73944	Right
74253	Right Inferior Oblique	73945	Left
74254	Left Superior Rectus	73946	Bilateral
74255	Left Inferior Rectus	49402	Without Bone Flap
74256	Left Inferior Oblique	49403	For Exploration
49389	Of Two Or More Vertical Muscles	49404	With Drainage Only
		49405	With Removal Of Lesion
74258	Right Superior Rectus	49406	With Removal Of Bone For Decompression
74259	Right Inferior Rectus		
74260	Right Inferior Oblique	49407	With Bone Flap Or Window (Lateral Approach)
74261	Left Superior Rectus		

SURGERY, CONT.

49408	For Exploration	74013	Right Upper Eyelid
49409	With Drainage	74270	Right Lower Eyelid
49410	With Removal Of Lesion	74271	Left Upper Eyelid
49411	With Removal Of Bone For Decompression	74272	Left Lower Eyelid
		49430	Under General Anesthesia
49412	Fine Needle Aspiration Of Orbital Contents	49431	Requiring Hospitalization
		49432	Correction Of Trichiasis
73947	Right	74061	Right Upper Eyelid
73948	Left	74062	Right Lower Eyelid
49413	Retrobulbar Injection	74063	Left Upper Eyelid
73949	Right	74064	Left Lower Eyelid
73950	Left	49433	Epilation
49414	Of Medication	49434	By Forceps Only
73951	Steroids	49435	By Electrosurgery
49415	Of Alcohol	74065	By Laser
49416	Injection Of Therapeutic Agent Into Tenon's Capsule	49436	By Cryotherapy
		49437	Incision Of Lid Margin
73952	Right	49438	With Free Mucous Membrane Graft
73953	Left		
73954	Steroids	49439	Excision Of ___ cm Lesion
73955	Antibiotics	73720	___ cm Lesion Of Right Upper Eyelid
49417	Orbital Implant		
73956	Right	73722	___ cm Lesion Of Right Lower Eyelid
73957	Left		
49418	Insertion	73721	___ cm Lesion Of Left Upper Eyelid
49419	Revision		
49420	Removal	73723	___ cm Lesion Of Left Lower Eyelid
49421	Optic Nerve Decompression		
73959	Right	49440	With Simple Direct Closure
73960	Left	49441	Destruction Of ___ cm Lesion Of Lid Margin
49376	Eyelids		
49422	Blepharotomy And Drainage Of Abscess	74066	___ cm Lesion of Right Upper Eyelid Margin
73961	Right Upper Eyelid	74067	___ cm Lesion of Right Lower Eyelid Margin
73968	Right Lower Eyelid		
73970	Left Upper Eyelid	74068	___ cm Lesion of Left Upper Eyelid Margin
73971	Left Lower Eyelid		
49424	Canthotomy	74069	___ cm Lesion of Left Lower Eyelid Margin
73972	Right		
73973	Left	49442	Temporary Closure By Suture
49425	Excision Of Chalazion	74070	Right
49426	Single	74071	Left
73974	Right Upper Eyelid	74072	Bilateral
73975	Right Lower Eyelid	49443	Construction Of Intermarginal Adhesions
73976	Left Upper Eyelid		
73977	Left Lower Eyelid	49446	Including Transposition Of Tarsal Plate
49427	Multiple		
49428	Same Lid	49444	Median Tarsorrhaphy
74008	Right Upper Eyelid	74073	Right
74009	Right Lower Eyelid	74074	Left
74010	Left Upper Eyelid	74075	Bilateral
74011	Left Lower Eyelid	49447	Including Transposition Of Tarsal Plate
49429	Different Lids		

SURGERY, CONT.

49423	Severing Of Tarsorrhaphy	74107	Right Upper Eyelid
74014	Right	74108	Right Lower Eyelid
74015	Left	74109	Left Upper Eyelid
74016	Bilateral	74110	Left Lower Eyelid
49445	Canthorrhaphy	49460	By Suture
74076	Right	49461	By Thermocauterization
74077	Left	49462	By Blepharoplasty Including
74078	Bilateral		Excision Of Tarsal Wedge
49448	Including Transposition Of Tarsal	49463	By Extensive Blepharoplasty
	Plate	49464	Repair Of Entropion
49449	Repair Of Brow Ptosis	74111	Right Upper Eyelid
74079	Right Upper Eyelid	74112	Right Lower Eyelid
74080	Left Upper Eyelid	74113	Left Upper Eyelid
74081	Both Upper Eyelids	74114	Left Lower Eyelid
49450	Repair Of Blepharoptosis	49465	By Suture
49451	By Suture Of Frontalis Muscle	49466	By Thermocauterization
74082	Right Upper Eyelid	49467	By Blepharoplasty, Including
74083	Left Upper Eyelid		Excision Of Tarsal Wedge
74084	Both Upper Eyelids	49468	By Extensive Blepharoplasty
49452	By Frontalis Muscle Fascial Sling	49469	Suture Of Recent Wound Involving
74085	Right Upper Eyelid		Lid Margin, Tarsus
74086	Left Upper Eyelid	74115	Right Upper Eyelid
74087	Both Upper Eyelids	74116	Right Lower Eyelid
49453	By Levator Resection And	74117	Left Upper Eyelid
	Advancement, Internal Approach	74118	Left Lower Eyelid
74088	Right Upper Eyelid	49470	And Palpebral Conjunctiva
74089	Left Upper Eyelid	49471	Partial Thickness
74090	Both Upper Eyelids	49472	Full Thickness
49454	By Levator Resection And	49473	Suture Of Recent Wound Involving
	Advancement, External Approach		Palpebral Conjunctiva
74091	Right Upper Eyelid	74119	Right Upper Eyelid
74092	Left Upper Eyelid	74120	Right Lower Eyelid
74093	Both Upper Eyelids	74121	Left Upper Eyelid
49455	By Superior Rectus Fascial Sling	74122	Left Lower Eyelid
74094	Right	49474	Partial Thickness
74095	Left	49475	Full Thickness
74096	Bilateral	49476	Removal Of Embedded Foreign
49456	By Conjunctivo-Tarso-Muller's		Body
	Muscle-Levator Resection	74123	Right Upper Eyelid
74097	Right Upper Eyelid	74124	Right Lower Eyelid
74098	Left Upper Eyelid	74125	Left Upper Eyelid
74099	Both Upper Eyelids	74126	Left Lower Eyelid
49457	Reduction Of Overcorrection Of	49477	Canthoplasty
	Ptosis	74127	Right Upper Eyelid
74100	Right Upper Eyelid	74128	Right Lower Eyelid
74101	Left Upper Eyelid	74129	Left Upper Eyelid
74102	Both Upper Eyelids	74130	Left Lower Eyelid
49458	Correction Of Lid Retraction	49478	Excision And Repair
74103	Right Upper Eyelid	74131	Right Upper Eyelid
74104	Right Lower Eyelid	74132	Right Lower Eyelid
74105	Left Upper Eyelid	74133	Left Upper Eyelid
74106	Left Lower Eyelid	74134	Left Lower Eyelid
49459	Repair Of Ectropion	49479	Up To One-Fourth Of Lid Margin

SURGERY, CONT.

49480	Over One-Fourth Of Lid Margin	49504	With Free Conjunctival Membrane Graft
49481	Full Thickness Reconstruction Of Eyelid	49505	With Free Buccal Mucous Membrane Graft
74135	Right Upper Eyelid	49506	By Division
74136	Right Lower Eyelid	49507	Including Insertion Of Conformer
74137	Left Upper Eyelid		
74138	Left Lower Eyelid	49508	Including Insertion Of Contact Lens
49482	Up To Two-Thirds Of Eyelid, One Stage		
		49509	Conjunctival Flap
49483	Total Lower Eyelid, One Stage	74156	Right
49484	Total Upper Eyelid, One Stage	74157	Left
49485	Second Stage	74158	Bilateral
49377	Conjunctiva	49510	Bridge
74139	Right	49511	Partial
74140	Left	49512	Total
74141	Bilateral	49513	Lacrimal System
49486	Incision And Drainage Of Cyst	49514	Incision And Drainage Of Lacrimal Gland
49487	Expression Of Follicles		
49488	Excision Of Lesion	74160	Right
49489	Up To One cm. (___cm)	74161	Left
49490	Over One cm. (___cm)	74162	Bilateral
73724	Superior Conjunctiva	49515	Incision And Drainage Of Lacrimal Sac
73725	Inferior Conjunctiva		
73726	Nasal Conjunctiva	74163	Right
73727	Temporal Conjunctiva	74164	Left
49491	With Adjacent Sclera	74165	Bilateral
49492	Destruction Of Lesion	49516	Snip Incision Of Lacrimal Punctum
74143	Superior Conjunctiva	74166	Right Upper Eyelid
74144	Inferior Conjunctiva	74167	Right Lower Eyelid
74145	Nasal Conjunctiva	74168	Left Upper Eyelid
74146	Temporal Conjunctiva	74169	Left Lower Eyelid
49493	Subconjunctival Injection	49517	Excision Of Lacrimal Gland
74147	Right	74170	Right
74148	Left	74171	Left
49494	Conjunctivoplasty	74172	Bilateral
74150	From ___ o'clock	49518	Total
74151	To ___ o'clock	49519	Partial
49495	With Conjunctival Graft	49520	Excision Of Lacrimal Gland Tumor
49496	With Extensive Rearrangement	74173	Right
49497	With Buccal Mucous Membrane Graft	74174	Left
		49521	By Frontal Approach
49498	Reconstruction Of Cul-de-Sac	49522	Involving Osteotomy
49499	With Conjunctival Graft	49523	Excision Of Lacrimal Sac
49500	With Extensive Rearrangement	74175	Right
49501	With Buccal Mucous Membrane Graft	74176	Left
		74177	Bilateral
49502	Repair Of Symblepharon	49524	Removal Of Dacryolith From Lacrimal Passage
74152	Right Superior Conjunctiva		
74153	Right Inferior Conjunctiva	74178	Right
74154	Left Superior Conjunctiva	74179	Left
74155	Left Inferior Conjunctiva	49525	Removal Of Foreign Body From Lacrimal Passage
49503	By Conjunctivoplasty		

SURGERY, CONT.

74180	Right		49548	Probing Of Lacrimal Canaliculi
74181	Left		74207	Right Upper Eyelid
49526	Plastic Repair Of Lacrimal		74208	Right Lower Eyelid
	Canaliculi		74209	Left Upper Eyelid
74182	Right Upper Eyelid		74210	Left Lower Eyelid
74183	Right Lower Eyelid		49549	Including Irrigation
74184	Left Upper Eyelid		41568	Oral
74185	Left Lower Eyelid		41569	Tooth Extraction
49527	Correction Of Everted Punctum,		41570	recent tooth extraction
	With Cautery		74364	Ear Surgery
74186	Right Upper Eyelid		74365	External
74187	Right Lower Eyelid		74366	Drainage Of Abcess
74188	Left Upper Eyelid		74549	Simple
74189	Left Lower Eyelid		74375	Complicated
49528	Fistulization Of Lacrimal Sac To		74367	Right Ear
	Nasal Cavity		74368	Left Ear
74190	Right		74369	Drainage Of Hematoma
74191	Left		74550	Simple
49529	Fistulization Of Conjunctiva To		74372	Complicated
	Nasal Cavity		74370	Right Ear
74192	Right		74371	Left Ear
74193	Left		74378	Piercing
49530	Without Tube Or Stent		74379	Right
49531	With Insertion Of Tube		74380	Left
49532	With Insertion Of Stent		74381	Simple Repair
49533	Closure Of The Lacrimal Punctum		74382	Right
74194	Right Upper Eyelid		74383	Left
74195	Right Lower Eyelid		74384	Amputation
74196	Left Upper Eyelid		74551	Right
74197	Left Lower Eyelid		74386	Left
49534	By Thermocauterization		74387	Otoplasty
49535	By Ligation		74385	Right
49536	By Laser		74388	Left
49537	By Plug		74553	External Auditory Canal
49538	Closure Of A Lacrimal Fistula		74556	Drainage Of Abcess
74198	Right		74554	Right
74199	Left		74555	Left
49539	Dilation Of The Lacrimal Punctum		74557	Exostosectomy
74200	Right Upper Eyelid		74558	Right
74201	Right Lower Eyelid		74559	Left
74202	Left Upper Eyelid		74560	Removal Of Lesion
74203	Left Lower Eyelid		74561	Right
49540	With Irrigation		74562	Left
49541	Bilateral		74563	Radical Excision Of Lesion
49542	Probing Of Nasolacrimal Duct		74566	With Neck Dissection
74204	Right		74564	Right
74205	Left		74565	Left
74206	Bilateral		74567	Removal Of Foreign Body
49543	Including Irrigation		74568	Under General Anesthesia
49544	Bilateral		74569	Right
49545	Requiring General Anesthesia		74570	Left
49546	With Insertion Of Tube		74571	Debridement Of Mastoidectomy
49547	With Insertion Of Stent			Cavity

SURGERY, CONT.

74572	Simple	74681	Radical
74573	Complex	74682	With Petrous Apicectomy
74574	Right	74683	Revision
74575	Left	74684	Complete
74576	Meatoplasty	74685	Modified Radical
74577	Right	74686	Radical
74578	Left	74687	With Tympanoplasty
74579	Repair Of Congenital Atresia	74688	With Apicectomy
74580	Right	74702	Aural Polyp Removal
74581	Left	74703	Right
74583	Middle Ear	74704	Left
74584	Eustachian Tube Inflation, Intranasal	74707	Aural Glomus Tumor Removal
74585	With Catheterization	74708	Transcanal Approach
74586	Without Catheterization	74709	Transmastoid Appraoch
74587	Right	74710	Extratemporal
74588	Left	74711	Tympanic Membrane Repair
74589	Eustachian Tube Catheterization, Transtympanic	74712	Right
		74713	Left
74590	Right	74714	Myringoplasty
74591	Left	74715	Right
74592	Application Of Phase Control Substance	74716	Left
		74717	Tympanoplasty
74593	Right	74718	With Ossicular Chain Reconstruction
74596	Left		
41561	Myringotomy	74719	& Synthetic Prosthesis
74598	With Aspiration	74720	With Antrotomy
74600	With Eustachian Tube Inflation	74721	& Ossicular Chain Reconstruction
74602	With Aspiration & Eustachian Tube Inflation	74722	& Synthetic Prosthesis
74604	Requiring General Anesthesia	74723	With Mastoidotomy
74605	Right	74724	& Ossicular Chain Reconstruction
74606	Left		
70607	Ear Pressure Equalization Tube	74725	& Synthetic Prosthesis
70608	Insertion	74726	With Mastoidectomy
70610	Under Local Anesthetic	74730	Complete
70611	Under General Anesthetic	74729	Radical
74676	Right	74728	With Intact Canal Wall
74677	Left	74727	& With Ossicular Chain Reconstruction
70609	Removal		
74667	Exploration	74732	Complete
74668	Right	74733	Radical
74669	Left	74731	With Intact Canal Wall
74670	Transcanal Tympanolysis	74734	Stapes Mobilization
74671	Right	74735	Right
74672	Left	74736	Left
74673	Transmastoid Antrotomy	74737	Stapedectomy
74674	Right	74738	Right
74675	Left	74739	Left
74678	Mastoidectomy	74744	With Footplate Drill Out
74689	Right	74746	Revision
74690	Left	74740	Stapedotomy
74679	Complete	74741	Right
74680	Modified Radical	74742	Left

SURGERY, CONT.

74743	With Footplate Drill Out	44474	Submucous Resection Of Turbinate
74745	Revision	44475	Rhinectomy
74747	Oval Window Fistula Repair	44476	Partial
74748	Right	44477	Total
74749	Left	44482	Intranasal Surgical Removal Of Foreign Body
74750	Round Window Fistula Repair		
74751	Right	44483	Surgical Removal Of Foreign Body By Rhinotomy
74752	Left		
74753	Mastoid Obliteration	41562	Rhinoplasty
74754	Right	44484	Conventional
74755	Left	44485	Complete (Bony Pyramid And Cartilages)
74756	Tympanic Neurectomy		
74757	Right	44486	Complete (With Major Septal Repair)
74758	Left		
74759	Postauricular Mastoid Fistula Closure	44487	Minor Revision
		44488	Intermediate Revision (Bony Work)
74760	Electromagnetic Bone Conduction Hearing Device	44489	Major Revision (Tip And Bony Work)
74761	Implantation	41567	Septoplasty
74762	Replacement	44490	Intranasal Choanal Atresia Repair
74763	Removal	44491	Transpalatine Choanal Atresia Repair
74764	Repair	44492	Lysis Of Intranasal Synechia
74765	Intratemporal Decompression Of Facial Nerve	44493	Oromaxillary Fistula Repair
		44494	Oronasal Fistula Repair
74766	Lateral To Geniculate Ganglion	44495	Intranasal Reconstruction
74767	Medial To Geniculate Ganglion	44496	Nasal Septal Perforation Repair
74768	Intratemporal Suture Of Facial Nerve	44497	Superficial Cauterization Of Turbinate Mucosa
74769	Lateral To Geniculate Ganglion	44498	Intramural Cauterization Of Turbinate Mucosa
74770	Medial To Geniculate Ganglion		
74691	Temporal Bone	44504	Surgical Control Of Nasal Hemorrhage
74692	External Approach	44505	Ligation Of Ethmoidal Arteries
74694	Resection	44506	Ligation Of Maxillary Artery
74705	Right	44507	Therapeutic Fracture Nasal Turbinate
74706	Left	44510	Sinusotomy
74693	Middle Fossa Approach	44511	Intranasal Maxillary Antrotomy
74695	Vestibular Nerve Section	44512	Radical
74696	Facial Nerve Decompression	44513	With Antrochoanal Polypectomy
74697	Facial Nerve Repair	44515	Sphenoid
74698	Facial Nerve Decompression And Repair	44516	With Mucosal Stripping
		44517	With Polypectomy
74699	Internal Auditory Canal Decompression	44518	Frontal
		44519	Simple, External
74700	Removal of Tumor	44521	Unilateral, Transorbital
74666	Rhinologic Surgery	44522	Obliterative, Brow Incision
41563	Extensive Excision Of Nasal Polyps	44523	Obliterative, Brow Incision With Osteoplastic Flap
44470	Excision / Destruction Of Intranasal Lesion (Internal Appr.)	44524	Non-obliterative, Brow Incision With Osteoplastic Flap
44471	Excision / Destruction Of Intranasal Lesion (External Appr.)	44525	Obliterative, Coronal Incision
44469	Complex Excision Of Dermoid Cyst (Under Bone Or Cartilage)	44526	Obliterative, Coronal Incision With Osteoplastic Flap
44473	Excision Of Turbinate		

632

SURGERY, CONT.

44527	Non-obliterative, Coronal Incision With Osteoplastic Flap	44636	Cervicothoracic
44528	Combined	44637	Excision Of Tracheal Tumor
44529	Ethmoidectomy	44638	Cervical
44530	Intranasal, Anterior	44639	Thoracic
44531	Intranasal, Total	44640	Suture Of External Tracheal Wound
44532	Extranasal, Total	44641	Cervical
44533	Maxillectomy	44642	Intrathoracic
44534	With En Bloc Exenteration Of Orbit	44643	Closure Of Tracheostomy / Fistula
44514	Pterygomaxillary Fossa Surgery	44644	With Plastic Repair
44540	Nasal Endoscopy	44645	Revision Of Tracheostomy Scar
44535	With Polypectomy	41577	Thyroid
44536	With Partial Ethmoidectomy	41578	Total Thyroidectomy
44537	With Total Ethmoidectomy	41579	Sub-Total Thyroidectomy
44538	With Maxillary Antrostomy	41580	Hemi-Thyroidectomy
44539	With Foreign Body Removal	41581	Thyroid lobectomy
44541	Maxillary Sinus Endoscopy	41582	Cistrunk Procedure
44542	With Foreign Body Removal	44115	Parathyroid
44543	With Removal Of Cyst	41583	Resection
44544	With Removal Of Mucous Membrane	41584	Single Tumor Removal
44545	With Polypectomy	41585	Sub-Total Parathyroidectomy
44546	With Fungus Ball Removal	41587	Breast
44547	Sphenoid Sinus Endoscopy	41588	Biopsy
44548	With Removal Of Mucous Membrane	41589	Lumpectomy
41560	Throat Surgery	41590	Simple Mastectomy
44549	Laryngotomy	41591	Radical Mastectomy
44550	With Removal Of Tumor	41592	Enlargement procedure
44551	With Removal Of Laryngocele	41593	Reduction procedure
44552	With Cordectomy	48834	Elective Surgery Augmentation
44553	Laryngectomy	48835	Elective Surgery Reduction
44554	Total	41594	Lung
44555	With Radical Neck Dissection	41602	Thoracentesis
44556	Subtotal, Supraglottic	44646	With Insertion Of Tube
44557	With Radical Neck Dissection	44748	Fluid Volume
41566	Partial	41596	Chest Tube Insertion
44558	Horizontal	40094	With Rib Resection
44559	Laterovertical	44647	With Open Flap Drainage For Empyema
44560	Anterovertical	41879	With Chemical Pleurodesis (non-chemotherapeutic)
44561	Antero-latero-vertical		
44562	Pharyngolaryngectomy With Radical Neck Dissection	41595	Bronchoscopy
		44615	With Central Airway Dilation
44563	With Reconstruction	44616	With Closed Reduction Of Fracture
44564	Arytenoidopexy	44617	With Stent Placement
44565	Arytenoidectomy	44618	With Foreign Body Removal
44631	Bronchoplasty	44619	With Excision Of Tumor
44632	Graft Repair	44620	Destruction Of Tumor
44633	Excision Of Stenosis And Anastomosis	44621	Relief Of Stenosis
		44622	With Therapeutic Aspiration
44634	Excision Of Tracheal Stenosis And Anastomosis	44623	Subsequent
		44624	Nasotracheobronchial Suctioning
44635	Cervical	44625	Using Flexible Fiberoptic Bronchoscope, Bedside
		41597	Mediastinoscopy

633

SURGERY, CONT.

44648	Thoracotomy	43588	Pericardial
44649	With Control Of Traumatic	43589	Tube Pericardiostomy
	Hemorrhage	43590	Pericardiotomy
44650	With Repair Of Lung Tear	43591	Creation Of Pericardial Window
44651	For Postoperative Complications	43592	Pericardiectomy
44652	With Open Intrapleural	43593	With Cardiopulmonary Bypass
	Pneumonolysis	43594	Excision Of Pericardial Cyst Or
44653	With Cyst Removal		Tumor
44654	With Excision-Plication Of Bullae	43595	Tumor Resection
44655	With Removal Of Intrapleural	43596	Of Intracardiac Tumor
	Foreign Body	43597	Of External Cardiac Tumor
44656	With Removal Of Intrapulmonary	43598	Wound Repair
	Foreign Body	43599	Cardiac
44657	With Cardiac Massage	43600	With Cardiopulmonary Bypass
44658	Pneumonostomy	43601	Exploratory Cardiotomy
44659	Pleural Scarification	43602	With Cardiopulmonary Bypass
44660	Decortication	43603	Suture Repair Of Great Vessels
44661	Partial	49578	With Shunt Bypass
44662	Parietal Pleurectomy	43604	With Cardiopulmonary Bypass
44663	Partial	43605	Insertion Of Graft, Great Vessels
44664	Decortication And Parietal	49579	With Shunt Bypass
	Pleurectomy	43606	With Cardiopulmonary Bypass
41599	Lobectomy	42608	Cardioverter-defibrillator
72908	With Bronchoplasty	42610	Pulse Generator
72907	Bilobectomy	49565	Insertion
72909	With Bronchoplasty	49571	With Leads
41826	Segmentectomy	49572	By Thoracotomy
72910	With Bronchoplasty	42609	Replacement
72911	Sleeve Lobectomy	42612	Repair
72913	Completion Pneumonectomy	49566	Removal
44669	Wedge Resection Of Lung	49568	By Thoracotomy
44670	Resection Of Lung And Chest Wall En	49569	Including Leads
	Bloc	49570	Insertion Of Leads
44671	With Chest Wall Reconstruction	49567	Replacement Of Leads
44672	With Prosthesis	42611	Insert Pads By Thoracotomy
44673	Extrapleural Empyemectomy	42613	Skin Pocket Revision / Relocation
44674	With Lobectomy	43608	Surgical Ablation Of Ventricular
41600	Pneumonectomy		Arrhythmogenic Focus
44665	Extrapleural	43612	Surgical Ablation Of S-V
44666	With Empyemectomy		Arrhythmogenic Focus
44814	Lung Transplant	43613	With Bypass
44675	Repair Lung Hernia	43614	Surgical Ablation Of S-V
44676	Closure Of Open Flap Drain For		Arrhythmogenic Pathway
	Empyema	43615	With Bypass
44677	Open Closure Of Bronchial Fistula	41608	Intra-Aortic Balloon
44678	Post-traumatic Chest Wall	49595	Percutaneous Insertion
	Reconstruction	42621	Insertion By Open Approach
44679	Extrapleural Rib Resection	42622	Removal
44680	Thoracoplasty	49673	Ventriclar Assist Device
44681	With Bronchopleural Fistula Closure	49674	Implantation For Single Ventricle
44682	Extraperiosteal Pneumonolysis		Support
44683	Therapeutic Pneumothorax	49675	Implantation For Biventricular
41603	Cardiovascular		Support

SURGERY, CONT.

49676	Removal Of Single Ventricle Support	74619	Of The right Atrium
49677	Removal Of Biventricular Support	44804	Ventricular Aneurysmorraphy
44815	Sternotomy	44805	Ventricular Pseudoaneurysm Repair
44816	Mid	70377	Patch Closure Of Myocardial Rupture
44817	Median	43636	Ventricular Septal Defect Repair
41611	Coronary Artery	43629	Repair Of Coronary Fistula
41612	Bypass Graft	49586	With Cardiopulmonary Bypass
43616	Single Venous Graft	43630	Repair Of Anomalous Coronary Artery
49589	In Combination With Arterial Graft	43631	Ligation
		43632	Graft
43617	Two Venous Grafts	43633	With Cardiopulmonary Bypass
49590	In Combination With Arterial Graft	49587	Construction Of Intrapulmonary Artery Tunnel
43618	Three Venous Grafts	49588	By Translocation From Pulmonary Artery To Aorta
49591	In Combination With Arterial Graft	41628	Cardiac Tumor Removal
43619	Four Venous Grafts	43655	Extended Extracorporeal Circulatory Support
49592	In Combination With Arterial Graft	49672	Each Additional 24 Hours
43620	Five Venous Grafts	43651	Cardiac Transplant Procedures
49593	In Combination With Arterial Graft	41627	Transplantation Of Heart
		43652	Donor Cardiectomy
43621	Six Or More Venous Grafts	43653	Heart-lung Transplant
49594	In Combination With Arterial Graft	43654	Donor Heart-Lung Removal
		43702	Aortic Valve Repair
45947	Saphenous Vein Graft (SVBG)	43703	Open Valvuloplasty
45948	Sequential Venous Grafts	43705	With Inflow Occlusion
45949	Y Graft	49580	Using Transventricular Dilation
45941	Single Arterial Graft		With Cardiopulmonary Bypass
45942	Two Arterial Grafts	44749	Decalcification
45943	Three Arterial Grafts	44826	Prolapse Repair
45944	Four Or More Arterial Grafts	44896	Resuspension
41615	Left Internal Mammary Artery Graft (LIMA)	44750	Insertion Of Aortic Valve Conduit
45945	Right Internal Mammary Artery Graft (RIMA)	43704	Construction Of Apical-Aortic Conduit
45946	Sequential Internal Mammary Artery Grafts	41624	Valvulotomy
		41622	Valve Replacement
43626	Reoperation (CABG) After One Month	49581	With Homograft
		43706	With Aortic Annulus Enlargement
43622	Nonautogenous Graft	43707	With Transventricular Annulus Enlargement
43623	Single Graft	49582	Translocation Of Autologous Pulmonary Valve With Homograft Replacement
43624	Two Grafts		
43625	Three Or More Grafts		
43627	Endarterectomy With Cardiopulmonary Bypass	49583	Repair Of LVOT By Patch Enlargement
43628	With Vascularization	43708	Of Subvalvular Aortic Stenosis
43634	Postinfarct Resection Of Myocardium	43709	Of Supravalvular Aortic Stenosis
43635	Aneurysmectomy	43711	Mitral Valve Repair
74616	Of The Left Ventricle	43714	Open Valvuloplasty
74617	Of The Right Ventricle	43715	With Prosthetic Ring
74618	Of The left Atrium	43716	With Radical Reconstruction

SURGERY, CONT.

44751	Chordal Shortening	43843	Repair Of One Valve, Replacement Of Two Valves
44752	Leaflet Repair		
44756	Annuloplasty	43844	Repair Of Three Valves
41621	Valve Replacement	43845	Replacement Of Three Valves
41618	Commissurotomy	44926	Leaflet Repair Procedure
43712	Closed	44832	McGoon
43713	Open	44833	Carpentier
43830	Pulmonary Valve Repair	44834	Merridino
44968	Open Valvuloplasty	44927	Annuloplasty Procedure
44969	Patch Closure	44827	Duran
43836	Outflow Tract Reinforcement	44828	Kaye
43837	Repair Of Infundibular Stenosis	44829	Carpentier
44761	Valve Replacement	44830	deVega
44762	Homograft	44723	Valve Prosthesis Type
44835	Heterograft	44724	Homograft
44839	Valvectomy	47657	Frame Mounted
43831	Commissurotomy	47658	Tube Mounted
43832	Transvenous Balloon	48976	With Coronary Reimplantation
43833	Closed	44725	Porcine
43834	Open, With Inflow Occlusion	44740	St. Jude
43835	Open, With Cardiopulmonary Bypass	44726	Starr-Edwards
		44730	Bjork-Shiley
43717	Tricuspid Valve Repair	44738	Carpentier-Edwards
49584	Valvectomy With Cardiopulmonary Bypass	44727	Braunwald-Cutter
		44728	Smeloff-Cutter
43719	Valvuloplasty	44729	McGovern-Cromie
49585	With Ring Insertion	44731	Lillehi-Kaster
44970	Patch Closure	44732	Hall-Medtronic
43720	Repositioning And Plication For Ebstein Anomaly	44733	Beall-Surgitool
		44734	Kaye-Shiley
44831	Leaflet Repair	44735	Hancock
44760	Annuloplasty	44736	Ionescu-Shiley
41623	Valve Replacement	44737	Angell-Shiley
43718	Open Commissurotomy	44739	Hufnagel
44840	Left A-V Valve Repair	44741	Hull
44841	Open Valvuloplasty	44824	Medtronic Intact
44842	Annuloplasty	44825	Carpentier-Edwards Low Pressure
44843	Valve Replacement	44821	Ball-Cage
44844	Right A-V Valve Repair	44822	Disc
44845	Open Valvuloplasty	44823	Tissue
44971	Patch Closure	47638	Xenograft
44846	Annuloplasty	41619	Heart Valve Replacement
44847	Valve Replacement	41620	Recent
48977	LV Conduit to Descending Aorta	41631	Cardiac Defect Repair
48978	LV Conduit to Ascending Aorta	49644	Closure of Mitral Valve
43838	Multiple Valve Procedures	49646	By Patch
43839	Repair Of Two Valves	49649	By Suture
43840	Repair Of One Valve, Replacement Of One Valve	49645	Closure of Tricuspid Valve
		49647	By Patch
43841	Repair Of Two Valves, Replacement Of One Valve	49650	By Suture
		48975	Closure of AV Valve
43842	Replacement Of Two Valves	49648	By Patch
		49651	By Suture

SURGERY, CONT.

49635	Closure Of Aortic Valve	44905	Suture Of Mitral Cleft
49636	By Patch	43647	Complete Tetralogy Of Fallot Repair
49637	By Suture	44908	Without Pulmonary Atresia
49638	Closure Of Pulmonary Valve	43648	With Transannular Patch
49639	By Patch	49632	With Pulmonary Atresia
49640	By Suture	43650	Pulmonary Artery Banding
49641	Closure Of Semilunar Valve	47655	Peak Systolic Gradient
49642	By Patch	47656	Mean Gradient
49643	By Suture	44898	Pulmonary Artery Closure
70376	Repair Of Cardiac Free Wall	49655	Repair Of Cor Triatriatum By
70378	Oversew Of Myocardial Tear		Resection Of Left Atrial Membrane
43637	Repair Of Congenital Septal Defect	49656	Repair Of Supravalvular Mitral Ring
44763	Atrial Defect		By Resection Of Left Atrial Membrane
41625	Secundum	43656	Transposition Repair
44764	Primum	44954	Auber Procedure
43642	Sinus Venosus Closure	44955	Jatene Procedure
44900	Direct Suture Closure	48963	Senning Procedure
44901	Patch Closure	48964	Mustard Procedure
44902	Surgical Enlargement	48965	With Biologic Material
46022	Balloon Enlargement	48966	With Synthetic Material
48869	Transcutaneous Enlargement	48967	With Pericardium
44956	Atrial Septation	44961	Great Arteries (TGA)
41626	Ventricular Septal Defect	49658	In Presence Of VSD And
44957	Common Ventricle Repair		Subpulmonary Stenosis
44958	Common Ventricle Repair - 1st	49659	In Presence Of Subpulmonary
	Stage		Stenosis With VSD Enlargement
44959	Common Ventricle Repair -	44962	1st Stage
	Complete	44963	Complete
44960	Septation	43662	With Pulmonary Band Removal
44897	Direct Suture Closure	43663	With VSD Closure
44906	Patch Closure	43664	With Subpulmonic Block Repair
44907	Surgical Enlargement	44964	Complete Transposition Of The
46023	Balloon Enlargement		Great Arteries
43638	With Valvulotomy	44965	1st Stage
43639	With Infundibular Resection	44966	Complete
43640	With Removal Of Pulmonary	43657	With Atrial Baffle
	Artery Band	43658	With Pulmonary Band Removal
43710	Myotomy For IHSS	43659	With VSD Closure
47639	Myectomy	43660	With Subpulmonic Block Repair
43641	Combined Atrial And Ventricular	44916	Corrective
43643	Tricuspid Atresia Repair	44917	Palliative
44812	Right Atrium To Pulmonary	44922	Right Atrium
	Artery Connection	44918	Revision Of Baffle
49634	Vena Cava To Pulmonary Artery	43661	With Artery Reconstruction
	Connection	48968	With Intraventricular Repair
44809	Repair Of Ebstein's Anomaly	48969	With Intraventricular Conduit
44810	Danielson Repair	48970	VSD to Aorta & RV to PT Conduit
44811	Ebstein's Repair		(Rastelli)
43644	Endocardial Cushion Defect Closure	48971	VSD to Pulmonary Artery & Arterial
43645	With VSD Repair		Switch
43646	Atrioventricular Canal Repair	48972	AP Window RV to PT Conduit
44903	Complete	48973	Double Conduit
44904	Partial	48974	Bi-Directional Caval Shunt

SURGERY, CONT.

43665	Shunting Procedures	43679	Fistula
43666	Atrial Septectomy	43680	With VSD Repair
43667	Closed	43681	Aneurysm
72916	Open With Bypass	49657	Closure Of Aortico-left Ventricular
43669	Balloon Transvenous Method		Tunnel
43668	Open, With Inflow Occlusion	43682	Total Anomalous Pulmonary Venous
43670	Blade Method		Drainage Repair
43671	Vascular Shunt	43683	Truncus Arteriosus Repair
43672	Subclavian To Pulmonary Artery	43684	Complete
44919	Subclavian To Right Pulmonary	44915	Conduit Replacement
	Artery	43685	Reimplantation Of Anomalous
44920	Subclavian To Left Pulmonary		Pulmonary Artery
	Artery	43686	Aortic Anomaly Repair
44921	Subclavian To Both Pulmonary	43687	Patent Ductus Arteriosus
	Arteries	43688	Primary Ligation
44951	Left Systemic To Pulmonary	43689	Division (Under 18)
	Artery	43690	Division (18 Or Over)
44952	Right Systemic To Pulmonary	43691	Performed With Another
	Artery		Procedure
44953	Bilateral Systemic To Pulmonary	43692	Coarctation Repair
	Artery	43693	With Direct Anastomosis
43673	Ascending Aorta To Pulmonary	44911	With Direct End-To-End
	Artery		Anastomosis
43674	Descending Aorta To Pulmonary	44912	With Direct End-To-Side
	Artery		Anastomosis
44909	Goretex Interposition	43694	With Graft
43675	Central, With Prosthetic Graft	44913	With Patch Aortoplasty
43676	Superior Vena Cava To	43695	With Gusset For Enlargement
	Pulmonary Artery	44914	With Subclavian Flap
47641	With Insertion Into The Right	43697	With Repair Of Hypoplastic Left
	Pulmonary Artery		Heart
47650	From A Left SVC	48959	Resection
47642	With Insertion Into The Left	48960	Left Subclavian Flap
	Pulmonary Artery	48961	Prosthetic Patch
47651	From A Left SVC	48962	Pericardial Patch
47640	With Conduit	43696	Repair Of Hypoplastic Aortic Arch
44813	Bidirectional	49660	With Cardiopulmonary Bypass
47643	Right Atrium To Pulmonary	49661	Repair Of Interrupted Aortic Arch
	Artery	49662	With Cardiopulmonary Bypass
47644	By Direct Anastomosis	43698	Vascular Ring Division
47645	With Conduit	43699	With Reanastomosis
47646	And Pericardial Patch	44935	Aortic Arch Reconstruction
47647	And Prosthetic Valve	43700	Aortopulmonary Septal Defect
47648	Using Homograft		Repair
47652	Intra-atrial Conduit To Pulmonary	43701	With Cardiopulmonary Bypass
	Artery	44939	Insertion Of Conduit From Right
47649	Right Atrium To Right Ventricle		Ventricle To Aorta
47653	Fistula From Residual Ventricle	44942	Double Outlet Right Ventricle
	To Pulmonary Artery		Repair
44910	Combination	49653	With Intraventricular Tunnel
44807	Intracardiac Shunt Repair (Non-septal)	49654	And Repair Of RVOT
44808	Extracardiac Shunt Repair		Obstruction
43678	Sinus Of Valsalva Repair	44943	1st Stage

SURGERY, CONT.

44944	Complete	44928	With Tissue Valve
43846	Thoracic Aortic Aneurysm Repair	44929	With Mechanical Valve
44785	Ascending Aorta	44838	Without Valve
43847	Graft	44936	Right Ventricle To Pulmonary Artery
49663	With Valve Suspension		
49664	With Coronary Reconstruction	44937	Left Ventricle To Pulmonary Artery
49665	And Aortic Root Replacement	44938	Morphologic Left Ventricle To Pulmonary Artery
43848	Graft With Valve Replacement		
44786	Resection	44940	Right Atrium To Pulmonary Artery
44848	Aortic Root Resection		
44787	Suture	44941	Aorta To Pulmonary Artery
44788	Transverse Arch	49652	Anastamosis Of Pulmonary Artery To Aorta
43849	Graft		
44789	Resection	44967	Unifocalization
44790	Suture	49671	Transection Of Pulmonary Artery With Cardiopulmonary Bypass
44791	Descending Aorta		
43850	Graft	44945	Right Ventricular Outflow Tract Reconstruction
44792	Resection		
44793	Suture	44946	Patch
44794	Thoracoabdominal	44947	Pericardial Tissue
43851	Graft	44948	Left Ventricular Outflow Tract Reconstruction
44795	Resection		
44796	Suture	44949	Patch
44765	Aneurysmorraphy	44950	Pericardial Tissue
44806	Aortic Dissection Repair	44766	Intracardiac Mass Removal
44849	Ascending	44767	Left Atrium
44923	Tube Graft	44768	Myxoma
44850	Aortic Arch	44769	Right Atrium
44924	Tube Graft	44770	Myxoma
44851	Descending	44771	Left Ventricle
44925	Tube Graft	44772	Right Ventricle
44852	Abdominal	49117	Intracardiac Thromboembolization
44934	Tube Graft	75221	Was Successful
43852	Pulmonary Artery Procedures	38168	Unsuccessful
43853	Embolectomy	44780	Intracardiac Thrombectomy
43854	With Bypass	44781	Left Ventricle
43855	Without Bypass	44782	Right Ventricle
43856	Endarterectomy	44783	Left Atrium
49666	Stenosis Repair	44784	Right Atrium
44930	Atresia Repair	41609	Arterial Embolectomy
49667	With VSD By Unifocalization Of Pulmonary Arteries	43367	By Neck Incision
		43368	By Thoracic Incision
49668	With Cardiopulmonary Bypass	43369	By Arm Incision
49669	With VSD By Conduit From LV To Pulmonary Arteries	43370	By Forearm Incision
		43371	By Abdominal Incision
49670	With VSD By Conduit From RV To Pulmonary Arteries	43372	By Femoral Incision
		43373	By Leg Incision
44931	1st Stage	43392	Thromboendarterectomy
44932	Complete	43393	Carotid
44933	Reconstruction	49682	Reoperation (At Least 1 Month Later)
44836	Pulmonary Conduit		
44837	With Valve	43394	Vertebral

SURGERY, CONT.

49793	Subclavian	43505	Brachiocephalic Trunk
43395	By Neck Incision	49683	And Branches
43396	By Thoracic Incision	49684	Tibioperoneal Trunk
43397	Innominate	49685	And Branches
43398	Axillary-Brachial	49881	With Radiologic Supervision And Interpretation Of Peripheral Artery
43399	Abdominal Aorta		
43400	Mesenteric	49884	Each Additional Artery
43401	Celiac	49686	Venous
43402	Renal	49888	With Radiologic Supervision And Interpretation
43403	Iliac		
43404	Iliofemoral	49694	Percutaneous Transluminal Atherectomy
43405	Combined Aortoiliac		
43406	Combined Aortoiliofemoral	49696	Renal Artery
43407	Common Femoral	49893	With Radiologic Supervision And Interpretation
43408	Deep Femoral		
43409	Combined Femoral, Popliteal, Tibioperoneal	49901	Each Additional Artery
		49697	Visceral Artery
45870	Percutaneous Transluminal Angioplasty	49894	With Radiologic Supervision And Interpretation
45871	Renal	49902	Each Additional Artery
45872	Radiologic Supervision And Interpretation	49698	Aortic
		49699	Iliac
49885	Each Additional Artery	49700	Femoral-popliteal
45873	Visceral Artery	49701	Brachiocephalic Trunk
49886	Radiologic Supervision And Interpretation	49702	And Branches
		49703	Tibioperoneal Trunk
49887	Each Additional Artery	49704	And Branches
49687	Aortic	49892	With Radiologic Supervision And Interpretation Of Peripheral Artery
49688	Iliac		
49689	Femoral-popliteal	49903	Each Additional Artery
49690	Brachiocephalic Trunk	49695	Intraoperative Transluminal Atherectomy
49691	And Branches		
49692	Tibioperoneal Trunk	49705	Renal Artery
49693	And Branches	49895	With Radiologic Supervision And Interpretation
49882	With Radiologic Supervision And Interpretation Of Peripheral Artery		
		49904	Each Additional Artery
49883	Each Additional Artery	49706	Visceral Artery
49889	Venous	49896	With Radiologic Supervision And Interpretation
49890	With Radiologic Supervision And Interpretation		
		49906	Each Additional Artery
43499	Intraoperative Transluminal Angioplasty	49707	Aortic
		49708	Iliac
43500	Renal Artery	49709	Femoral-popliteal
49897	Radiologic Supervision And Interpretation	49710	Brachiocephalic Trunk
		49711	And Branches
49898	Each Additional Artery	49712	Tibioperoneal Trunk
43501	Visceral Artery	49713	And Branches
49899	Radiologic Supervision And Interpretation	49891	With Radiologic Supervision And Interpretation Of Peripheral Artery
		49905	Each Additional Artery
49900	Each Additional Artery	43319	Arteriovenous
43502	Aortic	43320	Insertion Of External Cannula
43503	Iliac	43321	Revision Of External Cannula
43504	Femoral-popliteal		

SURGERY, CONT.

43322	Insertion Of Internal Cannula	43362	Temporal Artery
41630	Direct Anastomosis	43363	Major Artery of Neck
43323	Creation Of A-V Fistula	43364	Major Artery of Chest
43324	Autogenous Graft	43365	Major Artery of Abdomen
43325	Nonautogenous Graft	43366	Major Artery of Extremity
43326	Revision Of AV Fistula	49764	Angioaccess Arterioenous Fistula
43327	Insertion Of Cannula For	43507	Bypass Graft Using Vein
	Extracorporeal Circulation	43508	carotid (same side)
43328	Insertion Of Thomas Shunt	43509	carotid-subclavian
43329	Mandrin Insertion	43510	subclavian-carotid
43330	Mandrin Anastomosis	43511	carotid-vertebral
43331	Cannula Declotting	43512	carotid-carotid (right/left)
43332	With Balloon Catheter	43513	subclavian-subclavian
43357	Plastic Repair Of Arteriovenous	43514	subclavian-vertebral
	Aneurysm	43515	subclavian-axillary
43464	Repair Of Arteriovenous Fistula	43516	axillary-axillary
43465	Congenital	43517	axillary-femoral
43466	Of The Head And Neck	43518	aortic-subclavian
43467	In The Thorax	43519	aortic-carotid
43468	In The Abdomen	43520	aortic-celiac
43469	Of The Extremities	43521	aortic-mesenteric
43470	Traumatic	43522	axillary-femoral-femoral
43472	Of The Head And Neck	43523	splenic-renal
43473	In The Thorax	43524	aortic-iliac
43474	In The Abdomen	49790	aortobi-iliac
43475	Of The Extremities	43525	aortic-femoral or bifemoral
43476	Blood Vessel Repair	43526	aortic-iliac-femoral (unilateral)
43477	Direct	43527	aortic-iliac-femoral (bilateral)
43478	Neck	43528	aortic-femoral-popliteal
43479	Arm	43529	femoral-popliteal
43480	Hand Or Finger	43530	femoral-femoral
43481	Intrathoracic With Bypass	43531	aortic-renal
43482	Intrathoracic Without Bypass	43532	iliac-iliac
43483	Intra-abdominal	43533	iliac-femoral
43484	Leg	43534	femoral-tibial
43485	With Vein Graft	43535	femoral-peroneal
43486	Neck	43536	popliteal-tibial
43487	Arm	43537	popliteal-peroneal
43488	Intrathoracic With Bypass	43538	Bypass Graft (Non-Vein)
43489	Intrathoracic Without Bypass	43539	carotid
43490	Intra-abdominal	43540	carotid-subclavian
43491	Leg	43541	subclavian-subclavian
43492	With Nonvenous Graft	43542	subclavian-axillary
43493	Neck	43543	axillary-femoral
43494	Arm	49714	axillary-popliteal
43495	Intrathoracic With Bypass	49715	axillary-tibeal
43496	Intrathoracic Without Bypass	43544	aortic-subclavian
43497	Intra-abdominal	43545	aortic-carotid
43498	Leg	43546	aortic-celiac
43358	Arterial Ligation	43547	aortic-mesenteric
43359	External Carotid Artery	43548	aortic-renal
43360	Internal Or Common Carotid Artery	43549	splenic-renal
43361	With Gradual Occlusion	43550	vertebral-carotid transposition

SURGERY, CONT.

43551	vertebral-subclavian transposition		43463	Ulnar Artery Dilatation Or Occlusion
49718	subclavian-carotid transposition		43431	Abdominal Aorta
49719	carotid-subclavian transposition		41830	For Dilation or Occlusion
43552	aortic-iliac		43432	For Rupture
43553	carotid-vertebral		43433	Abdominal Aorta + Visceral Vessels
43554	subclavian-vertebral		43434	For Dilatation or Occlusion
41613	aortic-femoral or bifemoral		43435	For Rupture
43556	axillary-axillary		43436	Abdominal Aorta + Iliac Vessels
43557	aortic-femoral-popliteal		43437	For Dilatation or Occlusion
49716	aortic-femoral		43438	For Rupture
49717	aortic-bifemoral		43439	Splenic Artery
43558	axillary-femoral-femoral		43440	For Dilatation or Occlusion
41614	femoral-popliteal		43441	For Rupture
43560	femoral-femoral		43442	Hepatic Artery
43561	iliac-iliac		43443	For Dilatation or Occlusion
43562	iliac-femoral		43444	For Rupture
43563	femoral-tibial		43445	Celiac Artery
43564	femoral-peroneal		43446	For Dilatation or Occlusion
43565	popliteal-tibial		43447	For Rupture
43566	popliteal-peroneal		43448	Mesenteric Artery
43567	Composite		43449	For Dilatation or Occlusion
43568	In-Situ Vein Bypass		43450	For Rupture
43569	aortic-femoral-popliteal		43451	Renal Artery
43570	femoral-popliteal		43452	For Dilatation or Occlusion
43571	femoral-tibial		43453	For Rupture
43572	femoral-peroneal		43454	Iliac Artery
43573	popliteal-tibial		43455	For Dilatation or Occlusion
43574	popliteal-peroneal		43456	For Rupture
43410	For Aneurysm		43457	Femoral Artery
43411	Carotid Artery		43458	For Dilatation or Occlusion
43412	For Dilatation Or Occlusion		43459	For Rupture
43413	For Rupture		43460	Popliteal Artery
43414	Subclavian Artery (by neck incision)		43461	For Dilatation or Occlusion
43415	For Dilatation Or Occlusion		43462	For Rupture
43416	For Rupture		43575	Arterial Exploration
43424	Subclavian Artery (by thoracic incision)		43576	carotid
			43577	femoral
43425	For Dilatation Or Occlusion		43578	popliteal
43426	For Rupture		43579	Postoperative Arterial Exploration
43417	Vertebral Artery Dilatation Or Occlusion		43580	Of Neck
			43581	Of Chest
43418	Axillary Artery		43582	Of Abdomen
43419	For Dilatation Or Occlusion		43583	Of An Extremity
43420	For Rupture		43584	To Repair A Graft-enteric Fistula
43421	Brachial Artery		43585	Thrombectomy
43422	For Dilatation Or Occlusion		49720	With Repair Of Venous Graft
43423	For Rupture		43586	Excision Of Infected Graft
43427	Innominate Artery		49550	In The Neck
43428	For Dilatation Or Occlusion		49551	In An Extremity
43429	For Rupture		49552	In The Thorax
43430	Radial Artery Dilatation Or Occlusion		49553	In The Abdomen
			43587	With Revascularization

SURGERY, CONT.

44773	Venous Mass Removal	49876	With Radiologic Supervision And Interpretation
44774	Inferior Vena Cava		
44775	Superior Vena Cava	49752	Infusion (Non-Thromblytic)
43374	Venous Thrombectomy	49753	Retrieval Of Intravascular Foreign Body
43375	By Arm Incision		
43376	By Neck Incision	49880	With Radiologic Supervision And Interpretation
43377	By Abdominal Incision		
43378	By Combined Abdominal And Leg Incision	49754	Occlusion For Tumor Destruction
		49755	Embolization For Tumor Destruction
43379	By Combined Leg Incision	49873	Radiologic Supervision And Interpretation
44777	Inferior Vena Cava		
44778	Superior Vena Cava	49756	Occlusion To Achieve Hemostasis
44779	Post-Catheterization	49874	Radiologic Supervision And Interpretation
43380	Venous Reconstruction		
43381	Valvuloplasty Of Femoral Vein	49757	Embolization To Achieve Hemostasis
49678	Reconstruction Of Vena Cava		
49679	Superior Vena Cava	49877	With Angiographic Follow-Up Study
49680	Inferior Vena Cava		
49681	Both Vena Cava	49758	Intravascular Stent Placement
43382	Valve Transposition	49759	Percutaneous
43383	Vein Graft To Venous System	49761	Each Additional Vessel
43384	Saphenopopliteal Anastomosis	49760	By Cutdown
43297	Venous Interruption	49762	Each Additional Vessel
43299	Inferior Vena Cava	49879	With Radiologic Supervision And Interpretation
43298	Greenfield Filter Placement		
49878	with Radiologic Supervision And Interpretation	41616	Sympathectomy
		44797	Successful Surgical Result
43301	Common Iliac Vein	44044	Surgery Of The Spleen
43300	Femoral Vein	41656	Splenectomy
43288	Venous Ligation	44047	Total
43296	Internal Jugular Vein	44048	Partial
41617	Varicose Vein	49765	Total Enblock For Extensive Disease
43289	Short Saphenous Vein	44049	Repair Of Rupture
43290	Perforating Veins	41698	Lymphatic
43291	Long Saphenous Vein	44054	Drainage Of Node Abscess
43292	With Stripping	44055	Simple
43293	Saphenous Vein	44056	Extensive
43294	Saphenous Veins (Long & Short)	44057	Drainage Of Lymphadenitis
43295	With Skin Graft Or Venous Interruption	44058	Simple
		44059	Extensive
41679	Portosystemic Shunt	44060	Surgery On Channels
41680	Portocaval Shunt	44061	Closure Of Thoracic Duct
43353	Portorenal Shunt	44062	Cervical Approach
43354	Mesenteric-caval Shunt	44063	Thoracic Approach
43355	Proximal Splenorenal Shunt	44064	Abdominal Approach
43356	Distal Splenorenal Shunt	44188	Excision Of Cystic Hygroma
49750	Transcatheter Therapy	49791	Axillary
49751	Thrombolysis (Non-Coronary)	49792	Cervical
49875	With Radiologic Supervision And Interpretation	44189	Simple
		44190	With Deep Neurovascular Dissection
49763	With Exchange Of Previously Placed Catheter	41699	Lymphadenectomy
		44253	Suprahyoid
		44255	Axillary

SURGERY, CONT.

44256	Superficial		44205	Primary Bilateral, One-stage Procedure
44257	Complete		44206	Primary Bilateral, One Of Two Stages
49766	Thoracic			
49767	Abdominal		44207	Repeat
44258	Superficial Inguinofemoral		44208	With Cross Lip Pedicle Flap
44259	With Pelvic Extension		44209	Vestibule Of Mouth
44260	Pelvic		44263	Drain Lesion
44261	Extensive Retroperitoneal		44264	Simple
44262	Cannulation Of Thoracic (Lymphatic) Duct		44265	Complicated
			44266	Remove Foreign Body
41586	Radical Neck Dissection		44267	Simple
44254	Modified Radical Neck Dissection		44268	Complicated
49768	Mediastinum		44269	Frenotomy
49770	Mediastinotomy		44270	Excision Of Lesion
49772	By Cervical Approach		44271	Without Repair
49771	With Exploration		44272	With Simple Repair
49773	With Drainage		44273	With Complex Repair
49774	With Removal Of Foreign Body		44274	Complex, Deep
49775	By Transthoracic Approach		44275	Excision Of Mucosa For Donor Graft
49776	With Exploration		44276	Frenectomy
49777	With Drainage		44277	Obliteration Of Lesion
49778	With Removal Of Foreign Body		44278	Closure Of Laceration
49779	Excision Of Mediastinal Cyst		44279	Small
49780	Excision Of Mediastinal Tumor		44280	Large
49769	Diaphragm		44281	Plastic Repair
49781	Repair Of Diaphragmatic Laceration		44282	Anterior
49782	Repair Of Paraesophageal Hiatus Hernia		44283	Posterior
			44284	Unilateral
49783	Repair Of Neonatal Diaphragmatic Hernia		44285	Bilateral
			44286	Entire Arch
49784	Repair Diaphragmatic Hernia		44287	Complex
49785	By Thoracoabdominal Approach		44288	Floor Of Mouth
49786	With Dilation Of Stricture		44289	Incision And Drainage Of Intraoral Lesion
49787	Acute Traumatic			
49788	Chronic Traumatic		44290	Lingual
49789	Imbrication Of Diaphragm For Eventration		44291	Sublingual
			44292	Superficial
44191	Lip		44293	Deep, Supramylohyoid
44192	Shave (Vermilionectomy)		44294	Submental Space
44193	Excision		44295	Submandibular Space
44194	Transverse Wedge		44296	Masticator Space
44195	V-excision		44297	Lingual Frenotomy
44196	Reconstruction With Local Flap		44298	Incision And Drainage Of Extraoral Lesion
44197	Reconstruction With Cross Lip Flap			
44198	Major Resection, Without Reconstruction		44299	Sublingual
			44300	Submental
44199	Repair		44301	Submandibular
44200	Vermillion Only		44302	Masticator Space
44201	Simple		44303	Simple Excision Of Lingual Lesion
44202	Complex		44304	Excision Of Lingual Lesion With Closure
44203	Repair Of Cleft Lip			
44204	Primary Unilateral		44305	Anterior Two-thirds

644

SURGERY, CONT.

44306	Posterior One-third		44612	Tracheostoma Revision
44307	With Local Tongue Flap		44613	Simple
71036	Otolaryngologic		44614	Complex, With Flap Rotation
41564	Tonsillectomy		44626	Tracheoplasty
41565	Adenoidectomy		44627	Cervical
71037	Excision Of Palate		44628	Tracheopharyngeal Fistulization (Each Stage)
71038	With Simple Closure			
71039	With Flap Closure		44629	Intrathoracic
71040	Resection Of Palate		44630	Carinal Reconstruction
71043	Uvuloplasty		41632	Gastrointestinal
71044	Laser-assisted		41633	Ligation of Varices
71041	Uvulectomy		41634	Sclerosing of Varices
71042	Palatopharyngoplasty		41635	Esophagus
44566	Epiglottidectomy		42899	Esophageal Dilation
44572	Direct Laryngoscopy		42900	Single Pass
44579	With Aspiration		42901	Multiple Passes
44573	With Obturator Insertion		42902	With Guidance
44574	With Initial Dilation		42903	For Achalasia
44575	With Subsequent Dilation		42904	Retrograde
44576	With Foreign Body Removal		41637	Cricopharyngeal Myotomy
44577	Using Operating Microscope		42851	Esophagotomy By Cervical Approach
44580	Using Operating Microscope			
44581	With Excision Of Tumor		42852	With Removal Of Foreign Body
44584	Using Operating Microscope		42853	Esophagotomy By Thoracic Approach
44582	With Stripping Of Vocal Cords			
44585	Using Operating Microscope		42854	With Removal Of Foreign Body
44583	With Stripping Of Epiglottis		42885	Esophagostomy
44586	Using Operating Microscope		42886	Abdominal Approach
44587	With Arytenoidectomy		42887	Thoracic Approach
44588	Using Operating Microscope		42888	Cervical Approach
44589	With Injection Into Vocal Cords		42889	Esophagostomy Closure
44590	Using Operating Microscope		42890	Abdominal Approach
44594	Laryngoplasty		42891	Cervical Approach
44595	2-stage Laryngeal Web Repair		42892	Thoracic Approach
44596	For Laryngeal Stenosis		41643	Excision Of Lesion
44597	With Open Reduction Of Fracture		42855	Cervical Approach
44598	With Cricoid Split		42856	Thoracic Approach
44599	For Burns		42857	Wide Excision
44600	For Reconstruction After Partial Laryngectomy		41642	Esophagectomy
			42863	Total
44601	Laryngeal Reinnervation By Neuromuscular Pedicle		42858	With Pharyngogastrostomy
			42859	With Cervical Esophagogastrostomy
44602	Section Recurrent Laryngeal Nerve			
41601	Tracheostomy		42860	With Pyloroplasty
48842	Tracheostomy care requirement		41646	With Colonic Interposition
44605	Child Under 2 Years Old		42862	With Small Bowel Reconstruction
44606	Emergency		49619	Without Reconstruction, With Cervical Esophagostomy
44607	Transtracheal			
44608	Cricothyroid Membrane		49601	With Thoracotomy
44609	Fenestration With Skin Flaps		49602	With Pharyngogastrostomy
44610	Construct TE Fistula, Insert Speech Prosthesis		49604	With Cervical Esophagogastrostomy
44611	Transtracheal Aspiration		49603	With Pyloroplasty

SURGERY, CONT.

49605	With Colonic Interposition	42878	Thal-Nissen Procedure (Fundic
49606	With Small Bowel		Patch)
	Reconstruction	42879	With Gastroplasty
42861	With Second Stage	41638	Heller Myotomy
	Pyloroplasty	42880	Abdominal Approach
49607	Partial	42881	Thoracic Approach
49608	Cervical, With Graft	42882	Esophagojejunostomy
49609	Distal 2/3 With Thoracotomy	42883	Abdominal Approach
	And Thoracic	42884	Thoracic Approach
	Esophagogastrostomy	42893	Ligation Of Esophageal Varices
49610	Distal 2/3 With Thoracotomy	42894	Esophageal Transection For Varices
	And Colon Interposition	42895	Repair Of Wound / Injury
49611	Distal 2/3 With Thoracotomy	42896	Abdominal Approach
	And Small Bowel	42897	Cervical Approach
	Reconstruction	42898	Thoracic Approach
42864	Distal 2/3 With Thoracic	49627	Abdominal Approach
	Esophagogastrostomy	41647	Gastric Surgery
42865	With Pyloroplasty	42971	Gastrotomy
49612	Thoracoabdominal Approach	42972	With Foreign Body Removal
	With Esophagogastrostomy	42973	With Suture Of Bleeding Ulcer
49614	And Colon Interposition	42974	With Dilation Of Esophagogastric
49616	With Small Bowel		Junction
	Reconstruction	45760	Pyloromyotomy
49613	Abdominal Approach With	42975	Excision
	Esophagogastrostomy	41650	Total Gastrectomy
49615	And Colon Interposition	49620	With Esophagoenterostomy
49617	With Small Bowel	49621	With Roux-en-Y Reconstruction
	Reconstruction	42976	With Formation Of Intestinal
49618	Without Reconstruction, With		Pouch
	Cervical Esophagostomy	42978	Partial Gastrectomy
42866	Diverticulectomy Of Hypopharynx	42979	Distal
	By Cervical Approach	49622	With Gastroduodenostomy
42867	Diverticulectomy Of Esophagus By	49624	With Gastrojejunostomy
	Cervical Approach	49623	With Roux-en-Y
42868	Diverticulectomy Of Hypopharynx		Reconstruction
	By Thoracic Approach	49625	With Formation Of Intestinal
42869	Diverticulectomy Of Esophagus By		Pouch
	Thoracic Approach	42977	With Vagotomy
42870	Diverticulopexy Of Hypopharynx	42980	Proximal
42871	Esophagoplasty (Cervical)	41653	Hemigastrectomy
42872	With Repair Of	41657	Vagotomy
	Tracheoesophageal Fistula	42985	With Pyloroplasty
42873	Esophagoplasty (Thoracic)	42981	Parietal Cell Vagotomy (Highly
42874	With Repair Of		Selective)
	Tracheoesophageal Fistula	42986	Pyloroplasty
41644	Esophagogastrostomy	42987	Gastroduodenostomy
42875	Abdominal Approach	41651	Gastrojejunostomy
42876	Thoracic Approach	42989	With Vagotomy
42877	Esophagogastric Fundoplasty	42990	Temporary Gastrostomy
41639	Nissen Fundoplication	42991	Neonatal (For Feeding)
41640	Hill Repair	42992	Permanent Gastrostomy
41641	Belsey Mark IV	48843	Gastrostomy Care Requirement

SURGERY, CONT.

42993	Gastrorrhaphy (Suture Of Perforated Ulcer)	43740	With Coloproctostomy And Colostomy
42994	For Morbid Obesity	43749	With Terminal Ilectomy And Ileocolostomy
42996	By Vertical-banded Gastroplasty		
41845	By Gastric stapling	43741	Abdominal And Transanal Approach
42997	By Bypass With Roux-en-Y		
42995	With Small Bowel Reconstruction To Limit Absorption	43742	Total Abdominal Colectomy
		43743	With Ileostomy
49626	Revision	43744	With Ileoproctostomy
42998	Revision Of Gastroduodenostomy	43745	With Continent Ileostomy
42999	Without Vagotomy	43746	With Rectal Mucosectomy And Ileoanal Anastomosis
43000	With Vagotomy		
41652	Revision of Gastrojejunostomy	43747	With Rectal Mucosectomy And Creation Of Ileal Reservoir
43002	With Vagotomy		
43003	Closure Of Gastrostomy	41666	Total Proctocolectomy
43004	Closure Of Gastrocolic Fistula	43748	With Continent Ileostomy
43005	Anterior Gastropexy For Hiatal Hernia	41654	Roux-en-Y
		43722	Surgical Lysis Of Intestinal Adhesions
41648	Billroth I		
41649	Billroth II	43723	Laparoscopic Lysis Of Intestinal Adhesions
41655	Feeding gastrostomy		
41658	Intestinal Surgery	43724	Duodenotomy
43750	Enterostomy	43725	Percutaneous Radiologic Jejunostomy For Enteral Feeding
43751	Cecostomy		
43752	Ileostomy (Non-tube)	43726	Enterotomy
43753	Jejunostomy (Non-tube)	43727	Baker Tube Placement
48841	Ileostomy or other intestinal appliance	43728	Colotomy
		43729	Surgical Reduction Of Volvulus
41659	Ileostomy (Koch)	43730	Surgical Reduction Of Intussusception
48844	Ileostomy care requirement		
43754	Revision Of Ileostomy	43731	Surgical Reduction Of Internal Hernia
43755	Simple		
43756	Complex	43732	Correction Of Intestinal Malrotation
41660	Colostomy	41670	Local Resection
43757	With Multiple Biopsies	41694	Single Opening
48845	Colostomy care requirement	43721	Multiple Openings
41665	Afferent Loop Revision	41696	Excision Of Lesions
43758	Simple	41669	Small Bowel Resection
43759	Complex	43733	With Enterostomy
43760	With Paracolostomy Hernia Repair	49628	Each Additional Resection
		41676	Endoscopic Papillotomy
41663	Perineal resection	43761	Enteroscopic Procedures
41668	Enteroenterostomy, Anastomosis	41671	Foreign Body Removal
43734	With Cutaneous Enterostomy	41661	Polypectomy
49629	Take-down Of Splenic Flexure In Conjunction With Partial Colectomy	43762	Electrocoagulation
		43763	Laser Photocoagulation
41664	Partial Colectomy	43764	Ablation Of Lesion
43735	With Cecostomy	43765	By Laser Photocoagulation
43736	With Colostomy	43766	Hot Biopsy
43737	With End Colostomy & Closure Of Distal Segment	43767	PEJ Tube Placement
		43768	PEG Tube To PEJ Tube Conversion
43738	With Creation Of Mucofistula	43769	Colonoscopic Procedures Via Colostomy
43739	With Coloproctostomy		

SURGERY, CONT.

43770	Foreign Body Removal
43771	Electrocoagulation
43772	Laser Photocoagulation
43773	Heater Probe
43774	Polypectomy
43775	Ablation Of Lesion
43776	By Laser Photocoagulation
43777	Hot Biopsy
43778	Suture Of Small Intestine
43779	Single
43780	Multiple
49630	Suture Of Large Intestine
49631	Without Colostomy
43781	With Colostomy
43782	Closure Of Enterostomy
43783	With Resection And Anastomosis
43784	Closure Of Enterocutaneous Fistula
43785	Closure Of Enteroenteric Fistula
43786	Closure Of Enterocolic Fistula
43787	Closure Of Enterovesical Fistula
43788	With Intestinal Resection
43789	Without Intestinal Resection
43790	With Bladder Resection
43791	Without Bladder Resection
43792	Intestinal Plication
43793	Excision Of Meckel's Diverticulum
43795	Excision Of Omphalomesenteric Duct
43796	Excision Of Mesenteric Lesion
43797	Suture Of Mesentery
43798	Appendiceal Abscess I&D
41683	Appendectomy
43799	As Part Of Other Major Procedure
43800	For Ruptured Appendix
43801	Rectal Surgery
43802	Pelvic Abscess I&D, Rectal Approach
43803	Rectal Submucosal Abscess I&D
43804	Perirectal Muscle Abscess I&D
43805	Anorectal Myomectomy
43817	Repair Rectal Stricture
43818	Rectal Tumor Excision By Proctotomy
43819	Transanal Excision Of Rectal Tumor
43820	Destruction Of Rectal Tumor
43806	Proctectomy
43807	Complete
43808	Combined APR With Colostomy
43810	Partial Resection Of Rectum
43809	With Colectomy And Biopsies
41667	Combined Abdominoperineal Pull-Through Procedure

49812	Partial, Rectal Mucosectomy, Ileoanal Anastomosis & Creation Of Ileal Reservoir
43811	Partial, With Anastomosis
43812	Abdominal And Transacral Approach
43813	Transacral Approach (Kraske)
49813	Partial, Without Anastomosis, Perineal Approach
43814	Excision Of Rectal Procidentia
43815	Perineal Approach
43816	Abdominal And Perineal Approach
43955	Proctoplasty
43956	For Stenosis
43957	For Mucosal Prolapse
43958	Perirectal Sclerotherapy
43959	Proctopexy
43960	For Prolapse
43961	Abdominal Approach
43962	Perineal Approach
43963	With Sigmoid Resection
43964	Rectocele Repair
43965	Suture Of Rectal Laceration
43966	Closure Of Rectovesical Fistula
43967	With Colostomy
43968	Excision Of Rectovesical Fistula
43969	Closure Of Rectourethral Fistula
43970	With Colostomy
43971	Excision Of Rectourethral Fistula
43972	Reduction Of Procidentia Under Anesthesia
43973	Anal Sphincter Dilation Under Anesthesia
43974	Rectal Stricture Dilation Under Anesthesia
43975	Fecal Disimpaction Under Anesthesia
43978	Foreign Body Removal
43976	Anal Fistulotomy
43977	Removal Of Anal Seton
43979	Ischiorectal Abscess I&D
43982	With Submuscular Fistulectomy
43980	Perirectal Abscess I&D
43984	Perianal Abscess I&D (Superficial)
43981	Transanal I&D Of Abscess
43983	With Submuscular Fistulectomy
43986	Anal Sphincterotomy
43987	Incision Of External Thrombosed Hemorrhoid
43994	Anal Papillectomy
41684	Hemorrhoidectomy
43821	Simple Ligature
43822	Excision Of External Tags

SURGERY, CONT.

43823	Complete External Hemorrhoidectomy
43824	Simple Internal And External Hemorrhoidectomy
43825	With Fissurectomy
43826	With Fistulectomy
43827	Complex Internal And External Hemorrhoidectomy
43828	With Fissurectomy
43829	With Fistulectomy
43989	Excision Of External Thrombosed Hemorrhoids
43988	Sclerotherapy Of Hemorrhoids
44031	Destruction Of Hemorrhoids
44032	Internal
44033	External
44034	Internal And External
44035	Ligation Of Internal Hemorrhoids
44036	Single
44037	Multiple
41689	Fistula-in-ano Repair
43995	Subcutaneous
43996	Submuscular
43997	Complex / Multiple
43998	Second Stage
43990	Anal Fissurectomy
43991	Anal Cryptectomy
43992	Single
43993	Multiple
43999	Anoscopy
44000	For Dilation
44001	For Foreign Body Removal
44002	For Polyp Removal
44003	Multiple
44004	For Hemorrhage Control
44005	For Fulguration Of Lesion
43985	Incision Of Infantile Anal Septum
44006	Anoplasty Of Stricture
44007	Adult
44008	Infant
44009	Congenital Anovaginal Fistula Repair
44010	Perineal Transplant Of Anovaginal Fistula
44011	Construction Of Anus For Congenital Absence
44012	Perineal Approach
44013	Combined Abdominal & Perineal Approach
44014	With Urinary Fistula Repair
44015	Anal Sphincteroplasty
44016	Adult
44020	Muscle Transplant
44021	Park Procedure
44022	Implant Artificial Sphincter
44017	Child
44018	Thiersch Graft
44019	Remove Thiersch Wire
44023	Destruction Of Anal Lesions
44024	Simple
44025	By Chemical Means
44026	By Electrodesiccation
44027	By Cryosurgery
44028	By Laser Surgery
44029	By Surgical Excision
44030	Extensive
44038	Cryosurgery Of Rectal Neoplasm
44039	Benign
44040	Malignant
44041	Dilation And Cauterization Of Anal Fissure & Sphincter
44042	Initial
44043	Subsequent
41677	Liver
41678	Lobectomy
44068	Partial
44069	Total Left
44070	Total Right
44071	Trisegmentectomy
44065	Hepatotomy
44066	For Abscess Drainage
44067	For Drainage Of Cyst
44072	Donor Hepatectomy
49814	From Cadaver Donor
49815	Partial, From Living Donor
41968	Transplant
41969	Orthotopic
49816	Heterotopic
41970	Auxiliary Partial
44073	Marsupialization Of Liver Abscess Or Cyst
44074	Suture Of Laceration Of Liver
44075	Simple
44078	Complex
41672	Gallbladder / Biliary Tract
44079	Hepatic Duct Exploration
44080	Common Bile Duct Exploration
44081	With Sphincterotomy
44082	With Sphincteroplasty
44083	Common Bile Duct Incision Through Duodenum
44084	Transduodenal Sphincterotomy
44085	Transduodenal Sphincteroplasty
44086	Cholecystotomy
44087	Percutaneous
44088	Percutaneous Transhepatic Catheter Placement

SURGERY, CONT.

44089	Change Percutaneous Transhepatic Catheter	41690	Proximal Subtotal (Whipple Procedure)
44090	Revise Transhepatic T-tube	44124	Near-total With Preservation Of
44091	Intraoperative Biliary Endoscopy		Duodenum (Child-type Procedure)
44092	Percutaneous Biliary Endoscopy	44125	Total
44093	For Removal Of Stones	44126	With Transplant
44094	For Dilation	44127	Pancreaticojejunostomy (Puestow Procedure)
41673	Cholecystectomy		
44096	With Cholangiography	44128	Marsupialization Of Pancreatic Cyst
42334	Laparoscopic	44129	External Drainage Of Pancreatic Pseudocyst
44095	With Cholangiography		
41674	With Common Bile Duct Exploration	44130	Internal Drainage Of Pancreatic Pseudocyst
44097	With Choledochoenterostomy	44131	Direct
44098	With Transduodenal Sphincterotomy	44132	With Roux-en-Y
		44045	Abdominal / Peritoneal
44099	With Transduodenal Sphincteroplasty	44133	Reopen Recent Laparotomy
		44116	Surgical Drainage
44100	Bile Duct Stone Removal (Burhenne Procedure)	44135	Of Peritoneal Cavity
		44117	For Pancreatitis
44101	Exploration For Congenital Biliary Atresia	49821	With Cholecystostomy, Gastrostomy And Jejunostomy
44102	Portoenterostomy (Kasai Procedure)	44134	Of Peritoneal Abscess
44103	Excision Of Bile Duct Neoplasm	44136	Of Subdiaphragmatic Abscess
49817	Extrahepatic	44137	Of Subphrenic Abscess
49818	Intrahepatic	44138	Of Retroperitoneal Abscess
44104	Excision Of Bile Duct Cyst	41880	Abdominal Paracentesis
44105	Anastomosis Of Bile Duct Cyst	44139	Initial
44106	Bile Duct / Biliary Bypass	44140	Subsequent
44107	Direct	44141	Peritoneal Lavage
44108	With Gastroenterostomy	44142	Foreign Body Removal
44109	Roux-en-Y	44143	Excision Of Intra-abdominal Mass
41675	Extrahepatic Bile Duct Enterostomy	44144	Extensive
44111	Intrahepatic Bile Duct Enterostomy	44145	Excision Of Presacral Neoplasm
44110	Roux-en-Y of Extrahepatic Bile Duct Enterostomy	44146	Excision Of Sacrococcygeal Neoplasm
		44147	Staging Laparotomy For Hodgkin's Disease Or Lymphoma
49819	Roux-en-Y of Intrahepatic Bile Duct Enterostomy	44148	Excision Of Umbilicus
		44149	Resection Of Omentum
44112	Bile Duct Reconstruction	41695	Abdominoperineal resection
44113	Choledochal Stent Placement	44150	Insertion Of Intraperitoneal Catheter
44114	Hepaticoenterostomy (U-tube Technique)	44151	Temporary
		44152	Permanent
49820	Suture Of Extrahepatic Biliary Duct For Pre-existing Injury	44153	Peritoneal-venous Shunt
		44154	Denver
44046	Pancreatic	44155	LeVeen
44118	Removal Of Pancreatic Duct Calculus	49823	Insertion
49822	Resection / Debridement For Acute Necrotizing Pancreatitis	49825	Injection Procedure For Evaluation Of Previously Placed Shunt
44119	Excision	44156	Revision
44120	Pancreatectomy	49826	Ligation
44121	Distal	49827	Removal
44122	With Pancreaticojejunostomy	41685	Hernia Repair
44123	Ampulla Of Vater		

41686	Inguinal	
49828	Child Under 6 Months Old	
49829	Incarcerated	
49830	Strangulated	
44157	Child Between 6 Months And 5 Years Old	
49831	Incarcerated	
49832	Strangulated	
44158	Person Over Age 5	
49833	Incarcerated	
49834	Strangulated	
44162	Recurrent	
44164	Incarcerated	
44165	Strangulated	
44163	Sliding	
41687	Incisional	
49839	Incarcerated	
49840	Strangulated	
44166	Recurrent	
49841	Incarcerated	
49842	Strangulated	
49843	Implantation Of Mesh	
44167	Lumbar	
44168	Femoral	
44169	Via Groin Incision	
49835	Incarcerated	
49836	Strangulated	
44170	Via Henry Approach	
44171	Recurrent	
49837	Incarcerated	
49838	Strangulated	
44172	Epigastric	
44173	Reducible	
44174	Complex	
49844	Incarcerated	
49845	Strangulated	
44175	Umbilical	
44176	Child Under 5	
49846	Incarcerated	
49847	Strangulated	
44177	Person Over Age 5	
49848	Incarcerated	
49849	Strangulated	
44178	Spigelian	
44179	Omphalocele	
44180	Small	
44181	Large	
44182	Staged Closure	
44183	Stage One Gross Procedure	
44184	Stage Two Gross Procedure	
44185	Repeat Suture Of Abdominal Wall	
44186	For Evisceration	
44187	For Dehiscence	

41697	Recent Abdominal Surgery
41712	Genito-Urinary Tract
43920	Urological Procedures
43921	Renal Cyst Aspiration
43922	With Injection
43923	Renal Pelvis Aspiration
43924	With Injection
43925	Percutaneous Catheter Placement
43926	Into Renal Pelvis
43927	Into Ureter
43928	With Creation Of Nephrostomy Tract
43929	Change Of Nephrostomy Tube
43930	Renal Endoscopy Through Nephrostomy
43931	With Ureteral Catheterization
43932	With Fulguration
43933	With Incision
43934	With Radioactive Injection
43935	With Foreign Body Removal
43936	With Calculus Removal
43937	Renal Endoscopy Through Nephrotomy
43938	With Ureteral Catheterization
43939	With Fulguration
43940	With Incision
43941	With Radioactive Injection
43942	With Foreign Body Removal
43943	With Calculus Removal
44252	Ureterostomy Tube Replacement
44210	Ureteral Endoscopy Through Ureterostomy
44211	With Ureteral Catheterization
44212	With Fulguration
44213	With Incision
44214	With Radioactive Injection
44215	With Foreign Body Removal
44216	With Calculus Removal
44217	Ureteral Endoscopy Through Ureterotomy
44218	With Ureteral Catheterization
44219	With Fulguration
44220	With Incision
44221	With Radioactive Injection
44222	With Foreign Body Removal
44223	With Calculus Removal
44308	Bladder
44309	Aspiration
44310	By Needle
44311	By Trocar
44312	With Insertion Of Suprapubic Catheter
44313	Injection Procedure

SURGERY, CONT.

44314	For Cystography		43945	Cadaver Donor
44315	With Placement Of Chain For Cystourethrogram		43948	Recipient Nephrectomy
			43946	Homograft Implantation
44316	For Retrograde Cystourethrogram		43947	With Recipient Nephrectomy
44317	Of Cancer Treatment		43949	Transplant Removal
44318	Irrigation		43950	Autograft Reimplantation
44319	Cystostomy Tube Replacement		43857	Ureter
44320	Simple		44224	Ureterotomy
44321	Complicated		44225	For Insertion Of Stent
41681	Kidney		44226	Ureterolithotomy
43871	Nephrostomy With Drainage		44227	Upper Third Of Ureter
43872	Of Abscess		44228	Middle Third Of Ureter
43873	drainage of perirenal or renal abscess (separate procedure)		44229	Lower Third Of Ureter
			44230	Ureteroplasty
41724	Lithotomy		44231	Ureterolysis
43874	Repeat		44232	For Ovarian Vein Syndrome
43875	Complicated By Congenital Abnormality		44233	For Retrocaval Ureter
			44234	Ureteropyelostomy
43876	For Large Staghorn Calculus		44235	Ureterocalycostomy
41725	Percutaneous		44236	Ureteroureterostomy
43877	Percutaneous For Stone Over 2cm.		44237	Transureteroureterostomy
41726	Lithotripsy		44238	Ureteroneocystostomy
41727	Whole Body (Extracorporeal Shock Wave)		44239	With Bladder Flap
			44240	Ureteroenterostomy
43878	Pyelotomy		41722	Ureterosigmoidostomy
43879	With Drainage		44241	Ureterocolon Conduit
43880	With Lithotomy		44242	Ureteroileal Conduit
43881	Complicated By Congenital Abnormality		44243	Continent Ureteral Diversion
			44244	Revision Of Ureteral Diversion
43882	Repeat		41721	Ureterostomy
41719	Nephrectomy		44245	Replacement Of Ureter With Bowel Segment
41720	Bilateral			
43865	Complicated		44246	Ureterorrhaphy
43866	Radical		44247	Closure Of Ureterocutaneous Fistula
41718	With Total Ureterectomy		44248	Closure Of Ureterovisceral Fistula
43868	With Separate Ureterectomy		44249	Release Of Ureteral Ligation
43867	Partial		44250	Ureterectomy
43869	Cyst Excision		44251	Total, For Ectopic Ureter
43870	Perinephric Cyst Excision		43858	Bladder
43911	Pyeloplasty		44322	Cystotomy
43912	Complicated		44323	With Drainage
43913	Nephrorrhaphy		44324	With Insertion Of Ureteral Catheter
43914	Fistula Repair		44325	With Fulguration
43915	Nephrocutaneous		44326	With Cryosurgical Destruction Of Lesion
43916	Pyelocutaneous			
43917	Nephrovisceral - Abdominal Approach		44327	With Insertion Of Radioactive Material
43918	Nephrovisceral - Thoracic Approach		44328	With Basket Extraction Of Calculus
43919	Horseshoe Kidney Repair		44329	With Direct Removal Of Calculus
43883	Renal Vessel Revision		44335	Transvesical Ureterolithotomy
41682	Renal Transplant		44330	With Fragmentation Of Calculus
41993	Donor Nephrectomy		44331	For Excision Of Vesical Neck
43944	Living Donor		44332	For Excision Of Diverticulum

SURGERY, CONT.

44333	For Excision Of Neoplasm
44334	For Repair Of Ureterocele
44336	Drainage Of Perivesical Abscess
44337	Excision Of Urachal Cyst
41715	Cystectomy
44338	Partial
44339	Simple
44340	Complicated
44341	With Reimplantation Of Ureters
44342	Complete
44343	With Lymphadenectomy
44344	Complete With Ureterosigmoidostomy
44346	With Lymphadenectomy
44345	Complete With Cutaneous Ureterostomy
44347	With Lymphadenectomy
44348	Complete With Ureteroileal Conduit
44349	With Lymphadenectomy
44350	Complete With Sigmoid Bladder
44351	With Lymphadenectomy
44352	Complete With Continent Diversion
44353	Pelvic Exenteration For Malignancy
44354	Cystorrhaphy
44355	Simple
44356	Complicated
44357	Cystostomy Closure
44358	Fistula Repair
44359	Vesicouterine
44360	With Hysterectomy
44367	Enterocystoplasty
44368	Cutaneous Vesicostomy
44361	Exstrophy Repair
44362	Cystourethroplasty
44363	With Ureteroneocystostomy
44364	Anterior Vesicourethropexy
44365	Complicated
44366	Abdomino-Vaginal Vesical Neck Suspension
44408	Transurethral Resection Of Bladder Neck
41714	Cystoscopy
44369	With Fulguration
44370	Minor Lesion (Under 5mm)
44371	Small Lesion (5-20mm)
44372	Medium Lesion (2-5cm)
44373	Large Lesion (Over 5cm)
44374	With Dilation Of Bladder
44375	Under Local Anesthesia
44376	With Insertion Of Radioactive Substance
44377	With Internal Urethrotomy
44378	Female

44379	Male
44380	With Direct Vision
44381	With Resection Of External Sphincter
44382	For Urethral Stricture
44383	With Steroid Injection
44384	For Treatment Of Female Urethral Syndrome
44385	With Ureteral Meatotomy
44386	With Treatment Of Ureterocele(s)
44387	With Treatment Of Bladder Diverticulum
44388	With Removal Of Object
44389	Complicated
44390	With Fragmentation Of Bladder Calculus
44391	Complex Or Large (Over 2.5cm)
44392	With Removal Of Ureteral Calculus
44393	With Fragmentation Of Ureteral Calculus
44394	With Manipulation Of Ureteral Calculus
44395	With Insertion Of Ureteral Stent
44396	To Insert Guide Wire For Retrograde Nephrostomy
44397	With Ureteroscopy
44398	With Removal Of Calculus
44399	With Manipulation Of Calculus
44400	With Lithotripsy
44401	With Fulguration Of Lesion
44402	With Pyeloscopy
44403	With Removal Of Calculus
44404	With Manipulation Of Calculus
44405	With Lithotripsy
44406	With Fulguration Of Lesion
44407	With Surgical Procedure On Bladder Neck Or Posterior Urethra
43859	Urethra
44409	External Urethrotomy
44410	For Pendulous Urethra
44411	For Perineal Urethra
44412	Meatotomy
44413	In An Infant
44414	Drainage Of Deep Periurethral Abscess
44415	Drainage Of Skene's Gland
44416	Drainage Of Perineal Urinary Extravasation
44417	Complicated
44418	Total Urethrectomy
44419	Female
44420	Male
44421	Excision / Fulguration Of Urethral Carcinoma

SURGERY, CONT.

44422	Excision Of Urethral Diverticulum	42673	Ablation of Lesion(s)
44423	Female	42674	Extensive
44424	Male	42675	Vaginectomy
43860	Prostate	42676	Partial
41716	Prostatectomy (TURP)	42677	Complete
41717	Prostatectomy, Suprapubic	42678	Colpocleisis (Le Fort Procedure)
43861	Male Genitalia	42679	Excision Of Vaginal Septum
41713	Vasectomy	42680	Excision Of Vaginal Cyst Or Tumor
41728	Orchiectomy	42693	Colporrhaphy (Non-OB)
41729	Radical Orchiectomy	42694	Colpoperineorrhaphy (Non-OB)
41838	Penile Prosthetic Device	42695	Kelly Urethral Plication (Vaginal Approach)
41829	Sex Reassignment		
42501	Male to Female	42696	Plastic Repair Of Urethrocele (As Separate Procedure)
42502	Female to Male		
41700	Gynecologic	42697	Anterior Colporrhaphy, Repair Of Cystocele
42649	Perineal		
42650	Incision And Drainage Of Abscess (Nonobstetrical)	42635	Colporrhaphy
		42698	Anterior
42651	Perineoplasty (Nonobstetrical)	42699	Posterior
42652	Vulvar And Introitus	42700	Combined Anteroposterior
42653	Incision And Drainage	42701	Combined A-P With Enterocele Repair
42654	Bartholin's Gland Abscess		
42655	Marsupialization of Bartholin's Gland Cyst	42702	Enterocele Repair, Vaginal Approach (Separate Procedure)
42668	Excision of Bartholin's Gland or Cyst	42703	Enterocele Repair, Abdominal Approach (Separate Procedure)
42656	Lysis of Labial Adhesions	42704	Colpopexy, Abdominal Approach
42657	Ablation of Lesion(s)	42705	Sacrospinous Ligament Fixation For Posthysterectomy Prolapse
42658	Extensive		
42659	Vulvectomy	42706	Sling Operation For Stress Incontinence
42660	Partial		
42661	Complete	42707	Pereyra Procedure With Anterior Colporrhaphy
42662	Radical		
49852	Radical, Partial	42708	Construction Of Artificial Vagina
49853	With Inguinofemoral Lymphadenectomy	42709	With Graft (McIndoe Procedure)
		42710	Rectovaginal Fistula Repair
49854	Bilateral	42711	Vaginal Approach
49851	Radical, Complete	42712	Abdominal Approach
42663	With Inguinofemoral Lymphadenectomy	42713	Abdominal Approach With Colostomy
49850	Bilateral	42714	Urethrovaginal Fistula Repair
42664	Radical With Groin & Pelvic Lymphadenectomy	42715	with bulbocavernosus transplant
		42716	Vesicovaginal Fistula Repair
42665	Clitoridectomy	42717	Vaginal Approach
42666	Extensive	42718	Transvesical And Vaginal Approach
49855	Partial Hymenectomy		
49856	Revision Of Hymenal Ring	42719	Abdominal Approach
42667	Hymenotomy	42769	Cervix
42669	Plastic Repair Of Introitus	42770	Local Excision
42670	Vaginal	42771	Endocervical Curettage (Not D&C)
42767	Dilation Under Anesthesia	42772	Cervical Cauterization
42671	Colpotomy	42773	Cryosurgery
42672	With Drainage of Pelvic Abscess	42774	Laser Ablation

SURGERY, CONT.

42775	Cervical Conization
49857	By Cold Knife
49858	By Laser
49859	Loop Electrode Excision
42776	Trachelectomy (Cervicectomy)
42913	Excision Of Cervical Pregnancy With Evacuation
42777	Excision Of Cervical Stump, Abdominal Approach
42778	With Pelvic Floor Repair
42779	Excision Of Cervical Stump, Vaginal Approach
42780	With Colporrhaphy
42781	With Enterocele Repair
42782	Cerclage (Non-OB)
42919	Cerclage During Pregnancy
42920	Vaginal Approach
42921	Abdominal Approach
42783	Trachelorrhaphy
42784	Dilation Of Cervical Canal
42785	Dilation And Curettage Of Cervical Stump
42786	Uterus
41701	Dilation And Curettage
42917	Postpartum
42927	Following Medically Induced Abortion
49866	From Amniotic Injection(s)
49867	From Vaginal Suppositories
42937	For Hydatidiform Mole
42787	Myomectomy
42788	Abdominal Approach
42789	Vaginal Approach
42790	Uterine Suspension
42791	With Presacral Neurectomy
42792	Hysterorrhaphy (Non-OB)
42922	Hysterorrhaphy During Pregnancy
42793	Hysteroplasty (Repair Of Congenital Uterine Anomaly)
42905	Hysterotomy (Obstetrical)
42928	Following Medically Induced Abortion
49868	From Amniotic Injection(s)
49869	From Vaginal Suppositories
42912	Partial Resection For Interstitial Pregnancy
41702	Hysterectomy
42628	Total
42630	With Partial Vaginectomy And Lymph Node Biopsy
42911	For Interstitial Uterine Pregnancy
42925	After Cesarean Section
42634	Vaginal

42636	With Colpo-urethrocystopexy
42637	With Enterocele Repair
42638	With Colpectomy
42639	With Colpectomy And Enterocele Repair
42640	Radical
42629	With Colpo-urethrocystopexy
42631	Radical With Lymphadenectomy
42632	Supracervical
42633	Pelvic Exenteration
42794	Oviduct
42809	Fimbrioplasty
42810	Salpingostomy
41703	Tubal ligation
42641	After Vaginal Delivery
42642	During Cesarean Section
42795	Tubal Occlusion By Device
41706	Salpingectomy
42796	Unilateral
41707	Bilateral
42906	For Ectopic Pregnancy
42908	Surgical Excision Of Ectopic Pregnancy
42801	Adhesiolysis
42803	Tubotubal Anastomosis
42804	Tubocornual
42805	Isthmic-isthmic
42806	Isthmic-ampullary
42807	Ampullary-ampullary
42808	Tubouterine Implantation
42797	Salpingo-oophorectomy
42798	Unilateral
42799	Bilateral
42800	Ovary
42811	Drainage Of Ovarian Cyst
42812	Vaginal Approach
42813	Abdominal Approach
42814	Drainage Of Ovarian Abscess
42815	Vaginal Approach
42816	Abdominal Approach
42817	Ovarian Transposition
42818	Ovarian Wedge Resection
42909	Excision Of Ectopic Pregnancy
42802	Adhesiolysis
42819	Cystectomy
42648	Oophorectomy
41704	Unilateral
41705	Bilateral
42820	For Malignancy (With Biopsies & Washings)
42907	For Ectopic Pregnancy
42821	Resection Of Malignancy With BSO & Omentectomy

SURGERY, CONT.

42822	With TAH & Lymphadenectomy	45906	Incision And Drainage of Pilonidal Cyst
42823	With Radical Dissection For Debulking	45908	Simple
42824	Laparotomy	45909	Complicated
41708	Laparoscopy	45910	Incision And Removal of Subcutaneous Foreign Body
42643	With Fulguration of Oviducts		
42914	With Excision Of Ectopic Pregnancy	45911	Simple
42915	With Salpingectomy	45912	Complicated
42916	With Oophorectomy	45913	Incision And Removal of Hematoma
42831	With Occlusion Of Oviducts By Device	45914	Incision And Removal of Seroma
42832	With Fulguration Or Excision Of Lesions	45915	Incision And Removal of Loculated Fluid
42833	With Adhesiolysis	45916	Puncture Aspiration of Subcutaneous Abscess
42834	With Biopsy	45917	Puncture Aspiration of Bulla
42835	With Aspiration	45918	Puncture Aspiration of Cutaneous Cyst
42836	With Adnexectomy	41749	Skin Debridement
42837	Hysteroscopy	45920	Partial Thickness
42838	With Adhesiolysis	45921	Full Thickness
42839	With Resection	45922	With Subcutaneous Tissue
42840	With Removal Of Submucous Leiomyomata	45923	With Subcutaneous Tissue And Muscle
42841	With Endometrial Ablation	45924	With Subcutaneous Tissue, Muscle And Bone
42647	Obstetrical		
41842	Episiotomy	45925	Of Extensively Damaged / Diseased Skin
42918	By Other Than Attending Physician	45926	Up To 10% Of Body Surface Area
41711	Caesarean section	45927	Each Additional 10% Of Body Surface Area
41709	Surgical Treatment For Abortion		
42929	Spontaneous	49121	Burn Treatment
42930	Missed	49122	First Degree
42931	First Trimester	49123	Dressing / Debridement
42932	Second Trimester	49124	Small Area
42933	Septic	49125	Under Anesthesia
41710	Recent	49126	Medium Area
42934	Induced Abortion	49127	Under Anesthesia
42935	By Dilation And Curettage	49128	Large Area
42936	By Dilation And Evacuation	49129	Under Anesthesia
42910	Excision Of Abdominal Pregnancy	49130	Escharotomy
43006	Endocrine	49131	Excision Of Burn Wound
41691	Adrenalectomy	49132	Up To One Percent Of Body Surface
41692	Unilateral Adrenalectomy		
41693	Bilateral Adrenalectomy	49133	One To Nine Percent Of Body Surface
41745	Dermatological		
41688	Pilonidal Cyst Resection	49134	Each Additional Excision Of Up To Nine Percent Of Body Surface
72839	Simple		
72840	Extensive	41730	Orthopedic
72842	Complicated	41735	Hand surgery
41750	Skin Graft	41736	Prosthetic Device
45904	Incision And Drainage of Skin Abscess	41744	Cervical vertebral fusion
45907	Simple	41743	Lumbar vertebral fusion
45905	Complicated	41734	Scoliosis surgery
45919	Incision And Drainage of Postoperative Wound Infection, Complex	41732	Bone Graft

656

SURGERY, CONT.

41733	Open fracture reduction
41731	Local Resection
41738	Knee replacement
41739	Amputation
41742	Amputation of arm
48838	Fitting Artificial Arm
48839	Fitting Artificial Leg
45955	Head
49949	Right
49950	Left
49945	Fracture
45956	Closed Treatment Of Skull Fracture
45957	Closed Treatment Of Nasal Bone Fracture
45958	With Manipulation
45959	And Stabilization
48295	Open Treatment Of Nasal Bone Fracture
48296	Complicated
48297	With Open Treatment of Septal Fracture
45960	Closed Treatment Of Nasal Septal Fracture
48298	Open Treatment Of Nasal Septal Fracture
48299	Open Treatment Of Nasoethmoid Fracture
48300	With External Fixation
48301	Percutaneous Treatment Of Complex Nasoethmoid Fracture
48302	With Repair of Canthal Ligaments
48303	With Repair of Lacrimal Apparatus
48304	Open Treatment of Depressed Frontal Sinus Fracture
48305	Open Treatment of Complicated Frontal Sinus Fracture
48306	Closed Treatment of Complex Nasomaxillary Fracture with Fixation
48307	Open Treatment of Complex Nasomaxillary Fracture with Fixation
48308	With Multiple Open Approaches
48309	With Bone Grafting
48310	Percutaneous Treatment of Fracture of Malar Area
48311	Open Treatment of Depressed Malar Fracture
48312	Open Treatment of Depressed Zygomatic Arch Fracture
48313	Open Treatment of Complicated Malar Fracture(s) with Fixation with Bone Grafting
48314	Closed Treatment Of Orbital Fracture (non-"blowout")
45961	Closed Treatment Of Orbital Fracture (non-"blowout")
45962	With Manipulation
48487	Open Treatment Of Orbital Fracture (non-"blowout")
48488	With Implant
48489	With Bone Graft
48480	Open Treatment Of Orbital Fracture ("blowout")
48481	Transantral (Caldwell-Luc)
48482	Periorbital Approach
48485	With Implant
48486	With Bone Graft
48483	Combined Approach
48490	Closed Treatment Of Palatal Fracture (LeFort type I) with Fixation
48492	Open Treatment Of Palatal Fracture (LeFort type I)
48491	Closed Treatment Of Maxillary Fracture (LeFort type I) with Fixation
48493	Open Treatment Of Maxillary Fracture (LeFort type I)
48494	Complicated, Using Multiple Approaches
48495	Closed Treatment Of Craniofacial Separation (LeFort type III)
48496	Open Treatment Of Craniofacial Separation (LeFort type III)
48497	Complicated, Using Multiple Approaches
48498	Complicated, Using Fixation Using Multiple Approaches and Bone Graft
48499	
45963	Closed Treatment Of Maxillary Alveolar Ridge Fracture
48510	Open Treatment Of Maxillary Alveolar Ridge Fracture
70105	Excision
70110	Radical Resection Of Soft Tissue Tumor
70104	Benign Cyst / Tumor Of Facial Bone
70109	Malignant Tumor
70107	Of Facial Bone
70108	Contouring Of Facial Bone
70111	Of Torus Palatinus

SURGERY, CONT.

70500	Introduction	70677	Midface Reconstruction (not LeFort)
70501	Prosthesis Preparation		
70502	Obturator, Interim	70678	Segmental Maxillary Osteotomy
70503	Obturator, Definitive	70679	Facial Osteoplasty
70504	Palatal Augmentation	70680	Augmentation
70505	Palatal Lift	70681	Reduction
70506	Speech Aid	70682	Facial Bone Graft
70507	Oral Surgical Splint	70683	To Nasal Area
70508	Auricular	70684	To Malar Area
70509	Nasal	70685	To Maxillary Area
70510	Facial	70686	Facial Graft Using Rib Cartilage
70513	Application Of Maxilofacial Halo Appliance	70687	To Face
		70688	To Nose
70515	Application Of Maxillary Interdental Fixation Device	70689	To Ear
		70690	Facial Graft Using Ear Cartilage
70612	Repair	70691	To Nose
70651	Countouring Of Forehead	70692	To Ear
70652	With Application Of Prosthesis Or Graft	70693	Repair Of Zygomatic Arch And Glenoid Fossa
70653	With Setback Of Sinus Wall	70694	Repair Of Orbit With Osteotomies And Grafts
70654	Midface Reconstruction (LeFort I)		
72888	Without Bone Graft	70695	Repair Of Orbital Hypertelorism
70655	Single Piece	70696	By Extracranial Approach
72889	Two Pieces	70697	By Combined Approach
72895	Three Or More Pieces	70698	With Forehead Advancement
70656	With Bone Graft	70699	Unilateral Orbital Repositioning
70657	Single Piece	70700	By Combined Approach
70658	Two Pieces	70701	Prosthetic Malar Augmentation
70659	More Than Two Pieces	70702	Revision Of Orbito-cranio-facial Reconstruction
70660	With Multiple Osteotomies, Multiple Pieces		
		70703	Medial Canthopexy
70661	Midface Reconstruction (LeFort II)	70704	Lateral Canthopexy
		70705	Reduction Of Masseter
70662	Anterior Intrusion	70706	Intraoral Approach
70663	Requiring Bone Grafts	70707	Extraoral Approach
70664	Midface Reconstruction (LeFort III)	70094	Jaw
		45964	Closed Treatment Of Mandibular Alveolar Ridge Fracture
70665	With LeFort I		
70666	With Forehead Advancement	48511	Open Treatment Of Mandibular Alveolar Ridge Fracture
70667	And LeFort I		
70668	Reconstruction Of Superior-Lateral Orbital Rim	45965	Closed Treatment Of Mandibular Fracture
70669	Bifrontal	45966	With Manipulation
70670	Reconstruction Of Forehead	45967	With Interdental Fixation
70671	With Autograft	47606	On The Right
70672	Extracranial Countouring Of Cranial Bones	47607	On The Left
		48500	Open Treatment Of Mandibular Fracture
70673	Upper Facial Autografts Following Bone Tumor Excision		
		48501	With Interdental Fixation
70674	Of Less Than 40 cm2	48502	With External Fixation
70675	Of 40 to 80 cm2	48503	Complicated, With Multiple Approaches
70676	Of Over 80 cm2		

SURGERY, CONT.

48504	Open Treatment Of Mandibular Condylar Fracture	70632	With Sagittal Split And Internal Rigid Fixation
45968	Percutaneous Treatment Of Mandibular Fracture With External Fixation	70633	Repair Of Mandibular Body
		70634	With Sagittal Split
		70635	With Sagittal Split And Internal Rigid Fixation
45969	Closed Treatment Of Temporomandibular Dislocation	70636	Arthroplasty Of Temporomandibular Joint
45970	Complicated	70637	With Allograft
48505	Open Treatment Of Temporomandibular Dislocation	70638	With Prosthetic Joint Replacement
70093	Incision	70639	Repair Of Extraoral Mandible With Bone Plate
70095	TMJ Arthrotomy		
70096	Excision	70640	Repair Of Mandible With Subperiosteal Implant
70097	Benign Cyst / Tumor		
70098	Complex	70641	Partial
70099	Malignant Tumor	70642	Complete
70100	With Radical Resection	70643	Repair Of Mandible With Endosteal Implant
70101	Condylectomy Of The TMJ		
70102	Meniscectomy Of The TMJ	70644	Partial
70103	Coronoidectomy	70645	Complete
70106	Of Mandibular Bone	70646	Repair Of Mandibular Condyle With Autografts
70112	Of Torus Mandibularis		
70511	Introduction	70647	Segmental Osteotomy Of Mandible
70512	Preparation Of Mandibular Resection Prosthesis		
		70648	Mandibular Graft
70514	Application Of Mandibular Interdental Fixation Device	70650	Using Bone
		70649	Using Rib Cartilage
70613	Repair	72896	Unlisted Craniofacial And Maxillofacial Procedure
70614	Genioplasty		
70615	Augmentation	74819	Arthroscopy
70616	With Single Sliding Osteotomy	45976	Neck
70617	With Multiple Sliding Osteotomies	47608	On The Right
		47609	On The Left
70618	With Sliding Osteotomy And Augmentation	45971	Closed Treatment Of A Hyoid Fracture
70619	Mandibular Augmentation	45972	With Manipulation
70620	With Prosthetic Material	48506	Open Treatment Of A Hyoid Fracture
70621	With Bone Graft		
70622	Repair Of Mandibular Ramus	70006	Incision
70623	With Horizontal Osteotomy	70007	And Drainage
70624	With Horizontal Osteotomy And Bone Graft	70008	With Partial Ostectomy Of Rib
		70113	Excision
70625	With Vertical Osteotomy	45977	Soft Tissue Tumor
70626	With Vertical Osteotomy And Bone Graft	45978	Subcutaneous
		45979	Deep
70627	With A "C" Osteotomy	70114	Radical Resection Of Soft Tissue Tumor
70628	With A "C" Osteotomy And Bone Graft		
70629	With An "L" Osteotomy	70708	Repair
70630	With An "L" Osteotomy And Bone Graft	70709	Division Of Scalenus Anticus
		70710	With Cervical Rib Resection
70631	With Sagittal Split	70711	Division Of Sternocleidomastoid
		70712	With Application Of Cast

SURGERY, CONT.

45973	Thorax		45985	Closed Treatment Of Vertebral Body Fracture(s)
49946	Fracture		48512	Open Treatment Of Single Vertebral Body Fracture
45974	Closed Treatment Of A Single Rib Fracture		48513	Cervical
48508	Treatment of Rib Fracture with Fixation of Flail Chest		48514	Thoracic
48507	Open Treatment Of A Single Rib Fracture		48515	Lumbar
45975	Closed Treatment Of A Sternum Fracture		45986	Casting / Bracing Of Single Vertebral Body Fracture
48509	Open Treatment Of A Sternum Fracture		48516	Open Treatment Of Single Vertebral Body Dislocation
70010	Incision		48517	Cervical
70011	And Drainage		48518	Thoracic
70012	With Partial Ostectomy Of Rib		48519	Lumbar
70009	Deep, Of The Cortex		70132	Excision
70115	Excision		70133	Partial Resection Of Posterior Vertebral Component
70117	Soft Tissue Tumor		70134	Cervical Segment
70118	Subcutaneous		72900	Each Additional Cervical Segment
70119	Deep		70135	Thoracic Segment
70116	Radical Resection Of Soft Tissue Tumor		72901	Each Additional Thoracic Segment
70122	Of First Rib		70136	Lumbar Segment
70123	With Sympathectomy		72903	Each Additional Lumbar Segment
70124	Of Cervical Rib		70141	Partial Resection Of Vertebral Body
70125	With Sympathectomy		70142	Cervical Segment
70120	Partial Excision Of A Rib		72904	Each Additional Cervical Segment
70121	Costotransversectomy		70143	Thoracic Segment
70126	Sternal Debridement		72905	Each Additional Thoracic Segment
70127	Partial Ostectomy Of Sternum		70144	Lumbar Segment
70128	Radical Resection Of Sternum		72906	Each Additional Lumbar Segment
70129	With Mediastinal Lymphadenectomy		70717	Repair
45987	Of Subfascial Abdominal Wall Tumor		70728	Anterior Osteotomy Of Single Spine Segment
70713	Repair		70729	Cervical
70714	Of Pectus Excavatum		70730	Thoracic
70715	Of Pectus Carinatum		70731	Lumbar
70716	Of Sternotomy Separation		70732	Posterior Osteotomy Of Single Spine Segment
45980	Torso		70733	Cervical
45981	Excision Of Soft Tissue Tumor Of The Back		70734	Thoracic
45982	Excision Of Soft Tissue Tumor Of The Flank		70735	Lumbar
70130	Radical Resection Of Soft Tissue Tumor Of The Back		70736	Osteotomy Of Each Additional Spine Segment
70131	Radical Resection Of Soft Tissue Tumor Of The Flank		74879	Arthrodesis
45983	Spine		74880	Cervical
70092	Fracture			
45984	Closed Treatment Of Vertebral Process Fracure(s)			

SURGERY, CONT.

74883	Clivus-C1-C2 By Anterior Transoral Approach	46011	With Manipulation
74884	Clivus-C1-C2 By Anterior Extraoral Approach	48294	Open Treatment Of Humeral Greater Tuberosity Fracture
74885	C1-C2 By Posterior Approach	49948	Dislocation
74886	Below C2 By Anterior Interbody Technique	46002	Closed Treatment Of Sternoclavicular Dislocation
74887	Below C2 By Posterior Approach	46003	With Manipulation
74881	Thoracic	46004	Closed Treatment Of Acromioclavicular Dislocation
74888	By Anterior Approach	46005	With Manipulation
74895	Additional Interspace	46012	Closed Treatment Of Shoulder Dislocation With Manipulation
74889	By Posterior Approach	46013	Requiring Anesthesia
74896	Additional Vertebral Segment	49180	And Fracture Of Greater Tuberosity
74890	By Posterolateral Approach	49179	Open Treatment Of Acute Shoulder Dislocation
74897	Additional Vertebral Segment	49181	And Fracture Of Greater Tuberosity
74882	Lumbar	46014	Closed Manipulation Shoulder Dislocation & Fracture Anatomical Neck
74891	By Anterior Approach		
74898	Additional Interspace		
74892	By Posterior Approach	49182	Open Treatment Shoulder Dislocation And Fracture Anatomical Neck
74899	Additional Vertebral Segment		
74893	By Posterolateral Approach		
74900	Additional Vertebral Segment	70026	Incision
		70027	And Drainage
74894	By Posterior Interbody Technique	70028	Infected Bursa
		70029	Deep, Of The Cortex
45988	Of The Shoulder	70030	Arthrotomy With Exploration
47612	On The Right	70031	Of The Glenohumeral Joint
47613	On The Left	70032	Of The Acromioclavicular Joint
49947	Fracture	70033	Of The Sternoclavicular Joint
46000	Closed Treatment Of Clavicular Fracture	70516	Removal Of Implant
		70517	Subcutaneous
46001	With Manipulation	70518	Deep
47610	On The Right	70519	Removal Of "Total Shoulder"
47611	On The Left	70038	Open Removal Of Calcarious Deposits
48290	Open Treatment Of Clavicular Fracture	70039	Capsular Contracture Release
46006	Closed Treatment Of Scapular Fracture	70145	Excision
		70146	Soft Tissue Tumor
46007	With Manipulation	70147	Subcutaneous
48291	Open Treatment Of Scapular Fracture	70148	Deep
		70149	Radical Resection Of Soft Tissue Tumor
46008	Closed Treatment Of Proximal Humeral Fracture	70150	Arthrotomy
46009	With Manipulation	70151	With Biopsy
48292	Open Treatment Of Proximal Humeral Fracture	70152	Of The Glenohumeral Joint
		70153	Of The Acromioclavicular Joint
48293	With Prosthetic Replacement		
46010	Closed Treatment Of Humeral Greater Tuberosity Fracture	70154	Of The Sternoclavicular Joint
		70155	With Excision Of Cartilage

SURGERY, CONT.

70156	Of The Acromioclavicular Joint	70792	Tenodesis Of Long Biceps Tendon
70157	Of The Sternoclavicular Joint	70793	Transplantation Of Long Biceps Tendon
70158	With Exploration	70794	Resection Of Long Biceps Tendon
70159	Of The Glenohumeral Joint	70795	Anterior Capsulorraphy
70160	With Synovectomy	70796	Putti-Platt Capsulorraphy
70161	Of The Glenohumeral Joint	70797	Magnuson Capsulorraphy
70162	Of The Sternoclavicular Joint	70798	Bankart Capsulorraphy
70163	Claviculectomy	70799	With Bone Block
70164	Partial	70800	With Coracoid Process Transfer
70165	Total	70801	Posterior Capsulorraphy For Dislocation
70166	Acromioplasty	70802	Capsulorraphy For Multi-directional Instability
70167	Partial Acromionectomy	70803	Arthroplasty With Proximal Humeral Implant
70168	Curettage	70804	Arthroplasty With Total Shoulder Replacement
70169	Clavicle	70805	Osteotomy Of The Clavicle
70170	Scapula	70806	With Bone Graft
70171	Proximal Humerus	70807	Prophalactic Pinning Of The Clavicle
70172	Curettage With Autograft		
70173	Clavicle	74820	Arthroscopy
70174	Scapula	74821	With Removal Of Loose Body
70175	Proximal Humerus	74822	With Removal Of Foreign Body
70176	Curettage With Allograft	74823	With Partial Synovectomy
70177	Clavicle	74824	With Complete Synovectomy
70178	Scapula	74825	With Limited Debridement
70179	Proximal Humerus	74826	With Extensive Debridement
70180	Sequestrectomy	74827	With Lysis Of Adhesions
70181	Clavicle	74828	With Decompression Of Subacromial Space And Acromioplasty
70182	Scapula		
70183	Proximal Humerus		
70184	Partial Excision Of Bone	74829	With Coracoacromial Release
70185	Clavicle	74901	Arthrodesis
70186	Scapula	74902	With Local Bone Graft
70187	Proximal Humerus	74903	With Primary Autogenous Graft
70188	Radical Resection Of Bone	74772	Amputation
70189	Clavicle	74773	Forequarter
70190	Scapula	74774	Disarticulation
70191	Proximal Humerus	74775	With Secondary Closure
70192	With Autograft	74776	With Scar Revision
70193	With Prosthetic Replacement	45989	Humerus
70194	Partial Ostectomy Of The Scapula	46885	Fracture
70195	Resection Of The Humeral Head	49056	Shaft, Closed
70781	Repair	46893	With Manipulation
70782	Muscle Transfer	46892	Shaft, Open with Plate or Screws
70783	Multiple	49057	Shaft, Open with Medullary Implant
70784	Scapulopexy		
70785	Tenomyotomy	46894	Supracondylar, Closed
70786	Multiple	46895	With Manipulation
70787	Rotator Cuff Repair		
70788	Acute		
70789	Chronic		
70791	Chronic Rotator Cuff Avulsion		
70790	Coracoacromial Ligament Release		

SURGERY, CONT.

49058	Supracondylar, Percutaneous Fixation	74780	With Secondary Closure
49059	Supracondylar, Open	74781	With Scar Revision
49060	with Intercondylar Extension	74783	With Implant
49953	Incision	74785	Cineplastic
49951	And Drainage	74782	Re-amputation
49952	Infected Bursa	74784	Stump Elongation
49954	Deep, Of The Cortex	70584	Replantation
70520	Removal Of Implant	70585	Following Complete Amputation
70521	Subcutaneous	47614	On The Right
70522	Deep	47615	On The Left
70198	Excision	45990	Elbow
70199	Soft Tissue Tumor	46886	Fracture
70200	Subcutaneous	49076	Periarticular, Open
70201	Deep	49077	with Implant Arthroplasty
70202	Radical Resection Of Soft Tissue Tumor	46896	Transcondylar, Closed
		46897	With Manipulation
70213	Curettage	49061	Transcondylar, Percutaneous
70214	With Autograft	49062	Transcondylar, Open
70215	With Allograft	49063	with Intercondylar Extension
70223	Sequestrectomy Of The Shaft / Distal Humerus	46898	Medial Epicondylar, Closed
		46899	With Manipulation
70224	Partial Excision Of Bone	49064	Medial Epicondylar, Percutaneous Fixation with Manipulation
70225	Radical Resection Of Shaft / Distal Bone	49066	Medial Epicondylar, Open
		46900	Lateral Epicondylar, Closed
70226	With Autograft	46901	With Manipulation
70808	Repair	49065	Lateral Epicondylar, Percutaneous Fixation with Manipulation
70809	Muscle Transfer		
70810	Multiple	49067	Lateral Epicondylar, Open
70812	Tendon Transfer	49068	Medial Condylar, Closed
70813	Tendon Lengthening	49070	with Manipulation
70814	Open Tenotomy From Shoulder To Elbow	49069	Lateral Condylar, Closed
		49071	with Manipulation
70815	Tenoplasty And Muscle Transfer From Shoulder To Elbow	49072	Medial Condylar, Percutaneous Fixation
70816	Distal Reinsertion Of Ruptured Biceps Tendon	49073	Lateral Condylar, Percutaneous Fixation
70817	Distal Reinsertion Of Ruptured Triceps Tendon	49074	Medial Condylar, Open
		49075	Lateral Condylar, Open
70818	Osteotomy	46902	Proximal Ulna With Radial Dislocation, Closed
70819	Multiple Osteomotomies With Rod Realignment	49078	Proximal Ulna With Radial Dislocation, Open
70820	Osteoplasty	46903	Radial Head, Closed
70821	Repair Of Nonunion	46904	With Manipulation
70822	With Autograft	49183	Radial Head, Open
70823	Hemiepiphyseal Arrest	49184	With Prosthetic Replacement
70811	Prophalactic Pinning Of The Proximal Humerus	46905	Radial Neck, Closed
		46906	With Manipulation
70824	Prophalactic Pinning Of The Humeral Shaft	49185	Radial Neck, Open
		49186	With Prosthetic Replacement
74777	Amputation	46907	Olecranon, Closed
74778	With Primary Closure	46908	With Manipulation
74779	Open, Circular		

SURGERY, CONT.

49187	Olecranon, Open	70826	Muscle Transfer
49188	Dislocation	70827	Tendon Transfer
49189	Closed Treatment	70828	Tendon Lengthening
49190	Requiring Anesthesia	70829	Flexorplasty
49191	Open Treatment	70830	With Extensor Advancement
49118	Radial Head Subluxation	70831	Tenodesis Of Biceps Tendon
49119	With Manipulation	70832	Fasciotomy Of The Lateral
49955	Incision		Epicondyle
49956	And Drainage	70833	With Extensor Origin
49957	Infected Bursa		Detachment
49958	Deep, Of The Cortex Of The Bone	70834	With Annular Ligament
49959	Arthrotomy For Infection And		Resection
	Foreign Body	70835	With Stripping
49960	Arthrotomy With Capsular	70836	With Partial Ostectomy
	Excision	70837	Fasciotomy Of The Medial
70523	Removal Of Foreign Body From		Epicondyle
	Soft Tissue	70838	With Extensor Origin
70524	Subcutaneous		Detachment
70525	Deep	70839	With Annular Ligament
70547	Removal Of Implant From Elbow		Resection
	Joint	70840	With Stripping
70548	Removal Of Implant From Radial	70841	With Partial Ostectomy
	Head	70842	Arthroplasty
70203	Excision	70843	With Membrane
70204	Soft Tissue Tumor	70844	With Distal Humeral Prosthesis
70205	Subcutaneous	70845	With Implant And Ligament
70206	Deep		Reconstruction
70207	Radical Resection Of Soft Tissue	70846	With Total Elbow Replacement
	Tumor	70847	Of Radial Head
70208	Arthrotomy	70848	With Implant
70209	With Biopsy	74830	Arthroscopy
70211	With Exploration	74831	With Removal Of Loose Body
70210	With Synovectomy	74832	With Removal Of Foreign Body
70212	Excision Of The Olecranon Bursa	74833	With Partial Synovectomy
70222	Excision Of The Radial Head	74834	With Complete Synovectomy
70216	Curettage Of Head / Neck Of	74835	With Limited Debridement
	Radius	74836	With Extensive Debridement
70217	With Autograft	74904	Arthrodesis
70218	With Allograft	74905	With Local Bone Graft
70219	Curettage Of Olecranon	74906	With Autograft
70220	With Autograft	47616	On The Right
70221	With Allograft	47617	On The Left
70227	Sequestrectomy Of The Radial	45991	Forearm
	Head / Neck	46887	Fracture
70228	Partial Excision Of Radial Head /	46909	Radial Shaft, Closed
	Neck	46910	With Manipulation
70229	Radical Resection Of Radial Head	46911	With Distal Dislocation
	/ Neck	49079	Radial Shaft, Open
70230	With Autograft	49084	Multiple Fractures
70231	Sequestrectomy Of The Olecranon	49080	Open Treatment of Galeazzi
70232	Partial Excision Of Olecranon		Fracture/Dislocation
70233	Resection Of The Elbow Joint	49081	with Repair of Triangular
70825	Repair		Cartilage

SURGERY, CONT.

46912	Ulnar Shaft, Closed	70864	Secondary
46913	With Manipulation	70866	With Graft
49082	Ulnar Shaft, Open	70867	Tendon Lengthening
49083	Multiple Fractures	70868	Flexor
46914	Combined Radial And Ulnar	70869	Extensor
	Shafts, Closed	70870	Tendon Shortening
46915	With Manipulation	70871	Flexor
49085	Combined Radial and Ulnar	70872	Extensor
	Shafts, Open	70873	Open Tenotomy
49961	Incision	70874	Flexor
49962	And Drainage	70875	Extensor
49963	Infected Bursa	70876	Tenolysis
49964	Deep, Of The Cortex Of The Bone	70877	Flexor
70526	Removal Of Deep Implant	70878	Extensor
70043	Decompression Fasciotomy	71109	Tendon Transfer
70044	With Debridement	71110	Flexor
70234	Excision	71111	Extensor
70236	Soft Tissue Tumor	71112	With Graft
70238	Subcutaneous	71113	Flexor Origin Slide
70240	Deep	71114	With Tendon Transfer
70242	Radical Resection Of Soft Tissue	71115	Ulnar Osteotomy
	Tumor	71116	And Radius
70264	Curettage Of Radial Shaft	71117	Multiple Osteotomies With
70265	With Autograft		Realignment On Rod
70266	With Allograft	71118	Radius
70267	Curettage Of Ulnar Shaft	71119	Ulna
70268	With Autograft	71120	Of The Radius and Ulna
70269	With Allograft	71121	Shortening Osteoplasty
70276	Sequestrectomy	71122	Radius
70277	Partial Excision Of Radius	71123	Ulna
70278	Partial Excision Of Ulna	71124	Of The Radius and Ulna
70280	Radical Resection Of The Radius	71125	Lengthening Osteoplasty With
70279	Radical Resection Of The Ulna		Autograft
70263	Excision Of Lesion Of Tendon	71126	Radius
	Sheath	71127	Ulna
70270	Radical Excision Of Flexor Bursa	71128	Of The Radius and Ulna
70271	Radical Excision Of Extensor	71129	Nonunion Repair
	Bursa	71130	Radius
70849	Repair	71131	Ulna
70851	Flexor Muscle	71132	Of The Radius and Ulna
70852	Primary	71133	Nonunion Repair With Autograft
70853	Secondary	71134	Radius
70854	With Free Graft	71135	Ulna
70855	Extensor Muscle	71136	Of The Radius and Ulna
70856	Primary	71137	Repair Of Defect With Autograft
70857	Secondary	71138	Radius
70865	With Graft	71139	Ulna
70858	Flexor Tendon	71140	Of The Radius and Ulna
70859	Primary	71141	Prophylactic Pinning
70860	Secondary	71144	Radius
70861	With Free Graft	71145	Ulna
70862	Extensor Tendon	71146	Of The Radius and Ulna
70863	Primary	71142	Prophylactic Plating

SURGERY, CONT.

71147	Radius	49966	And Drainage
71148	Ulna	49967	Infected Bursa
71149	Of The Radius and Ulna	49968	Deep, Of The Cortex Of The Bone
71143	Prophylactic Wiring	49969	Arthrotomy For Infection And
71150	Radius		Foreign Body
71151	Ulna	70527	Removal Of Deep Implant
71152	Of The Radius and Ulna	70528	Removal Of A Prosthesis
71159	Osteotomy Of Radius	70529	Complicated
71160	Distal Third	70530	"Total Wrist"
71161	Middle Third	70040	Of The Tendon Sheath At The
71162	Proximal Third		Radial Styloid
70850	Decompression Fasciotomy With	70041	Decompression Fasciotomy
	Brachial Artery Exploration	70042	With Debridement
74786	Amputation	70235	Excision
74788	Open, Circular	70237	Soft Tissue Tumor
74789	With Secondary Closure	70239	Subcutaneous
74790	With Scar Revision	70241	Deep
74791	Re-amputation	70243	Radical Resection Of Soft Tissue
70587	Replantation		Tumor
70588	Following Complete Amputation	70244	Capsulotomy
47618	On The Right	70245	Arthrotomy
47619	On The Left	70246	With Biopsy
45992	Wrist	70247	With Exploration
46888	Fracture	70248	With Synovectomy
46916	Distal Radial, Closed	70249	For Repair Of Triangular
46917	With Manipulation		Cartilage Complex Of Distal
49086	Distal Radial, Percutaneous		Radioulnar Joint
	Fixation/Manipulation	70250	Curettage Of Carpal Bones
49087	Distal Radial, Open	70251	With Autograft
46920	Carpal Bone, Closed (Each)	70252	With Allograft
46921	With Manipulation	70253	Sequestrectomy
49192	Carpal Bone, Open (Each)	70254	Excision Of Ganglion
49089	Carpal Scaphoid, Open	70255	Primary
46918	Carpal Scaphoid, Closed	70256	Recurrent
46919	With Manipulation	70257	Excision Of Lesion Of Tendon
49088	Carpal Scaphoid, Open		Sheath
46922	Ulnar Styloid, Closed	70258	Carpectomy
49193	Dislocation	70259	Of One Bone
49194	Radiocarpal, Closed Manipulation	70260	Of All Bones Of A Proximal
49195	Radiocarpal, Open		Row
49196	Intercarpal, Closed Manipulation	70261	Radial Styloidectomy
49197	Intercarpal, Open	70262	Excision Of The Distal Ulna
49199	Distal Radioulnar, Closed	70272	Radical Excision Of Flexor Bursa
	Manipulation	70273	Radical Excision Of Extensor
49198	Distal Radioulnar, Open		Bursa
	Treatment	70274	Synovectomy Of Extensor Tendon
49200	Lunate, Closed Manipulation		Sheath
49201	Lunate, Open Treatment	70275	With Resection Of The Distal
49202	Trans-Scaphoperilunar Fracture,		Ulna
	Closed Manipulation	71106	Repair
49203	Trans-Scaphoperilunar Fracture,	71105	Tenodesis
	Open Treatment	71107	Flexors
49965	Incision	71108	Extensors

SURGERY, CONT.

71153	Capsulorrhaphy for Carpal Instability	46889	Fracture
		46923	Single Metacarpal, Closed
71154	Arthroplasty	46924	With Manipulation
71155	With Implant	46925	With Fixation
71156	Pseudoarthrosis Type With Internal Fixation	49090	Single Metacarpal, Percutaneous Fixation
71157	Centralization Of Wrist On Ulna	49091	Single Metacarpal, Open
71158	Soft Tissue Stabilization Of Distal Ulna	46926	Proximal Phalanx Of One Finger, Closed
71163	Repair Of Nonunion Of The Scaphoid	46927	With Manipulation
		49096	Proximal Phalanx Of One Finger, Percutaneous Fixation
71164	Arthroplasty With Prosthesis		
71165	Distal Radius	49100	Proximal Phalanx Of One Finger, Open
71166	Distal Ulna		
71167	Scaphoid	46928	Middle Phalanx Of One Finger, Closed
71168	Lunate		
71169	Trapezium	46929	With Manipulation
71170	Distal Radius And Wrist	49097	Middle Phalanx Of One Finger, Percutaneous Fixation
71171	Revision Of Arthroplasty, Implant Removal	49101	Middle Phalanx Of One Finger, Open
71172	Interposition Arthroplasty	46930	Distal Phalanx Of One Finger, Closed
71173	Intercarpal Joint		
71174	Carpometacarpal Joint	46931	With Manipulation
71175	Epiphyseal Arrest	49099	Distal Phalanx Of One Finger, Percutaneous Fixation
71176	Distal Radius		
71177	Distal Ulna	49098	Distal Phalanx Of One Finger, Open
71178	Distal Radius And Ulna		
74837	Arthroscopy	46932	Finger Joint, Closed
74838	For Lavage And Drainage	46933	MCP
74839	With Partial Synovectomy	46934	PIP
74840	With Complete Synovectomy	46935	DIP
74841	With Excision/Repair Of Triangular Fibrocartilage	46936	With Manipulation
		49102	Single Finger Joint, Open
74842	And Joint Debridement	49103	MCP
74843	With Internal Fixation	49105	PIP
74844	With Release Of Transverse Carpal Ligament	49104	DIP
74907	Arthrodesis	49093	Thumb, Carpometacarpal
74908	With Sliding Graft	49092	Closed, With Manipulation
74909	With Autograft	49094	Percutaneous Fixation with Manipulation
74910	By Intercarpal Fusion		
74911	With Autograft	49095	Open
74912	Distal Radioulnar And Segmental Ulnar Resection	49204	Dislocation
		49205	Carpometacarpal, Closed Manipulation (Not Thumb)
74792	Amputation		
74793	Krukenberg Procedure	49206	Requiring Anesthesia
74794	Disarticulation	49207	Carpometacarpal, Percutaneous Fixation & Manipulation (Not Thumb)
74795	With Secondary Closure		
74796	With Scar Revision		
74797	Re-amputation	49208	Carpometacarpal, Open Treatment (Not Thumb)
47620	On The Right		
47621	On The Left	49209	Difficult Reduction
45993	Hand		

SURGERY, CONT.

49210	Metacarpophalangeal, Closed Manipulation (Single)	70292	Partial, With Release Of A Single Digit Including The PIP
49211	Requiring Anesthesia	70293	Partial, With Release Of An Additional Digit Including The PIP
49212	Metacarpophalangeal, Percutaneous Fixation And Manipulation (Single)	70294	Synovectomy
49213	Metacarpophalangeal, Open Treatment (Single)	70295	Of A Carpometacarpal Joint
		70296	Of An MCP Joint With Intrinsic Release And Hood Reconstruction
49214	Interphalangeal, Closed Manipulation (Single)		
49215	Requiring Anesthesia	70297	Of A PIP Joint With Extensor Reconstruction
49216	Interphalangeal, Percutaneous Fixation And Manipulation (Single)	70299	Excision Of A Tendon Cyst
		70300	Excision Of A Palmar Flexor Tendon
49217	Interphalangeal, Open Treatment (Single)	70301	Excision Of A Finger Flexor Tendon
70045	Incision		
70046	Drainage Of Finger Abscess	70298	Radical Synovectomy Of A Tendon Sheath - Palm or finger
70047	Complicated		
70048	Drainage Of Tendon Sheath	70302	Curettage Of A Metacarpal Bone
70049	Drainage Of Palmar Bursa	70303	With Autograft
70050	Multiple	70304	Curettage Of A Proximal Phalanx Of A Finger
70051	Complicated		
70034	Arthrotomy With Exploration	70305	With Autograft
70035	Of The Carpometacarpal Joint	70306	Curettage Of A Middle Phalanx Of A Finger
70036	Of The Metacarpophalangeal Joint		
		70307	With Autograft
70037	Of The Interphalangeal Joint	70308	Curettage Of A Distal Phalanx Of A Finger
70052	Deep, Of The Cortex Of The Bone		
70531	Removal Of Implant	70309	With Autograft
70053	Decompression Fasciotomy Of The Hand	70310	Partial Excision Of A Metacarpal Bone
70054	For Injection Injury	70311	Partial Excision Of A Proximal Phalanx Of A Finger
70055	Palmar Fasciotomy For Dupuytren's Contracture	70312	Partial Excision Of A Middle Phalanx Of A Finger
70056	Open	70313	Partial Excision Of A Distal Phalanx Of A Finger
70058	Subcutaneous Tenotomy		
70057	Tendon Sheath Of A Finger	70314	Radical Resection Of A Metacarpal Bone
70281	Excision		
70287	Soft Tissue Tumor	70318	With Autograft
70288	Subcutaneous	70315	Radical Resection Of A Proximal Phalanx Of A Finger
70289	Deep		
70290	Radical Resection Of Soft Tissue Tumor	70319	With Autograft
		70316	Radical Resection Of A Middle Phalanx Of A Finger
70282	Arthrotomy		
70283	With Biopsy	70320	With Autograft
70284	Of The Carpometacarpal Joint	70317	Radical Resection Of A Distal Phalanx Of A Finger
70285	Of The Metacarpophalangeal Joint	71179	Repair
70286	Of An Interphalangeal Joint	71180	Flexor Tendon
70291	Palmar Fasciectomy	71181	With Free Graft

SURGERY, CONT.

71182	Flexor Tendon In "No Man's Land"	71226	Flexor
		71227	Extensor
71183	Primary	71228	Finger Tendon Lengthening
71184	Secondary	71229	Flexor
71185	Secondary, With Free Graft	71230	Extensor
71186	Profundus Tendon Repair (Intact Sublimis)	71231	Hand Tendon Shortening
		71232	Flexor
71187	Primary	71233	Extensor
71188	Secondary	71234	Finger Tendon Shortening
71189	Secondary, With Free Graft	71235	Flexor
71190	Tendon Excision, Rod Implantation For Delayed Graft	71236	Extensor
		71525	Dorsal Tendon Transfer
71191	Flexor	71526	With Free Tendon Graft
71192	Extensor	71527	Palmar Tendon Transfer
71193	Removal Of Rod And Insertion Of Tendon Graft	71528	With Free Tendon Graft
		71529	Tendon Transfer To Restore Intrinsic Function
71194	Flexor		
71195	Extensor	71530	Ring And Little Finger
71196	Dorsal Extensor Tendon Of Hand	71531	All Four Fingers
71197	With Free Graft	71532	Correction Of Claw Finger(s)
71198	Dorsal Extensor Tendon Of A Finger		Without Tendon Transfer
		71533	Opponensplasty
71199	With Free Graft	71534	Sublimis Tendon Transfer
71200	Secondary Extensor Tendon, Central Slip (Boutonniere deformity)	71535	Tendon Transfer With Graft
		71536	Hypothenar Muscle Transfer
		71537	Tendon Pulley Reconstruction
71201	With Free Graft	71538	With Local Tissues
71202	Extensor Tendon Repair (Mallet Finger)	71539	With Tendon Graft
		71540	With Fascial Graft
71203	Closed	71541	With Tendon Prosthesis
71204	Open	71542	Thenar Muscle Release For Thumb Contracture
71205	Open, With Free Graft		
71206	Extensor Tendon Realignment In The Hand	71543	Cross Intrinsic Muscle Transfer
		71544	Cross Intrinsic Tendon Transfer
71207	Simple Tenolysis, Flexor Tendon	71545	Capulodesis For M-P Joint Stabilization
71208	Palm		
71209	Finger	71546	Single Digit
71210	Palm And Finger	71547	Two Digits
71211	Tenolysis, Extensor Tendon	71548	Three Or Four Digits
71212	Dorsum Of Hand	71549	Capsulotomy For Single MCP Contracture
71213	Finger		
71214	Including Hand And Forearm	71550	Capsulotomy For Single IP Contracture
71215	Tenotomy		
71216	Flexor	71551	Arthroplasty Of Single MCP Joint
71217	Palm	71552	With Prosthetic Implant
71218	Finger	71553	Arthroplasty Of Single IP Joint
71219	Extensor	71554	With Prosthetic Implant
71220	Dorsum Of Hand	71555	Primary Repair Of MCP Collateral Ligament
71221	Finger		
71222	Tenodesis For Joint Stabilization	71556	With Tendon Graft
71223	Proximal Interphalangeal Joint	71557	With Fascial Graft
71224	Distal Interphalangeal Joint	71558	With Local Tissue
71225	Hand Tendon Lengthening		

SURGERY, CONT.

71559	Reconstruction Of Single IP Collateral Ligament	71592	Abductor Minimi Digiti, Right Hand
71560	Repair Of Finger, Volar Plate, IP Joint	71593	Flexor Brevis Minimi Digiti, Right Hand
71561	Pollicization Of A Finger	71594	Opponens Minimi Digiti, Right Hand
71562	Thumb Reconstruction Using Toe		
71563	Positional Change Of A Finger	71595	1st Dorsal Interosseous Muscle, Left Hand
71564	Toe To Finger Transfer		
71565	1st Stage	71596	2nd Dorsal Interosseous Muscle, Left Hand
71566	2nd Stage		
71567	Each Delay	71597	3rd Dorsal Interosseous Muscle, Left Hand
71568	Repair Of A Syndactaly Web Space	71598	4th Dorsal Interosseous Muscle, Left Hand
71569	With Skin Flaps		
71571	With Skin Flaps And Grafts	71599	1st Palmar Interosseous Muscle, Left Hand
71570	Involving Bone Or Nails		
71572	Osteotomy For Metacarpal Deformity	71600	2nd Palmar Interosseous Muscle, Left Hand
71573	Osteotomy For Phalangeal Deformity Of Finger	71601	3rd Palmar Interosseous Muscle, Left Hand
71574	Osteoplasty For Metacarpal Lengthening	71602	1st Lumbrical Muscle, Left Hand
71575	Osteoplasty For Lengthening Of Finger Phalanx	71603	2nd Lumbrical Muscle, Left Hand
71576	Repair Of Cleft Hand	71604	3rd Lumbrical Muscle, Left Hand
71577	Repair Of Bifid Finger		
71578	Reconstruction Of Supernumerary Finger	71605	4th Lumbrical Muscle, Left Hand
71579	Repair Of Macrodactylia	71606	Abductor Minimi Digiti, Left Hand
71580	Repair Of Intrinsic Hand Muscles		
71581	1st Dorsal Interosseous Muscle, Right Hand	71607	Flexor Brevis Minimi Digiti, Left Hand
71582	2nd Dorsal Interosseous Muscle, Right Hand	71608	Opponens Minimi Digiti, Left Hand
71583	3rd Dorsal Interosseous Muscle, Right Hand	71609	Release Of Intrinsic Hand Muscles
71584	4th Dorsal Interosseous Muscle, Right Hand	71610	1st Dorsal Interosseous Muscle, Right Hand
71585	1st Palmar Interosseous Muscle, Right Hand	71611	2nd Dorsal Interosseous Muscle, Right Hand
71586	2nd Palmar Interosseous Muscle, Right Hand	71612	3rd Dorsal Interosseous Muscle, Right Hand
71587	3rd Palmar Interosseous Muscle, Right Hand	71613	4th Dorsal Interosseous Muscle, Right Hand
71588	1st Lumbrical Muscle, Right Hand	71614	1st Palmar Interosseous Muscle, Right Hand
71589	2nd Lumbrical Muscle, Right Hand	71615	2nd Palmar Interosseous Muscle, Right Hand
71590	3rd Lumbrical Muscle, Right Hand	71616	3rd Palmar Interosseous Muscle, Right Hand
71591	4th Lumbrical Muscle, Right Hand	71617	1st Lumbrical Muscle, Right Hand

SURGERY, CONT.

71618	2nd Lumbrical Muscle, Right Hand	71649	Flexor
71619	3rd Lumbrical Muscle, Right Hand	71650	With Skin Grafts
		71651	With Rearrangement Flaps
71620	4th Lumbrical Muscle, Right Hand	71652	With Z-plasties
		71653	Extensor
71621	Abductor Minimi Digiti, Right Hand	71654	With Skin Grafts
		71655	With Rearrangement Flaps
71622	Flexor Brevis Minimi Digiti, Right Hand	71656	With Z-plasties
		75164	Arthrodesis
71623	Opponens Minimi Digiti, Right Hand	75165	Thumb In Opposition, With Graft
		75166	Thumb Carpometacarpal Joint
71624	1st Dorsal Interosseous Muscle, Left Hand	75167	With Autograft
		75168	Carpometacarpal Joint
71625	2nd Dorsal Interosseous Muscle, Left Hand	75169	With Autograft
		75170	MCP Joint
71626	3rd Dorsal Interosseous Muscle, Left Hand	75171	With Autograft
		75172	Hand IP Joint
71627	4th Dorsal Interosseous Muscle, Left Hand	75173	With Autograft
		75174	Each Additional Joint
71628	1st Palmar Interosseous Muscle, Left Hand	75175	With Autograft
		74798	Amputation
71629	2nd Palmar Interosseous Muscle, Left Hand	74799	Transmetacarpal
		74800	With Secondary Closure
71630	3rd Palmar Interosseous Muscle, Left Hand	74801	With Scar Revision
		74802	Re-amputation
71631	1st Lumbrical Muscle, Left Hand	74803	Metacarpal
		74804	And Thumb
71632	2nd Lumbrical Muscle, Left Hand	74805	And Index Finger
		74806	And Middle Finger
71633	3rd Lumbrical Muscle, Left Hand	74807	And Ring Finger
		74808	And Little Finger
71634	4th Lumbrical Muscle, Left Hand	74809	Finger, With Neurectomy
		74811	Thumb
71635	Abductor Minimi Digiti, Left Hand	74812	Index Finger
		74813	Middle Finger
71636	Flexor Brevis Minimi Digiti, Left Hand	74814	Ring Finger
		74815	Little Finger
71637	Opponens Minimi Digiti, Left Hand	74810	And Flaps
		70593	Replantation
71638	Excision Of Constricting Ring With Z-plasties	70590	Of The Hand Following Complete Amputation
71639	Release Of Finger Scar Contracture	70594	Of The Proximal Thumb Following Complete Amputation
71640	Flexor	70595	Of The Distal Thumb Following Complete Amputation
71641	With Skin Grafts	70597	Of A Proximal Finger Following Complete Amputation
71642	With Rearrangement Flaps		
71643	With Z-plasties	70599	Of A Distal Finger Following Complete Amputation
71644	Extensor		
71645	With Skin Grafts	47622	On The Right
71646	With Rearrangement Flaps	47623	On The Left
71647	With Z-plasties	45994	Pelvis
71648	Release Of Hand Scar Contracture	46890	Fracture

SURGERY, CONT.

46937	Pelvic Ring, Closed	70353	Deep
46938	With Manipulation And	70358	Radical Resection
	Anesthesia	70357	Of Wing Of Ilium
49107	Pelvic Ring, Posterior,	70359	Of One Pubic Ramus
	Percutaneous Fixation	70360	Of One Ischial Ramus
49108	Pelvic Ring, Posterior, Open with	70361	Of Symphysis Pubis
	Fixation	70362	Of The Ilium, Including
49112	Pelvic Ring, Anterior, Open with		Acetabulum
	Fixation	70363	And Both Pubic Rami
49106	Coccygeal, Open	70364	And The Ischium
46939	Coccygeal, Closed	70365	Of The Entire Innominate Bone
49114	Iliac Spine, Open	70366	Of The Ischial Tuberosity And
49115	Iliac Wing, Open		Greater Trochanter
49116	Ileal Tuberosity Avulsion, Open	70367	With Skin Flaps
49109	Dislocation	70368	Primary Coccygectomy
49110	Pelvic Ring, Posterior,	71657	Repair
	Percutaneous Fixation	71659	Proximal Hamstring Recession
49111	Pelvic Ring, Posterior, Open with	71660	Adductor Transfer To Ischium
	Fixation	71661	Bilateral Osteotomy
49970	Incision	71662	Iliac Osteotomy
49971	And Drainage	71663	With Open Reduction Of The
49972	Infected Bursa		Hip
49973	Deep, Of The Cortex Of The Bone	71664	With Femoral Osteotomy
70532	Removal Of Implant	71665	With Open Reduction Of The
70533	Subcutaneous		Hip And Femoral Osteotomy
70534	Deep	71666	Osteotomy Of Innominate Bone
70321	Excision	71667	With Open Reduction Of The
70323	Soft Tissue Tumor		Hip
70325	Subcutaneous	71668	With Femoral Osteotomy
70327	Deep	71669	With Open Reduction Of The
70329	Radical Resection Of Soft Tissue		Hip And Femoral Osteotomy
	Tumor	71672	Acetabular Osteotomy
70331	Arthrotomy Of Sacroiliac Joint,	71673	With Open Reduction Of The
	With Biopsy		Hip
70335	Excision Of Ischial Bursa	71674	With Femoral Osteotomy
70336	Excision Of Benign Lesion Of	71675	With Open Reduction Of The
	Wing Of Ilium		Hip And Femoral Osteotomy
70337	Superficial	71676	Acetabuloplasty
70338	Deep	71677	With Femoral Head Resection
70339	With Separate Incision For	75176	Arthrodesis
	Autograft	75177	Sacroiliac Joint
70340	Excision Of Benign Lesion Of	75178	Right
	Symphysis Pubis	75179	Left
70341	Superficial	75180	Symphysis Pubis
70342	Deep	47624	On The Right
70343	With Separate Incision For	47625	On The Left
	Autograft	45995	Treatment Of Hip
70348	Partial Excision Of Wing Of Ilium	46891	Fracture
70349	Superficial	46940	Acetabulum, Closed
70350	Deep	46941	With Manipulation
70351	Partial Excision Of Symphysis	49135	Acetabulum, Open
	Pubis	49136	Wall Fracture
70352	Superficial	49137	Two-part Fracture

49138	Three-part Fracture	70537	Deep
46942	Proximal Femoral Neck, Closed	70538	Removal Of A Prosthesis
46943	With Manipulation	70539	Complicated
49139	Proximal Femoral Neck, Percutaneous Fixation	70540	"Total Hip"
		70059	Subcutaneous Tenotomy Of Hip Adductor
49140	Proximal Femoral Neck, Open		
46944	Intertrochanteric, Closed	70060	Closed
46945	With Manipulation	70069	Single
49141	Intertrochanteric, Open	70070	Multiple
49142	With Intramedullary Implant	70061	Open
46946	Pertrochanteric, Closed	70062	With Obturator Neurectomy
46948	With Manipulation	70063	Iliopsoas Tenotomy
49143	Pertrochanteric, Open	70064	Open Tenotomy Of Hip Abductor
49144	With Intramedullary Implant	70065	Fasciotomy
46947	Subtrochanteric, Closed	70066	Denervation
46949	With Manipulation	70322	Excision
49145	Subtrochanteric, Open	70324	Soft Tissue Tumor
49146	With Intramedullary Implant	70326	Subcutaneous
46950	Greater Trochanter, Closed	70328	Deep
49147	Greater Trochanter, Open	70330	Radical Resection Of Soft Tissue Tumor
71774	Dislocation		
71772	Closed Treatment Of Traumatic Dislocation	70332	Arthrotomy Of The Hip Joint
		70333	With Biopsy
71773	Requiring Anesthesia	70334	With Synovectomy
71775	Open Treatment Of Traumatic Dislocation Without Internal Fixation	70344	Excision Of Benign Lesion Of The Greater Trochanter
		70345	Superficial
71776	Open Treatment Of Dislocation, Fracture Acetabular Wall & Femoral Head	70346	Deep
		70347	With Separate Incision For Autograft
71777	Closed Treatment Of Spontaneous Dislocation	70354	Partial Excision Of Greater Trochanter
71778	By Abduction	70355	Superficial
71779	With Splint	70356	Deep
71780	With Traction	71658	Repair
71781	With Manipulation Under Anesthesia	71670	Transfer Of Iliopsoas Muscle To Greater Trochanter
71782	Open Treatment Of Spontaneous Dislocation	71671	Transfer Of Iliopsoas Muscle To Femoral Neck
71783	With Femoral Shaft Shortening	71678	Transfer Of External Oblique Muscle To Greater Trochanter
71784	Closed Treatment Dislocation Post-arthroplasty	71679	Transfer Of Paraspinal Muscle To Hip
71785	Under Anesthesia		
49974	Incision	71680	Partial Hip Replacement With Prosthesis
49975	And Drainage		
49976	Infected Bursa	41737	Total hip replacement
49977	Deep, Of The Cortex Of The Bone	71681	Conversion Of Previous Surgery To "Total Hip" Replacement
49979	Arthrotomy For Infection With Drainage		
		71682	Revision Of Total Hip Arthroplasty
49978	Arthrotomy For Infection And Foreign Body	71683	Acetabular Component Only
		71684	Femoral Component Only
70535	Removal Of Implant	71685	Osteotomy Of The Femoral Neck
70536	Subcutaneous		

SURGERY, CONT.

71686	Osteotomy And Transfer Of Greater Trochanter	45879	Shaft, Open With Plate And Screws
71687	Intertrochanteric Osteotomy	45880	Supracondylar, Closed
71688	Subtrochanteric Osteotomy	45881	With Manipulation
71689	Bone Graft	45882	Supracondylar, Open
71690	Femoral Head	45883	With Intercondylar Extension
71691	Femoral Neck	45884	Transcondylar, Closed
71692	Intertrochanteric Area	45885	With Manipulation
71693	Subtrochanteric Area	45886	Transcondylar, Open
71757	Traction For Slipped Femoral Epiphysis	45887	With Intercondylar Extension
71758	In Situ Pinning Of Slipped Femoral Epiphysis	45888	Distal End, Closed
		45889	With Manipulation
71759	Open Treatment Of Slipped Femoral Epiphysis	45890	Distal End, Percutaneous Skeletal Fixation
71760	By Pinning	45891	Distal End, Open
71761	With Bone Graft	45892	Medial Condyle, Closed
71762	By Closed Manipulation And Pinning	45893	With Manipulation
		45894	Medial Condyle, Percutaneous Skeletal Fixation
71763	By Osteoplasty Of Femoral Neck	45900	Supracondylar, Percutaneous Skeletal Fixation
71764	By Osteotomy And Internal Fixation	45895	Medial Condyle, Open
		45896	Lateral Condyle, Closed
71765	Arrest Of Femoral Epiphysis	45897	With Manipulation
71766	By Epiphysiodesis	45901	Transcondylar, Percutaneous Skeletal Fixation
71767	By Stapling		
71768	Prophylactic Pinning Of The Femoral Neck And Proximal Femur	45898	Lateral Condyle, Percutaneous Skeletal Fixation
		45899	Lateral Condyle, Open
71769	Prophylactic Nailing Of The Femoral Neck And Proximal Femur	49980	Incision
		49981	And Drainage
		49982	Infected Bursa
71770	Prophylactic Wiring Of The Femoral Neck And Proximal Femur	49983	Deep, Of The Cortex Of The Bone
		70541	Removal Of Deep Implant
		70071	Closed Subcutaneous Tenotomy Of Hamstring Adductor
71771	Prophylactic Plating Of The Femoral Neck And Proximal Femur	70072	Multiple
		70067	Fasciotomy
75181	Arthrodesis	70073	Neurectomy Of Hamstring Muscle
75183	Right	70379	Excision
75184	Left	70380	Soft Tissue Tumor
75182	With Subtrochanteric Osteotomy	70381	Subcutaneous
74816	Amputation	70382	Deep
74817	Hindquarter	70383	Radical Resection Of Soft Tissue Tumor
74818	Disarticulation		
47626	On The Right	70404	Curettage of Femur
47627	On The Left	70405	With allograft
45874	Treatment Of Femur	70406	With Autograft
45875	Fracture	70407	Including Internal Fixation
45876	Shaft, Closed	70408	Partial Excision of Femoral Bone
45877	With Manipulation	70402	Radical Resection Of Femoral Bone
45878	Shaft, Open With Implant		
		71786	Repair

SURGERY, CONT.

71788	Suture Of The Quadriceps Muscle	71836	Shortening
71789	Primary	71837	Lengthening
71790	Secondary	71838	Combined Lengthening And Shortening With Segment Transfer
71797	Rectus Femoris		
71798	Vastus Internus		
71799	Vastus Externus	71839	Repair Malunion Of Femoral Shaft
71800	Crureus		
71791	Suture Of Hamstring Muscle	71840	With Graft
71792	Primary	71841	Epiphyseal Arrest Of The Distal Femur
71793	Secondary		
71794	Biceps Flexor Cruris	71842	With Proximal Tibia And Fibula
71795	Semitendinosus		
71796	Semimembranosus	71846	Prophylactic Pinning Of The Femoral Shaft
71801	Tenotomy Of Hamstring Muscle		
71802	Single	71847	Prophylactic Nailing Of The Femoral Shaft
71803	Multiple, Right Leg		
71804	Multiple, Left Leg	71848	Prophylactic Wiring Of The Femoral Shaft
71805	Multiple, Both Legs		
71806	Biceps Flexor Cruris	71849	Prophylactic Plating Of The Femoral Shaft
71807	Semitendinosus		
71808	Semimembranosus	71850	Decompression Fasciotomy Of The Thigh
71809	Lengthening Of Hamstring Tendon		
		71851	With Debridement
71810	Single	71852	Flexor Compartment
71811	Multiple, Right Leg	71853	Extensor Compartment
71812	Multiple, Left Leg	71854	Adductor Compartment
71813	Multiple, Both Legs	71855	Decompression Fasciotomy Of Multiple Compartments Of The Thigh
71814	Biceps Flexor Cruris		
71815	Semitendinosus		
71816	Semimembranosus	71856	With Debridement
71817	Transplant Of Hamstring Tendon To Patella	41741	Amputation Of Leg Above Knee
		72063	Immediate Fitting Technique With First Cast
71818	Single		
71819	Multiple	72064	Open, Circular
71820	Biceps Flexor Cruris	72065	Secondary Closure
71821	Semitendinosus	72066	Scar Revision
71822	Semimembranosus	72067	Re-amputation
71823	Transplant Of Hamstring Tendon To Femur	47628	Of The Right Leg
		47629	Of The Left Leg
71824	Biceps Flexor Cruris	45996	Knee
71825	Semitendinosus	46851	Fracture
71826	Semimembranosus	46852	Patellar, Closed
71827	Transplant Of Hamstring Muscle To Femur	47710	Patellar, Open
		46853	Tibial Plateau, Closed
71828	Biceps Flexor Cruris	46854	With Skeletal Traction
71829	Semitendinosus	47711	Tibial Plateau, Open
71830	Semimembranosus	47712	Bicondylar
71831	Quadricepsplasty	47714	Intercondylar Spine(s), Closed
71832	Osteotomy Of The Femoral Shaft	47715	Intercondylar Spine(s), Open
71833	With Fixation	47713	Tibial Tuberosity, Closed
71834	Multiple, With Realignment On Rod	47716	Tibial Tuberosity, Open
		49984	Incision
71835	Femoral Osteoplasty	49985	And Drainage

SURGERY, CONT.

49986	Infected Bursa	71880	Anterior Tibial Tubercleplasty
49987	Deep, Of The Cortex Of The Bone	71881	Reconstruction For Recurrent Patellar Dislocation
49988	Arthrotomy For Infection And Foreign Body	71882	With Muscle Transfer
70542	Removal Of Deep Implant	71883	With Patellectomy
70068	Fasciotomy	71884	Lateral Retinacular Release
70074	Popliteal Neurectomy Of Gastrocnemius Muscle	71885	Ligamentous Reconstruction
		71886	Extra-articular
70386	Excision	71887	Intra-articular (Open)
70387	Soft Tissue Tumor	71888	Extra- And Intra-articular (Open)
70388	Subcutaneous		
70389	Deep	71889	Posterior Capsular Release
70390	Radical Resection Of Soft Tissue Tumor	71890	Patellar Arthroplasty
		71891	With Prosthesis
70409	Partial Excision of Proximal Tibial Bone	71892	Arthroplasty Of The Tibial Plateau
70410	Partial Excision of Proximal Fibula	71893	Multiple
		71894	With Synovectomy
70391	Arthrotomy Of The Knee	71895	Arthroplasty Of The Femoral Condyles
70385	With Biopsy		
70384	With Joint Exploration	71896	With Synovectomy
70392	With Medial Meniscectomy	71897	Arthroplasty With Constrained Prosthesis
70393	With Lateral Meniscectomy		
70394	With Medial and Lateral Meniscectomy	71898	Combined Arthroplasty Of Condyle & Plateau
70395	With Anterior Synovectomy	71899	Medial Compartment
70396	With Posterior Synovectomy	71900	Lateral Compartment
70397	With Anterior and Posterior Synovectomy	71901	Medial And Lateral Compartments
70398	Excision Of Prepatellar Bursa	71902	Proximal Tibial And Fibular Osteotomy
70399	Excision Of Baker's Cyst		
70400	Patellectomy	71903	Before Epiphyseal Closure
70401	Hemipatellectomy	71904	After Epiphyseal Closure
70403	Radical Resection Of Bone of Knee Joint	71905	Revision Of Total Knee Arthroplasty
		71906	One Component
71787	Repair	71907	All Components
71864	Suture Of Infrapatellar Tendon	71908	Removal Of Knee Prosthesis
71865	Primary	71843	Epiphyseal Arrest Of The Proximal Tibia And Fibula
71866	Secondary		
71867	Arthrotomy With Open Meniscus Repair	71844	Hemiepiphyseal Arrest Of The Distal Femur
71868	Primary Repair Of Ligament	71845	Hemiepiphyseal Arrest Of The Proximal Leg
71869	Collateral		
71872	Medial	71857	Decompression Fasciotomy Of The Knee
71873	Lateral		
71870	Cruciate	71858	With Debridement
71874	Anterior	71859	Flexor Compartment
71875	Posterior	71860	Extensor Compartment
71871	Collateral And Cruciate	71861	Adductor Compartment
71876	Medial Collateral	71862	Decompression Fasciotomy Of Multiple Compartments Of The Knee
71877	Lateral Collateral		
71878	Anterior Cruciate		
71879	Posterior Cruciate		

SURGERY, CONT.

71863	With Debridement	49149	With Fibular Fracture
74845	Arthroscopy	49151	Tibial Shaft, Open Treatment
74853	With Lavage And Drainage		With Plate / Screws
74854	With Removal Of Loose Body	49152	With Fibular Fracture
74855	With Removal Of Foreign Body	49153	Tibial Shaft, Open Treatment
74856	With Limited Synovectomy		With Implant
74857	With Extensive Synovectomy	49154	With Fibular Fracture
74858	With Debridement Of Articular	46858	Proximal Fibula, Closed
	Cartilage	46859	With Manipulation
74859	With Abrasion Arthroplasty	49155	Proximal Fibula, Open
74860	With Multiple Drilling	46860	Fibular Shaft, Closed
74861	With Medial Meniscectomy	46861	With Manipulation
74862	With Lateral Meniscectomy	49156	Fibular Shaft, Open
74863	With Medial And Lateral	49989	Incision
	Meniscectomy	49990	And Drainage
74864	With Medial Meniscus Repair	49991	Infected Bursa
74865	With Lateral Meniscus Repair	49992	Deep, Of The Cortex Of The Bone
74866	With Medial And Lateral	70075	Decompression Fasciotomy
	Meniscus Repair	70076	Anterior Compartment
74867	With Lysis Of Adhesions	70077	Lateral Compartment
74868	With Drilling For Osteochondritis	70078	Posterior Compartment
	And Bone Grafting	70079	Anterior And Posterior
74869	With Drilling For Intact		Compartments
	Osteochondritis Lesion	70080	Lateral And Posterior
74870	With Internal Fixation		Compartments
74871	With Anterior Cruciate Ligament	70411	Excision
	Repair	70415	Soft Tissue Tumor
74872	With Posterior Cruciate Ligament	70416	Subcutaneous
	Repair	70417	Deep
74846	With Repair Of Intercondylar	70439	Excision of Cyst of Tendon
	Spine(s)		Sheath
74848	And Fixation	70413	Radical Resection of Soft Tissue
74847	With Repair Of Tuberosity		Tumor
	Fracture	70425	Curettage of Tibia
74849	And Fixation	70431	With allograft
74850	With Repair Of Proximal Tibial	70432	With Autograft
	Fracture	70426	Curettage of Fibula
74851	Unicondylar	70429	With Allograft
74852	Bicondylar	70430	With Autograft
75185	Arthrodesis	70433	Partial Excision of Tibial Bone
75186	Right	70434	Partial Excision of Fibula
75187	Left	70435	Radical Resection Of Tibial Bone
72068	Amputation Of Leg By	70436	Radical Resection Of Fibula
	Disarticulation At The Knee	70437	Radical Resection Of Talus
47630	On The Right	70438	Radical Resection Of Calcaneus
47631	On The Left	71925	Repair
45997	Leg	71928	Fascial Defect
46855	Fracture	71929	Flexor Tendon Repair
46856	Tibial Shaft, Closed	71930	Primary
46857	With Manipulation	71931	Secondary
49150	With Fibular Fracture	71932	Extensor Tendon Repair
49148	Tibial Shaft, Percutaneous	71933	Primary
	Fixation	71934	Secondary

SURGERY, CONT.

71935	Repair For Peroneal Dislocating Tendons	46862	Fracture
		46863	Medial Malleolus, Closed
71936	With Fibular Osteotomy	46864	With Manipulation
71937	Gastrocnemius Recession	49157	Medial Malleolus, Open
71938	Osteotomy	46865	Lateral Malleolus, Closed
71939	Tibial	46866	With Manipulation
71940	Fibular	49158	Lateral Malleolus, Open
71941	Tibia And Fibula	46867	Bimalleolar, Closed
71942	Multiple, With Rod Realignment	46868	With Manipulation
		49159	Bimalleolar, Open
71943	Lengthening Osteoplasty Of The Tibia And Fibula	46869	Trimalleolar, Closed
		46870	With Manipulation
71944	Repair Of Tibial Nonunion	49160	Trimalleolar, Open
71945	With Sliding Graft	49161	With Fixation Of Posterior Lip
71946	With Autograft	49162	Weight Bearing Distal Tibia, Closed
71947	By Synostosis With Fibula		
71948	Repair Of Congenital Tibial Pseudarthrosis	49163	With Traction / Manipulation
		49164	Weight Bearing Distal Tibia, Open
71949	Epiphyseal Arrest		
71950	Of The Distal Tibia	49165	Weight Bearing Distal Fibula, Open
71951	Of The Distal Fibula		
71952	Of The Distal Tibia And Fibula	49166	Weight Bearing Distal Tibia And Fibula, Open
71953	Of The Combined Proximal And Distal Tibia And Fibula		
		49993	Incision
71954	And Distal Femur	49994	And Drainage
71955	Prophylactic Pinning Of The Tibia	49995	Infected Bursa
71956	Prophylactic Nailing Of The Tibia	49996	Arthrotomy For Infection And Foreign Body
71957	Prophylactic Wiring Of The Tibia		
71958	Prophylactic Plating Of The Tibia	49997	Arthrotomy With Posterior Capsular Release
71968	Tendon Lengthening		
71969	Multiple Through The Same Incision	70081	Subcutaneous Tenotomy Of Achilles Tendon
71970	Tendon Shortening	70082	Requiring General Anesthesia
71971	Multiple Through The Same Incision	70412	Excision
		70418	Soft Tissue Tumor
75191	Arthrodesis Of Tibiofibular Joint	70419	Subcutaneous
75192	Right Proximal	70420	Deep
75193	Right Distmal	70440	Excision of Cyst of Tendon Sheath
75194	Left Proximal		
75195	Left Distmal	70414	Radical Resection of Soft Tissue Tumor
41740	Amputation Of Leg Below Knee		
72069	Immediate Fitting Technique With First Cast	70422	Arthrotomy Of The Ankle
		70421	With Joint Exploration
72070	Open, Circular	70423	With Synovectomy
72071	Secondary Closure	70424	Including Tenosynovectomy
72072	Scar Revision	71926	Repair
72073	Re-amputation	71959	Primary Repair Of Ruptured Achilles Tendon
72075	Through Malleoli With Plastic Closure And Nerve Resection		
		71960	With Graft
70601	Replantation	71961	Secondary Repair Of Ruptured Achilles Tendon
47632	On The Right		
47633	On The Left	71962	Tenolysis Of Ankle Flexor
45998	Ankle		

SURGERY, CONT.

71963	Multiple Through The Same Incision	46879	With Manipulation
		49172	Tarsal Bone, Percutaneous Fixation And Manipulation (Each)
71964	Tendon Lengthening		
71966	Multiple Through The Same Incision	49173	Tarsal Bone, Open (Each)
		46876	Metatarsal Bone, Closed (Each)
71965	Tendon Shortening	46877	With Manipulation
71967	Multiple Through The Same Incision	49174	Metatarsal Bone, Percutaneous Fixation And Manipulation (Each)
71972	Tendon Transfer	49175	Metatarsal Bone, Open (Each)
71973	Superficial	46880	Toe, Closed
71974	Deep	46881	With Manipulation
71975	Each Additional Tendon	49178	Toe, Open
71976	Primary Suture Of Collateral Ligament	46882	Great Toe, Closed
		46883	With Manipulation
71977	Medial	49176	Great Toe, Percutaneous Fixation And Manipulation
71978	Lateral		
71979	Both	49177	Great Toe, Open
71980	Secondary Suture Of Collateral Ligament	46884	Sesamoid Bone, Closed
		49998	Incision
71981	Medial	49999	And Drainage Of Infected Bursa
71982	Lateral	70000	Deep, Of The Cortex Of The Bone
71983	Arthroplasty	70001	Arthrotomy For Infection And Foreign Body
71984	With Implant ("Total Ankle")		
71985	Secondary Reconstruction, Total Ankle	70004	Of A Metatarsophalangeal Joint
		70005	Of An Interphalangeal Joint
71986	Removal Of Implant	70543	Removal Of Foreign Body
74873	Arthroscopy	70545	Subcutaneous
74874	With Removal Of Loose Body	70544	Deep
74875	With Removal Of Foreign Body	70546	Complicated
74876	With Partial Synovectomy	70083	Deep Dissection Below Fascia Of Bursal Space
74877	With Limited Debridement		
74878	With Extensive Debridement	70084	Multiple
75188	Arthrodesis	70085	Fasciotomy Of The Foot
75189	Right	70086	Fasciotomy Of A Toe
75190	Left	70087	Subcutaneous Tenotomy Of A Toe
72074	Amputation Of The Foot By Disarticulation At The Ankle		
		70088	Multiple
47634	On The Right	70089	Neurectomy Of Intrinsic Musculature Of The Foot
47635	On The Left		
45999	Foot	70090	Tarsal Tunnel Release
46871	Fracture	70427	Excision
46872	Calcaneus, Closed	70428	Soft Tissue Tumor
46873	With Manipulation	70441	Subcutaneous
49167	Calcaneus, Percutaneous Fixation And Manipulation	70442	Deep
		70443	Radical Resection Of Soft Tissue Tumor
49168	Calcaneus, Open		
49169	With Autogenous Bone Graft	70444	Arthrotomy And Biopsy
46874	Talus, Closed	70457	Intertarsal Joint
46875	With Manipulation	70446	Tarsometatarsal Joint
49170	Talus, Percutaneous Fixation And Manipulation	70447	Metatarsophalangeal Joint
		70448	Interphalangeal Joint
49171	Talus, Open	70449	Plantar Fasciectomy
46878	Tarsal Bone, Closed (Each)	70450	Partial

SURGERY, CONT.

70451	Radical	70496	Radical Resection Of Foot Bone Tumor
70452	Of Single Morton's Neuroma		
70456	Synovectomy	70497	Smaller Tarsal Bone
70445	Of A Single Intertarsal Joint	70498	Metatarsal
70458	Of A Single Tarsometatarsal Joint	70499	Toe Phalanx
		71927	Repair
70459	Of A Single Metatarsophalangeal Joint	71987	Primary Flexor Tendon Repair
		71988	Secondary Flexor Tendon Repair
70453	Synovectomy, Tendon Sheath	71989	With Free Graft
70454	Flexor	71990	Primary Extensor Tendon Repair
70455	Extensor	71991	Secondary Extensor Tendon Repair
70460	Excision Of Cyst Of Tendon Sheath	71992	With Free Graft
70461	Of Foot	71993	Tenolysis Of Foot Flexor
70462	Of Toes	71994	Multiple, Through The Same Incision
70469	Curettage Of Calcaneus		
70470	With Autograft	71995	Tenolysis Of Foot Extensor
70471	With Allograft	71996	Multiple, Through The Same Incision
70466	Curettage Of The Talus Bone		
70467	With Autograft	71997	Open Tenotomy Of Foot Flexor
70468	With Allograft	71998	Open Tenotomy Of Foot Extensor
70463	Curettage Of Other Tarsal Bones	71999	Open Tenotomy Of Toe Flexor
70464	With Autograft	72000	Open Tenotomy Of Toe Extensor
70465	With Allograft	72001	Advancement Of Posterior Tibial Tendon With Navicular Excision
70472	Curettage Of Metatarsal Bones		
70473	With Autograft	72002	Tenotomy Of Abductor Hallucis Muscle
70474	With Allograft		
70475	Curettage Of Phalanges Of Foot	72003	Division Of Plantar Fascia And Muscle
70476	Partial Excision Of Calcaneus		
70477	Partial Excision Of Talus	72004	Midfoot Capsulotomy And Medial Release
70478	Partial Excision Of Other Tarsal Bones		
		72005	With Tendon Lengthening
70479	Partial Excision Of Metatarsal Bone	72006	Midfoot And Posterior Capsulotomy With Tendon Lengthening
70480	Partial Excision Of Phalanx Of Toe		
		72007	Midtarsal Capsulotomy
70482	Partial Excision Fifth Metatarsal Head (Bunionette)	72008	Metatarsophalangeal Capsulotomy
		72009	Interphalangeal Capsulotomy
70481	Complete Excision	72010	Webbing Operation
70483	First Metatarsal Head	72011	Hammertoe Operation
70484	Second, Third or Fourth Metatarsal	72012	Cock-Up Fifth Toe Operation With Plastic Closure
70485	Fifth Metatarsal Head	72013	Partial Ostectomy, Each Metatarsal Head
70486	All Metatarsal Heads		
70487	Excision of Tarsal Coalition	72014	Hallux Valgus (Bunion) Correction
70488	Ostectomy Calcaneus		
70489	For Spur	72015	Simple Exostectomy (Silver Procedure)
70490	Talectomy		
70491	Metatarsectomy	72016	Keller Procedure
70492	Resection Single Phalangeal Base	72017	McBride Procedure
70493	Single Phalangectomy, Toe	72018	Mayo Procedure
70494	Resection Head of Phalanx, Toe	72019	Lapidus Procedure
70495	Hemiphalangectomy, Single Toe		

SURGERY, CONT.

72020	With Tendon Transplants (Joplin Procedure)	75199	Triple
		75200	Midtarsal
72021	Resection Of Joint With Implant	75205	Single
		75206	Multiple
72022	With Metatarsal Osteotomy	75201	With Osteotomy
72023	By Phalanx Osteotomy	75202	Tarsometatarsal
72024	By Double Osteotomy	75207	Single
72025	Tarsal Osteotomy	75208	Multiple
72026	Of The Calcaneus	75203	With Osteotomy
72027	Of The Talus	75204	Navicular-Cuneiform
72029	Of The Tarsal Scaphoid	75209	MTP Great Toe
72034	With Autograft	75210	IP Great Toe
72030	Of The Cuboid	75211	With Extensor Hallucis Transfer
72035	With Autograft		
72031	Of The Internal Cuneiform	72076	Amputation
72036	With Autograft	72077	Midtarsal
72032	Of The Middle Cuneiform	72078	Transmetatarsal
72037	With Autograft	72079	Metatarsal And Toe
72033	Of The External Cuneiform	72080	Toe At The MTP Joint
72038	With Autograft	72081	Toe At The IP Joint
72039	Metatarsal Osteotomy	70604	Replantation
72040	Of The First Metatarsal	70605	Following Complete Amputation
72041	With Autograft	47636	On The Right
72042	Of The Second Metatarsal	47637	On The Left
72043	Of The Third Metatarsal	46951	Orthopedic Casting
72044	Of The Fourth Metatarsal	46952	Halo Body Cast
72045	Of The Fifth Metatarsal	46953	Risser Body Jacket
72046	Multiple Metatarsal Osteotomies For Cavus Foot	46954	Including Head
		46955	Turnbuckle Body Jacket
72047	Proximal Phalangeal Osteotomy	46956	Including Head
72048	Of The Great Toe	46957	Shoulder To Hip Body Cast
72049	Of The Second Toe	46958	Including Head, Minerva Type
72050	Of The Third Toe	46959	Including One Thigh
72051	Of The Fourth Toe	46960	Including Both Thighs
72052	Of The Fifth Toe	46961	Plaster Figure-Of-Eight
72053	Soft Tissue Reconstruction, Angular Deformity Of Toe	46962	Shoulder Spica
		46963	Plaster Velpeau
72054	Sesamoidectomy Of The First Toe	46964	Long Arm
72055	Repair Of Malunion Of Tarsal Bones	46965	Short Arm
		46966	Gauntlet
72056	Repair Of Malunion Of Metatarsal Bones	46967	Hip Spica
		46968	One Leg
72057	Soft Tissue Reconstruction Of Toe For Macrodactyly	46969	One And One-half Spica
		46970	Both Legs
72058	Requiring Bone Resection	46971	Long Leg Cast
72059	Reconstruction Of Toes For Polydactyly	46972	Walking Type
		46973	Long Leg Cast Brace
72060	Reconstruction Of Toes For Syndactyly (Each Web)	46974	Thigh-To-Ankle Cylinder Cast
		46975	Short Leg
72061	Reconstruction Of Cleft Foot	46976	Walking Type
75196	Arthrodesis	49120	Rigid Total Leg Contact
75197	Pantalar	46977	Patellar Tendon Bearing Cast
75198	Subtalar	46978	Clubfoot Cast

SURGERY, CONT.

46979	Adding A Walker To A Previously Applied Cast	49923	Insertion Of Pin
		49924	Removal Of Pin
47680	Removal Of Cast (Applied Here)	49925	Application Of Cranial Tongs
47682	Gauntlet	49926	Removal Of Cranial Tongs
47684	Boot	49927	Application / Removal Of Halo
47685	Body	49928	Cranial
47686	Full Arm	49929	Pelvic
47687	Full Leg	49930	Femoral
47688	Shoulder Spica	49931	Removal Of Tongs (Applied By
47689	Hip Spica		Another Physician)
47690	Minerva Jacket	49932	Removal Of Implant
47691	Risser Jacket	49933	Superficial
47692	Turnbuckle Jacket	49934	Deep
47681	Removal Of Cast (Applied Elsewhere)	49937	External Fixation Device
47683	Gauntlet	49935	Application Of A Uniplane, Unilateral, External
47693	Boot		
47694	Body	49936	Application Of A Multiplane, Unilateral, External
47695	Full Arm		
47696	Full Leg	49938	Adjustment Of External Fixation Device Reguiring Anesthesia
47697	Shoulder Spica		
47698	Hip Spica	49939	Revision Of External Fixation Device Reguiring Anesthesia
47699	Minerva Jacket		
47700	Risser Jacket	49940	Removal Of External Fixation Device Under Anesthesia
47701	Turnbuckle Jacket		
47703	Repair Of Cast	70013	Grafts
47704	spica	70014	Bone
47705	body cast	70015	Minor
47706	jacket	70016	Large
47707	Windowing of Cast	70017	Cartilage
47708	Wedging of Cast	70018	Costochondral
47709	Wedging of a Clubfoot Cast	70019	Nasal Septum
47660	Orthopedic Splinting	70020	Fascia Lata
47661	Long Arm	70021	By Stripper
47662	Short Arm	70022	By Incision And Area Exposure
47663	Dynamic	70023	Distant Tendon
47664	Finger	41752	Neurological
47665	Dynamic	44867	Cranial Tap
47666	Long Leg	44868	Subdural
47667	Short Leg	44869	Initial
47659	Orthopedic Strapping	44870	Subsequent
47668	Thorax	44871	Ventricular
47669	Lower Back	44872	With Injection
47670	Shoulder	44873	Cisternal (C1-C2), With Injection
47671	Elbow	44874	Lateral Cervical (C1-C2), With Injection
47672	Wrist		
47673	Hand	44875	Of Shunt Tubing
47674	Finger	44876	For Injection
47675	Hip	44877	Of Reservoir
47676	Knee	44878	For Injection
47677	Ankle	41761	Burr Holes
47678	Toes	44879	Without Other Surgery
40058	Unna boot	44880	With Other Surgery
47679	Denis-Browne Splint	44881	Subdural

SURGERY, CONT.

44882	Evacuation Of Hematoma	45021	Suboccipital
45056	Implant Strip Electrodes For Long Term Seizure Monitoring	45023	With Cervical Laminectomy
		45022	Decompression Of Medulla And Spinal Cord With Dural Graft
44883	Evacuation Of Extradural Hematoma	45024	Decompression Of Medulla And Spinal Cord Without Dural Graft
44884	Ventricular		
44885	For Catheter Implantation	45025	Cranial Nerve Exploration
44886	With Injection	41770	Suboccipital Cranial Nerve Decompression
44887	With Injection For Surgery		
44894	Intracranial	45027	Section Of Cranial Nerve(s)
41767	Abscess Drainage	45028	Medullary Tractotomy
44888	With Aspiration Of Abscess	45029	Mesencephalic Tractotomy
44889	With Aspiration Of Cyst	45030	Mesencephalic Pedunculotomy
44890	Intracerebral	45045	Excision Of Brain Tumor
44891	With Aspiration Of Hematoma	45046	Excision Of Meningioma
44892	With Aspiration Of Cyst	45047	Excision Of Cerebellopontine Angle Tumor
44893	With Device Implantation		
44895	Insertion Of Subcutaneous Infusion System	45048	Excision Of Midline Tumor Base Of Skull
41762	Craniotomy	41773	Frontal Lobotomy
44983	Supratentorial	42128	Leucotomy
44984	Extradural Hemorrhage Removal	45031	Section Of Tentorium Cerebelli
44985	Subdural Hemorrhage Removal	45032	Subtemporal
41768	Intracerebral Hemorrhage Removal	45033	Section Of Sensory Root Of Gasserian Ganglion
44986	Drainage Of Intracranial Abscess	45034	Compression Of Sensory Root Of Gasserian Ganglion
45036	Excision Of Brain Tumor		
45037	Excision Of Meningioma	45035	Decompression Of Sensory Root Of Gasserian Ganglion
45038	Excision Of Brain Abscess		
45039	Excision Of Cyst	45053	Transtemporal
45040	Fenestration Of Cyst	45054	Excision Of Cerebellopontine Angle Tumor
44987	Infratentorial		
44988	Extradural Hemorrhage Removal	45055	And Middle/Posterior Fossa For Tumor Excision
44989	Subdural Hemorrhage Removal		
44990	Intracerebellar Hemorrhage Removal	45057	Subdural Electrode Array
		45058	For Long Term Seizure Monitoring
44991	Drainage Of Intracranial Abscess		
45051	Excision Of Brain Abscess	45059	Excision Of Epileptogenic Focus Without Electrocorticography
41769	Excision Of Cyst		
45052	Fenestration Of Cyst	45060	Excision Of Epileptogenic Focus With Electrocorticography
45041	Excision Of Brain Tumor		
45042	Excision Of Meningioma	45061	Lobectomy With Electrocorticography
45043	Excision Of Cerebellopontine Angle Tumor		
		41771	Temporal Lobectomy With Electrocorticography
45044	Excision Of Midline Tumor Base Of Skull		
		41772	Corpus Callosum Section
44992	Transcranial Approach	45062	Total Hemispherectomy
44993	Decompression Of Orbit	45063	Partial Hemispherectomy
44994	Removal Of Lesion	45064	Excision Of Choroid Plexus
44995	Removal Of Foreign Body	45065	Coagulation Of Choroid Plexus
45017	Cranial Decompression	45066	Excision Of Craniopharyngioma
45018	Subtemporal	45067	Removal Of Array
45019	Supratentorial	45081	Transoral To Skull Base
45020	Suboccipital		

SURGERY, CONT.

45082	For Decompression	41757	Carotid Endarterectomy
45083	For Excision Of Lesion	45120	Intracranial And Cervical Occlusion Of Carotid Artery
45084	Requiring Splitting Of Tongue		
45085	Requiring Splitting Of Mandible	45121	For An Aneurysm
45086	Transoral To Brain Stem	45122	For A Vascular Malformation
45087	For Decompression	45123	For A Carotid-Cavernous Fistula
45088	For Excision Of Lesion	45124	Intracranial Electrothrombosis
45089	Requiring Splitting Of Tongue	45125	For An Aneurysm
45090	Requiring Splitting Of Mandible	45126	For A Vascular Malformation
45091	Transoral To Upper Spinal Cord	45127	For A Carotid-Cavernous Fistula
45092	For Decompression	45128	Extracranial-Intracranial Arterial Anastomosis
45093	For Excision Of Lesion		
45094	Requiring Splitting Of Tongue	41751	Pituitary Ablation
45095	Requiring Splitting Of Mandible	45129	Intracranial Microdissection
41764	Tumor Removal - Partial	45130	Spinal Microdissection
41763	Tumor Removal - Complete	45131	Intracranial Stereotaxis
45049	Excision Of Bone Lesion Of Skull	45132	Globus Pallidus
45050	For Osteomyelitis	41788	Stereotactic Thalamotomy
45069	Intracranial Hypophysectomy	45133	Subcortical Structure
41780	Transsphenoidal Hypophysectomy	45134	For Aspiration Of Intracranial Lesion
41779	Transsphenoidal Tumor Removal		
45068	Craniosynostosis	45135	For Excision Of Intracranial Lesion
45070	Single Suture	45136	CT-Guided
45071	Multiple Sutures	45137	To Implant Depth Electrodes For Seizure Monitoring
45072	Frontal Bone Flap		
45073	Parietal Bone Flap	45138	Catheter Insertion For Brachytherapy
45074	Bifrontal Bone Flap		
45075	Extensive, Not Requiring Bone Grafts	45139	Gamma Radiosurgery
		45140	Focused Proton Beam
45076	Extensive With Bone Autografts	45141	Stereotactic Ablation
45077	Excision Of Benign Cranial Bone Tumor	45142	Gasserian Ganglion
		45143	Alcohol
45078	With Optic Nerve Decompression	45144	Thermal
45079	Excision Of Foreign Body	41759	Percutaneous Electrocoagulation
45080	Treatment Of Penetrating Wound	45146	Radiofrequency
45173	Intracranial Repair Of Dural / CSF Leak	45147	Trigeminal Medullary Tract
		45148	Alcohol
45178	Repair Of Encephalocele, Skull Base	45149	Thermal
41766	A-V Malformation Repair	45150	Percutaneous Electrocoagulation
45111	Supratentorial	45151	Radiofrequency
45112	Simple	45152	Implantation Of Intracranial Neurostimulator
45113	Complex		
45114	Infratentorial	45153	Cortical
45115	Simple	45154	By Burr Holes
45116	Complex	45155	By Craniectomy
45117	Dural	45156	By Craniotomy
45118	Simple	45157	Subcortical
45119	Complex	45158	By Burr Holes
41765	Aneurysm Repair, Intracranial Approach	45159	By Craniectomy
		45160	By Craniotomy
45109	Carotid Circulation	45161	Revision Of Electrodes
45110	Vertebral-Basilar Circulation	45162	Removal Of Electrodes
41760	Aneurysm repair, Cervical Approach	45163	Placement Of Pulse Generator

SURGERY, CONT.

45165	Removal Of Pulse Generator	45211	Replacement Of Ventricular CSF Catheter
45164	Placement Of Pulse Receiver		
45166	Removal Of Pulse Receiver	45207	Revision Of CSF Shunt
41865	Neural Transplantation	45208	Replacement Of Obstructed CSF Shunt Valve
45167	Elevation Of Depressed Skull Fracture		
45168	Simple, Extradural	45209	Replacement Of Distal CSF Catheter
45169	Compound, Extradural	45212	Removal Of Complete CSF Shunt System
45170	Comminuted, Extradural		
45171	With Repair Of Dura	45213	With Replacement
45172	With Debridement Of Brain	41774	Laminectomy
45174	Reduction Of Craniomegalic Skull	45241	For Exploration
45175	With Simple Cranioplasty	45242	Up To Two Cervical Segments
45176	Requiring Craniotomy And Reconstruction	45243	More Than Two Cervical Segments
45179	Cranioplasty	45244	Up To Two Thoracic Segments
45177	For Repair Of Encephalocele, Skull Vault	45245	More Than Two Thoracic Segments
45180	Of Skull Defect Up To 5 cm.	45246	Up To Two Lumbar Segments
45181	Of Skull Defect Over 5 cm.	45247	More Than Two Lumbar Segments
45182	Of Skull Defect, With Reparative Brain Surgery	45248	Up To Two Sacral Segments
45183	With Autograft Up To 5 cm.	41776	Decompressive
45184	With Autograft Over 5 cm.	45249	Up To Two Cervical Segments
45185	Removal Of Skull Bone Flap	45250	More Than Two Cervical Segments
45186	Removal Of Skull Prosthetic Plate		
45187	Replacement Of Skull Bone Flap	45251	Up To Two Thoracic Segments
45188	Replacement Of Skull Prosthetic Plate	45252	More Than Two Thoracic Segments
41756	Temporal Artery - Middle Cerebral Bypass	45253	Up To Two Lumbar Segments
45200	Ventriculocisternostomy	45254	More Than Two Lumbar Segments
45201	Torkildsen Procedure		
45202	Third Ventricle	45255	Up To Two Sacral Segments
45203	By Stereotaxis	45256	With Removal Of Abnormal Facets
41755	Ommaya Reservoir Placement		
45189	Creation Of CSF Shunt	45257	Pars Inter-Articularis
45190	Subarachnoid-Atrial	45270	Decompressive With Facetectomy And Foraminotomy
45191	Subarachnoid-Jugular		
45192	Subarachnoid-Auricular	45271	Cervical Segment
45196	Subarachnoid-Peritoneal	45272	Thoracic Segment
45197	Subarachnoid-Pleural	45273	Lumbar Segment
45193	Subdural-Atrial	45274	Additional Segment
45194	Subdural-Jugular	45309	With Myelotomy
45195	Subdural-Auricular	45310	Cervical
45198	Subdural-Peritoneal	45311	Thoracic
45199	Subdural-Pleural	45312	Thoracolumbar
41753	Ventriculo-Atrial	45313	With Drainage Of Intramedullary Cyst
45204	Ventriculo-Jugular		
45205	Ventriculo-Auricular	45314	To Subarachnoid Space
41629	Ventriculo-Venous (CSF)	45315	To Peritoneal Space
41754	Ventriculo-Peritoneal	45316	With Drainage Of Intramedullary Syrinx
45206	Ventriculo-Pleural		
45210	Irrigation Of Ventricular CSF Catheter	45317	To Subarachnoid Space
		45318	To Peritoneal Space

SURGERY, CONT.

45319	Section Of Cervical Dentate Ligaments	45345	Sacral
		45258	Hemilaminectomy
45320	Up To Two Segments	45259	Decompressive With Partial Facetectomy
45321	More Than Two Segments		
45322	With Rhizotomy	45260	One Cervical Interspace
45323	Up To Two Segments	45261	One Lumbar Interspace
45324	More Than Two Segments	45262	Additional Interspace
45325	With Section Of Spinal Accessory Nerve	45263	Cervical Re-Exploration
		45264	Lumbar Re-Exploration
41785	With Cordotomy	41775	With Disc Removal
41786	Percutaneous	45265	One Cervical Interspace
41787	Open	45266	One Lumbar Interspace
45327	One Tract, One Stage, Cervical	45267	Additional Interspace
45326	One Tract, One Stage, Thoracic	45268	Cervical Re-Exploration
45328	Both Tracts, One Stage, Cervical	45269	Lumbar Re-Exploration
45329	Both Tracts, One Stage, Thoracic	45275	Transpedicular Spinal Decompression
45330	Both Tracts, Two Stages, Cervical	45276	Thoracic
45331	Both Tracts, Two Stages, Thoracic	45277	Lumbar
45332	With Ablation Of Spinal Cord Arteriovenous Malformation	45278	Additional Segment
		45279	Costovertebral Thoracic Decompression
45333	Cervical		
45334	Thoracic	45281	Additional Segment
45335	Thoracolumbar	45280	Anterior Spinal Diskectomy With Osteophytectomy
45346	Excise Intraspinal Tumor		
41835	Extradural	45282	Cervical Interspace
45347	Extradural, Cervical	45283	Single
45348	Extradural, Thoracic	45284	Additional
45349	Extradural, Lumbar	45285	Thoracic Interspace
45350	Extradural, Sacral	45286	Single
41836	Intradural	45287	Additional Segment
45351	Intradural, Extramedullary, Cervical	45288	Vertebral Body Resection With Diskectomy
45352	Intradural, Extramedullary, Thoracic	45289	Cervical Segment
		45290	Single
45353	Intradural, Extramedullary, Lumbar	45291	Additional Segment
		45292	Thoracic Segment
45354	Intradural, Sacral	45293	Single
42129	Intramedullary	45294	Additional Segment
45355	Intramedullary, Cervical	45295	Thoracolumbar Approach
45356	Intramedullary, Thoracic	45296	Lower Thoracic Segment
45357	Intramedullary, Thoracolumbar	45297	Lumbar Segment
45358	Combined Extra-Intradural	45298	Additional Segment
45336	For Excision Of Extradural Intraspinal Lesion	45299	Transperitoneal Approach
		45300	Lower Thoracic Segment
45337	Cervical	45301	Lumbar Segment
45338	Thoracic	45302	Sacral Segment
45339	Lumbar	45308	Additional Segment
45340	Sacral	45303	Retroperitoneal Approach
45341	For Excision Of Intradural Intraspinal Lesion	45304	Lower Thoracic Segment
		45305	Lumbar Segment
45342	Cervical	45306	Sacral Segment
45343	Thoracic	45307	Additional Segment
45344	Lumbar		

SURGERY, CONT.

41866	Vertebral Body Resection For Excision Of Intraspinal Lesion	45412	Under 5cm.
		45413	Over 5cm.
45374	Extradural	45414	Repair Of Myelomeningocele
45375	Cervical	45415	Under 5 cm.
45376	Thoracic (Transthoracic Approach)	45416	Over 5 cm.
		45420	Repair Of Pseudomeningocele With Laminectomy
45377	Thoracic (Thoracolumbar Approach)	45417	Repair Of CSF Leak
45378	Lumbar (Transperitoneal Approach)	45418	Without Laminectomy
		45419	With Laminectomy
45379	Lumbar (Retroperitoneal Approach)	45421	Spinal Dural Graft
		45422	Spinal CSF Shunt
45380	Sacral (Transperitoneal Approach)	45423	Creation Of Lumbosubarachnoid-Peritoneal Shunt
45381	Sacral (Retroperitoneal Approach)		
45382	Intradural	45424	With Laminectomy
45383	Cervical	45425	Percutaneous
45384	Thoracic (Transthoracic Approach)	45426	Creation Of Lumbar-Subarachnoid-Peritoneal-Pleural Shunt
45385	Thoracic (Thoracolumbar Approach)	45427	With Laminectomy
		45428	Percutaneous
45386	Lumbar (Transperitoneal Approach)	45430	Irrigation Of Lumbosubarachnoid Shunt
45387	Lumbar (Retroperitoneal Approach)	45429	Revision Of Lumbosubarachnoid Shunt
45388	Sacral (Transperitoneal Approach)	45431	Replacement Of Lumbosubarachnoid Shunt
45389	Sacral (Retroperitoneal Approach)		
45390	Additional Segment	45432	Removal Of Lumbosubarachnoid Shunt System
45391	Spinal Stereotaxis		
45392	Creation Of Cord Lesion	45477	Peripheral Nerve Neurostimulator
45393	Stimulation Of Cord	45478	Transcutaneous
45394	Aspiration Of Cord Lesion	45479	Percutaneous
45395	Excision Of Cord Lesion	45480	Cranial Nerve
45396	Implantation Of Spinal Neurostimulator	45481	Peripheral Nerve
		45482	Autonomic Nerve
45397	Percutaneous	45483	Neuromuscular
45398	Epidural	45484	By Incision
45399	By Laminectomy	45485	Cranial Nerve
45400	Epidural	45486	Peripheral Nerve
45403	Revision	45487	Autonomic Nerve
45404	Remove Electrodes	45488	Neuromuscular
45405	Subcutaneous Placement Of Spinal Neurostim. Pulse Generator	45489	Revision
		45490	Removal Of Electrodes
45406	Subcutaneous Placement Of Spinal Neurostimulator Receiver	45491	Subcutaneous Placement Of Pulse Generator
45407	Revision Of Implanted Spinal Neurostimulator Pulse Generator	45492	Subcutaneous Placement Of Receiver
45408	Removal Of Implanted Spinal Neurostimulator Pulse Generator	45493	Revision Of Pulse Generator
		45494	Removal Of Pulse Generator
45409	Revision Of Implanted Spinal Neurostimulator Receiver	45495	Revision Of Receiver
		45496	Removal Of Receiver
45410	Removal Of Implanted Spinal Neurostimulator Receiver	45497	Nerve Ablation
		45498	Trigeminal
45411	Repair Of Meningocele	45499	Supraorbital Branch

SURGERY, CONT.

45500	Infraorbital Branch	45543	Intrapelvic Obturator Nerve
45501	Mental Branch	45544	Cranial Nerve Avulsion
45502	Inferior Alveolar Branch	45545	Supraorbital Nerve
45503	2nd and 3rd Division Branches At Foramen Ovale	45546	Infraorbital Nerve
		45547	Mental Nerve
45504	2nd and 3rd Division Branches At Foramen Ovale + Rad Monitor	45548	Inferior Alveolar Osteotomy
		45549	Lingual Nerve
45505	Facial	45550	Facial Nerve
45506	Cervical Spine	45551	Spinal Nerve Avulsion
45507	Intercostal Nerve	45552	Greater Occipital Nerve
45508	Paravertebral Facet Joint, Single Lumbar Level	45553	Phrenic Nerve
		45554	Pudendal Nerve
45509	Paravertebral Facet Joint, Additional Lumbar Level	45555	Extrapelvic Obturator Nerve
		45556	Intrapelvic Obturator Nerve
45510	Pudendal Nerve	45557	Excision Of Neuroma
45511	Celiac Plexus	45558	Cutaneous Nerve
45512	Neuroplasty	45559	Digital Nerve
45513	Digital	45560	Additional
45514	Hand	45561	Hand
45515	Foot	45562	Additional
45516	Median Nerve	45563	Foot
45517	Ulnar Nerve	45564	Additional
45518	Radial Nerve	45565	Median Nerve
45519	Tibial Nerve	45566	Ulnar Nerve
45520	Posterior Tibial Nerve	45567	Radial Nerve
45521	Peroneal Nerve	45568	Tibial Nerve
45522	Sciatic Nerve	45569	Posterior Tibial Nerve
41778	Brachial Plexus	45570	Peroneal Nerve
45523	Lumbar Plexus	45571	Sciatic Nerve
45524	With Transposition	45572	Implantation Of Nerve End Into Bone
45525	Cranial Nerve	45573	Implantation Of Nerve End Into Muscle
41783	Ulnar Nerve		
45526	Ulnar Nerve - At Elbow	45574	Excision Of Neurofibroma
45527	Ulnar Nerve - At Wrist	45575	Cutaneous Nerve
70091	Decompression Of Median Nerve At Carpal Tunnel	45576	Peripheral Nerve
		45577	Extensive
41782	Median Nerve At Carpal Tunnel	45578	Excision Of Neurolemmoma
45529	Decompression	45579	Cutaneous Nerve
45528	Plantar Nerve	45580	Peripheral Nerve
45530	Internal Neurolysis With Operating Microscope	45581	Extensive
		45582	Surgical Sympathectomy
45531	Cranial Nerve Transection	45583	Cervical
45532	Supraorbital Nerve	45584	Cervicothoracic
45533	Infraorbital Nerve	45585	Thoracolumbar
45534	Mental Nerve	45586	Lumbar
45535	Inferior Alveolar Osteotomy	45587	Neurorrhaphy
45536	Lingual Nerve	45588	Of The Hand
45537	Facial Nerve	45589	One Digital Nerve
45538	Spinal Nerve Avulsion	45591	Common Sensory Nerve
45539	Greater Occipital Nerve	45592	Median Nerve
45540	Phrenic Nerve	45593	Ulnar Nerve
45541	Pudendal Nerve	45594	Of The Foot
45542	Extrapelvic Obturator Nerve	45595	One Digital Nerve

SURGERY, CONT.

45596	Repair Additional Digital Nerve	72585	Unusual Anesthesia
45597	Repair Additional Distal Nerve	44999	Professional Component
45600	Radial Nerve	45000	Mandated Services
45601	Tibial Nerve	45001	Anesthesia By Surgeon
45602	Posterior Tibial Nerve	45002	Bilateral Procedure
45603	Peroneal Nerve	45003	Multiple Procedures
45604	Sciatic Nerve	45004	Reduced Services
45605	Brachial Plexus	45005	Surgical Care Only
45606	Lumbar Plexus	72614	Decision For Surgery
45607	Repair Additional Peripheral Nerve	45006	Postoperative Management Only
45608	Repair Peripheral Nerve Without Transposition	45007	Preoperative Management Only
		45008	Two Surgeons
45590	Facial Nerve	45009	Surgical Team
45609	Extracranial	45010	Repeat Procedure By Same Physician
45610	Intratemporal	45011	Repeat Procedure By Another Physician
45614	Requiring Secondary Suture		
45615	Requiring Extensive Mobilization	45012	Postoperative Return To The O.R. For Related Procedure
45616	Requiring Distal Shortening Of Bone		
		45013	Unrelated Postoperative Procedure By Same Physician
45611	Facial-Spinal Anastomosis		
45612	Facial-Hypoglossal Anastomosis	72616	Related Postoperative Procedure By Same Physician
45613	Facial-Phrenic Anastomosis		
45598	With Nerve Graft	45014	Assistant Surgeon
45599	Head - Up To 4 Cm.	45015	Minimum Assistant Surgeon
45617	Head - Over 4 Cm.	45016	Assistant Surgeon - Resident Surgeon Unavailable
45622	Neck - Up To 4 Cm.		
45623	Neck - Over 4 Cm.	72607	Prolonged Evaluation and Management Services
45618	Hand - Single Strand Up To 4 Cm.		
		72609	Unrelated Post-Op E&M Services By The Same MD
45619	Hand - Single Strand Over 4 Cm.		
45628	Hand - Cable Up To 4 Cm.	72612	Separate E&M Service By Same MD On Same Date
45629	Hand - Cable Over 4 Cm.		
45624	Foot - Single Strand Up To 4 Cm.	72619	Use Of Outside Laboratory
45625	Foot - Single Strand Over 4 Cm.	72620	Multiple Modifiers
45630	Foot - Cable Up To 4 Cm.	**75134**	**Transfusions, Transplantation**
45631	Foot - Cable Over 4 Cm.	75214	See, Also: Specific Organ System
45620	Arm - Single Strand Up To 4 Cm.	41791	Transfusions
45621	Arm - Single Strand Over 4 Cm.	41792	Blood
45632	Arm - Cable Up To 4 Cm.	41794	Packed RBCs
45633	Arm - Cable Over 4 Cm.	41795	Washed Red Blood Cells
45626	Leg - Single Strand Up To 4 Cm.	42000	Irradiated
45627	Leg - Single Strand Over 4 Cm.	43270	Child Under 2 - (Push)
45634	Leg - Cable Up To 4 Cm.	43271	Exchange
45635	Leg - Cable Over 4 Cm.	43272	Newborn
45636	Additional Nerve, Single Strand	43273	Intrauterine
45637	Additional Nerve Cable	41793	Recent
45638	Nerve Pedicle Transfer, 1st Stage	41796	Fibrinogen
45639	Nerve Pedicle Transfer, 2nd Stage	41797	Plasma
41789	Surgical Drainage, NOS	41798	Albumin Infusion
41790	Needle Aspiration, NOS	41800	Plasmapheresis
44996	Modifying Circumstance	43275	Photopheresis
44997	Microsurgery	43274	Cellular Apheresis
44998	Unusual Procedural Services	41801	Platelets

SURGERY, CONT.

41802	White Blood Cells
49749	Intraosseous Infusion
43352	Hypervolemic Hemodilution
74945	Transfusion-Related Physician Services
74946	For Difficult Cross Match
74947	For Investigation Of Transfusion Reaction
74948	For Investigation Of Possible Disease Transmission
74949	For Authorization To Use Outdated Blood
74950	For Authorization To Use Rh Incompatible Unit
44050	Transplantation Services
44051	Bone Marrow Collection For Transplant
41803	Bone Marrow Transplant
44052	Allogenic
44053	Autologous
41921	Fetal Tissue Transplant
41922	Thymic
41923	Lymphatic
41924	Hepatic
41925	Splenic
41990	Gene Therapy
41991	Somatic Cell
41992	Germline Cell
42075	Photochemotherapy
42076	Ultraviolet B + Tar or Petrolatum
42077	Psoralens + Ultraviolet A (PUVA)
42729	Prolonged Direct Physician Supervision (4-8 Hours)
41544	Radiation Therapy
41545	Head
41546	Whole Brain
41547	Base of Skull
41548	Chest
41549	Spine
41550	Neck
41551	Pituitary Gland
41552	Abdomen
41553	Kidney
41554	Pelvis
49800	**Disposition Of Patient**
70771	No Action Taken
40083	Hospitalization
43334	In The CCU
43335	In The MICU
70756	In The Detoxification Unit
49806	Medical Therapy
49801	Surgery
49802	Cardiac
49803	Operative Death
49804	In Hospital Death

49805	Non-cardiac
74973	Scheduled For Home Visit
43391	Referred to Emergency Room
70759	Sent Ambulance To Home
70758	Sent Mobile Crisis Unit To Home
70757	Referred To Local Mental Health Center
70572	Referred To Hospital Burn Center
70565	Consultation With A Specialist
70566	Allergist
70567	Audiologist
70766	Cardiologist
70767	For Same Day Appointment
70768	For Next Day Appointment
70769	For Next Available Appointment
70568	Dermatologist
70745	Dentist
71513	Endocrinologist
70569	ENT
70777	Family Practioner
70570	Gastroenterologist
70575	Pediatric
70763	For Same Day Appointment
70764	For Next Day Appointment
70765	For Next Available Appointment
70779	Gerontologist
70571	Hematologist
70776	Internist
70578	Nephrologist
70579	Pediatric
70573	Neurologist
70774	Ob/Gyn
70576	Ophthalmologist
70778	Pediatrician
70775	Podiatrist
70738	Psychiatrist
70772	Child
70760	For Same Day Appointment
70761	For Next Day Appointment
70762	For Next Available Appointment
70742	Psychologist
71512	Pulmonogist
70580	Surgeon
70577	Orthopedic
70581	Pediatric
70574	Neurosurgeon
70780	Plastic Surgeon
70582	Urologist
71514	Telephone Consultation With Specialist
71515	Allergist
70739	Consultation With A Paraprofessional
70740	Physical Therapist
70741	Respiratory Therapist

DISPOSITION OF PATIENT, CONT.

70773	Optometrist
70743	Social Worker
70744	Psychiatric Nurse
70746	Mental Health Counselor
70747	Addictions Counselor
70748	Nutritionist
70753	Sex Therapist
48263	Referred By Workplace
48264	To A Physician
48265	To A Hospital
70750	Alcoholism-related
70751	Weight-watching
70752	Addictions
70754	Alzheimer's Association
70755	The National Alliance for the Mentally Ill
43386	Discharged Home
70770	Referred For Second Opinion
43390	Transferred to another hospital
48847	Occupational Therapy and Vocational Rehabilitation
43385	Placement In An Extended Care Facility
70737	For Residential Treatment
43387	Left Facility Against Medical Advice
43388	Patient Died
43389	Autopsy
19467	Free Text (Plan):
80566	Care Plan:
82186	Discharge Summary:
43338	Follow-up
43345	Pre-Visit Lab Work
44460	Free Text (Notes):
46015	Patient Information Sheets:
49941	Correspondence Sent:
49942	Patient Care Reviewed. Signed:
70024	Signed:
70025	Reviewed For Quality Assurance: Signed:
70583	User Finding:
75133	**Medical Supplies And Equipment**
75132	Supplies
40054	Wrappings
49920	Ace Bandage
40046	Elastic Stockings
40055	Warm Compresses
40056	Wet to Dry Dressings
40059	Tourniquet
40047	Arch Support
40048	Heel Lift
40068	Splint
49921	Ankle Control
49922	Knee, Pneumatic
49809	Immobilizer
49810	Forearm

49811	Knee
40070	Cast
40071	Body Cast
43346	Diabetic
43347	Insulin Syringes (U-100)
43348	Low Dose
43349	Stylets For Fingerstick
43350	Glucose Monitoring Strips
43351	Alcohol Swabs
72176	Durable Medical Equipment
74356	Ambulation Devices
42312	Canes
72115	Single Prong
72116	Quad or Three Prong
74974	Replacement Supplies
74975	Handgrip
74976	Tip
42311	Crutches
72117	Forearm
72118	Single
72119	Pair
72120	Underarm
72121	Single
72122	Wood
72123	Aluminum
72124	Pair
72125	Wood
72126	Aluminum
74977	Replacement Supplies
74978	Underarm Pad
74979	Handgrip
74980	Tip
72127	Walker
72128	Rigid
74051	Adjustable Or Fixed Height
74052	Wheeled With Seat
74056	With Wheel Attachment
72129	Folding
74053	Wheeled Without Seat
74357	Adjustable Or Fixed Height
72130	Wheeled
72131	With Seat
72134	Crutch Attachments
72132	Without Seat
74054	Heavy Duty
74055	Variable Wheel
72138	With Attachments
72139	Platform
72140	Seat
72141	Crutch
72142	Leg Extensions
74981	Replacement Supplies
74982	Handgrip

DME, CONT.

74983	Tip	74335	With Side Rails
72177	Bed Equipment	72191	With Mattress
72160	Decubitus Care	74058	Without Mattress
72161	Pressure Pad	74341	Without Side Rails
73728	Alternating With Pump	74342	With Mattress
73729	Heavy Duty	74343	Without Mattress
73730	Pump For	72196	Semielectric
72171	Air	74336	With Side Rails
72172	Dry	72198	With Mattress
72173	Water	74059	Without Mattress
72162	Gel	74344	Without Side Rails
72163	Synthetic Sheep Skin	74345	With Mattress
72164	Lambswool Sheep Skin	74346	Without Mattress
72165	Low Pressure And Positioning	72203	Electric
	Equalization	74337	With Side Rails
72166	Mattress	72205	With Mattress
72167	Dry Pressure	74060	Without Mattress
72168	Air Pressure	74347	Without Side Rails
72169	Water Pressure	74348	With Mattress
72170	Gel Pressure	74349	Without Mattress
73731	Bed	74322	Institutional Type
72174	Powered Air Flotation	74323	With Mattress
72175	Air-Fluidized	74329	Mattress
73732	Heel Or Elbow Protector	74330	Innerspring
74032	Heat/Cold Application	74331	Foam Rubber
74033	Heat Lamp	74332	Alternating Pressure
74034	With Stand	72212	Accessories
74035	Without Stand	72213	Bed Side Rails
74036	Phototherapy (Bilirubin) Light	72214	Half Length
74037	Heat Pad	72215	Full Length
74044	Electric	72216	Boards
74038	Standard	73750	Tables
74039	Moist	72217	Urinal, Jug Type
74045	Nonelectric	72218	Male
74046	Moist	72219	Female
74040	Hot Water Bottle	72220	Electronic Bowel
74041	Hydrocollator Unit		Irrigation/Evacuation System
74042	With Pads	72221	Control Unit
74043	Portable	72222	Disposable Pack
74047	Ice Cap Or Collar	74324	Bed Board
74048	Paraffin Bath Unit, Portable	74325	Over-Bed Table
74049	Pump For Water Circulating Pad	74326	Bed Pan
74050	Water Circulating Heat/Cold Pad,	74327	Standard
	W/ Pump	74328	Fracture
72179	Hospital Beds	74333	Bed Cradle
72182	Fixed Height	72223	Oxygen and Respiratory Equipment
74334	With Side Rails	72224	Stationary Oxygen System
72184	With Mattress	73908	Gaseous
74057	Without Mattress	72225	Rental
74338	Without Side Rails	72226	Purchase
74339	With Mattress	72232	Liquid
74340	Without Mattress	72233	Rental
72189	Variable Height	72234	Purchase

DME, cont.

72229	Portable Oxygen System	72772	488 Cu. Ft.
73909	Gaseous	72773	732 Cu. Ft.
72230	Rental	72776	976 Cu. Ft.
72231	Purchase	72777	1220 Cu. Ft.
72235	Liquid	72779	1464 Cu. Ft.
72236	Rental	72780	1708 Cu. Ft.
72237	Purchase	72782	1952 Cu. Ft.
72239	Oxygen	72784	Over 1952 Cu. Ft.
73910	Liquid	72791	At 85 Percent Or Greater
72241	Portable		Concentration
72240	Gaseous	74350	With Specified Maximum Flow
72242	Portable		Rate
72246	Ventilator	74351	Not Greater Than 2L/Min
72243	Volume	74352	Greater Than 2L/Min
72244	Therapeutic	74353	Greater Than 3L/Min
72247	Negative Pressure	74354	Greater Than 4L/Min
72245	Oxygen tent	74355	Greater Than 5L/Min
72248	Percussor	72813	Oxygen And Water Vapor
72249	Chest Shell		Enriching System
72250	Chest Wrap	72815	With Heated Delivery
73914	Intermittent Assist Device	72816	Without Heated Delivery
73921	Rocking Bed With Side Rails	72927	Bath And Toilet Aids
73936	IPPB Machines	73751	Bath Tub Rail
72252	Related Equipment	72928	Wall
72253	Humidifier	72930	Floor Base
73941	Extensive	73752	Transfer Attachment
73942	Glass/Autoclavable Plastic	72932	Toilet Rail
	Bottle	72933	Raised Toilet Seat
73943	Supplemental	72934	Tub Stool Or Bench
72257	Compressor	73753	Pad For Water Circulating Heat Unit
72258	Nebulizer	72448	Wheelchairs
72259	With Compressor	72454	Standard
72260	Ultrasonic	72455	With Fixed Full Length Arms
72261	Glass/Autoclavable Plastic	72457	With Footrests
	Bottle	72463	With Leg Rests
72262	With Compressor, Heater	72459	With Detachable Arms
72263	Suction Pump/Room Vaporizers	72458	With Footrests
73757	Portable Suction Pump	72460	With Leg Rests
72265	Continuous Airway Pressure	72482	Motorized
	Device (CPAP)	72484	With Fixed Full Length Arms
72266	Room Vaporizer	72487	With Footrests
72267	Postural Drainage Board	72488	With Leg Rests
72756	Oxygen Delivery Equipment	72486	With Detachable Arms
72757	Regulator	72490	With Footrests
72759	Stand/Rack	72489	With Leg Rests
72760	Nebulizer	72514	Heavy Duty
72762	Immersion External Heater For	72515	With Fixed Full Length Arms
	Nebulizer	72516	With Footrests
72764	Portable With Small Compressor	72517	With Leg Rests
72767	Oxygen Concentrator	72519	With Detachable Arms
72769	High Humidity System Equivalent	72521	With Footrests
	To	74226	With Leg Rests
72771	244 Cu. Ft.	72522	With Special Seat

DME, cont.

72524	Height From Floor	74264	Deep Cycle
72525	Depth	72429	Power Attachment
72526	By Upholstery	72491	Special Size
72527	By Construction	72492	Special Sized Or Constructed
72505	Lightweight	72493	Customized
72506	With Fixed Full Length Arms	72494	Semi-Reclining
72507	With Footrests	74244	Fully Reclining
72509	With Leg Rests	72497	Power-Operated
72508	With Detachable Arms	72496	With Special Height Arms
72512	With Footrests	74245	With Special Back Height
72511	With Leg Rests	72499	With Fixed Arms
72464	Amputee	72500	With Footrests
72465	With Fixed Full Length Arms	72501	With Leg Rests
72467	With Footrests	72502	With Detachable Arms
72480	With Leg Rests	72503	With Footrests
72476	Without Footrests Or Leg Rests	72504	With Leg Rests
72481	With Detachable Arms	72364	Accessories
72470	With Footrests	72414	Single Wheel
72471	With Leg Rests	72365	Tray
72473	Without Footrests Or Leg Rests	72366	Loop
72449	Semireclining	72367	Toe
72451	With Fixed Full Length Arms	72368	Heel
72452	With Leg Rests	72395	Tire
72453	With Detachable Arms	74295	Solid
74243	With Leg Rests	74296	With Pneumatic Cast
72417	Fully Reclining	74297	Pneumatic
72426	With Fixed Full Length Arms	74298	With Wheel
74249	With Leg Rests	72398	Safety Device
72427	With Detachable Arms	74292	Belt
72428	With Leg Rests	72399	With Airplane Buckle
74257	With Footrests	72400	With Velcro Closure
72418	High Strength Lightweight	74293	Vest
72424	With Fixed Full Length Arms	72370	Caster
72423	With Footrests	72402	Semipneumatic
74277	With Leg Rests	72403	With A Fork
72422	With Detachable Arms	72404	Without A Fork
74279	With Footrests	72405	Rest
74278	With Leg Rests	72408	Arm
72441	Hemiwheelchair	72409	Calf
74268	With Fixed Full Length Arms	72406	Elevating Leg
74269	With Footrests	72371	Attachment For One Arm Drive
74273	With Leg Rests	72410	Seat
74274	With Detachable Arms	72411	Solid Insert
74275	With Footrests	74294	Upholstery
74276	With Leg Rests	72372	Amputee Adapter
72443	Wide Heavy Duty	72373	Brake Extension
72444	With Detachable Desk Or Full	72374	Hook On Head Rest Extension
	Length Arms	72375	Cushion
74281	With Footrests	72376	1"
74282	With Leg Rests	72377	2"
74280	Youth	72378	3"
72432	Battery	72379	4"
72430	Charger	74291	Wedge

DME, CONT.

72380	Hand Rims W/ 8 Vertical Rubber Tipped Projections
72381	Commode Seat
72383	No. 2 Footplates, Except For Elevating Leg Rest
72384	Anti-Tipping Device
72385	Transfer Board Or Device
72386	Adjustable Height, Detachable Arms
72389	"Grade-Aid" Device
72390	Upholstery
72393	Reinforced
72391	Seat
72392	Back
72394	Back
72382	Narrowing Device
74321	Rollabout Chair
72146	Commodes And Accessories
40053	Sitz Bath
72143	With Faucet Attachments
72144	Chair
72145	Commode Chair
72147	Stationary
72148	With Fixed Arms
72149	With Detachable arms
72150	Mobile
72151	With Fixed Arms
72152	With Detachable Arms
72153	With Pail or Pan
72154	With Footrest
72155	Pressure Pad Or Cushion
72156	Air
72157	Water
72158	Gel
72159	Dry
72750	Whirlpool Equipment
72751	Portable (Overtub Type)
72753	Nonportable
72273	Patient Lifts
72274	Sling
72275	Kartop
72276	Combination Lift
72277	Electric Seat Lift Mecahanism
72278	Nonelectric Seat Lift Mecahanism
73754	With Seat Or Sling
72279	Hydraulic
72280	Electric
72281	Pneumatic Compressor/ Appliances
73986	Pneumatic Compressor
73987	Nonsegmental
73988	Segmented
73989	With Calibrated Gradient Pressure

73990	Without Calibrated Gradient Pressure
73991	Pneumatic Appliance
73992	Nonsegmental Used W/ Compressor
73997	Arm
73993	Half
73995	Full
73998	Leg
73994	Half
73996	Full
73999	Segmental Used With Compressor
74000	Arm
74001	Full
74002	Leg
74003	Half
74004	Full
74005	Segmental Gradient Pressure
74006	Arm
74007	Full
74012	Leg
74018	Half
74019	Full
74020	Ultraviolet Cabinet
72326	Traction Equipment
72327	Cervical
72329	Frame, Attached To Headboard
72330	Stand, Freestanding
72337	Extremity
72335	Frame, Attached To Footboard
73755	Stand, Freestanding
72340	Pelvic
72341	Frame, Attached To Footboard
72328	Stand, Freestanding
72333	Overdoor
73756	Cervical
72354	Gravity Assisted Traction Device
72344	Trapeze Bar
72352	Freestanding
72353	Attached To Bed
72346	Fracture Frame
74024	Freestanding With Weights
74025	Attached To Bed
74026	With Weights
74027	Dual With Cross Bars
74028	Attachments
74029	For Pelvic Traction
74030	For Cervical Traction
74021	Safety Equipment
74022	Restraints
72706	Dressings
72707	Surgical
72708	Paste

DME, CONT.

72709	Powder	72898	Nonelastic
72710	Granules	72774	Hydrocolloid
72711	Beads	72775	Without Adhesive Border
72712	Wound Pouch	72778	Pad Size 16 sq. in. Or Less
72714	Alginate	72785	Pad Size 16-48 sq. in.
72715	Pad size 16 sq. in or less	72786	Pad Size More Than 48 sq. in.
72716	Pad Size 16-48 sq. in.	72787	With Adhesive Border
72718	Pad Size More Than 48 sq. in.	72790	Pad Size 16 sq. in. or Less
72717	Wound filler	72793	Pad Size 16-48 sq. in.
72719	Composite	72798	Pad Size More Than 48 sq. in.
72720	Pad Size 16 sq. in. Or Less	72801	Wound Filler
72721	Pad Size 16-48 sq. in.	72808	Paste Per Fluid Ounce
72722	Pad Size More Than 48 sq. in.	72811	Dry Foam Per Gram
72723	Contact Layer	72814	Hydrogel
72724	Pad Size 16 sq. in. or Less	72817	Without Adhesive Border
72725	Pad Size 16-48 sq. in.	72818	Pad Size 16 sq. in. Or Less
72726	Pad Size More Than 48 sq. in.	72823	Pad Size 16-48 sq. in.
72727	Foam	72825	Pad Size More Than 48 sq. in.
72728	Without Adhesive Border	72827	With Adhesive Border
72729	Pad Size 16 sq. in. Or Less	72828	Pad Size 16 sq. in. Or Less
72730	Pad Size 16-48 sq. in.	72830	Pad Size 16-48 sq. in.
72731	Pad Size More Than 48 sq. in.	72832	Pad Size More Than 48 sq. in.
72732	With Adhesive Border	72834	Wound Filler
72733	Pad Size 16 sq. in. or Less	72843	Gel Per Fluid Ounce
72734	Pad Size 16-48 sq. in.	72845	Dry Foam Per Gram
72735	Pad Size More Than 48 sq. in.	72860	Specialty Absorptive
72736	Wound Filler	72871	Without Adhesive Border
72737	Gauze	72872	Pad Size 16 sq. in. Or Less
72738	Nonimpregnated Dressing	72874	Pad Size 16-48 sq. in.
72739	Without Adhesive Border	72877	Pad Size More Than 48 sq. in.
72740	Pad Size 16 sq. in. Or Less	72878	With Adhesive Border
72741	Pad Size 16-48 sq. in.	72879	Pad Size 16 sq. in. Or Less
72742	Pad Size More Than 48 sq. in.	72882	Pad Size 16-48 sq. in.
		72884	Pad Size More Than 48 sq. in.
72743	With Adhesive Border	72887	Transparent Film
72745	Pad Size 16 sq. in. Or Less	72891	16 sq. in. Or Less
72746	Pad Size 16-48 sq. in.	72893	16-48 sq. in.
72747	Pad Size More Than 48 sq. in.	72894	More Than 48 sq. in.
		74984	Ostomy Supplies
72748	Impregnated	74985	Faceplate
72749	Other Than Water/Normal Saline	74986	Skin Barrier
		74987	Solid
72758	Pad Size 16 sq. in. Or Less	74988	Liquid
72761	Pad Size 16-48 sq. in.	74989	Adhesive
72763	Pad Size More Than 48 sq. in.	74990	Belt
		74991	Irrigation Supply
72899	Any Width Per Linear Yard	74992	Sleeve
72765	Water/Normal Saline	74993	Bags
72766	Pad Size 16 sq. in. Or Less	74994	Cone/Catheter
72768	Pad Size 16-48 sq. in.	74995	Set
72770	Pad Size More Than 48 sq. in.	74999	Pouch
		75000	Closed
72897	Elastic	75003	With Barrier Attached

DME, CONT.

75004	Without Barrier Attached	72997	Thermoplastic Foam
75005	For Use On Faceplate	72998	Thermoplastic Foam With
75006	For Use On Barrier With		Thoracic Extension
	Flange	72999	Multiple Post Collar
75001	Drainable	73000	Adjustable
75007	With Barrier Attached		Occipital/Mandibular Supports
75008	Without Barrier Attached	73001	Adjustable Cervical Bars
75009	For Use On Barrier With	73002	Thoracic Extension
	Flange	72356	Head Harness/Halter
75010	With Faceplate Attached	72357	Pillow
75011	For Use On Faceplate	72924	Thoracic
75002	Urinary	72925	Rib Belt
75012	With Barrier Attached	72926	Custom Fitted
75013	Without Barrier Attached	72929	Custom Fabricated
75014	For Use On Barrier With	72931	Thoracic-Lumbar-Sacral (TLSO)
	Flange	72936	Flexible
75015	With Faceplate Attached	72937	Custom Fitted
75016	For Use On Faceplate	72938	Custom Fabricated
74996	Lubricant	72939	Elastic Type
75017	Continent Device	72941	Anterior-Posterior Control
75018	Plug	72942	Taylor Type
75019	Catheter	72943	Knight-Taylor Type
74997	Ring	72944	Anterior-Posterior-Lateral-Rotary
74998	Miscellaneous		Control
75020	Incontinence Appliances/Supplies	72945	Arnold, Magnuson, Steindler
75021	Bedside Drainage Bottle		Types
75022	Rigid	72946	Jewett, Lennox, Baker, Cash
75023	Expandable		Types
75024	Urinary Suspensory	72947	With Extensions
75025	Urinary Leg Bag	72948	Molded To Patient Model
75026	Leg Strap	73003	Custom Fitted Flexion
75027	Latex		Compression Jacket
75028	Foam Or Fabric	73004	Molded Flexion Compression
75029	Intermittent Urinary Catheter		Jacket
75030	Straight Tip	73005	Molded With Interface Material
75031	Curved Tip	73006	2 Piece Molded
72914	Orthotic Devices	73007	2 Piece Molded With Interface
72358	Pelvic Belt/Harness/Boot		Material
72359	Extremity Belt/Harness	73008	Interface Material Custom
74023	Passive Motion Exercise Device		Fitted
72917	Cervical	73009	Overlapping and Spring Steel
72918	Craniostenotic Helmet		Front Sxn
72919	Molded	72949	Lumbar-Sacral (LSO)
72920	Unmolded	72950	Flexible
72921	Flexible Collar	72951	Custom Fitted
72922	Foam	72952	Custom Fabricated
72923	Thermoplastic	72953	Elastic type
72993	Semirigid Collar	72954	Anterior-Posterior-Lateral Control
72994	Adjustable Plastic	72955	Knight, Wilcox Types
72995	Plastic With Adjustable Chin	72956	Anterior-Posterior Control
	Cup	72957	Macausland Type
72996	Wire Frame	72958	Lumbar Flexion
	Occipital/Mandibular Support	72959	Williams Flexion Type

DME, CONT.

73010	Molded Ant-Pstr-Ltrl Control	73269	Sternal
73011	Molded Ant-Pstr-Ltrl Control	73270	Thoracic
	With Interface Material	73271	Trapezius Sling
73012	Cstm Fitted Ant-Pstr-Ltrl	73272	Outrigger
	Control	73273	Outrigger With Vertical
72961	Sacroiliac		Extensions
72962	Flexible	73274	Lumbar Sling
72963	Custom Fitted	73275	Plastic Or Leather Ring
72964	Custom Fabricated		Flange
72965	Semirigid	73276	Plastic Or Leather Molded
72966	Goldthwaite, Osgood Types		Ring Flange
73296	CTLSO Halo Procedure	73277	Cover For Upright
73297	Anterior-Posterior-Lateral Control	73278	Thoracic-Lumbar-Sacral (TLSO)
73298	Molded		Low Profile
73299	Minerva Type	73279	Inclusive Of Furnishing Initial
73300	Halo Procedure		Orthosis
73301	Incorporated Into Jacket Vest	73295	Thoracic Extension
73302	Incorporated Into Plaster Body	73281	Lateral
	Jacket	73282	Anterior
73303	Incorporated Into Milwaukee	73283	Milwaukee Type Superstructure
	Type Orthosis	73284	Lumbar Derotation Pad
73304	MRI Compatible System	73285	Anterior Asis Pad
73102	Torso Supports	73286	Anterior Thoracic Derotation
73103	Ptosis		Pad
73104	Custom Fitted	73287	Abdominal Pad
73105	Custom Fabricated	73288	Elastic Rib Gusset
73106	Pendulous Abdomen	73289	Lateral Trochanteric Pad
73107	Custom Fitted	73290	Other Scoliosis Procedures
73108	Custom Fabricated	73291	Body Jacket
73109	Postsurgical	73292	Molded
73110	Custom Fitted	73293	Post-Operative
73111	Custom Fabricated	73294	Unlisted Procedure For Spinal
73112	Pads		Orthosis
73305	Additions To Spinal Orthoses	73113	Lower Limb
73306	TLSO	73114	Hip (HO)
73307	Corset Front	73115	Frejka Type With Cover
73308	Full Corset	73116	Frejka Cover Only
73309	LSO Full Corset	73117	Pavlik Harness
73310	Axillary Crutch Extension	73118	Von Rosen Type
73311	Peroneal Straps	73119	Static Thigh Cuffs
73312	Stocking Supporter Grips	73120	Ilfled Type
73313	Protective Body Sock	73121	Plastic
73261	Scoliosis Procedures	73122	Dynamic Rancho Type
73262	Cervical-Thoracic-Lumbar-Sacral	73123	Postoperative Custom
	(CTLSO)		Fabricated
73280	Inclusive Of Furnishing Initial	73124	Postoperative Custom Fitted
	Orthosis	73125	Legg Perthes
73263	Correction Pads	73126	Toronto Type
73264	Axilla Sling	73127	Newington Type
73265	Kyphosis	73128	Tachdijan Type
73266	Floating Kyphosis	73129	Scottish Rite Type
73267	Lumbar Bolster	73130	Sam Brown Rite Type
73268	Lumbar Or Lumbar Rib	73131	Patten Bottom Type

DME, CONT.

73132	Knee (KO)	73180	Molded
73146	Elastic	73181	Soft
73133	With Stays	73182	Semi-Rigid
73134	With Joints	73183	Rigid
73135	With Condylar Pads	73184	KAFO
73136	With Condylar Pads And	73185	Plaster
	Joints	73186	Synthetic
73137	Knee Cap	73187	Thermoplastic
73138	Immobilizer	73188	Molded
73139	Adjustable Knee Joints	73189	Soft
73140	Without Adjustable Knee Joints	73190	Semi-Rigid
73141	Swedish Type	73191	Rigid
73143	Molded Supracondylar	73192	Additions
	Prosthetic Socket	73193	Plastic Shoe Insert With
73142	Pneumatic Knee Pads (CTI)		Ankle Joints
73144	Molded Thigh And Calf Lacers	73194	Drop Lock Knee Joint
73145	Nonmolded Thigh And Calf	73195	Limited Motion Knee Joint
	Lacers	73196	Lerman Type
73147	Ankle-Foot (AFO)	73197	Quadrilateral Brim
73148	Dorsiflexion Assist Calf Band	73198	Waist Belt
73149	Anklet Gauntlet	73199	Hip Joint
73150	Molded Anklet Gauntlet	73200	Pelvic Band
73151	Multiligamentus Ankle Support	73201	Thigh Flange
73152	Single Bar Clasp	73202	Pelvic Belt
73153	Phelps Or Perlstein Type	73236	Additions To Lower Extremity
73154	Custom Fitted		Orthosis
73155	Molded	73203	Shoe-Ankle-Shin-Knee
73156	Rigid Anterior Tibial Section	73204	Limited Ankle Motion
73157	Spiral	73205	Dorsiflexion Assist
73158	Posterior Solid Ankle	73206	Dorsiflexion And Plantar
73159	With Ankle Joints		Assist/Resist
73160	Single Bar Stirrup	73207	Split Flat Caliper Stirrups
73161	Double Bar Stirrup		And Plate Attachment
73162	Hip-Knee-Ankle Foot (Or Any	73208	Round Caliper And Plate
	Combination)		Attachment
73163	Double Upright	73209	Molded Foot Plate With
73164	Single Upright		Stirrup Attachment
73165	Multi-Axis Ankle Without	73210	Scott-Craig Type
	Knee Joint	73211	Long Tongue Stirrup
73166	Torsion Control (HKAFO)	73212	Varus/Valgus Correction
73167	Bilateral Rotation Straps		Strap
73168	Bilateral Torsion Cables	73213	Plastic Varus/Valgus
73169	Hip Joint		Correction
73170	Ball Bearing Hip Joint	73214	Molded Inner Boot
73171	Unilateral Rotation Straps	73215	Abduction Bar
73172	Unilateral Torsion Cable	73216	Abduction Bar-Straight
73173	Hip Joint	73217	Nonmolded Lacer
73174	Ball Bearing Hip Joint	73218	Molded Lacer
73175	Fracture Orthoses	73219	Anterior Swing Band
73177	AFO	73220	Molded Pretibial Shell
73176	Plaster	73221	Prosthetic Type (BK) Socket
73178	Synthetic	73222	Extended Steel Shank
73179	Thermoplastic	73223	Patten Bottom

DME, CONT.

73224	Ankle Joint And Half Solid Stirrup	73319	Drop Lock Retainter
73225	Straight Knee Joint	73320	Full Kneecap
73226	Heavy Duty Straight Knee Joint	73321	Medial Or Lateral Pull Kneecap
73227	Offset Knee Joint	73322	Condylar Pad
73228	Heavy Duty Offset Knee Joint	73323	Soft Interface Below Knee Section
73229	Suspension Sleeve	73324	Soft Interface Above Knee Section
73230	Straight Knee Or Offset Knee Joints	73325	Tibial Length Sock
73231	Drop Lock	73326	Femoral Length Sock
73232	Cam Lock (Swiss, French, Bail Types)	73327	Concentric Adjustable Torsion-Style Mechanism
73233	Disc or Dial Lock For Adjustable Knee Flexion	73328	Unlisted Procedures
73234	Polycentric	73329	Upper Limb
73235	Lift Loop For Drop Lock Ring	73330	Shoulder (SO)
73237	Additions To Lower Extremity	73331	Figure 8 Design Abduction Restrainer
73238	Thigh/Weight Bearing-Gluteal/Ischial Weight	73332	Canvas And Webbing Abduction Restrainer
73239	Ring	73333	Acromio/Clavicular
73240	Molded Quadrilateral Brim	73334	Elbow (EO)
73241	Custom Fitted Quadrilateral Brim	73335	Elastic
73242	Molded Containment/Narrow M-L Brim	73336	With Stays
		73337	With Metal Joints
73243	Custom Fitted Containment/Narrow M-L Brim	73338	Double Upright With Forearm/Arm cuffs
73244	Nonmolded Lacer	73339	Free Motion
73245	Molded Lacer	73340	Extension/Flexion Assist
73246	High Roll Cuff	73341	Adjustable Position Lock With Active Control
73247	Pelvic And Thoracic Control	73342	Wrist-Hand-Finger (WHFO)
73248	Clevis Type Two Position	73343	Short Opponens
73249	Pelvic Sling	73344	Long Opponens
73250	Heavy Duty	73345	Shoulder-Elbow-Wrist-Hand (SEWHO)
73251	Adjustable Flexion	73346	Abduction Positioning-Custom Fitted
73252	Plastic Molded	73347	Airplane Design
73253	Metal Frame	73348	Erbs Palsy Design
73256	Unilateral Band And Belt	73349	Molded With Articulating Elbow Joint
73255	Bilateral Band And Belt	73350	Mobile Arm Support (SEO)
73257	Gluteal Pad	73351	Adjustable
73258	Thoracic Band	73352	Reclining
73259	Paraspinal Uprights	73354	Friction
73260	Lateral Support Uprights	73355	Yoke Type
73314	General	73353	Radial Arm Support (SEO)-Adjustable Rancho Type
73315	Plating Chrome Or Nickel Bar	73356	Additions to Mobile Arm Supports (SEO)
73316	Extension Bar	73357	Elevating Proximal Arm
73317	Any Material Bar or Joint		
73318	Non-Corrosive Finish		

DME, CONT.

73358	Offset Or Lateral Rocker Arm With Elastic Balance Control	72971	Spenco
		72972	Plastazote Or Equal
		72973	Silicone Gel
73359	Supinator	72974	Longitudinal Arch Support
73360	Fracture Orthoses	72975	Longitudinal/Metatarsal Support
73361	Humeral		
73362	Radius/Ulnar	72977	Formed To Patient Foot
73363	Forearm, Hand With Wrist Hinge	72978	Arch Support
		73101	Removable
73364	Humeral, Radius/Ulnar, Wrist Combination	72979	Longitudinal
		72980	Metatarsal
73365	Unlisted Procedures	72981	Longitudinal/Metatarsal
73366	Replace Orthotic Device	73013	Nonremovable
73367	Girdle For Milwaukee Orthosis	73015	Longitudinal
73368	Trilateral Socket Brim	73016	Metatarsal
73371	Quadrilateral Socket Brim	73014	Longitudinal/Metatarsal
73369	Molded	73017	Hallus-Valgus Night Dynamic Splint
73370	Custom Fitted		
73372	Thigh Lacer	73018	Abduction And Rotation Bars
73373	Molded	73019	Including Shoes
73374	Unmolded	73020	Without Shoes
73375	Calf Lacer	73021	Adjustable Shoe-Styled Positioning Device
73376	Molded		
73377	Unmolded	73022	Plastic Heel Stabilizer
73378	High Roll Cuff	73023	Shoes
73379	Proximal And Distal Upright (KAFO)	73024	Orthopedic Oxfords
		73025	Infant
73380	Metal Bands	73026	Child
73382	Proximal Thigh (KAFO)	73027	Junior
73383	Calf Or Distal Thigh (KAFO-AFO)	73028	Orthopedic Hightops
		73029	Infant
73384	Leather Cuff	73030	Child
73385	Proximal Thigh (KAFO)	73031	Junior
73386	Calf Or Distal Thigh (KAFO-AFO)	73032	Surgical Boot
		73033	Infant
73387	Pretibial Shell	73034	Child
73388	Repair Orthotic Device	73035	Junior
73389	Hourly Rate	73036	Benesch Boot
73390	Repair Or Replace Minor Parts	73037	Infant
73391	Ancillary Orthotic Services	73038	Child
73392	Multipodus Or Equal Orthotic Preparatory Management System For Lower Extremities	73039	Junior
		73040	Ladies' Shoes
		73041	Oxford
73393	Flexible Foot Positioner For an AFO	73042	Depth Inlay
		73043	Hightop and Depth Inlay
73394	Pneumatic Splint	73044	Surgical Boot
73395	Ankle Control	73050	Oxford Used As Part Of A Brace
73396	Walking		
73397	Full Leg	73045	Men's Shoes
73398	Knee	73046	Oxford
72967	Orthopedic Footwear	73047	Depth Inlay
72969	Insert	73048	Hightop and Depth Inlay
72970	Berkeley Shell	73049	Surgical Boot

DME, CONT.

73051	Oxford Used As Part Of A Brace	74953	Of Off-The-Shelf Depth Inlay Shoe
73052	Nonstandard Size Or Width	74954	Of Shoe Molded From Casts Of Patient's Foot
73053	Nonstandard Size Or Length		
73054	Additional Charge For Split Size	74955	Modification
		74956	With Roller Or Rigid Rocker Bottom
73055	Ambulatory Surgical Boot		
73056	Plastazote Sandal	74957	With Wedge(s)
73058	Orthopedic Shoe Lifts	74958	With Metatarsal Bar
73059	Heel Tapered To Metatarsals	74959	With Off-Set Heel
73060	Neoprene Heel And Sole	74960	Not Otherwise Specified
73061	Cork Heel And Sole	74961	Multiple-Density Insert(s)
73062	Metal Extension (Skate)	73399	Prosthetic Devices
73063	Tapered And Inside The Shoe	73400	Lower Limb
73064	Heel	74634	Partial Foot
73065	Orthopedic Shoe Wedges	74635	Shoe Insert With Longitudinal Arch
73066	Heel Wedge, SACH		
73067	Heel Wedge	74636	Molded Socket
73068	Outside Sole Wedge	74637	Ankle Height
73069	Wedge Between Sole	74638	Tibial Tubercle Height
73070	Clubfoot	74639	Ankle
73071	Outflare	74651	Symes
73072	Metatarsal Rocker Bar	74652	Molded Socket
73073	Betweeen Sole Metatarsal Bar	74653	Metal Frame
73074	Full Sole And Heel	74640	Below Knee
73075	Orthopedic Heels	74654	Molded Socket
73076	Plastic Reinforced	74655	Plastic Socket
73077	Leather Reinforced	74641	Knee Disarticulation
73078	SACH Cushion Type	74656	External Knee Joints
73079	New Leather	74657	Bent Knee Configuration
73080	New Rubber	74642	Above Knee
73081	Thomas With Wedge	74658	Molded Socket
73082	Thomas Extended To Ball	74659	Short Prosthesis
73083	Pad And Depression For Spur	74660	With Foot Blocks
73084	Pad Removable For Spur	74662	With Articulated Ankle/Foot
73085	Shoe Additions	74661	For Proximal Femoral Focal Deficiency
73086	Leather Insole		
73087	Rubber Insole	74643	Hip Disarticulation
73088	Felt Covered With Leather	74663	Canadian Type
73089	Half Sole	74664	Tilt Table Type
73090	Full Sole	74644	Hemipelvectomy
73091	Standard Toe Tap	74665	Canadian Type
73092	Horseshoe Toe Tap	74645	Endoskeletal
73093	Extension To Instep (Leather With Eyelets)	74646	Below Knee
		74647	Knee Disarticulation
73094	Convert Instep To Velcro Closure	74648	Above Knee
		74649	Hip Disarticulation
73095	Convert Firm Counter To Soft Counter	74650	Hemipelvectomy
		73401	Upper Limb-Additions
73096	March Bar	73409	Hinge
74951	Diabetics Only	73403	Polycentric
74952	Fitting	73404	Single Pivot
		73405	Flexible Metal

DME, CONT.

73406	Wrist Unit	73452	Model #6
73410	Disconnect Locking	73453	Model #7
73411	Additional Disconnect Insert	73454	Model #7lo
	For Locking	73455	Model #8
73412	Flexion-Friction	73456	Model #8x
73413	Spring Assisted Rotational	73457	Model #88x
73414	Rotation With Cable Lock	73458	Model #10p
73415	Quick Disconnect Hook	73459	Model #10x
	Adapter	73460	Model #12p
73416	Quick Disconnect Lamination	73461	Model #99x
	Collar	73462	Model #555
73417	Stainless Steel On Any Wrist	73463	Model #SS555
73418	Latex Suspension Sleeve	73465	Accu, Or Equal
73419	Lift Assist For Elbow	73466	2 Load, Or Equal
73420	Nudge Control Elbow Lock	73467	Aprl VC, Or Equal
73421	Shoulder Abduction Joint	73468	Modifier Wrist Flexion Unit
73422	Excursion Amplifier	73469	TRS Grip, VC
73423	Pulley Type	73470	TRS Adept, VC
73424	Lever Type	73471	Child
73425	Shoulder Flexion-Abduction	73472	Infant
	Joint	73473	TRS Super Sport, Passive
73426	Shoulder Univeral Joint	73474	Otto Bock/Equal Pincher Tool
73427	Control Cable	73476	Terminal Devices-Hands
73428	Standard	73477	Dorrance, VO
73429	Heavy Duty	73478	Aprl, VC
73430	Teflon/Equal Cable Lining	73479	Sierra, VO
73431	Hook To Hand Cable Adapter	73484	Becker
73432	Harness	73480	Imperial
73433	Chest or Shoulder-Saddle	73481	Lock Grip
	Type	73485	Plylite
73434	Single Control	73482	Robin-Aids
73435	Dual Control	73483	VO
73436	Test Socket	73486	VO Soft
73437	Wrist Disarticulation Or	73487	Passive
	Below Elbow	73488	Detroit Infant (Mechanical)
73438	Elbow Disarticulation Or	73489	Passive Infant (Steeper,
	Above Elbow		Hosmer, Equal)
73439	Shoulder Disarticulation Or	73490	Child Mitt
	Interscapular Thoracic	73491	NYU Child
73440	Suction Socket	73492	Steeper/Equal Mechanical
73441	Frame Type Socket		Infant
73442	Below Elbow Or Wrist	73493	Bock
	Disarticulation	73494	VC
73443	Shoulder Disarticulation	73495	VO
73444	Interscapular-Thoracic	73496	Gloves For Above Hands
73445	Removable Insert	73497	Production
73446	Silicone Gel Insert Or Equal	73498	Custom
73475	Terminal Devices-Hooks	73500	External Power-Terminal Devices
73464	Dorrance Or Equal	73501	Electronic Hand, Switch
73450	Model #5x		Controlled
73448	Model #3	73502	Otto Bock
73449	Model #5	73503	Steeper Or Equal
73451	Model #5xa	73505	System Teknik

DME, CONT.

73506	Variety Village Or Equal	73628	Heavy Weight
73508	Electronic Hand Greifer	73629	Surgical Weight
73516	Otto Bock Or Equal	73630	Full Length
73509	Switch Controlled	73631	Medium Weight
73510	Myoelectronically Contolled	73632	Heavy Weight
73507	Electronic Hand, Myoelectrically	73633	Surgical Weight
	Controlled	73634	Leotards
73511	Otto Bock Or Equal	73635	Medium Weight
73512	System Teknik	73636	Surgical Weight
73513	Variety Village Or Equal	73637	Custom Made
73514	Hosmer Or Equal Prehensile	73638	Lymphedema
	Acutator	73639	Garter Belt
73515	Michigan Or Equal Electronic	73549	Trusses
	Hook	73555	With Standard Pad
73517	External Power-Elbow	73550	Single
73518	Boston Or Equal	73551	Double
73519	Switch Controlled	73552	Addition To Standard Pad
73520	Myoelectronically Controlled	73553	Water Pad
73521	Hosmer Or Equal	73554	Scrotal Pad
73522	Utah Or Equal	73556	Prosthetic Socks
73523	Variety Village Or Equal	73557	Sheath
73529	Switch Controlled	73558	Below Knee
73524	Adolescent	73559	Above Knee
73525	Child	73560	Upper Limb
73526	Myoelect Controlled	73561	Wool Sock
73527	Adolescent	73562	Below Knee
73528	Child	73563	Above Knee
73530	External Power-Control Modules	73564	Upper Limb
73531	Electronic Wrist Rotator	73565	Shrinker
73532	Otto Bock Or Equal	73566	Below Knee
73533	For Utah Arm	73567	Above Knee
73534	Control	73568	Upper Limb
73535	Servo-Steeper Or Equal	73569	Stump Sock
73536	Analogue-UNB Or Equal	73570	Below Knee
73537	Proportional-Utah Or Equal	73571	Above Knee
73538	External Power-Battery Components	73572	Upper Limb
73539	6V Battery-Otto Bock Or Equal	73573	Addit To Sheath/Sock-Air Seal
73543	12V Battery-Utah Or Equal		Suction Retention System
73540	Battery Charger	73574	Unlisted Procedure For Miscell
73541	6V Otto Bock Or Equal		Services
73542	12V Utah Or Equal	73575	Prosthetic Implants
73544	Breast Prostheses	73576	Artificial Larynx
73545	Mastectomy Bra	73577	Tracheostomy Speaking Valve
73546	Mastectomy Sleeve	73578	Integumentary System
73547	Mastectomy Form	73579	Silicone/Equal Breast
73548	Silicone Or Equal	73580	Urinary Tract-Collagen Implant
73621	Elastic Supports	73581	Tissue Expander
73622	Below Knee	73582	Head (Skull, Facial Bones and
73623	Medium Weight		Temporomandibular Jt)
73624	Heavy Weight	73583	Ocular
73625	Surgical Weight	73584	Orbit
73626	Above Knee	73585	Aqueous Shunt
73627	Medium Weight	73586	Ossicula

DME, CONT.

73587	Cochlear Device/System	72824	Heparin Infusion Pump
73588	Temporomandibular Joint	72826	Air Bubble Detector
73589	Maxilla	72829	Pressure Alarm
73590	Mandible	72831	Bath Conductivity Meter
73591	Palate	72833	Blood Leak Detector
73592	Cochlear-External Speech Processor	72844	Unipuncture Control System
		72846	Hemodialysis Machine
73593	Upper Extremity	72854	Blood Pump
73594	Radial Head	74149	Peritoneal Dialysis
73595	Distal Humerus	72847	Automatic Intermittent System
73596	Proximal Ulna/Radius	72857	Reciprocating System
73597	Distal Ulna	72848	Cycler Dialysis Machine
73598	Distal Radius	72875	Dynamic Adjustable
73599	Trapezium		Extension/Flexion Device
73600	Wrist	72876	Elbow
73601	Lunate	72880	Wrist
73602	Carpus	72881	Knee
73603	Scaphoid	72883	Ankle
73604	Metacarpophalangeal Joint	72886	Soft Interface Material
73605	Lower Extremity (Joint: Knee, Ankle, Toe)	72890	Finger
		72892	Toe
73606	Patella	72850	Delivery/Install Charges
73607	Metatarsal Joint	74159	Water Purification System
73608	Hallux Implant	72852	Reverse Osmosis
73609	Muscular-Skeletal	72853	Deionizer
73610	Flexor Tendon (Hand, Finger)	72856	Water Softening System
73611	Extensor Tendon (Hand, Finger)	72858	Wearable Artificial Kidney
		72859	Compact Travel Hemodialyzer System
73612	Tendon (Other Than Hand, Finger)	72866	Sorbent Cartridges
73613	Interphalangeal Joint	72868	Replacement Components
73614	Cardiovascular System	72869	Jaw Motion Rehabilitation System
73615	Synthetic Vascular Graft Material	72870	Replacement Cushions
		72873	Replacement Measuring Scales
73616	Genital	72841	Transducer Protectors/Fluid Barriers
73617	Biliary Stent (Permanent)	72838	Adjustible Chair, ESRD Patient
73618	Testicle	41837	Transcutaneous/Neuromuscular
73619	Taxes		Electrical Nerve Stimulators
73620	Orthotic/Prosthetic/Other	73978	TENS
72314	Infusion Supplies	72301	Two Lead
72315	IV Pole	72302	Four Lead
72316	Infusion Pump	72303	Conductive Garment
72323	Stationary	73979	Pelvic Floor Stimulator
72324	Single/Multiple Channel	73980	Incontinence Treatment System
72317	Ambulatory	73981	Neuromuscular Stimulator
72318	Single/Multiple Channels	72305	For Scoliosis
72319	Insulin	72306	Electric Shock Unit
72320	Implantible	72307	Electromyography Biofeedback Device
72321	Nonprogrammable		
72322	Programmable	73982	Osteogenesic Stimulator
72821	Artificial Kidney Machines And Accessories	72308	Nonspinal Applications
		73983	Spinal Applications
74142	For Dialysis	73984	Surgically Implanted

DME, CONT.

73985	Implantable Neurostimulator
72311	Pulse Generator/Receiver
72312	Electrodes/Leads
72313	Electronic Salivary Reflex Stimulator

Appendix A - Additional Data Components Used with MEDCIN

Each finding in MEDCIN may have a set of components attached to it, in order to indicate the history status, modifier, course, or result of that finding.

Status

The history status of a finding is designated by a blank, one or two letters/characters, or a number.

	(blank) Current Finding	SC	Scheduled for
O	Ordered	FU	Follow-Up for
H	Personal History	E	Evaluate Preoperatively for
F	Family History	AL	Allergy to
RI	Risk of	IN	Intolerant to
?	Possible	UN	Unresponsive to
?+	Probable	IO	Intra-operative
W	Working Diagnosis	PO	Post-operative
A	Admission Diagnosis	PE	Perioperative
P	Primary Diagnosis	IP	Intraprocedural
S	Secondary Diagnosis	PP	Postprocedural
DS	Discharge Diagnosis	PS	Post
RO	Rule Out	D	Cause of Death
RD	Referral Diagnosis	1 - 9	Group Designator[1]
RF	Referred Elsewhere for		

---

[1] Group Designator: findings may be specified as part of a group. For example, a patient may have multiple heart murmurs. The findings associated with "murmur 1" are designated as being in Group 1; findings with "murmur 2" are in Group 2; and so forth.

Modifier

This is an adjective phrase that is used to further describe or modify the finding.

	blank (no entry)		
	blank (no entry)	SV	severe
TI	tiny, insignificant	BO	borderline
T	tiny	PA	partial
S	small	CO	complete
SM	small-moderate	UN	upper normal
M	moderate	ST	stable
ML	moderate-large	TK	thick
L	large	TN	thin
MK	marked	EP	episodic
MN	minimal	FL	fluctuating
TR	trivial	C	constant
TC	trace	IN	increasing
MI	mild	SE	seasonal
MM	mild-moderate	RE	recent
MS	moderate-severe		

Course

This is also an adjectival phrase, and enables the description of the course or progression of a condition.

I	improving	E	expanding
W	worsening	L	louder
U	unchanged	S	softer

Result of a Finding

A result indicator may be linked to an item which is a measurable physical finding or a test.

	blank (no entry)
A	abnormal or positive
H	high
N	normal or negative
L	low

Appendix B - Using MEDCIN to Build Applications

MEDCIN and its supplemental files and tools are designed to support clinical applications. The information below should help to show how a coded and hierarchial nomenclature can be used to provide software features.[i]

EMR Database Components

In addition to the descriptive text of the nomenclature, each finding may be associated with additional components in order to be more descriptive or detailed. There are seven data components which are specifically designed to complement the nomenclature. These are: status, result, modifier, and course, as denoted in Appendix A, as well as onset, duration, and value.

Status

The status codes can be used to attach a particular status to a finding. The complete status code supplemental file is applicable to all findings. Since these codes change the clinical interpretation of a finding, they are integrated in supplemental decision support files.

Result

The results file includes the information needed to calculate a numeric result as high, low, normal or abnormal. It also has elements that contain information necessary to evaluate results by age and sex using seven levels of significance. This permits the construction of decision support algorithms based on six levels of variation from the normal range.

Modifier

Additional modifier information can be attached to any finding.

Course

A set of additional descriptors is available to describe the continuing course of a finding.

Value

Many findings have values which are associated with common units of measurement such as pounds or kilograms for weight, mg/dL, IU/L, etc. A supplemental file includes the standard and alternate units of measure for every applicable finding, and the mechanism for arithmetic conversion of values into alternate units, such as pounds to kilograms, inches to centimeters, etc. This is necessary because analytical functions require measurements to be in consistent units.

Additional Information for a Finding

Since findings are unique and independent of each other, additional information can be linked to any finding. This can include graphics, images, voice files, free-text, prescription, test order information, etc.

Use of Clinical Data for Reporting and Analysis

Having clinical information available as discrete data elements, rather than as free-text, enables the building of powerful search, reporting and analytical capabilities. A brief description of search and reporting functions is presented below and on the following pages.

Differential Diagnosis - An Example of Clinical Analysis

MEDCIN EXPERT (see Appendix C) has tables so that for any finding, all related diseases can be located and for any disease, all related findings can be located. The significance of the relation between findings and diseases can be quantified by points based on tables that consider age, sex, race, ethnicity, measurement (value), onset, duration, expiration and delay.

A differential diagnosis can be performed by adding each finding's points toward each disease to rank the relative probability (risk) of each disease. Then each disease probability can be adjusted for age, sex, race, and then adjusted for findings that are not present. Finally the probability can be adjusted by applying logic for discovering constellations of findings. The end result would be a ranked list of diseases, relatively weighted.

As an application, this logic could feed a statistics program with the top three diseases of an entire patient group and, combined with demographics, relationships could be studied. Other uses of differential diagnosis include risk analysis, early detection of disease based on patient history and symptomatology, population disease state management, etc.

Searching for Findings by Disease

MEDCIN has a table linking diseases to findings. For any disease or group of diseases, all related findings can be identified, grouped into six major categories by finding type, and subdivided into hierarchical groups. The relative significance of the disease-finding link can be evaluated to allow control over the level of generality of the search results.
This is a good source for creating problem-oriented protocols for data entry.

Searching for Findings by Vocabulary Words

MEDCIN has tables to support the location of findings based on vocabulary word searches, using both the vocabulary word and the hierarchical sequence. As the findings are hierarchical, so are the words used to describe them.

In the example of "heart murmur", the words "heart" and "murmur" would be in the vocabulary table, associated with the hierarchical sequence for the finding of "heart murmur." The approximately 1,000 other "heart murmur" findings do not need to have entries with the words "heart" and "murmur" because, being a subset, they inherit the words from the higher level "heart murmur" finding.

Vocabulary linked to a higher level finding is automatically inherited by all lower-level findings under it. Thus, each finding has only words unique to its level in the vocabulary table. This significantly reduces the number of entries in the table, yielding much faster searches and reporting.

Developer's note: once the hierarchical sequence structure is found for each word, they can be compared using "and" logic. The intersecting ranges yield the hierarchical sequences that are linked to the findings that are the search results.

Searching for Findings for Intelligent Prompting [1]

Using differential diagnosis logic, a list of findings can be suggested for entry. Following is an example of how this can be implemented:

> Apply diagnostic logic to the clinical data entered thus far in a patient's visit to get a list of potential assessments. Then using the capability described in "Searching for findings by disease", a resulting list of findings can be obtained and used to select additional physical findings or symptoms for entry, or to order tests and therapy.

Cohort Studies

Cohort studies identify a group of patients based on selective criteria. Further analysis of the clinical data in each patient's record may show what findings or medical history the group of patients has in common.

Searching for selected findings is straightforward because each finding has its own unique identifying code. Searching is further enhanced by the hierarchical structure. For example, if searching for all patients that have some form of heart murmur, it would be tedious to setup a search which identifies all of the approximately 1,000 unique murmur findings. Instead a search based on the hierarchical sequence would only have to identify the top level heart murmur finding to include all the lower level findings.

Searches can be made more specific by including the following criteria for each finding: finding status, age at onset, onset date, duration, results, value and modifier. Searches can be made to use Boolean selection logic. An example of such as search would be to find all male patients, who at age 12-20 years had severe mumps, and had a heart problem within five years after the onset of mumps.

---

[1]   Patent pending

Reporting to External Systems

Coded patient records are difficult to transfer between computer systems using dissimilar coding structures. In addition to providing text output in either professional or lay terminology, MEDCIN has code translation tables for numerous other coding systems in its CODE LINKS files. Use of protocols such as HL7 will facilitate transfers.

---

[i] For more information on MEDCIN implementation contact Kirby Trump at kirby@medicomp.com, (703) 803-8080, Medicomp Systems, Inc., 14500 Avion Parkway, Suite 175, Chantilly, Virginia 20151.

Appendix C - Supplemental Files and Tools for MEDCIN

MEDCIN, and several complementary files and tools, are available on computer media through Medicomp Systems, Inc.

These files and tools are arranged under five major categories:
MEDCIN NOMENCLATURE
MEDCIN SEARCH
MEDCIN CHART
MEDCIN EXPERT
Additional Tools

MEDCIN NOMENCLATURE

The MEDCIN NOMENCLATURE includes the MEDCIN finding identification number, hierarchical sequence, and hierarchical phrasing (as in this publication) for every finding in the MEDCIN nomenclature.

The nomenclature can be displayed by utilizing the accompanying browser, a Windows95 program with a branching tree display format.

MEDCIN SEARCH

MEDCIN SEARCH combines MEDCIN NOMENCLATURE with the addition of vocabulary words, synonyms, and standalone phrasing for each MEDCIN finding. The browsing capability is enhanced by the utilization of vocabulary words and synonyms to locate matching findings in the nomenclature.

The MEDCIN NOMENCLATURE uses hierarchical phrasing for each finding as presented in this publication, while MEDCIN SEARCH uses standalone phrasing. The example below shows the difference between hierarchical phrasing and standalone phrasing for three findings:

Finding ID:	Hierarchical Phrasing:	Standalone Phrasing:
279	chest pain	chest pain or discomfort
288	radiating	chest pain which radiates
292	to the left arm only	chest pain which radiates to the left arm only

MEDCIN CHART

MEDCIN CHART combines MEDCIN SEARCH with the following additional resources that permit the construction of electronic patient chart applications based on the MEDCIN nomenclature.

Several data files are included that enable a narrative engine[1] to use syntactical rules to generate sentences and paragraphs from MEDCIN findings. The data files include insertion points and phrase manipulation to incorporate any finding's value, onset, status, modifier and course into a sentence. Phrasing in professional and lay terminology includes the appropriate positive/negative (or normal/abnormal) terms for each finding.

MEDCIN CHART also includes age and sex sensitive numerical ranges for physical findings and tests, common and alternate units of measure, prescription information including common dosages and formulations, basic contraindications for drugs and tests, and alerts for life-threatening test results.

MEDCIN EXPERT

MEDCIN EXPERT combines MEDCIN CHART with an expert system database including a 420,000 planar element , multidimensional matrix of MEDCIN findings and 3,100 diagnoses, syndromes and conditions. This matrix provides templates from which users can construct clinical protocols to suit their own individual practice needs, create decision support protocols (such as differential diagnosis and triage) and perform risk analysis.

---

[1]   Patent pending

Additional Tools

MEDCIN CODE LINKS provides a mapping table to other commonly used coded nomenclatures. Each record in this file contains a MEDCIN finding identification number and the codes for associated findings in the following nomenclatures: ICD-9-CM, ICD-10, ICD-O, CPT, ACC, HCPCS, DSM-IV and CAS[2].

Additional function-specific tools are also available, including cohort search capabilities, decision support engines, etc.

---

[2] ICD-9-CM, ICD-10, ICD-O are trademarks of the World Health Organization. CPT is a trademark of the American Medical Association. ACC is a trademark of the American College of Cardiology. HCPCS is a trademark of the Health Care Financing Administration. DSM-IV is a trademark of the Psychiatric Association. CAS is a trademark of the Chemical Abstract Service.